BH.

SURGERY

A Monthly Journal Devoted to the Art and Science of Surgery

VOLUME 35 √
JANUARY—JUNE, 1954

ST. LOUIS
THE C. V. MOSBY COMPANY
1954

Printed in the
United States of America

Press of
The C. V. Mosby Company
St. Louis

SURGERY

VOL. 35 | JANUARY, 1954 | NO. 1

Original Communications

Society for Vascular Surgery (concluded)

AN EVALUATION OF "HIGH" LUMBAR SYMPATHECTOMY IN ARTERIOSCLEROTIC CIRCULATORY INSUFFICIENCY OF THE LOWER EXTREMITIES

GEORGE D. LILLY, M.D., DONALD W. SMITH, M.D.,
CHARLES F. BIGGANE, JR., M.D., AND JOSEPH T. JANA, JR., M.D.,
MIAMI, FLA.

SEVERAL years ago we[1] made the observation that individuals upon whom thoracolumbar sympathectomies had been performed for hypertension seemed to have more complete sympathectomies of the lower extremities than did individuals on whom the classical lumbar sympathectomies had been performed for peripheral vascular disease of the lower extremities. This caused us to change our technique for performing lumbar sympathectomies, and since 1948 we have, routinely, performed lower extremity sympathectomies by resecting the distal two-thirds of the twelfth rib and, through the bed of this rib, extending an incision forward and downward toward the umbilicus to expose the sympathetic trunk (Fig. 1), retroperitoneally, where it emerges from the diaphragm. Through such an incision, we are able to remove the upper three lumbar ganglia and, by splitting the crus of the diaphragm (Fig. 2), the twelfth thoracic ganglion can be removed. The removal of these four ganglia can be accomplished quickly without undue retraction and with clear visualization of the entire area through such an incision.

We are of the opinion that such a procedure accomplishes a complete sympathetic denervation of the entire lower extremity. We feel that the better exposure affords a much greater degree of protection against hemorrhage and that the avoidance of excessive retraction, which is necessary in the usual type of lumbar sympathectomy, reduces the incidence of postsympathectomy causalgia and genitofemoral neuralgia.

In recent weeks we have learned that Coldwater, Cox, Randall, Alexander, and Hertzman[2] have been employing a similar approach. They have found

Read at the seventh annual meeting of the Society for Vascular Surgery, New York, N. Y., May 31, 1953.

that by stimulating the various ganglia at the time of surgery they were able to demonstrate that sympathetic innervation to all parts of the lower extremity is frequently derived from as high as the first lumbar ganglion, and as low as the fifth lumbar ganglion. Their clinical results, both in primary operation and in secondary operation where previous "low" sympathectomy had proved to be unsatisfactory, have been most gratifying, and their enthusiam for total lumbar sympathectomy seems to compare with our own. They[4] have shown by animal investigation that such variations in sympathetic pathways do exist.

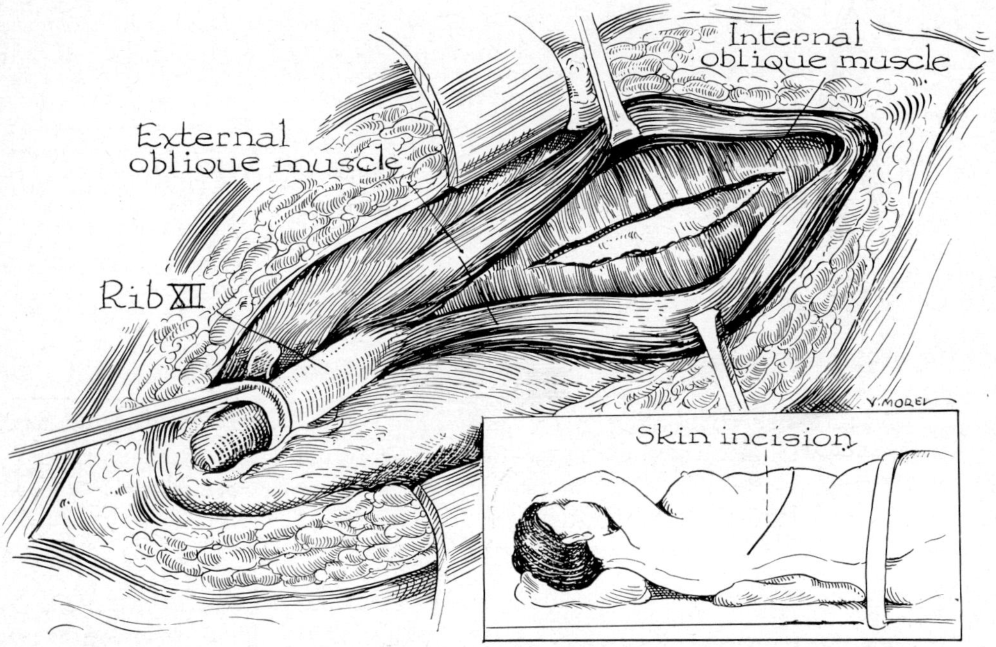

Fig. 1.—The patient is placed on a sandbag with the operative side up at an angle of forty-five degrees. Immobilization is assured by a wide adhesive strip across the hips.

The incision is made in the line of the twelfth rib and carried forward toward the umbilicus to the lateral edge of the rectus muscle.

The distal two-thirds of the twelfth rib is resected subperiosteally, and the oblique muscles are divided in the same line. Care is exercised to avoid injury to the intercostal nerves. The retroperitoneal space is entered. The peritoneum and, on the right side, the vena cava are retracted anteriorly.

Francioli,[5] also, has recently advocated approaching the lumbar sympathetic ganglia from a "high" incision through the bed of the twelfth rib.

Since Royle[3] first described his approach to the lumbar ganglia, various modifications have been described.[6, 7] Longitudinal, transverse, oblique, and curved skin incisions have been employed, and various techniques of muscle splitting and muscle cutting have been advocated. All of these entail an approach to the sympathetic trunk at the level of the fourth lumbar vertebral body; then, by retraction upon the renal pedicle and, on the right side, the vena cava, some of the upper ganglia are removed. In the obese "short-coupled" individual it is difficult to expose any part of the sympathetic trunk through such an incision and, under the most ideal circumstances, it is frequently impossible to remove the second lumbar ganglion by this approach. When the upper lumbar ganglia are exposed, or removed blindly,[6] through such an incision, there is great danger of tearing a large lumbar vein where it enters the vena cava, particularly since the first and second lumbar veins frequently pass anterior to the sympathetic trunk on the right side. Injury to the vena cava, or even the renal vessels, is another definite danger.

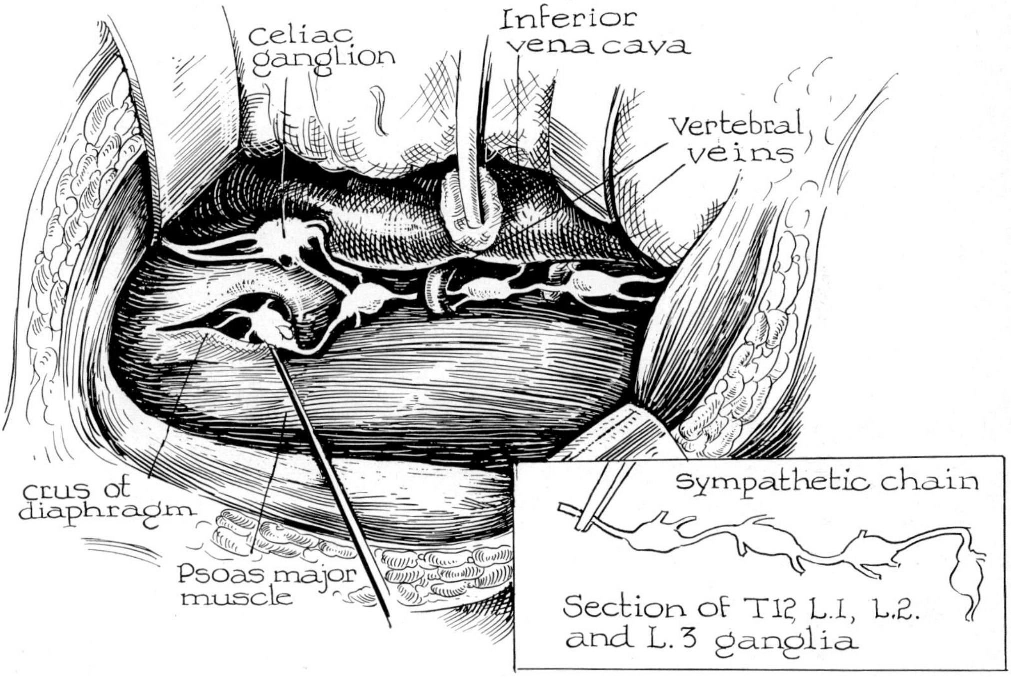

Fig. 2.—The lumbar sympathetic trunk is palpated against the vertebral bodies at the medial edge of the psoas muscle. The trunk and first, second, and third lumbar ganglia are freed under direct viualization, thereby avoiding injury to the lumbar veins which may course anterior to the trunk. The trunk is followed to the diaphragm and, if desirable, the diaphragm may be opened extrapleurally and the twelfth thoracic ganglia removed.

Yeager and Cowley[8] and Edwards[9] have emphasized the many variations which may occur in the sympathetic distribution to the extremity. Our experience has been similar to theirs. We have encountered many "double trunks" and other anomalies in which most of the sympathetic innervation of the lower extremities originated from the first or second ganglia.

Recently, Reed and Kirgis[10] have evaluated the clinical application of Cannon's law of denervation[11] and have concluded that the consideration of preganglionic versus postganglionic sympathectomy is not of value, clinically. We might point out, however, that excision of the twelfth thoracic ganglion and the first, second, and third lumbar ganglia constitutes a practical preganglionic sympathectomy.

The tendency toward regeneration of severed sympathetic pathways has been stressed by Langley[12] and many others during the past one-half century.

Without doubt, regeneration does play a part in the long-term clinical benefit of sympathectomy. We feel that regeneration can be avoided most successfully by performing an extensive sympathetic ganglionectomy, and we agree with Edwards[9] that "the removal of rather long segments of the sympathetic trunk" is advisable. Thompson, Brose, and Smithwick[13] have shown that removal of the first lumbar ganglion affords the best chance of removing existing collateral sympathetic pathways, and we feel that resection of the twelfth thoracic ganglia, with subsequent closure of the diaphragm, is the best insurance against regeneration. In regard to regeneration, we believe that most clinical failures to accomplish permanent sympathectomy of the lower extremity may be attributable to an incomplete operation, rather than to regeneration.

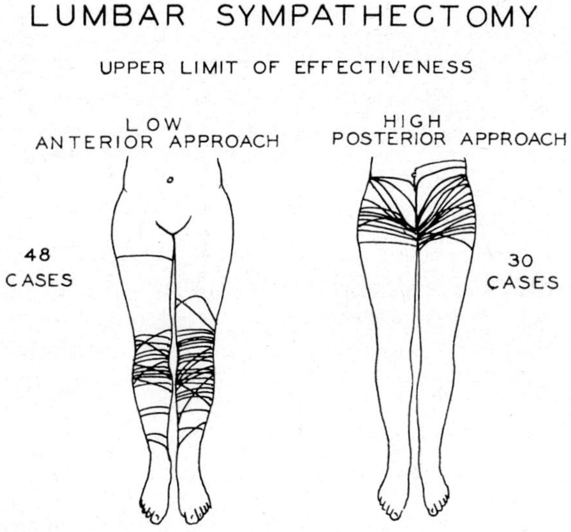

Fig. 3.—Starch-iodine studies were made on seventy-eight patients. Black lines designate lower margin of sudomotor activity, indicating a much more complete sympathectomy in those cases operated upon through a high posterior approach.

Reoperation upon those individuals who, obviously, have had inadequate sympathectomy has presented an exceedingly difficult problem when an attempt is made at exploration through the same low incision. We have encountered many such cases and have found that in them an approach through the upper part of the field is simple and safe.

One valid objection to this high operation is that simultaneous bilateral lumbar sympathectomy may be impractical where rib resection has to be carried out. We feel that it is probably better to operate on the second side at a later date, but there is no great objection to carrying out a bilateral procedure at one operation.

The question of sexual disturbances following the removal of the first lumbar ganglia may arise. Many of these individuals are in an age group in which such difficulties occur through the normal changes of senescence; for this reason, we refrain from making direct inquiry for fear of increasing the difficulties by the power of suggestion. We have had only two voluntary complaints in a series of forty male patients. Alnor[14] has made a careful and scientific study of this problem, and has concluded that the age of the patient and the underlying disease which makes sympathectomy necessary play a much greater role in any impotence which may occur than does the surgical procedure.

Lindstrom[15] has reported on a series of fourteen patients in whom the classical lumbar sympathectomy failed to relieve symptoms and on whom reoperations were performed to resect the first lumbar ganglion. One-half of these were benefited, and no disturbances in sexual function were encountered.

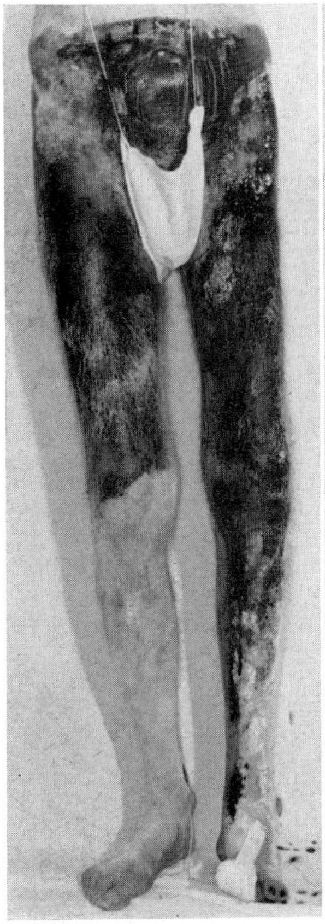

Fig. 4.

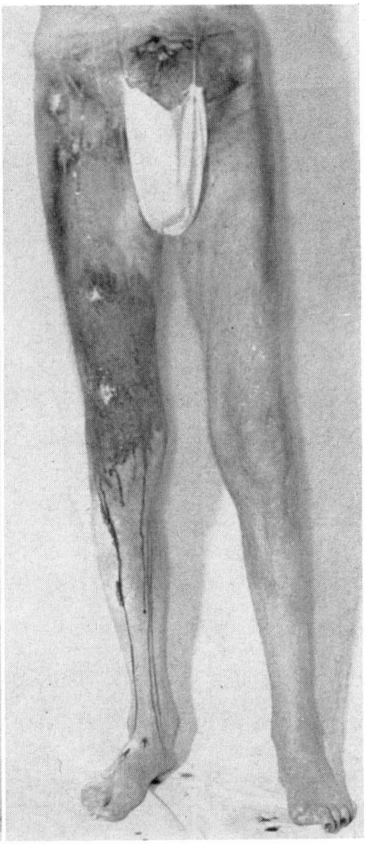

Fig. 5.

Fig. 4 (Case A. D.).—Starch-iodine test after bilateral low lumbar sympathectomy indicating inadequate sympathectomy on left, persistence of symptoms, and failure to heal at the site of amputated digit.

Fig. 5 (Case A. D.).—Starch-iodine test following reoperation through high posterior approach indicating complete sympathectomy and healing of amputated stump.

Starch-iodine tests were carried out on seventy-eight of our patients to evaluate the effectiveness of the sympathectomies on a basis of sudomotor activity (Fig. 3). Very few of those operated upon through a low anterior approach showed signs of sympathetic interruption above the knee. All of those operated upon through the high posterior approach showed complete loss of sweating below the inguinal ligament, and many of these were dry up to the umbilicus.

A single case is presented as being a typical illustration of the results obtained in our series.

CASE REPORT

A. D., a 47-year-old white man, developed symptoms of thromboangiitis obliterans in 1950. Because of multiple gangrenous digits and painful ischemia, quadrilateral sympathectomies were performed, elsewhere, in May, 1951. The patient was relieved of symptoms until April, 1952, when he was admitted to the Surgical Service of the Veterans Administration Hospital in Coral Gables, Fla., with gangrene of the left great toe. This digit was amputated on June 4, 1952, but the operative area did not heal and pain persisted. The patient insisted on holding the foot in a dependent position, which caused edema.

A starch-iodine test (Fig. 4) revealed sweating on the medial aspect of the left leg. It was felt that reoperation for high left lumbar sympathectomy would be beneficial. This was performed on Aug. 6, 1952. The twelfth thoracic and the first and second lumbar ganglia were removed. Postoperatively there was immediate relief of pain, with obvious warming of the foot. Healing of the previous amputation site was complete within two weeks (Fig. 5). The patient is working and is free of complaints.

In an attempt to evaluate the results of a lumbar sympathectomy, we have reviewed all lumbar sympathectomies performed on patients with arterial circulatory insufficiency at the Jackson Memorial Hospital in Miami and the Veterans Administration Hospital in Coral Gables, Fla., during a four-year period ending Dec. 31, 1952.

Material Studied (Table I).—A total of eighty-five patients were operated upon one hundred fifteen times. Forty of these were in the Veterans Administration Hospital and forty-five were in the Jackson Hospital. Seventy-two of these could be located for review. There were no operative or postoperative deaths in this series, and there were no serious complications as the result of sympathectomy. Twenty-one had died of unrelated causes. Fifty-one were interviewed and evaluated.

TABLE I. MATERIAL REVIEWED

	VETERAN'S ADMINISTRATION HOSPITAL	JACKSON HOSPITAL	TOTAL
Total patients	40	45	85
Total operations	51	64	115
Operative deaths	0	0	0
Operative complications	0	0	0
Patients followed	31	41	72
Living	24	27	51
Dead	7	14	21
Cause of death			
Heart disease	4	4	8
Malignancy	2	3	5
Cerebral hemorrhage	1	3	4
Suicide	0	1	1
Undetermined	0	3	3

Type of Operation and Age (Table II).—Of the 115 operations, eighty-one were of the low type performed through an anterior approach and twenty-three were of the high type performed through a posterior subdiaphragmatic approach. Eleven of these were reoperations in which the first low sympathectomy had been unsatisfactory and a second high lumbar sympathectomy was carried out. The average data on these patients are shown in Table II.

TABLE II. TYPE OF OPERATION AND AGE

	VETERANS ADMINISTRATION HOSPITAL	AVERAGE AGE (YR.)	JACKSON HOSPITAL	AVERAGE AGE (YR.)	TOTAL
Classical (low anterior approach)	31	48	50	57	81
Complete (high posterior approach)	10	51	13	60	23
Reoperation, first low, second high	3	39	8	54	11

Type of Disease (Table III).—Of the fifty-one patients operated upon, thirty-seven were diagnosed as having arteriosclerosis, and in this group twenty-one had diabetes. Twelve were diagnosed as having thromboangiitis obliterans. There was one with Leriche syndrome, and one case of traumatic vasospasm.

TABLE III. TYPE OF DISEASE

	VETERANS ADMINISTRATION HOSPITAL	JACKSON HOSPITAL	TOTAL
Arteriosclerosis	17	20	37
With diabetes	8	13	21
Thromboangiitis obliterans	6	6	12
Leriche syndrome	1	0	1
Traumatic vasospasm	0	1	1

Results in Living Patients (Table IV).—Sixty-eight operations were evaluated in the cases of those living patients who were located. There were fifty low lumbar sympathectomies in this group; 54 per cent showed improvement. Sixteen per cent were unimproved and 30 per cent experienced questionable results. There were eighteen high lumbar sympathectomies. Seventy-eight per cent were improved, 17 per cent were unimproved, and in one case there was a questionable result. Nine high reoperations were performed on individuals who had been operated upon through a low anterior approach, either by us or elsewhere, with unsatisfactory results. Eighty-nine per cent of these experienced improvement. The remaining eleven per cent experienced equivocal results.

TABLE IV. RESULTS OF SYMPATHECTOMY IN LIVING PATIENTS

	LOW	HIGH	REOPERATION HIGH
Improved	27 (54%)	14 (78%)	8 (89%)
Unimproved	8 (16%)	3 (17%)	0
Equivocal	15 (30%)	1 (5%)	1 (11%)
Total	50	18	9
Dead	31	4	2

CONCLUSIONS

1. Complete sympathectomy affords a practical method for improving arterial circulation to the lower extremity.

2. It is impractical, and often impossible, to attempt complete lumbar sympathectomy through the usual anterior incision.

3. Removal of the twelfth thoracic and the upper three lumbar sympathetic ganglia through a posterior subdiaphragmatic incision is a simple and safe method of accomplishing a complete sympathetic interruption to the lower extremity.

REFERENCES

1. Lee, R. M., Krauskoph, F. F., and Lilly, G. D.: Evaluation of Lumbar Sympathectomy, South. M. J. **42**: 864, 1949.
2. Coldwater, K. B., Cox, J. W., Randall, W. C., Alexander, W. F., and Hertzman, A. B.: Sweating Patterns and Vascular Responses in the Lower Extremity of Man Elicited by Stimulation of the Sympathetic Trunk, Proc. Surg. Forum, Clin. Congress Am. Coll. Surgeons, 1953, Philadelphia, 1953, W. B. Saunders Company.
3. Royle, N. D.: The Treatment of Spastic Paralysis by Sympathetic Ramisection, Surg., Gynec. & Obst. **39**: 701, 1924.
4. Randall, W. C., Alexander, W. F., Cox, J. W., and Hertzman, A. B.: Functional Analysis of the Vasomotor Innervation of the Dog's Hind Foot Pad, Circulation Res. **1**: 63 (Jan.) 1953.
5. Francioli, P.: The Surgical Approach in Lumbar and Lumbo-Thoracic Sympathectomies, Kelvet. Chir. Acta **18**: 536, 1951; Abstracted in Internat. Abstr. Surg. **331**: (Oct.) 1952.
6. Pratt, G. H.: The Present Status of Sympathectomy in the Treatment of Vascular Diseases, Angiology **1**: 9 (Feb.) 1950.
7. Flothow, P. G.: Observations on Twenty Years of Experience in Surgery of the Sympathectic Nervous System, West. J. Surg. **59**: 110, 1951.
8. Yeager, G. H., and Cowley, A.: Anatomical Observations on the Lumbar Sympathectics With Evaluation in Organic Peripheral Vascular Disease, Ann. Surg. **127**: 953, 1948.
9. Edwards, E. A.: Operative Anatomy of the Lumbar Sympathetic Chain, Angiology **2**: 184 (June) 1951.
10. Reed, A., and Kirgis, H.: Some Problems of Sympathectomy, Bull. Tulane M. Fac. **11**: 157 (May) 1952.
11. Cannon, W. B.: A Law of Denervation, Am. J. M. Sc. **198**: 737, 1939.
12. Langley, J. N.: On the Regeneration of Preganglionic and Postganglionic Nerve Fibers, J. Physiol. **22**: 215, 1898.
13. Thompson, J. E., Brose, N. A., and Smithwick, R. H.: Patterns of Electrical Skin Resistance Following Sympathectomy, Arch. Surg. **60**: 431, 1950.
14. Alnor, P.: The Influence of Lumbar Sympathetic Chain Resection Upon Sexual Functions, Ztschr. Chir. **269**: 506, 1951; Abstracted in Internat. Abstr. Surg. **95**: 331 (Oct.) 1952.
15. Lindstrom, B. L.: The Effect of High Lumbar Sympathectomy in Patients With Organic Arterial Disease of the Lower Limb Previously Treated With Low Lumbar Sympathectomy, Acta chir. Scandinav. **103**: 370, 1952.

PULMONARY VALVULOTOMY

Results of Operation in Twenty-Five Cases

George H. Humphreys, II, M.D., Samuel Powers, M.D., Hugh Fitzpatrick, M.D., and Ben Marr Lanman, M.D., New York, N. Y.

(From the Department of Surgery, College of Physicians and Surgeons, Columbia University, and the Surgical Services of the Babies and Presbyterian Hospitals)

SINCE the first introduction by Brock[1] of an operative procedure designed to overcome pulmonary valvular obstruction and since its further development by Brock[2, 3] and Blalock,[4] pulmonary valvulotomy has become established as a successful method. Refinements of technique have since been added by Potts and his co-workers,[5] but the sound physiologic principle of direct surgical relief of obstruction to blood flow into the lungs remains unaltered. There is still, however, a good deal of uncertainty as to how widely this technique can be applied to the various cardiac anomalies which include an element of pulmonic stenosis[6] and as to what results can be expected, both clinically and physiologically. Because the method is relatively new, and few series have been reported which include follow-up data,[7, 8] it seems worth while to present results of studies in a group of twenty-five consecutive patients operated upon at the Columbia-Presbyterian Medical Center between June, 1950, and December, 1952. In observing the results of operation we have attempted to determine the effectiveness of valvulotomy in producing changes in the circulation of patients with various closely related anomalies and to evaluate the clinical effects of these changes.

The group is limited to those cases in which a stenosis at the pulmonary valve was found at operation and in which incision and dilatation according to the Brock technique[3] were carried out. The age of the patient at operation varied from 4 months to 24 years, with twelve (or about one-half) in the age group between 6 and 10 years. The patients were equally divided between both sexes (Tables I and II).

Table I. Sex

	MALE	FEMALE	TOTAL
Valvular stenosis only	5	4	9
With auricular defect	2	3	5
With ventricular defect	5	6	11
Totals	12	13	25

Of the twenty-five patients, in nine (36 per cent), the anomaly was limited to the stenotic pulmonary valve. In seven of these, the valve was symmetrically stenosed into a conical diaphragm with narrowed central orifice

Supported in part by grants from the American Heart Association and by a research grant, PHS No. H-819, from the National Heart Institute, National Institutes of Health, United States Public Health Service.

Read at the seventh annual meeting of the Society for Vascular Surgery, New York, N. Y., May 31, 1953.

through which a strong jet of blood could be felt to flow during systole. In two, the valve was irregularly and asymmetrically stenosed. In all, the pulmonary artery showed poststenotic dilatation, twice described as "aneurysmal" but, in one, this was not apparent on frontal roentgenogram.

TABLE II. AGE (YEARS)

	0-5	6-10	11-15	16-20	21-25	TOTAL
Valvular stenosis only	0	4	1	3	1	9
With auricular defect	1	3	0	1	0	5
With ventricular defect	3	5	2	0	1	11
Totals	4	12	3	4	2	25

In five patients (20 per cent) with valvular stenosis there was, in addition, a defect in the interauricular septum. In three of these, the valve was symmetrically stenosed as in the cases without other anomaly and, in two, it was asymmetrical and irregular. All showed poststenotic dilatation of the pulmonary artery at operation, but this was evident on roentgenogram in only three.

In eleven patients (44 per cent) the pulmonary valvular stenosis was combined with an interventricular septal defect and varying degrees of dextroposition or overriding of the aorta. In one patient, the aortic arch and descending aorta lay on the right, and in one there was a true dextrocardia. These patients represent a variety of tetralogy of Fallot but vary widely within the group between a situation almost indistinguishable from the first group to one practically identical with tetralogy with infundibular stenosis. In only four was there a typical conical valvular stenosis, and in only three was a poststenotic dilatation of the pulmonary artery present. The single death in the entire series was in this group (Table III).

TABLE III

	VALVE		PULMONARY ARTERY		
	CONICAL	IRREGULAR	DILATED	NORMAL OR SMALL	TOTAL
Valvular stenosis only	7	2	9	0	9
With auricular defect	3	2	5	0	5
With ventricular defect	5	6	3	8	11
Totals	15	10	17	8	25

A variety of studies were carried out on these patients before, during, and after operation. These were designed to demonstrate the circulatory abnormality not only in order to determine the anatomic anomaly, but also to define the degree of physiologic disturbance and the extent to which the procedure succeeded in restoring a more nearly normal situation. More information was obtained by catheterization studies than by any other method. Venous catheterization of the right heart by the method of Cournand and associates[9] was successful in fourteen cases.* The findings are in agreement with previous studies reported by others.[10-12]

*These studies were carried out in the cardiorespiratory laboratory of the Department of Medicine at the College of Physicians and Surgeons by Dr. John West and his associates.

In addition, direct catheterization of the right ventricle and pulmonary artery before and immediately after valvulotomy, as described by Fitzpatrick and associates,[13] was carried out in ten cases, in seven of which venous catheterization had either failed or had not been attempted. This method permits pressure recordings which correlate well with the first, but does not permit sampling for blood gas analysis. Thus, preoperative right ventricular pressure records are available in twenty-one of the twenty-five cases. Immediate postvalvulotomy pressures are available in nine, and venous catheterization has been carried out at periods up to two years after operation in four. It is unfortunate that the reluctance of parents to consent to postoperative studies once their child has been relieved of symptoms has hampered the obtaining of adequate late studies.

In addition to catheterization, radioactive isotope flow studies by the method of Powers and co-workers[14] have yielded valuable information. By this method it has been found possible not only to obtain a curve quite characteristic of pulmonary stenosis, but also to determine in many instances the direction and degree of intracardiac shunting. In some cases, small shunts were demonstrated by this method which could not otherwise be detected and which proved to be present at operation. Shifts in direction of shunting following vulvulotomy were also well shown.

VALVULAR STENOSIS WITHOUT SEPTAL DEFECT

In eight of the nine cases, catheterization studies were obtained before valvulotomy. The ninth case involved a patient whose true anomaly was not recognized before operation, since it had been mistakenly thought that he had a patent ductus arteriosus. Four of the nine were catheterized before operation. Two patients were catheterized both before and during operation, the resulting readings correlating well. Two were catheterized on the operating table immediately before valvulotomy and again immediately thereafter, without preoperative catheterization. The striking finding in this group was the high right ventricular systolic pressure, averaging 125 mm. including one reading of 32 mm. which seemed inconsistent with the patient's clinical handicap and subsequent improvement. The highest individual reading (217/9) was also in this group (Table IV).

Six patients were catheterized after valvulotomy: four, immediately; one, one year later; and one, two years later. Striking falls in right ventricular

TABLE IV. RIGHT VENTRICULAR PRESSURES BEFORE AND AFTER VALVULOTOMY: PURE VALVULAR STENOSIS

PATIENT	BEFORE	AFTER	RESULT	FOLLOW-UP PERIOD
L. C.	147/19, 149/0*	65/0*	+++	1½ yr.
R. E.	217/9	69/2	++++	1 yr.
W. F.	32/6		+++	2½ yr.
L. G.	195/8		++++	3 yr.
J. K.	92/6*	60/0*	++++	2 yr.
T. M.	104/2*	58/8*	++++	2¾ yr.
J. R.	162/12	78/15	++++	2½ yr.
A. S.			+++	1 yr.
A. S.	94/10, 85/10*	40/8*	+	6 mo.

*Direct catheterization at operation.

systolic pressure were noted in all cases, although in every case a pressure slightly in excess of accepted normal persisted. In the case studied two years after valvulotomy (J. R.) the pressure remains substantially below the preoperative level. The average was 61 mm.

The tracings, especially those obtained on the operating table, also showed striking returns toward normal, not only in the mean pulmonary arterial pressure, but also in the pulse contour, which changed from a low, damped curve to one with characteristic dicrotic notch, demonstrating restoration of valvular function (Figs. 1 and 3).

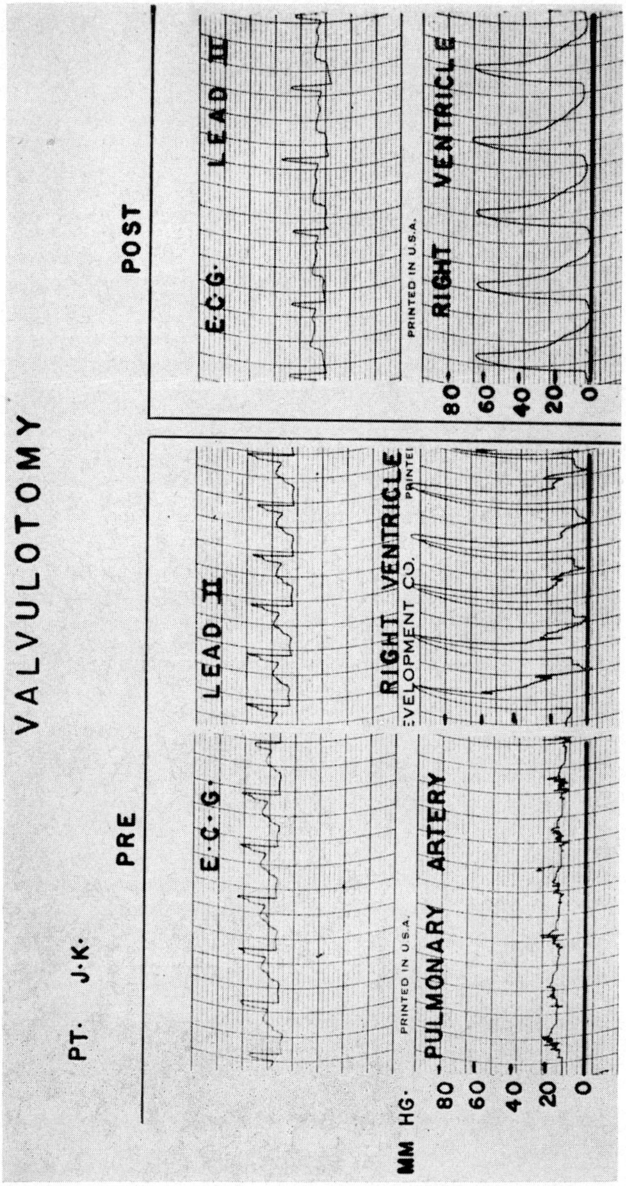

Fig. 1.—Tracings obtained by direct cardiac catheterization at operation on a patient with isolated pulmonary valvular stenosis (J. K.).

The upper tracing is a Lead II electrocardiographic record. The lower tracing shows on the left the low, damped pulmonary artery pressure contrasting with the high right ventricular pressure before valvulotomy. On the right the ventricular pressure is shown to be substantially lower immediately after valvulotomy.

Isotope dilution curves showed a characteristic slow rise in the wave, presumably due to the eddying beyond the jet of blood, which holds some of the isotope in the dilated pulmonary artery causing greater dilution. This effect has also been well demonstrated in angiocardiograms (Fig. 2).

Clinically, all of these patients showed a characteristic picture. Dyspnea was the chief complaint and varied from mild to severe. None showed cyanosis, and only one was physically retarded, a condition possibly related to concomitant bilateral cryptorchidism. In age, the patients ranged between 5½ and 24 years, the average being 13. This is distinctly older than the other groups, probably because of the absence of cyanosis and the relatively milder handicap of dyspnea only. None had shown evidence of failure.

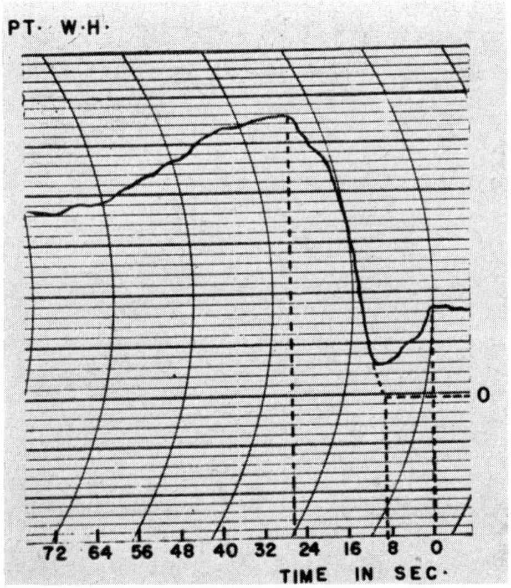

Fig. 2.—A typical curve of isotope dilution obtained in a patient with isolated pulmonary valvular stenosis (W. H.). From the injection point, *O*, on the right end of the record, the dye appears in normal time, 8 seconds (showing no right-to-left shunt). The rise to a peak at twenty-five seconds is approximately twice normal (showing delay in the passage of dye through the stenotic pulmonary valve).

Nevertheless, all but one (the most recent) were markedly improved following operation, five being able to carry out entirely normal activities and three being restricted only on vigorous exertion. However, the murmur persists with varying degrees of softening in all cases and, in all, the roentgen evidence of pulmonary artery dilatation is not noticeably changed.

VALVULAR STENOSIS WITH AURICULAR SEPTAL DEFECT

In four of the five cases, catheterization studies were obtained before valvulotomy. Two patients were successfully studied before operation; in two, attempted preoperative catheterization was technically unsuccessful; in one, a very sick infant of 4 months, it was not considered wise to attempt it. Catheterization on the operating table was performed both before and immediately after operation in two of the three patients in whom preoperative studies were not obtained and in one of the other two. The high average right ventricular pressure (125 mm.) corresponds to that found in valvular stenosis without septal defect. In one instance, the pressure was over 200. In this child (B. C.), the valve opening was so small that the catheter occluded it, with a resultant alarming increase in cyanosis (Table V).

TABLE V. RIGHT VENTRICULAR PRESSURES BEFORE AND AFTER VALVULOTOMY: VALVULAR STENOSIS WITH AURICULAR SEPTAL DEFECT

PATIENT	BEFORE	AFTER	RESULT	FOLLOW-UP PERIOD
B. C.	201/16	77/13	++++	2½ yr.
C. M.			++	1 yr.
D. P.	122/4, 120/10*	65/10*	?	9 mo.
C. R.	125/10*	60/8*	+++	1 yr.
G. T.	100/0*	40/0,* 77/4	++++	1½ yr.

*Direct catheterization at operation.

Four of the five patients were catheterized after valvulotomy, four immediately, one six months later, and one a year and one-half after operation. In one patient (C. R.), pressure tracings taken immediately after valvulotomy indicated an inadequate fall in ventricular pressure. A second dilatation of the pulmonary valve was then performed, after which the ventricular pressure fell to a satisfactory level, with corresponding improvement in the pulmonary artery pressure curve. This case demonstrates the usefulness of immediate studies after valvulotomy and the possibility that persistent elevations of ventricular pressures found in postoperative studies may represent a technically inadequate operation rather than recurrence of stenosis. In another patient (G. T.), comparison of the immediate with the later postoperative result is possible and shows only a slight late rise in ventricular systolic pressure, to a level corresponding to that found postoperatively in cases of valvular stenosis without septal defect.

As in the previous group, the pressure curves obtained in this group postoperatively show a striking return toward normal. It is to be expected that these two groups should show similar findings, since the right ventricle, in the absence of tricuspid insufficiency, can empty only through the stenotic valve (Fig. 3).

The isotope dilution curve in this group, however, contrasts with that in isolated valvular stenosis, because of the shunting of blood across the auricular septum. Before valvulotomy, this shunt is both from right to left and from left to right, presumably varying with the phase of the cardiac cycle. The magnitude of each varies with the degree of pulmonic stenosis. After valvulotomy, the change in direction to a predominantly left-to-right shunt is well shown on these curves, which also permit an estimate of its volume (Fig. 4).

Angiocardiograms have not been successful in distinguishing these patients from those with valvular stenosis only. Presumably the shunt from the right auricle to the left is, in most cases, too small in volume to permit early appearance of contrast medium in the left heart. Prolonged visualization of the pulmonary artery is present in both.

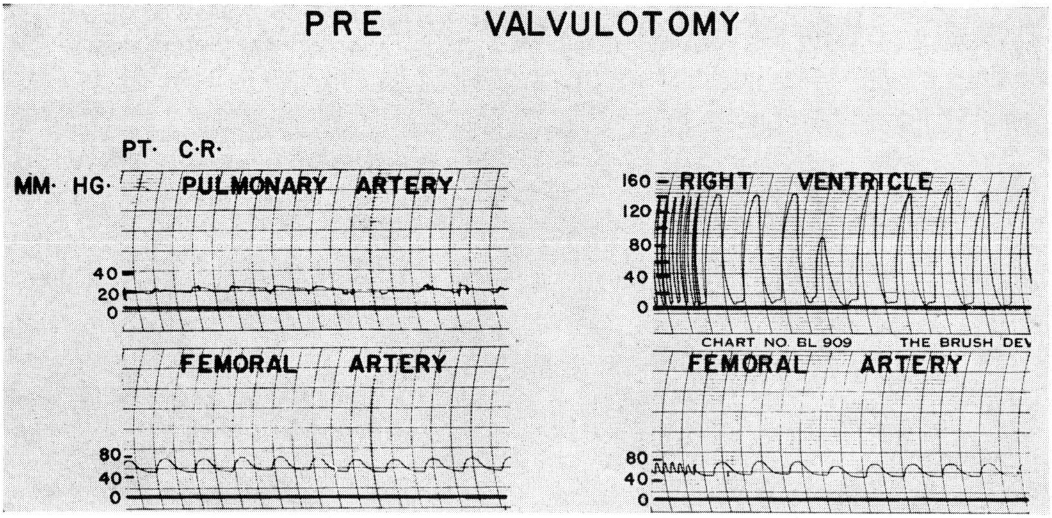

A.

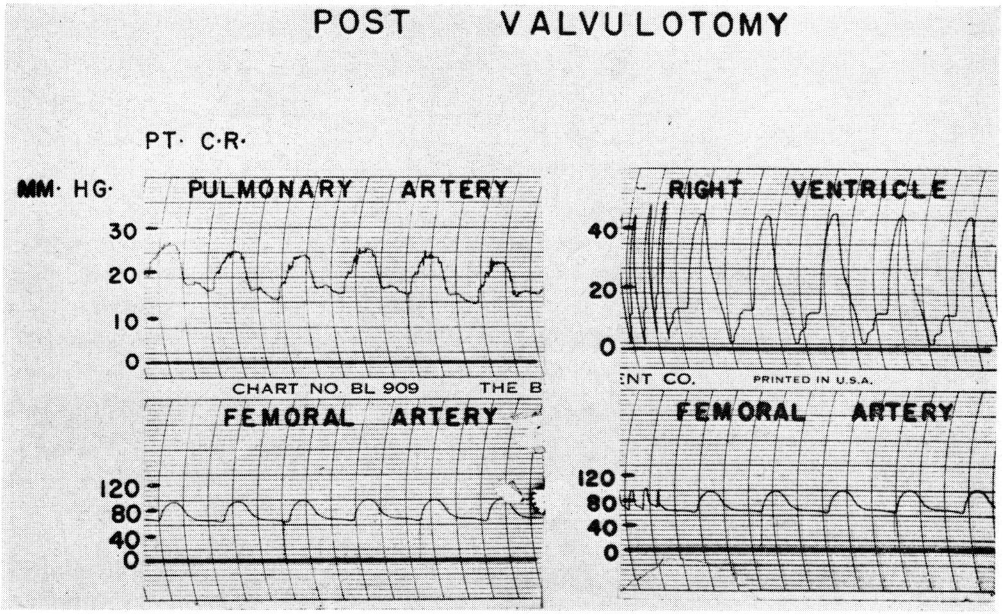

B.

Fig. 3.—*A,* Tracings obtained by direct cardiac catheterization at operation on a patient with pulmonary valvular stenosis and interauricular septal defect (C. R.). These are substantially the same as those in isolated pulmonary stenosis (Fig. 1). A low damped pulmonary arterial pressure on the left contrasts with the high right ventricular pressure on the right.

B, Tracings obtained immediately after valvulotomy on the same patient (C. R.). The rise in pulmonary arterial pressure and restoration to normal contour with dichrotic notch (indicating restoration of valve function) as well as the marked lowering of ventricular pressure are evident.

Clinically, this group of patients showed a more variable picture than the first. Cyanosis was present on exertion in three of the five, one to a very slight degree, one to an obvious degree, and in one it became progressively more conspicuous with age, being moderate even at rest at the time of operation. In the latter two, mild polycythemia and clubbing were present. In the other two cases, cyanosis was not noted, but one of these was a swarthy 4-month-old infant in whom it may have been overlooked. Dyspnea was moderate to severe in all, and two showed marked retardation in development. In age, the group was widely scattered. Only the infant showed evidence of failure.

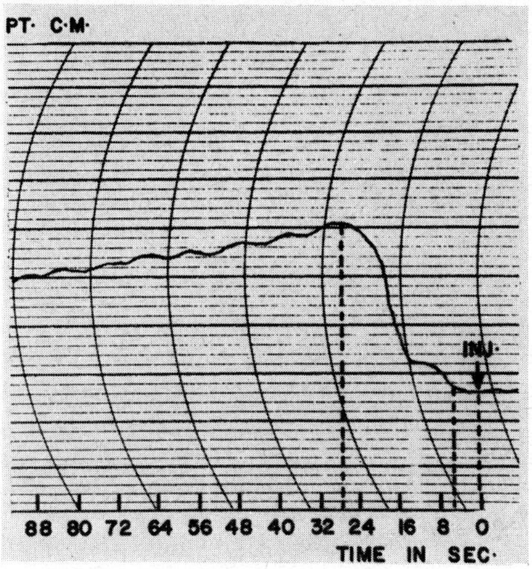

Fig. 4.—Isotope dilution curve obtained in a patient (C. M.) with pulmonary valvular stenosis associated with interauricular septal defect. Evidence of right-to-left shunt is shown by the short period of five seconds after injection at which dye first appears, although the major peak is delayed to twenty-six seconds. Evidence of left-to-right shunt is shown by the early secondary peak after the major peak, indicating recirculation through the lungs.

The operation was successful in eliminating cyanosis in all cases in which it had been present. Two patients were restored to essentially normal exercise tolerance and a third shows only slightly more dyspnea on exertion than normal. The infant, whose auricular defect is presumably large, has shown no further evidence of failure but is still markedly retarded both physically and mentally. The fifth patient developed rheumatic fever six months after operation, so the result is questionable. Murmurs persist in all, with less change than was noted in the group without septal defect.

VALVULAR STENOSIS WITH VENTRICULAR SEPTAL DEFECT

In nine of the eleven cases catheterization studies were obtained before valvulotomy. In one, catheterization was unsuccessful, and in the other, catheterization was not performed because the patient was thought to have a classical case of tetralogy of Fallot, the valvular stenosis being found at operation. Five were catheterized before operation, two both before and during operation and two at operation only. The characteristic feature in this group was the finding of right ventricular pressures at or below the systemic arterial level, whereas in the two previous groups it frequently exceeded aortic pressure. The average was only 92 mm. In only three were postoperative readings obtained, and these demonstrated a less striking fall in pressure than in the previous groups, a finding to be expected since the ventricular defect permits the left ventricular pressure to be transmitted to the right (Table VI).

TABLE VI. RIGHT VENTRICULAR PRESSURES BEFORE AND AFTER VALVULOTOMY: VALVULAR STENOSIS WITH VENTRICULAR SEPTAL DEFECT

PATIENT	BEFORE	AFTER	RESULT	FOLLOW-UP PERIOD
J. A.	105/5, 110/0*	90/20*	++	1½ yr.
J. B.	67/8, 68/0*	40/0*	++++	1½ yr.
R. C.	114/11		+	2 yr.
S. C.	–		Died	
I. DeR.	–		++	8 mo.
B. K.	128/8		++++	2½ yr.
S. P.	98/7		±	2½ yr.
L. R.	50/0*		±	1½ yr.
R. S.	88/0*	65/0*	++	1 yr.
F. S.	90/9		+	6 mo.
R. S.	75/2		+++	2½ yr.

*Direct catheterization at operation.

The pressure tracings varied with the anatomic variation of the anomalies. Where the defect was small and overriding of the aorta was not present, they took a form similar to that seen with isolated pulmonary stenosis before valvulotomy, but the return toward normal was not as striking postoperatively because of the persistent ventricular hypertension (Fig. 5). Where the anomaly included overriding of the aorta while the pulmonary artery curve took on a more nearly normal form, the right ventricular curve was scarcely altered. Some apprehension was felt, in such cases, that the result might lead to an actual pulmonary arterial hypertension with resultant conversion to a form of Eisenmenger's syndrome, and vigorous stretching of the pulmonic ring was, therefore, not carried out.

As in the group with auricular septal defects, intracardiac shunting of blood both in direction and volume is directly reflected in the isotope dilution curves. For this reason these curves demonstrate well the variations in anatomy of the anomaly. Where no aortic overriding is present, right and left ventricular pressures may be so well balanced that the shunt is negligible before operation and the presence of a small ventricular defect may go undetected even on gas analysis of the right ventricular outflow tract blood. Yet a small early secondary peek in the isotope curve will suggest re-entry of the left ventricular blood into the lesser circulation well before the normal secondary rise of systemic recirculation. After valvulotomy, this peak is more obvious, as the ventricular pressure balance is altered and a larger left-to-right shunt occurs (Fig. 6). On the other hand, with aortic overriding and consequent entrance of right ventricular blood into the aorta, the early peak in the isotope curve will demonstrate its presence and extent; after valvulotomy this peak may disappear almost completely as the shunt becomes predominantly left to right (Fig. 7). The curve is not helpful, however, in distinguishing this group from classical tetralogy with infundibular stenosis. Similarly, angiocardiograms may demonstrate early aortic filling in this group but will rarely demonstrate the site of obstruction to pulmonary flow.

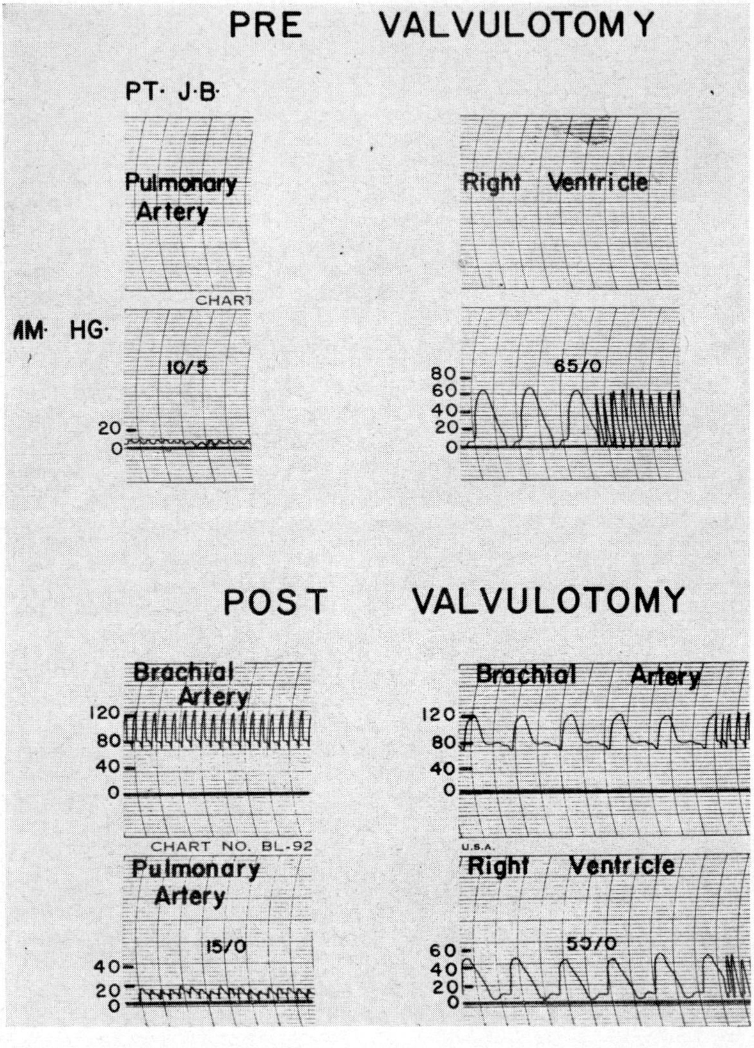

Fig. 5.—Tracings obtained by ventricular catheterization before and immediately after valvulotomy in a patient (J. B.) with pulmonary valvular stenosis and associated ventricular septal defect, but little or no overriding. The pulmonary artery tracing has improved but the right ventricular pressure, which was not excessively high even before valvulotomy, has not changed significantly.

Clinically, this is an interesting but often disappointing group. It is extremely variable. In only one patient (J. B.), whose defect was so small that it was detected only by isotope curve and proved to be present at operation, was there no cyanosis at any time. On the other hand, only two of the remaining ten were cyanotic from birth. Three developed cyanosis during the first year of life, and in five it appeared after the first year. In all ten, cyanosis became increasingly severe with age but in one-half of these, it was apparent only on exertion. While the other five showed some cyanosis even at rest, only one (S. P.) was constantly deeply cyanotic, and he had a complex anomaly with dextrocardia and a high degree of overriding of the aorta. As

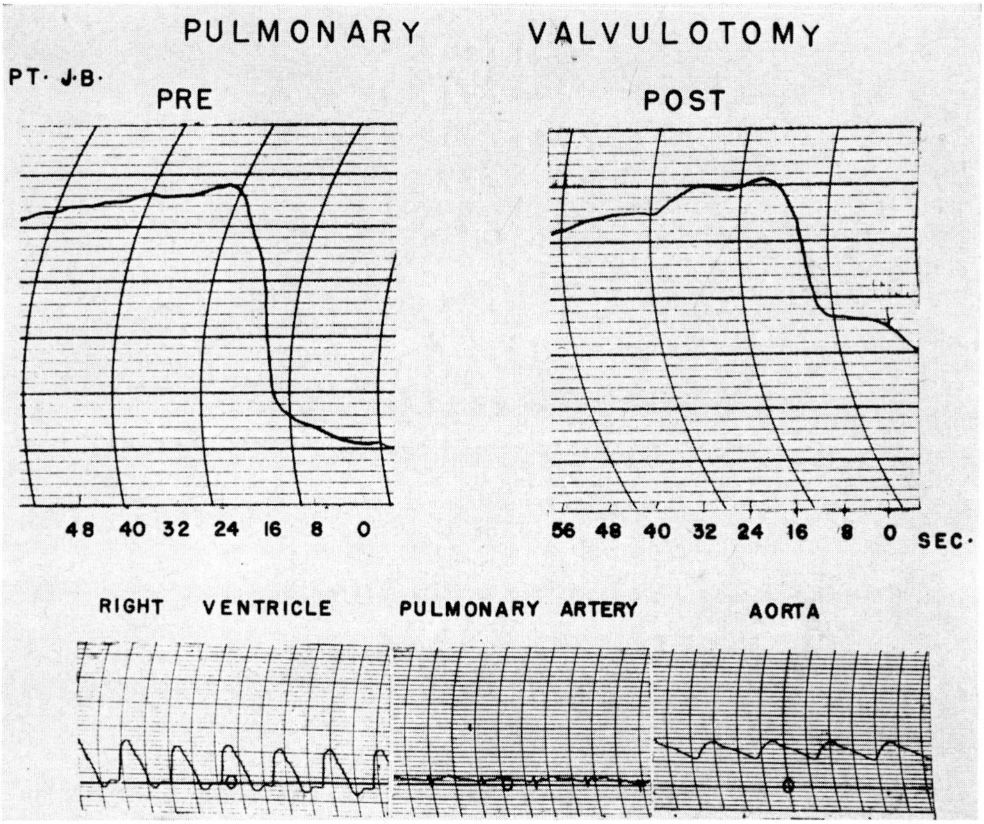

Fig. 6.—Isotope dilution curves in patient (J. B.) with pulmonary valvular stenosis and associated ventricular septal defect, unsuspected until this tracing was obtained. A small early secondary peak in the curve before valvulotomy indicates a left-to-right shunt. Immediately after valvulotomy this secondary peak is much more conspicuous, indicating considerable increase in volume of the same shunt, following relief of obstruction at the pulmonary valve.

Below are shown pressure curves on the same patient from right ventricle, pulmonary artery, and aorta, into which the catheter passed from the right ventricle, thus proving directly the presence of an interventricular defect.

would be expected, moderate clubbing of the fingers was present in three of the five who were cyanotic at rest, and slight clubbing in the other two, whereas clubbing was present in only two of the five who showed cyanosis only on exertion. The habit of assuming a squatting position was usual, being present in all but two of the cyanotic group. In these two, significant cyanosis was late in appearing.

Other evidences of congenital somatic inadequacy were also more frequent in this group. One was severely retarded physically, one was mentally defective although normal in development, and one was retarded both mentally and physically. A right aortic arch was present in one, dextrocardia in another, a left vena cava in a third, and one had an associated imperforate anus. The patient who died was found at autopsy to have also an infundibular stenosis and a patent foramen ovale.

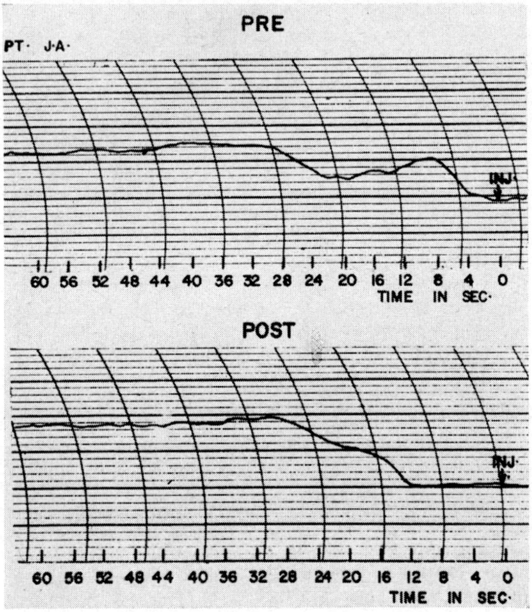

Fig. 7.—Isotope dilution curves in a patient (J. A.) with pulmonary valvular stenosis associated with ventricular septal defect and overriding aorta. The top curve, before valvulotomy, shows an early sharp peak of considerable magnitude, indicating a significant right-to-left shunt. The bottom curve, immediately after valvulotomy, shows that this shunt has been almost completely eliminated. Both curves show the early secondary peaks which indicate the rapid recirculation of left-to-right shunting.

As would be expected in such a variable group, the result of operation has been inconstant. One patient (B. K.), a woman of 23 years who had been cyanotic since birth with progression to severe exercise restriction, now shows no cyanosis and has normal exercise tolerance. One other patient (R. S.) is no longer cyanotic but occasionally squats when tired. The other seven surviving patients who were cyanotic still show some cyanosis on exertion and in two of these, there is no appreciable change. The patient without cyanosis before operation (J. B.), on the other hand, has had an excellent result comparable to the patient with valvular stenosis alone. The single operative mortality occurred in this group in a cyanotic child (S. C.) thought to have classical tetralogy of Fallot. An operation was performed one year before his death with the intention of creating a surgical ductus arteriosus, but his condition became alarming when the pulmonary artery was temporarily occluded, and the operation was terminated. One year later, on a second attempt, a conical value and jet were found to be present and a valvulotomy was performed. At the close of the procedure, ventricular fibrillation occurred. At autopsy both a valvular and infundibular stenosis were found, as well as a patent foramen ovale. It seems probable that creation of a surgical ductus would have been a more suitable choice in this case, in spite of the failure on the first attempt.

SUMMARY

The results of physiologic studies on twenty-five consecutive cases of valvular stenosis treated by valvulotomy according to the technique of Brock are presented. Some significant findings on catheterization before, during, and after operation are presented, as well as selected examples of isotope dilution curves to demonstrate the usefulness of that method in such cases. Twenty-one of the twenty-five were catheterized before valvulotomy, and thirteen after the procedure. In nine patients, the anomaly was limited to the pulmonary valve, and in all but one of these, clinical results have been excellent. In five patients, a defect in the auricular septum was also present. Clinical results are excellent in two, good in two, and questionable in the other one. In eleven patients, a defect in the ventricular septum was also present. Reasons for the variable results in this group, which includes the only operative mortality, are discussed.

REFERENCES

1. Brock, R. C.: Pulmonary Valvulotomy for the Relief of Congenital Pulmonary Stenosis, Brit. M. J. **1**: 1121, 1948.
2. Brock, R. C.: The Surgery of Pulmonary Stenosis, Brit. M. J. **22**: 399, 1949.
3. Brock, R. C., and Campbell, M.: Valvulotomy for Pulmonary Valvular Stenosis, Brit. Heart J. **12**: 37, 1950.
4. Blalock, A., and Kieffer, R., Jr.: Valvulotomy for the Relief of Congenital Valvular Pulmonic Stenosis With Intact Ventricular Septum, Ann. Surg. **132**: 496, 1950.
5. Potts, W. J., Gibson, S., Riker, W. L., and Leininger, C. R.: Congenital Pulmonic Stenosis With Intact Ventricular Septum, J. A. M. A. **144**: 8, 1950.
6. Glover, R. P., Bailey, C. P., O'Neil, T. J. E., Downing, D. F., and Wells, C. R. E.: The Direct Intracardiac Relief of Pulmonary Stenosis in Tetralogy of Fallot, J. Thoracic Surg. **23**: 114, 1952.
7. Brock, R. C.: Direct Cardiac Surgery in the Treatment of Congenital Pulmonary Stenosis, Ann. Surg. **136**: 63, 1952.
8. Muller, W. H., Jr., and Longmire, W. P., Jr.: The Surgical Treatment of Cardiac Valvular Stenosis, SURGERY **30**: 29, 1951.
9. Cournand, A., Riley, R. L., Breed, E. S., Baldwin, E. DeF., and Richards, D. W., Jr.: Measurement of Cardiac Output in Man Using the Technique of Catheterization of the Right Auricle or Ventricle, J. Clin. Investigation **24**: 106, 1945.
10. Greene, D. G., Baldwin, E. DeF., Baldwin, J. S., Himmelstein, A., Roh, C. E., and Cournand, A.: Pure Congenital Pulmonary Stenosis and Idiopathic Congenital Dilatation of the Pulmonary Artery, Am. J. Med. **6**: 24, 1949.
11. Engle, M. A., and Taussig, H. B.: Valvular Pulmonic Stenosis With Intact Ventricular Septum and Patent Foramen Ovale, Circulation **2**: 481, 1950.
12. Maraist, F., Daley, R., Draper, A., Jr., Heimbecker, R., Damman, F., Jr., Kieffer, R., Jr., King, J. T., Ferencz, C., and Bing, R. J.: Physiological Studies in Congenital Heart Disease: X. Physiological Findings in 34 Patients with Isolated Pulmonary Valvular Stenosis, Bull. Johns Hopkins Hosp. **88**: 1, 1951.
13. Fitzpatrick, H. F., Weissman, S. G., Deterling, R. A., Papper, E. M., Blakemore A. H., and Humphreys, G. H., II: Observations on the Alterations in Cardiovascular Dynamics Resulting From Surgical Procedure on the Heart and Great Vessels in Man, Proc. Surg. Forum, Clin. Congress Am. Coll. Surgeons, 1951, Philadelphia, 1952, W. B. Saunders Company, p. 262.
14. Powers, S. R., Rossi, H. H., and Papper, E. M.: An Instrument for the Measurement of Cardiac Output, Rev. Scient. Instruments **23**: 178, 1952.

CARDIAC OUTPUT: A CLINICAL COMPARISON OF THE DIRECT FICK, DYE, AND BALLISTOCARDIOGRAPHIC METHODS*

William A. Neely, M.D., Frank C. Wilson, Jr., M.D.,** J. Pervis Milnor, M.D., James D. Hardy, M.D., and Harwell Wilson, M.D.,
Memphis, Tenn.

(From the Department of Surgery and Surgical Laboratories and the Department of Medicine, Medical College of The University of Tennessee, and the John Gaston Hospital)

THE accurate measurement of cardiac output has wide applicability in the field of vascular surgery. For this reason we have examined three of the methods in current use with a view to assessing the relative accuracy and clinical usefulness of the several methods. It has seemed particularly important to check the accuracy of the dye method. In the most seriously ill patients, the ballistocardiographic record is often so abnormal as to preclude interpretation, and in certain other patients the arms may not be available for the introduction of the cardiac catheter to obtain samples of mixed venous blood from the pulmonary artery for the direct Fick measurements.

The Direct Fick Method.—In 1870, Fick[1] proposed the principle that the rate of blood flow through an organ could be determined by measuring the arteriovenous difference of a metabolite and by measuring the amount of the metabolite consumed over a definite period of time. Grehant[2] later applied the Fick principle to the measurement of cardiac output in dogs. Forssmann[3] in 1928, in a series of experiments on himself, was the first to catheterize the right heart in man, and in recent years Cournand[4] and his associates have developed this technique to an extent which has made the direct Fick method applicable in man.

The direct Fick method suffers from certain disadvantages, however. To measure cardiac output by this method, it is necessary to cut down on a vein in the antecubital fossa. This obviously limits the number of separate catheterizations which can be accomplished in any one patient, and in certain patients the antecubital fossae may not be available. Moreover, there are occasions when the catheterization is unsuccessful, and in other instances it is inconvenient, if not clinically inadvisable, to remove the seriously ill patient to the fluoroscopic room for the catheterization procedure. Therefore, although the direct Fick method is often accepted as possibly the most accurate method available, it has its limitations.

The Ballistocardiographic Method.—As early as 1905, Henderson[5] realized that the ballistic impulses of the human body were somehow related to cardiac

---

Read at the seventh annual meeting of the Society for Vascular Surgery, New York, N. Y., May 31, 1953.

*This work has been conducted under Army Contract No. DA-49-007-MD-296 between the University of Tennessee and the Office of the Surgeon General, Department of the Army, and has been aided by a grant from the Memphis Heart Association.

**Public Health Service Research Fellow of the National Cancer Institute.

output, as he observed that breath-holding reduced the magnitude of the impulses recorded by his machine. In 1939, Starr[6] developed the ballistocardiograph to a point of clinical usefulness and derived a formula relating the magnitude of the impulses to stroke volume. The Starr ballistocardiograph is the one used in the present study.

Without entering into the controversy regarding the value of the ballistocardiographic method in patients who are not critically ill, we merely wish to restate a fact which is accepted by all workers, namely, that in the most critically ill patients, in whom cardiac output data would be most desirable, the ballistocardiographic complexes are frequently so abnormal as to preclude accurate interpretation. Particularly is this true in the severely burned patient. Therefore, while the ballistocardiographic method does permit rapid and repeated measurements in the same normal subject, in the abnormal subject this method is often not applicable.

The Blue Dye Method.—Disappointed with the limitations of first the Fick and later the ballistocardiographic methods for the study of critically ill patients, we have examined the blue dye method for the measurement of cardiac output. In 1897, Stewart[7] proposed that cardiac output could be measured if a substance were infused at a constant rate into a vein so that a concentration plateau could be achieved in the peripheral blood. He realized that the measurements had to be made before significant recirculation had taken place. It was apparent that, by knowing the amount of the substance infused per second and the concentration level of the plateau, a figure related to cardiac output could be obtained. In 1928, Hamilton,[8] while studying circulation times by the single-injection method, realized that the mean concentration of the injected substance in arterial blood was inversely related to cardiac output. Later Kinsman[9] demonstrated that following a single injection of a substance it was possible to correct for the recirculation by plotting the concentrations of timed arterial samples on semilogarithmic paper. This is essentially the method that is in use today.

To apply the dye injection principle, one can use either the kymographic method of Hamilton and associates[8] or a more elaborate automatic recording device as advocated by Friedlich, Heimbecker, and Bing.[10] It is possible to purchase parts for the manufacture of a constant-flow cuvette for approximately eighty dollars. The cost of this item, if purchased assembled, is many times this amount. Certain auxiliary parts, such as a direct current amplifier and a sensitive recording galvanometer, are required. These items are costly.

The advantages of the constant-flow cuvette are mainly those of convenience. As the blood flows through the cuvette, an automatic record is made of the light transmission through the flowing blood. Multiple records can be made, and it is not necessary to read each individual sample in a spectrophotometer as in the Hamilton method.

The disadvantages of the constant-flow cuvette are numerous. A calibration curve must be plotted for each patient and more than one for the same patient if the oxygen content of arterial blood changes. Change in the rate of flow of blood through the cuvette influences the transmission readings; therefore, adequate precaution must be taken to insure constant flow. The apparatus is elaborate, and as much blood is shed as with the Hamilton method. For these reasons we have used the kymographic method of Hamilton.

If the dye method can be shown to have an accuracy comparable to that obtained by the use of the Fick method or the ballistocardiograph, it may become the clinical method of choice, for it offers certain advantages which the other two methods do not. Multiple measurements may be performed on the same patient without the necessity of moving the patient to the fluoroscopic room. Moreover, the method can be used in the seriously ill patients whose ballistocardiographic tracings are frequently unreadable, and it can often be used in patients who have been severely burned and whose antecubital fossae may not be available for catheterization.

PROCEDURE USED IN THE PRESENT STUDY

The patient was allowed nothing but water for eight hours preceding the study. Thirty minutes before the skin was incised for the introduction of the cardiac catheter into the antecubital vein, the patient received 0.18 Gm. of Sodium Amytal orally. The patient was then moved to the ballistocardiographic table, and a tracing was taken after fifteen minutes. Following this he was placed upon the fluoroscopic table in a quiet room where, under sterile conditions, the cardiac catheter was introduced into an antecubital vein and passed into the pulmonary artery under fluoroscopic control. The next step consisted of introducing a special indwelling needle with stylet into the femoral artery under local anesthesia for the collection of the blood samples necessary for both the Fick and dye determinations. After a five-minute period the patient was allowed to begin breathing pure oxygen through a Sanborn basal metabolism rate machine. The kymograph assembly was placed beside the patient in such a manner as to permit the polyethylene tubing to reach readily the indwelling needle in the femoral artery (Fig. 1). Ten minutes after the patient started breathing pure oxygen, the first blood sample was collected from the pulmonary artery, the second sample from the femoral artery, the third sample from the pulmonary artery, and the last sample from the femoral artery. Immediately following the collection of the direct Fick samples for arterial and venous oxygen analyses, the kymograph assembly was started by one operator. Thirty seconds later, the polyethylene tubing with Luer Lok adaptor was connected to the indwelling needle by one operator while another operator started the kymograph timer and rapidly injected 1 c.c. of 0.5 per cent blue dye (T 1824) into the indwelling intravenous needle. Forty seconds after the time of injection, the kymograph was stopped, the polyethylene tubing was disconnected, and the stylets were replaced in both the intra-arterial and the intravenous needles.

Both the dye and the Fick measurements were then repeated as soon as a second kymograph drum with mounted fresh tubes could be substituted for the one which contained arterial blood from the first dye measurement. Mean-

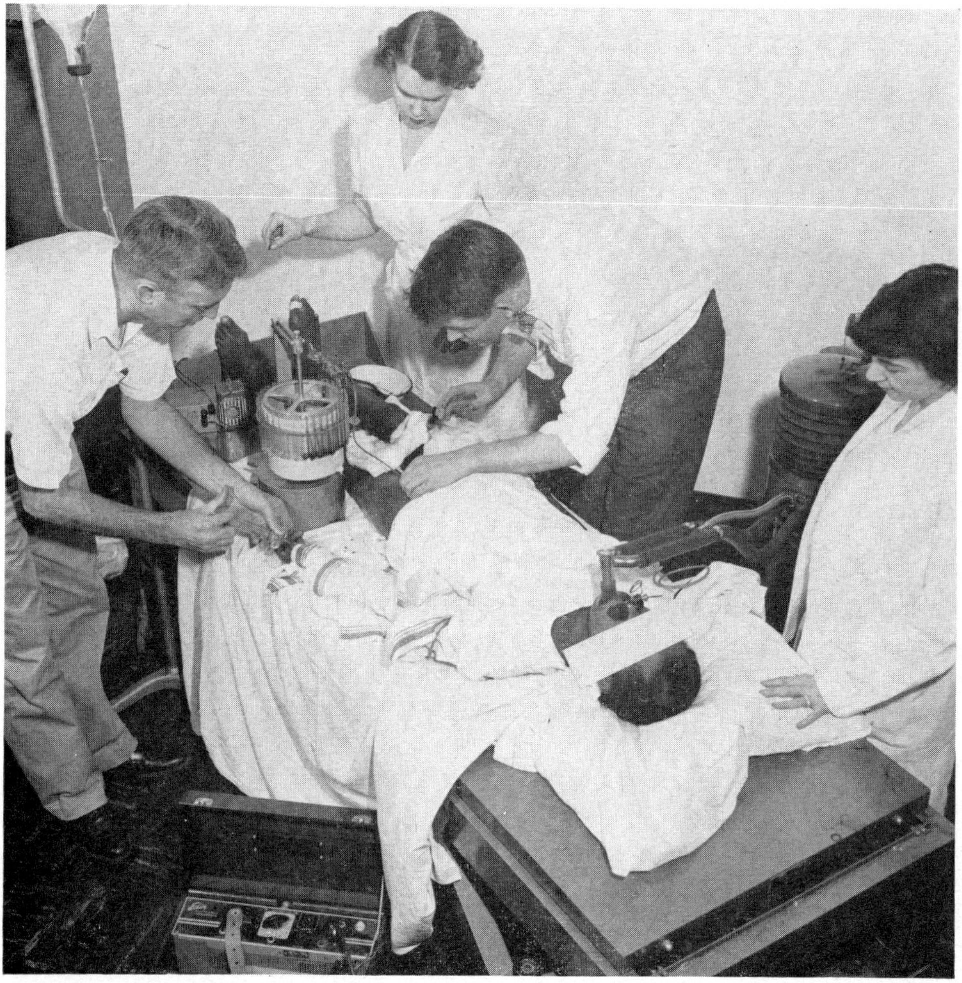

Fig. 1.—Measurement of cardiac output by the direct Fick, dye, and ballistocardiographic methods. This figure shows a patient lying on the ballistocardiographic table, the cardiac catheter protruding from beneath the sterile drapes covering the left arm, and the dye method in operation. The photograph was taken during a dye determination. One operator can be seen holding the polyethylene tubing that has been connected to the indwelling arterial needle. Blood can be seen flowing through the polyethylene tubing into the revolving tubes. The other operator has previously injected the blue dye into the catheter and can be seen holding the syringe containing 15 c.c. of saline solution that was injected rapidly to wash the blue dye into the pulmonary artery through the indwelling cardiac catheter. In about one-third of our cardiac output determinations the dye has been injected into the cardiac catheter and rapidly washed into the circulation with 15 c.c. of saline solution. The catheter is used for this injection when a large vein is not readily available in the other arm, which was the case with this patient. The ballistocardiographic tracing and the Fick arterial and mixed venous blood samples have already been obtained. A second series of determinations by both methods (Fick and dye) is made as rapidly as possible after the first. The oxygen consumption is measured by the Sanborn basal metabolism rate machine shown at the far right of the photograph. Normally the patient is placed upon the ballistocardiograph, a tracing is taken, and then he is moved to the fluoroscopic table, where he remains for the duration of the procedure. For the purpose of illustration, however, we have here placed the patient back upon the ballistocardiograph after the cardiac catheter has been introduced into the pulmonary artery under fluoroscopy.

TABLE I. CARDIAC OUTPUT DETERMINATIONS BY THE FICK, DYE, AND BALLISTOCARDIOGRAPHIC METHODS

PT.	SEX	AGE (YR.)	HT. (CM.)	WT. (KG.)	DIAGNOSIS	EXP. NO.	O_2 USED	A-V DIFF. VOL. %	CARDIAC OUTPUT FICK	CARDIAC OUTPUT DYE	CARDIAC OUTPUT BALLISTOGRAPH	SURF. AREA (SQ. M.)	CARDIAC INDEX FICK	CARDIAC INDEX DYE
W. G.	M	57	180	54.5	Ca. of rectum	1	226	5.70	3.97	4.84	3.58	1.63	2.44	2.97
R. L.	M	49	178	84.5	Inguinal hernia	1	338	4.66	7.25	5.63	7.17	2.00	3.62	2.82
J. H.	M	28	173	71.0	Burn	1	254	4.89	5.20	8.30		1.83	2.84	4.54
						2	300	5.71	5.25		7.60		2.87	
R. M. B.	F	37	165	62.7	Lipoma	1	250	4.81	5.19	4.78		1.68	3.09	2.85
						2	250	4.68	5.33		5.12		3.18	
M. J. G.	F	40	152	55.0	Nodular goiter	1	170	4.37	3.90	4.50		1.50	2.60	3.00
						2	153	3.91	3.90		5.68		2.60	
R. T.	M	18	170	77.0	Pilonidal sinus	1	280	4.74	5.90	8.10		1.87	3.25	4.33
						2	305	5.34	5.70	7.55	6.36		3.00	4.03
A. M.	F	42	162	54.1	Granuloma of vulva	1	221	3.00	7.37	6.40		1.36	5.41	4.71
						2	218	4.11	5.38	7.00			3.95	5.15
O. K.	M	46			Postoperative hernia	1	266	7.11	5.40	6.00	6.37			
L. T.	M	20			Laceration of tendon	1	300	3.83	7.83	5.22				
						2	295	3.50	8.44	5.38	7.80			
E. J.	M	24			Stab wound of thorax	1	317	3.51	9.03	8.65	6.38			
L. C.	M	57	180	81.8	Hypertension	1	217	5.84	3.72			2.00	1.86	
						2	200	5.72	3.50	4.94	3.35		1.75	2.73
A. M.	F	57	169	50.0	Ca. of esophagus	1	193	4.61	4.20	4.20		1.55	2.71	3.29
						2	205	3.99	5.20	6.00	5.30		2.71	3.87
M. W.	F	39			Lymphopathia venereum	1	171	3.35	5.10	3.80				
L. H.	M	24	158	51.4	Perirectal abscess	1	193	4.19	4.60	5.20		1.33	3.46	3.90
						2	191	4.40	4.35	5.20			3.27	3.90
C. B.	F	40	156	62.2	Hemorrhoids	1	199	6.04	3.30			1.61	2.05	
						2	206	6.05	3.40	6.43			2.15	4.00
R. T.	M	49	147	52.0	Inguinal hernia	1	197	4.43	4.44	4.50		1.43	3.10	3.14
						2	198	4.44	4.50	4.90			3.14	3.43
W. M. W.	F	44	168	60.8	Pheochromocytoma	1	190	4.17	4.55	4.97		1.68	2.71	2.96
						2	170	4.13	4.10				2.46	
E. B.	M	23	180	88.6	Hernia	1	285	3.03	9.40	8.30		2.09	4.50	3.97
						2	270	2.54	11.60	6.60			5.55	3.16
F. S.	M	20	179	82.7	Hernia	1	308	5.31	5.80	11.80		2.00	2.90	5.90
						2	330	5.03	6.50				3.25	
K. B.	F	44	168	65.5	Lipoma	1	295	3.96	7.45	8.10		1.73	4.30	4.68
						2	241	3.88	6.20	7.65			3.59	4.42
C. P.	M	24	167	70.0	Gunshot of thigh	1	338	5.06	6.70	7.33		1.78	3.76	4.12
						2	330	4.84	6.82	8.10			3.83	4.56
J. I.	M	23	185	91.0	Laceration of thigh	1	410	4.32	9.50			2.14	4.44	
						2	368	4.27	8.60	9.60			4.02	4.49

while, the patient had been breathing pure oxygen, and the oxygen consumption was measured at the time of the taking of the Fick samples.

By this technique, two measurements of cardiac output by both the Fick and the dye method were obtained in only a few minutes. The blood oxygen analyses were made by the micromethod of Roughton and Scholander,[11] which has been checked previously with the manometric procedure of Van Slyke. Normally, determinations would be thrown out if duplicate blood samples did not check within 0.2 volume per cent. In this paper, however, no determinations were thrown out because of a lack of agreement greater than 0.2 volume per cent. Further details concerning the dye method are to be reported elsewhere,[12] but basically the Steward-Hamilton technique was employed in the calculation of cardiac output by the dye method.

RESULTS

The data are shown in Table I. The numerals 1 and 2 refer to the first and second measurements, respectively, taken on each patient. The samples for the dye measurements were collected first in Patients 1 through 13, and the samples for the Fick measurements were collected first in Patients 14 through 22. The initial Fick sample, F1, and initial dye sample, D1, were collected as nearly simultaneously as possible, as were F2 and D2. Moreover, the collection of the samples for the second paired measurements (Fick and dye) followed the collection of the samples for the first pair of measurements as closely as possible. Thus, the two dye measurements and the two Fick measurements were all accomplished in only a few minutes' time, in an effort to minimize the differences due to variations in actual cardiac output.

The results of the statistical analysis, including the mean, standard deviation, and the degree of freedom, are given in Table II. Essentially, the study would seem to indicate the following points. First, in these "normal" patients the ballistocardiograph gave consistently good results and on the surface might appear to be quite useful clinically; actually, this is not the case,

TABLE II. ANALYSIS OF DATA FROM TABLE I

Cardiac Output

	FICK 1	DYE 1	FICK 2	DYE 2	BALLISTOGRAPH 2
Mean	5.75	6.22	5.99	6.81	5.88
Standard deviation (±)	1.80	2.05	2.20	1.44	1.47
Degrees of freedom	20	17	17	12	10
Coefficient of variation	.314	.331	.367	.212	.250

F = 0.723, not significant at the 5 per cent level

Cardiac Index

	FICK 1	DYE 1	FICK 2	DYE 2
Mean	3.305	3.718	3.268	3.976
Standard deviation (±)	0.947	0.955	0.903	0.687
Degrees of freedom	16	13	14	10
Coefficient of variation	0.286	0.256	0.276	0.172

F = 1.908, not significant at the 5 per cent level

since in many seriously ill patients the ballistocardiograph is unsatisfactory. Second, there is no particular advantage of the Fick method over the dye method from the point of view of accuracy (Table II). Third, both methods have a standard deviation of almost 2 L. or approximately 30 per cent. Fourth, and most important, multiple measurements with any one of the three methods, performed on the same patient at the same time, agree to within approximately 10 per cent. Since, therefore, either the dye or the Fick method is acceptable for comparing alterations of cardiac output in the same patient, the more easily performed dye method would appear to have certain advantages for clinical use.

DISCUSSION

Our results compare well with those of Hamilton and associates.[13] If variations in the body surface area of the patients are taken into consideration, both the standard deviation and the mean are diminished, as may be observed from the cardiac index in Table I, and the coefficient of variation becomes slightly less. The correlation coefficient between the Fick and the dye methods is 0.455, which is statistically significant at the 5 per cent level. The absence of a higher degree of correlation may be due to a number of factors. First, it is possible that the cardiac output actually changed in the short time which elapsed between the Fick and the dye measurements, but it is considered unlikely that a change of significant magnitude occurred. Second, the Fick method includes the measurement of the oxygen concentration in samples of venous and arterial blood and of oxygen consumption with the basal metabolism rate machine. The analytic error in the oxygen determinations is ±6 per cent, and the magnitude of the error incurred in measuring the oxygen consumption with the Sanborn machine is unknown. If a leak around the face mask should occur and remain constant, the error can be common to both the Fick measurements which were made for each patient. Third, the Fick method measures average cardiac output over a period of many minutes, whereas the dye method measures cardiac output over a period of only a few seconds. In the Fick method, brief variations in cardiac output would be "averaged out," but these variations could substantially alter the result obtained in any single dye measurement. Therefore, respiratory and other clinical physiologic variations could play a role in the observed variations in cardiac output. Fourth, if an unsuspected cardiac shunt were present, further discrepancies in the results obtained by either method could be expected.

CONCLUSIONS

1. The direct Fick, dye, and ballistocardiographic methods have been compared in eleven patients, and the first two methods have been compared in twenty-two patients.

2. Although the direct Fick method has been the "reference standard" for many years, its use in the clinic is limited.

3. The ballistocardiograph is easily the most convenient of the three methods and, in "normal" patients, the results obtained with this method

compare favorably with those obtained with the Fick. However, in severely ill patients the ballistocardiographic tracings are frequently so abnormal as to defy accurate interpretation.

4. The dye method is simple and is readily applicable clinically. It compares favorably with the Fick in accuracy, and serial (duplicate) measurements in the same individual have been found to vary less than 10 per cent. One disadvantage is that in patients with intracardiac shunts or auriculoventricular fistulas a very abnormal dye curve may be obtained.

The statistical analyses herein reported were generously performed by Dr. R. V. Brown, Department of Pharmacology, Medical College of The University of Tennessee.

REFERENCES

1. Fick: Sitzungsb. d. phys.-med. Gesellsch. zu Würzb. **16:** 1780, Quoted From Marshall, E. K., Jr.: Cardiac Output of Man, Medicine **9:** 175, 1930.
2. Grehant, M. M., and Quinquad: Recherches expérimentales sur la mesure du volume de sang qui traverse les poumons en un temps donné, Compt. rend. Soc. de biol., Par. **38:** 159, 1886.
3. Forssmann, W.: Die Sondierung des rechten Herzens, Klin. Wchnschr. **8:** 2085, 1929.
4. Cournand, A., and Ranges, H. A.: Catheterization of the Right Auricle in Man, Proc. Soc. Exper. Biol. & Med. **46:** 462, 1941.
5. Henderson, Y.: The Mass-Movements of the Circulation as Shown by a Recoil Curve, Am. J. Physiol. **14:** 287, 1905.
6. Starr, I., Rawson, A. J., Schroeder, H. A., and Joseph, N. R.: Studies on the Estimation of Cardiac Output in Man and of Abnormalities in Cardiac Function, From the Heart's Recoil and the Blood's Impacts; The Ballistocardiogram, Am. J. Physiol. **127:** 1, 1939.
7. Stewart, G. N.: Researches on the Circulation Time and on the Influences Which Affect It. IV. The Output of the Heart, J. Physiol. **22:** 159, 1897.
8. Hamilton, W. F., Moore, J. W., Kinsman, J. M., and Spurling, R. G.: Simultaneous Determination of the Pulmonary and Systemic Circulation Times in Man and of a Figure Related to the Cardiac Output, Am. J. Physiol. **84:** 338, 1928.
9. Kinsman, J. M., Moore, J. W., Hamilton, W. F.: Studies on the Circulation. I. Injection Method: Physiol. and Mathematical Considerations, Am. J. Physiol. **89:** 322, 1929.
10. Friedlich, A., Heimbecker, R., and Bing, R. J.: A Device for Continuous Recording of the Concentration of Evans Blue Dye in Whole Blood and Its Application to Determination of Cardiac Output, J. Appl. Physiol. **3:** 12, 1950.
11. Roughton, F. J. W., and Scholander, P. F.: Micro Gasometric Estimation of the Blood Gases. I. Oxygen, J. Biol. Chem. **148:** 541, 1943.
12. Wilson, F. C., Jr., Neely, W. A., and Hardy, J. D.: The Blue Dye Method for Cardiac Output, Fundamental Forum, Am. Coll. Surgeons, 1954, Philadelphia, W. B. Saunders Company. To be published.
13. Hamilton, W. F., Riley, R. L., Attyah, A. M., Cournand, A., Fowell, D. M., Himmelstein, A., Noble, R. P., Remington, J. W., Richards, D. W., Jr., Wheeler, N. C., and Witham, A. C.: Comparison of the Fick and Dye Injection Methods of Measuring the Cardiac Output in Man, Am. J. Physiol. **153:** 309, 1948.

THE INFLUENCE OF ACUTE HYPERVOLEMIA ON THE FREEZE-DRY HOMOLOGOUS AORTIC GRAFT

Thomas O. Gentsch, M.D., Levin L. Waters, M.D., and William W. L. Glenn, M.D., New Haven, Conn.

(From the Departments of Surgery and Pathology, Yale University School of Medicine)

SEVERAL types of material have been utilized by investigators to maintain the continuity of the lumen of a major artery, a portion of which has been interrupted during development or by disease or trauma. These materials include glass tubes,[2] plastic tubing,[7] Vitallium tubes with a vein lining,[1] tubes fashioned from autologous tissue,[16, 19] segments of veins,[10] and, finally, segments of arteries.[3, 5, 6, 11, 13, 15, 17, 18, 20] Perhaps the most promising graft material tested thus far is fresh autologous artery.[9, 13, 18] This material, however, is rarely available in sufficient quantity or adequate size to be of value clinically, although short segments may sometimes be made available for use as described by Potts and associates.[18]

During recent years the use of homologous arterial grafts has been extensively studied, and a number of methods for preservation of the tissue prior to use have been investigated. Debate has centered around the question of whether viability of the graft at the time of implantation was necessary for success of the grafting operation. It has been shown that nonviable grafts preserved by the freeze-dry method have healed to the normal adjacent artery,[11, 15] and continuity of the vessel lumen has been maintained. Other studies suggest that viable cells in homologous arterial grafts preserved by other methods do not maintain viability after implantation into a host.[4, 20]

Whereas the immediate success of the homologous arterial graft is encouraging, unless some form of acute stress can be brought to bear on the implanted homografts, years may elapse before an appraisal can be made of the degenerative changes to which the graft may be susceptible. The purpose of this study is to report the results of a series of experiments in which an attempt was made to test the susceptibility of implanted arterial homografts to an acute injury. After considering several methods of stress, it was decided to attempt the production of lesions in these grafts by the administration of large infusions of lipid emulsions.

The freeze-dry method of preservation of arteries was selected because of the advantages of being able to store preserved arteries for a prolonged period at room temperature and the apparently low incidence of thrombosis after implantation in the host.[15, 21]

Aided in part by a grant from the Connecticut Heart Association, a contract from the Office of Naval Research, United States Navy, and a grant from the Life Insurance Medical Research Fund.

Read at the seventh annual meeting of the Society for Vascular Surgery, New York, N. Y., May 31, 1953.

METHOD

Healthy mature dogs were sacrificed and utilized as a source of aortic tissue. Sterile segments of the thoracic aorta were rapidly frozen immediately after death by dropping each section into an individual dry centrifuge bottle partially submerged in liquid air. After freezing, drying of the aortic segments was accomplished in a lyophilizer at a pressure of 0.1 to 4.0 μ of mercury. After a drying period of from thirty-six to seventy-two hours, the specimens were sealed in their glass containers at a pressure of approximately 30 μ of mercury.

Freeze-dry aortic homografts were implanted in a series of twelve normal adult dogs. A small segment of the host thoracic aorta was removed between Potts ductus clamps and a reconstituted homograft sutured in place by a continuous everting mattress suture, posteriorly, and interrupted everting mattress sutures, anteriorly. Ischemia of the spinal cord was prevented during the period of aortic occlusion by the establishment of a shunt between the proximal end of the left subclavian artery and the proximal end of the left femoral artery through a long polyethylene tube with an internal diameter of approximately 1.5 mm. (Fig. 1). Following implantation of the aortic graft, the animal was allowed to recover and was placed on standard kennel care. Approximately eight to nine weeks following implantation of the graft, one-half of the series of animals, usually alternates, were subjected to hypervolemic-lipid stress.

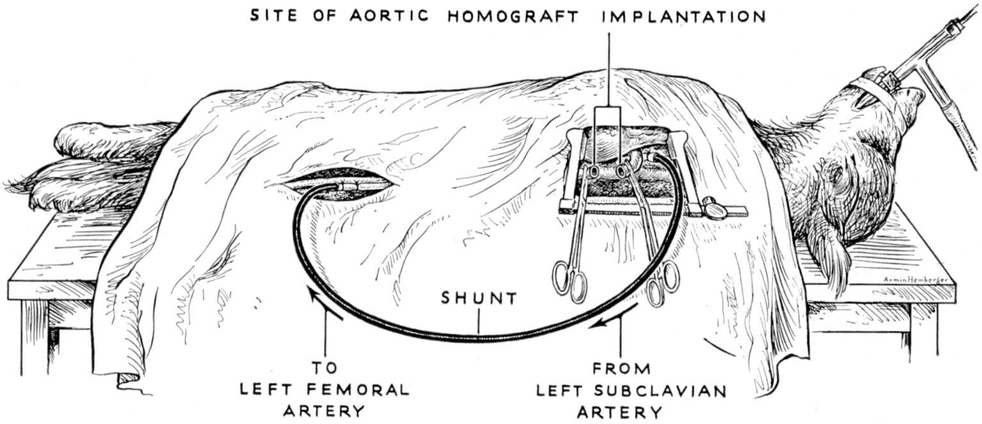

Fig. 1.

To effect the desired hypervolemia a saline emulsion of egg yolk was infused intravenously into the dogs once daily for varying periods (Table I). The egg yolk emulsion was prepared by mixing egg yolks with twice their volume of sterile normal saline solution and then filtering through sterile gauze. The total volume of each infusion was 17 c.c. per kilogram. This amount of egg yolk is usually well tolerated by normal animals and produces a marked and persistent lipemia. All fractions of blood lipids rise progressively, and by the third injection the total blood cholesterol is about 500 mg. per cent, and it usually remains at this level. Three of the six animals so treated died after

TABLE I

HOST		GRAFT			STRESS		RESULTS				
EXPERIMENT NUMBER	LENGTH OF SURVIVAL (DAYS)	DONOR	LENGTH OF PROCESSING (HOURS)	LENGTH OF STORAGE (DAYS)	NUMBER OF INFUSIONS	NUMBER OF DAYS	CALCIFICATION	HEMORRHAGE	SUBENDOTHELIAL MURAL THROMBI	FAT INFILTRATION	INFLAMMATORY AND FOAM CELLS
1	71	L–1	72	82	9	10	None	None	Present	Heavy	Many
3	78	L–4	72	44	4	8	Diffuse	None	Present	Heavy	Many
5	73	L–6	72	12	4	5	None	Medial	Present	Heavy	Many
8	76	L–7	48	32	7	11	Diffuse	None	Present	Slight	Slight
10	79	L–10	72	21	7	14	Diffuse	Intimal	Present	Heavy	Many
11	63	L–9	72	32	1	1	None	None	Present	Heavy	None
2	72	L–4	72	37			None	None	Present	None*	None*
4	28	L–6	72	5			Localized	None	Absent	None*	None*
6	78	L–7	48	18			None	None	Present	None*	None*
7	86	L–7	72	22			None	None	Present	None*	None*
9	78	L–9	36	14			None	None	Absent	None*	None*
12	56	L–10	72	56			None	None	Present	None*	None*

*Some fat, inflammatory cells, and foam cells only seen around sutures in control group.

hypervolemia was produced but before completion of the contemplated course of infusions. Three animals were sacrificed after receiving a complete course of infusions. Six animals with implanted freeze-dry aortic grafts received no stress and were sacrificed at approximately the same time following implantation as the stressed group of animals.

A.

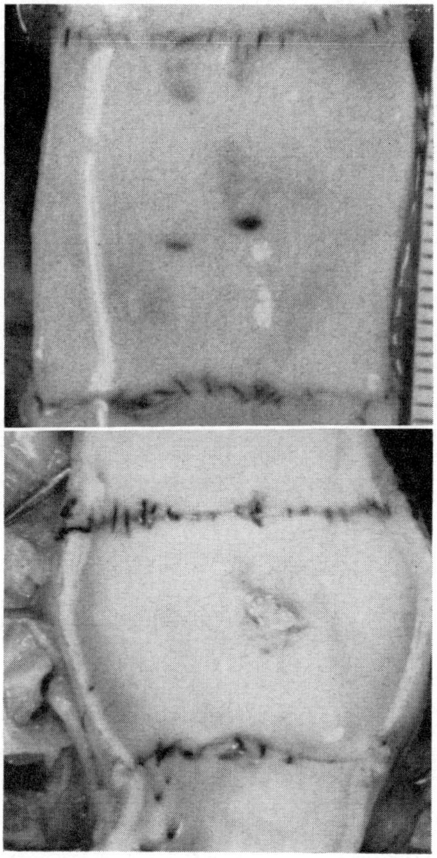

B.

Fig. 2, *A* and *B*.—Gross specimen of implanted aortic freeze-dried homografts.
A, Control group (Experiment 2), seventy-two days after implantation, showing soft, pliable graft with several small mural thrombi.
B, Control group (Experiment 3), seventy-eight days after implantation, illustrating stiffened graft due to medial calcification. Also note mural thrombus.

At necropsy the aorta was removed en bloc and fixed in 10 per cent formalin. Frozen sections of the fixed tissue were stained for fat with sudan IV. Masson's trichrome stain was also made of the same and additional blocks .

RESULTS

Despite the fact that aortic occlusion sometimes exceeded two hours while the graft was sutured in place, the small polyethylene shunts functioned well,

C.

D.

E.

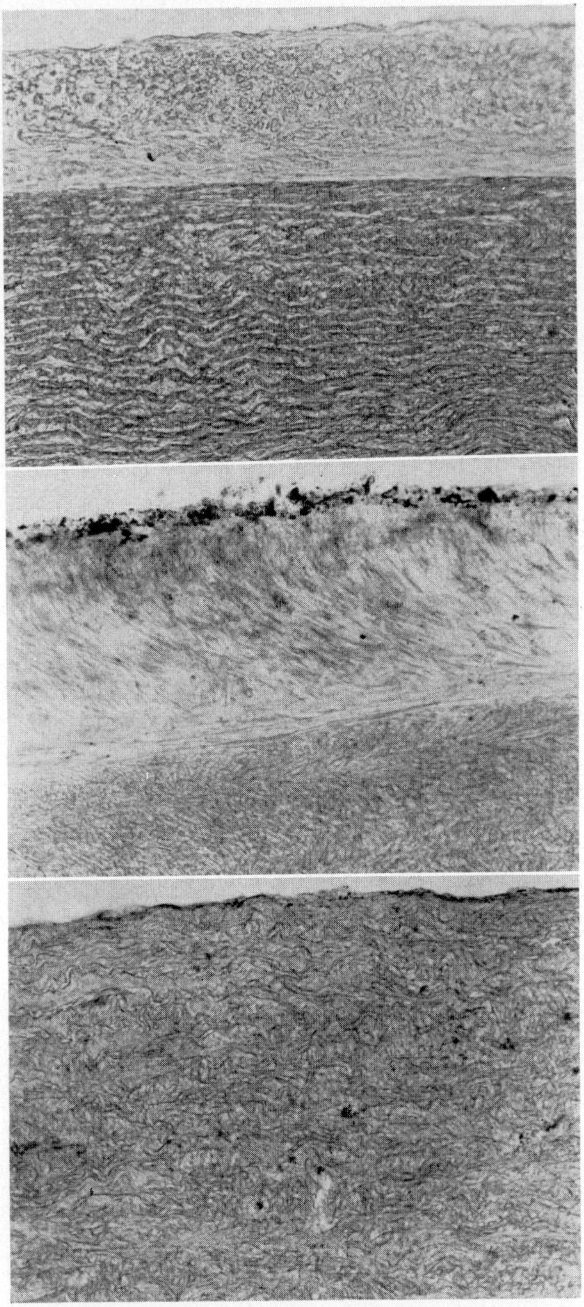

Fig. 2, *C, D,* and *E.*—Microscopic sections.

C, Control group (graft of Experiment 2), note thickened intima but absence of fat, inflammatory cells, and foam cells. Sudan IV. (×285, reduced one-third.)

D, Stressed group (graft of Experiment 3), illustrating a thickened intima with many subendothelial foam cells and diffuse fat infiltration of intima and inner media. Sudan IV. (×285, reduced one-third.)

E. Stressed group (host aorta in Experiment 3), note diffuse but minimal fat infiltration. No foam cells were seen. Note also that intima is a single endothelial-cell layer. Sudan IV. (×285, reduced one-third.)

and there was no evidence of paraplegia in any animal. At necropsy the implanted grafts were patent and appeared grossly and microscopically similar to other homologous aortic grafts as described by other investigators.[3, 15] A thickened intima had grown in from the host aorta covering the entire inner surface of the graft. Muscle fibers in the media had disappeared and the elastic fibers were condensed and slightly fragmented. There was evidence of ingrowth of fibroblasts and capillaries from the host into the wall of the graft. Subintimal mural thrombi were seen in all six of the grafts in the stressed group and in four of the six grafts in the control group (Fig. 2, *A* and *B*, and Fig. 3).

Several important changes not apparent in the adjacent host aorta were noted in the grafts of the stressed animals. These grafts showed a diffuse infiltration of fat with frequent foam cells and inflammatory cells, especially in the intimal layer (Fig. 2, *C* through *F*). Diffuse calcification was present in three of these grafts (Figs. 2 and 3). In addition, two grafts in the stressed group showed large areas of hemorrhage, in the medial layer in one case and in the intimal layer in the second. There was a heavy concentration of fat in each of these areas of hemorrhage. In the control group of nonstressed animals only one of the grafts showed any of these changes, this being in the form of a single plaque of calcium. A summary of these findings will be found in Table I.

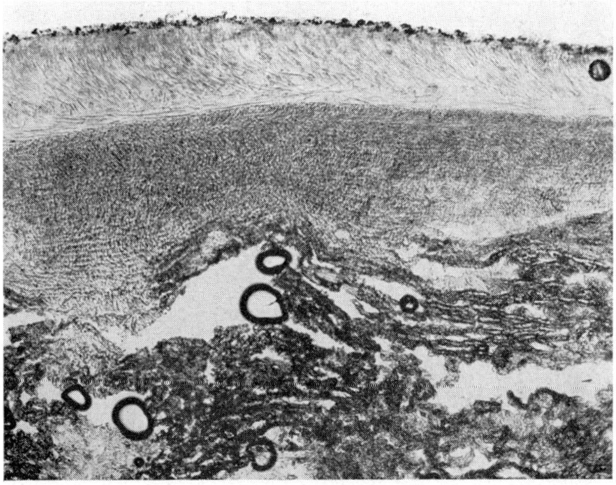

Fig. 2, *F*.—Stressed group (graft of Experiment 3), note destruction of media by calcification. Sudan IV. (×120, reduced one-third.)

DISCUSSION

There is no convincing evidence that any of the cellular elements of an arterial homograft survive or grow following implantation. As pointed out earlier, other investigators have demonstrated that viability of the graft at the time of implantation in the host is not a requirement for success of the graft when judged by healing of the graft to the artery of the host and by the patency of the vessel lumen. From the point of view of long-term survival of a functioning graft, it is important to determine if the method of preservation will influence the eventual development of degenerative changes in the graft. There is already some evidence[8, 12] to suggest that the electron radiation method of sterilization of the graft may predispose the graft to excessive calcification. There is also evidence that a high percentage of grafts preserved by formalin

A.

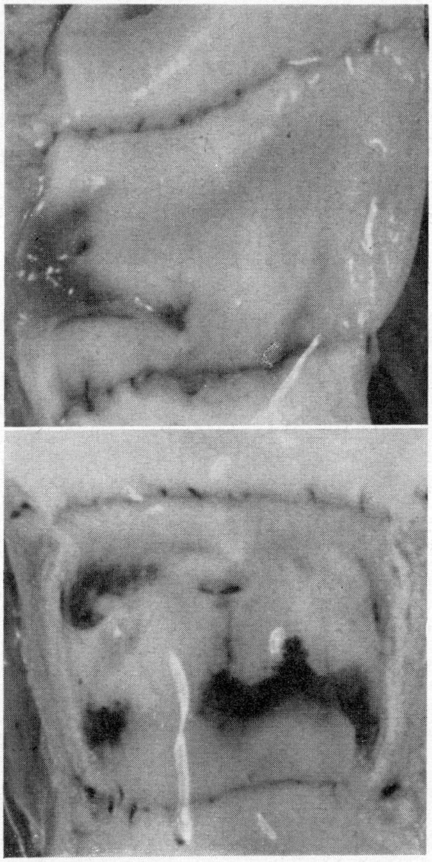

B.

Fig. 3.—Gross specimens of implanted aortic freeze-dry homografts.
A, Control group (Experiment 7), eighty-six days after implantation. A subendothelial mural thrombus is seen. Graft was soft and pliable.
B, Stressed group (Experiment 8), seventy-six days after implantation. Several subendothelial mural thrombi are seen, and the walls of the graft are thickened and calcified.

fixation develop calcification after implantation.[17] On the other hand, studies using homologous arterial grafts preserved by the freeze-dry method[13, 14] and in nutrient media[4, 5] have been carried out for two years after implantation of the grafts and have shown a low incidence of degenerative changes in the artery wall. To complete the evaluation of the influence of age on the development of degenerative changes in these grafts, however, it may be necessary to follow these animals for much longer periods.

Waters and deSuto-Nagy[23] have found that when hypervolemia is produced in dogs by the rapid infusion of compatible dog plasma, there is acute intimal injury of the aorta and coronary arteries. This injury consists of subendothelial edema and leukocytic infiltration, giving rise within a few days to a thin subendothelial scar. Waters[22] has extended these observations to the lesions that follow hypervolemia produced in dogs by the rapid intravenous injection of lipid emulsions and has found that lipid localizes in the arterial wall selectively at areas of injury. Furthermore, he has noted the similarity of site of location of these lesions to those of arteriosclerosis in man and also striking morphologic similarities between the experimental lesions and those of early arterioclerosis.

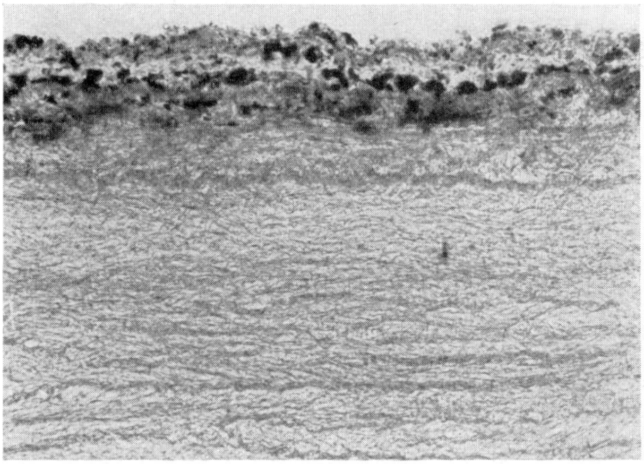

Fig. 4.—Early arteriosclerotic changes found in the aorta of an 8-year-old boy. (Accidental death.) Note fat infiltration of the thickened intima, with many foam cells. Lesion is similar to that found in stressed homograft (Fig. 2, *D*). Sudan IV. (×285, reduced one-third.)

The healed aortic homograft was considered to represent an area of lessened resistance in the aortic wall, subject throughout the life of the host to various conditions of stress. The hypervolemic stress described, combining a factor of hyperlipemia, proved to be a convenient method of testing this hypothesis. The excessive fat deposits, inflammatory cells, foam cells, hemorrhage, and calcification seen in some of these grafts following hypervolemia-lipid stress suggest that the aortic homograft preserved by the freeze-dry method is more susceptible to injury than the adjacent normal host aorta. The changes found in the wall of the grafts in the stressed group may not be progressive, but at the time of sacrifice of the animals they present many similarities to early arteriosclerotic changes in the human artery (Fig. 3). It remains to be determined whether grafts preserved by other methods are affected in a similar way by this form of stress.

The organizing mural thrombi which were observed in the implanted grafts in these experiments appeared more severe in the stressed group, although in no case did they interfere with the patency of the graft. The high incidence of these lesions in the control group of animals, higher than reported by other investigators,[11, 14, 15] suggests that what appears to be minor differences in the technique of processing of the freeze-dry graft may be responsible for these lesions.

SUMMARY

Aortic homografts preserved by the freeze-dry technique were subjected after eight to ten weeks of implantation in a host to a stress in the form of multiple infusions of an egg yolk saline mixture. All grafts so treated showed extensive infiltration with fat, foam cells, and inflammatory cells. These changes were much more marked in the graft than in the adjacent normal host aorta. Diffuse calcification of the graft was evident in one-half of the grafts in the stressed group of animals. In a control group of animals receiving no stress, fat deposits were rarely seen in the graft. Diffuse calcification and inflammatory and foam cells were not observed in the control group of grafts, although a single plaque of calcium was found in one of these grafts. The findings indicate that grafts preserved by the freeze-dry method, when subjected to appropriate stress, show changes in the vessel wall similar to those seen in degenerative arterial disease in the human being. The results of these experiments suggest that this method of stress, applied a relatively short time after implantation of the graft, may be of value in the investigation of the influence of methods of preservation on the ultimate development of the degenerative type of lesion in the wall of a grafted segment of artery.

Acknowledgments.—We gratefully acknowledge the assistance in this work of Mr. Armand Negri, Mr. Peter Integlia, and Mr. Edward Iannucci. We are also indebted to Dr. Hayes Cluxton, Dr. William E. Bloomer, and Dr. Donald P. Shedd for their valuable technical assistance.

REFERENCES

1. Blakemore, A. H., and Lord, J. W., Jr.: A Non-Suture Method of Blood Vessel Anastomosis, Ann. Surg. **121:** 435, 1945.
2. Carrel, A.: Permanent Intubation of the Thoracic Aorta, J. Exper. Med. **16:** 17, 1912.
3. Coleman, C., Deterling, R. A., and Parshley, M.: Experimental Studies of Preserved Aortic Homografts, Ann. Surg. **134:** 686, 1951.
4. Deterling, R. A.: Personal communication.
5. Deterling, R. A., Parshley, M., and Blunt, J. W.: A Critical Study of Present Criteria Governing Selection and Use of Blood Vessel Grafts, SURGERY **33:** 213, 1953.
6. Gross, R. E., Bill, H., and Pierce, D.: Methods of Preservation and Transplantation of Arterial Grafts, Surg., Gynec. & Obst. **88:** 689, 1949.
7. Hufnagel, C. A.: Permanent Intubation of the Thoracic Aorta, Arch. Surg. **54:** 382, 1947.
8. Hui, K. L., Keefer, E. B. C., Deterling, R. A., Parshley, M. S., Humphrey, G. H., II, and Glenn, F.: Early Results of Experimental Studies of the Action of High Intensity Electrons on Aortic Homografts, Proc. Surg. Forum, Clin. Congress Am. Coll. Surgeons, 1951, Philadelphia, 1952, W. B. Saunders Company, p. 255.
9. Johnson, J. C., Kirby, C. K., Allam, M. W., and Hagan, W.: Growth of Vena Cava and Aortic Grafts, SURGERY **29:** 726, 1951.
10. Johnson, J. C., Kirby, C. K., Greifenstein, F. E., and Castillo, A.: The Experimental and Clinical Use of Vein Grafts to Replace Defects in Large Arteries, SURGERY **26:** 945, 1949.
11. Marrangoni, A., and Cecchini, L.: Homotransplantation of Arterial Segments Preserved by the Freeze-dry Method, Ann. Surg. **134:** 977, 1951.
12. Meeker, I., and Gross, R. E.: Sterilization of Frozen Arterial Grafts by High Voltage Cathode Ray Irradiation, SURGERY **30:** 19, 1951.

13. Miller, H. H., Callow, A. D., Welch, C. S., and MacMahon, H. E.: The Fate of Arterial Grafts in Small Arteries (Experimental Study), Surg., Gynec. & Obst. **92**: 581, 1951.
14. Pate, J. W.: Personal communication.
15. Pate, J. W., and Sawyer, P. N.: Freeze-Dried Aortic Grafts—A Preliminary Report of Experimental Evaluation, Research Report, Naval Medical Research Institute **11**: 49, 1953.
16. Peirce, E. C., II: Autologous Tissue Tubes for Aortic Grafts in Dogs, SURGERY **33**: 648, 1953.
17. Peirce, E. C., II, Rheinlander, H. F., Moritz, A. R., Gross, R. E., and Merrill, K.: Transplantation of Aortic Segment Fixed in 4 per cent Neutral Formalin, Am. J. Surg. **78**: 314, 1949.
18. Potts, W. J., Alberts, H., and Fischer, H. W.: Autogenous Aortic Grafts Fashioned From a Smaller Artery, SURGERY **33**: 518, 1953.
19. Sako, Y.: Prevention of Dilatation in Autogenous Venous and Pericardial Grafts in the Thoracic Aorta, SURGERY **30**: 148, 1951.
20. Sauvage, L. R., and Harkins, H. H.: Experimental Vascular Grafts: An Evaluation Relating to Types, Means of Preservation and Methods of Suture in the Growing Pig, SURGERY **33**: 587, 1953.
21. Sawyer, P. N., and Pate, J. W.: A Study of Electrical Potential Differences Across the Normal Aorta and Aortic Grafts of Dogs, Research Report, Naval Medical Research Institute **11**: 69, 1953.
22. Waters, L. L.: Foam Cellular Lesions of the Aorta and Coronary Arteries in the Dog, Circulation **6**: 457, 1952.
23. Waters, L. L., and deSuto-Nagy, G. I.: Circulatory Factors in the Pathogenesis of Experimental Arteriolar Necrosis, Yale J. Biol. & Med. **22**: 751, 1950.

THE MANAGEMENT OF RECURRENT VARICOSE VEINS

Josephus C. Luke, M.D., Montreal, Quebec, Canada

(From the Surgical Service, Royal Victoria Hospital)

It is an admitted fact that there is no guaranteed long-term cure for varicose veins. However the trends of treatment are gradually producing an increasing incidence of good results. The general acceptance of the basic principle that, as a primary requisite, the great and/or small saphenous vein should be ligated and divided flush with the deep vein has produced many cures, or considerable improvement, to the unfortunate possessors of these abnormal veins. Ten years ago, the operation of high ligation, with or without multiple lower ligations and the use of sclerosing injections, was thought to be the answer to the problem. In the interval, however, the large number of recurrences which have followed this procedure have greatly shaken this opinion. Surgical opinion has now turned to other more radical measures in an attempt to produce better results. At the present time it is the consensus of opinion of the majority of vascular surgeons that the operation of flush saphenous ligation (including the small saphenous vein where indicated) with stripping of each vein to the dorsum of the foot is the procedure of choice. Again, no promise of permanent freedom from recurrence can be offered.

This presentation concerns a relatively large group of patients who have already undergone vein ligation but whose varicose veins have recurred. On examination they can readily be separated into two main categories. The first group contains those in whom the initial surgery obviously did not conform to the basic principles mentioned previously. Examples are still encountered of relatively recent surgery performed by those with little understanding of the problem, where the ligation was performed well below the groin or where the surgeon contented himself with a local excision of a mass of varices. Such cases present no problem in management. It is the second category which presents a more difficult solution where, apparently, a proper proximal ligation was carried out but nevertheless recurrence has taken place. The operations in this group have been performed by competent surgeons during the past twelve years. As a rule, subsequent to the return of these veins, multiple local injections have been given, and the existing vein pattern becomes definitely bizarre.

As the result of a study of thirty-two cases belonging to the second category where reoperation has been carried out, certain reasons for recurrence can be cited. It is difficult to be specific in all cases as to the exact cause of the recurrences, and therefore the subsequent list contains only those in which the causative factor was relatively definite.

Read at the seventh annual meeting of the Society for Vascular Surgery, New York, N. Y., May 31, 1953.

1. Despite an adequately high position of the groin incision, it was obvious in four cases that the saphenous ligation was made one inch or more distal to the saphenofemoral junction. The tributary veins remaining attached to the saphenous stump showed marked dilatation, and presumably allowed reconnection with this stump and the distal saphenous vein. This type of recurrence can be surmised from inspection of the groin area. Multiple new subcutaneous veins can be seen which the patient states have arisen since the operation.

2. On re-exploration of the saphenofemoral area, it becomes obvious that the initial surgeon has ligated only one limb of a high division of the saphenous vein into the relatively common inverted-Y anomaly. The other limb of the Y remains patent. This cause was found in three cases. The patient usually states that some early benefit followed this operation but that, after a period of months, the veins were about as obvious as before the operation.

3. Failure of the surgeon to identify and ligate an accessory saphenous vein is another cause. This abnormal branch, present in only 2 to 3 per cent of individuals and seen in this series on three occasions, usually joins the great saphenous vein at its concavity just before its entrance into the common femoral vein. However, in one instance it was found to join the common femoral vein one inch above the normal saphenofemoral junction. A proper dissection of this junction and exposure of the common femoral vein at the initial operation will prevent this oversight as well as those mentioned in Types 1 and 2.

4. Two cases were encountered in which the area of scarring about the saphenofemoral junction and the lack of the usual tributaries indicated that the surgeon had performed a proper ligation. A segment of vein had not been resected, and patency of the saphenous vein had again appeared. Catgut sutures had been used, and it is likely that this reopening was the result of absorption of the catgut ligature. Such a phenomenon is usual when a major artery has been ligated in continuity, and consequently it is entirely a possibility here, where pressures up to 400 mm. of water can be produced when the patient strains.

5. An incompetent small saphenous vein is too frequently missed in the initial assessment of the patient. It should be remembered that in 15 to 20 per cent of patients with primary varicose veins, this vein is involved either solely or in conjunction with great saphenous incompetence. Failure to ligate and remove this vein allows for continuing varices in the calf and lateral ankle region and a so-called recurrence.

6. The great majority of recurrences, twenty in this series, are the result of the missing, or the subsequent opening, of incompetent communicating veins between the saphenous systems and the deep venous circulation. The incompetent communicating veins result in recanalization of the original thrombosis, or dilatation and the production of varicosities in hitherto small superficial collateral channels. Attempts to locate accurately such incompetent communicators by the comparative or multiple tourniquet tests have,

in my hands, been far from successful. The majority connect relatively directly with the two saphenous systems, but others appear independently. It is the existence of this latter type which makes it impossible to promise cure in any case of primary varicose veins despite every known type of treatment.

In this catalogue of the causes of recurrent varicose veins, it is taken for granted that the varices associated with a previous deep phlebitis, congenital or acquired arteriovenous fistula, and cirrhosis of the liver have been ruled out. I have not found the type described as arterial varices except in conjunction with a localized or generalized congenital arteriovenous fistula.

TREATMENT

Further attention to these recurrent varicose veins is demanded by the patient for several reasons. The appearance of these deforming veins may be a primary factor, there may have been recurrence of eczema or ulceration, or the return of the symptoms originally experienced may bring the patient for further therapy.

The decision as to whether this further treatment should be conservative or radical depends, as originally, on whether a positive Trendelenburg test can be demonstrated. When this test is negative or doubtful for reverse flow on standing, then local injections of sclerosing fluid are all that is indicated. When it is obvious that the original valvular incompetence has recurred or persisted, local injections are merely temporary in benefit, and further surgery is indicated.

This secondary surgery should consist of a re-exploration of the saphenofemoral junction to correct the possible faults in this area and a stripping of the existing principal superficial veins. Prior to operation, the small saphenous vein should be carefully inspected in the popliteal area. When dilated, this vein can be palpated when the patient is erect. When doubt exists as to its state of incompetency, exploration of this area is indicated. Re-exploration of the saphenofemoral junction can be a most difficult procedure. Scar obliterates the landmarks and especially the areolar tissue which ensheaths the veins, making the dissection next to impossible. The recurrent veins in the scar are thin-walled, friable, and tortuous. Resulting troublesome bleeding harasses the surgeon. The following technique is offered to facilitate this religation and to ensure a proper high ligation of the saphenous vein.

The previous incision is reopened if it is placed in the fold of the groin. If the original scar is lower in the thigh, a new incision in the fold is made.

Following division of the scarred subcutaneous fat, the dissection is carried centrally, beneath the upper skin flaps, through normal fatty tissue toward the inguinal ligament. The common femoral vein is sought just distal to this ligament, and its position can be quickly determined lying medial to the readily palpable femoral artery. During this phase of the operation and during the subsequent stripping, the Trendelenburg position will be of assistance by reducing venous pressures. The femoral sheath is opened and the anterior half of the common femoral vein exposed. The usual surrounding areolar tissue about this vein has been undisturbed by the original operation and permits easy dissection downward of the femoral vein to the saphenofemoral junction. If a proper high ligation had been made previously, scarring is again encountered at the fossa ovalis but, by keeping close to the sides of the femoral vein in this areolar envelope, the exposure can be carried below this junction. The common femoral vein is now exposed both above and below the saphenous junction, and it is a simple matter to pass a silk ligature about the saphenous vein for a proper flush ligation. This exposure also allows for detection of any accessory saphenous veins which join the main veins in this area. The saphenous tributaries can be disregarded once a proper proximal ligation has been carried out.

The remainder of the surgical procedure consists in isolating the great saphenous vein at the knee level or any other level where it can be seen or palpated with passage of an appropriate stripper toward the groin. In most cases it will be found to halt just distal to the previous scar, and the head of the stripper can be isolated by dissection through the lower part of the groin incision. Stripping of the vein downward from the medial knee incision is next carried out, and as large a segment of vein as possible is removed through another small incision. The lower end of the great saphenous vein is isolated just distal and anterior to the medial malleolus, and the stripper is passed upward as far as possible. It frequently follows an entirely different venous channel than that discovered at the medial knee and emphasizes the finding that reduplication of the great saphenous vein is not uncommon.

Stripping of a vein segment which has recanalized following a previous thrombosis from sclerosing fluids is not as easy as stripping a virgin vein. Perivenous thrombosis causes tethering, and considerable pull on the stripper is necessary. The vein may come out in fragments, and the job is not as clean-cut as in an uncomplicated case. The surgeon should not hesitate to excise segments which cannot be removed by the stripper. As mentioned previously, the saphenous tributaries are usually numerous and bizarre in these cases, and several postoperative visits are necessary as a rule to clear up these branches by local injections.

Thirty-two patients of Category 2 type of recurrent varicose veins have been reoperated upon in the past three years by this method. Twenty-four have been treated over one year ago and have reported, to date, complete to partial satisfaction with the result. Postoperative injections which were required ranged in all cases from a minimum of two to a maximum of eleven. With a follow-up of three years at the longest, it is difficult to be dogmatic about the eventual results. Undoubtedly more varices will appear in some of these patients, but it is likely that they can be held in check by the occasional injection given at the yearly visits which these patients are requested to make. Four of the thirty-two patients have required further injections to date, but the veins were small and readily responded to sclerosing therapy.

CONCLUSIONS

1. The causes of major recurrence in thirty-two patients with primary varicose veins previously operated upon who underwent further surgery are

discussed. Persistent or new incompetent communicating veins are the greatest single cause.

2. A new technique is described for religation of the saphenous vein at the femoral junction which obviates the difficulties and dangers of secondary surgery in this area.

3. The importance of the small saphenous vein as a cause of recurrence is stressed.

4. The results of a three-year follow-up have been satisfactory in the great majority, but the need for yearly visits and possible further local sclerosing injections is indicated.

THE USE OF INTRAVENOUS TRYPSIN IN EXPERIMENTAL PULMONARY EMBOLISM

H. David Roach, M.D., and Harold Laufman, M.D., Ph.D., Chicago, Ill.

(From the Department of Surgery, Northwestern University Medical School)

TRYPSIN is an enzyme which is known to hydrolyze (digest) certain proteins including fibrin and fibrinogen.[1] There occurs normally in the circulating blood of animals and man a small quantity of a proteolytic enzyme, fibrinolysin (plasmin),[2] which will also hydrolyze fibrin and fibrinogen. The precursor to fibrinolysin, profibrinolysin (plasminogen), also occurs normally in the circulating blood and in much larger amounts. There are many drugs, conditions, and disease states which will activate profibrinolysin to fibrinolysin[2-4] and increase the fibrinolytic activity of the blood. The amount of activation exhibits a species variation for some of the activators studied.[5-7] Streptokinase will activate this precursor a barely perceptible amount in sera of dogs[8] and a larger amount in sera of man.

In the search for a thrombolytic agent, enzymes known to hydrolyze fibrin have been studied. Johnson and Tillett[9] made use of the fibrinolytic enzyme occurring in the circulating blood. They administered streptokinase to rabbits intravenously. This enzyme activated the profibrinolysin to fibrinolysin and caused a gross increase in the fibrinolytic activity of the blood. They reported the complete lysis of clots in ear veins of rabbits twenty-three out of twenty-five times, resulting from the increased lytic activity. Innerfield and associates[10, 11] gave trypsin intravenously to dogs and rabbits after producing intravascular clots, and they reported the complete lysis of clots in some cases. They also reported the lysis of thrombi in patients with acute and chronic thrombophlebitis.

We[12] found that the administration of 130,000 U. of trypsin per kilogram intravenously in dogs would not cause lysis of an experimentally produced thrombus. Also, we found that the administration of 3,000 U. of trypsin per kilogram in human beings had no apparent effect upon the thrombi. However, our in vitro experiments[13] showed that if trypsin was added to blood before it was clotted, a small amount was required to lyse this clot as compared to the amount required to lyse a clot containing no trypsin.

The present experiments were conducted to determine whether intravenous trypsin administered prior to the production of experimental pulmonary emboli and again afterward would cause lysis of the emboli. A standard technique of production of pulmonary emboli was first established. Trypsin was administered intravenously after production of experimental pulmonary emboli in one series of dogs. In another series of dogs, trypsin was administered intravenously before, and again after, production of experimental pulmonary emboli.

Read at the seventh annual meeting of the Society for Vascular Surgery, New York, N. Y., May 31, 1953.

METHODS

Fifty-two healthy adult mongrel dogs weighing from seven to fifteen kilograms were used. A modification of the method of Holden and co-workers[14] was used. The external jugular veins were exposed on both sides for a distance of 8 to 10 cm. A rubber-shod bulldog clamp was applied to the proximal end of the exposed segment. The vein was gently milked toward the clamp to overcome spasm in the vein and to distend the vein with blood. A total of 500 U. of thrombin* (0.5 c.c.) was injected through a 27 gauge needle using three different sites along the vein. Bleeding from the puncture site was prevented by slowly injecting while the needle was being withdrawn from the vein. The vein segment was then massaged gently four or five times to insure mixing of the thrombin and blood. An immediate clot was formed and could be palpated and fractured between the index finger and thumb. Time from production of clots until their release into the circulation varied from five to forty-five minutes. The surviving dogs were sacrificed forty-eight hours later. The heart and lungs were quickly removed and examined immediately. The right ventricle was opened and inspected for emboli and mural thrombi, recent or old, and any recent extension of clots. The pulmonary arterial tree was carefully dissected and inspected for emboli. Specimens were taken from areas containing emboli for microscopic study.

Using this basic technique, certain variations were employed on twenty-six animals comprising the control group. In eight dogs the clot was produced in only one jugular vein. In six of these dogs the clots were released into the circulation forty minutes after formation and in one dog, five minutes after formation. The eighth dog received an injection of thrombin into one jugular vein without clamping off the segment. In eighteen other dogs the clots were produced in both jugular veins. The bilateral clots were released almost simultaneously into the circulation twenty minutes after formation in six dogs, and forty-five minutes after formation in eight dogs. In one dog, one clot was released after ten minutes. In three dogs the bulldog clamps were replaced with partially constricting ligatures ten minutes after clot formation.

Twenty-six dogs were treated with intravenous trypsin† at various times before and after clots were produced in both jugular veins. The thrombi were released into the circulation as in the control animals.

RESULTS

Control Series.—In the first six untreated animals with clots produced in only one jugular vein and released after forty minutes, the only effect was a slight increase in respiratory rate and depth shortly afterward, returning to normal after ten minutes. These animals were sacrificed after forty-eight hours. Post-mortem examination revealed pulmonary emboli in three of the six dogs.

*Thrombin, Topical (bovine origin), Parke, Davis & Company, 1,000 U vial.

†Enzar, developed, manufactured, and supplied by the Armour Laboratories, Chicago, consists of 90 per cent pure trypsin, 5 per cent ash (mostly magnesium), 4 per cent traces of ribonuclease plus cathepsin and alpha, beta, and gamma chymotrypsin, 1 per cent undetermined.

If the clot from one external jugular vein was released into the circulation five minutes after formation, death occurred in ten minutes. In one such experiment the right ventricle was found to contain a large, soft recent clot attached to an older clot cast in the shape of the jugular vein. In another animal, .025 c.c. (250 U.) of thrombin was injected into the unclamped external jugular vein. This also resulted in death in ten minutes and post-mortem findings of a large, soft clot in the right ventricle.

In the eighteen untreated animals with clots in both jugular veins, the results were as follows. Release of one or both jugular vein clots into the circulation ten minutes after formation resulted in death of each of four dogs within ten minutes after release. This was true even when partial occlusion was substituted for the bulldog clamps ten minutes after clot formation. All these animals had soft clots in the right ventricle, with or without pulmonary embolism. Simultaneous release of the clots into the circulation twenty minutes after formation resulted in death in ten minutes in two of the six dogs. The right ventricle contained recent soft clots, and large emboli were found in the pulmonary arterial tree (Fig. 1). The four surviving dogs were sacrificed at forty-eight hours, and in each instance large emboli were found in the pulmonary arterial tree. In one of these dogs, a mural thrombus was present in the right ventricle.

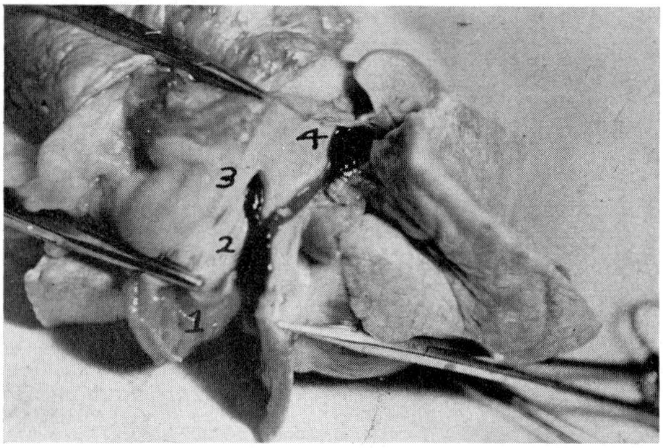

Fig. 1.—Fatal pulmonary embolism in control animal. The clots produced in the external jugular veins were released into the circulation twenty minutes after they were produced. The dog died ten minutes later. Large soft clot in right ventricle (*1*) extends into pulmonary trunk (*2*) and to ostia of right pulmonary artery (*3*) and left pulmonary artery (*4*), where it was attached to the emboli which almost occluded the ostia.

If the bilateral jugular vein clots were allowed to remain in place for forty-five minutes before release into the circulation, the animals survived, but at sacrifice forty-eight hours later they were found to have large emboli in the pulmonary arterial tree without intracardiac thrombi (Fig. 2). This result was consistent in eight dogs.

It was obvious from this series that jugular vein clots had to be produced bilaterally in order to result in the consistent formation of pulmonary emboli. Furthermore, release of the clots before they had an opportunity to inactivate the thrombin resulted in death of the animals more from soft ventricular thrombi than from pulmonary embolism. Consistent production of firm pulmonary emboli in eight out of eight dogs was accomplished by releasing bilateral jugular vein thrombi into the circulation forty to forty-five minutes after formation. Death proved to be a poor criterion for the presence of pulmonary embolism in the dog. Only by sacrifice of the animal and dissection of the pulmonary arterial tree and heart chambers could the presence and extent of the embolizations be determined.

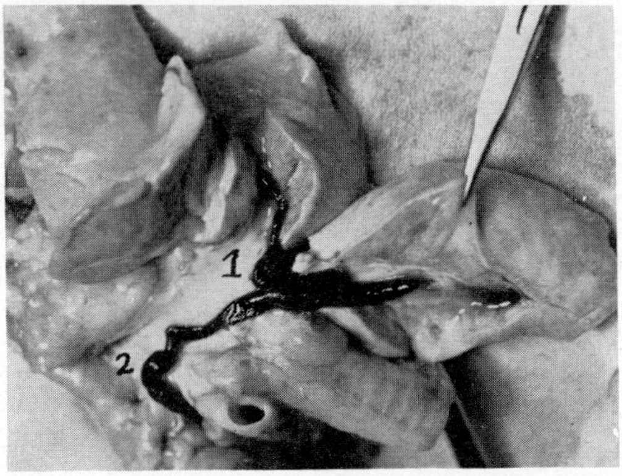

Fig. 2.—Standard pulmonary emboli in control animal. The dog was sacrificed forty-eight hours later. There is a large saddle embolus at branching of left pulmonary artery into arteries to the left upper and middle lobes (*1*) and extending into the right pulmonary artery (*2*). The emboli are firm and red, and have a nonshiny surface.

Series of Trypsin-Treated Animals.—Twenty-six dogs comprised this series. In five dogs, trypsin was given intravenously after pulmonary emboli were produced by releasing thrombi from both jugular veins. Trypsin was given in dosages varying from 25,000 to 120,000 U. per kilogram and in periods of time ranging from one minute to five hours. When as little as 25,000 U. per kilogram of trypsin was injected in one minute, death of the animal followed in from fifteen to forty-five minutes after injection. Two dogs died in shock, interpreted as peptone shock, resulting from the rapid injection of trypsin. In the remaining three animals, the trypsin was administered over a two- to four-hour period in the dosage of 120,000 U. per kilogram. One dog died in three hours and another dog in twenty-four hours; the third dog survived and was sacrificed at the end of forty-eight hours. Pulmonary emboli were found in all three of these animals (Fig. 3). Thus, the administration of trypsin, almost regardless of dosage, after a pulmonary embolism had been produced had no effect on the embolus.

Our next step was to administer trypsin before the clots were produced in both external jugular veins. In order to determine the size of trypsin dosage we performed certain in vitro experiments. We found that 100 U. of trypsin per cubic centimeter of oxalated blood would allow the blood to clot, but the clot would undergo subsequent lysis if kept at 37.5° C. in a water bath. Thus, assuming that the circulating blood volume of a dog was 12 per cent of its body weight, a ten kilogram dog would have a total blood volume of 1,200 c.c. Therefore, the proper dosage would be roughly 12,000 U. of trypsin per kilogram as a preliminary administration of trypsin. To test this calculation, we injected 13,000 U. of trypsin per kilogram rapidly into dogs, and five minutes later a sample of blood was drawn. In each instance the blood clotted in the tube but the clot underwent lysis within twenty-four hours at water-bath temperature.

Employing this plan, six dogs were given 13,000 U. of trypsin per kilogram in 30 c.c. of saline solution intravenously in one minute. This resulted in an

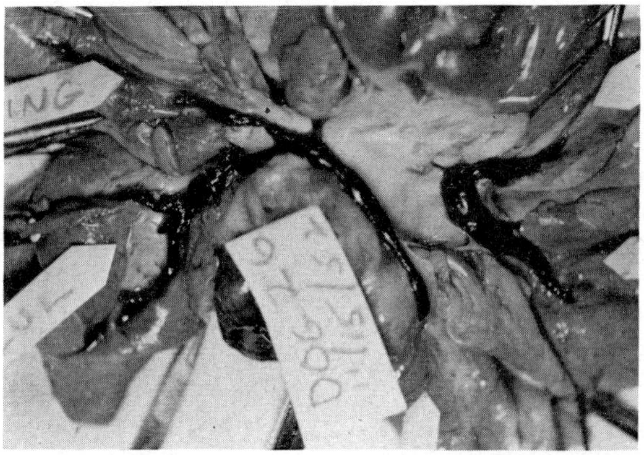

Fig. 3.—Emboli in dog treated with trypsin after production of standard pulmonary embolism. Trypsin, 33,000 U. per kilogram, was given intravenously in five hours, and the animal was sacrificed forty-eight hours later. There is no gross evidence of digestion of the emboli. The emboli are black and have a shiny glistening surface.

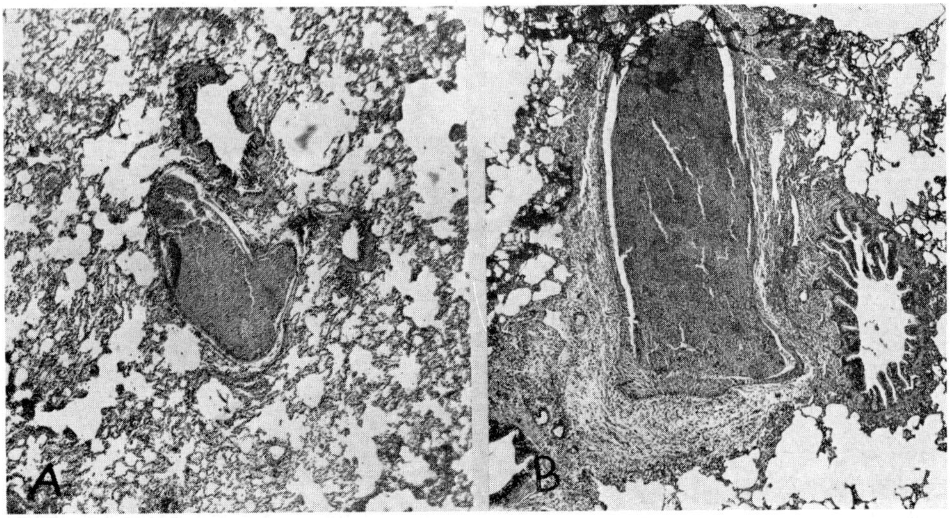

A. *B.*

Fig. 4.—Photomicrographs of pulmonary emboli in control animal and in animal treated with trypsin.

A, Control section from lungs shown in Fig. 2; *B,* treated with trypsin after production of emboli. Section from lungs shown in Fig. 3. There is no microscopic evidence of digestion of the embolus in the trypsin-treated animal as compared to the control.

almost immediate drop in blood pressure to about 40 mm. Hg with return to control levels in about ten minutes. Bilateral jugular vein clots were then produced. In five dogs the clots were released into the circulation forty-five minutes later. Four of these dogs received an additional intravenous injection of 13,000 U. of trypsin per kilogram five minutes after release of the clots. Blood drawn five minutes after this injection did not clot, even after the addition of thrombin to the sample. The blood of these animals was now considered to be afibrinogenemic. This state lasted from two to four hours, after which there was gradual spontaneous restitution to normal clotting.

One of the four dogs so treated was found dead the morning after the experiment. Post-mortem examination revealed no clots in any of the pulmonary vessels or in the right ventricle. The other three dogs were sacrificed after forty-eight hours, and in none of these animals was there any evidence of pulmonary or ventricular emboli (Fig. 5). The fifth pretreated dog whose jugular vein clots were released forty-five minutes after formation did not receive the second injection of trypsin. It was found dead the following morning. Examination revealed no emboli in this animal, but the lungs showed a massive pneumonia with large amounts of mucus in the bronchi.

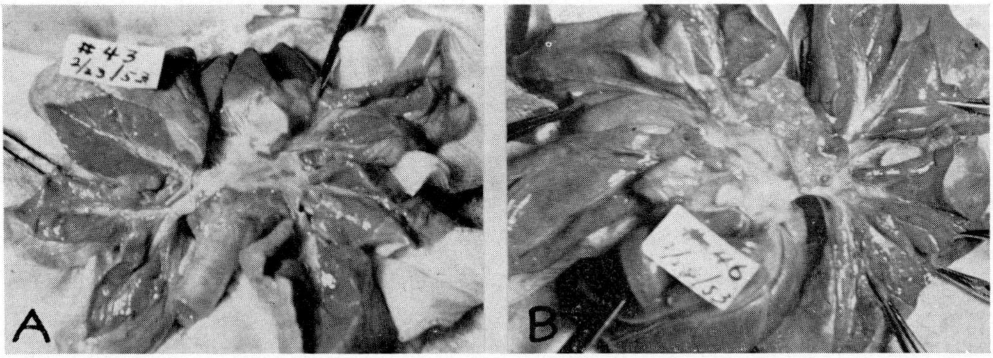

Fig. 5.—Dissection of the pulmonary arterial tree showing absence of pulmonary emboli.

A, Animal was given 13,000 U. of trypsin per kilogram intravenously in one minute. Pulmonary embolism was produced and an additional 13,000 U. of trypsin per kilogram was given. Animal was sacrificed forty-eight hours later.

B, Animal was given 19,000 U. of trypsin per kilogram in 175 c.c. of saline solution intravenously in one hour, ten minutes. Pulmonary embolism was produced, and an additional 16,000 U. of trypsin per kilogram in 125 c.c. of saline solution was given in fifty minutes. Animal was sacrified forty-eight hours later.

By error, the jugular vein clots in the sixth dog of this series were released just five minutes after formation. This dog died in ten minutes and was found to have a large, soft recent clot in the right ventricle and emboli in the pulmonary arteries (Dog 44, Table I).

In the next series of ten dogs, slower infusions of trypsin were given in an attempt to obviate the shock caused by rapid injection. We found that 19,000 U. of trypsin per kilogram in 175 c.c. of saline solution, infused over a period of one hour, ten minutes, usually resulted in the same degree of autolysis of a clot of drawn blood as did the one-minute injection of 13,000 U. per kilogram without lowering the blood pressure. Preinfusion and postinfusion circulating fibrinogen levels were determined in some animals, and antitrypsin titers* were calculated. Seven of these dogs received only pretreatment, while three received an additional infusion of 16,000 U. of trypsin per kilogram in 125 c.c. of saline solution over a fifty-minute period after release of the jugular vein clots. Results in these animals are summarized in Table II. All animals survived and were sacrificed after forty-eight hours.

TABLE I. PRE-EMBOLISM DOSE OF 13,000 U. OF TRYPSIN PER KILOGRAM ADMINISTERED INTRAVENOUSLY IN 30 C.C. OF SALINE SOLUTION IN ONE MINUTE; POSTEMBOLISM DOSE THE SAME

DOG	AUTOLYSIS CLOT*	AFIBRINOGENEMIA	EMBOLI PRESENT
44	Complete	No	Yes; dog died ten minutes after clots released
45	Complete	After second injection	No
46	Complete	After second injection	No
47	Complete	After second injection	No; dead in cage next day
48	Complete	No; second injection not given	No; dead in cage next day

*Blood sample drawn, allowed to clot, and observed for autolysis after initial dose of trypsin.

TABLE II. PRE-EMBOLISM DOSE OF 19,000 U. OF TRYPSIN PER KILOGRAM IN 175 C.C. OF SALINE SOLUTION ADMINISTERED INTRAVENOUSLY IN SEVENTY MINUTES; NO ADDITIONAL TRYPSIN GIVEN

DOG	PLASMA FIBRINOGEN (MG. PER CENT) PRE-INFUSION	POST-INFUSION	TRYPSIN TITRATION OF PROTHROMBIN-FREE PLASMA (UNITS OF TRYPSIN)	AFIBRINOGENEMIA	AUTOLYSIS CLOT	EMBOLI PRESENT
51	390	Not done	Not done	No	Complete	None
52	280	159	450	No	Complete	None
53	402	411	909	No	No	Present (see Fig. 6)
54	Not done	Not done	525	No	Complete	None
55	Not done	Not done	450	No	Complete	Small embolus
56	Not done	Not done	675	No	Complete	Small embolus
57	Not done	Not done	650	No	Complete	None

TABLE III. PRE-EMBOLISM DOSE OF 19,000 U. OF TRYPSIN PER KILOGRAM IN 175 C.C. OF SALINE SOLUTION ADMINISTERED INTRAVENOUSLY IN SEVENTY MINUTES. POSTEMBOLISM DOSE OF 16,000 U. OF TRYPSIN PER KILOGRAM IN 125 C.C. OF SALINE SOLUTION ADMINISTERED INTRAVENOUSLY IN FIFTY MINUTES

DOG	AUTOLYSIS CLOT	AFIBRINOGENEMIA	EMBOLI PRESENT
42	Complete	After second infusion	No
43	Complete	After second infusion	No
50	Complete	After second infusion	No

Four of the seven dogs with pretreatment alone had no evidence of cardiac or pulmonary embolism (Fig. 5, *B*). Two of the dogs were found to have small recent pulmonary emboli, and one had pulmonary emboli no different from those found in untreated animals. It is interesting that this dog (Fig. 6, No. 53

*Trypsin titration of prothrombin-free plasma determined the antitrypsin titer.[13] Prothrombin-free plasma was prepared by the method of Frommeyer and Epstein.[15] Varying small quantities of trypsin were added to 0.5 c.c. samples of prothrombin-free plasma. Thrombin was then added. The end point was taken as the concentration of trypsin in the tube in which a soft clot formed in one minute, provided the contents of the tube with the next higher concentration of trypsin remained liquid.

in Table II) had rather high fibrinogen levels, pre- and postinfusion, and an extremely high antitrypsin titer.

The three dogs in this group receiving an additional infusion of 16,000 U. of trypsin per kilogram after the release of the clots exhibited afibrinogenemia at the conclusion of this infusion. None of these animals had any evidence of pulmonary embolism when sacrificed forty-eight hours later (Table III).

Our subsequent experiments were concerned with variations in dosage of the trypsin before and after emboli were produced, with parallel determinations of pre- and postinfusion fibrinogen levels and antitrypsin titers, and observation of drawn blood for lysis of clots.

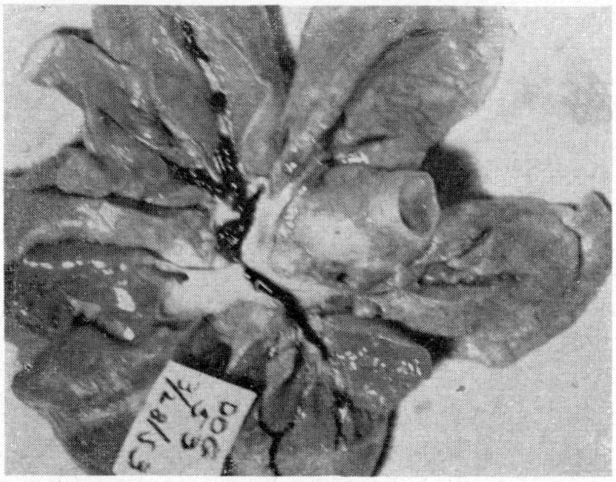

Fig. 6.—Dissection of the pulmonary arterial tree showing emboli present after treatment with trypsin. Animal was given 19,000 U. of trypsin per kilogram in 175 c.c. of saline solution in one hour, ten minutes. Pulmonary embolism was produced and no additional trypsin given. Animal was sacrificed forty-eight hours later.

Trypsin, 16,000 U. per kilogram in 175 c.c. of saline solution infused for one hour, ten minutes prior to formation of the jugular vein clots and 19,000 U. per kilogram after embolization, resulted in the absence of pulmonary emboli in one dog, but did not prevent the formation of two very small emboli in another dog. Blood drawn at the time of jugular vein clot production in the latter dog showed lysis of only two-thirds of the clot in the test tube in twenty-four hours. This indicated to us that the initial dose of trypsin by slow infusion was borderline to or below adequate levels, and therefore emboli could sometimes be expected almost regardless of the amount of the second dose. Fibrinogen levels and antitrypsin determinations were noncontributory in these animals (Table IV).

In two dogs the pre-embolism dose of trypsin was cut to 13,000 U. per kilogram, but the dose after release of the bilateral jugular vein thrombi was increased to 22,000 U. per kilogram. Both dosages were given by slow infusion. Clotted blood samples drawn after the first infusion did not completely lyse after twenty-four hours in the water bath. After the second infusion, a state of afibrinogenemia existed in each dog. Yet pulmonary emboli were found in each case, although they were not as large as those seen in control dogs. Antitrypsin levels were high in these dogs (Table V).

TABLE IV. PRE-EMBOLISM DOSE OF 16,000 U. OF TRYPSIN PER KILOGRAM IN 175 C.C. OF SALINE SOLUTION ADMINISTERED INTRAVENOUSLY IN SEVENTY MINUTES; POSTEMBOLISM DOSE OF 19,000 U. OF TRYPSIN PER KILOGRAM IN 125 C.C. OF SALINE SOLUTION IN FIFTY MINUTES

DOG	PLASMA FIBRINOGEN (MILLIGRAMS PER CENT)		TRYPSIN TITRATION OF PROTHROMBIN-FREE PLASMA (UNITS OF TRYPSIN)	AFIBRINOGENEMIA	AUTOLYSIS CLOT	EMBOLI PRESENT
	PRE-INFUSION	AFTER FIRST INFUSION				
61	397	327	750	After second infusion	Not complete	None
62	336	280	350	After second infusion	Not complete	Two small emboli

It would appear from these four experiments that the initial dosage of trypsin before embolization must be great enough to cause lysis of a sample of clotted blood drawn after the infusion in order to prevent the persistence of pulmonary emboli.

TABLE V. PRE-EMBOLISM DOSE OF 13,000 U. OF TRYPSIN PER KILOGRAM IN 175 C.C. OF SALINE SOLUTION ADMINISTERED INTRAVENOUSLY IN SEVENTY MINUTES; POSTEMBOLISM DOSE OF 22,000 U. OF TRYPSIN PER KILOGRAM IN 125 C.C. OF SALINE SOLUTION IN FIFTY MINUTES

DOG	PLASMA FIBRINOGEN (MILLIGRAMS PER CENT)		TRYPSIN TITRATION OF PROTHROMBIN-FREE PLASMA		TRYPSIN TITRATION OF PLASMA		AFIBRINOGENEMIA	AUTOLYSIS CLOT	EMBOLI PRESENT
	PREINFUSION	AFTER FIRST INFUSION	PREINFUSION	AFTER FIRST INFUSION	PREINFUSION	AFTER FIRST INFUSION			
63	468	412	400	350	600	400	No	No	Massive emboli; dog died after release of clots
64	468	280	1,000	350	1,250	750	After second infusion	No	Three small emboli
65	465	224	950	650	1,350	1,150	After second infusion	No	Two small emboli

One additional dog deserves special mention. This animal was given 13,000 U. of trypsin per kilogram as the pre-embolism dose. The animal was supposed to have received the 22,000 U. dosage after embolization, similar to the last two animals mentioned previously. However, the dog died ten minutes after release of the bilateral forty-five minute jugular vein thrombi and before the second trypsin infusion had been completed. Immediate post-mortem examination revealed large soft recent clots in both ventricles in addition to an older clot in the right ventricle shaped like the external jugular vein. The pulmonary arterial tree was completely cast with soft recent clotted blood containing several older clots (Dog 63, Table V). This unexpected finding might be explained on the basis of the persistence of some free thrombin around the embolus at the time of release or of an unusual amount of activation of prothrombin to thrombin by the trypsin.

SUMMARY AND DISCUSSION

In order for these experiments to be considered valid, it must be assumed that the method of producing pulmonary embolism in the control series of animals was valid. The size of our control series is small. Yet the fact that we found emboli in each instance by actual dissection of the sacrificed animals, rather than by the use of symptoms or survival as the criterion for the presence of pulmonary embolism, lends validity to the method. We found it necessary to produce clots in both external jugular veins in order to be assured of consistent pulmonary emboli. In order to allow survival for at least forty-eight hours, the jugular vein clots had to remain in place for forty-five minutes. If the clots were released into the circulation much sooner, there was apparently enough free thrombin in the embolized segment to cause rapid soft clot formation in the right ventricle and pulmonary arterial tree, and death. Evidence for this was seen in the animal in the control series in which thrombin was injected into the unclamped jugular vein. Death occurred in ten minutes, and a large soft clot was found in the right ventricle extending into the pulmonary artery.

Trypsin administered in almost any dosage after the production of pulmonary embolism had no effect on the emboli. This substantiates our previous work[12] which contradicted that of Innerfield and associates.[10, 11]

Infusions of trypsin before emboli were produced and again afterward usually prevented their persistence. Determination of dosage for the pretreatment infusion was based mainly on the observation of lysis of a clot of blood drawn five minutes after injection. A somewhat larger quantity of trypsin was necessary with slow infusion than with rapid injection to accomplish the same effect on the blood, which may be explained partially by the deterioration rate of trypsin solution. Rapid injections caused shock and were therefore undesirable.

At the time blood was drawn after the initial injection of trypsin, some delay in clotting was observed provided the dosage was adequate. Observation of drawn clotted blood for lysis revealed different rates of lysis occurring in the samples from various dogs given the same dosage by weight. Possible explanations for this finding include the variants involved in administering a drug on a weight basis, and perhaps differences in antitrypsin levels. As a rule, optimum infusion dosages caused the first postinfusion blood sample clot to undergo lysis over a period of eight to ten hours at 37.5° C. If more trypsin was infused, lysis occurred as rapidly as ten minutes after the clot formed in the tube. Further administration resulted in blood which was incoagulable and afibrinogenemic. An intravascular clot, released into the circulation at a time when lysis is demonstrated in drawn clotted blood, will be lysed by an additional dosage of trypsin. We found that the pre-embolism dosage is more important than the second dosage of trypsin. In our dogs, at least 19,000 U. per kilogram infused slowly as a pre-embolism dosage, followed by a similar postembolism dosage, was necessary to prevent embolism. However, rapid injections of 13,000 U. per kilogram were just as effective, although they caused temporary shock.

COMMENT

Great caution must be exercised in any attempt to project our experimental work to possible application in the human being, for two main reasons which are: (1) there is known to be a species difference in the fibrinolytic effect of trypsin,[3] and (2) the afibrinogenemia occurring in our successful experiments after the second infusion of trypsin would be a most undesirable postoperative consequence in human surgery.

REFERENCES

1. Northrop, J. H.: Crystalline Enzymes, New York, 1948, Columbia University Press.
2. MacFarlane, R. G., and Biggs, R.: Fibrinolysis: Its Mechanism and Significance, Blood **3**: 1167, 1948.
3. Kocholaty, W., Ellis, W. W., and Jensen, H.: Activation of Plasminogen by Trypsin and Plasmin, Blood **7**: 882, 1952.
4. Tagnon, H. J., Levenson, S. M., Davidson, C. S., and Taylor, F. H. L.: The Occurrence of Fibrinolysis in Shock With Observations on the Prothrombin Time and the Plasma Fibrinogen During Hemorrhagic Shock, Am. J. M. Sc. **211**: 88-96, 1946.
5. Gerheim, E. B., and Ferguson, J. H.: Species Reactivity to Staphylokinase, Proc. Soc. Exper. Biol. & Med. **71**: 261, 1949.
6. Clifton, E. E., and Cannamela, D. A.: Variations in Proteolytic Activity of Serum of Animals Including Man, Proc. Soc. Exper. Biol. & Med. **77**: 305, 1951.
7. Clifton, E. E.: Variations in the Proteolytic and the Anti-proteolytic Reactions of Serum: Effects of Disease, Trauma, X-ray, Anaphylactic Shock, ACTH and Cortisone, J. Lab. & Clin. Med. **39**: 105, 1952.
8. Downee, G. R., and Clifton, E. E.: A Method of Assay of Serum Proteolytic Activity, Proc. Soc. Exper. Biol. & Med. **71**: 138, 1949.
9. Johnson, A. J., and Tillett, W. S.: The Lysis in Rabbits of Intravascular Blood Clots by the Streptococcae Fibrinolytic System (Streptokinase), J. Exper. Med. **95**: 449, 1952.
10. Innerfield, I. F., Schwartz, A. W., and Angrist, A. A.: Fibrinolytic and Anticoagulant Effects of Intervenous Trypsin, Bull. New York Acad. Med. **28**: 537, 1952.
11. Innerfield, I. F., Schwartz, A. W., and Angrist, A. A.: Intravenous Trypsin; Its Anticoagulant, Fibrinolytic and Thrombolytic Effects, J. Clin. Investigation **31**: 1049, 1952.
12. Laufman, H., and Roach, H. D.: Intravenous Trypsin in the Treatment of Thrombotic Phenomena, Arch. Surg. **66**: 552, 1953.
13. Roach, H. D.: Unpublished data.
14. Holden, W. D., Shaw, B. W., Cameron, D. B., Shea, P. J., and Davis, J. H.: Experimental Pulmonary Embolism, Surg., Gynec. & Obst. **88**: 23, 1949.
15. Frommeyer, W. B., and Epstein, R. D.: Hemorrhagic Diseases (Concluded), New England J. Med. **241**: 743, 1949.

THE EMPIRIC USE OF GASTRIC RESECTION IN THE TREATMENT OF UPPER GASTROINTESTINAL HEMORRHAGE

E. T. THIEME, M.D., ANN ARBOR, MICH.

IN RECENT years the problem of upper gastrointestinal hemorrhage has received much attention in both the medical and surgical literature. Whether authors are inclined toward the conservative nonoperative treatment or surgical intervention, the fact stands out that timely and adequate blood replacement has greatly reduced the mortality of either method of treatment. From many such reports the consensus would seem to be that there is a group of patients who require emergency surgery if they are to survive. The size and importance of the group of patients requiring emergency surgery for the control of upper gastrointestinal hemorrhage differ greatly from one article to the next. It is not the purpose of this paper to indicate how to select these patients but, rather, once the decision to operate has been reached, to advocate the empiric use of gastric resection.

When operating for gastrointestinal hemorrhage, there is general agreement that with a lesion palpable in the duodenum or stomach, gastric resection is the operation of choice. Simple ligation of the bleeding point, gastroenterostomy, and/or vagotomy are a poor compromise at best. However, there are always a few instances in which no lesion can be felt. If the liver and spleen are normal, with few exceptions authors advocate a wide gastrotomy to locate the bleeding point but frequently have been unable to find one. It is our contention that gastrotomy not only prolongs the operation in a poor-risk patient but also is frequently futile. This contention is based both on the experience previously reported in the literature and the cases here reported.

Opinions vary greatly as to the extent to which preoperative studies should be made to establish the etiology of the bleeding. Some feel that surgery should not be undertaken without good proof of peptic ulceration. Other authors feel that these patients are in no condition to undergo gastrointestinal x-ray examinations and that if surgery is delayed to obtain x-ray pictures the patient will be lost. Certainly, the patient requiring emergency surgery for the control of hemorrhage is not a good candidate for x-ray studies. Also, inconclusive x-ray pictures have all too frequently been reported when taken during active bleeding. Normal gastrointestinal x-ray pictures taken after the bleeding has stopped have been reported in as high as 25 per cent of the cases studied. Relatively little has been written to explain the normal stomach and duodenum found either by x-ray examination or at gastrotomy. The role of minute gastric erosions in this problem has been emphasized by Wangensteen,[7] Crohn,[2] Ives,[5] and recently by Cooper and Ferguson.[1] These lesions cannot be shown by x-ray picture. In the fresh

Received for publication, April 7, 1953.

specimen they cannot be palpated and usually can be seen only after fixation. When demonstrated after fixation the erosion is a clear-cut entity following the expected pattern of location of gastric ulcers and not possibly confused with hemorrhagic gastritis. It is a common experience to find that at operation the bleeding has ceased and that the stomach and duodenum are empty. This situation coupled with a gastric erosion always too small to be seen explains the failure of gastrotomy.

In 1884, in a widely quoted report, Dr. Gallard[3] gave a classic description of two patients who died of exsanguination despite cold white wine, ergot, and rum. At autopsy the gastric erosion was overlooked at first but later demonstrated after fixation. A third case would have been described but the "seance" closed. Since that time little attention has been given to superficial gastric erosions other than by the authors mentioned. Unfortunately, from those cases previously reported elsewhere and those cases to be reported here, no clear-cut clinical picture can be drawn which will point to the diagnosis of gastric erosion. Sudden, painless, catastrophic bleeding in a previously healthy patient is suggestive, but perhaps 20 per cent of peptic ulcers first manifest themselves by such a hemorrhage. Because the medical treatment of hemorrhage from a peptic ulcer or a superficial gastric erosion is the same, no importance can immediately be attached to the differential diagnosis. The matter of prime importance is that this diagnosis be in the mind of the surgeon after the decision to operate has been reached. There is insufficient recorded experience to compare the prognosis following surgery for these two conditions. Because the diagnosis of gastric erosion cannot be made with certainty, except at operation, there is no information concerning the prognosis or instance of recurrence following medical care. However, in each of the four articles mentioned, the discussion of this condition would seem to have been initiated by recurrent hemorrhage when a gastrotomy alone was done.

During a three-year period, eleven patients from one surgical service at St. Joseph's Mercy Hospital were operated upon because of uncontrolled gastrointestinal hemorrhage. A gastric ulcer was found in four cases, a duodenal ulcer in three cases, and no lesion was palpated in four cases. This is about the same proportion of cases as that reported in the series of Cooper and Ferguson. They reported eighteen patients operated upon as emergencies, in six of whom no lesion was palpated in the stomach or duodenum. They performed the gastric resection as a "blind gastric resection." Here it is preferred to consider this a gastric resection on an "empiric basis."

Brief case summaries of four patients in whom no lesion could be palpated follow.

Case 1.—A 30-year-old, single woman, a shoe clerk, was attending a customer when she suddenly felt ill and vomited a large amount of clotted blood. This she attributed to the fact that the customer's small daughter had recently vomited liberally about the store. She herself had never had stomach trouble. She rested at home during that day but early next morning she passed large clots of blood by rectum and vomited blood once again. She was admitted to the hospital as an emergency. Blood pressure was 90/60, pulse 108, hemoglobin 7½ Gm., red blood count 2.01 million. In the next thirty hours she received

4,000 c.c. of blood, but the blood counts were essentially unchanged and the bleeding from the rectum continued. Emergency operation was advised and accepted. At operation the stomach and duodenum were empty and no lesions could be palpated. As the liver and spleen were normal, immediate gastric resection was undertaken. As the Von Petz clamp was being put in place, the stomach was seen to be filling up with blood. It was opened and a small artery was seen to be spurting on the lesser curvature just at the point where the Von Petz clamp was to be applied. Resection was completed and the patient made an uneventful recovery. She received a total of 7,000 c.c. of blood in thirty-six hours. She is alive and well three years later.

CASE 2.—A 68-year-old retired businessman was admitted to the medical service complaining of anorexia, weight loss, and tarry stools. X-ray pictures elsewhere had been reported as normal for the gastrointestinal tract. He admitted the abuse of alcohol for many years. On admission the liver and spleen were not palpably enlarged. The hemoglobin was 8.4 Gm., the red blood count was 3,000,000, and liver function studies were normal except for a lowered prothrombin time. X-ray pictures demonstrated a diverticulosis of the sigmoid colon and a diverticulum of the second portion of the duodenum. Esophagoscopy failed to demonstrate esophageal varices. During the ten days of hospitalization he received 5,500 c.c. of blood with unmaintained improvement. Tarry stools continued, but no vomiting.

The early morning of the eleventh hospital day he awakened his private nurse by having three large bloody bowel movements in bed. One thousand cubic centimeters of blood was given rapidly because of the marked drop in blood pressure and rise in pulse. There seemed little improvement with this, therefore an additional 2,000 c.c. of blood was given and surgical consultation obtained. As his condition was not improving, emergency surgery was advised and accepted. At operation the liver and spleen were normal, the stomach and duodenum were empty. No lesion could be palpated in either bowel or stomach. Gastric resection was performed immediately with an uneventful recovery. He received 4,500 c.c. of blood in this thirty-hour period. The patient is alive and well two years later. When the stomach was seen in the fresh state no lesion could be seen or palpated. However, after fixation two-minute gastric erosions were demonstrated on the lesser curvature. Considering this, the normal x-ray pictures are easily understood and it is doubted that gastrotomy would have demonstrated these lesions unless they could have been made to bleed.

CASE 3.—A 70-year-old farmer was admitted to the hospital for the Phenylbutizon therapy of a gouty arthritis. During the nine days of treatment he received 200 mg., four times a day. This produced a remarkable improvement in the arthritis and he was ready for discharge. On admission a secondary anemia had been noted which responded to a transfusion. During the afternoon of the tenth hospital day he passed large tarry stools and became very weak despite 1,500 c.c. of blood. During the subsequent night he received an additional 4,000 c.c. of blood and the next morning when seen in surgical consultation he appeared as well as his 7 Gm. of hemoglobin indicated. Emergency surgery was advised and accepted but before he could be taken to the operating room he had several large bloody stools and went into shock. Cut-downs were placed at each arm and 1,000 c.c. of blood was given quickly and he was taken to the operating room. At operation the liver and spleen were normal, the stomach and duodenum were empty, and no lesion could be palpated in the bowel, duodenum, or stomach. Gastric resection was performed immediately. Recovery seemed satisfactory but the patient died on the fourteenth postoperative day without preceding elevation of pulse, temperature, or respiration except during the last twelve hours of life. No autopsy was granted. Examination of the fresh specimen revealed no ulcer, but after fixation a small erosion was seen low on the lesser curvature of the stomach. This lesion not found by careful inspection of the stomach out of the body could never have been seen by gastrotomy unless bleeding had been started. Unsatisfactory side reactions have been reported in as many as 35 per cent of the patients

Fig. 1.

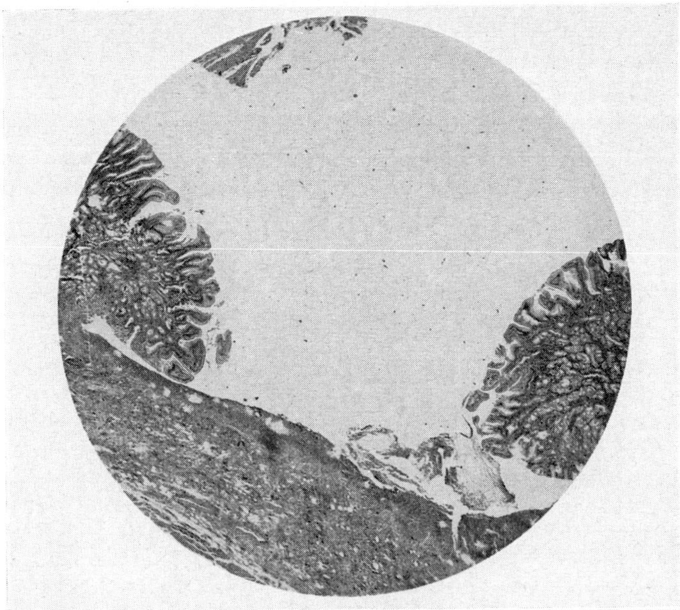

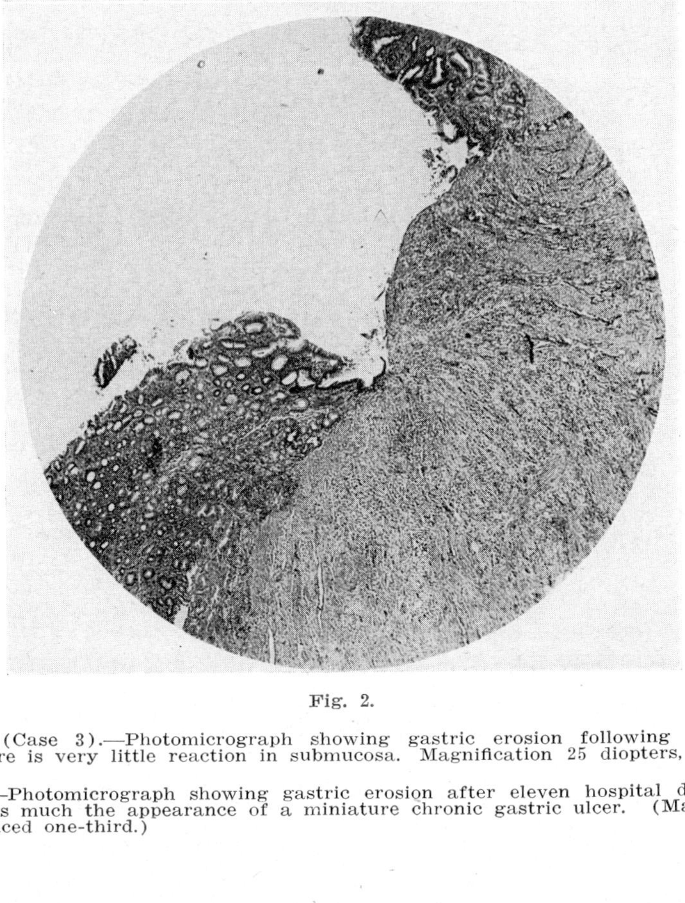

Fig. 2.

Fig. 1 (Case 3).—Photomicrograph showing gastric erosion following Phenylbutizon therapy. There is very little reaction in submucosa. Magnification 25 diopters, reduced one-third.)

Fig. 2.—Photomicrograph showing gastric erosion after eleven hospital days of bleeding. This has much the appearance of a miniature chronic gastric ulcer. (Magnification 25 diopters, reduced one-third.)

treated with Phenylbutizon.[4-6] These usually take the form of agranulocytosis or toxic reaction, but occasionally a duodenal ulcer has been activated or gastric hemorrhage has followed the use of Phenylbutizon.

CASE 4.—A 47-year-old professor was admitted as an emergency because he had suddenly vomited a large amount of blood. In 1935, a diagnosis of duodenal ulcer was first made for this patient, by x-ray examination. He was treated by diet and x-ray therapy. In 1944, he had a serious exacerbation, with a prolonged period of hemorrhage. In 1951, he had a minor exacerbation and at that time x-ray pictures showed some old scarring of the duodenum. Since then he has felt unusually well and has been very active. He had, however, had back pain the week prior to this illness and had taken an undisclosed amount of aspirin by mouth. On admission the patient soon passed several large bloody stools. During the next eighteen hours he received 3,500 c.c. of blood with a slow dropping in the hemoglobin and red blood count. He continued to have bloody stools by rectum, so emergency surgery was advised and accepted. Again at operation the liver and spleen were normal, and the stomach and duodenum were empty. No lesion could be felt in the stomach or duodenum but the gastric resection was performed without gastrotomy. The postoperative course was very satisfactory and he was discharged the ninth postoperative day. He received 5,500 c.c. of blood during a period of thirty-six hours. Again when the specimen was examined in the fresh state no lesion could be palpated or seen. However, after fixation a small superficial gastric erosion was demonstrated on the posterior aspect of the stomach. It was felt that a smaller erosion was seen higher up in the stomach but the microscopic examination failed to confirm this impression. There was no evidence of the so-called hemorrhagic gastritis that has been reported following the excessive use of aspirin.

The decision to operate on any of the eleven patients, and specifically in the four cases just detailed, may be questioned. It can only be stated that in each instance the situation seemed desperate and the prognosis poor without surgical intervention. However, once the decision to operate had been made the decision for gastric resection without demonstrating the bleeding point would seem to have been justified by the pathology that was demonstrated. Also, this decision would seem to be the logical answer to the situation in which no lesion is palpated in the stomach or duodenum.

There are two obvious weaknesses to this statement as presented here. First, in only one case was bleeding actually seen to come from a gastric erosion. However, in none of the other cases was there any evidence of hemorrhagic gastritis or other sources of hemorrhage seen by the pathologist. Second, no evidence has been given in this paper to show that gastrotomy alone is followed by recurrent hemorrhage. As previously mentioned recurrent hemorrhage has been reported in other series of cases and had drawn the attention of those authors to the existence of superficial gastric erosion.

SUMMARY

Once the decision to operate for uncontrolled gastrointestinal hemorrhage has been made, immediate gastric resection is the operation of choice if the liver and spleen are normal and a lesion is palpable in the stomach or duodenum. In those cases in which no lesion is palpated in the stomach or duodenum, gastric resection is advocated without gastrotomy to prove a bleeding point. Gastrotomy prolongs the operation in a poor-risk patient and frequently fails to show the bleeding point. Superficial gastric erosions, which can neither be felt nor seen in the fresh specimen but which can be the source of exsanguination, are offered as the explanation of the hemorrhage when no lesion can be demonstrated by gastrotomy or later by x-ray picture. Four such cases are presented.

REFERENCES

1. Cooper, D. R., and Ferguson, L. K.: Gastric Resection for Upper Gastrointestinal Hemorrhage of Undetermined Cause, J. A. M. A. 879-884 (March), 1953.
2. Crohn, B. B.: Repeated Gastro-duodenal Hemorrhages Without Discoverable Explanation, Gastroenterology **10**: 120-128 (Jan.), 1948.
3. Gallard, M.: Altérations peu connues de la nuqueuse de l'estomac, Gaz. d. hôp. 196-198 (Feb.), 1884.
4. Granirer, L.: Untoward Effects of Phenylbutizone, J. A. M. A. **150**: 1332 (Nov.), 1952.
5. Ives, L.: Emergency Gastrectomy for Haematemesis, Lancet **2**: 644-646 (Oct.), 1949.
6. Stevens, C., et al.: Benefits and Toxicity of Phenylbutizone in Rheumatoid Arthritis, J. A. M. A. **150**: 1084-1086 (Nov.), 1952.
7. Wagensteen, O. H.: The Ulcer Problem; (1) Etiology, With Special Reference to an Inter-Relationship Between the Vascular and Acid-Peptic Digestive Factors; (2) Characterization of a Satisfactory Operation Which Will Protect Against Recurrent Ulcer (Listerian Oration), Canad. M. A. J. **53**: 309-331 (Oct.), 1945.
8. Wangensteen, O. H.: The Ulcer Problem; (1) Etiology, With Special Reference to an Inter-Relationship Between the Vascular and Acid-Peptic Digestive Factors; (2) Characterization of a Satisfactory Operation Which Will Protect Against Recurrent Ulcer (Listerian Oration), Journal Lancet **66**: 31-49 (Feb.), 1946.

MALIGNANT LESIONS OF THE THYROID

Morley Cohen, M.D.,* and George E. Moore, M.D.,** Minneapolis, Minn.

(From the Department of Surgery, University of Minnesota, Medical School)

INTRODUCTION

THE last decade has brought forth an increased interest in malignant diseases of the thyroid, partly because of the relative increased safety of radical head and neck surgery in the elderly, and particularly since radioactive materials have become available as an adjunct to diagnosis and therapy. Undoubtedly further strides will be made, and the present report concerns a review of the primary malignant lesions of the thyroid which were observed, treated, and followed at the University of Minnesota Hospitals over a twenty-eight year period, from June, 1924, to June, 1952. In order to give the figures significance, only those 101 cases in which the patients had histologically confirmed cancers were included in this study. The data were gathered from hospital files, tumor clinic follow-ups, x-ray therapy files, letters to local physicians, and reports from the Bureau of Vital Statistics.

It has long been recognized that one of the chief sources of difficulty in the management of thyroid lesions is the establishment of the clinical and, particularly, the pathologic diagnoses, of benignancy or malignancy. For this reason the incidence of malignancy in thyroid disease is not definitely known.[1] An average figure, derived from cumulative reports in the literature, has been quoted at about 3 per cent of all thyroid lesions. In 1946, 0.4 per cent of all cancer deaths were due to thyroid malignancy, a figure which equals that of cancer of the mouth. The average incidence in the state of Connecticut, from 1940 to 1946 was 1 per 100,000 population. There is recent increasing evidence that some thyroid cancers, particularly those that are less well differentiated, are in reality secondary lesions rather than primary thyroid malignancies.[1] The pathologist's responsibility is indeed a heavy one. Because many thyroid malignancies differentiate to such a high degree that the microscopic features closely simulate normal thyroid tissue, it is often extremely difficult to make a definitive diagnosis, particularly on frozen section. His responsibility is further weighted by the well-documented fact that any thyroid tumor which can be diagnosed clinically as being malignant is almost invariably beyond the stage of being resectable. It is the recognition of this fact that has served to increase the index of diagnostic suspicion. However, as a result of the increased surgical material presented to him in the past twenty years, the pathologist is now in a less vulnerable position except for a few lesions, particularly those classed as "metastasizing struma," which continue to be confusing.

Received for publication, March 3, 1953.

*Medical Fellow, Department of Surgery.

**Associate Professor, Department of Surgery. Director, Roswell Park Memorial Institute, Buffalo, N. Y.

The statement is not infrequently made that patients with thyroid disease have a strong family history of some thyroid disorder. In this group of 101 cases there were 21 instances in which an immediate relative had had a goiter, and, in 6 of these 21, there was reason to suspect that the "goiter" was a cancer, in that the said relative subsequently died of cancer of the neck or throat.

Twelve patients of the entire group had had previous thyroid surgery. In 9 of these 12 the original material was available for review by our pathologists. In 6 cases the original diagnosis of a benign lesion was confirmed. In the remaining 3 the original diagnosis was reversed as having actually been malignant. In the 3 cases in which the original slides were not available, although the interval between the original surgery and the onset of the present lesion was quite long (mean of eleven years), one cannot say with certainty that the original lesion was benign, for a slow-growing papillary carcinoma can recur as long as twenty-five years postoperatively.[2]

Of the entire group of 101 patients, in 89 instances there was a clinical diagnosis or impression available from the chart. In only 52 instances (58 per cent) there was mention of a diagnosis or suspicion of malignancy; in the remaining 37 cases (42 per cent) the diagnosis was that of benign disease which at operation or on pathologic report was found to be malignant. It should also be pointed out that 36 cases had metastases either regional or distant when first seen. Actually, therefore, in only 16 cases (18 per cent) was the clinical diagnosis in any way astute! Further review of the charts showed 44 cases in which adequate clinical description was available for comparison with the gross operative or pathologic report. In 24 instances, or slightly more than one-half of this latter group, was there any reasonable correspondence of these descriptions. This strongly suggests that the attitude toward all thyroid swellings, clinically single, diffuse, or multiple, should assume the same index of suspicion which we now hold for swellings in the breast. Many studies have attempted to determine the incidence of malignancy in single nodules of the thyroid. Ward[3] found that 22 per cent of clinically solitary nodules were malignant. Others have found higher and lower incidences; Lahey[4] found 10.04 per cent of single nodules and 0.64 per cent of multiple nodules; Cole[5] reports 24.4 per cent of single nodules and 9.8 per cent of multiple nodules. The wide discrepancies between studies are interesting per se. Suffice it to say that such factors as the geographic region (goiter belt), variances in definitions, controversial pathologic diagnoses, etc., still do not completely resolve these discrepancies in the incidence of malignancy. For teaching purposes and as a general policy we have adopted the average figure of a 7 per cent incidence of malignancy in single nodules. This is the approximate incidence of malignancy of single clinically benign nodules in the breast and, therefore, the necessity of surgical excision can be emphasized. Actually the higher incidence of malignancy reported by some authors, even of multiple nodules, would suggest that this dictum of excision of thyroid nodules be extended to include all nodular goiters.

A factor which may partly explain the relatively large number of patients (36 of 101) who had metastases when first seen, was the long interval between the time the patient first noticed the goiter and treatment. In 86 patients this period was available from the medical history chart. It ranged from less than one month up to forty-five years, with a mean duration of sixty-eight months. This approximates Cole's[5] figure of seventy-three months. This long interval serves to reinforce the impression that most carcinomas of the thyroid arise in benign nodules or adenomas. In 12 of the 86 cases the patients had been under the observation of a physician for a period of years and had been given Lugol's solution or advised to do nothing despite suggestive symptoms of neoplasm.

The age of the patients is shown in Table I. It can be seen from this table that the majority (82 per cent) occurred in the older age groups, yet almost one patient in five was under the age of forty. The average age of this group was 55.5 years, which is a little older than that of other reported series.[5-7] It has been generally appreciated, however, that the average age for thyroid carcinoma is lower than that of most other malignancies because it is relatively common in adolescents.

TABLE I. AGE DISTRIBUTION

	AGE IN YEARS								
	0-10	10-20	20-30	30-40	40-50	50-60	60-70	70-80	80-90
Number of cases	0	4	2	12	15	21	24	22	1

Sex.—The sex distribution (Table II) is in agreement with other reported series in being predominantly female. Seventy-three of the cases occurred in women, a ratio of approximately 3:1. Ward[3] has repeatedly stressed the comparatively high incidence of carcinoma in the male nontoxic multinodular goiter. Of this series of 101 patients, 29 had adenomatous goiters. Of these, 10 were men, indicating a slight definite preponderance in this group.

TABLE II. SEX DISTRIBUTION

SEX	NUMBER OF CASES	PER CENT
	101	100
Male	28	27.7
Female	73	72.3

TABLE III. PRESENTING COMPLAINT

Swelling in neck	57
Pressure	
Hoarseness, Dysphagia, Dyspnea, Cough or hemoptysis	19
Weight loss	2
Pain	7
Weakness	3
Symptons of thyrotoxicosis	6
Not available	7
Total	101

Signs and Symptoms.—The presenting symptom, that is the outstanding complaint bringing the patient to his doctor, was available in 94 patients in the series. These are listed in Table III. As shown in the table the majority had a simple swelling of the neck and sought advice mainly because of the cosmetic deformity. Nineteen had pressure symptoms as a leading complaint. Six of the group presented with thyrotoxic symptoms; however, only 1 had a typical picture of Graves' disease. Pain was not a common complaint and when present was almost invariably the result of regional or distant metastases.

The over-all nature of the symptoms and signs, as obtained from physical examination of the patient, is shown in Table IV. Ninety-six of the entire group of 101 had a palpable lesion, and in almost one-half of the cases pressure symptoms were experienced. As noted, there is a relatively high incidence of thyrotoxicosis. These were judged on the basis of history and physical findings, basal metabolism rate (BMR) studies, and, in 2 patients, a significantly reduced serum cholesterol level. In only 1 of the 11 thyrotoxic patients was there reason to feel that the increased BMR was due to widespread metastases to bone and soft tissues. Crile[10] has suggested this occurrence as a plausible explanation for the variance in the incidence of thyrotoxicosis in reported series of thyroid malignancy. In 5 of these patients the BMR was over 40 on repeated determinations. As mentioned, one case was classically Graves' disease. In the literature, the highest incidence of thyrotoxicosis and malignancy is that of Pemberton and Lovelace, their figure being 33.5 per cent.[8, 9] McSwain and Diveley[11] quoted an incidence of 10 per cent in their series. However, in spite of these figures, the prevalent opinion is that one should make the diagnosis of malignancy with extreme caution in the presence of frank hyperthyroidism. There is general agreement that the carcinomatous tissue itself usually does not have a hyperthyroid function.

TABLE IV. TOTAL PHYSICAL SIGNS ON ADMISSION

Thyroid swelling	
Single	57
Nodular	29
Diffuse	10
Pressure	
Hoarseness, Dysphagia, Dyspnea, Cough	47
Weight loss	11
Pain	7
Weakness	3
Thyrotoxicosis	11
Metastases	
Regional	16
Distant	20
Not available	1

As indicated in Table IV, 36 patients presented with metastases; 16 were regional, and 20 were more widely disseminated. Included in the 16 regional cases are 5 cases of so-called "aberrant" thyroid carcinoma. Although the 20 patients with distant metastases were considered incurable, in a few instances the primary lesion was resectable and radon implantation carried out. This served to relieve pressure upon the trachea and was felt to be advisable in those cases which might be suitable for radioiodine therapy. In addition to these 36 cases, 23 patients developed metastases during their follow-up. Of these, 8 were regional (not uncommonly in the thyroid scar), and 15 were distantly disseminated. The distribution of all metastases is shown in Fig. 1.

This distribution parallels the experience of most investigators[8, 14] who have emphasized the predilection of thyroid metastases for lungs and bones.

Pathology.—Of the entire series, 3 patients were classified as having lymphoblastomas (1 Hodgkins, 2 lymphosarcomas), adenocarcinoma being diagnosed in the remainder. Of the latter, 5 were not classified because of their extremely uncharacteristic microscopic picture. The pathologic diagnoses are listed in Table V.

It should be emphasized that relatively few cases show a histologic picture which is uniform in type. If enough sections are reviewed from any one case, many features are seen which would justify a multiplicity of diagnostic terms. In the described classification, a given lesion was named according to the predominating structural form as described in the pathologic report. The real purpose of dividing any group of thyroid cancers in this way is the significantly different clinical prognosis of the various forms, and the necessity of planning the over-all therapy, whether by surgery, x-ray, hormones, radioactive iodine, or a combined approach, that will afford the best possible chance for cure to each patient. The recognized tendency of the more differentiated forms to take up radioactive iodine has been noted by many.[12]

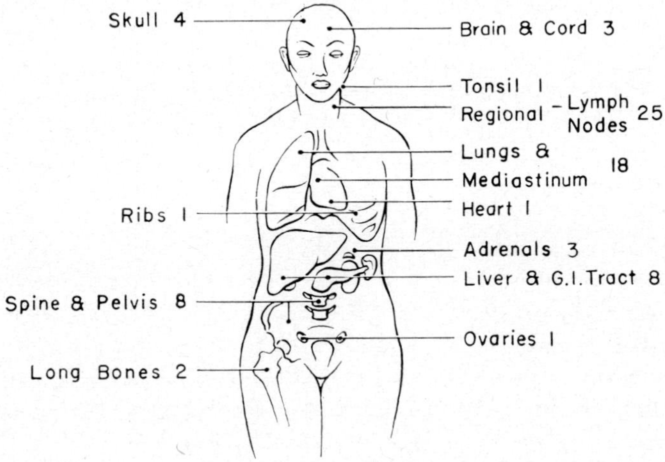

Fig. 1.—Distribution of metastasis-thyroid carcinoma.

Treatment.—In many instances the diagnosis of carcinoma was not made until the paraffin sections had been reviewed and, therefore, the primary treatment was based upon the clinical diagnosis and the appearance of the gland at the time of surgery. Where the clinical diagnosis of a widespread rapidly growing lesion was obvious, nothing save a tracheotomy and biopsy could, as a rule, be carried out. Significant treatment data were available in 96 cases and are outlined in Table VI.

TABLE V. PATHOLOGIC CLASSIFICATION OF THYROID MALIGNANCIES

Metastasizing struma	2
Papillary	37
Follicular and alveolar	18
Solid adenocarcinoma	23
Hürthle cell	2
Spindle or giant cell	8
Anaplastic	3
Lymphoblastoma	3
Unclassified	5
Total	101

TABLE VI. TREATMENT OF MALIGNANT LESIONS OF THE THYROID

Number of cases		96
Metastases when first seen—regional or distant		36
Biopsy only (usually with radiation)		32
Patients submitted to surgery		64
Patients operated on for cure	44	
Patients operated on for palliation	20	

TABLE VII. SURGICAL PROCEDURE

PROCEDURE	NODULECTOMY	SUBTOTAL BILATERAL LOBECTOMY	TOTAL LOBECTOMY	TOTAL LOBECTOMY AND RADICAL NECK DISSECTION	TOTAL THYROIDECTOMY	TOTAL THYROIDECTOMY AND RADICAL NECK DISSECTION
For cure (44)	8	8	13	6	6	3
For palliation (20)	0	13	3	1	3	0

The type of surgical procedure carried out is listed in Table VII.

Of the entire group, 64 were submitted to a major surgical procedure. This represents an operability rate of 63.3 per cent. This is higher than many reported series which average about 50 per cent. Of these 64 cases, 46 received a full course of radiation therapy immediately or very soon after they recovered from the operative procedure. Eighteen patients were treated by surgery alone, either because they refused radiation therapy or did not survive long enough to obtain a full course of treatment. Almost all of the 37 patients who were treated nonoperatively received some radiation therapy. Thirty-two of these 37 had distant metastases or else the lesion was so locally invasive that resection was not feasible. Admittedly, most of the latter group were hopeless cases. Those patients who were treated surgically and listed as palliative were classified as such, mainly for two reasons. In some cases a subtotal thyroidectomy had been performed and malignancy was not discovered until the report on the paraffin section was returned. In others, although all gross tumor was removed, the lesion had invaded the tracheal cartilages or the muscular esophagus and had to be cut away by sharp dissection for removal of the primary tumor.

Isotope Therapy.—Twenty-six patients were given tracer doses of radioactive iodine (I^{131}). Of these, only 7 received a trial with a therapeutic dose. Among these 7 cases the highest uptake was 29 per cent, so it can be seen that, at best, the results could not be expected to be dramatic; moreover, many of these cases were far advanced and hopeless. The reports in the literature[12] state that 15 to 20 per cent of thyroid malignancies will take up significant amounts of radioiodine. This is consistent with our experience. Histologic grading of these lesions and their affinity for iodine expressed as measured uptake are shown in Table VIII. As might be expected, all but one of these tumors was well differentiated. Of several interesting cases 2 deserve further mention.

TABLE VIII. THERAPEUTIC RADIOIODINE THERAPY

PATIENT	PATHOLOGIC DIAGNOSIS	RADIOIODINE UPTAKE (PER CENT)	RESPONSE
E. B.	Papillary adenocarcinoma	22.0	Satisfactory
M. F.	Spindle cell adenocarcinoma	4.6	Poor
A. H.	Follicular adenocarcinoma	29.0	Poor*
J. M.	Papillary adenocarcinoma	22.0	Good
M. M.	Metastasizing struma	22.0	Satisfactory
S. W.	Alveolar adenocarcinoma	19.0	Satisfactory
C. C.	Follicular adenocarcinoma	9.8	Satisfactory

*Died of concomitant cancer of breast with metastases.

CASE 1 (O. C., University Hospitals, No. 799726).—This 43-year-old farmer was referred to the University Hospitals for treatment in February, 1949. Since the age of 18 years, he had noticed a continuously enlarging nodule in the neck which caused no symptoms and was described by his doctor as being a goiter. Between 1938 and 1940 he was treated by daily medication with iodine and pills. In 1946 the mass had involved the entire right side of the neck and interfered with his ability to sleep on the right side. In December, 1946, his local physician performed a subtotal thyroidectomy, removing in addition a nodule from behind the right ear which was diagnosed as metastatic thyroid carcinoma. He was given twenty-three x-ray treatments over the entire right cervical area. Six months later, two other lumps appeared on the right side of the neck, one in front of the ear and one over the collar bone. In March, 1948, excision of these lumps was attempted under local anesthesia by his physician, and the biopsy reports were again reported as metastatic thyroid carcinoma. These nodules did not disappear entirely after surgery, and in October, 1948, the patient was referred to the University Hospitals for further treatment. Review of his slides showed a follicular adenocarcinoma. On Oct. 19, 1948, a tracer dose of radioactive iodine was given orally, and approximately 21 per cent uptake was retained by the normal thyroid. The metastatic masses also toop up an appreciable amount of iodine (9.8 per cent). For this reason it was decided to thyroidectomize the patient with large doses of radioactive iodine. This was accomplished with 20 mc. of I^{131} administered a few days later. One month later the patient complained of a feeling of tiredness, weakness, slight weight increase, loss of appetite, and susceptibility to temperature changes.

On Dec. 17, 1948, the patient was admitted to the hospital and 23 mc. of I^{131} was given orally. A second dose of 77 mc. was administered on Jan. 3, 1949. The symptoms of myxedema became worse and he was placed on 3 gr. of thyroid a day. The large metastatic masses, which were previously considered inoperable by reason of their fixation and extension through the deep tissues below the attachment of the sternomastoid to the mastoid, and the posterior surface of the clavicle, were now found to have decreased markedly in size.

On March 4, 1949, the patient was taken to surgery with a view to resecting the residual tumor masses. Surgical excision* included the medial two-thirds of the clavicle, a radical

*Performed by Dr. R. L. Varco and Dr. G. E. Moore.

neck dissection, removal of the sternomastoid muscle from its origin at the mastoid with ligation of the internal jugular vein at the base of the skull. The dissection was made difficult by much capillary oozing, likely the result of the previous irradiation, both deep x-ray therapy and the radioiodine.

The pathologic report stated that both tumor masses consisted of metastatic carcinoma of the thyroid, the acini containing colloid material, while others showed papillary projections with lesser amounts of colloid. Mitotic figures were scarce. Subsequent examination of the patient in September, 1949, revealed no recurrence of tumor. At present the patient is engaged in farm work and, except for some disability as a result of the removal of his clavicle, has had no recurrence. He requires 3 gr. of thyroid daily.

It is too early to predict the final outcome in Case 1, yet the palliation afforded by a combination of isotope therapy and surgical excision of residual tumor is encouraging. Certainly at the time surgery was contemplated on the patient's original visit to the hospital, the size and fixation of the metastatic masses were such as to discourage the most aggressive surgeon.

CASE 2 (M. M., University Hospitals, No. 817908).—This 62-year-old man first noticed a solitary lump in the left thyroid region in 1943. It enlarged very slowly until 1947, when his local physician advised a thyroidectomy. An enucleation of the nodule was carried out and the pathologic report read as a "benign colloid adenoma."

The patient remained well until July, 1949, when he noted the onset of pain and swelling in the left axillary region. X-ray examination revealed an expanding lesion of the left sixth rib in the anterior axillary area. This was biopsied and reported as adult thyroid tissue, the diagnosis being that of "benign metastasizing struma." He was subsequently referred to the University Hospitals for further treatment. When seen here in May, 1950, he had a small nodule in the lower pole of the left lobe of the thyroid and a healed biopsy incision over a 4 cm. mass in the left sixth rib at the axilla. A bone survey was negative except for the destructive lesion in the left sixth rib. A tracer dose of radioiodine revealed a normal (22.2 per cent) uptake in the thyroid area, but none over the rib lesion.

On May 11, 1950, a total thyroidectomy was carried out. Pathologic examination showed both lobes to contain numerous small circumscribed adenomas which were histologically benign, and identical with the original adenoma removed in 1947. The diagnosis was that of multiple well-differentiated malignant adenomas.

A tracer study carried out on June 15, 1950, revealed no uptake over the rib lesion and a 4 per cent uptake in the thyroid area. A relative protein-bound iodine determination (seventy-two hours) was 65 to 70 per cent. This was interpreted as indicating the presence of functioning thyroid, likely in the form of the metastases. At this time, planographic studies of the chest showed a second destructive lesion in the body of the manubrium. Because pain was becoming a prominent symptom, it was decided to admit him and excise the rib and sternal metastases. On Aug. 1, 1950, a second tracer study was carried out, and at this time the uptake over the manubrium and rib lesion was 7 per cent, indicating that functioning thyroid tissue was now present. It was therefore decided to give him a therapeutic trial of radioiodine; 100 mc. was administered in two doses over a five-day period. He was also treated with external radiation following his discharge from the hospital, receiving a total of 4,200 roentgens in air over the manubrium. In November, 1950, the rib lesion was noted to be smaller, but the manubrial metastasis remained unchanged. A tracer uptake revealed the presence of active tissue in the neck, manubrium, and sixth left rib. At this time it was elected to employ a preliminary dose of thyroid-stimulating hormone and then to administer a further therapeutic dose of I^{131} as well as external radiation therapy. Follow-up study showed a slight decrease in the size of the metastases.

In February, 1951, the patient returned with recurrence of pain in the region of the left sixth rib, and it was elected to excise the rib lesion and intercostal bundle. This was done on Feb. 23, 1951, and pathologic examination disclosed a well-differentiated colloid containing metastasis. The postoperative course was uneventful. The patient was placed on desiccated thyroid and discharged.

Frequent follow-ups in the Tumor Clinic showed that the patient gained weight and felt well except for a mild cough. When he was last seen it was felt that no further therapy was necessary.

Case 2 is cited to stress the peculiar biologic nature of many thyroid cancers. The problems facing the pathologist, as well as the complexities involved in employing radioiodine, cannot be overemphasized.

Morbidity and Mortality.—
Morbidity:

A. Surgical (8 cases): There were 7 cases of recurrent laryngeal nerve injury which occurred at surgery and persisted after the

TABLE IX. SURGICAL MORTALITY

CAUSE	NUMBER OF CASES	TIME OF OCCURRENCE
Tracheal collapse	1	Fourth postoperative day
Tracheal obstruction	3	Second to tenth postoperative day
Common carotid ligation	1	At operation
Coronary insufficiency	1	Third postoperative day
Pneumonia	1	Sixth postoperative day

TABLE X. OVER-ALL SURVIVAL FOR THYROID CARCINOMA

YEAR	NUMBER OF CASES	SURVIVAL (YEARS) 1	2	3	4	5	6	7	8	9	10	11	12	13	14	15	16	17	18
1924	1	1	1	1	1	1	1	1	1	1	0	0	0	0	0	0	0	0	0
1925	0	0	0	0	0	0	0	0	0	0	0	0	0	0	0	0	0	0	0
1926	1	1	1	1	1	1	1	1	1	1	1	1	1	1	0	0	0	0	0
1927	0	0	0	0	0	0	0	0	0	0	0	0	0	0	0	0	0	0	0
1928	1	1	0	0	0	0	0	0	0	0	0	0	0	0	0	0	0	0	0
1929	2	2	2	2	1	1	0	0	0	0	0	0	0	0	0	0	0	0	0
1930	1	0	0	0	0	0	0	0	0	0	0	0	0	0	0	0	0	0	0
1931	1	1	1	1	1	1	1	0	0	0	0	0	0	0	0	0	0	0	0
1932	0	0	0	0	0	0	0	0	0	0	0	0	0	0	0	0	0	0	0
1933	2	2	2	1	0	0	0	0	0	0	0	0	0	0	0	0	0	0	0
1934	4	3	3	1	1	1	1	1	1	1	1	1	1	1	1	1	1	1	1
1935	4	2	2	2	2	2	1	1	1	1	1	1	1	1	1	1	1	1	
1936	7	4	4	4	4	4	4	4	4	4	4	3	3	3	3	3	3		
1937	7	3	3	3	3	2	2	1	1	1	1	1	0	0	0	0			
1938	3	2	2	2	2	2	2	2	2	2	1	1	1	1	1				
1939	2	2	2	2	2	2	2	2	2	2	2	2	2	1					
1940	3	1	1	1	1	1	1	1	1	1	1	0	0						
1941	6	4	4	4	4	3	3	3	3	1	1	1							
1942	7	3	3	2	1	1	1	0	0	0	0								
1943	2	1	1	1	1	0	0	0	0	0									
1944	3	2	2	2	2	2	2	2	0										
1945	7	3	3	1	1	1	1	1											
1946	5	5	3	3	3	3	3												
1947	4	2	2	1	1	1													
1948	11	8	8	6	2														
1949	4	2	2	2															
1950	3	1	1																
1951	6	5																	
1952	1	1																	
Cases	98	98	97	91	88	84	73	69	64	57	54	52	45	39	36	34	31	24	17
Survivals		62	53	43	34	29	26	20	17	15	13	11	9	8	6	5	5	2	1
Per cent survivals		63	54	47	38	34	35	29	26	26	24	21	20	20	16	14	16	8	6
Corrected per cent survival		63	54	48	40	37	37	30	28	29	26	23	20	23	19	17	19	12	11

operation. One of these was bilateral. The other surgical complication was a severe wound hematoma.

B. X-ray: There were 4 cases of severe x-ray dermatitis. Three of these were followed by extensive scarring.

Mortality: Seven patients died of causes consequent to a surgical procedure. These are listed in Table IX.

As 64 patients were treated surgically this results in an operative mortality of 10 per cent. Portmann noted a mortality of 8.5 per cent. Such figures are a reflection of the increased technical difficulties of dealing with a malignancy in the thyroid area, of the use of more radical procedures, as well as of the advanced age of many of these patients. As has been stressed repeatedly, this should be considered one of the strongest arguments for prophylactic removal of all thyroid nodules at a time when this is easily accomplished and when the mortality and morbidity are each well under 1 per cent.[4]

Results.—The over-all survival rate for 98 patients of the entire group of 101 is shown in Table X. Three cases of lymphoblastomas are not included. In addition 4 patients who were lost to follow-up are presumed dead of their disease. In terms of percentage, the three-, five-, ten-, and fifteen-year survivals are 47 per cent, 34 per cent, 24 per cent, and 14 per cent, respectively. Five

TABLE XI. OVER-ALL SURVIVAL OF CASES TREATED WITH SURGERY*

YEAR	NUMBER OF CASES	SURVIVAL (YEARS)																	
		1	2	3	4	5	6	7	8	9	10	11	12	13	14	15	16	17	18
1924	1	1	1	1	1	1	1	1	1	1	0	0	0	0	0	0	0	0	0
1925	0	0	0	0	0	0	0	0	0	0	0	0	0	0	0	0	0	0	0
1926	0	0	0	0	0	0	0	0	0	0	0	0	0	0	0	0	0	0	0
1927	0	0	0	0	0	0	0	0	0	0	0	0	0	0	0	0	0	0	0
1928	1	1	1	0	0	0	0	0	0	0	0	0	0	0	0	0	0	0	0
1929	2	2	2	2	1	1	0	0	0	0	0	0	0	0	0	0	0	0	0
1930	1	1	0	0	0	0	0	0	0	0	0	0	0	0	0	0	0	0	0
1931	1	1	1	1	1	1	1	0	0	0	0	0	0	0	0	0	0	0	0
1932	0	0	0	0	0	0	0	0	0	0	0	0	0	0	0	0	0	0	0
1933	0	0	0	0	0	0	0	0	0	0	0	0	0	0	0	0	0	0	0
1934	2	2	2	1	1	1	1	1	1	1	1	1	1	1	1	1	1	1	1
1935	2	2	2	2	2	2	1	1	1	1	1	1	1	1	1	1	1	1	0
1936	4	3	3	3	3	3	3	3	3	3	3	2	2	2	2	2	2	0	
1937	5	3	3	3	3	2	2	1	1	1	1	1	0	0	0	0	0		
1938	1	1	1	1	1	1	1	1	1	1	1	1	1	1	1	1			
1939	2	2	2	2	2	2	2	2	2	2	2	2	2	1	0				
1940	2	1	1	1	1	1	1	1	1	0	0	0	0	0					
1941	3	3	3	3	3	2	2	2	2	0	0	0	0						
1942	1	1	1	1	0	0	0	0	0	0	0	0							
1943	1	1	1	1	1	0	0	0	0	0	0								
1944	2	2	2	2	2	2	2	2	2	0									
1945	5	3	3	1	1	1	1	1	0										
1946	5	4	3	3	3	3	3	0											
1947	4	2	2	1	1	1	0												
1948	7	7	7	6	2	0													
1949	3	2	2	2	0														
1950	2	1	1	0															
1951	6	3	0																
1952	1	0																	
Cases	64	64	63	57	55	52	45	41	36	31	29	28	27	24	22	20	19	14	10
Survivals		48	44	35	29	24	21	16	15	10	9	8	7	6	5	5	4	2	1
% Survival		75	70	61	52	46	46	39	41	32	31	29	29	25	23	25	28	14	10

*Forty-six had additional radiation.

patients who died of unrelated causes and were apparently free of disease at the time are included in these figures. If we correct for this latter group, the survival rates are slightly higher, 48 per cent, 37 per cent, 26 per cent, and 17 per cent, respectively.

Of the 64 cases treated surgically, the results are shown in Table XI. Forty-six of this number received a full course of radiation therapy. In the remaining 18, x-ray treatment was not given, was incomplete, or else the patient succumbed after the surgical procedure. The three-, five-, ten-, and fifteen-year figures are better than the over-all survival rate, but not strikingly so. These are 61 per cent, 46 per cent, 31 per cent, and 25 per cent, respectively.

As indicated in the discussion on the pathology of these thyroid cancers, one of the main reasons for attempting to classify them is the recognized variations in behavior of the different histologic types. For example, the papillary tumors are moderately radiosensitive, they invade neighboring structures, and they spread slowly to the regional lymph nodes, but practically never to distant organs by the blood stream. The alveolar adenocarcinomas are more rapidly growing and prone to cause bulky tumors exerting pressure on the trachea and

TABLE XII. OVER-ALL SURVIVAL OF "WELL-DIFFERENTIATED"* THYROID CARCINOMA

YEAR	NUMBER OF CASES	SURVIVAL (YEARS) 1	2	3	4	5	6	7	8	9	10	11	12	13	14	15	16	17	18
1924	1	1	1	1	1	1	1	1	1	1	0	0	0	0	0	0	0	0	0
1925	0	0	0	0	0	0	0	0	0	0	0	0	0	0	0	0	0	0	0
1926	1	1	1	1	1	1	1	1	1	1	1	1	1	1	0	0	0	0	0
1927	0	0	0	0	0	0	0	0	0	0	0	0	0	0	0	0	0	0	0
1928	1	1	0	0	0	0	0	0	0	0	0	0	0	0	0	0	0	0	0
1929	1	1	1	1	0	0	0	0	0	0	0	0	0	0	0	0	0	0	0
1930	0	0	0	0	0	0	0	0	0	0	0	0	0	0	0	0	0	0	0
1931	1	1	1	1	1	1	1	0	0	0	0	0	0	0	0	0	0	0	0
1932	0	0	0	0	0	0	0	0	0	0	0	0	0	0	0	0	0	0	0
1933	0	0	0	0	0	0	0	0	0	0	0	0	0	0	0	0	0	0	0
1934	2	2	2	1	1	1	1	1	1	1	1	1	1	1	1	1	1	1	1
1935	3	2	2	2	2	2	1	1	1	1	1	1	1	1	1	1	1	1	
1936	4	4	4	4	4	4	4	4	4	4	4	3	3	3	3	3	3		
1937	4	3	3	3	3	2	2	1	1	1	1	1	0	0	0	0			
1938	1	1	1	1	1	1	1	1	1	1	1	1	1	1	1				
1939	2	2	2	2	2	2	2	2	2	2	2	2	2	1					
1940	2	2	2	2	2	2	2	2	2	1	1	0	0						
1941	3	3	3	3	3	2	2	2	2	1	1	1							
1942	2	2	2	1	0	0	0	0	0	0	0								
1943	1	1	1	1	1	1	0	0	0	0									
1944	2	2	2	2	2	2	2	2	2										
1945	3	1	1	1	1	1	1	1											
1946	3	3	3	3	3	3	3												
1947	3	2	2	1	1	1													
1948	7	6	6	6	2														
1949	2	2	2	2															
1950	2	1	1																
1951	4	3																	
1952	1	0																	
Cases	56†	56	55	51	49	47	40	37	34	31	29	28	26	23	21	19	18	14	10
Survival		47	43	39	31	27	24	19	18	14	13	11	9	8	6	5	5	2	1
% Survival		84	78	76	63	57	60	51	53	45	44	39	34	34	28	27	27	14	10

*Benign metastasizing struma, papillary adenocarcinoma, follicular and alveolar adenocarcinoma.

†Fifty-seven cases of well-differentiated thyroid carcinomas, 1 not followed.

esophagus; they are only slightly radiosensitive and metastasize through both lymphatic and blood channels. The spindle or giant cell tumors are consistently radioresistant, metastasize widely, early, and are rapidly fatal. With these facts in mind, it was felt desirable to compare the survival of the well-differentiated lesions in this study with the more poorly or undifferentiated ones. These are shown in Tables XII and XIII. It will be seen immediately that those cases generally considered to be of low malignancy have a prognosis which is vastly more favorable than that of the undifferentiated, highly malignant group. This comparison should serve to remind one of at least two important points. First, in reading about operative results, one must, with carcinoma of the thyroid in particular, consider the histologic frequency of the well-differentiated lesions in any given series. Second, and as a corollary, it would appear that with thyroid cancer, the histology is still the most important factor in prognosis. One cannot deny that many of those cases in the undifferentiated group were well advanced and inoperable when they were first seen. However, in reality many of these cases came to the physician sooner than the slower-growing lesions.

TABLE XIII. OVER-ALL SURVIVAL OF "POORLY DIFFERENTIATED"* CARCINOMA OF THYROID

YEAR	NUMBER OF CASES	SURVIVAL (YEARS)								
		1	2	3	4	5	6	7	8	9
1924	0	0	0	0	0	0	0	0	0	0
1925	0	0	0	0	0	0	0	0	0	0
1926	0	0	0	0	0	0	0	0	0	0
1927	0	0	0	0	0	0	0	0	0	0
1928	0	0	0	0	0	0	0	0	0	0
1929	1	1	1	1	1	1	0	0	0	0
1930	1	0	0	0	0	0	0	0	0	0
1931	0	0	0	0	0	0	0	0	0	0
1932	0	0	0	0	0	0	0	0	0	0
1933	1	1	1	1	0	0	0	0	0	0
1934	2	1	1	0	0	0	0	0	0	0
1935	1	0	0	0	0	0	0	0	0	0
1936	3	0	0	0	0	0	0	0	0	0
1937	3	0	0	0	0	0	0	0	0	0
1938	2	1	1	1	1	1	1	1	1	1
1939	0	0	0	0	0	0	0	0	0	0
1940	2	0	0	0	0	0	0	0	0	0
1941	3	1	1	1	1	1	1	1	1	0
1942	5	1	1	1	1	1	1	0	0	0
1943	1	0	0	0	0	0	0	0	0	
1944	1	0	0	0	0	0	0	0		
1945	4	2	2	0	0	0	0			
1946	2	2	0	0	0	0				
1947	1	0	0	0	0					
1948	4	2	2	0						
1949	2	0	0							
1950	1	0								
1951	2	0								
1952	0	0								
Cases	42	42	42	40	39	37	33	32	30	26
Survival		12	10	5	4	4	3	2	2	1
% Survival		28	24	12	10	10	9	6	6	4

*Solid adenocarcinoma, Hürthle cell, spindle or giant cell, anaplastic unclassified.

There remains in the literature considerable variation of opinion regarding the best surgical management of the most common thyroid cancer precursor, the solitary adenoma. Ward[3] has strongly advocated unilateral total lobectomy for all solitary adenomas. Lahey,[4] on the other hand, although less dogmatic, feels that simple excision of the nodule is initially sufficient, unless malignancy is suspected either clinically or at surgery. It is a difficult point to settle, and with these ideas in mind 8 cases of solitary adenoma treated by enucleation, but which turned out to be adenocarcinomas on microsection, were followed. No further surgery was performed on these patients either because they refused it or because the pathologist felt that the carcinoma was very small and well circumscribed, and had likely been completely removed. These are tabulated in Table XIV. It will be seen that 3 of the 8 are alive and well. Of these 3, 2 are possibly cured, having each survived sixteen years. All were so-called "low grade tumors." Two additional patients are still alive but have metastases. Admittedly 3 cases are far too few for any conclusion, but nevertheless, might possibly lend support to Ward's contention.

TABLE XIV. RESULTS OF NODULECTOMY FOR MALIGNANT ADENOMAS

PATIENT	DATE	TREATMENT	PATHOLOGIC DIAGNOSIS	FOLLOW-UP
R. N	1931	Nodulectomy	Benign colloid adenoma	
	1936	Nodulectomy and radiation	Papillary adenocarcinoma	February, 1952, alive and well
F. P.	1936	Nodulectomy and radiation	Papillary adenocarcinoma	February, 1952, alive and well
M. M.	1947	Nodulectomy	Metastasizing struma	
	1950	Total thyroidectomy and excision of rib metastasis and radiation	Metastasizing struma	May, 1952, probable lung metastases
B. B.	1948	Nodulectomy and radiation	Papillary cystadenocarcinoma	January, 1952, alive and well
L. A.	1928	Nodulectomy and radiation	Papillary carcinoma	Died January, 1930, due to widespread metastases
H. S.	1952	Nodulectomy and radiation	Follicular adenocarcinoma	September, 1952, alive with metastases
L. O.	1945	Nodulectomy and radiation	Follicular adenocarcinoma	Died, 1946, with carcinomatosis
A. L.	1948	Nodulectomy and radiation	Papillary cystadenocarcinoma	Died, 1951, with metastases

Table XV shows some figures drawn from the literature for comparison. The wide variation is immediately obvious. In 421 patients followed for five years at the Mayo Clinic, Pemberton reported a 61 per cent five-year survival. At the opposite extreme, Watson and Pool reported only a 7.8 per cent five-year survival. Our own figures parallel those of Cole who reported a 38 per cent survival in 1948. The explanation for this variation is difficult to find. In Pemberton's series, 60 per cent of his cases were unsuspected preoperatively or at the time of surgery. Thus in only 40 per cent of his series was the diagnosis made preoperatively. Obviously it would be more difficult to demonstrate satisfactory end results if the clinical diagnosis was more evident in a higher percentage of cases. In our own series, the diagnosis of malignancy was suspected in 58 per cent before surgery. In Watson and Pool's report[14] 70 per cent of their cases were inoperable. A second possibility that suggests itself is that certain observers might be more lenient in classifying borderline cases as malignant. Finally, one should again recall the rather favorable prognosis in the papillary lesions, which, if constituting a larger proportion of any given series, will certainly boost the five-year survival figure.

TABLE XV. COMPARATIVE[5] RESULTS, FIVE-YEAR SURVIVAL IN THYROID CARCINOMA

AUTHOR	NUMBER OF PATIENTS FOLLOWED FIVE YEARS	FIVE-YEAR SURVIVAL (PER CENT)
Pemberton, Rochester, Minn., 1938	421	61.0
Horn and associates, Philadelphia, Pa., 1947	42	55.0
Cole and associates, Chicago, Ill., 1948	36	38.0
Portmann, Cleveland, Ohio, 1940	149	35.5
De Quervain, Switzerland, 1935	108	17.5
D'Argent, Lyon, France, 1941	135	9.6
Watson and Pool, New York, N. Y., 1940	167	7.8
University of Minn. Hospitals, Minneapolis, Minn., 1952	84	37.0

As regards comparative figures in those cases where patients were treated by thyroidectomy, those reported by Pemberton[8] should be mentioned. Thus, of patients who underwent a thyroidectomy with or without radiation, he reported a three-, five-, and ten-year survival of 77 per cent, 70 per cent, and 58 per cent, respectively. Our own figures as shown in Table XI were 61 per cent, 46 per cent, and 31 per cent, respectively, for the same time intervals.

SUMMARY

1. One hundred one cases of thyroid malignancy seen and treated at the University Hospitals from June, 1924, to June, 1952, are reviewed.

2. Over one-third (35 per cent) of the cases presented with metastases on their initial visit.

3. In a high percentage of those cases where the diagnosis of malignancy was not obvious, the clinical description and assessment of the lesion were inaccurate.

4. The mean duration from onset of the lesion to treatment was sixty-eight months.

5. Ten per cent of the patients showed clinical and laboratory evidence of hyperthyroidism.

6. The manner in which these patients were treated is outlined. The operability rate for the entire group was 63.3 per cent. A majority of the patients received deep x-ray therapy.

7. The percentage of cases suitable for isotope therapy was similar to that of other reported series.

8. The over-all survival for rates for three, five, ten, and fifteen years was 47 per cent, 34 per cent, 24 per cent, and 14 per cent, respectively.

9. Of those patients who underwent thyroid surgery (usually with irradiation) the three-, five-, ten-, and fifteen-year survival rates were 61 per cent, 46 per cent, 31 per cent, and 25 per cent, respectively.

10. The histologic nature of the tumor remains an important factor in the prognosis.

REFERENCES

1. Perloff, W. H., and Schneeberg, N. G.: The Problems of Thyroid Carcinoma, Surgery **29:** 572-580, 1951.
2. Crile, G., Jr.: Papillary Tumors of Thyroid of Lateral Aberrant Thyroid Origin, Surg., Gynec. & Obst. **69:** 39-47, 1939.
3. Ward, R.: Malignant Goiter, Surgery **16:** 783-803, 1944.
4. Lahey, F. H., and Hare, H. F.: Malignancy in Adenoma of the Thyroid, J. A. M. A. **145:** 689-695, 1951.
5. Cole, W. H., Slaughter, D. P., and Majarakis, J. D.: Carcinoma of the Thyroid Gland, Surg., Gynec. & Obst. **89:** 349-356, 1949.
6. Lahey, F. H.: Carcinoma of the Thyroid Gland, Am. J. Roentgenol. **46:** 469, 1941.
7. Lahey, F. H., Hare, H. F., and Warren, S.: Carcinoma of the Thyroid, Ann. Surg. **112:** 977, 1941.
8. Pemberton, J. De J.: Malignant Lesions of the Thyroid Gland, Surg., Gynec. & Obst. **69:** 417, 1939.
9. Pemberton, J. De J., and Lovelace, W. R., Jr.: Malignant Lesions of the Thyroid Gland, S. Clin. North America **21:** 1037, 1941.
10. Crile, G., Jr.: Hyperthyroidism Associated With Malignant Tumors of the Thyroid Gland, Surg., Gynec. & Obst. **62:** 995-999, 1936.
11. McSwain, B., and Diveley, W.: Malignant Tumors of the Thyroid Gland, Surgery **23:** 525, 1948.
12. Symposium on Radioiodine, Brookhaven Conference Report, July 28 to 30, 1948. United States Atomic Energy Commission, Oak Ridge, Tenn.
13. Portmann, U. V.: Malignant Tumors of the Thyroid Gland, Surg., Gynec. & Obst. **70:** 185, 1940.
14. Watson, W. L., and Pool, J. L.: Cancer of the Thyroid, Surg., Gynec. & Obst. **70:** 1037-1050, 1940.

VILLOUS PAPILLOMAS OF THE COLON AND RECTUM

A Study of Twenty-Eight Cases With End Results of Treatment Over a Five-Year Period

Harry E. Bacon, M.D., Edward J. Lowell, Jr., M.D.,* and Howard D. Trimpi, M.D., Philadelphia, Pa.

(From the Department of Proctology, Temple University Hospital)

THE distinctive morphology of a group of tumors has resulted in their descriptive classification as "villous papillomas" of the colon and rectum. Holmes,[1] a British pathologist, originated use of the term "villous tumor" in 1860, thus dividing benign epithelial tumors of the large bowel into two categories, the villous papilloma and the adenomatous polyp. This concept has proved useful to the clinician as an aid in classification, and the concept is believed to be substantiated by morphologic, pathologic, and clinical features which tend to demarcate this type of intestinal neoplasm from the more commonly appreciated adenomatous polyp to which it is closely related.

Villous papillomas are not confined entirely to the large bowel, although the colon and rectum constitute the site of most common occurrence. Hauser[2] in 1890 described villous tumors of the stomach. Villiform papillomas of the gall bladder have been encountered. Among the earliest to describe villous papillomas of the rectum were Quenu and Landel,[3] Lambling,[4] and Bensaude.[5]

As Dukes[6] has pointed out, both varieties of benign epithelial tumor arise from mucous membrane, but the adenoma is typically a compact, spherical, pedunculated mass while the villous papilloma is typically a soft, sessile tumor without pedicle. The adenoma is common, occurring in 7 per cent of adults, according to Helwig,[7] while the papilloma is a rare tumor. Villous papillomas are often referred to as papillary adenomas, but differences in cancer potential, morphology, and clinical behavior tend to differentiate true papilloma and true adenoma. All villous papillomas may be described as papillary, but not all adenomas are papillary, for the adenomas have preponderantly a typical, pedunculated configuration, except for the smooth embryonic forms recognized as mammillations of only several millimeters in size. The soft, velvetlike consistency and broad sessile arrangement of villiform projections identify the villous papilloma in striking contrast to all other tumors of the distal bowel.

The purpose of this study is to present differential criteria which have been useful in diagnosis and managment of villous papillomas over a five-year period.

Received for publication, March 26, 1953.

*Resident, Department of Proctology, Temple University School of Medicine and Hospital.

MATERIAL AND METHODS

The twenty-eight cases* were selected from a total of 1,144 tumors of the colon and rectum treated during a five-year period from November, 1946, to December, 1951. This series excluded all tumor-simulating lesions of the colon and rectum which were of inflammatory or granulomatous nature unassociated with neoplasm. For comparative purposes, it may be stated that of these 1,144 tumors, the most common was adenocarcinoma, comprising 69 per cent of the total, while benign epithelial tumors, or "polyps," made up 23.7 per cent of the total. The remaining 7.3 per cent included uncommon tumors such as lymphoma, sarcoma, carcinoid, fibroma, endometrioma, hemangiopericytoma, and others.

Of the benign epithelial tumors, consisting of 272 cases, it was found that the adenoma accounted for 21.4 per cent of the total (243 adenomas) while the villous papilloma was found in 28 cases, or 2.3 per cent of the total number of 1,144 tumors.

Determination of the incidence of villous papilloma was based on these primary considerations: (1) villous configuration, (2) broad, sessile base without pedicle, (3) predominantly benign morphology, (4) soft consistency, free of ulceration or induration, and (5) freedom of fixation to the underlying muscularis layer of the bowel. Additional secondary considerations excluded those tumors whose surface was only coarsely lobular or those tumors having a gross papillary surface but failing on microscopic examination to possess true villous processes. Only those tumors were included which did not appear clinically to present any evidence of carcinoma, or microscopically did not show diffuse carcinomatous change. Tumors were included whose structure, except for microscopic foci of cytologic carcinoma (in situ), was otherwise benign.

Thus it was found that 28 of 1,144 tumors sufficiently satisfied these criteria to permit their classification as villous papillomas in contradistinction to either adenomatous polyps or well-differentiated papillary adenocarcinomas. Adenomatous polyps having a variable papillary appearance of their outer pole, away from their pedunculated base, were similarly excluded. Features of the architectural pattern of villous papillomas described by Dukes,[6] Gabriel,[8] and Ewing[9] have been helpful in differentiating these tumors. Sunderland and Binkley[10] and recently Fisher and Castro[11] have described a group of papillary adenomas, and it has been reiterated that papillary adenomas are growth variants of the same process that produces the adenomatous polyp. Which term better identifies these varieties of epithelial bowel tumors is a matter of individual preference, as long as appreciation exists that the villous papillomas present a striking morphologic pattern apart from the more common adenoma.

*Two additional patients, making a total of 30 cases, have recently undergone resection for villous papilloma, but too recently to be included in the follow-up of this series.

PATHOLOGY

The identifying gross pathologic features of the villous papilloma include (1) villous configuration, (2) broad, sessile base without pedicle, (3) soft, velvety consistency without ulceration or induration, and (4) mobile, superficial disposition without fixation. The tumor is pale and reddish gray in color, and usually extends over a wide area of bowel mucosa ranging from 4 to 5 cm. in area to complete circumferential involvement as shown in Figs. 1 and 2. Frequently there is a viscid coat of mucus, secreted in liberal amounts by the tumor and accounting for its most classic symptom.

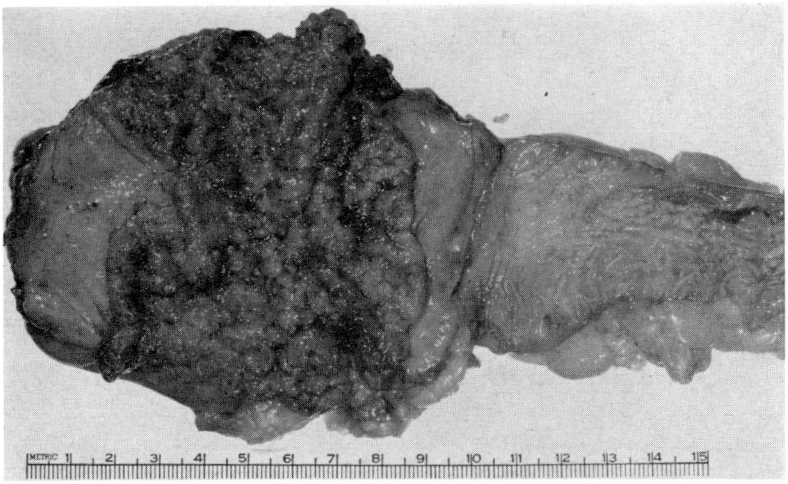

Fig. 1.—Villous papilloma of rectosigmoid in A. M., a 58-year-old woman.

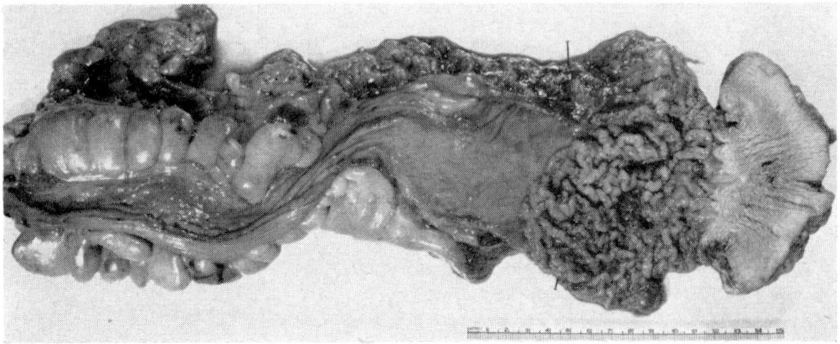

Fig. 2.—Villous papilloma of rectum with carcinomatous change in A. H., a 69-year-old woman.

The identifying microscopic features found most helpful in diagnosis are (1) innumerable elongated fingerlike projections, covered by surface epithelium and having a core of connective tissue stroma, small vessels, and occasional nerve fibers, (2) typical goblet cells of mucosa, although there is no remarkable increase in their number and there is no striking increase of dense glandular acini, (3) normal-staining nuclear and cytoplasmic components, unless there are isolated, focal areas of what is described as "carcinoma in situ." Thus, the histologic structure is essentially and predominantly benign, in the classic example, without increased mitoses, hyperchromaticity, architectural derangement, lack of differentiation, or depolarization, and (4) a characteristic limitation to the superficial mucosal layer without evidence of cellular invasion through the lamina propria to the muscularis.

The histopathologic factor of greatest aid in diagnosis of this tumor is the presence of elongated villous processes with the relative absence of compactly arranged glandular elements, as demonstrated in Fig. 3; when these features are apparent, as in the typical case, distinction may be made from the typical adenomatous polyp, which is being detected and removed with increasing frequency.

The increased mucoepithelial surface, rather than the glandular elements, as reflected in the villous configuration, illustrates the theory advanced by Dukes[6] that the villous papilloma is the end result of a growth pattern which has affected mainly the superficial epithelium in contrast to the adenoma which is the result of a growth pattern affecting mainly those cells at a deeper level.

Metastases to the reginal lymph nodes or extension to other viscera appear to be uncommon, even when isolated foci of the villous tumor demonstrate malignant change.

CLINICAL FEATURES

Symptomatically, villous papilloma may be confused with "mucous colitis," for in the classic example of this tumor, elaborating increased mucus, the patient notes mucus discharges from the rectum, unassociated with other complaints. Other symptoms include rectal bleeding, altered bowel habit, more frequently toward diarrhea than toward constipation, and protrusion of tissue fragments.

Of the twenty-eight patients studied, bleeding occurred in 78.5 per cent, diarrhea in 46.4 per cent, mucoid discharges in 31.4 per cent, and protrusion of tumor in 21.4 per cent. Constipation occurred in 17.8 per cent and weight loss in 14.3 per cent, while 7.1 per cent complained of pruritus and 3.6 per cent complained of rectal pain. Of the twenty-eight patients, 17.8 per cent were free of symptoms, indicating that the villous papilloma may be a silent tumor; in these asymtomatic patients, almost one-fifth of the series, discovery of the lesion was made as a result of routine proctosigmoidoscopy.

Length of symptoms varied from one week to fifteen years, the average being fifteen months. One patient having symptoms of fifteen years' duration had been erroneously treated for mucous colitis.

Age of the patients ranged from 23 to 74 years, the average age being 55.4 years. Sunderland and Binkley[10] reported the average age of forty-eight patients having papillary adenomas to be 62.9 years, while adenomatous polyps are variously reported in the range of from 45 to 54 years. Thus, it would appear that villous papillomas tend to occur in a slightly older age group than the adenomas.

Sex incidence paralleled that of adenomas, being 56 per cent for male patients and 44 per cent for women, in this study.

Fig. 3.

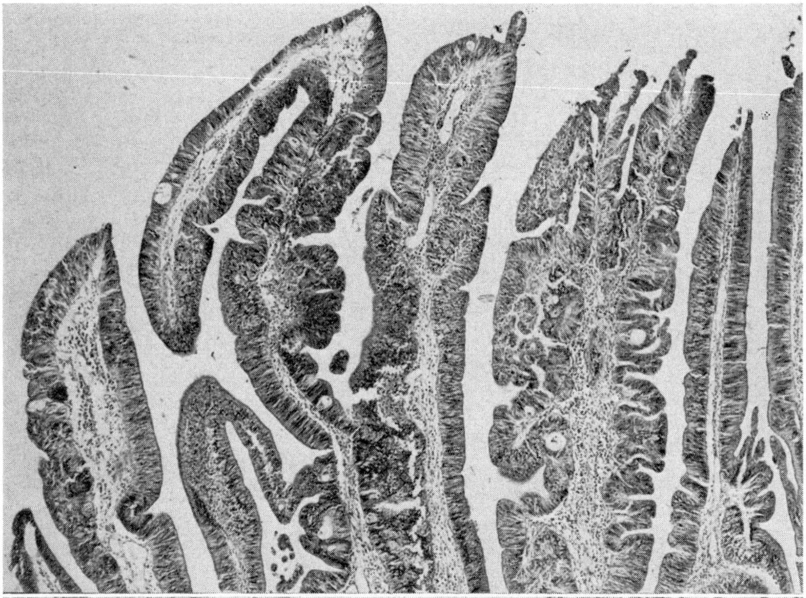

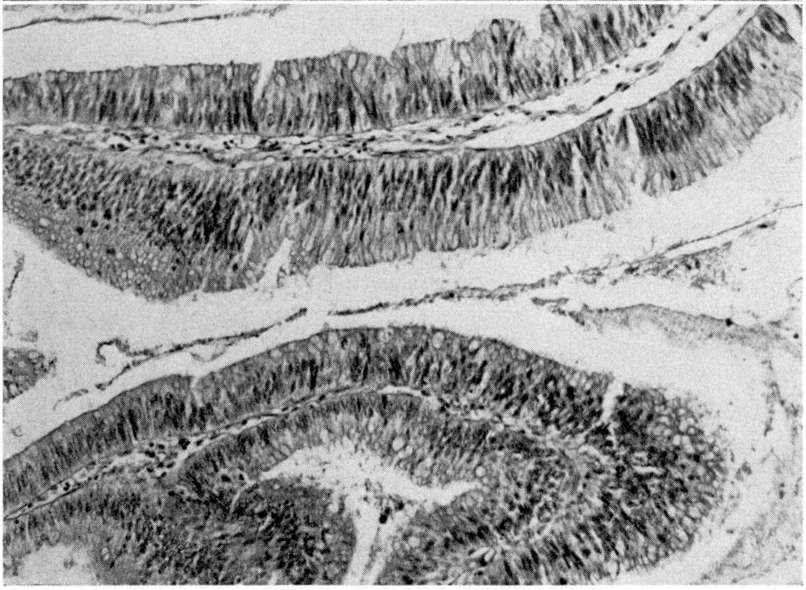

Fig. 4.

Fig. 3.—Typical microscopic appearance of villous papilloma (×40, reduced ⅓) in O. L., a 59-year-old man.

Fig. 4.—Villous papilloma with areas of atypism in C. H., a 71-year-old man.

The appearance of the tumor is that of a villiform, sessile configuration composed of pale, reddish gray rows of mucosa. When within reach of the examining finger, the classical villous papilloma frequently escapes notice because of its innocuously soft texture, as emphasized by Gabriel[8] and others, and even on direct sigmoidoscopic visualization it may escape attention as the sigmoidoscope flattens its pliable, resilient pattern.

Size varied from 2 by 5 cm. to 10 by 18 cm., the largest in circumference; the average size was found to be approximately 6 by 12 cm.

Site of occurrence for the majority of these tumors was below the level of the peritoneal reflection, for example, in the rectum, twenty-two of the twenty-eight tumors occurring at or below the rectosigmoid junction (78.5 per cent) and 6, or 21.5 per cent, occurring above the level of the peritoneal reflection, for example, the sigmoid colon or higher.

Position of the tumor with reference to the lumen of the bowel was found to be almost or completely circumferential in 39.2 per cent or eleven of the twenty-eight cases, mainly anterior in 21.5 per cent (six cases), mainly anterolateral in 25 per cent (seven cases), posterolateral and lateral, respectively, in 7.1 per cent (two cases), demonstrating a preference for origin in the anterior and lateral phases of the lumen.

The proximalmost tumor occurred in the transverse colon, although Fisher and Castro[11] have reported occurrence of villous papilloma in the ascending colon.

Associated, incidental, typically pedunculated adenomatous polyps were found in three of the twenty-eight patients, or 10.7 per cent, the adenomas being located an appreciable distance away from the villous tumor; associated, separate adenocarcinoma, occurring synchronously with the villous papilloma, was found in two of the twenty-eight patients, or 7.1 per cent.

Liver involvement, as noted on abdominal exploration, was demonstrable in 7.1 per cent, or two of the twenty-eight patients; in these two patients areas of low-grade papillary adenocarcinoma were found on subsequent pathologic study of the lesion; both occurred in the lower rectum, and both of these patients are alive two and one-half years following a Miles-type procedure, with abdominal colostomy. Lymph-node involvement was present in one of the twenty-eight cases, or 3.6 per cent.

HISTOPATHOLOGIC FEATURES

The twenty-eight villous papillomas were analyzed with respect to histologic patterns. Fig. 3 illustrates the representative pattern found in eighteen of the twenty-eight lesions, or 64.3 per cent, classified as benign villous papilloma. The remaining 35.7 per cent were classified as showing malignant changes.

Further analysis revealed the following: seven of the twenty-eight tumors (25 per cent) were designated as classical benign villous papilloma without evidence of cellular changes; six of the twenty-eight tumors (21.5 per cent) were designated as showing "adenoma malignum" change in addition to the basic architecture, while five of the twenty-eight, or 17.1 per cent, received the analogous term now in use—atypism. These two qualifications, adenoma malignum and atypism, have been employed to designate the near-malignant changes of hyperchromatism, stratification, nuclear and cytoplasmic irregularities without actual immaturity, and lack of differentiation or of invasiveness. The term adenoma malignum was used formerly to designate changes which are now being described as atypism and represent the same histologic findings, which, however, do not qualify as actual carcinomatous change, whether diffuse or in situ. Thus eleven of the twenty-eight lesions, or 38.6 per cent, showed changes of atypism if the later terminology were applied to all of such cases as illustrated in Fig. 4.

However, in five of the twenty-eight tumors, or 17.1 per cent, one or more focal, limited areas were found satisfying the qualification of localized adenocarcinoma in situ, as illustrated in Fig. 5, and in four of the twenty-eight tumors, areas of unconfined papillar, well-differentiated "low-grade," or Grade I, adenocarcinoma were present (14.3 per cent), as illustrated in Fig. 6. Thus, nine of the twenty-eight villous papillomas, or 35.7 per cent, without gross or preoperative evidence to biopsy or other means, were found to contain either focal adenocarcinoma or proliferating areas of well-differentiated, papillary adenocarcinoma. The percentage of malignant degeneration found in villous tumors has been reported by Sunderland and Binkley[10] as 68 per cent, and by Ewing[9] as from 10 to 20 per cent. More recently, Fisher and Castro[11] by serial section reported four cases of papillary adenoma to have demonstrable areas of adenocarcinoma in 100 per cent, while Welch, McKittrick, and Behringer[12] have shown that malignancy is demonstrable in 22 per cent of papillary villous tumors as compared to 17 per cent in pedunculated adenomas.

TREATMENT AND RESULTS

Wide removal of the lesion was carried out in twenty-six of the twenty-eight patients (92.9 per cent), while in two patients of the twenty-eight (7.1 per cent) a localized Bevan-type excision of rectal mucosa was employed. Specific types of procedure were based on location of the lesion and routes of lymphatic spread for malignant lesions of the large bowel. Thus lesions occurring at or below the lateral ligaments of the rectum, corresponding to Kohlrausch's plica, that is, 7 cm. above the anus, were treated by extended Miles excision of the rectum with abdominal colostomy, while lesions occurring above the zone of lateral spread but below the lower sigmoid (that is, 7 to 15 cm. above the anus) were treated by abdominoperineal proctosigmoidectomy with sphincter preservation, as shown by the abbreviation APPS in Table I. Lesions in the sigmoid colon, presenting adequate segment of bowel for anticipated cure without recurrence by resection, were treated by sigmoidectomy; the APPS has proved to result in removal of more extensive length of bowel in the treatment of upper rectal or "rectosigmoidal" lesions than permitted by low anterior resection, which is admittedly accompanied by the risk of malignant cytologic exfoliation and greater possibility of recurrence than with a more radical procedure, when performed for other than palliative purpose. Resection, then, was mainly restricted to lesions above the upper rectum, for example, sigmoid, and, for one lesion occurring in the transverse colon, with end-to-end anastomo-

Fig. 5.

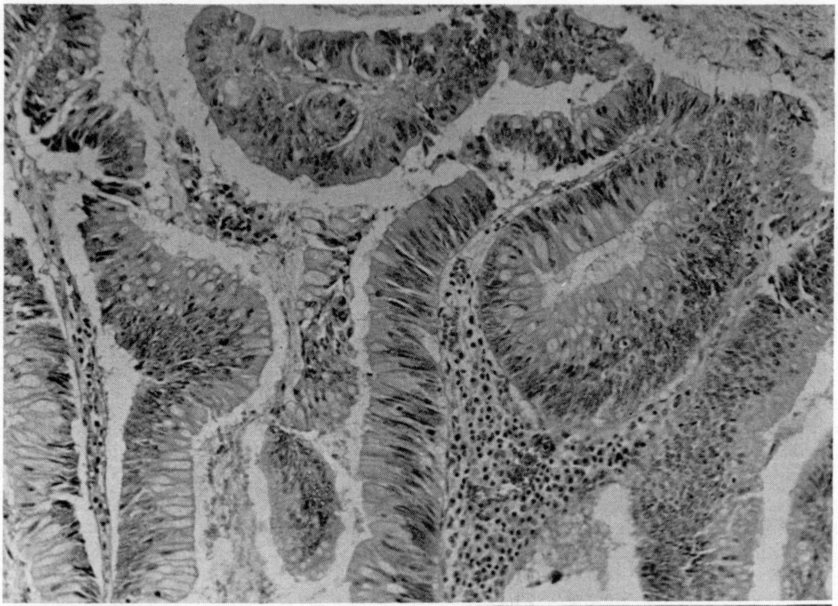

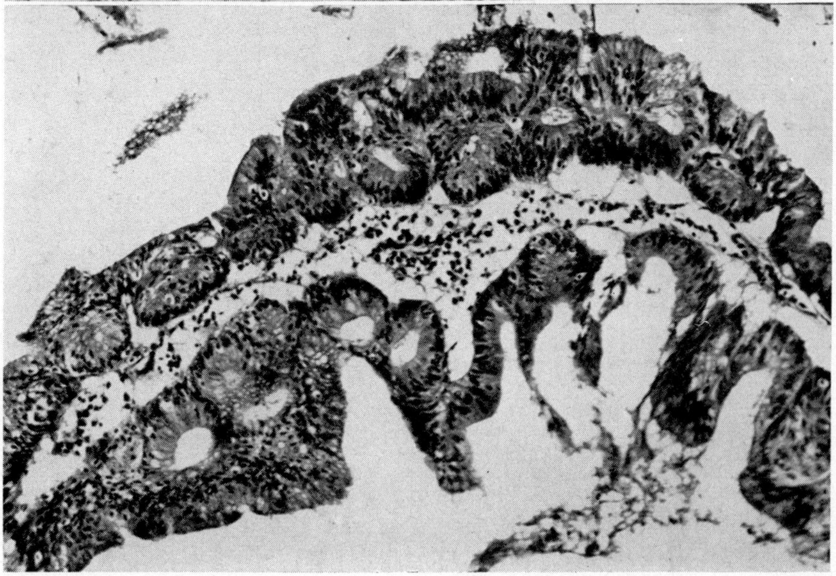

Fig. 6.

Fig. 5.—Villous papilloma with area of adenocarcinoma in situ (×200, reduced ⅓) in A. M., a 58-year-old woman.

Fig. 6.—Villous papilloma with carcinomatous change but without invasion of muscularis; superficial adenocarcinoma, well differentiated in A. H., a 69-year-old woman.

sis; all procedures included removal of contiguous mesentery, including lymph nodes and vascular pedicle ligation up to the origin of the inferior mesenteric artery from the aorta, except for the two instances where Bevan excision was indicated. The treatment is summarized in Table I, along with results.

TABLE I. TREATMENT AND RESULTS

PERIOD OF TIME FOLLOWING SURGERY IN WHICH PATIENTS ARE ALIVE AND WELL (YEARS)	TYPE OF PROCEDURE EMPLOYED AND NUMBER OF PATIENTS				
	APPS*	MILES	SIGMOID-ECTOMY	RESECTION TRANSVERSE COLON	BEVAN EXCISION
1-2	3	2	2	0	1
2-3	1	1	0	1	1
3-4	3	1	1	0	0
4-5	2	1	0	0	0
5-6	5	1	1	0	0
6-7	1	0	0	0	0
Known liver involvement	0	2	0	0	0
Deaths	1†	1	0	0	0
Unavailable for follow-up	1‡	0	0	0	0
Known recurrence	1§	0	0	0	0
Total of patients living	14	5	4	1	2
Total patients	15	6	4	1	2

*Abdominoperineal proctosigmoidectomy.

†Death due to recurrent gastric carcinoma as revealed by autopsy.

‡Alive at last follow-up two years previously; moved to another state.

§Patient had multiple malignancy, adenocarcinoma of rectum, causing recurrence, in addition to villous papilloma of splenic flexure, with carcinomatous degeneration; lymph-node studies had revealed unfavorable prognosis following surgery, despite any procedure.

Of the twenty-eight patients treated, and followed for a period of time ranging from two to seven years, there have been no deaths attributable to the tumor per se; two patients have died from incidental causes; one patient died from cerebrovascular accident eight months following discharge from the hospital, while in the other patient death occurred ten months following gastrectomy for an adenocarcinoma of the stomach discovered and treated incident to removal of the rectum for a villous papilloma with carcinomatous change; autopsy in this instance revealed death due to recurrence of gastric carcinoma.

The prognosis in three patients now living is unfavorable because of liver involvement noted at the time of surgery in two patients and known recurrence from a simultaneously occurring and treated adenocarcinoma of the rectum in addition to a villous papilloma of the splenic flexure. Of the two patients with liver involvement, one is alive two and one-half years following surgery, and the other now living three and one-half years following surgery, both patients having had a Miles operation for a villous papilloma with carcinomatous degeneration in the lower rectum, of Dukes or Bormann Type 1 lesion.

SUMMARY AND CONCLUSIONS

Benign epithelial tumors, arising from mucous membrane, represent the most common tumors of the colon and rectum and may be classified into two groups. The more common, originating as a mucosal mammillation, is recognized as the adenomatous polyp, which is typically a compact, pedunculated mass, usually smooth but often having a papillary arrangement of the luminal pole and which occurs in approximately 7 per cent of all adults. The other less commonly occurring lesion appears as a broad, sessile velvetlike tumor with soft villous projections in striking morphologic contrast to all other benign or malignant tumors of the large bowel. The descriptive classification of villous papillomas, often referred to as papillary adenomas, has been useful to the clinician in recognizing certain morphologic, pathologic, and clinical features tending to demarcate this tumor from the closely related adenomatous polyp. Villous papillomas often present a problem, for repeated biopsies may be consistently benign and the lesions present no opportunity for well-defined local excision or electrodesiccation commonly presenting with the adenomatous polyp or mammillation.

Based on the study of 1,144 benign and malignant tumors of the large bowel, over a five-year period from 1946 to 1951, twenty-eight villous papillomas were encountered, representing an incidence of 2.3 per cent of the total, compared to adenomatous polyps having an incidence of 21.4 per cent. In this series, adenomatous polyps were ten times as common as the villous papilloma. Criteria for the villous papilloma have been described. According to Dukes, the villous papilloma is the end result of a growth pattern affecting mainly the superficial epithelium rather than cells at a deeper layer giving rise to the adenoma.

Symptomatology and clinical features have been presented. Analysis of the histopathologic features reveals that evidence of adenocarcinoma was present in 35.7 per cent of villous papillomas in this series, in the absence of any induration or other finding to suggest malignancy. In contrast, adenocarcinomatous change is found in 15 to 19 per cent of adenomatous polyps.

Follow-up study on twenty-eight having undergone surgery from 1946 to 1951 reveals the over-all survival rate to be 92.9 per cent over a period ranging from two to seven years at the time of concluding this study. Eleven patients, or 39.3 per cent, have survived five or more years, while the remainder are at present in the two- to five-year group. The prognosis has been found more favorable in those patients in whom no evidence of carcinomatous foci was demonstrable, and more favorable in those patients whose lesions were above the level of Kohlrausch's plica or lateral ligaments of the rectum.

Recognition of villous papilloma, from the criteria described, and appreciation of its tendency toward malignant behavior present indication for adequate extirpation of involved large bowel and areas of lymphatic drainage despite ostensibly benign pathology.

Acknowledgment is made to Edwin S. Gault, M.D., Professor of Pathology, Temple University School of Medicine, Philadelphia, Pa., in appreciation of photomicrographs and cooperation in this study.

REFERENCES

1. Holmes, T.: Tr. Path. Soc. Lond. **12:** 120, 1860.
2. Hauser, G.: Das Cylinderepithel Karcinom des Magens und des Dickdarms, Sweden, 1890, Iena.
3. Quenu, E., and Landel, G.: Des tumeurs villeuses ou epitheliomas superficiels vegetants du rectum, Rev. de gynéc. et de chir. abd. **3:** 95-126, 1899.
4. Lambling, A.: Les tumeurs villeuses du rectum, Paris, 1928, Masson & Cie.

5. Bensaude, R., Cain, A., and Lambling, A.: Les tumeurs villeuses du rectum, Presse méd. **38**: 1713, 1930.
6. Dukes, C.: An Explanation of the Difference Between a Papilloma and an Adenoma of the Rectum, Proc. Roy. Soc. Med. **40**: 829-830 (Nov.), 1947.
7. Helwig, E. B.: Evolution of Adenomas of Large Intestine and Their Relation to Carcinoma, Surg., Gynec. & Obst. **84**: 36-49, 1947.
8. Gabriel, W. B.: Surgical Management of Large Villous Tumours of the Rectum, Proc. Roy. Soc. Med. **45**: 696-700 (Oct.), 1952.
9. Ewing, M. R.: Villous Tumours of the Rectum, Ann. of Roy. Coll. Surgeons England **6**: 413-441 (June), 1950.
10. Sunderland, D. A., and Binkley, G. E.: Papillary Adenomas of Large Intestine; a Study of Forty-eight Cases, Cancer **1**: 184-207 (July), 1948.
11. Fisher, E. R., and Castro, A. F.: Diffuse Papillomatous Polyps (Villous Tumors) of the Colon and Rectum, Am. J. Surg. **85**: 146-151 (Feb.), 1953.
12. Welch, C. E., McKittrick, J. B., and Behringer, G.: Polyps of the Rectum and Colon and Their Relation to Cancer, New England J. Med. **247**: 959-965 (Dec.), 1952.

CONSECUTIVE SURVIVAL OF OPEN-CHEST, HYPOTHERMIC DOGS AFTER PROLONGED BY-PASS OF HEART AND LUNGS BY MEANS OF A PUMP-OXYGENATOR

FRANK GOLLAN, M.D., EDWARD C. HAMILTON, M.D., AND GEORGE R. MENEELY, M.D., NASHVILLE, TENN.

(From the Research Laboratory and Radioisotope Unit, Thayer Veterans Administration Hospital, and the Department of Medicine and Surgery, Vanderbilt University School of Medicine)

THE idea of substituting a mechanical device for the function of the heart and lungs is by no means new. Le Gallois wrote in 1812: "If one could substitute for the heart a kind of injection of arterial blood, either natural or artificially made, one would succeed easily in maintaining alive indefinitely any part of the body whatsoever."[1] In spite of the great interest and definite advances in this field in recent years, the statement must still be considered overoptimistic since the most enthusiastic investigator of today would hardly state that he succeeds "easily" in keeping animals alive even for short periods of time by artificial devices.

The literature has been extensively reviewed by Björk,[2] Dennis,[3] and Miller,[4] but many substantial contributions from abroad[5-9] have not been given sufficient attention in this country.

The first mammal, a cat, which survived clamping of the pulmonary artery for thirty minutes, was reported by Gibbon in 1937.[10] The first series of consecutive survivals of thirteen dogs in which the entire blood flow was diverted from the heart and the lungs was achieved by Gibbon and his associates last year.[11] These investigators have been pioneers in the perfection of a blood-film-type oxygenator, and the continuity of at least sixteen years of experimental effort has been rewarded by the first successful clinical application.[12]

The present communication describes experiences with a pump-oxygenator based on the principle of gas dispersion.[13, 14] The efficiency and safety of this instrument have been tested previously in the prevention of acute anoxic anoxia[15] and in the exclusion of heart and lungs from the circulation of hypothermic "closed-chest" dogs.[16] Although all dogs whose chests were not opened survived the by-pass of heart and lungs, dogs with thoracotomies showed a high mortality when subjected to the same procedure.[17] It seemed probable that inadequate neutralization of the heparin effect after thoracic surgery was the major obstacle to survival.

MATERIALS AND METHODS

Operative Procedure.—Dogs are anesthetized with 50 mg. of Nembutal per kilogram, and the right jugular vein and both femoral arteries and veins are prepared for cannulation. After the injection of 10 mg. of heparin per kilogram, polyethylene catheters with longitudinal slits are introduced into the

This work was supported by a grant-in-aid from the American Heart Association.
Received for publication, June 26, 1953.

veins for the withdrawal of blood from the caval system to the pump-oxygenator. Long polyethylene tubes for the return of the oxygenated blood from the instrument are introduced into the femoral arteries and advanced far enough to reach the aortic arch. The right carotid artery is connected to a mercury manometer.

A thoracotomy through the right fourth intercostal space is performed under strictly aseptic conditions. Cutting, as well as meticulous hemostasis, is performed with the Bovie electrosurgical unit exclusively. No delay of wound healing and no increased incidence of morbidity have been noted. Positive pressure aeration of the lungs is achieved with an endotracheal tube and a mechanical air respirator, employing an air-tight system.

The vena azygos is ligated, and the superior and inferior venae cavae are mobilized for later occlusion with rubber-dam tapes. When satisfactory blood flow, oxygenation, and hypothermia are achieved by the pump-oxygenator the respirator is shut off, and the venae cavae are occluded by tightening the rubber tapes and holding them in place with bulldog clamps. Hypothermia can be rapidly produced by cooling the blood in the extracorporeal circulation by means of a silver or stainless steel coil immersed in ice water.[18]

When the perfusion is over the occlusive tapes are released, the respirator is started, and the pump-oxygenator is stopped. This can be done abruptly since the heart takes over from one beat to another without any evidence of electrocardiographic change.

The thoracotomy incision is carefully closed in anatomic layers about a thoracotomy tube connected to constant water suction, and the animal remains on the table under observation for the next four to five hours. Observation of the blood pressure is continued until normal coagulation time is restored, and artificial respiration is continued until shivering appears (at a rectal temperature of about 30° C.). The thoracotomy tube is also removed at this time. It is preferable to raise the body temperature slowly by means of heating pads in order to prolong the period of hypothermic low-oxygen requirement immediately following the closure of the chest cavity. The rate and volume of the respirator should be reduced during this time in order to avoid respiratory alkalosis. When shivering has begun, the animal may be placed in the cage. Subsequent postoperative care consists of the administration of antibiotics for five days and the maintenance of adequate nutrition.

Neutralization of Heparin.—Two to five milligrams of heparin are sufficient to keep the blood incoagulable in any of the blood-film-type oxygenators, but a minimum of 10 mg. of heparin per kilogram is needed to prevent fibrin embolism in the gas-dispersion-type oxygenator used in these experiments.

In sixty-eight heparinized dogs, clotting-time determinations in siliconed tubes and protamine-heparin titrations were carried out during the first two postoperative hours. Six different routines of immediate postoperative management of the heparin-induced clotting defect were tested: (1) administration of a dose of Protamine Sulfate equivalent to the heparin which had been given; (2) administration of one-half the equivalent amount of protamine; (3) slow transfusion with 300 to 500 ml. of citrated blood; (4) administration of one-half the equivalent amount of protamine followed by a transfusion of citrated blood; (5) administration of one-half the equivalent amount of protamine, slow intravenous injection of 1 Gm. of calcium gluconate, and then a transfusion of citrated blood; and (6) administration of one-half the equivalent dose of heparin followed by a transfusion of fresh or decalcified blood.

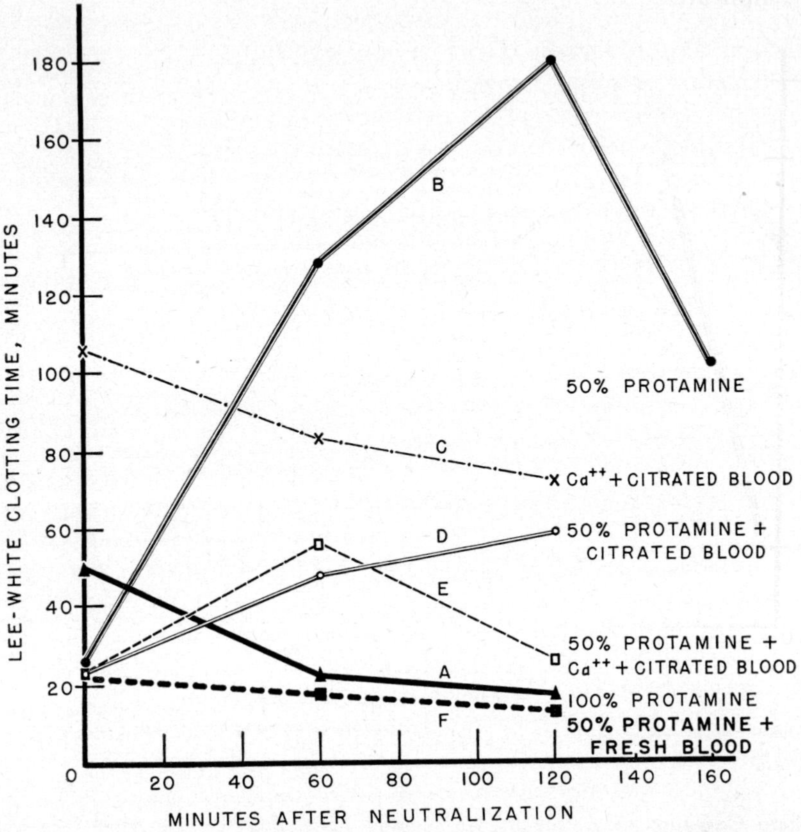

Fig. 1.—Neutralization procedures of heparin after the use of a pump-oxygenator.

If each milligram of heparin is covered with an equal amount of protamine, clotting time remains prolonged for about one hour (Fig. 1, *A*). Covering one-half of the injected amount of heparin with protamine rapidly restores the clotting time to normal. This situation, however, is not stable under our experimental conditions, and a prolongation of clotting time occurs again which reaches its maximum after one to two hours (Fig. 1, *B*). During this time increasing amounts of protamine are needed to bring the clotting time back to normal in heparin-protamine titrations (Fig. 2). Such titrations were found too cumbersome for routine use. Attempts were therefore made to preserve the initial benefit of the one-half dose of protamine by the transfusion of blood. The results of this procedure (Fig. 1) show that neither calcium gluconate and citrated blood (*C*) nor one-half the dose of protamine followed by a transfusion of citrated blood with (*E*) or without (*D*) calcium gluconate is capable of restoring normal blood clotting at all times after the experiment.

The only procedure which achieves this goal is the administration of one-half the equivalent dose of protamine followed by a transfusion of 300 to 500 ml. of fresh or decalcified blood (*F*). With this technique of heparin neutralization, postoperative prolongation of clotting time was prevented and all hemorrhagic complications were eliminated.

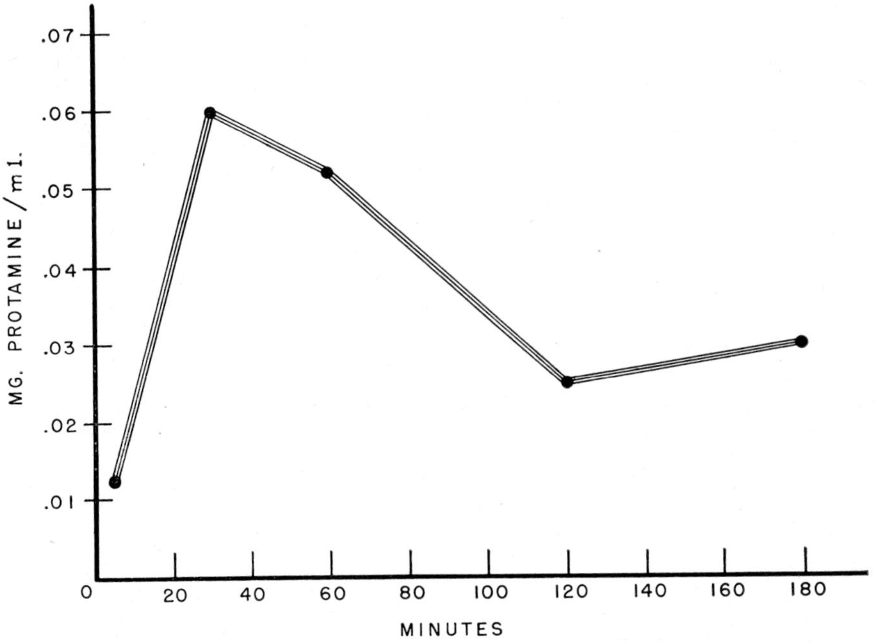

Fig. 2.—Fifty per cent protamine titration of heparinized blood to five minutes' clotting time. (Each point represents the average of ten experiments.) Heparin-protamine: Titration in 1 ml. blood samples after intravenous administration of one-half the equivalent amount of protamine.

Blood Changes During Perfusion.—The maintenance of satisfactory oxygen saturation, pH, and carbon-dioxide content by the use of this instrument has been reported previously.[13, 17] Hemolysis is minimal even after prolonged pumping.[14] The present study encompasses changes in the hematocrit, red blood count, white blood count, platelet count, eosinophil count, and vitamin C blood level. Changes in the corpuscular elements are due to the effect of filling the instrument with heparinized donor blood diluted with 5 per cent glucose in saline solution and to destruction of cells that has occurred during the perfusion (Fig. 3). Hematocrit and red cell count show the dilution effect at the end of the perfusion, but the transfusion of fresh or decalcified blood raises their level somewhat higher than the preperfusion value. The destruction of platelets during the procedure is evident from reduction to less than one-half the original value at the end of the perfusion. The blood transfusion, however, returns the platelet count to a safe level. Even more severe is the drop in the white cell count at the end of the perfusion to about one-fourth of the original count. Again, the blood transfusion at the end of the procedure returns the total white blood count to a normal level. In contradistinction to all other cell elements studied, the eosinophil cell reduction after the perfusion is not brought back to normal by a subsequent blood transfusion. Table I shows the mean percentage change from the control value, as well as the difference from the red cell count.

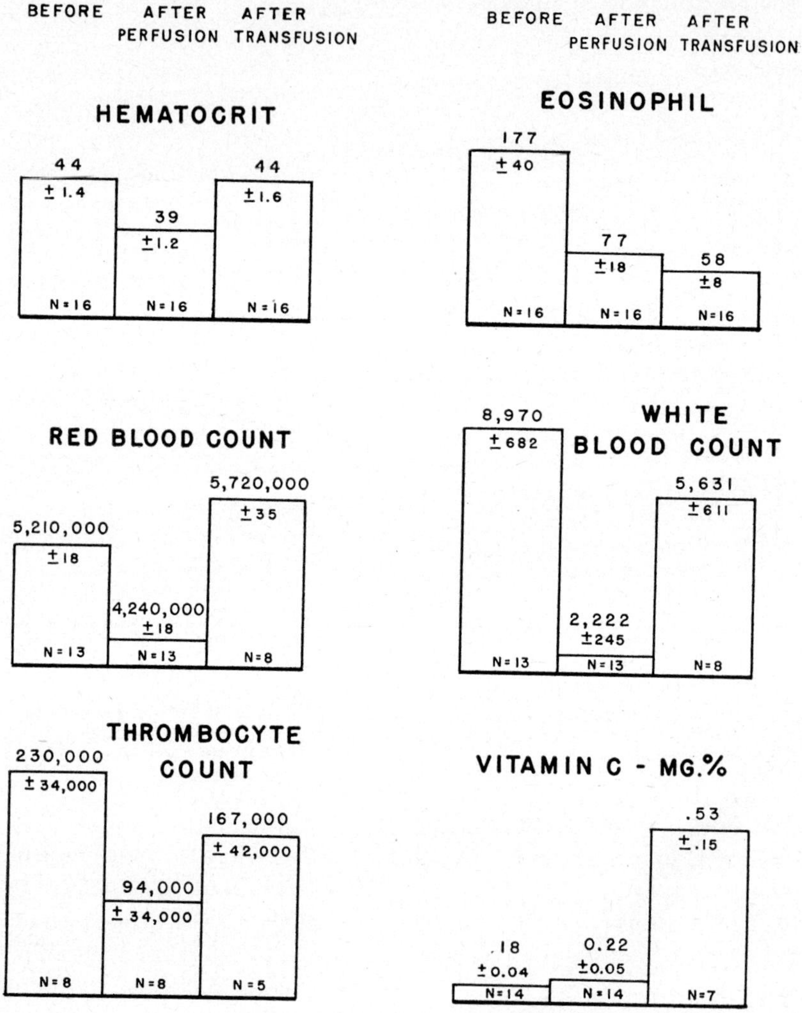

Fig. 3.—Blood changes after perfusion and after transfusion.

Preliminary tests have shown that vitamin C disappears from blood in about fifteen minutes when oxygen dispersed by sintered glass bubbles through it. The question arose as to whether the hemorrhagic manifestations after the perfusion might be due to an acute deficiency of ascorbic acid produced by the prolonged dispersion of fine oxygen bubbles in blood. The results of blood vitamin C determinations in these animals show that the changes during the perfusion are insignificant and that transfusion of fresh or decalcified blood raises the vitamin C to about three times the control level.

TABLE I. MEAN PERCENTAGE OF CHANGE FROM CONTROL VALUE TO VALUE AT END OF THIRTY-MINUTE PERFUSION

	NUMBER OF DOGS	MEAN PERCENTAGE ± STANDARD ERROR	DIFFERENCE FROM RED BLOOD COUNT (MEAN PERCENTAGE OF CHANGE)	PROBABILITY
Red blood count	13	−17 ± 3		
White blood count	16	−72 ± 4	55	.001
Platelet	8	−54 ± 7	37	.001
Eosinophils	16	−48 ± 7	33	.01

Physiologic Observations.—Measurement of carotid blood pressure, blood flow through the instrument, respiratory rate, and rectal temperature during the exclusion of heart and lungs are recorded in Table II. Seventeen consecutive dogs of 15 to 28.7 kilograms in weight were perfused from twenty-seven to sixty minutes. Fifteen survived the procedure without any ill effects and were observed for about one month. Dog 2 died of acute anoxia due to a leak in the rubber cuff of the endotracheal tube during the closure of the thoracotomy. Dog 11 walked around the day after the experiment, but appeared weak and did not drink. A subcutaneous infusion of 5 per cent glucose was given at a rapid rate by the addition of hyaluronidase. At the end of the infusion the animal collapsed and died. An autopsy was negative and no blood was found in the chest cavity; the cause of death was attributed to electrolyte shock due to too rapid subcutaneous infusion of glucose.[19]

TABLE II

DOG	WEIGHT (KG.)	BLOOD FLOW (C.C./KG./MIN.)	RECTAL TEMPERATURE (° C.)	BLOOD PRESSURE (MM. HG)	RESPIRATORY RATE (PER MIN.)	DURATION OF BY-PASS (MIN.)	OUTCOME	LENGTH OF OBSERVATION (DAYS)
1	19.0	55	27.5	100/60	4	27	Lived	32
2	20.0	50	26.5	100/50	2	30	Died	1
3	15.5	45	25.0	40/35	0	30	Lived	23
4	21.5	40	26.5	90/60	0	32	Lived	33
5	27.3	41	27.0	90/50	–	35	Lived	29
6	23.6	35	25.0	80/40	–	30	Lived	28
7	18.6	47	26.0	90/50	0	35	Lived	28
8	16.4	50	27.0	90/50	8	31	Lived	27
9	28.7	46	27.0	70/40	2	31	Lived	31
10	19.5	45	27.0	100/50	0	30	Lived	27
11	15.0	54	24.0	55/20	10	30	Died	1
12	22.2	38	24.0	40/20	0	60	Lived	28
13	21.3	33	25.0	80/50	0	31	Lived	32
14	16.8	68	24.0	100/50	0	30	Lived	28
15	21.3	53	25.0	90/40	2	60	Lived	28
16	18.1	65	27.0	90/40	0	32	Lived	30
17	23.0	35	26.0	80/40	0	57	Lived	32

Blood pressure, blood flow, and respiratory rate at the prevailing low body temperature can be evaluated only if compared with the physiologic values for the corresponding degree of hypothermia. Fig. 4 indicates that the blood flow reached corresponded in most cases to the cardiac output of hypothermic animals as determined by Bigelow and associates.[20] Even such low flow rates as 30 to 40 c.c. per kilogram per minute at 25° C., as compared with 130 to 150 c.c. per kilogram per minute at normal body temperature, are sufficient to supply the brain with enough oxygen. It should be added, however, that this holds true only if the blood pressure in the cerebral circulation is kept at a much higher level than is physiologic at these low body temperatures. Fig. 5 shows that the location of the arterial catheters high up in the aorta resulted generally in carotid blood pressure materially higher than in dogs of the same degree of hypothermia with the catheters placed more distally.[20] In previous experiments, for example, we have seen brain damage result if, at such a low blood flow rate, the arterial cannulae were placed in the femoral arteries. In such instances, the carotid blood pressure equaled the ''physiologic'' hypothermic values as reported by Bigelow and co-workers.[20]

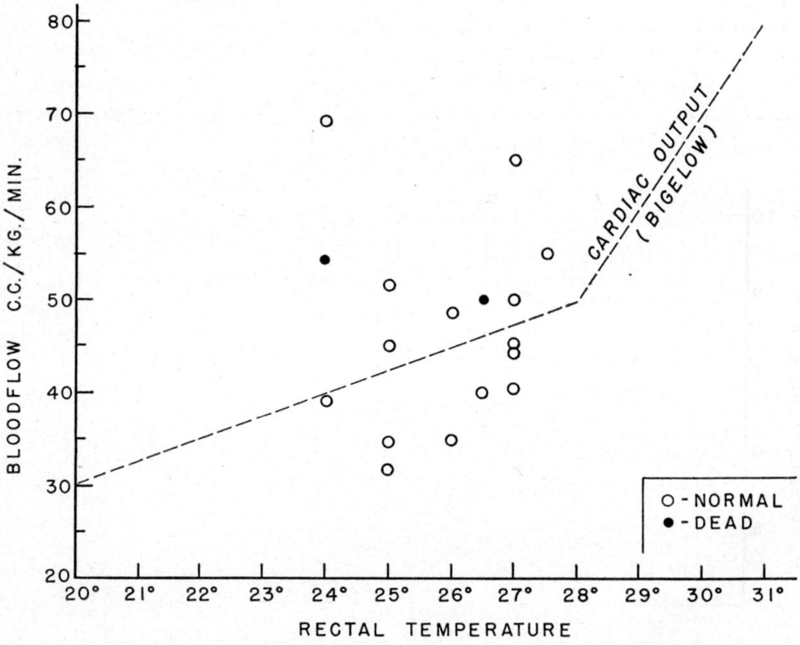

Fig. 4.—Blood flow in the pump-oxygenator during total by-pass of heart and lungs in hypothermic, open-chest dogs.

The fact that we actually overoxygenated the brains of all but two animals can be seen in Fig. 6 where the recorded respiratory rates are compared with those found in nembutalized dogs immersed in ice water.[21] In most experiments, the open-chest dogs did not exhibit any respiratory movements while the respirator was stopped during the perfusion. This phenomenon is attributed to depression of the respiratory center resulting from cerebral overoxygenation. In corroboration of this hypothesis, it was observed that blood from the vena cava superior was materially lighter in color than the blood from the vena cava inferior and that the tongues of these animals remained light pink due to the presence of "arterialized" blood in the superficial veins of the heads.

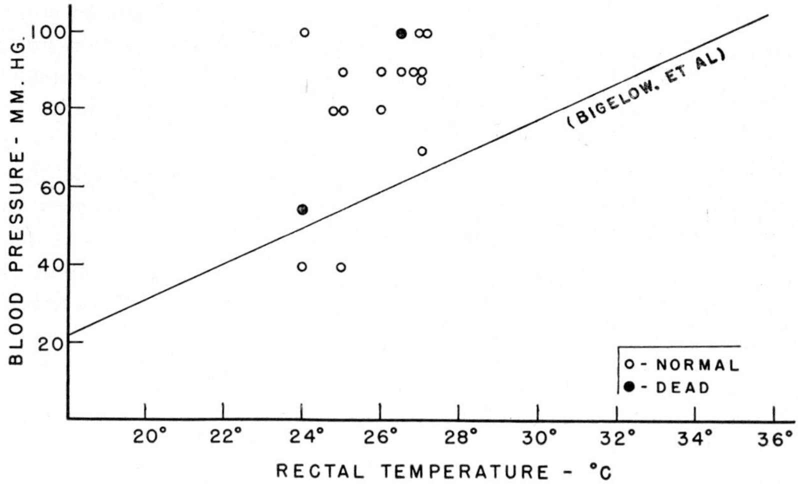

Fig. 5.—Carotid blood pressure during total by-pass of heart and lungs in hypothermic, open-chest dogs.

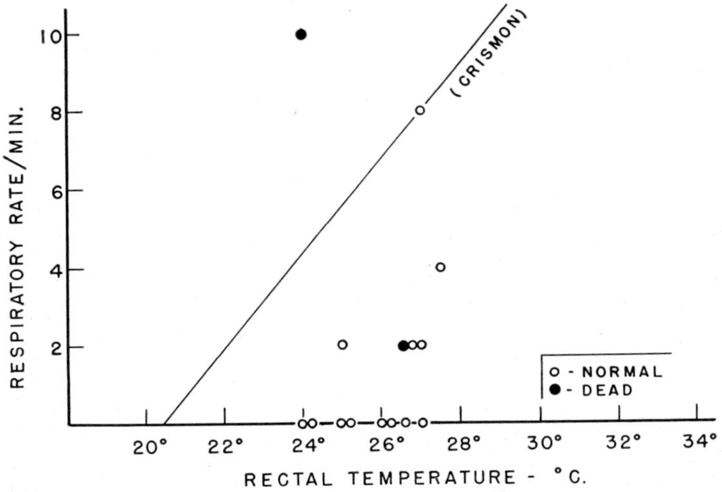

Fig. 6.—Respiratory rate during total by-pass of heart and lungs in hypothemic, open-chest dogs.

DISCUSSION

Although it has been shown that a gas dispersion pump-oxygenator can be used safely and efficiently for providing artificial circulation and oxygenation in closed-chest dogs, its application in open-chest animals has been limited, and its use in human intracardiac surgery prohibited, by the high mortality due to postoperative complications. The exclusive use of electrocautery in all surgical procedures, as well as the described method of restoration of normal clotting time after the administration of large amounts of heparin, has permitted these difficulties to be overcome.

The delayed prolongation of clotting time after neutralization of the heparin effect by Protamine Sulfate has been observed previously.[6] The heparin-protamine titrations carried out during this period indicate that a larger amount of protamine is needed to reduce this delayed prolongation to normal. The explanation for this phenomenon is not clear at present. It seems, however, that the chemical conditions for a stable heparin-protamine complex are not present in the postoperative period. Studies[22] on the effect of pH have shown that alkalinity inhibits the heparin-protamine linkage, and it is possible that overventilation by the respirator during the postoperative period might have produced the same effect.

Since hemolysis is minimal, the drop in hematocrit and red cell count can be attributed to dilution of the donor blood by 5 per cent glucose in saline solution. We have gained the impression that the relatively high concentration of glucose is essential in the prevention of hemolysis. By comparing the percentages of reduction of various cell elements with the fall of erythrocytes, an estimation of the destruction of these cells during the procedure can be made. The destruction of the fragile platelets is marked, but a thrombopenic bleeding tendency after the experiment can be excluded since the transfusion of fresh blood raises the platelet count to higher levels.

The marked reduction of leukocytes during the perfusion is probably due to adherence of the white cells to the large surface of the extracorporeal circuit. The continuing drop of eosinophilic leukocytes is of interest and may be due to an effect upon the pituitary gland and/or the adrenal gland. Since we have not provided any evidence for such an assumption a speculative discussion of this point would be fruitless.

The constancy of the vitamin C blood level during the oxygenation by gas dispersion may indicate that the dog produces vitamin C at the same rate as it is destroyed. The high ascorbic-acid content of the blood after the transfusion eliminates the possibility of an acute vitamin C deficiency as a cause of a hemorrhagic diathesis.

The marked hypothermia induced by rapid cooling of the blood reduces the amount of blood necessary to be pumped and oxygenated by the instrument to the low cardiac output values found in hypothermia. This low blood flow can be reduced further by raising the blood pressure in the cerebral circulation so that only about one-fifth of the cardiac output requirement at normal body temperature is sufficient to supply the oxygen requirement of the brain and thereby prevent cerebral damage. The oxygen requirement of the rest of the body and of the heart, which is beating slowly and pumping coronary blood only, seems to be so low that the small amount of oxygenated blood pumped at low pressure is sufficient to preserve normal function of all organs.

SUMMARY

1. After the use of large amounts of heparin during the employment of a gas-dispersion-type pump-oxygenator, postoperative hemorrhagic manifestations

could be eliminated by the exclusive use of electrosurgical technique and the restoration of normal clotting time by a combination of Protamine Sulfate and fresh or decalcified blood.

2. Hematologic changes during the perfusion are due partly to dilution of blood with 5 per cent glucose in physiologic saline solution and partly to destruction and can be restored to normal by blood transfusions. The blood vitamin C level does not change during the oxygenation procedure.

3. By maintaining a high carotid blood pressure at 25° C. body temperature, as little as 30 to 40 c.c. of oxygenated blood per kilogram per minute is sufficient to cover the oxygen consumption of the body and to prevent anoxic brain damage in a one-hour by-pass of heart and lungs. Under these conditions consecutive survival of fifteen dogs has been achieved.

Acknowledgments.—We are greatly indebted to Mrs. Con Ball for statistical evaluation of the data and for criticism of the manuscript, to Mr. Raymond Jones for technical assistance, and to Dr. W. R. Kirtley, Ely Lilly & Company, Indianapolis, Ind., for Protamine Sulfate.

REFERENCES

1. Le Gallois, quoted by Björk.[2]
2. Björk, V. O.: Brain Perfusions in Dogs With Artificially Oxygenated Blood, Acta chir. scandinav. **96**: 1, 1948.
3. Dennis, C., Spreng, D. S., Jr., Nelson, G. E., Karlson, K. E., Nelson, R. M., Thomas, J. V., Eder, W. P., and Varco, R. L.: Development of a Pump-Oxygenator to Replace the Heart and Lungs, Ann. Surg. **134**: 709, 1951.
4. Miller, B. J., Gibbon, J. H., Jr., and Gibbon, M. H.: Recent Advances in the Development of a Mechanical Heart and Lung Apparatus, Ann. Surg. **134**: 694, 1951.
5. Mondini, P.: Pneumectomia totale bilaterale con sopravvivenza dell' animale mediante l'uso d'un nuovo ossigenatore del sangue, Acta chir. patavina **4**: 3, 1948.
6. Kolff, W. J., and Dubbelman, C. P.: Het kunstmatig hart, ''Geneeskundige Gids'' van 30 Juni 1949.
7. Tosatti, E.: Ulteriori studi sulla macchina cardio-pulmonare, Atti e Memorie della Soc. Romana di Chirurg. **7**: 3, 1949.
8. Dogliotti, A. M., and Constantini, A.: Primo caso di applicazione all'uomo di un apparecchio di circulazione sanguigna extracorporea, Minerva chir. **6**: 1, 1951.
9. Thomas, J. A., and Beauduin, P.: Caractéristiques physiologiques du coeur-poumon artificiel pour la perfusion au sang du corps humain, J. physiol., Paris **43**: 311, 1951.
10. Gibbon, J. H., Jr.: Artificial Maintenance of Circulation During Experimental Occlusion of the Pulmonary Artery, Arch. Surg. **34**: 1105, 1937.
11. Gibbon, J. H., Jr.: Discussion note, J. Thoracic Surg. **24**: 18, 1952.
12. New York Times, May 8, 1953, p. 31.
13. Clark, L. C., Jr., Gollan, F., and Gupta, V. B.: The Oxygenation of Blood by Gas Dispersion, Science **111**: 85, 1950.
14. Clark, L. C., Jr., Hooven, F., and Gollan, F.: A Large Capacity, All-glass Dispersion Oxygenator and Pump, Rev. Scient. Instruments **23**: 748, 1952.
15. Gollan, F., Clark, L. C., Jr., and Gupta, V. B.: The Prevention of Acute Anoxic Anoxia by Means of a Pump-Oxygenator, Am. J. M. Sc. **222**: 76, 1951.
16. Gollan, F., Blos, P., and Schuman, H.: Exclusion of Heart and Lung From the Circulation of Hypothermic, Closed-chest Dogs by Means of a Pump-Oxygenator, J. Appl. Physiol. **5**: 180, 1952.
17. Helmsworth, J. A., Clark, L. C., Jr., Kaplan, S., Sherman, R. T., and Largen, T.: Artificial Oxygenation and Circulation During Complete By-pass of the Heart, J. Thoracic Surg. **24**: 117, 1952.
18. Gollan, F., Blos, P., and Schuman, H.: Studies on Hypothermia by Means of a Pump-Oxygenator, Am. J. Physiol. **171**: 331, 1952.
19. Webb, W. R.: Effect of Hyaluronidase on Rate of Absorption of Subcutaneous Fluids, Arch. Surg. **65**: 77, 1952.
20. Bigelow, W. G., Lindsay, W. K., and Greenwood, W. F.: Hypothermia, Ann. Surg. **132**: 849, 1950.
21. Crismon, J. M.: Resuscitation From Deep Hypothermia, Army Air Forces, Aero-Med. Lab., Memorandum Report No. TSEAA-695-56 A. (Dec. 21) 1945.
22. Burstein, M., and Loeb, J.: Sur l' effet antithrombinique de l' héparine. Rôle du pH, de la concentration saline et des ions alcalino-terreux, Compt. rend. Soc. de biol. **146**: 250, 1952.

A TECHNIQUE FOR THE PRODUCTION OF HYPOTHERMIA

Preliminary Report

Charles B. Ripstein, M.D., Charles E. Friedgood, M.D., and Nathan Solomon, Ph.D., Brooklyn, N. Y.

(From the Department of Surgery, Maimonides Hospital, and the State University of New York, College of Medicine at New York)

THE production and maintenance of a hypothermic state is potentially of great value in cardiac surgery. Because of the decreased metabolic needs of the tissues at lower temperatures, the heart can be excluded from the circulation for prolonged periods without producing irreversible brain damage.[1, 2] This permits clamping the venae cavae, opening the bloodless heart, and performing surgical procedures under direct vision. Such a technique lends itself well to the repair of septal defects and the correction of valvular abnormalities. Successful cases have already been reported in the literature.[3]

The methods used to lower body temperature have involved the application of cold to the skin surface or cooling of the inspired air. A prolonged period of exposure and deep anesthesia are usually necessary to overcome the heat-maintaining mechanism in a warm-blooded animal and to achieve a satisfactory hypothermic state (Fig. 1). This is an exhausting process and it leaves the animal in poor condition to withstand a major surgical procedure. Liver and cardiac muscle glycogen are decreased and a severe stress reaction occurs. In addition, once the defense mechanism has been overcome the temperature may continue to drop and rewarming is then difficult. This "overshooting" phenomenon has been the cause of many serious complications. Recent work by Laborit,[5] Huguenard,[4] and others[6] in France has indicated that certain antihistaminic drugs exert an inhibitory effect on the thermoregulatory center in warm-blooded animals. One of these compounds (Chlorpromazine) developed by Rhone-Poulenc of France has been made available to us for experimental use* and, after preliminary trials, the following technique has been evolved.

The subject, in the fasting state, is anesthetized with Pentothal Sodium and curare, and an endotracheal tube is inserted to maintain adequate pulmonary ventilation. The sensing bulb of a recording thermometer[7] is inserted into the rectum and a continuous record of body temperature is maintained.

The subject is placed in refrigeration blankets and an alcohol solution at 30° F. is circulated through the coils of the blanket (Fig. 3). Chlorpromazine is given in the dosage of 50 mg. intravenously and 100 mg. intramuscularly initially supplemented by 50 mg. intramuscularly every one to two hours dur-

Received for publication, April 7, 1953.

*Through the courtesy of Dr. Ernest Brown of Smith, Kline & French Laboratories, Philadelphia, Pa.

ing the period of hypothermia. No other medication is used and light anesthesia is maintained by Pentothal Sodium curare.

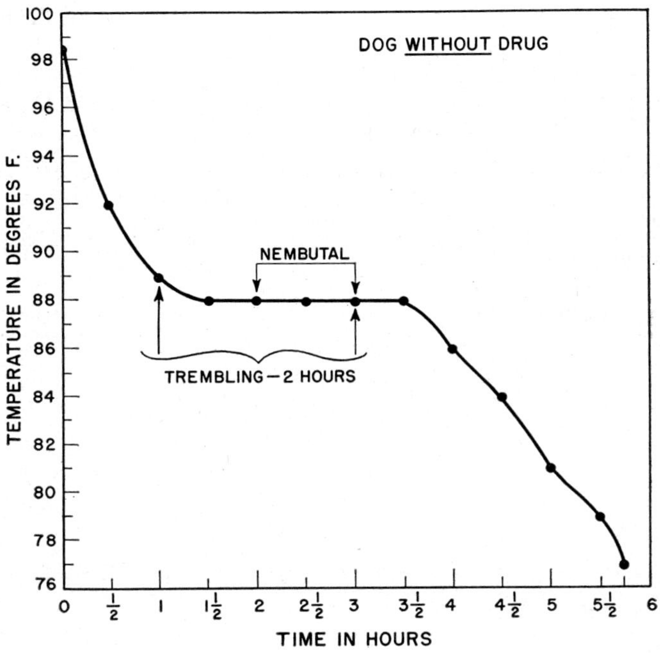

Fig. 1.—Temperature curve of dog refrigerated without Chlorpromazine. There is a prolonged period of shivering before the final drop of temperature occurs.

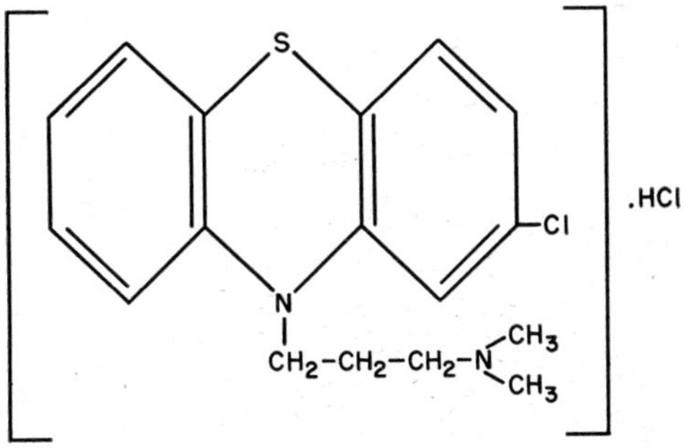

DIMETHYLAMINOPROPYL—N—CHLOROPHENOTHIAZINE HYDROCHLORIDE

Fig. 2.—Structural formula of Chlorpromazine.

When the body temperature reaches 80° F. the temperature of the refrigerant fluid is raised to 70° F. so as to maintain the hypothermic state at this level. All of the complications which we have encountered in the human being have occurred below 80° F., and, at the moment, we feel that this represents the limit of safety. Rewarming can be accomplished at any time by injecting 50 mg. of Chlorpromazine intramuscularly and raising the fluid temperature of the blanket to 110° F.

RESULTS

In the dog and in man, the body temperature begins to fall immediately and continues to drop in a smooth curve reaching 80° F. in fifteen to forty-five minutes. Shivering does not occur and there is no evidence of undue stress (Fig. 4). A minimal amount of anesthetic agent is required and thus the exhausting effect of prolonged deep anesthesia is avoided. If Chlorpromazine is given without the use of the refrigeration blanket, the temperature drops to from 92 to 94° F. and stabilizes at that level. Figs. 5 and 6 show a comparison of the effects of refrigeration with and without the drug in the dog and in man. It is apparent that with Chlorpromazine the temperature drops more rapidly and reaches a lower level with the same degree of refrigeration and anesthesia.

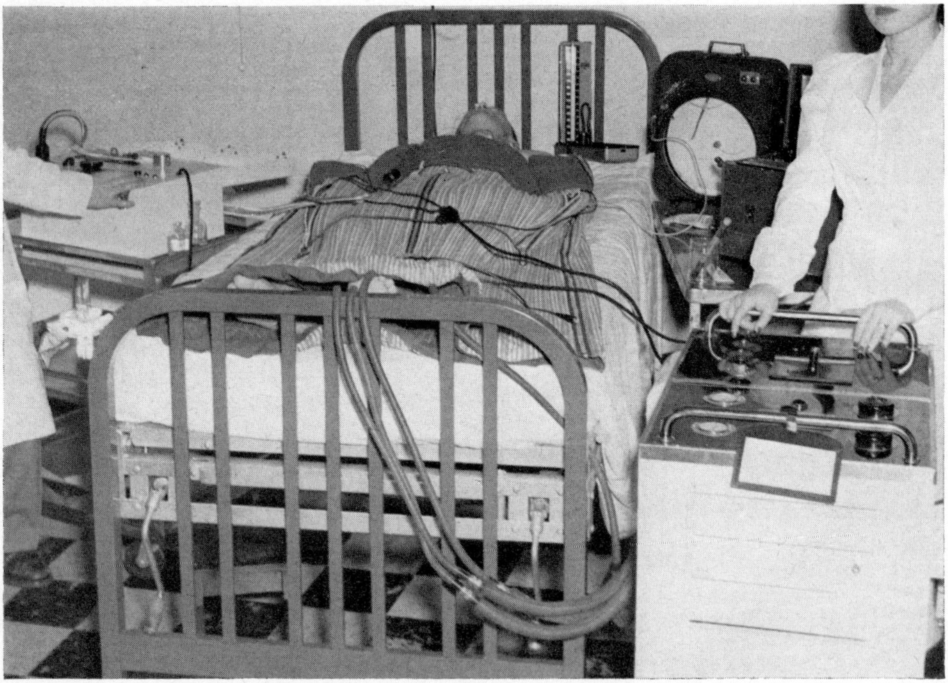

Fig. 3.—Refrigeration apparatus used in this experiment.

In the dog, the heart has been excluded from the circulation for periods up to fifteen minutes and the animals have recovered with no evidence of cerebral damage. The right atrium has been opened and interatrial septal defects have been created and repaired. Direct suture has been used for small defects, and a pedicle flap of the auricular appendage for large openings. This procedure has carried a 25 per cent mortality rate chiefly because of irreversible ventricular fibrillation. Because of this, it has been our feeling that cardiac surgery under hypothermia should be attempted only in desperate cases of patients with no chance of survival without operation and in whom operation is not feasible without the help of this technique. Three patients have had exploratory cardiotomy, one adult for an intracardiac tumor visualized on angiocardiography which proved to be a thrombus at operation and

Fig. 4.

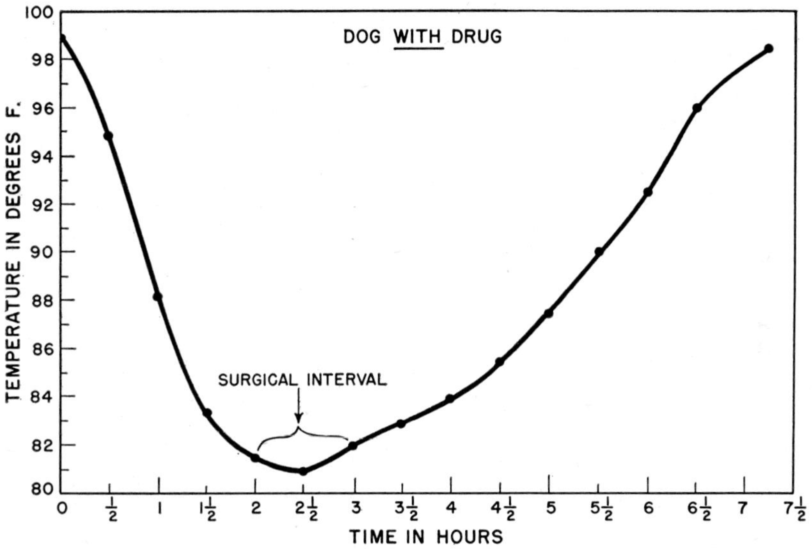

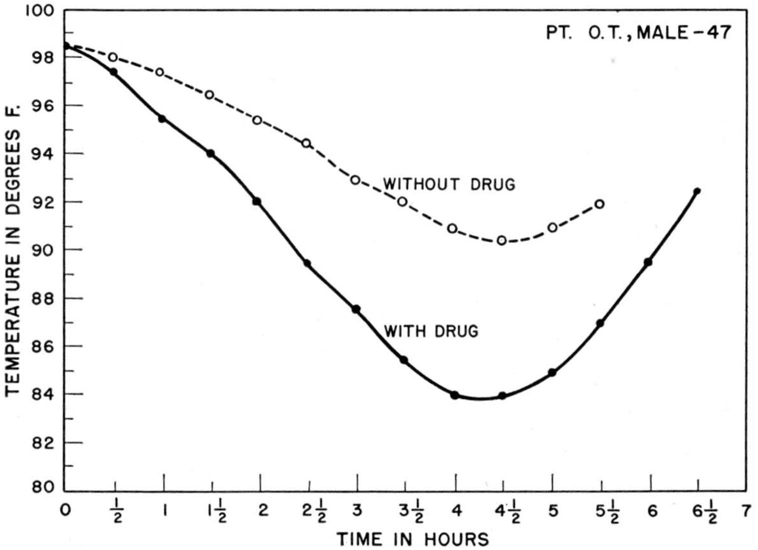

Fig. 5.

Fig. 4.—Temperature curve of dog refrigerated with Chlorpromazine. The smooth drop in temperature is obvious and there is no period of shivering.

Fig. 5.—Temperature curves in a patient refrigerated with and without Chlorpromazine. There is a more rapid drop to a lower temperature level with the drug.

two infants in terminal heart failure from septal defects. None survived operation, two developing ventricular fibrillation and one cardiac standstill.

In order to study the effects of hypothermia in the human being, seventeen patients have been subjected to artificial hibernation to control the hyperpyrexia in severe sepsis or to alleviate intractable pain due to inoperable carcinoma. All have recovered, but two developed cardiac irregularities (one, auricular fibrillation and one, ventricular extrasystoles) which reversed on rewarming. The other fifteen patients showed electrocardiographic changes related to decreased body temperature[8] but all reversed with no evidence of residual cardiac damage. It is noteworthy that in all patients developing significant arrhythmias the body temperature fell below the "safe level" of 80° F. Electroencephalographic studies revealed no abnormalities, and studies of renal function, liver function, and the circulating blood elements have shown no deleterious effects attributable to hypothermia.

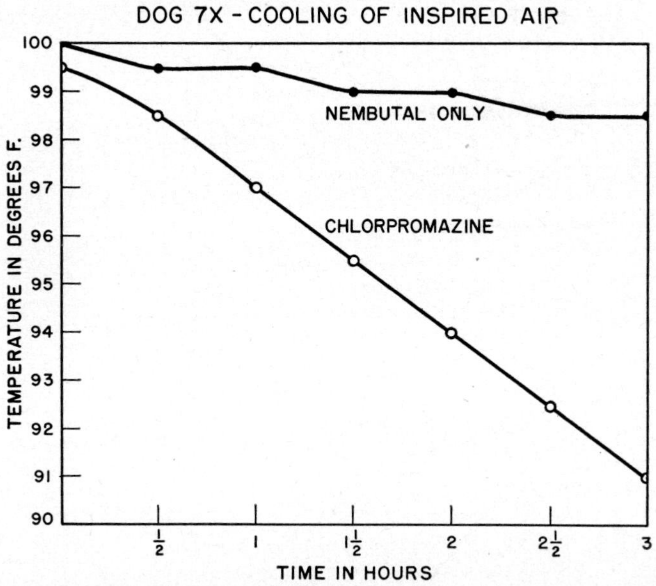

Fig. 6.—Temperature curves in a dog refrigerated by cooling the inspired air. With Chlorpromazine the temperature drops to a lower level.

The high incidence of cardiac complications is a limiting factor to the widespread use of the hypothermia technique in cardiac surgery at the present time. Further experimental work on the effect of cold on heart muscle and the mechanism of ventricular fibrillation is now being carried out in an attempt to obviate these complications. We feel, however, that this technique offers great possibilities for the future.

SUMMARY

1. A new technique for the production of a hypothermic state in the dog and in man has been described. This involves the use of refrigerated blankets

and a drug, Chlorpromazine, which exerts an inhibitory effect on the thermoregulatory center in mammals.

2. The only serious complication has been the high incidence of cardiac irregularities which have developed at low temperature levels (below 80° F.).

3. Hypothermia has a limited application at the present time and further experimental work is necessary to make this a safe procedure.

REFERENCES

1. Cookson, B. A., Neptune, W. B., and Bailey, C. P.: Hypothermia as a Means of Performing Intracardiac Surgery Under Direct Vision, Dis. Chest. **22:** 245, 1952.
2. Bigelow, W. G., Callahan, G. C., and Hopps, J. A.: General Hypothermia for Experimental Intracardiac Surgery, Ann. Surg. **132:** 531, 1950.
3. Lewis, F. J., and Taufic, M.: Closure of Atrial Septal Defects With the Aid of Hypothermia, SURGERY **33:** 52, 1953.
4. Huguenard, P.: Artificial Hibernation, Anesth. et analg. **9:** 240, 1952.
5. Laborit, H., Jaulmes, C., and Benitta, A.: Certain Experimental Aspects of Artificial Hibernation, Anesth. et analg. **9:** 232, 1952.
6. Alluaume, R.: Various Degrees of Artificial Hibernation, Anesth. et analg. **9:** 261, 1952.
7. Weiss, R., and Ripstein, C. B.: An Instrument for the Continuous Recording of Body Temperature, J. A. M. A. In press.
8. Wayburn, E.: Immersion Hypothermia, Arch. Int. Med. **79:** 77, 1947.

CLINICAL USE OF LEVO-ARTERENOL DURING CYCLOPROPANE ANESTHESIA

SYLVAN N. SURKS, M.D.,* AND NORTON M. LUGER, M.D.,** BROOKLYN, N. Y.

(From the Anesthesiology Section and Medical Service, Veterans Administration Hospital)

CARDIAC arrhythmias occur not infrequently with all the general anesthetic agents.[1, 2] In the presence of a heightened irritability of the myocardium occasioned by use of anesthetic drugs, small doses of epinephrine may cause such arrhythmias as premature beats, auriculoventricular block, slow ectopic rhythms, ventricular tachycardia, abnormal QRS complexes, and ventricular fibrillation.[3] These effects are more frequently noted in connection with the use of cyclopropane anesthesia.[4-6] For this reason most anesthesiologists prohibit the use of epinephrine during the administration of cyclopropane. Because of the structural similarity between epinephrine and levo-arterenol (l-norepinephrine) this interdiction has also been transferred to the latter drug.

In the course of our work in the treatment of shock with levo-arterenol,[7] forty-five patients were anesthetized with cyclopropane while receiving levo-arterenol by intravenous infusion. In none was there clinical evidence of toxicity.

Many of our patients were poor surgical risks in profound shock who had proved refractory to the usual blood- and fluid-replacement therapy and levo-arterenol was used to help treat the shock state. Without its use, a number of the operative procedures could not have been undertaken or would have had to be greatly curtailed. For these reasons, it was felt justified to try the supposedly dangerous combination of cyclopropane and levo-arterenol.

Clinical Material.—The clinical material on which we are reporting consisted of forty-five patients. Seven of these, in shock preoperatively, received levo-arterenol prior to and during the induction and maintenance of cyclopropane anesthesia. The operations involved consisted of:

1. Intra-abdominal procedures
   - (a) Perforated viscus (two cases)
   - (b) Intestinal obstruction (three cases)
   - (c) Total gastrectomy for bleeding carcinoma (one case)
2. Urologic procedure
   - (a) Suprapubic cystostomy for massive intravesical hemorrhage (one case).

Sponsored by the Veterans Administration and published with approval of Chief Medical Director. The statements and conclusions published by the authors are a result of their own study and do not necessarily reflect opinion or policy of Veterans Administration.

The levo-arterenol (l-norepinephrine) used in this study was supplied by the Department of Medical Research, Winthrop-Stearns, Inc., New York City.

Received for publication, March 2, 1953.

*Chief, Anesthesiology Section. Present address: Department of Anesthesiology, State University of New York, College of Medicine at New York City, Brooklyn, N. Y.

**Attending physician.

Thirty-eight other patients went into shock while undergoing operation and levo-arterenol therapy was initiated during the maintenance of cyclopropane anesthesia. The types of operative procedures included:

1. Intrathoracic procedures
   (a) Pneumonectomy (seven cases)
   (b) Lobectomy (four cases)
   (c) Repair of myocardial laceration (one case)
   (d) Thoracolumbar sympathectomy (ten cases)
2. Thoracoabdominal procedures
   (a) Splenorenal vein anastomosis (one case)
   (b) Esophagogastrectomy (one case)
   (c) Splenectomy (one case)
3. Intra-abdominal procedures
   (a) Abdominoperineal resection (two cases)
   (b) Colostomy (one case)
   (c) Revision of ileostomy (one case)
   (d) Resection of ileum for regional enteritis (one case)
   (e) Anterior resection for carcinoma of the sigmoid (one case)
   (f) Transverse colostomy for perforated rectum (one case)
4. Urologic procedures
   (a) Nephrectomy for carcinoma (three cases)
   (b) Nephrostomy for carcinoma of the bladder (one case)
   (c) Radical retropubic prostatectomy for carcinoma (one case)
5. Patient anesthetized but operation canceled because of persistent hypotension.

Administration of Levo-arterenol.—Levo-arterenol was administered by constant intravenous infusion, the rate (usually 1 to 3 c.c. per minute) depending on the adequacy of restoration of blood pressure. The concentration of the drug used was usually 8 μg per cubic centimeter. However, on rare occasions, concentrations as high as 16 μg per cubic centimeter were used.

Anesthetic Technique.—Twenty-three patients received cyclopropane with small amounts of ether and twenty-two received cyclopropane alone. Only small amounts of either anesthetic agent given infrequently were required by these patients, and depth of anesthesia was at no time judged to be below upper second plane. In all but three patients, anesthetics were administered via cuffed endotracheal tubes.

Results.—Continuous electrocardiographic observations were made in seven of the forty-five cases and at no time were changes of rhythm or contour noted. It is realized that cardiac arrhythmias which escape clinical detection may occur, but in none of our patients was there any clinical evidence of arrhythmia. No sudden deaths occurred. In twenty-three cases direct observation of the exposed heart disclosed no irregularity.

Nineteen patients had preoperative clinical and electrocardiographic evidence of moderate-to-severe myocardial disease. In several of these the surgical shock was so profound that hypoxia must have been present. After institution of levo-arterenol therapy, this group, like the others, did not show evidence of arrhythmia.

DISCUSSION

Of all the potent general anesthetics, cyclopropane appears to have the least deleterious effect on the peripheral circulation. Indeed, its central and peripheral circulatory effects are such as to be helpful in shock.[8-11] For this reason cyclopropane was chosen for these cases.

Since levo-arterenol became available for clinical use there has been hesitation in administering this pressor drug during cyclopropane anesthesia.[12] This hesitancy is based on experimental work done with laboratory animals. Garb and Chenoweth[6] used a dose of 30 μg per kilogram in a 2 c.c. volume administered as a single intravenous injection over a period of twenty seconds in cats deeply anesthetized with cyclopropane. They produced ventricular fibrillation with epinephrine in fourteen of twenty animals and with levo-arterenol in two of five cats.

Orth and associates,[5] in similar experiments on dogs, used single doses of 10 μg per kilogram in a 5 c.c. volume given intravenously over fifty seconds with deep cyclopropane anesthesia. They produced ventricular tachycardia in every one of twenty epinephrine-treated animals and in four of five levo-arterenol treated animals.

It should be noted that these doses are massive when compared to those we have used clinically. Our dosage of levo-arterenol usually ranges between 0.2 and 0.4 μg per kilogram per minute and rarely is higher while in Garb and Chenoweth's experiments the dose was 90 μg per kilogram per minute and in Orth's it was 12 μg per kilogram per minute. These represent 450 and 60 times, respectively, the dose we have used clinically. In addition, these laboratory experiments were carried out in deeply anesthetized animals.

Other workers, using the same laboratory animals, compared the effects of light and deep planes of cyclopropane anesthesia in the experimental production of ventricular fibrillation by epinephrine.[13, 14] They found that doses of intravenous epinephrine which produced ventricular fibrillation under deep anesthesia failed to do so during light cyclopropane anesthesia. It should be noted that all our patients were maintained in light planes of anesthesia.

There is one fully reported fatality in man from the combined use of epinephrine and cyclopropane.[4] This resulted from the injection of 2 c.c. of 1:1,000 epinephrine (2,000 μg) into four quadrants of the cervix for the purpose of producing an avascular field prior to a vaginal plastic operation. Waters[15] makes brief reference to a clinical case in which "accidental intravenous injection of 400 μg of epinephrine during cyclopropane anesthesia produced cardiac death." In another publication[16] he mentions one case in which intracardiac epinephrine during cyclopropane anesthesia caused death possibly due to ventricular fibrillation. The dose used in the latter case is not given. In these reported cases the amount of epinephrine used was of the order of magnitude injected experimentally to produce ventricular fibrillation.

It therefore seems reasonable to assume that these deaths resulted from the administration of unusually large doses of epinephrine during cyclopropane anesthesia.

It has been shown that the action of levo-arterenol is short lived and disappears within one to four minutes after termination of the infusion. For this reason, the appearance of arrhythmia would not seem to be as serious as with epinephrine, the cardiac effects of which may last as long as twenty-three minutes.[17, 18]

While the number of observations is small, we believe that the theoretical objections to the simultaneous use of levo-arterenol and cyclopropane, based on animal experiments and a few case reports, are not analogous to our clinical usage. When the combination of epinephrine and light cyclopropane anesthesia is used in animal experiments, arrhythmias are not produced. This more accurately reflects our clinical experience with cyclopropane and levo-arterenol. The combination appears to be safe and deserves further trial and study.

SUMMARY AND CONCLUSIONS

1. Forty-five patients in shock were given levo-arterenol by constant intravenous infusion during light cyclopropane anesthesia.

2. No untoward cardiocirculatory effects from this combination were noted. (Despite this, it is felt that the technique should be employed cautiously and discontinued in the event cardiac irregularities develop.)

3. The simultaneous administration of light cyclopropane anesthesia and a continuous intravenous infusion of dilute levo-arterenol does not appear to be as dangerous as hitherto believed.

REFERENCES

1. Kurtz, C. M., Bennett, J. H., and Shapiro, H. H.: Electrocardiographic Studies During Surgical Anesthesia, J. A. M. A. **106**: 434, 1936.
2. Meek, W. J., Hathaway, H. R., and Orth, O. S.: The Effects of Ether, Chloroform and Cyclopropane on Cardiac Automaticity, J. Pharmacol. & Exper. Therap. **61**: 240, 1939.
3. Burstein, C. L.: Misuse of Adrenalin and Coramine, Altered Drug Effects During Anesthesia, Am. J. Surg. **73**: 102, 1947.
4. Adelman, M. H.: Sudden Death During Cyclopropane-Ether Anesthesia Following the Administration of Epinephrine, Anesthesiology **2**: 657, 1941.
5. Orth, O. S., Leigh, M. D., Mellish, C. H., and Stutzman, C. H.: Action of Sympathomimetic Amines in Cyclopropane, Ether and Chloroform Anesthesia, J. Pharmacol. & Exper. Therap. **67**: 1, 1939.
6. Garb, S., and Chenoweth, M. B.: Studies on Hydrocarbon-Epinephrine Induced Ventricular Fibrillation, J. Pharmacol. & Exper. Therap. **94**: 12, 1948.
7. Fremont, R., Luger, N. M., Surks, S. N., and Kleiman, A.: Treatment of Surgical Shock With Levo-Arterenol. To be published.
8. Beecher, H. K.: Choice of Anesthesia for Seriously Wounded Patients, J. A. M. A. **121**: 899, 1943.
9. Hershey, S. G., and Rovenstine, E. A.: The Value of Cyclopropane in the Anesthetic Management of Patients With Recent Severe Hemorrhage, Anesthesiology **5**: 149, 1944.
10. Brace, D. E., Scherf, D., and Spire, L. J.: The Effect of Cyclopropane on the Blood Pressure, Stroke Volume and Heart Size of the Dog, Anesthesiology **2**: 261, 1941.
11. Hershey, S. G., and Zweifach, B. W.: Peripheral Vascular Hemeostasis in Relation to Anesthetic Agents, Anesthesiology **11**: 145, 1950.

12. Deterling, R. A., and Apgar, V.: The Use of Nor-Epinephrine (L-Arterenol) as a Pressor Drug With Special Reference to Thoraco-Lumbar Sympathectomy, Ann. Surg. **133**: 37, 1951.
13. Waters, R. M.: Present Status of Cyclopropane, Lancet **2**: 629, 1936.
14. Hutcheon, D. E.: Susceptibility to Ventricular Fibriilation During Chloroform and Cyclopropane Anesthesia, Brit. J. Pharmacol. **6**: 31-34, 1951.
15. Seevers, M. H., and Waters, R. M.: Pharmacology of the Anesthetic Gases, Physiol. Rev. **18**: 447, 1938.
16. Waters, R. M.: Present Status of Cyclopropane, Brit. M. J. **2**: 1013, 1936.
17. Fremont, R. E., Zelman, S., and Hart, R. W.: The Effect of L-Arterenol on Patients With Coronary Artery Disease. To be published.
18. Goldenberg, M., Pines, K. L., Baldwin, D. de F., Green, D. A., and Roh, C. H.: The Hemodynamic Response of Man to Nor-Epinephrine and Epinephrine and Its Relation to the Problem of Hypertension, Am. J. Med. **5**: 792, 1948.

COMPLICATIONS FOLLOWING THE USE OF EFOCAINE

DANIEL C. MOORE, M.D., SEATTLE, WASH.

(From the Department of Anesthesiology, The Mason Clinic and Virginia Mason Hospital)

DURING the past year and one-half, all reports reviewed in medical literature concerning the use of Efocaine have been favorable.[1-9] The drug has likewise been highly advertised by mail and at medical meetings. Comments such as the following have led to wider use of Efocaine: "Efocaine is a safe and effective local anesthetic that is indicated in the control of postoperative pain"[1]; "Local anesthesia with Efocaine may be advantageously used for intercostal nerve block as a means of postoperative pain control in upper abdominal surgery"[2]; "Efocaine, the aqueous, miscible, anesthetic agent is a safe, effective and highly desirable agent for the control of postoperative pain in ano-rectal surgery"[3]; "This drug is an effective means of pain control and is worthy of routine use in ano-rectal surgery"[6]; "Clinical study of this drug in more than 75 patients revealed that this agent was highly effective in the control of postoperative pain. There were no local or systemic toxic reactions; tissue sloughs or gross necrosis were not encountered."[7]

Judging from numerous inquiries I have received, many of the physicians who have not actually used Efocaine have read or heard about it. In our community, the public has been made aware by the newspapers and radio that a drug is now available which will render the postoperative period free of pain.

Despite the literature extolling Efocaine as a safe mixture, many isolated serious complications have arisen following its use. Evidently, these have not received wide enough attention, and not all have been reported. In view of all the favorable reports in the literature, physicians in whose practices these unfortunate problems have occurred may conclude that the complications were due to personal inexperience with the technique of regional analgesia employed and were not the fault of the drug. My associates and I might have reached the same conclusion except for the fact that in our institution in the past five years we have performed intercostal nerve blocks for surgical procedures and postoperative pain in over 2,000 patients, using one of the common local anesthetic agents, namely, Pontocaine (tetracaine) hydrochloride. Most of these patients had six or more intercostal nerves blocked at approximately the angles of the ribs. Our percentage of successful blocks in these patients is over 96 per cent.

Until we started to use Efocaine we did not encounter intercostal neuritis or paralysis following the blocks, although an occasional patient had tenderness at the site of the needle punctures. Of forty-one patients who received an intercostal Efocaine block for postoperative pain, the majority were free or partially relieved of pain and in eight instances the patients stated that they did not know

Received for publication, March 2, 1953.

where the incision was located. However, the first four patients in whom an intercostal block with Efocaine was performed, received 4 to 5 c.c. of the mixture, and three of these developed a severe intercostal neuritis.

When this occurred, we wrote Dr. R. W. Bartlett[10] since his experience with Efocaine in intercostal block was more extensive than ours. He answered that in their earlier cases he and his associates used 3 c.c. of Efocaine to each intercostal space but that this dose invariably caused local pain lasting up to four weeks. He also stated that with 1 to 1.5 c.c. doses of Efocaine he had gotten excellent relaxation and no instance of postoperative local pain. We then reduced our dose as recommended and never placed more than 2 c.c. of Efocaine under any one rib, yet in the next thirty-seven patients there still developed six severe cases of intercostal neuritis.

All of the nine patients with intercostal neuritis had identical reports. For the first two weeks following operation they were completely or relatively free of pain. They required little if any sedation. Most of them left the hospital in seven to ten days. After they had been home for from seven to ten days they noted pain which followed the course of one or all of the blocked intercostal nerves. The pain occurred not only at the site where the Efocaine was deposited, but radiated to the abdominal wall, and was characterized by burning which resembled a causalgia. The patients complained that contact with clothing or bed linen caused pain of a burning nature. This type of pain lasted for from two to six weeks before completely disappearing. Two of these patients consulted lawyers and intimated the possibility of legal action.

Because of our sizable previous experience with intercostal nerve blocks we did not believe our technique was faulty. However, our interest was stimulated, and from inquiries from colleagues at medical meetings we were able to find that we were not alone in having difficulties. Bonica[11] had six cases of postinjection neuritis in "over 100 cases." It is interesting to note that four of these cases of neuritis occurred in a series of twenty-five patients blocked intercostally for postoperative pain.[12] Eastwood[13] in a recent communication stated, "We have been using this drug and are beginning to have complications which may preclude its use on somatic nerves."

Four documented cases of transverse myelitis with varying degrees of severe paralysis were accumulated.[14-17]

Hubbard's[14] case occurred following a paravertebral lumbar sympathetic block with 3 c.c. of Efocaine at the level of the second lumbar vertebra. Three hours after the block the patient became partially paralyzed, retaining some motor power in her legs, mainly in the quadriceps and anterior tibials. Bladder control was lost but rectal control was retained. The patient's condition has not markedly improved in the last year.

Berg's[15] case followed a left decortication of the lung in which an intercostal block of the fifth, sixth, and seventh thoracic vertebrae for postoperative pain control was performed under direct vision using between 1 and 2 c.c. of Efocaine in each intercostal nerve, two to three inches from the intervertebral foramina. About six hours postoperatively, complete motor and sensory loss from approximately the level of the eighth thoracic vertebra caudad was noted. Twenty days postoperatively there was no appreciable change in the patient's condition. The patient died approximately two months following the operation from tuberculosis without great change in his paralyzed condition at the time of death. Autopsy revealed an area of avascular myelomalacia at about the fifth thoracic vertebra in the spinal cord. The dura and the meninges showed no evidence of arachnoiditis. The cord above and below the fifth thoracic vertebra was normal, as was the cauda equina.

Griffith's[16] case occurred following repair of a diaphragmatic hernia by the transthoracic approach. The ninth rib was resected during the procedure. Three c.c. of Efocaine were injected under direct vision into the eighth, ninth, and tenth intercostal nerves just distal to the tubercle of the ribs. The left phrenic nerve was also injected with 1 c.c. of Efocaine. On the first postoperative day the patient began to complain of urinary difficulty. He was made to get up to stimulate the desire to void. On the second postoperative day the patient was up and about but could not urinate and required catheterization. On the third postoperative day the patient complained of not being able to move his legs. Physical examination revealed (1) sensory loss below the level of the eighth thoracic vertebra, (2) complete motor paralysis of the left leg with positive Babinski reflex, and (3) almost complete motor loss of the right leg, but the patient could still weakly extend and flex toes on the right and the Babinski reflex was negative. The Efocaine was injected Nov. 10, 1952, and I saw the patient Dec. 13, 1952. At that time, Dr. Griffith demonstrated the fact that the patient was showing very slow improvement with return of sensation and partial return of the motor function of both legs. The patient is able to elevate slightly both legs, the right leg better than the left, but there is still a marked weakness and hypotonia of all muscles of the legs. Cystometrograms made Nov. 21, 1952, were consistent with atonic bladder. On repetition, Nov. 28, 1952, there was some evidence of improvement, and the patient had a desire to void when 400 c.c. were present in the bladder. Dr. Griffith feels that improvement will continue, but the prognosis for complete recovery is very poor.

During a discussion of Efocaine on a recent visit to Minneapolis, Dr. Knight and Dr. Luth[17] told me of a case of transverse myelitis following the use of Efocaine. The patient had been operated upon for a lesion which turned out to be a small tuberculoma of the lung. The fourth rib was resected during the operation. At the completion of the resection of the lesion 2 c.c. of Efocaine were injected intraneurally at the transverse processes of the second, third, fourth, fifth, and sixth thoracic vertebrae. On first postoperative day the patient exhibited the signs and symptoms of a transverse myelitis. The lesion was judged to be at the level of the sixth thoracic dermatome. It has been approximately two months since the injection, and the patient is showing some return of motion in the quadriceps and tibial group of muscles.

At first, it was difficult for us to understand how a solution placed two to three inches away from the spinal cord could cause a transverse myelitis. Dr. Ward[18] and Dr. Johnson,[19] Professor of Neurosurgery and Professor of Anatomy, respectively, at the University of Washington, were consulted, and they emphasized the fact that the perineural spaces of any peripheral nerve, while essentially filled with loose areolar tissue and so forth, are still continuous with those of their roots at least as far centrally as the spinal cord (Figs. 1 and 2). Dr. Ward[18] elucidated the subject by saying that if an adequate quantity of India ink is injected intraneurally into the sciatic nerve at the sciatic notch,

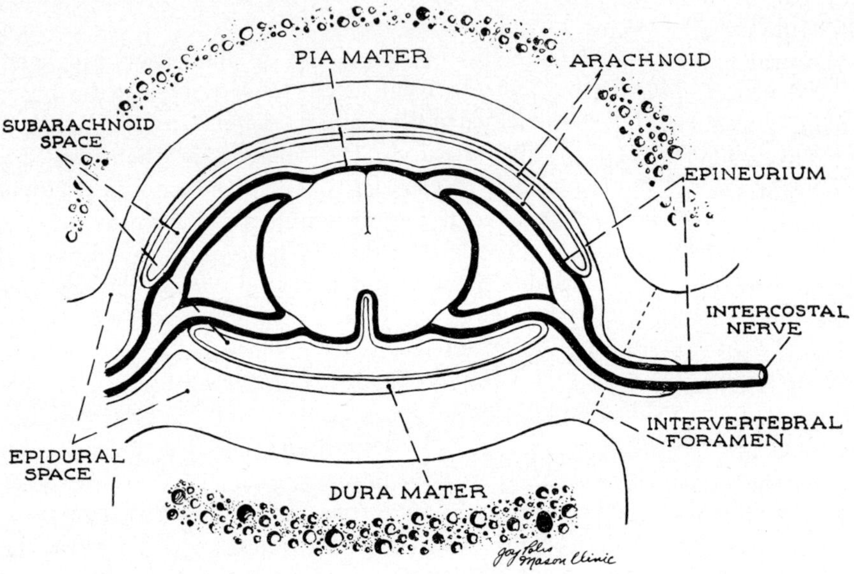

Fig. 1.—Cross section of the spinal cord. Note that the epineurium of the nerve is a continuation of the pia mater. This essentially makes a pathway for fluid injected intraneurally to undergo retrograde diffusion and reach the spinal cord.

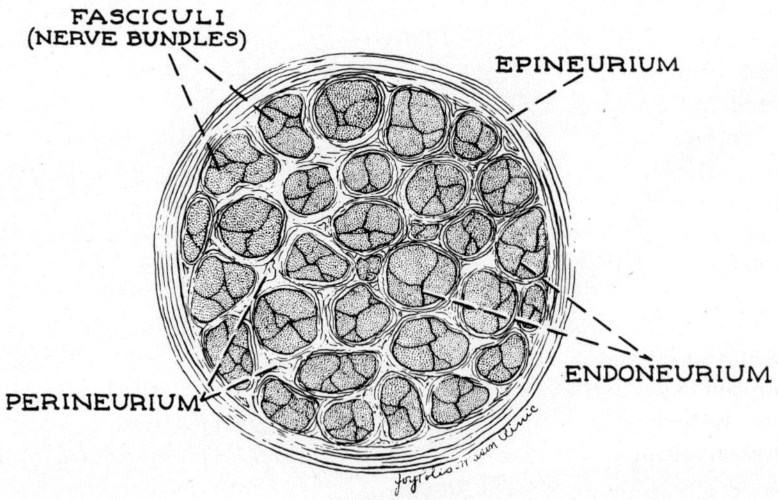

Fig. 2.—Cross section of an intercostal nerve. Note that while the interstices between the nerve bundles (fasciculi) are filled with connective tissue called perineurium, they are potential avenues for retrograde diffusion of materials injected intraneurally.

the ink can be found in the subarachnoid space from minutes to hours later. This retrograde diffusion could be the explanation of the transverse myelitis which has occurred with Efocaine.

In addition to transverse myelitis and intercostal neuritis from Efocaine, cellulitis and sloughs have been noted, although to date I have not seen any. However, Hubbard[14] has seen severe cellulitis following block of the facial nerve with 2 c.c. of Efocaine, block of the coccygeal nerves bilaterally with 2 c.c. of Efocaine on each nerve, block of the perirectal area with 4 c.c. of Efocaine, and bilateral block of the perineum with 3 c.c. of Efocaine on each side. The signs and symptoms of cellulitis lasted from seven to ten days in these cases. Dr. Knight and Dr. Luth[17] also told me of a slough of the tissue around the anus. This occurred in a doctor, following the injection of 1 c.c. of Efocaine on each side of the rectum to relieve postoperative pain of a hemorrhoidectomy. The slough necessitated additional hospitalization of approximately five weeks. Spano[20] has had three cases of ischiorectal abscesses following the injection of Efocaine into the rectal sphincter to relieve the postoperative pain of a hemorrhoidectomy.

The exact cause of these reactions where Efocaine has been used is to date not solved. Efocaine is a mixture composed of "1 per cent Procaine and 0.25 per cent Procaine hydrochloride as the anesthetic base, 5 per cent butyl-p-amino-benzoate, 2 per cent polyethylene glycol-300, and 78 per cent propylene glycol as the aqueous-miscible solvent, and 0.1 per cent sodium metabisulfate and 1:2,500 phenyl mercuric borate as the preservatives."[21] Weinberg[22] states, "The subcutaneous, intramuscular and perineural injection of Efocaine produces no significant permanent damage to the tissue involved and is the same order as that seen following the injection of procaine or penicillin-in-oil. The injection of Efocaine does not result in a foreign body giant cell reaction. There is no apparent permanent storage of Efocaine at the site of injection."

It must be pointed out that Weinberg's experiments were conducted using rabbits, guinea pigs, and rats, and the tissue reactions may not be identical with those in man. He attributed the focal degeneration of the myelin sheath in injected brachial plexuses of rabbits as being caused by the injection of a large volume of the drug rather than by the drug itself. Perhaps in view of the side results of Efocaine in the human being, this should be reinvestigated. It is interesting to note in our patients with neuritis that the neuritis did not occur until a period of two weeks elapsed, and then its characteristics resembled those which are often seen when a peripheral nerve is regenerating.

SUMMARY

Cases of neuritis, transverse myelitis, cellulitis, tissue slough, and abscess following the use of Efocaine are cited.

How Efocaine injected paravertebrally and intercostally can result in transverse myelitis has been proposed.

CONCLUSIONS

Some of the complications observed may only be coincidental with the use of Efocaine rather than be caused by the mixture itself, but nevertheless they have occurred often enough so that Efocaine as the responsible factor cannot be disregarded. Perhaps before injecting Efocaine it is best to consider this question: When a drug or mixture is capable of producing transverse myelitis, intercostal neuritis, or a tissue slough, should it be used routinely in patients whose pain is only temporary in nature, for example, postoperative pain, and in whom surgery for a curable disease such as diaphragmatic hernia is being performed?

REFERENCES

1. Iason, A. H., and Shaftel, H. E.: A New Approach to the Problem of Postoperative Pain, Am. J. Surg. **83**: 549-555, 1952.
2. Puderbach, W. J., and Shaftel, H. E.: Prolonged Intercostal Nerve Block in Upper Abdominal Surgery, Lancet **72**: 203-208, 1952.
3. Raicus, E.: Postoperative Anesthetics in Anorectal Surgery, Med. Times, March, 1952.
4. Gross, J. M., and Shaftel, H. E.: The Role of Efocaine in Anorectal Anesthesia and Analgesia, New York State J. Med. **52**: 1413-1417, 1952.
5. Deaton, W. R., and Bradshaw, H. H.: A Long-lasting Local Anesthetic Solution—Use in Thoracic Surgery, Am. Surgeon **18**: 616-620, 1952.
6. Tucker, C. C.: The Control of Postoperative Pain in Ano-Rectal Surgery, J. Kansas M. Soc. **52**: 230-235, 1952.
7. Ansboro, F. P., Iason, A. H., Shaftel, H. E., Halpern, A., Latteri, F. S., and Bodell, B.: A New Approach to Prolonged Local Anesthesia, the Development of Efocaine, Anesthesiology **13**: 306-319, 1952.
8. Bartlett, R. W., and Eastwood, D. W.: Long-acting Bilateral Intercostal Nerve Block for Upper Abdominal Surgery, Surgery **32**: 956-960, 1952.
9. Bartlett, R. W.: Prolonged Anesthesia for Upper and Lower Abdominal Surgery With Bilateral Intercostal Nerve Block. Brief of paper from the program of the Western Surgical Meeting, Houston, Texas.
10. Bartlett, R. W.: Personal communication.
11. Bonica, J. J.: Management of Intractable Pain, J. A. M. A. **150**: 1581-1586, 1952.
12. Bonica, J. J.: Personal communication.
13. Eastwood, D. W.: Personal communication.
14. Hubbard, S. T.: Personal communication.
15. Berg, R.: Personal communication.
16. Griffith, C. A.: Personal communication.
17. Knight, R. T., and Luth, D. V.: Personal communication.
18. Ward, A.: Personal communication.
19. Johnson, R.: Personal communication.
20. Spano, J. P.: Personal communication.
21. E. Fougera and Co., Inc. (Brochure).
22. Weinberg, T.: A Study of the Effects of Efocaine Upon Nerves, Muscles, Skin and Subcutaneous Tissue, Fougera Scientific Research Bulletin **2**: (Jan.) 1952.

THORACIC NEURENTERIC CYST

George W. Holcomb, Jr., M.D., and Donald D. Matson, M.D., Boston, Mass.

(From the Surgical and Neurosurgical Services of the Children's Medical Center and the Department of Surgery, Harvard Medical School)

RECENTLY a large retropleural thoracic cyst resulting from persistence of an accessory neurenteric canal was encountered in a child who complained of persistent cough and wheezing. Because of its rarity, embryologic interest, and suitability for satisfactory surgical treatment if properly recognized, its diagnostic, pathologic, and therapeutic features seemed worthy of description.

CASE REPORT

P. P. (A379247), a 4½-year-old boy, entered the Children's Medical Center Nov. 2, 1951, because of severe cough and wheezing respirations of nine months' duration. His father complained that because of the wheezing it was impossible for anyone to sleep in the same room with him. He remained afebrile and the cough was productive only rarely of small amounts of mucus. However, one week prior to admission he did cough up two teaspoonsful of bright blood following a prolonged paroxysm.

Family history was not contributory and the delivery was uneventful. He had whooping cough as an infant. Mental development was commensurate with the other eleven children of the family, although he was somewhat small for his age.

Physical examination revealed a pale underdeveloped boy who was dyspneic and obviously in acute respiratory distress. Temperature was 101° and pulse 100. The trachea was deviated to the left. His neck was short, suggesting a Klippel-Feil syndrome, and there was mild kyphoscoliosis most pronounced at the third dorsal vertebra. There was no irregularity of the overlying skin in this area. Respiratory excursions were labored but equal bilaterally and there was no sternal retraction. Coarse rales were audible over both lung fields. Neurological examination elicited no motor, sensory, or reflex abnormalities. The patient had normal rectal and bladder sphincter control.

Roentgenologic examination revealed multiple congenital anomalies of the spine extending from the fifth cervical vertebra to the fifth dorsal vertebra characterized by unmatched hemivertebrae and spina bifida. The vertebral bodies of the first dorsal vertebra through the fourth dorsal vertebra appeared fused. In the region of the third dorsal vertebra there was an anterior circular defect measuring 1.6 cm. in diameter (Fig. 1). A soft tissue mass in the superior-posterior mediastinum projected toward the right and produced forward displacement of the trachea.

Myelography showed deflection but no obstruction to the passage of the opaque medium in this region and none of it entered the extraspinal mass. It was concluded that the lesion was an anterior meningocele which protruded through the large vertebral defect into the right hemithorax and that the neck of the sac had probably become sealed off from the subarachnoid space.

On Nov. 9, 1951, laminectomy was performed at the third and fourth dorsal vertebrae (by D. D. M.). The spinal canal was markedly widened in the area of the spina bifida. The dorsal dura was intact and normal in appearance but almost twice normal width. It was opened revealing a normal-appearing spinal cord except for atrophy of nerve roots on the right. After dividing the dentate ligaments and two or three of the atrophic dorsal rootlets, the cord was rotated to expose a stalk approximately 5 to 6 mm. in diameter which

Received for publication, Feb. 9, 1953.

emerged from the middle of the anterior surface of the cord and passed through a circular defect in the anterior dura and vertebral body. The stalk was solid and appeared to be fibrous tissue which merged intimately with the ventral surface of the cord. Adhesions to the stalk were divided, following which it was doubly ligated with silk and divided. A patch, 1.5 by 1.5 cm., of the redundant dorsal dura was used as a free graft to close the defect in the anterior dura, and routine closure of the rest of the wound carried out. Convalescence was uneventful and the patient was discharged on Dec. 2, 1951.

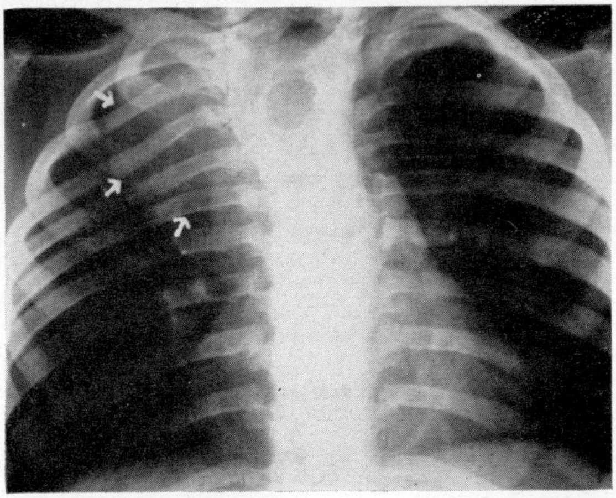

Fig. 1.—Anteroposterior chest roentgenogram which reveals a mass at the right apex (outlined by arrows). Note multiple anomalies of vertebral bodies fifth cervical through fourth dorsal vertebrae and the 1.6 cm. defect which was traversed by a stalk extending from the neurenteric cyst to the anterior spinal cord surface.

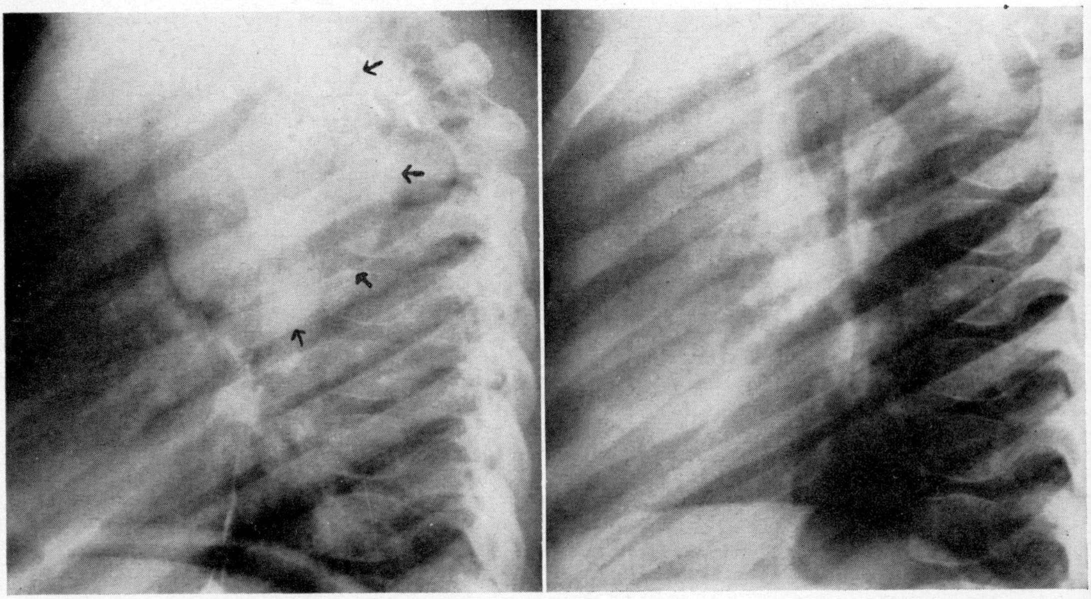

A. *B.*

Fig. 2.—*A,* Lateral chest roentgenogram prior to thoracotomy showing forward tracheal displacement produced by the large intrathoracic mass.

B, The same view five months after thoracotomy illustrating return of trachea to normal position.

Symptoms of tracheal compression persisted and roentgen examination revealed no significant decrease in size of the intrathoracic mass (Fig. 2, *A*). Therefore, the patient was readmitted to the hospital and thoracotomy was performed on Feb. 1, 1952 (by G. W. H.). The pleural cavity was entered through the right fourth intercostal space cutting the fifth and fourth ribs posteriorly. A smooth rounded mass which occupied the posterior apical portion of the right hemithorax (Fig. 3) was easily seen. Following division of the azygos vein the pleura was incised and the cystic mass exposed. Palpation indicated that this was probably not a meningocele because it had a very thick wall. Viscid mucoid material, which bore no resemblance to spinal fluid, was aspirated. The cyst wall measured from 0.5 to 1.0 cm. in thickness, and its lining resembled intestinal mucosa suggesting the possibility that this was an esophageal duplication. Dissection of the mass was accomplished except for its posterior attachments to the vertebral bodies and ribs. Following excision of the redundant cyst wall, the resultant small cavity was obliterated by folding in the remaining tissue with three layers of silk. The dural graft previously placed over the circular vertebral defect was intact. Pleura was approximated and the chest was closed without drainage. The postoperative course was uncomplicated and symptoms of tracheal compression disappeared entirely (Fig. 2, *B*). Eleven months later the patient continues to be symptom free.

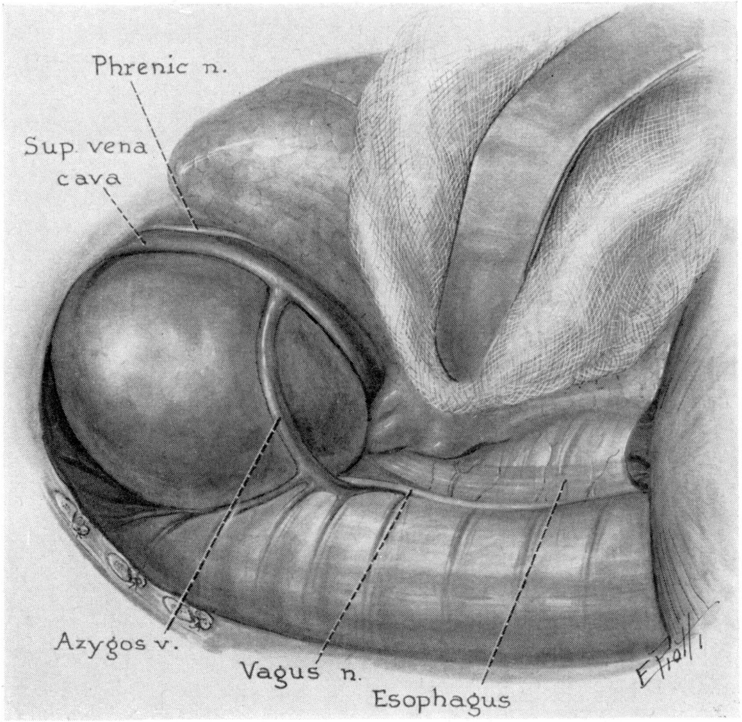

Fig. 3.—Appearance of the retropleural mass at operation.

The cyst wall showed no evidence of inflammation. Microscopically the mucosa varied from pseudostratified columnar epithelium to a single layer of cuboidal cells. Deep to a loose submucosa were two thick layers of interwoven muscle fibers. Nerve bundles and blood vessels were scattered throughout the muscle fibers.

It would be impossible to distinguish this lesion from a duplication of the esophagus by microscopic examination. Grossly, however, there were two important features which suggested another origin: (1) a duplication is usually intimately fused with the esophageal muscle layer whereas this anomaly had no such relationship; (2) the presence of a fistulous tract extending from the cyst through the vertebral defect and dura to the anterior surface of the cord strongly suggested that the etiology was related to an accessory neurenteric canal.

EMBRYOLOGY

Early in the development of the human embryo there is a small connection between the yolk sac and surface of the embryo called the neurenteric canal. This fistulous structure traverses the primitive knot and connects the future enteric cavity with the neural groove in the region of the coccyx. Bremer[1] drew a distinction between this short lasting neurenteric canal and any patent or solid tract which might occur between the alimentary tract and the dorsal midline structures cephalad to the coccygeal tip. He stated that the latter condition represents an ectopic or accessory neurenteric canal because the primitive knot is not traversed. He cited the experimental work of Lereboullet,[1] who, in 1868, following artificial insemination of pike embryos, noticed that some specimens had longitudinal clefts extending between normal heads and normal tails thus exposing the yolk-sac surfaces. By delaying fertilization until frog ova were overripe, Hertwig,[2] in 1892, was able to produce similar conditions. These experimentally produced open clefts have all characteristics of the minute human neurenteric canal but differ from it in the large size and more cephalad location of the former. Bremer[1] referred to reports in the literature of three stillborn infants each with wide-open clefts between the spinal cord and different portions of the alimentary tract (pharynx, esophagus, stomach, and intestine) which provided direct communication from the lumen of these structures to the dorsal cutaneous surfaces.

Just as it is possible to find vitelline-duct remnants varying from a patent tube connecting the ileum and umbilicus, to a cyst in the center with a patent tract either to the skin or to the ileum, or to a solid fibrous band, and most often there is no remnant at all, so will the dorsal neurenteric fistula occasionally persist in one of these many forms. The outstanding difference is that while the vitelline duct traverses a cavity, no evidence of its former presence can be found after it disappears. The neurenteric fistula, on the other hand, passes through all the dorsal midline structures and usually leaves some permanent evidence of its former presence such as: (1) a widened vertebral body resulting from bony proliferation in an attempt to fill the gap following disappearance of the tract; (2) a circular defect in the body of a vertebra produced by persistence of a tract which forces bone to form around it; (3) a bony or cartilaginous spur which projects into the spinal canal delaying union of the vertebral halves to the extent that independent pedicular processes form. When these finally do unite, following disappearance of the dorsal fistula at a time later than normal, the pedicular processes fuse to form a median spur. This condition is known as diastematomyelia. Recalling its embryologic origin, it is possible that the entire neurenteric sinus might persist rather than only a segement as occurred in this case. Keen and Coplin[3] reported such a lesion, in 1906, which was found in the sacral region of a 2-year-old girl. This tube measured 4 to 5 mm. in diameter and extended from the dorsal rectal wall through a sacral vertebral defect and the nerve roots of the cauda equina to the skin.

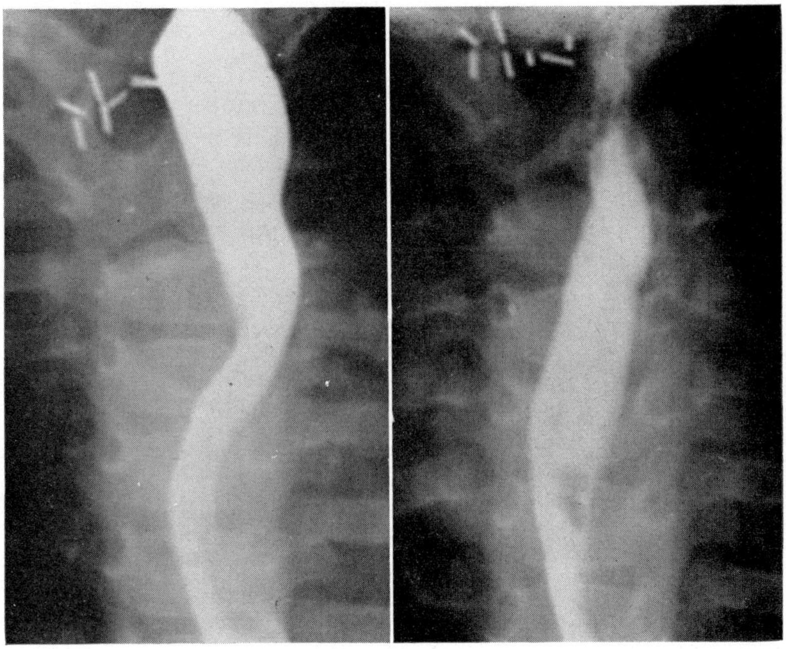

A. *B.*

Fig. 4.—*A*, Anteroposterior roentgenogram of barium-filled upper esophagus indicating deviation to left produced by the expanding retropleural neurenteric cyst. Note the normal esophageal indentation on the left side below this level produced by the aortic arch.

B, Roentgenogram five months following operation illustrating normal position of the esophagus.

SYMPTOMATOLOGY

Symptoms produced by such an anomaly naturally will depend upon the anatomic location of the persisting embryologic tract. In this case, there was no esophageal or cutaneous connection and the spinal cord itself was not actually malformed although the stalk did merge into its anterior surface. The expanding cyst produced tracheal compression which resulted in severe cough accompanied by a loud, wheezing type of respiration. There was not sufficient obstruction of the esophagus to interfere with deglutition. Had the fetal type of pseudostratified epithelium progressed to form gastric mucosa, a severe inflammatory process might have resulted from secretion of hydrochloric acid and pepsin. Mucosal ulceration with inflammation spreading to the surrounding structures could produce marked irritation and symptoms even in the absence of a large expanding mass. Perforation into the pleural cavity, the trachea, or the esophagus with disastrous results might follow such an intense chemical reaction. A simple fistula from the esophagus to the back would allow liquids to flow out the external orifice and would call attention to the abnormality early in life. Meningitis might appear any time after birth if such an esophageal fistula terminated in the subarachnoid space.

ROENTGEN EXAMINATION

Roentgen examination of such a patient usually will be informative but not always diagnostic. In this case, the circular defect in the body of the third dorsal vertebra, associated with a mass projecting into the right thoracic cavity, suggested the presence of an anterior meningocele. Barium swallow indicated displacement of the esophagus to the opposite side although the obstruction was not sufficient to produce symptoms (Fig. 4). A tracheogram did not seem indicated because it was obvious from the symptoms and the location of the lesion that this structure was being compressed (Fig. 2). Myelogram revealed widening of the neural canal in the cervical and upper dorsal regions. No dye passed anteriorly into the cyst. The dye distributed itself around this defect in such a manner as to outline quite sharply its circumscribed margin, all of which suggested that there was some connection between the anterior mass and the subarachnoid space although not necessarily a patent one. There does not appear to be any method by which this lesion could positively be differentiated from an anterior meningocele on roentgen examination.

TREATMENT

Persistence of any portion of a dorsal intestinal fistula (accessory neurenteric canal) should be treated by surgical excision as soon as symptoms call attention to its presence. It may be impossible to remove the outer cyst wall entirely because of adhesion to other structures although this is certainly desirable. In such instances it is permissible to excise the redundant portion and fold the remaining wall in to obliterate the cavity. However, if aspiration reveals the cyst contents to be acid or bloody, the importance of completely excising the lesion or of stripping away any remaining mucous membrane cannot be overemphasized. When a stalk penetrates the spinal canal, dura, and subarachnoid space, meticulous care must be taken to close the meningeal defect either directly or by grafting or approximation of the overlying soft tissues. This obviously implies division of any connections with the spinal cord itself. Great care should be exercised to manipulate the spinal cord as little as possible and to avoid injury to any intraspinal structure which might contain functioning neural tissue.

SUMMARY

The case of a 4½-year-old boy complaining of repeated upper respiratory infections, persistent cough, and loud wheezing is described. Examination revealed multiple spinal anomalies including a circular defect of the vertebral body of the third dorsal vertebra associated with a right intrathoracic mass. This was incorrectly diagnosed preoperatively as an anterior meningocele. Laminectomy was first performed, a fibrous stalk attached to the anterior-cord surface was severed, and the anterior dural defect was closed. Thoracotomy with subtotal excision of the retropleural cyst wall and complete obliteration of the remaining cyst cavity was performed three months later. Microscopic examination of the specimen revealed fetal intestinal epithelium and layers of smooth muscle which resembled duplication of the esophagus. We are indebted to Bremer[1] who clarified the embryologic origin of this interesting lesion. He stated that it is a cyst of neurenteric origin which retained its dorsal spinal connection but lost both remaining distal segments (esophageal and cutaneous). The patient had a successful recovery and remains symptom free.

REFERENCES

1. Bremer, J. L.: Dorsal Intestinal Fistula; Accessory Neurenteric Canal; Diastematomyelia, Arch. Path. **54**: 132-138, 1952.
2. Hertwig, O.: Urmund und Spina bifida; eine vergleichend morphologische, teratologische Studie an missgebildeten Froscheiern. Arch. f. mikr. Anat. **39**: 353-530, 1892.
3. Keen, W. W., and Coplin, W. M. L.: Sacrococcygeal Tumor (Teratoma) With an Opening Entirely Through the Sacrum, and a Sinus Passing Through This Opening and Communicating With the Rectum, the Sinus Resembling a Bronchus, Surg., Gynec. & Obst. **3**: 661-671, 1906.

Editorial

Dangers of Conservative Surgery in Abdominal Emergencies*

IN THE era before antibiotics, modern anesthesia, and the blood bank, many surgeons were fearful of performing extensive and definitive operations on patients who were desperately ill as a result of abdominal catastrophes. Shock was interpreted as a contraindication to surgical intervention, localized peritonitis was considered a reason for avoiding exploration, and the philosophy of the surgeon was to do as little as possible and to hope for the best.

Developments in surgical technique, in anesthesia, and in the physician's ability to control hypotension and infection have resulted in a reversal of the age-old policy of conservative treatment in certain types of desperately ill patients. It is now being recognized that a definitive operation, although extensive and perhaps prolonged, is safer than a smaller operation which does not accomplish its purpose. Surgeons now realize that it is not the operation which causes the death of critically ill patients but the disease for which the operation is being performed. If the operation does not correct the pathology, the patient is doomed and might as well have had no operation at all.

Several examples of this new type of thinking can be found in the field of abdominal surgery. For many years surgeons have believed that a loop ileostomy was the safest treatment for a patient with fulminating or acutely toxic ulcerative colitis. They disregarded the fact that the ileostomy did not remove the source of the toxicity, that the danger of perforation was not removed, and that the patients still could bleed to death or lose enormous quantities of protein from defunctionalized colons. Fear that the friable bowel might be perforated during its removal and that fatal peritonitis might ensue prevented them from performing ileostomy and simultaneous colectomy. Today we recognize that the mortality rate of operations for acute toxic ulcerative colitis is lower if the colon is removed and the disease eradicated. Since the discovery of the antibiotics, we have lost our fear of contamination peritonitis and no longer view a perforation of the colon at operation as an irrevocable tragedy. A leak that continuously pours the contents of the bowel into the peritoneal cavity, as may happen after ileostomy, is still as fatal as ever, but contamination, if followed by an adequate peritoneal toilet, is likely to be of little consequence.

Perforations of the colon, such as occasionally occur with carcinoma or diverticulitis, are sometimes managed by inadequate operations which fail to deal directly and completely with the perforation itself. In the past, it was considered good practice to treat a patient with a free perforation of the

*From the Cleveland Clinic and the Frank E. Bunts Educational Institute.

sigmoid by transverse colostomy. This diversion of the fecal stream was supposed to limit the amount of contamination and result in a localization of the peritonitis. Surgeons were afraid to attack the cause of the peritonitis directly for fear of spreading the infection. Today, with the protection afforded by antibiotics, there is little excuse for such half-hearted measures, even in patients who are desperately ill. It appears that a direct attack on the source of the contamination, with exteriorization or resection of the involved segment, drainage of abscesses, and aspiration of as much as possible of the pus and feces in the peritoneal cavity, affords the patient the best chance of survival.

The wheel of surgical practice threatens to make a complete turn toward the days when surgeons eviscerated patients with peritonitis and lavaged their intestines in antiseptic solutions. Valueless as the antiseptics have proved, nevertheless a thorough peritoneal lavage with removal of as much pus and foreign material as possible is today practicable and worth while. Any contamination of clean parts of the cavity can be controlled by antibiotic therapy. Most important is the elimination of the source of contamination. If this is done, the patient has a better chance of recovery than he does following a small operation which diverts the fecal stream but leaves a leaking column of stool below the colostomy.

The same principles apply to the treatment of acute gastroduodenal hemorrhage and other abdominal emergencies. The surgeon, the anesthetist, and the blood bank should be prepared not to sustain the patient for a minimum procedure but to support him during a definitive operation. It is the disease, not the operation, that causes death, and the first responsibility of the surgeon is to eradicate the disease.

—*George Crile, Jr.*

Recent Advances in Surgery

CONDUCTED BY ALFRED BLALOCK, M.D.

TREATMENT OF TUMORS OF THE PAROTID SALIVARY GLAND

IRVING M. ARIEL, M.D., ANTHONY P. JEROME, M.D., AND GEORGE T. PACK, M.D., NEW YORK, N. Y.

(From the Pack Medical Group)

INTRODUCTION

THE inadequacy of past methods of treating parotid tumors has produced a high rate of recurrences and treatment failures, which has resulted in confusion concerning the natural history of parotid neoplasms. Many physicians believed that parotid tumors originated from multicentric foci, and they attributed the high recurrence rate to the concept that new tumors developed after the treated ones had been cured. Another empiric and fallacious practice was that advanced by McFarland, who believed that the recurrence rate was lower when the larger parotid tumors were excised; therefore, he advocated the practice of watchful waiting until the tumor became "ripe" before excising it.[27, 28]

It has been determined that most tumors arise as a single nidus and gradually grow to infiltrate the glandular parenchyma and sometimes to compress or infiltrate the facial nerve. The high recurrence rate is the result of inadequate removal because of fear of damaging the nerve. After a period of growth, malignant parotid tumors will invade contiguous cervical tissues, infiltrate into the pterygomandibular space, produce metastases to regional lymph nodes, or disseminate by way of the blood stream to distant organs.

The purpose of this review is to present criteria for treating parotid neoplasms and to describe surgical techniques which will permit their resection without damaging the facial nerve unless the nerve has been invaded by cancer, in which case it is sacrificed. The technique to be described has been utilized in a large number of patients with gratifying results. Histologic features and nosology of parotid neoplasms have been adequately described and will not be labored in this review.[20, 31, 42] One hundred patients with parotid tumors treated at the Pack Medical Group are analyzed to glean an insight into those factors by which an early diagnosis can be established, the type of anatomic structure determined, and the results of the therapy analyzed.

CLASSIFICATION OF PAROTID TUMORS

For determining the type and extent of treatment for different parotid neoplasms the simplest and most adequate classification into which the majority fit is arrived at by merely subdividing the group into (1) benign epithelial tumors (mixed tumors are the most frequent), (2) malignant epithelial

Received for publication, Nov. 9, 1952.

tumors (carcinoma), and (3) miscellaneous, which includes a heterogeneous group comprised of other than epithelial elements.

Complete classifications have been presented recently by Rawson and associates,[42] Kirklin and co-workers,[20] Marshall and Miles,[31] and Stein and Geschickter.[47] Such a complete classification is of importance in understanding the pathologic development of the salivary gland cellular elements and in determining the radiosensitivity of certain tumors, and is of prognostic value.

CLASSIFICATION OF PAROTID TUMORS*

- A. Benign epithelial tumors
  - 1. Mixed tumor
  - 2. Papillary cystadenoma lymphomatosum (Wharton's tumor)
  - 3. Sebaceous gland tumor
  - 4. Adenoma
    - a. Ordinary adenoma
    - b. Oncocytic adenoma
- B. Malignant epithelial tumors
  - 1. Cylindroma
  - 2. Malignant papillary cystadenoma
  - 3. Adenocarcinoma
  - 4. Squamous-cell carcinoma
  - 5. Undifferentiated carcinoma
  - 6. Mixed carcinoma (mucoepidermoid carcinoma)
- C. Miscellaneous tumors
  - 1. Benign
    - a. Cysts
    - b. Lipoma
    - c. Neurofibroma
    - d. Lymphocytic tumor
    - e. Hemangioendothelioma
  - 2. Malignant
    - a. Neurosarcoma
    - b. Fibrosarcoma
    - c. Melanoma
    - d. Lymphosarcoma
    - e. Hodgkin's disease

It is difficult at times to establish the exact pathologic type because salivary gland tumors may develop rather bizarre formations or combinations to preclude a clear-cut classification of type. Not infrequently, an apparently benign tumor will show infiltration of the capsule while others will have one locus which is malignant and will produce distant blood-borne metastases. Such unusual behavior of parotid neoplasms makes essential a complete understanding of the natural history of this oncologic entity in order that proper criteria for therapy be established and exact techniques developed.

CLINICAL FEATURES

Incidence.—There have been approximately 20,000 patients with tumors observed at the Pack Medical Group of which 100 were of the parotid gland.

*After Rawson, Howard, Royster, and Horn.[42]

Thus, parotid neoplasms represent 0.5 per cent of all neoplasms. Hellwig[15] described an incidence of 2 per cent of 4,352 tumors at Wichita, Kan. Schreiner and Mattick[44] noted an incidence of salivary tumors of 1 per cent at the State Institute for Maligant Diseases at Buffalo, N. Y. Its rarity is stressed by McFarland,[27] who collected only 310 mixed tumors in the course of twenty-five years in Philadelphia. Ahlbom[1] observed only 254 tumors of the salivary gland during twenty years at the Radiumhemmet, which institute treats patients with neoplasms from the entire country of Sweden.

It is difficult to compare the true incidence in relationship to other neoplasms since certain treatment centers have disproportionate numbers of patients bearing parotid tumors referred to them. These larger series treated by certain standard regimes have become available for comparative purposes and supply data for understanding the natural history and methods of treatment of parotid neoplasms.

Etiology.—There is no definite factor or group of factors in this series which could account for the production of these tumors. Analysis of the data does not reveal any correlation between such factors as poor oral hygiene, previous infection, associated diseases such as syphilis or tuberculosis, or repeated trauma to account for the development of the neoplasm.

Age.—In this series the average age of the 100 patients with tumors of the parotid gland was 45.2 years. The average age for patients with benign tumors was 36.1 years, the youngest patient was 7.5 years old, and the oldest was 62 years old. In the 44 patients with carcinoma of the parotid gland the average age was 52.9 years, the youngest being 15 years and the oldest 78 years of age. It is of interest that a malignant parotid tumor was observed in a newborn infant,[29] and Duthoit[11] described one in a child 6 weeks of age. Wood[51] described a tumor of the parotid in a child 7 months old. The peak incidence for patients with benign tumors is less than that for patients with carcinoma.[42] There is so much overlapping, however, in the ages of the two groups that the age of a given patient cannot be utilized to determine if the given tumor be benign or malignant.

Sex.—Of the 100 patients with parotid tumors, 56 were men and 44 were women. The sex distribution of patients with benign tumors was similar for the two types: 28 patients were men and 26 were women. Men bore cancer somewhat more frequently than women. Of the 46 patients with parotid cancer, 28 were men and 18 were women.

Symptoms.—The constant history related to the presence of a slowly growing, painless mass in the vicinity of either ear. The mass continued to grow in size over a period of years, and the majority of patients presented themselves because of cosmetic disfigurement.

Five patients, on admission, presented evidence of facial nerve paralysis. In each case the histologic examination of the tumor revealed carcinoma, and in all instances the patients died of the cancer.

An asymptomatic mass was uniformly the symptom of patients with benign tumors, while in patients bearing carcinoma, in addition to the mass, some also complained of pain, dysphagia, facial nerve paralysis, or a cervical tumor. When the latter symptoms and signs were present, the diagnosis was carcinoma.

Culpability for Delay in Seeking Therapy.—Of 100 patients with parotid tumors, in all but 5 a history was available of the duration from the patient's observation of the mass until the time he first sought medical attention. Of these 95 patients, only 3 sought immediate medical attention. The others delayed from 6 months to 304 months. The average delay of all patients with tumors of the parotid gland was forty-two months (three and one-half years). Patients with benign tumors of the parotid gland delayed an average of forty-eight months (four years); patients with carcinoma delayed an average of thirty-eight and one-half months (three and two-tenths years). Of the group with carcinoma, only 2 patients sought immediate medical attention; delays in the others varied from two months to twenty-five years. Other authors have observed similar delays.[4, 42, 51] Thus a tumor of long duration may be a carcinoma, and the period of its presence may be no indication of its morbid anatomy.

The culpability in most instances lay with the patient who delayed excessively before seeking medical attention. Although most physicians instituted early treatment, their failure to understand the natural history of parotid neoplasms resulted in only partial excision of the tumor, frequently as an office procedure.

Location of Tumors.—There were 50 tumors on the right side and 50 on the left. Of the benign tumors there were 23 on the right side and 31 on the left; of the carcinomas there were 27 on the right side and 19 on the left side. These data demonstrate that there is no selectivity for either side in the benign or malignant tumors of the parotid gland. No instance of bilateral parotid involvement by tumor occurred.

Clinical Course.—Tumors of the parotid gland, both benign and malignant, are characterized by their slow growth; it usually takes one year or more before the average tumor reaches a size of 2 cm. The average duration of forty-two months before the patients seek medical attention characterizes the benign clinical course manifested by these tumors. In this series, in only 5 cases was there a history of rapid growth. Most of the patients complained of no symptoms other than the cosmetic deformity. However, 8 patients presented cervical metastases in addition to the primary tumor on admission. In most instances the tumors were located at the angle of the jaw, usually directly in front of the lobe but occasionally posterior to the lobe. Because of the embryologic development of the parotid gland (discussed later) with glandular projections in several directions, and because of the thin capsule about the gland in certain locations (retromandibular), parotid tumors may present in different locations. They may occur along the zygoma and at any locus in a region extending from the zygoma in a semicircular manner to the angle of the jaw and posteriorly to the mastoid process in addition to the pharynx. On physical examination the characteristic finding was a smooth, ovoid, firm mass which in many of the benign tumors was movable, and the overlying skin moved over the tumor. Attempts to discern by physical examination whether the tumor was benign or malignant were very frequently misleading. Thus, carcinomas of the parotid gland may present a smooth, firm, freely movable mass within the parotid gland, which suggests benignity. The converse is also encountered where, because of an associated sialadenitis around a benign tumor, the presumptive diagnosis will usually be carcinoma. The size of the tumor, likewise, is no criterion in distinguishing a benign from a malignant tumor. The average size of the benign tumors studied here was 3.3 cm. in diameter, whereas the average size of the carcinomas of the parotid was 5.4 cm. in diameter. Although the average size for carcinomas was larger, mixed tumors may be massive (Fig. 1).

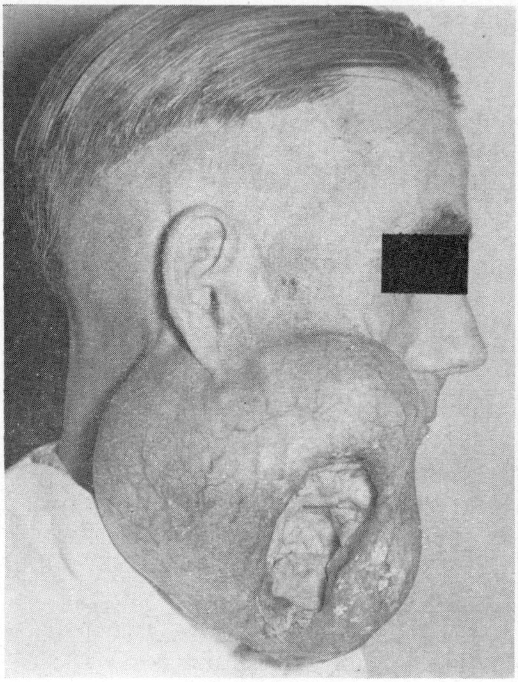

Fig. 1.

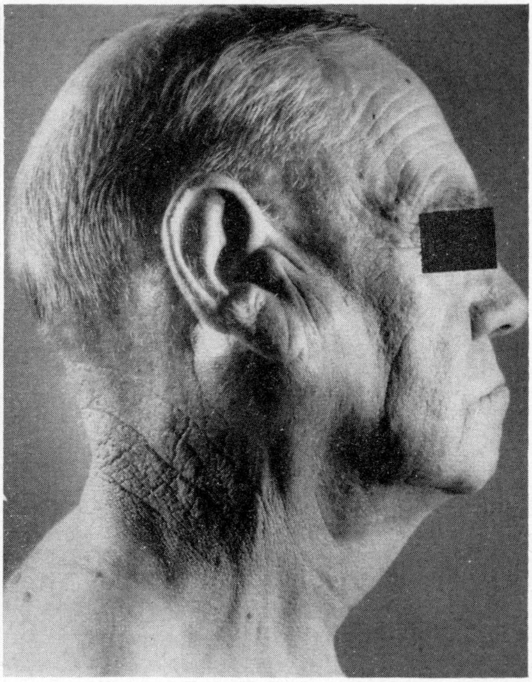

Fig. 2.

Fig. 1.—Clinical photograph of a massive mixed tumor which had been present for twelve years. It was resected by Dr. John Conley of the Head and Neck Department.

Fig. 2.—Carcinoma of the parotid gland which has extended into the pterygomandibular fossa and is fixed to the overlying skin.

In 6 patients the tumor arose from the retromandibular portion of the parotid gland, became localized between the posterior edge of the ascending ramus of the mandible and the mastoid process, and presented clinically as a poorly defined fullness rather than a discrete mass. Previous physicians had not suspected that this poorly delineated fullness was neoplastic. Thus, one must consider the possibility of a parotid tumor in all instances of fullness in this region.

GROSS PATHOLOGIC ANATOMY

Parotid tumors present a firm, grayish white, rounded mass, usually with a definite capsule. As the tumors grow the capsule may become thinned or become invaded by tumor cells. If the tumor is superficial, it may grow into the subcutaneous tissue, being attached to the parotid gland by a rather narrow base. Certain benign parotid tumors in the superficial location may grow to massive sizes and present as a large pedunculated mass with thinned-out skin and often necrosis and secondary infection (Fig. 1). Tumors situated within the depths of the parotid gland will, with continued growth, compress the branches of the facial nerve. Benign tumors may grow to large sizes with consequent marked pressure against the facial nerve branches, but no instance has been encountered in which paralysis or paresis developed from this type of pressure. On the other hand, malignant tumors may infiltrate the nerve with ensuing facial paralysis. Whereas benign tumors tend to remain discrete, carcinomas will invade contiguous structures and, in advanced cases, will present a brawny fixed mass which is adherent to the parotid, overlying skin, and surrounding cervical tissues. They might become fungating and ulcerating. A neuralgia of the trigeminal nerve can occur from infiltration into the nerve. Extension of the tumor into the pterygomandibular fossa produces interference with jaw motion. Cervical metastases may occur. Although malignant tumors usually differ in gross appearance from the benign ones, it is frequently difficult to distinguish between the two types either clinically or at the time of operation. The presence of a definite capsule is no assurance of the benignity of the tumor. Careful microscopic examination not infrequently reveals infiltration of the capsule by tumor cells at one or more foci with extension of the cancer into the surrounding glandular tissue.

In several instances at the time of exploration the tumor was considered to be malignant because of marked induration about a solid tumor mass. In these instances the indurated gland was resected with the tumor mass and the benign nature of the tumor was established by microscopic examination, with the induration found to be due to an associated sialadenitis. In most instances it is clinically impossible to distinguish between a benign parotid neoplasm and one which is malignant (Fig. 2). In certain benign tumors such as papillary cystadenoma lymphomatosum the clinical and gross picture is such that a diagnosis of a benign tumor can usually be established.

DIAGNOSIS

Because of the difficulty in establishing a preoperative correct diagnosis, recourse must be had to additional data.

Sialography.—The instillation of Lipiodol into the parotid ducts and roentgenographic visualization of the gland give evidence of a mass within the gland. An anteroposterior view indicates its location (superficial or deep). Although Blady and Hocker[5] described how benign and malignant tumors could be identified by this technique, it has been found most difficult to distinguish one from the other. The technique is a distinct aid in identifying the nature of a mass in the parotid region and in distinguishing those which are extrinsic to the gland. Intrinsic masses can be further subdivided into inflammatory reactions with dilatation of the entire ductal system from a solid mass within the gland containing no ducts but producing distortion of the surrounding ducts. This visualization indicates the location of the tumor and its relation to the facial nerve (whether superficial or deep) and aids in formulating the operative plan.

Cervical Lymph Nodes.—The presence of cervical adenopathy may indicate metastases from a parotid carcinoma, but caution must be exercised so that the nature of the cervical adenopathy is accurately determined. In several instances cervical adenopathy associated with a parotid mass was later found to be chronic lymphadenitis due to an intraoral infection which subsided with antibiotic therapy.

Another diagnostic pitfall is the presence of a small mass situated at the anteroinferior aspect of the parotid gland which is frequently mistaken for a primary parotid neoplasm. This may represent metastases from a silent intraoral primary cancer to the subfascial, extra glandular parotid lymph nodes. In other instances, lymphomas (Hodgkin's disease, and so forth) may present as a tumefaction in this locality.

Technique for Histologic Diagnosis.—The premise is accepted that a clinical diagnosis is often misleading; hence it cannot be utilized as criteria for therapy. In every instance a histologic diagnosis is obtained. The first attempt is an aspiration biopsy. This expedient procedure is performed rapidly as part of the physical examination and usually establishes the diagnosis. The aspiration biopsy is repeated if the first attempt is unsuccessful.

It is considered unwise to perform an incisional biopsy preceding operative intervention for fear of rupturing the capsule and inducing exophytic extension. Therefore, an exploratory incision into the parotid is made and a frozen section is performed. If this test is not diagnostic and the resection would involve sacrifice of the nerve, it is believed that the patient could be best benefited by closing the wound and awaiting the diagnosis from paraffin sections before proceeding with the radical operation.

METASTASES

Malignant parotid neoplasms metastasize by means of the lymphatics and the blood stream. In this series, metastases had occurred in 25 per cent of the cases when the patients were first observed. Eight patients had metastases to the cervical lymph nodes. The lungs were a frequent site of metastatic deposits, and occasionally many organs were diffusely invaded. Metastases from parotid cancer may sometimes adopt rather bizarre manifestations. In one observed patient the first metastasis to a lymph node occurred in the inguinal chain after which the patient demonstrated numerous discrete subcutaneous metastatic nodules. Another patient developed a subungual metastasis of the right middle finger, followed by metastases to the right axilla. The patient then developed pulmonary and cerebral metastases and died.

Another interesting feature of the behavior of metastases from parotid cancer is that in certain instances the metastases may grow wildly and the patient may die within a very short period. In other instances, especially the cylindroma type, massive metastatic deposits may be observed in the lungs over a period of years and produce minimal symptoms (Fig. 3).

A subject of much speculation is the nature of metastases from so-called benign mixed tumors of the parotid gland. Brunschwig[8] and Kornblith[22] reported such instances; Mulligan[37] reviewed the literature and noted 21 instances of metastases arising from apparently benign tumors of the parotid gland. No such occurrence was observed in this series.

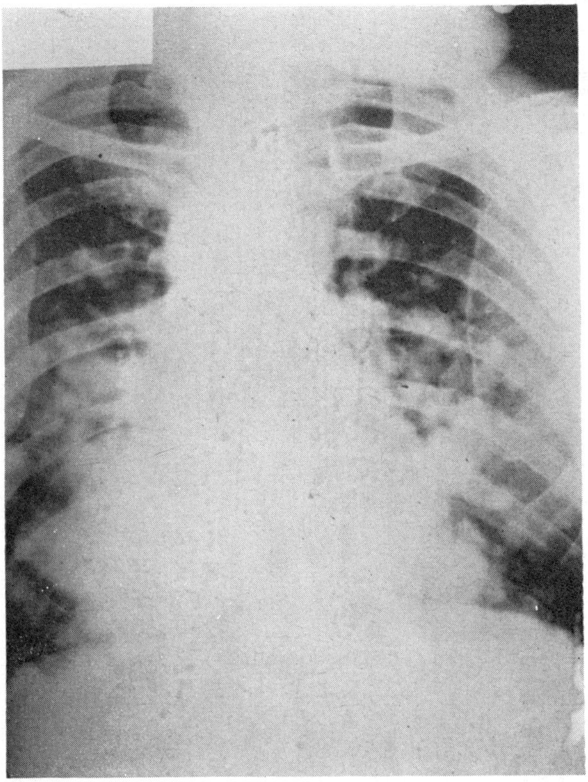

Fig. 3.—Roentgenogram of pulmonary metastases from a carcinoma (cylindroma type) of the parotid gland. Both lungs were diffusely involved but the patient had no symptoms when the roentgenogram was taken.

RECURRENCE OF THE TUMORS

Benign Tumors.—Of the 54 patients with benign parotid tumors, 34 were treated initially at the Pack Medical Group. Of these, 1 patient died postoperatively of a pulmonary embolus, 1 died from other causes one year after treatment with no evidence of parotid neoplasia, and 1 was lost to follow-up immediately after operation. Only 1 patient developed a recurrence three years after initial treatment here which had consisted of local excision and postoperative x-ray therapy. The recurrence was widely excised and interstitial gold radon seeds were inserted. This patient has remained free of disease for thirteen years. Of the remaining 30 patients, 17 were treated within the past five years; thus 13 patients have remained free of recurrence for over five years.

Of the 20 patients whose referrals were subsequent to treatment elsewhere, in only 4 was the treatment adequate with the patients remaining free of tumor. The additional 16 were referred to this clinic manifesting recurrences an average of 4.2 years after the initial treatment (ranging from two months to ten years). Those recurrences which appeared early were undoubtedly persistence of tumor after inadequate treatment. Those whose clinical onset was delayed may possibly have had second primary neoplasms, but because of their indolent growth characteristics, the delayed recurrences may represent persistence of tumor after incomplete excisions. Recurrences were treated at the Pack Medical Group by wide surgical excision and usually postoperative irradiation. Two of this group developed a second recurrence which was adequately controlled by more radical surgical extirpation. In no instance was the facial nerve permanently damaged. These data attest to the adequacy of radical surgical extirpation and serve to develop criteria for treating primary mixed parotid tumors and their recurrences.

Carcinoma.—Of the 46 patients bearing carcinoma, 17 (37 per cent) presented evidence of recurrence an average of two and seven-tenths years from the time of attempted therapy; the range was from four months to ten years. Of this group of 46 patients, 33 had been treated elsewhere before referral, and of the 13 patients treated initially at this institution, 9 were referred with the neoplasm operable. There was a recurrence in 1 patient 15 months after operation.

There was nothing in the material studied to correlate a recurrence with the age of the patient, delay before therapy was instituted, the size of the tumor, or any feature of its histologic picture. The bulk of the evidence indicates that a recurrence is the result of inadequate extirpation.

Another factor of interest is the observation that recurrences usually retained the same histologic pattern as did the primary tumor. On occasion, however, a recurrence of a mixed tumor may be malignant. One such interesting occurrence was observed. A mass was removed from the base of the left parotid gland of a 33-year-old woman and was reported as a benign mixed parotid tumor. She was given postoperative radium therapy. A recurrence six years later revealed a mixed tumor of the parotid with suspicious malignant areas. She received postoperative x-ray therapy. Seven years after the excision of the first recurrence, a second recurrence presented itself and was widely excised. This recurrent tumor was a fully malignant adenocarcinoma. The patient has remained well and free of recurrence for sixteen years after resection of the parotid cancer.

Kirklin[20] reported that 34.3 per cent of the patients treated for a recurrence developed a second recurrence. This would seem to indicate that the distored tissue subsequent to an initial surgical attack hinders adequate dissection of residual tumor tissue.

It is stressed that because of the indolent nature of the growth of many of these tumors, long periods must elapse before a treated tumor can be considered cured, for recurrences have been observed ten years and more after treatment.

In no patient of this series was the opposite parotid gland involved by neoplasia, suggesting that parotid tumors most frequently arise from a solitary nidus, and recurrences indicate renewed growth after ineffectual extirpation rather than a proclivity of salivary gland to develop tumors. In an occasional case, multicentric foci can be observed in a given gland, but this is unusual.

Another cause for recurrences is spillage at the time of extirpation with seeding of tumor cells in the area. The presence of several small tumor nodules in the operative scar demonstrates such means of tumor propagation.

PROGNOSIS OF PAROTID TUMORS

It is difficult to evaluate the results of therapeutic attempts with parotid tumors because many of the tumors grow slowly and recur late, and because, as a result of the long interim necessary to observe these patients, many may be lost to follow-up. Furthermore, many patients are first seen in a state of extensive neoplasia (in this series, 35.7 per cent of patients with carcinoma), and nothing but palliation can be offered. In addition, previous attempts at treatment will have distorted the anatomic structures, and the treatment of a recurrence cannot be compared with the initial treatment of a primary tumor. The outlook is worsened with each recurrence.

The end results of the patients treated at this institution are tabulated in Table I. It will be noted that 39 patients were treated within the past five years. Of the 61 patients treated over five years ago, 25 of the 30 patients with benign tumors are alive and free of disease, an absolute survival rate of 83.3 per cent, and 10 of the 31 patients with carcinoma are free of cancer, an absolute survival rate of 32.3 per cent.

TABLE I. FIVE-YEAR END RESULTS IN 100 CASES OF PAROTID GLAND TUMORS*

		BENIGN TUMOR	CARCINOMA
Total number of patients	100	54	46
Number used for five-year survival (39 patients were treated too recently)	61	30	31
Number alive and free of disease five years or more		25	10
Absolute five-year survival rate		83.3 per cent	32.3 per cent
Number of patients lost to follow-up before five-year period		4	7
Relative five-year survival rate		96.2 per cent	41.7 per cent
Number on whom curative procedures were attempted (12 patients with carcinoma presented themselves too late)		30	19
Number used to compute therapeutic five-year survival rate (does not include 11 lost to follow-up and 12 on whom no curative procedure was attempted)		26	12
Therapeutic five-year survival rate		96.2%	83.3%

*Seen at the Pack Medical Group, New York, N. Y.

To evaluate the relative five-year survival rates, those patients who were lost to follow-up and were free of tumor at the time are subtracted from the total group. Since there is no way of ascertaining the fate of these people, the relative five-year survival rate is of value; in this series it is 96.2 per cent for the patients with benign tumors and 41.7 per cent for the patients with carcinoma.

Inasmuch as a certain number of patients present themselves with far-advanced cancer, including distant metastases, and since no curative procedure can be attempted on them, it is essential to subtract that group if an evaluation is to be made of the accomplishments of any therapeutic regime. In this series there were 13 patients with carcinoma who when first seen were considered incurable. If this group is subtracted in order to compute the therapeutic five-year survival rate, there are 12 patients with carcinoma on whom a therapeutic attack was made and who were followed for over five years. The therapeutic five-year survival rate for carcinoma of the parotid gland is then 83.3 per cent. Table II presents graphically the total experience of 41 patients treated for parotid cancer who were followed after treatment. Thirteen patients were treated too recently for five-year evaluation, and of the 28 patients followed for five years or longer, 11 survived (39 per cent). The discrepancy between this value and the 41.7 per cent relative five-year survival of Table I is due to the fact that patients who were followed for shorter periods are used for computation in Table II. The difference is not significant.

Table II. Survival Rates of 41 Patients With Parotid Carcinoma Treated Between 1933 and 1950 Inclusive

YEAR	NUMBER OF CASES	YEARS OF SURVIVAL 1	2	3	4	5	6	7	8	9	10	REMARKS
1933	1	0										
1934	3	3	3	2	2	2	2	2	2	2	2	Two patients alive and well 10 and 16 years after treatment
1936	2	1	1	1	1	1	1	1	1	1	1	Well 14 years after treatment
1937	2	1	1	1	1	1	1	1	1	1	1	Well 13 years. (Other patient died 10 years after onset)
1939	2	2	2	2	1	1	1	1	1	1	1	Well 13 years after treatment
1940	4	4	2	2	2	2	2	2	1	1		One patient died at 7 years after treatment of other causes
1941	2	1	0	0	0	0	0	0	0	0		
1942	2	2	1	1	1	1	1	1	0			
1943	6	2	1	1	1	1	1					One patient died immediately after treatment (27 years after onset). Another was immediately lost to follow-up and presumed dead
1944	1	1	1									Lost to follow-up after 2 years
1945	3	3	2	2	2	2						One patient died of other causes at 1 year
1946	4	2	2	2	2							
1947	4	4	2	2								One patient died of lymphosarcoma at 16 months
1949	2	1										
1950	3	1										
Total cases	41	41	38	36	32	28	25	24	18	16	14	
Survival		28	18	16	13	11	9	8	5	6	5	
Per cent		68	47	44	41	39	36	33	33	37	36	

CLINICAL COURSE OF PATIENTS WITH CARCINOMA ANALYZED ACCORDING TO PATHOLOGIC TYPE

Malignant Mixed Tumor.—Eight such patients were treated at the Pack Medical Group. Of these, 2 are alive and well for eight and thirteen years, respectively. In two additional cases the period of treatment was too recent for evaluation. One patient is apparently free of tumor two years after treatment and another, one year after therapy. The malignant nature of this tumor is demonstrated in the case of 2 patients who died eight and fifteen months after treatment. In a third instance the patient died sixteen months after treatment because of malignant lymphoma. One additional patient died of heart failure postoperatively.

The exact nosology of malignant mixed tumors is not completely understood. The long history of 2 of these patients with presence of a mass of three years' duration followed by rapid growth for one year with pain of two to three months' duration suggests that malignant transformation within a mixed tumor had occurred. The clinical course may either be very slow (one patient presented a thirty-seven-year history with recurrences at ten- to twenty-year intervals) or extremely rapid, death occurring within one year after the onset of symptoms.

These tumors have a tendency to invade locally and sometimes grow to large size. Two of our patients presented the ominous symptom of facial nerve paralysis.

Some authors (Kirklin and associates[20]) do not believe in classifying such tumors as malignant mixed tumors but rather under the heading of the predominant cell type, such as squamous-cell carcinoma, adenocarcinoma, and so forth. The designation of malignant mixed tumor or carcinoma (squamous, adenocarcinoma and so forth) within a mixed tumor indicates the natural history of the specific neoplasm. The treatment, of course, should be radical surgical extirpation combined with neck dissection when a carcinoma is more than Grade I malignancy. Although these tumors are relatively radioresistant, postoperative gold radon seeds are indicated whenever infiltration into contiguous structures has occurred. If there is a possibility of residual tumor, the interstitial irradiation may be supplemented with external deep x-ray therapy.

Cylindroma.—There was only one patient bearing cylindroma observed here, and he was lost to follow-up. In other reported series cylindromas have constituted 4.7 per cent[20] and 3.2 per cent[42] of parotid tumors. They grow slowly but relentlessly. They invade locally, metastasize to regional lymph nodes (23.6 per cent), and also produce distant metastases. These tumors are relatively resistant, and although the initial response to x-ray therapy is good, recurrence is the rule.

Adenocarcinoma.—These tumors are more malignant. Of the 9 patients treated here, 5 have died from the neoplasms (55 per cent mortality), and death occurred rather rapidly (four and five months after treatment in 2

cases). Two patients presented the ominous symptom of facial nerve paralysis when first seen. These patients responded poorly to irradiation.

Squamous Carcinoma.—Of the 6 patients in this series 3 (50 per cent) died from the cancer. The course of patients bearing them is somewhat prolonged. One patient of this group died four years after the initial manifestation of the neoplasm and another, twenty-five years after the onset. The additional 3 patients are well four, six, and fourteen years, respectively, after the initial manifestation. Metastases develop early, and are frequently to the regional lymph nodes, less frequently to distant localities. Squamous carcinomas of the parotid gland, like epidermoid carcinoma elsewhere, are of moderate radiosensitivity and respond well initially to irradiation.

One patient in this series with squamous carcinoma of the parotid gland was treated exclusively by irradiation and has remained free of disease for sixteen years. He received 200 r. each day to a 7 cm. port (198 kv., 0.5 mm. Cu filter, 63 cm. target-skin distance) for a total of 4,000 r., after which he received interstitial radon seeds for a total dosage of 2,926 mc. hours. A small plastic operation was recently performed for a radiation ulcer.

Mucoepidermoid Carcinoma.—There were 4 patients bearing this interesting tumor first identified by Stewart, Foote, and Becker,[48] who described them as being either of very low-grade or very high-grade malignancy. These extremes in clinical course were observed in our 4 cases. One patient died seven months after treatment while the other 3 are apparently free of disease for three, four, and five years, respectively. These tumors are relatively radioresistant although Rawson and co-workers[42] describe beneficial effects in one such patient receiving x-ray therapy.

Undifferentiated Carcinoma.—This is a highly malignant form of cancer, and of the 12 patients observed here, 6 have died. Only 1 patient has survived four years; 2 died of other causes, 1 postoperatively and 1 seven years after treatment; 2 were lost to follow-up; 1 was treated too recently for follow-up study. Massive growths and regional lymph node metastases, as well as distant metastases to varied locations, are produced by this malignant neoplasm. The most radical attack, including both surgical extirpation plus interstitial gold radon seeds and external radiation therapy, must be administered to effect a cure.

Miscellanaeous.—The miscellaneous groups vary in malignancy from very benign lipomas and lymphocytic tumors to highly malignant adenosarcomas. The clinical behavior of sarcoma and melanoma in the parotid is similar to that of these neoplasms elsewhere.

TREATMENT

The data of this series demonstrate some lamentable shortcomings in the over-all treatment of parotid tumors and indicate routes of attack to overcome these shortcomings. Some of these are enumerated.

Errors in the Management of Mixed Tumors.—1. The slow growth of mixed tumors has lulled both patients and physicians into a false sense of security concerning the benignity of these tumors. Thus, patients are first seen for treatment after long delays. During the delay a certain definite number of the tumors may have undergone malignant transformation and may be inoperable when first observed. In other instances the tumor may extend into the retromandibular portion of the parotid gland, making resection more difficult, or the tumors may grow externally (Fig. 1) to massive proportions. Although the latter are usually technically resectable with good end results, they do present a frightful appearance.

2. The belief that mixed parotid tumors are well encapsulated has led to the performance of local enucleation with resultant frequent recurrences. Some believe that there is no real capsule about the tumors and that the pseudocapsule consists of compressed parotid parenchyma. Regardless of the nature of the capsule it has been amply demonstrated that infiltration of the capsule by tumor cells occurs frequently. Accordingly, the capsule must be removed in every instance.

3. The previous fallacious teachings that larger tumors respond better to surgical extirpation have led to the dangerous practice of watchful waiting. All parotid tumors, as all tumors in every part of the body, should be removed with dispatch.

4. The performance of excisional biopsy without definitive treatment accounted for spillage and seeding of new foci of growths in certain instances.

5. The diffuse fullness of certain tumors (papillary cystadenoma lymphomatosum or retromandibular tumors) was not suspected of being neoplastic, and no treatment was instituted.

6. Lack of knowledge of the anatomy of the parotid gland and fear of dealing with the facial nerve have led to inadequate surgical excision. Recurrence is the rule. Past teaching indicates that this is a natural characteristic of mixed parotid tumors and that a recurrence should be expected. Parotid tumors exemplify an instance where inadequate medical efforts have camouflaged the natural history of a neoplasm, which false knowledge has more or less endorsed the inadequate treatment. It is our strong conviction that except in very few instances (mixed tumors with multicentric foci) a recurrence of a mixed parotid tumor reflects the inadequacy of the surgical attempt.

7. Certain soft parotid tumors, especially those which have undergone cystic degeneration, are misdiagnosed as cysts and are simply drained.

8. Small tumors are misdiagnosed as preauricular lymph nodes and no treatment is instituted.

9. Fear of producing salivary fistula has resulted in limited surgery. Only one such fistula was observed in this series.

10. Failure of certain surgeons to appreciate the limitations of irradiation for parotid tumors will cause them to leave residual tumor and to depend on postoperative irradiation to control the residuum. There are definite indications for radiation therapy for parotid tumors, but it should not be used as a crutch for inadequate surgery.

Errors in the Management of Parotid Carcinomas.—The major faults in the treatment of parotid carcinoma have been long delays before the institution of treatment, inadequate resection due to fear of damaging the seventh nerve, and a failure to recognize the malignant nature of the neoplasm. Furthermore, a lack of understanding of the lymphatic drainage of the parotid gland and the high incidence (25 per cent) of metastases to regional lymph nodes from parotid carcinoma have accounted for certain treatment failures.

Accordingly, the simple tenet for treating all parotid tumors is that they be adequately excised by sharp dissection. To accomplish this, a knowledge of the anatomy of the parotid gland and the facial nerve and of lymphatic drainage of the parotid is essential. Specific circumstances call for individual criteria for the extent of the resection. Each of these shall be discussed, including the role of irradiation for treating parotid neoplasms.

SURGICAL ANATOMY OF THE PAROTID GLAND

Embryologically the parotid gland develops as an outpushing from the angle of the mouth which extends toward the ear. When it reaches the vicinity of the mandible it sends buds superiorly, laterally, medially, and posteriorly, the primordial ductal system about which develop the glandular elements. Thus, in the adult the parotid salivary gland is irregular in shape. It extends superiorly along the zygoma, inferior to the angle of the jaw, and over the masseter muscle in a superficial position. The anterior surface is grooved by the posterior margin of the ascending ramus of the mandible, and the posterior extension protrudes between the pterygoid muscles toward the pharynx in the so-called retromandibular (pterygomandibular) space. The inner surface drops deeply into the neck by two large processes; one goes behind the styloid process toward the mastoid process and may attach to the sternomastoid muscle, and the other process extends behind the articulation of the lower jaw.

It is thus evident that parotid neoplasms may develop anywhere on the side of the face: along the zygoma, on the cheek, in front of or below the ear, in the retromandibular fossa, in the stylomastoid recess, about the mastoid at the sternocleidomastoid origin, and into the pharynx. This description further illustrates the difficulty in attempting to remove each vestige of parotid tissue.

An extension of the superficial cervical fascia envelops the parotid gland and is continuous with the fascia of the masseter and the sternomastoid muscles. From the viewpoint of tumors, several characteristics of the fascia are important. (1) It varies in thickness in different positions. The retromandibular part of the gland is almost devoid of fascia, permitting tumors of this region to grow readily toward the pharynx and giving those tumors which present in the pterygomandibular fossa an appearance of diffuse fullness rather than that of a discrete mass. (2) The capsule is thickened over the anteroinferior aspect, thus producing a sense of tenseness of tumors of this location. (3) Some tumors grow beyond the capsule and are attached to the gland by a narrow stalk. (4) The enveloping fascia sends small fibrous strands throughout the gland, dividing the glandular elements into myriads of tiny lobulations interconnected by innumerable fibrous septa. The importance of this will be discussed in relationship to the surgical anatomy of the seventh nerve.

THE SURGICAL ANATOMY OF THE FACIAL NERVE

The surgical anatomy of the facial nerve has dominated every attempt directed at treating parotid tumors. It is of interest that the change in thinking pertaining to the relationship of the facial nerve to the parotid gland has been from one school of teaching which taught that the nerve was so intimately imbedded in the gland that it defied efforts to extricate the gland from the nerve, to the present trend which attempts to attribute an oversimplification of the relationship of the nerve to the gland. McWhorter,[30] McCormick, Cauldwell, and Anson,[25] and more recently State[46] have described the parotid gland as consisting of superficial and deep lobes connected by a narrow isthmus. They described the nerve as passing between the two lobes, but not actually penetrating the parotid capsule, and lying within the parotid parenchyma. The nerve was described by these authors as having the same relationship to the two parts of the parotid gland as a bookmark has to the two pages of a book it separates (State[46]) or as the "meat in a sandwich" (Bailey[2]). Our numerous dissections have failed to confirm this concept. In every instance the nerve was found to have passed through the parotid fascia and to lie directly within the parotid parenchyma. Martin[32] has also described this relationship. In no instance were separate lobes of parotid encountered separated by fascial envelopes with the nerve traversing this hypothetical space. If one unfamiliar with the relationship of the facial nerve to the parotid gland attempts to dissect the parotid neoplasm expecting to find the nerve lying between two separated parotid lobes, he will be uniformly disappointed, and the further progress of the dissection may be affected.

It may be mentioned that ontogenetically the nerve, after emerging from the stylomastoid foramen, separates into two branches at a point where a small nubbin of parotid tissue exists. With the development of the parotid gland, two superficial projections, one growing inferiorly and the other superiorly, and two deep projections, growing superiorly and inferiorly, respectively, develop and fuse intimately at about the eighth week of prenatal life, thus completely embedding certain portions of the facial nerve within the parotid parenchyma.

The parotid gland can readily be dissected away from the seventh nerve, essentially because of the differences in consistence. The flaccid, yielding, spongelike consistence of the parotid glandular tissue, which is bound together by innumerable tiny fibrous septa, can readily be peeled away from the firm, taut nerve which traverses it. One might envision the pouring of a sticky wax over the nerve which on hardening could have its superficial portion easily removed. Likewise, the deeper portion posterior to the nerve and those trabeculations which extend into the various anatomic recesses of this location could only be removed piecemeal.

The facial nerve emerges from the stylomastoid foramen and runs anteriorly with a slight inferior inclination through a small potential space anterior to the mastoid process, at which point it traverses the parotid gland (Fig. 4). Shortly after traversing the gland it bifurcates into the temporofacial and cervicofacial divisions. Occasionally this bifurcation will occur before the nerve enters the parotid substance (Fig. 5). Numerous divisions then occur within the parotid gland. Whereas the main trunk of the nerve measures about 3 mm. in diameter when it enters the gland, about five to seven small filamentous branches take exit from the anterior border extending over the masseter muscle to their various points of innervation. The small mandibular marginal branch takes exit from the inferior border of the gland and travels within the platysma swinging inferior to or beyond the horizontal ramus of the mandible to innervate the lower lip. Whereas most of the other branches have numerous cross-anastomoses and damage to one branch will frequently be corrected by an anastomotic branch, the marginal branch has no such anastomoses, and its severance will always result in paralysis of the corresponding half of the lower lip.

LYMPH NODES OF THE PAROTID GLAND*

The parotid nodes are divided into three principal groups: (1) superficial-suprafascial, (2) subfascial-extraglandular, and (3) deep intraglandular (Fig. 6).

1. *The Suprafascial Parotid Nodes.*—These nodes exist in one-third of the cases; their number varies from one to four, and the size is in inverse proportion to their number. They are always preauricular and placed in the neighborhood of the tragus. The nodes are sometimes situated opposite the notch which separates tragus from antitragus, or else above the tragus. In the latter case, the nodes are always placed against the superficial temporal blood vessels, sometimes behind, sometimes lateral to, but rarely in front of, these blood vessels.

2. *The Subfascial-extraglandular Nodes.*—In this group are included the lymph nodes contained in the parotid sheath and placed immediately below the fascia. Some of these nodes are placed anteriorly, in front of the auricle, (a) the anterior or preauricular. The others, (b) inferior or infra-auricular, lie at the inferior extremity of the parotid gland.

(a) *The subfascial preauricular nodes:* There are usually one or two, but there may be as many as four. They are placed between the fascial covering and the external surface of the parotid gland, sometimes near the tragus and sometimes rather at a distance from it in front of the auricle. Normally there exists but one subfascial node near the tragus, whereas the neighboring subfascial nodes are frequently absent. The parotid gland occasionally partially conceals certain subfascial preauricular nodes; in that case, the latter are always placed at some distance in front of the auricle, along the anterior limit of the

*After Rouviere.[43]

Fig. 4.

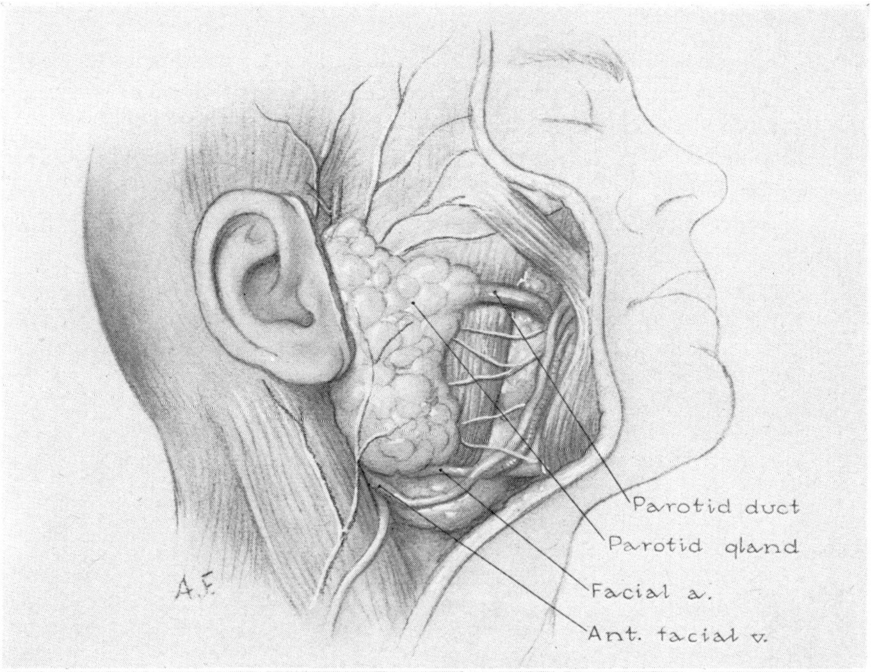

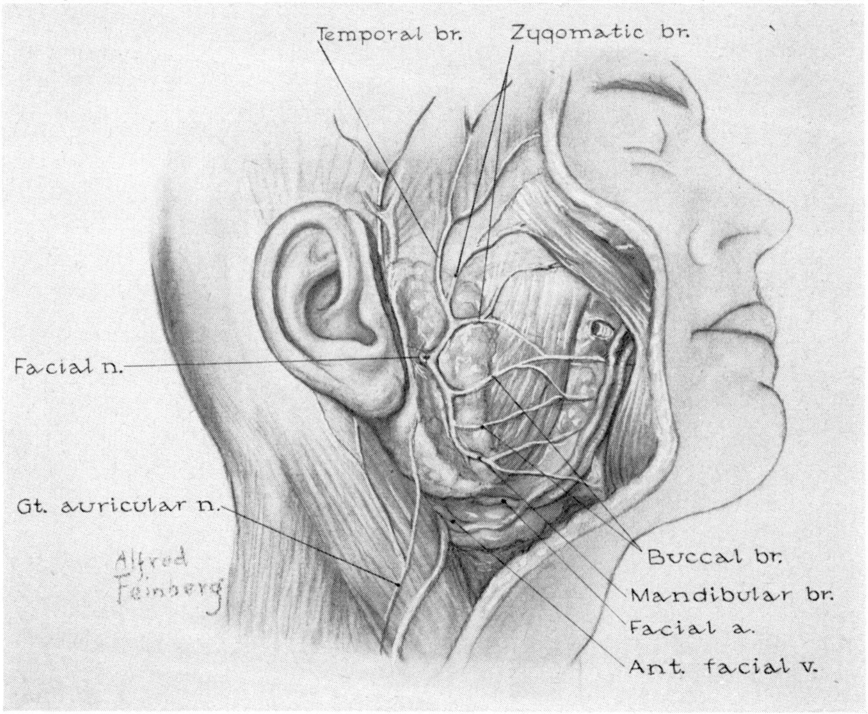

Fig. 5.

Fig. 4.—Illustration demonstrating the relationship of the parotid salivary gland to the facial nerve. The posterior portion of the nerve is buried within the gland. The terminal branches of the facial nerve emerge superficially from the anterior border of the parotid gland to their various sites of innervation. The great auricular nerve can be observed ascending over the sternocleidomastoid muscle and coursing over the superficial surface of the parotid gland.

Fig. 5.—Illustration demonstrating the course of the facial nerve through the parotid gland. The nerve, shortly after emerging from the stylomastoid process, penetrates the parotid gland and is intimately bound by the glandular parenchyma. The superficial portion of the gland can be easily dissected away from the nerve, but the deeper portion must be removed piecemeal.

superficial lobe of the parotid gland. This disposition of the nodes is due to the mode of development of the parotid gland. In fact, before the gland is completely developed, the external surface of these lymph nodes is in contact with the fascial covering of the parotid gland, but because of the manner in which the superficial lobe of the parotid gland extends during its development in nearly all directions, and particularly in front, the glandular tissue insinuates itself between the fascial covering of the parotid and the external surface of the lymph nodes, concealing the latter totally or partially. In the first instance, the lymph nodes become the deep intraglandular parotid nodes, and in the latter case they assume the location referred to previously.

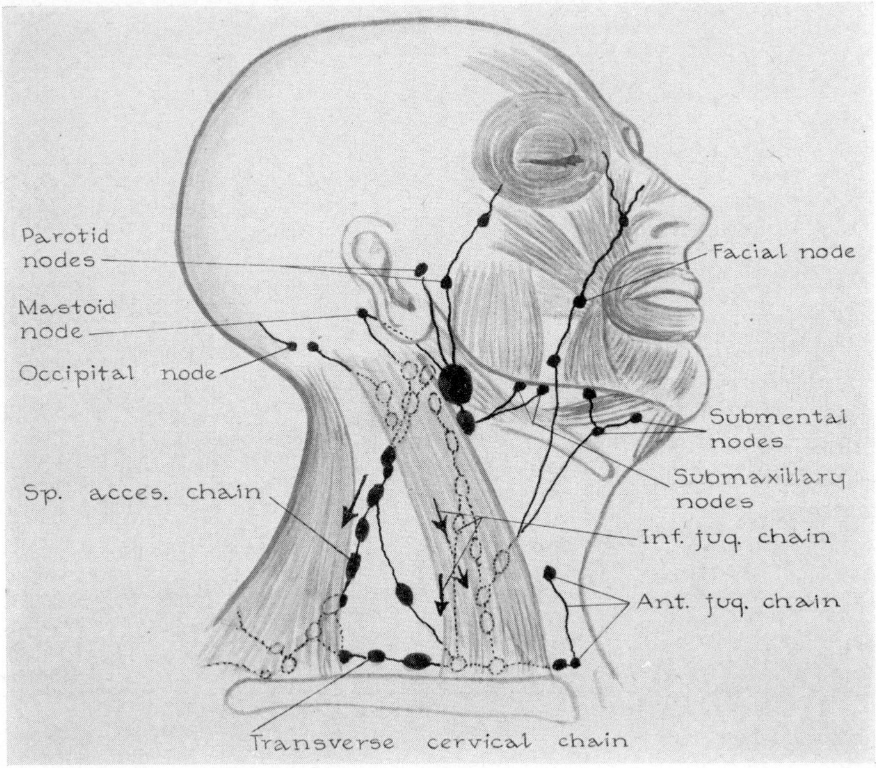

Fig. 6.—The cervical lymph nodes, indicating the routes of drainage from the parotid gland and demonstrating the need for a radical neck dissection to treat metastases from parotid carcinoma to the cervical lymph nodes (after Rouviere).

(b) *The inferior parotid infra-auricular nodes:* These are a group of one to three nodes situated in the region of the external jugular vein, at the point at which this blood vessel leaves the parotid gland. They are covered by the superficial layer of the deep cervical fascia and are placed between the inferior extremity of the parotid and the anterior border of the sternocleidomastoid muscle, from which they are separated by the sheath of the latter muscle, while above and below the nodes are separated from the parotid glandular tissue by a thin layer of fibrocellular tissue only. This fine layer of tissue is sometimes thickened, particularly in the adult and the aged person, and may assume the aspects of a fibrous membrane, in which case the nodes appear enclosed in a reduplication of fascia. In the newborn child, this group of nodes ascends, like the parotid gland, behind the lobule of the ear.

3. *Deep Intraglandular Nodes.*—In the fine cellular tissue which unites the superficial with the deep lobes of the parotid gland, four to ten lymph nodes are always found. This number does not include the minute nodes nor the periacinar lymph elements which can be revealed on microscopic examination only. The deep nodes are grouped around the external jugular and posterior fascial veins in the region, chiefly, where the facial crosses the external jugular vein. They are placed sometimes on the inner and sometimes on the outer side of the nerve rami and also more often and in greater number on the outer than on the inner side of the nerve. It is not uncommon to find a few nodes at some distance from, and in front of, or behind, the external jugular vein. The deep nodes are located most often in the cellular tissue which separates the two lobes of the parotid gland, but they are sometimes partly or wholly surrounded by the glandular tissue of one or the other lobe. At times there exist one or two nodes along the external carotid artery, either before this artery enters the parotid gland or in the tissue of the deep lobe.

OPERATIVE TECHNIQUE FOR RESECTING PAROTID NEOPLASMS

The amount of tissue to be removed surgically will depend on many factors and will vary from a simple extracapsular local excision to a total parotidectomy with sacrifice of the facial nerve and radical neck dissection in continuity. The various indications will be discussed.

Two fundamental processes considered essential for any operative procedure are (1) that the histologic nature of the tumor be determined and (2) that wide surgical exposure be obtained for every case, with the possible exception of certain subcutaneous tumors arising from the periphery of the gland and which are 1 cm. in diameter or less. In such instances a small incision over the tumor may be made with local excision of the tumor, including its capsule. In all other cases the operative exploration to be described is utilized, and the decision as to the extent of the procedure is determined on the basis of the histologic picture and the morbid anatomy encountered (Figs. 7 to 17).

It is advisable always to forewarn the patient concerning the possibilities of facial nerve paresis or paralysis. In no instance of our experience has the facial nerve been accidentally severed. The existence of temporary facial paresis is common, and unless the patient has been forewarned of its occurrence, its recognition will be alarming.

Anesthesia.—Endotracheal general anesthesia is routinely employed. The choice of anesthetic agents is a matter of individual preference. The patient is draped in such a manner that the entire half of the face on the involved side is visible. This permits visualization of the muscle contractions when the nerve branches are stimulated. General anesthesia permits this observation, and since local anesthesia does not, it should never be used except in the most unusual cases although its use is technically feasible.

Incision.—The Y incision is used almost exclusively (Figs. 7 and 8). The lobe of the ear is retracted upward. The posterior component of the incision permits adequate exposure for dissecting the main branch of the facial nerve, entrance into the pterygomandibular space, and removal of the mastoid tip and sternocleidomastoid muscle where indicated, and facilitates the completion of a radical neck dissection when performed. The anterior component of the incision facilitates the dissection and isolation of the terminal seventh nerve branches. These two incisions join under the tip of the lobe, and the incision is continued inferiorly parallel to the stenocleidomastoid muscle for a variable

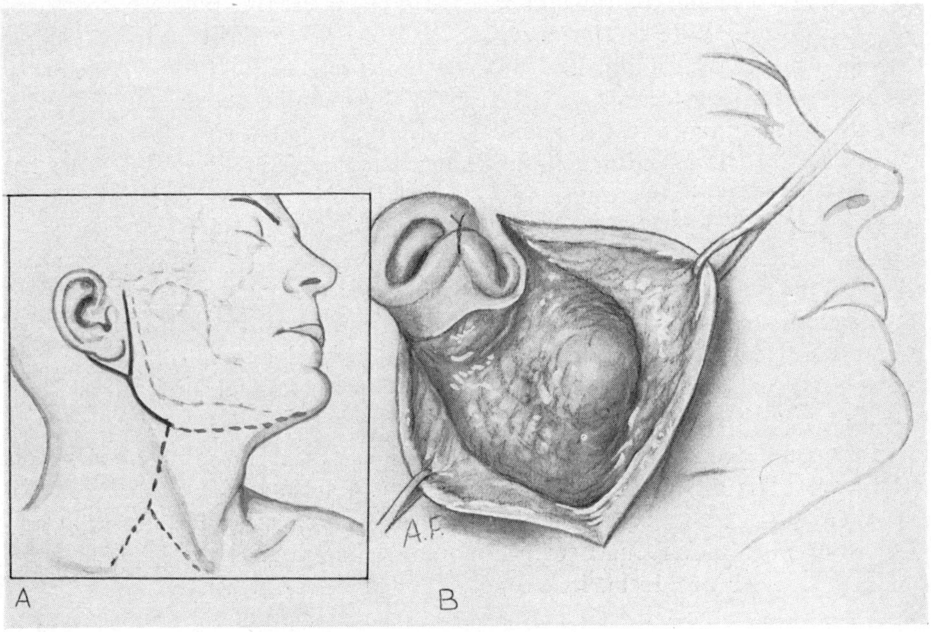

Fig. 7.—*A*, The Y-shaped incision utilized for practically all parotid gland explorations. The broken lines indicate the incision extended to perform a radical neck dissection in continuity with a parotidectomy. *B*, The ear is dissected superiorly and sutured away from the operative field. The skin flaps are being developed.

distance, depending on the location and extent of the neoplasm, usually one fingerbreadth (1½ cm.) inferior to the angle of the mandible. This has been a convenient landmark for exposing the external carotid artery shortly after its bifurcation, and frequently in parotid resections its ligation helps to minimize bleeding. Skin flaps are developed (Fig. 7). The facial flaps are thin and continue anteriorly to the location where the facial branches emerge from the parotid gland. The posterior flap is dissected to expose adequately the mastoid process and the tip of the sternomastoid muscle. The posterior portion of the parotid gland occasionally presses intimately against the upper portion of the sternomastoid muscle. The gland is easily separated from the muscle unless involved by cancer, and by retracting the gland anteriorly a potential space is developed in the depths of which is the main branch of the seventh cranial nerve.

At this point the decision can usually be made as to the nature and extent of the operative procedure required. It may consist of (1) a simple extracapsular excision of a mixed tumor, (2) excision of that portion of the gland superficial to the facial nerve (so-called superficial lobectomy[46]), (3) a subtotal parotidectomy with excision of the deeper portion of the gland for certain recurrent tumors, (4) a parotidectomy with preservation of the facial nerve combined with a radical neck dissection, (5) a radical parotidectomy with sacrifice of the facial nerve, and (6) radical parotidectomy with resection of a portion of the ascending ramus of the mandible.

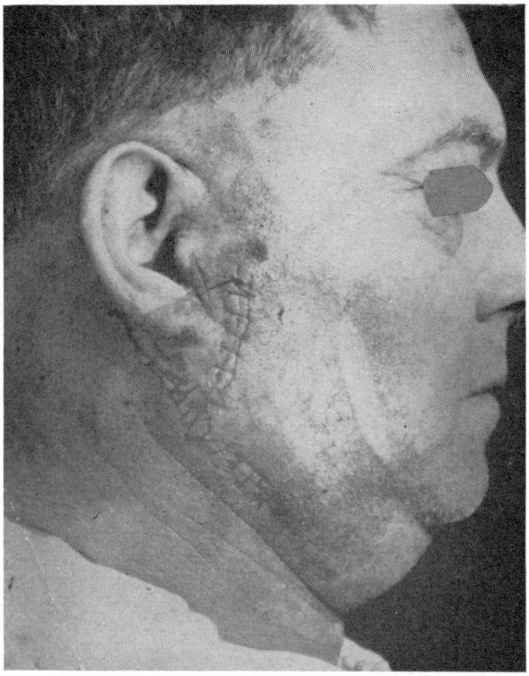

Fig. 8.—Clinical photograph showing the Y incision sutured.

There are some who may believe that this exposure is too extensive for mixed tumors of the parotid which appear small on clinical examination. When it is recalled that many parotid tumors are like icebergs with only a small portion of the total presenting superficially and the main mass being present in the depths of the gland, the need for adequate exposure becomes apparent. Dissection under direct observation will permit complete extirpation of the tumor regardless of how deep it extends and will further permit preservation of the seventh nerve. When one further recalls the high recurrence of mixed parotid tumors, usually the result of inadequate surgery, and the ensuing difficulty of resecting a recurrent tumor, the somewhat larger exposure is definitely warranted.

A modification of this incision must be utilized for certain parotid cancers which have infiltrated the skin. In these instances the skin and subcutaneous tissue must be excised in continuity with the parotid gland, and radical neck dissection performed. The resulting defect is closed with skin graft (Figs. 16 and 17).

Fig. 9.

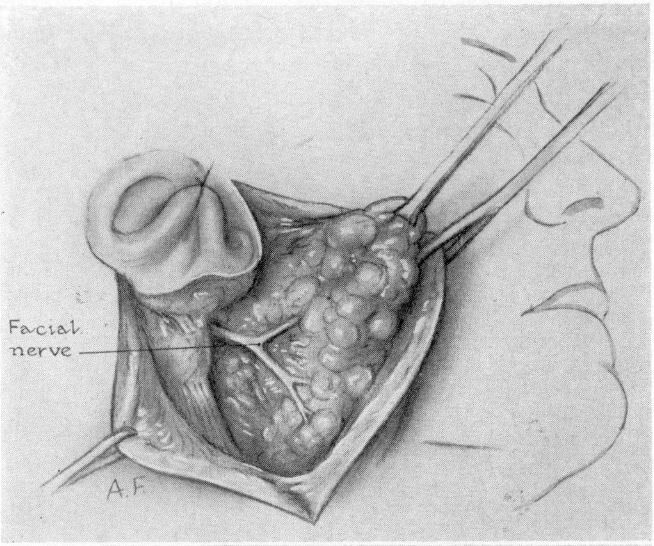

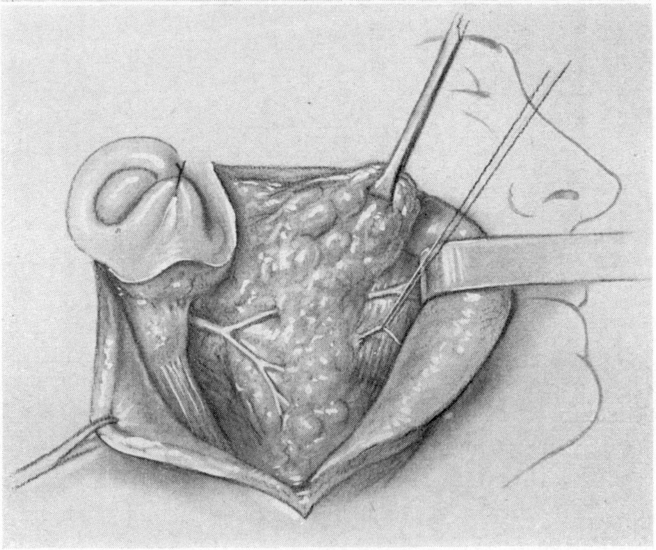

Fig. 10.

Fig. 9.—The parotid gland has been dissected away from the mastoid process and sternocleidomastoid muscle. The nerve is quite deep (1.25 to 2 cm. from the skin) and is the only nerve bisecting the plane of the incision and traversing the operative field from a posterior origin, anteriorly. It measures from 2 to 3 mm. in diameter. By gently teasing the gland anteriorly the main branch of the seventh nerve and its divisions can be brought into view.

Fig. 10.—Technique utilized in separating an associated sialadenitis about a parotid tumor from the facial nerve. A piece of silk suture or a nerve hook is placed around the main trunk and around the terminal branches of the nerve, which permits dissecting between the immobilized nerve. The gland can be separated by blunt dissection if adherence is due to an inflammatory reaction. In our experience it could not be freed by blunt dissection if adherence is due to cancer, in which case it is sacrificed.

Exposure of the Facial Nerve.—Three methods have been described for exposing the seventh nerve. They consist of (1) first isolating the marginal mandibular branch and tracing it to the main stem, or (2) tracing one of the branches as it emerges from the anterior border of the parotid back to the main branch, or (3) identifying the main branch first as it comes out of the stylomastoid foramen. After having utilized all three methods we are convinced that the easiest and most direct way is first to isolate the main branch. The easiest method of exposing the facial nerve is to deepen the incision along the upper portion of the sternocleidomastoid muscle at its origin in the mastoid process. By dissecting in this plane it is almost impossible to damage the nerve. The origin of the posterior belly of the digastric muscle into the mastoid is an additional aid in identifying the nerve, for it presents itself just superior to this point. As the dissection continues for a distance of 1½ cm. the nerve will be encountered extending at almost right angles from the stylomastoid foramen, swinging beneath the external auditory canal to extend superficially to the anterior surface of the ascending ramus.

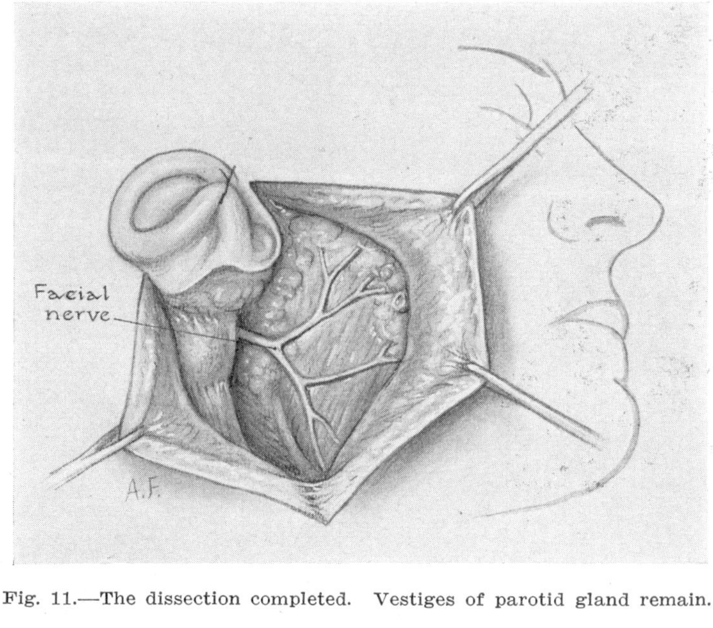

Fig. 11.—The dissection completed. Vestiges of parotid gland remain.

Practically all nerves in this vicinity travel in a more or less vertical direction, while the facial nerve travels almost at right angles to the vertical plane of the incision. By following the anterior border of the sternomastoid and deepening the incision by gently dissecting the posterior portion of the parotid gland anteriorly, the nerve will be encountered extending in the direction of the dissection, that is, from posterior, anteriorly (Fig. 9).

An aid which has been found helpful in certain short-necked patients with long overhanging mastoid processes is to remove a portion of the mastoid with the osteotome, which affords additional room for dissection.

Dissection of Tumor.—The superficial portion of the parotid gland can now be dissected free of the nerve with relative ease. The peculiar pliable consistence renders it dissectible. The gland is dissected anteriorly, and as the dissection continues the nerve will be found to divide into its component branches. By continuing the dissection to the anterior margin, the entire portion of the gland superficial to the facial nerve can easily be removed. Since most of the

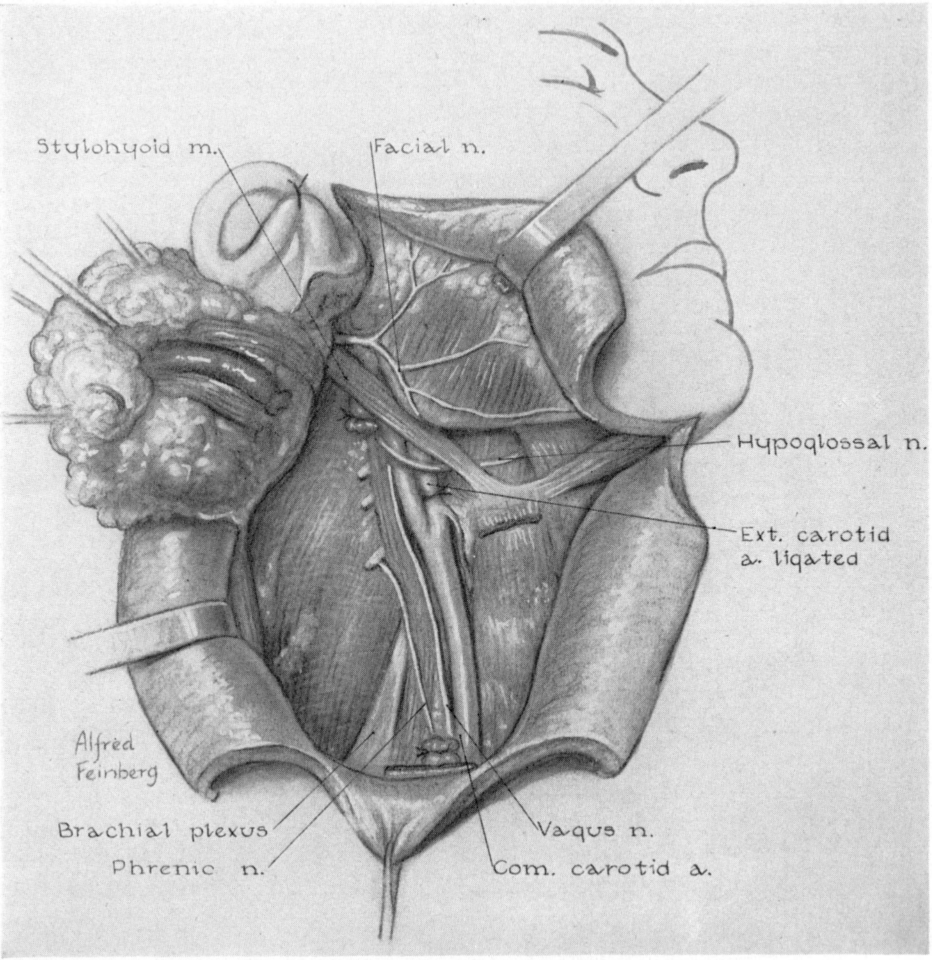

Fig. 12.—Combined parotidectomy and radical neck dissection in continuity. The nerve may be spared in occasional instances of low-grade carcinoma which had produced metastases to cervical lymph nodes.

mixed tumors occur in this location, this procedure will permit adequate resection of the majority of mixed parotid tumors. If it is not desired to remove the entire superficial gland, an extracapsular local excision of the tumor can be performed adequately under direct vision. If the tumor extends posteriorly between the branches of the nerves (we have never seen mixed tumors infiltrate the facial nerve; instead they distort the nerve by pushing it aside as tumor growth continues), the tumor can be readily dissected into the posterior portions of the parotid gland.

In certain instances the presence of a mixed tumor may induce an associated sialadenitis which may present a clinical picture of cancer. When operating on recurrent mixed tumors, the associated inflammation and adhesions so distort the tissues that it is difficult to distinguish where the tumor

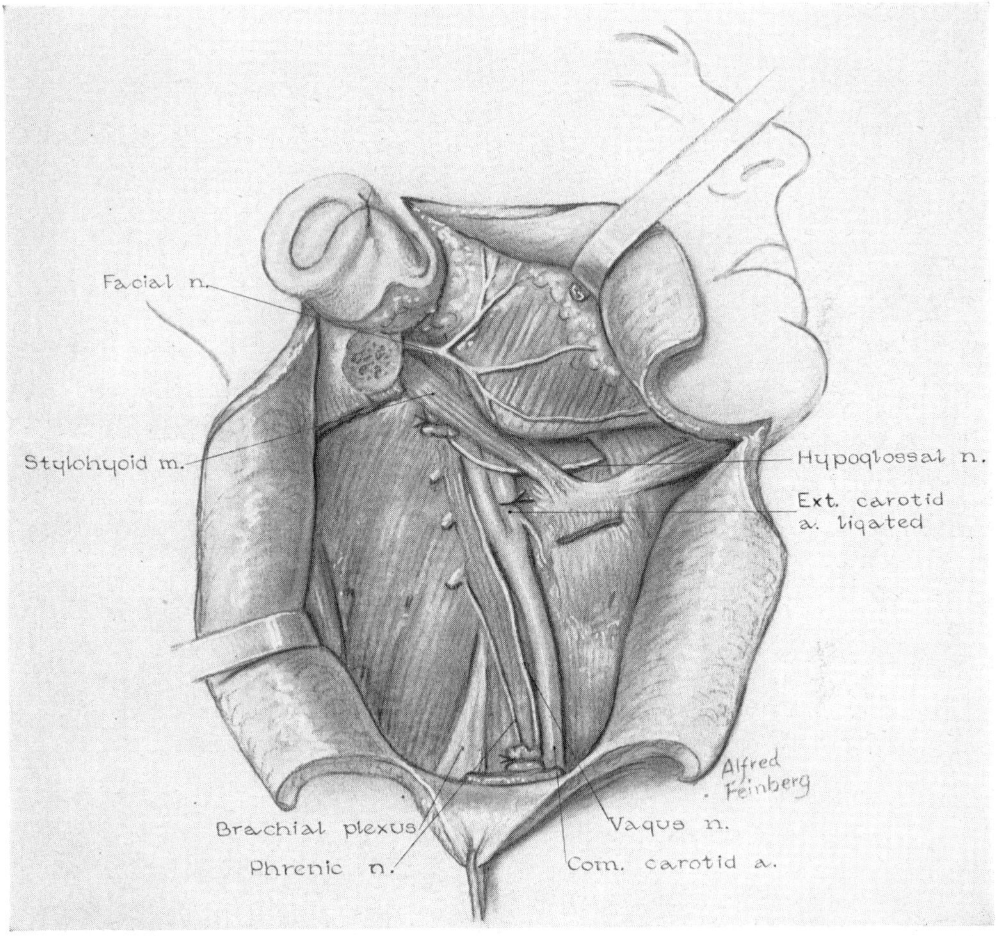

Fig. 13.—Combined parotidectomy and radical dissection completed. Note the ligated external carotid artery to help minimize bleeding. This is performed at the beginning of the operation. A portion of the mastoid process has been removed to afford better exposure. The stylohyoid muscle may be removed.

ends and scarring begins. Certain of these cases give a mistaken impression of carcinoma invading the nerve. A useful technique for dealing with these situations is to identify the nerve branches as they emerge from the gland by keeping these branches taut by either a nerve hook or a small piece of silk and placing a similar piece of silk under the proximal branch, thus immobilizing the nerve. Each branch can then be dissected separately, free of the surrounding tissue. In every instance where this was performed and where the distorted parotid tissue could be dissected free by blunt dissection, the pathologic report was always sialadenitis. Contrariwise, when the nerve branches could not be isolated by blunt dissection, cancer was always present. This simple technique has been found most useful in deciding if the nerve should be severed, or which of its branches should be severed, in the presence of parotid cancer (Fig. 10).

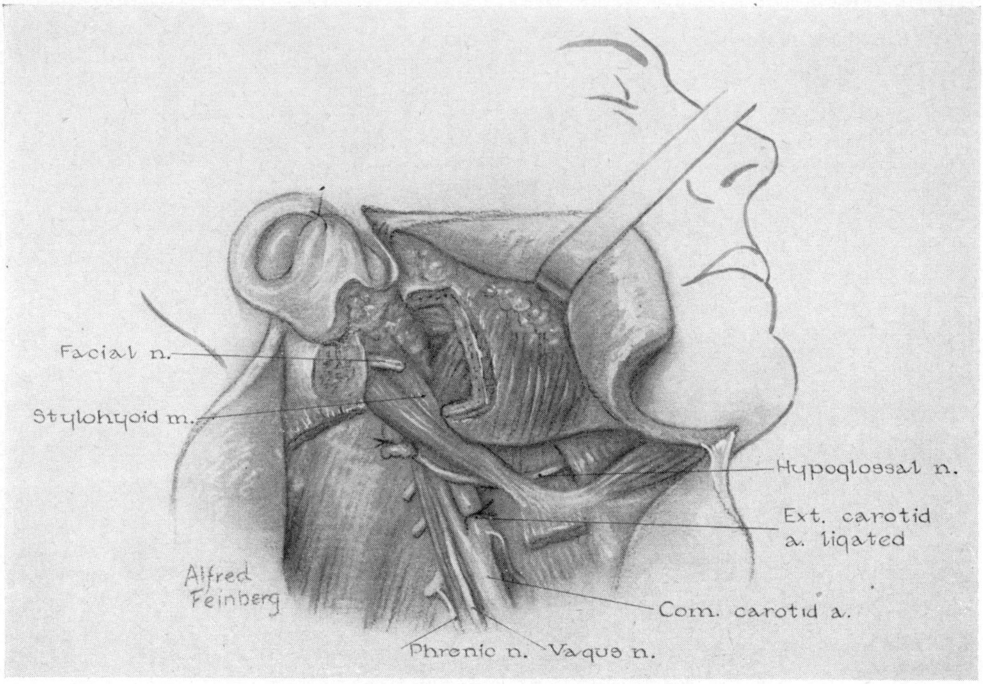

Fig. 14.—Combined parotidectomy and radical neck dissection with a portion of the ascending ramus removed to permit entering into the pterygomandibular fossa and removing the posterior portion (deep lobe) of the parotid gland. The facial nerve has been sacrificed.

Treatment of Parotid Carcinoma.—Admittedly, the best method of treating cancer of any organ is radical extirpation of that organ, sacrificing any intervening structures which interfere with a block dissection and removing the regional lymph nodes in continuity. The parotid gland lends itself well to such extirpation except for certain prolongations of the gland within anatomic recesses. The sacrifice of the facial nerve certainly facilitates the resection, and theoretically this should be accomplished for all cases of cancer. The resultant deformity is great, and in certain instances, especially in younger patients, we have violated the tenets of cancer surgery and have performed the parotidectomy leaving the seventh nerve in situ. This procedure seems warranted in certain low-grade carcinomas developing in mixed tumors (the so-called malignant mixed tumor), in certain discrete cylindromas, and in squamous-cell, adeno-, and mucoepidermoid carcinomas of low-grade malignancy. The technique of separating the parotid tissue from the nerve by blunt dissection is utilized, and if it can be accomplished, the nerve is not sacrificed. However, if any branch cannot be so dissected free, that branch is severed. If the main trunk cannot be easily freed, the entire nerve is resected.

The seventh nerve is never spared for undifferentiated carcinoma or any carcinoma which is diffusely infiltrative. Usually no attempt is made to spare the nerve for recurrent cancer except for very low-grade carcinoma. The failure of recurrence when this technique has been practiced is encouraging, but it must be realized that it is a clinical compromise with the disciplines of cancer surgery, and continued critical observation of these patients must be maintained for proper evaluation and a possible change in the practiced technique, if indicated.

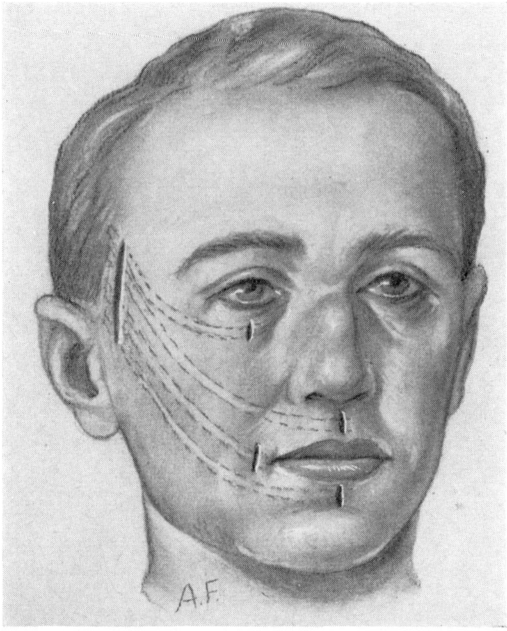

Fig. 15.—Technique of reconstructing the paralyzed face after severance of the seventh nerve (after Brown). Temporal fascial slings are utilized.

Neck Dissection.—The high incidence of metastases to regional lymph nodes from parotid cancer (25 per cent of this series) emphasizes the need of resecting these nodes in continuity with the primary tumor. The parotid gland lends itself well to this procedure.

The lymph node distribution is presented in Fig. 6. The rich network of nodes in the vicinity of the parotid gland favors rapid dissemination to this chain. The dissection should always include all the preauricular and subauricular lymph nodes. It should extend posteriorly to excise the mastoid node, and it is advisable to extend the dissection further posteriorly to include the occipital nodes. An occasional metastasis to this site has been noted. The abundance of lymph nodes about the parotid facilitates dissemination to all cervical nodes, and then nothing short of a complete radical neck dissection should be accomplished.

It may be mentioned that the lymph nodes to be excised during a complete neck dissection for a primary tumor of any location of the head and neck should include the suprafascial, glandular, and subfascial parotid nodes. To accomplish their removal it is necessary to resect the inferior portion of the parotid gland and the contiguous tissue, which includes this group of lymph nodes.

Technique of Combined Parotidectomy and Radical Neck Dissection.—The essential steps are graphically shown in Figs. 12 and 13. The incision is extended as shown by the dotted line in Fig. 7. The contents of the submaxillary triangle, the jugular vein, and spinal accessory nerves are routinely removed. The external carotid artery is usually ligated at the beginning of the operation; the stylohyoid muscle is usually removed but may be preserved. The sternocleidomastoid muscle must be removed at its origin, and frequently the mastoid process is removed with an osteotome.

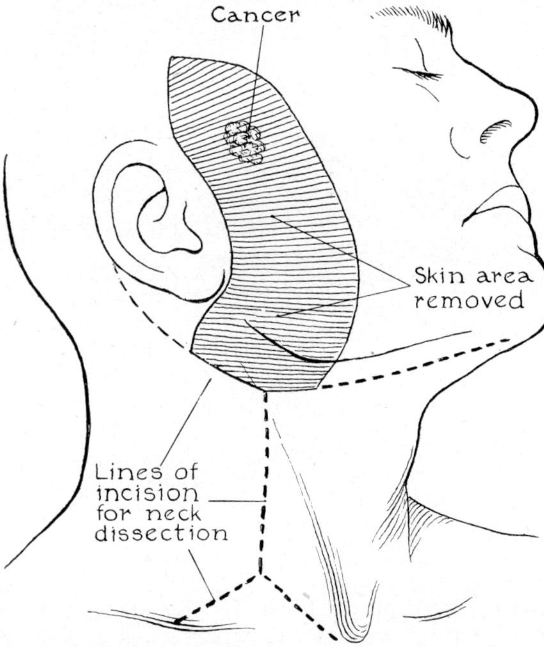

Fig. 16.—Combined parotidectomy and neck dissection necessitating, in addition, removal of a large portion of skin because of dermal infiltration of a parotid cancer.

The Mandible and Tumors of the Parotid Gland.—The mandible frequently presents a formidable obstacle in treating certain parotid tumors. The parotid gland is visualized hugging the posterior border of the ascending mandibular ramus with extension anterior (forming the superficial lobe, the site of most tumors) and a posterior extension into the retromandibular fossa. The mandible must be surgically manipulated for (1) parotid tumors which arise from the posterior portion of the parotid gland when the possibility exists that they have extended posterior to the mandible; (2) any tumor arising from that portion of the parotid gland in back of the mandible (so-called deep lobe). These tumors fill the retromandibular (pterygomandibular) space and require special surgical consideration; (3) carcinomas which invade the mandible.

Surgical Techniques for Operation on the Mandible in Its Relationship to Parotid Neoplasms.—

1. *Tumors extending posterior to the mandible:* A simple method of exploring this region is to remove a block of bone from the posterior portion of the ascending ramus. Frequently the tumor will be exposed and its excision effected (Fig. 14). If the tumor should extend beyond the area exposed, it is necessary to sever the ascending ramus with a Gigli saw, and by retracting the severed portion of bone, access is afforded to the pterygomandibular space. The severed bone ends are wired or plated together at the finish of the operation. Very little functional incapacity is experienced by the patient.

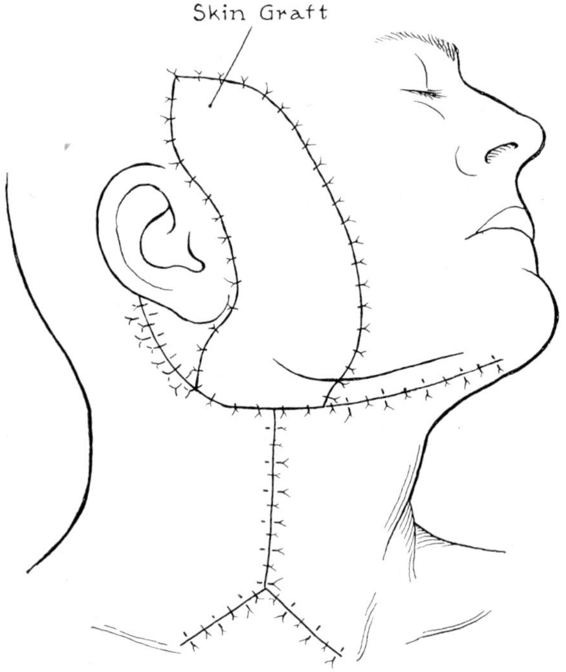

Fig. 17.—The operation described in Fig. 16 completed with a split-thickness skin graft utilized to cover the defect.

2. *Tumors of the retromandibular (pterygomandibular) space:* This potential space, bounded by the mastoid proces, the ascending ramus of the mandible, the vertebral column, and the pharynx, is relatively inaccessible to the surgeon. The important structures which traverse this space are the parotid gland, internal carotid artery, internal carotid vein, and the ninth, tenth, eleventh, and twelfth cranial nerves. Since this space is almost entirely encased in bone, tumors which arise here either present in the space between the posterior border of the ramus and the mastoid or they bulge into the pharynx. If a mixed tumor of the retromandibular portion of the parotid

gland presents into the pharynx, it may be removed by the intraoral route as described by Ehrlich.[12] If the tumor is malignant or if it presents posteriorly, it must be resected by the external approach.

The incision is the same as previously described. The mandible is skeletonized and transected with a Gigli saw, and separation of the ends affords access to this space. If the tumor is not adherent to the mandible, it may be removed in toto by this exposure.

3. *If the mandible is invaded by the neoplasm* a hemimandiblectomy combined parotidectomy and radical neck dissection is accomplished. If roentgenographic evidence of mandibular destruction is apparent, then it is best to disarticulate the involved side of the mandible and perform a complete hemimandiblectomy combined with radical parotidectomy and neck dissection.

IRRADIATION OF PAROTID TUMORS

The role of irradiation has not been truly assessed as a therapeutic agent for treating parotid neoplasms. Although most of the parotid tumors are radioresistant, cures have been obtained by treating parotid cancer exclusively by irradiation. The picture has been confused by the fact that radiotherapy has been applied to neoplasms after they have become widespread, infiltrating contiguous structures, and as a crutch for inadequate surgery. If there was a recurrence after this regime the surgeon was not blamed because it was usually agreed that the irradiation was not great enough, and if there was no recurrence it would be impossible to assess the role of irradiation in effecting the cure. It is impossible to compare the results of excision alone to those obtained by surgery combined with irradiation because in most instances the practiced surgery was not complete. Nothing can be gained by comparing an inadequate surgical procedure to results obtained from surgical treatment combined with irradiation. Thus, Smith and Stenstrom[45] quoted the poor results obtained from surgical resection by Benedict and Meigs (96.7 per cent failure), MacFee (81 per cent failure), and others. In contrast they purported to show that better results have been obtained by Ahlbom, who used irradiation either exclusively or combined with surgical excision and obtained a 25 per cent five-year survival, and Cade, who obtained a 27 per cent five-year survival for carcinomas treated by radical surgery plus postoperative irradiation.

It is believed that irradiation (both interstitial and external) has a definite place in the treatment of parotid neoplasms, but it is necessary to define that place accurately and to use irradiation intelligently and aggressively whenever indicated. Conversely, it is believed that sole reliance upon irradiation for operable parotid tumors should be condemned.

In this series, of the 13 patients with primary carcinoma of the parotid gland who received initial treatment here, 1 patient was treated exclusively by interstitial gold radon seeds, and he remained well and free of disease for seven years after which time he died from other causes. One other patient was treated by external x-ray therapy and interstitial radon seeds, and he has survived for over sixteen years with no signs of recurrence. These data demonstrate that parotid cancer can be cured by irradiation in certain instances. Two other patients who are apparently cured were treated by radical excision alone, and 2 others were treated by excision plus postoperative irradiation. In past years, irradiation had been used quite frequently; at present, most reliance is placed on surgical removal, and as more time elapses the results of surgical intervention can be evaluated.

It is believed that in the treatment of benign tumors sole reliance should be placed upon adequate surgical extirpation. However, because the parotid gland may have projections into areas which are relatively inaccessible (such as the depths of the stylomastoid notch and certain recesses of the pterygomandibular space) gold radon seeds are always available in the operating room. If the tumor is in the vicinity of one such recess, it is considered advisable to insert interstitial gold radon seeds into these sites. Gold seeds 0.3 mm. in diameter and containing 1 to 1.5 mc. of radon are inserted into the proper site. The total dose depends on the size of the sphere to be irradiated and varies from 600 to 2,200 mc. hours. No additional irradiation is given.

The indications for x-ray therapy for mixed tumors are: (1) operable tumor for which the patient refuses surgical intervention, or if operation is contraindicated for other reasons; (2) postoperatively after incomplete excision, especially after an attempted surgical excision of a recurrence; (3) inoperable tumors. After numerous recurrences the tumor may be so mutilated that operation is contraindicated. In such instances response to irradiation is usually poor.

Ahlbom advocates preoperative irradiation, believing that it facilitates operation by making the capsule firmer. We cannot subscribe to this policy.

The x-ray factors usually employed were 200 to 250 kv., 15 to 30 Ma., 0.5 mm. Cu filter, 30 to 50 cm. target-skin distance; the size of the portal varied with the tumor in question and averaged 6 by 9 cm. One hundred fifty roentgens were given to each of two portals daily for a total dosage of 1,500 to 1,800 r., measured in air, to each of three ports.

Irradiation of Parotid Cancer.—Most parotid carcinomas are radioresistant. However, cures may on occasion be obtained by this type of therapy.

Indications for irradiation of parotid cancer: (1) operable cancer for which the patient refuses operation, or if operation is contraindicated for other reasons; (2) if the complete resection would involve sacrifice of the facial nerve and the patient refuses this defect. As much of the tumor as possible should be resected and a combination of interstitial radon and external x-ray therapy applied. The surgeon should not advocate this practice but must resort to it as a compromise regime; (3) after a radical parotidectomy certain remnants of parotid tissue remain in inaccessible anatomic recesses which were not too distant to the cancer. These areas should receive interstitial gold radon seeds and a course of postoperative deep external x-ray therapy; (4) inoperable carcinoma; (5) postoperatively for all instances of undifferentiated carcinoma. The results of this group by surgical intervention alone are poor; (6) the presence of distant metastases. Both the primary site as well as the metastases should be irradiated.

It is believed that reliance should be placed on surgical removal for parotid tumors. This group of neoplasms, although resistant to irradiation, does respond to radiation therapy sufficiently to warrant its use whenever surgical intervention is contraindicated or inadequate. The role of this form of treatment has not yet been exactly determined.

SUMMARY AND CONCLUSIONS

1. The clinical features of 100 patients bearing tumors of the parotid salivary gland are presented.

2. Parotid tumors comprised 0.5 per cent of all patients bearing neoplasms treated at the Pack Medical Group. Of the 100 patients, 54 bore benign tumors, and 46 suffered from carcinoma.

3. The average age of all patients was 45.2 years. Although the peak incidence of patients with benign tumors was less (36.1 years) than patients with carcinoma (52.9 years), there is so much overlapping in the ages of the two groups that the age of a given patient cannot be utilized as a diagnostic criterion.

4. The most frequent presenting symptom is the presence of an asymptomatic mass in the vicinity of either ear.

5. The diagnosis of benign or malignant tumor cannot be made clinically (except in advanced cases), and a biopsy must be taken to determine the type and extent of the surgical intervention required.

6. Indications and techniques for surgical extirpation of parotid neoplasms are described which have been developed on the basis of the surgical anatomy of the parotid salivary gland, the anatomy of the facial nerve, the lymphatic drainage of the parotid salivary gland, and the natural history of neoplasms arising from this organ.

7. The role of irradiation in the treatment of parotid neoplasms is described, and it is emphasized that radiation therapy should not be used as a crutch for inadequate surgical removal but should be used for its specific indications.

8. The data are analyzed to discern the cause for frequent recurrences in the past, and these features are discussed.

9. Of the 54 patients with mixed parotid tumors, 31 per cent developed recurrences. Of the 34 patients treated initially at this institution, only 1 developed a recurrent tumor. Of the 46 patients with carcinoma, 37 per cent presented a recurrence an average of 2.7 years from the time of attempted treatment.

10. The absolute five-year survival rate for the benign tumors is 83.3 per cent and for carcinoma, 32.2 per cent. The relative five-year survival rate for benign tumors is 96.2 per cent, and for the malignant neoplasms it is 41.7 per cent. The therapeutic five-year survival rate for patients with parotid cancer is 83.3 per cent.

REFERENCES

1. Ahlbom, H. E.: Mucous and Salivary Gland Tumors; Clinical Study With Special Reference to Radiotherapy, Acta Radiol., supp. 23, 1-452, 1935.
2. Bailey, H.: Treatment of Tumours of the Parotid Gland, Brit. J. Surg. **28**: 337, 1941.
3. Bailey, H.: Parotidectomy: Indications and Results, Brit. M. J. **1**: 404, 1947.
4. Benedict, E. B., and Meigs, J. V.: Tumors of Parotid Gland, Surg., Gynec. & Obst. **51**: 626, 1930.
5. Blady, J. V., and Hocker, A. F.: Application of Sialography in Non-neoplastic Diseases of Parotid Gland, Radiology **32**: 131, 1939.
6. Brown, J. B., McDowell, F., and Fryer, M. P.: Direct Operative Removal of Benign Mixed Tumors of Anlage Origin in the Parotid Region, Surg., Gynec. & Obst. **90**: 257, 1950.
7. Brown, J. R.: Papillary Cystadenoma Lymphomatosum, Arch. Surg. **63**: 185, 1951.
8. Brunschwig, A.: Mixed Tumors of Tongue and Sublingual Gland, Surg., Gynec. & Obst. **50**: 407, 1930.
9. Buxton, R. W., Maxwell, J. H., and Cooper, D. R.: Tumors of the Parotid Gland, Laryngoscope **59**: 565, 1949.
10. Dockerty, M. B., and Mayo, C. W.: Primary Tumors of the Submaxillary Gland With Special Reference to Mixed Tumors, Surg., Gynec. & Obst. **74**: 1033, 1942.
11. Duthoit, cited by Ahlbom.[1]
12. Ehrlich, H.: Mixed Tumors of the Pterygomaxillary Space; Operative Removal: Oral Approach Oral Surg. **3**: 1366, 1950.
13. Favata, B. V.: Characteristics of Mixed Tumors of the Parotid Growing in Vitro, Surg., Gynec. & Obst. **86**: 659, 1948.
14. Halpert, B., and Hackney, V. C.: Anlage Tumors of the Salivary Gland Type in Unusual Sites, SURGERY **27**: 609, 1950.
15. Hellwig, C. A.: Mixed Tumors of the Salivary Glands, Arch. Path. **40**: 1, 1945.
16. Hempelmann, L. H., Jr., and Womack, N. A.: The Pathogenesis of Mixed Tumors of the Salivary Gland Type, Ann. Surg. **116**: 34, 1942.
17. Hendrick, J. W., Ward, G. E., and Lacy, M. M.: Salivary Tissue Neoplasms, Am. J. Surg. **81**: 373, 1951.
18. Howard, J. M., Rawson, A. J., Koop, C. E., Horn, R. C., and Royster, H. P.: Parotid Tumors in Children, Surg., Gynec. & Obst. **90**: 307, 1950.
19. Janes, R. M.: Treatment of Tumors of Salivary Glands by Radical Excision, Canad. M. A. J. **43**: 554, 1940.
20. Kirklin, J. W., McDonald, J. R., Harrington, S. W., and New, G. B.: Parotid Tumors, Surg., Gynec. & Obst. **92**: 721, 1951.
21. Klopp, C. T., and Winship, T.: Treatment of Mixed Tumors of the Parotid Gland by Subtotal Parotidectomy, Arch. Surg. **61**: 477, 1950.
22. Kornblith, A. B.: Zur Frage der Bösartigkeit der sog. Mischgewächse der Mundspeicheldrüsen, Virchows Arch. f. path. Anat. **286**: 74, 1932.
23. Levin, I.: Pathogenesis and Radium Therapy of Mixed Tumors of the Salivary Glands, Radiology **34**: 69, 1940.
24. MacFee, W. F.: Malignant Tumors of the Salivary Glands, Ann. Surg. **109**: 534, 1939.
25. McCormack, L. J., Caudwell, E. W., and Anson, B. J.: The Surgical Anatomy of the Facial Nerve, Surg., Gynec. & Obst. **80**: 620, 1945.
26. McCune, W. S.: Total Parotidectomy in Tumors of the Parotid Gland, Arch. Surg. **62**: 715, 1951.
27. McFarland, J.: The Histopathologic Prognosis of Salivary Gland Tumors, Am. J. M. Sc. **203**: 502, 1942.
28. McFarland, J.: The Mysterious Mixed Tumors of the Salivary Glands, Surg., Gynec. & Obst. **76**: 23, 1943.
29. McKnight, H. A.: Malignant Parotid Tumor in the Newborn, Am. J. Surg. **45**: 128, 1939.
30. McWhorter, G. L.: The Relations of the Superficial and Deep Lobes of the Parotid Gland to the Ducts and to the Facial Nerve, Anat. Rec. **12**: 149, 1917.
31. Marshall, S. F., and Miles, G. O.: Tumors of Submaxillary and Parotid Gland Areas, S. Clin. North America **27**: 501, 1947.
32. Martin, H.: The Operative Removal of Tumors of the Parotid Salivary Gland, SURGERY **31**: 670, 1952.
33. Martin, H., and Ehrlich, H. E.: Papillary Cystadenoma Lymphomatosum of the Parotid Salivary Gland, Surg., Gynec. & Obst. **79**: 611, 1944.
34. Martin, J. D.: Mixed Tumors of the Parotid Gland, New Orleans M. & S. J. **99**: 99, 1946.
35. Mohs, F. E.: Chemosurgical Treatment of Tumors of the Parotid Gland, Ann. Surg. **129**: 381, 1949.

36. Moyse, P.: Report of 72 Cases of Parotid Tumors Treated Surgically, Extrait du Bulletin du Cancer **36:** 18, 1949.
37. Mulligan, R. M.: Metastasis of Mixed Tumors of the Salivary Glands, Arch. Path. **35:** 357, 1943.
38. Patey, D. H.: Treatment of Mixed Tumours of the Parotid Gland, Brit. J. Surg. **28:** 29, 1940.
39. Perrin, T. L.: Mixed Tumor of the Parotid With Metastases, Arch. Path. **33:** 930, 1942.
40. Quattlebaum, F. W., Dockerty, M. B., and Mayo, C. W.: Adenocarcinoma, Cylindroma Type, of the Parotid Gland, Surg., Gynec. & Obst. **82:** 342, 1946.
41. Rawson, A. J., and Horn, R. C.: Sebaceous Glands and Sebaceous Gland-containing Tumors of the Parotid Salivary Gland, SURGERY **27:** 93, 1950.
42. Rawson, A. J., Howard, J. M., Royster, H. P., and Horn, R. C., Jr.: Tumors of the Salivary Glands, Cancer **3:** 445, 1950.
43. Rouviere, H.: Anatomy of the Human Lymphatic System, Ann Arbor, Mich., 1938, Edwards Brothers, Inc.
44. Schreiner, B. F., and Mattick, W. L.: Tumors of the Salivary Glands Based on a Study of 66 Cases, Am. J. Roentgenol. **21:** 541, 1929.
45. Smith, M. J., and Stenstrom, K. W.: Parotid Tumors, Radiology **52:** 655, 1949.
46. State, D.: Superficial Lobectomy and Total Parotidectomy With Preservation of the Facial Nerve in the Treatment of Parotid Tumors, Surg., Gynec. & Obst. **89:** 237, 1949.
47. Stein, I., and Geschickter, C. F.: Tumors of the Parotid Gland, Arch. Surg. **28:** 492, 1934.
48. Stewart, F. W., Foote, F. W., and Becker, W. F.: Muco-epidermoid Tumors of Salivary Glands, Ann. Surg. **122:** 830, 1945.
49. Swinton, N. W., and Warren, S.: Salivary Gland Tumors, Surg., Gynec. & Obst. **67:** 424, 1938.
50. Taylor, G. W., and Garcelon, G. G.: Tumors of Salivary-gland Origin, New England J. Med. **238:** 766, 1942.
51. Wood, F. C.: Mixed Tumors of Salivary Glands, Ann. Surg. **39:** 57, 207, 1904.

Surgical Technique

CHOLEDOCHOJEJUNOSTOMY EN ROUX Y

RALPH F. BOWERS, M.D., MEMPHIS, TENN.

(From the General Surgical Service, Veterans Administration Medical Teaching Group Hospital)

CHOLEDOCHOJEJUNOSTOMY en Roux Y has proved to be a satisfactory surgical procedure for control of chronic recurring pancreatitis.[6-8] Eleven patients have received the operation at Kennedy Veterans Administration Hospital. All except one have remained free of attacks. The eleventh patient suffered one slight attack during an alcoholic bout, but has been symptom-free since 1948. Several cases have been followed for as long as four to five years.

The control of pancreatitis achieved by this operation strongly suggests that Opie's[1] concept of the etiology is correct. This concept involves regurgitation of bile into the pancreatic duct under pressure. Experimental production[3] of pancreatitis also presents evidence in favor of this theory. The benefits from sphincterotomy, advocated by Doubilet, Mulholland,[2] and others, are gained by avoidance of this regurgitation. Choledochojejunostomy severely tests the validity of this concept because the operation cannot possibly permit any change of function except deviation of bile from the pancreatic duct and duodenum.

The operation, however, has not been universally accepted because of assumed technical difficulties, and it is considered "too radical" by many surgeons, who would otherwise employ the procedure. Consequently, these operators seek a more simple procedure. The main criticism concerns the formation of stricture at the site of the common-duct intestinal anastomosis, which in effect would produce common-duct stricture, a dreaded and obstinate anatomic deformity. Another unfounded criticism involves surgical work in the face of enlarged, indurated, edematous pancreas and peripancreatic inflammation. Actually, the occasional small size of the unobstructed duct is the only threatening difficulty. One stricture occurred twenty-two months after the operation. This stricture was easily corrected by resection of the strictured anastomosis, and reanastomosis was performed. The ease of the reanastomosis was evident because the obstruction had induced dilatation of the common duct. This patient has remained free of trouble for more than one year, which suggests that the duct will probably remain free of stricture formation.

It should not be necessary to call attention to the fact that this type of anastomosis must be used in all pancreaticoduodenectomies and has been

Received for publication, July 29, 1953.

successfully used by many[4, 5] for correction of common-duct strictures and accidental injury of the common duct during gastric resection for ulcer or tumor. Recent reports of stricture formation for this operation in the previously mentioned conditions are notably lacking, particularly if the Roux Y principle is employed. The Roux Y principle establishes a defunctioned loop, which creates a situation where infection around the anastomotic area and in the common duct is either minimal or entirely absent.

I have received numerous requests for a description of the technique of this operation by surgeons who hesitate, but who are eager, to employ it. It must be stated that I claim no originality in the technique briefly described later; although minor variations may be present, these are regarded as variants existing in the maneuvers of different surgeons. One routine rule can be stated however: the choledochojejunal anastomosis must be accomplished by the insertion of very few sutures. It is believed that numerous silk sutures, many of which are unnecessary, will invoke a local foreign-body fibrosis extensive enough to lead to stricture formation. Reinforcement must not be achieved by "piling on" interrupted silk sutures. If a suture is not accomplishing a job, it is better to remove it.

When choledochojejunostomy has been selected for control of pancreatitis, we proceed as follows:

1. Dissect common duct and place tape around lower end. It is not necessary to trace the duct under or into pancreatic tissue because the length of common duct is sufficient.

2. Perform cholecystectomy in usual manner.

3. Transect jejunum between Kocher clamps about ten to twelve inches below Treitz's ligament.

4. Close end of upper jejunal segment with interrupted fine black silk sutures.

5. Partially close end of lower jejunal segment allowing opening large enough to "fit" lumen of common duct.

6. Transport lower end of jejunum through an opening in transverse mesocolon.

7. Transect common duct as low as possible and ligate or transfix lower end.

8. Begin choledochojejunal anastomosis by placing a posterior row of interrupted atraumatic 00 catgut sutures between the common duct and jejunum. Make certain that there is mucosa-to-mucosa suturing. These are drawn up and tied so that the knots reside in the lumen. Four or five sutures will suffice.

9. Make small stab wound in anterior jejunum about one and one-half inches below choledochojejunal anastomosis. Place T tube as indicated in diagram (Fig. 1).

10. Close anterior part of anastomosis with interrupted fine black silk sutures. Knots are obviously outside of lumen. Stitches do not include mucosa, if possible.

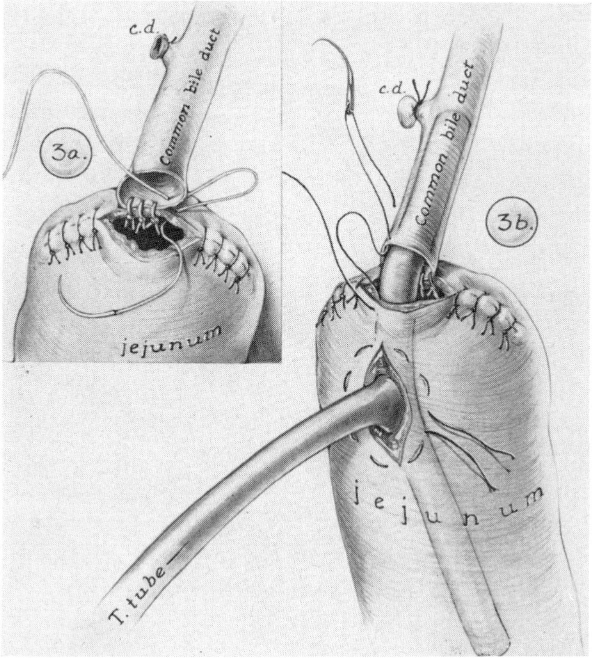

Fig. 1.—Sketch showing details of anastomosis and method of placing T tube.

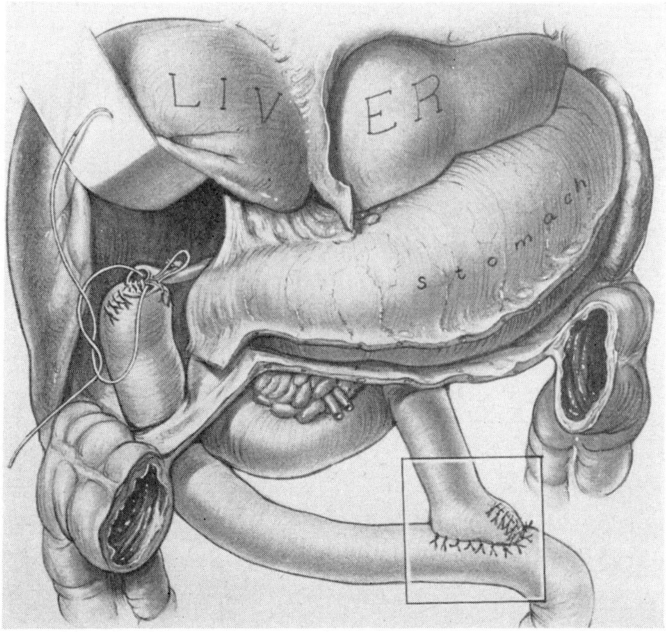

Fig. 2.—Sketch showing general plan of operation.

11. Suture jejunum to liver or round ligament or any available structure which pulls jejunum toward liver to relieve any possible tension on suture line.

12. Suture transverse mesocolon to jejunum to prevent herniation of intestinal loops.

13. Perform enteroenterostomy at site twelve to eighteen inches below choledochojejunal anastomosis.

Lateral anastomosis has been used in our cases, but end-to-side is proper if preferred by operator.

14. Reapproximate mesenteries.

15. Place drain lateral to choledochojejunal anastomosis.

The postoperative care is the same as for common-duct exploration. The T tube is allowed to remain in place for three months. It must be gently irrigated once daily to prevent collection of "mud." Cholangiogram is taken before removal to assure soundness of anastomosis.

It may not be necessary to leave the T tube in place for three months. There is a difference in thickness of the wall of the common duct compared to that of the jejunum, and perhaps the T tube permits more uniform luminal formation. One patient removed the tube on the thirteenth postoperative day without ill effect. The drain is usually removed in stages from the fourth to seventh day.

The procedure requires two to three hours of operating time.

REFERENCES

1. Opie, E. L.: The Etiology of Acute Hemorrhagic Pancreatitis, Bull. Johns Hopkins Hosp. **12**: 182, 1901.
2. Doubilet, H., and Mulholland, J. H.: The Surgical Treatment of Recurrent Acute Pancreatitis by Endocholedochal Sphincterotomy, Surg., Gynec. & Obst. **86**: 295, 1948.
3. Archibald, E.: The Experimental Production of Pancreatitis in Animals as a Result of the Resistance of the Common Duct Sphincter, Surg., Gynec. & Obst. **28**: 529, 1919.
4. Allen, A. W.: A Method of Re-establishing Continuity Between the Bile Ducts and the Gastro-Intestinal Tract, Ann. Surg. **121**: 412, 1945.
5. Cole, W. H., Reynolds, J. T., and Ireneus, C., Jr.: Strictures of the Common Duct, Ann. Surg. **128**: 332, 1948.
6. Bowers, R. F.: Surgical Procedures for Pancreatic Lesions, Arch. Surg. **60**: 817, 1950.
7. Bowers, R. F., and Greenfield, J.: Choledochojejunostomy—Its Role in the Treatment of Pancreatitis, Ann. Surg. **134**: 99, 1951.
8. Bowers, R. F.: Surgical Therapy for Chronic Pancreatitis, SURGERY **30**: 116, 1951.

Book Reviews

Anatomy of the Autonomic Nervous System. By G. A. G. Mitchell. Pp. 356. Edinburgh and London, 1953, E. & S. Livingstone.

Professor Mitchell, director of the anatomic laboratories at the University of Manchester, has been publishing descriptions of the autonomic plexuses for nearly twenty years in the British journals. To this reviewer, who has followed his work from the beginning, Mitchell's illustrations and text have been pre-eminent in this field of neuro-anatomy. Now, happily, these studies have been expanded into a book. This volume contains a singularly simple, clear description of the complicated peripheral pathways of the craniosacral and thoracolumbar plexuses, together with chapters on their embryologic development and central representation within the brain and spinal cord. At a random sampling from the index, it is seen that practically nothing that the surgeon would want to ask the neuro-anatomist has been omitted. The 131 figures comprise a series of superb colored and half-tone illustrations, photomicrographs, and photographs of the author's dissections. Apart from the manifest skill with which these were made, their accuracy is attested to by Sir James Learmouth, who states in his foreword that even in the finest branches no doubtful strand was accepted "as nervous unless its nature was proved by microscopic examination."

The bibliography contains over 800 references. Professor Mitchell deserves high praise for the way he has done justice to the extensive and often conflicting literature that has grown up in this complex field, especially regarding the central nuclei and fiber tracts. In view of the especially confusing problems concerned with the hypothalamus, the reader will relish the following admission from so distinguished an anatomist: "Anyone who suffers from the delusion that anatomy is an effete subject with no problems left to solve is advised to read even a tithe of the bewildering conglomeration of literature on the hypothalamus and its connections. If he does, delusion will be replaced by disillusion."

In the opinion of the reviewer this book is a stimulating product of the British school of anatomy at its best and should appeal particularly to American readers.

Pathologische Physiologie der frischen geschlossenen Hirnverletzungen, insbesondere Hirnerschütterung: klinische, anatomische und experimentelle Befünde. By Dr. R. Wanke, Professor of Surgery at the Universität Kiel. Pp. 196, with 90 colored illustrations. Stuttgart, 1948, Georg Thieme Verlag.

This book is a relatively complete treatise on the pathologic physiology of head injuries. The author has included considerable clinical data along with experimental material in an attempt to understand better the physiologic processes produced by various types of brain lesions. He has included pathologic changes in the liver, in the lungs, in the kidneys, and of the blood, as well as those of the brain. He has attempted to interpret many of the clinical manifestations of such lesions in the light of the pathologic physiology found. Throughout the book there are many charts and graphs explaining these variations, and as an addendum there are color illustrations of the pathologic processes found in the lung and in the brain. Many of his final conclusions are similar to those generally accepted; for example, he believes that blood pressure changes are the most constant clinical findings in patients with increasing intracranial pressure. However, there are considerable data regarding blood sugar levels, porphyrin studies, body temperature regulation, and so forth, in patients and experimental animals with cerebral lesions. The book is written in an involved literary style and is very difficult to translate from the German. To be certain the translation was correct, the book was offered to, and read by, a physician trained in Germany. He also had difficulty, at times, in establishing the author's intent. It is felt that the book is of no particular asset to the average investigator or clinician, but would be of distinct value to anyone willing to spend long hours at translation in order to obtain a few pertinent points of the pathologic physiology of the brain.

Shoulder Lesions. By H. F. Moseley, D.M., F.R.C.S., F.A.C.S. Ed. 2. New York, 1953, Paul B. Hoeber, Inc. $12.00.

Every author should have a publisher like this one, and every publisher, such an author. This book sets a standard in medical publishing. The type, illustrations, and arrangement make the book a pleasure to read. Contained within it are many of the colored plates on the shoulder previously distributed by the drug houses. Many of these beautiful drawings could be used to great advantage in other medical books. In spite of the quality of the book, its price has remained reasonable. The author's material, selected almost entirely from his own experience, gives the work a tone of quiet assurance. By limiting the scope of the book, the author remains in command of the subject throughout. The final chapter is the weakest and emphasizes the faults of many of the recent "regional" books without detracting from this one. This is probably the best book on the shoulder to be published since Codman's classic.

Reconstruction Surgery and Traumatology. Edited by Max Lange, Vol. 1. Basel, Switzerland, 1953, S. Karger.

This marks the first of a series of annual volumes in the field of reconstructive surgery and traumatology. The Editorial Board contains outstanding surgeons throughout Europe, several from South America, and from the United States. It is an attempt to bring together a variety of opinions based on widely divergent experience.

The initial volume deals with three subjects: intramedullary nailing, the late results of fractures of the neck of the femur, and reconstructive operation for nerve paralyses. The high caliber of the presentations can be judged by a partial list of authors: Küntscher, d'Aubigné, Böhler, Scaglietti, Bunnell, Steindler, and Lange. If such a group of presentations can be assembled each year, this will undoubtedly become one of the more important annual publications in its field.

Tumors of Bone, A Roentgenographic Atlas. Annals of Roentgenology, Vol. 21. By Bradley L. Coley and Norman L. Higinbotham. New York, 1953, Paul B. Hoeber, Inc. $10.00.

This volume contains a well-selected and well-reproduced sample of x-ray pictures of bone tumors and of bone diseases simulating bone tumors. There are occasional photographs of gross pathologic specimens. A histologic diagnosis has been made in each case. The accompanying text detracts from the x-ray pictures; the pictures speak for themselves, and the editors were better silent. It is unfortunate that a brief history and clinical appraisal do not accompany each case with a differential diagnosis and final diagnosis following on the next page. With all of the cases mixed indiscriminately together, the book would then be more of a challenge for the reader.

Die gesunde und die kranke Wirbelsäule in Röntgenbild und Klinik. By Dr. Georg Schmorl and Dr. Herbert Junghanns. Ed. 3. Stuttgart, Germany, 1953, Georg Thieme Verlag, Agent for U. S. A.: Grune & Stratton, Inc., New York, N. Y.

It is surprising to see a third edition following so rapidly on the heels of the second. However, for those who have not already obtained a copy, this newer edition is to be preferred. This book is probably the outstanding work on the pathology of the spine and its correlation with the accompanying x-ray changes. It should find wide use among roentgenologists and orthopedists as a reference work. The information obtained from the systematic examination of over 10,000 spines removed at autopsy is invaluable from the point of view of determining the frequency of normal variations and the incidence of various pathologic processes.

The Temporomandibular Joint. Edited by Bernard G. Sarnat, M.D., M.S., D.D.S., F.A.C.S. Springfield, Ill., 1951, Charles C Thomas, Publisher. $4.75.

Maxillofacial surgeons and orthodontists will find this book invaluable. Within its pages, is the present sum and total knowledge of the temporomandibular joint and its relation to the growth and development of the face. It is an excellently printed book written by a group of specialists.

Roentgen Examinations in Acute Abdominal Diseases. By J. Frimann-Dahl, M.D., Ph.D., chief of Roentgen Department, Ulleval Hospital, Oslo, Norway. Pp. 323, with 305 illustrations. Springfield, Ill., 1951, Charles C Thomas, Publisher. $12.50.

This splendid book, prepared by an eminent European radiologist, deserves a wide audience. It should appeal both to the radiologist who must read films of acute abdominal diseases and to surgeons and internists who have the responsibility of handling these patients, often without benefit of immediate radiologic consultation.

In the introductory chapter the author stresses that cooperative endeavor is necessary to gain the maximum benefit from x-ray study of these illnesses. Full information about the patient's history and physical findings, careful fluoroscopy, and roentgen technique varied according to different lesions are stressed as important features in the author's methods, through which his death rate has fallen from 50 per cent to 10 per cent. This result, due largely to improvement in diagnosis, has not been achieved by routine examination and indifferent quality films.

A chapter on normal findings is followed by one on general pathologic findings, in which are considered absorption and production of intestinal gas, fluid in intestine, pneumoperitoneum, free fluid in peritoneal cavity, and lesions in chest. Then the special findings in a wide variety of diseases, twenty-eight in all, are described and portrayed in accompanying sketches and x-ray reproductions, which the American reader will be glad to know are reproduced as negative prints. Most of the x-ray pictures are well done, an important consideration in soft tissue radiography which the author is accentuating. Contrast studies, made when necessary, are also given full place. Surgeons will be interested to note that many of the diagnostic advances were the result of basic surgical experiment.

In summary, this is a very worth-while monograph, thoughtful, well constructed, and concerning an important and somewhat neglected field.

Rötgenuroscopie. By G. W. Günther. Pp. 45, with 86 illustrations. Paper covers. Stuttgart, 1953, Georg Thieme Verlag, Agent for U. S. A.: Grune & Stratton, Inc., New York, N. Y.

Called pyeloscopy by Harris in Australia and by Herbst in this country, the fluoroscopic observation of the renal pelvis and ureter filled with contrast agent gives a better idea of the dynamics of the upper urinary tract than do the conventional methods of urography with films. This is particularly true of the differentiation of stricture from spasm, and of detecting aberrations of peristalsis. However, the same information can be secured by the judicious use of serial exposures in connection with excretory urography, and by delayed exposures after retrograde pyelography.

The trouble with uroscopy is that it ties up the patient, the observer, and the equipment for long periods in order to secure information otherwise available just as accurately and much more expeditiously, and without the danger of overexposure of patient and operator inherent in fluoroscopy.

Uroscopy seems to the reviewer to be a technique for the study of the function of the urinary collecting apparatus rather than a method for widespread clinical application. The book should be read with this in mind. The illustrations are excellent, and the bibliography, with one exception, is strictly German.

ANNOUNCEMENTS

Sixth International Cancer Congress

Physicians and scientists are invited to present papers at the Sixth International Cancer Congress to be held in São Paulo, Brazil, July 23 to 29, 1954, under the sponsorship of the International Union Against Cancer. The program will include sections on fundamental cancer research, on clinical studies on cancer, and on cancer control. Registration blanks are available from the Chairman, National Committee on the International Union Against Cancer, National Research Council, 2101 Constitution Avenue, N.W., Washington 25, D. C.

It is expected that round trip transportation by air from Miami to São Paulo will be available for about $480. Detailed information regarding travel arrangements and hotel reservations may be obtained from Dr. Brewster S. Miller, American Cancer Society, Inc., 47 Beaver Street, New York 4, N. Y.

In accordance with similar arrangements being made in other countries to coordinate participation in the Congress, residents of the United States who desire to present papers must send *five* copies of an abstract of each paper proposed for presentation to the Chairman, National Committee on the International Union Against Cancer, at the Washington address by Jan. 15, 1954. Abstracts are not to exceed 250 words and must be accompanied by a title and the name, address, academic or professional title, and institutional affiliation of the investigator or physician. These requirements do not apply to people who have been invited to participate by the President of the Congress unless application is made for travel allotments as described later.

Travel allotments of approximately $600 each will be available to a limited number of individuals requiring such assistance. Applications for travel allotments must be submitted in quintuplicate to the Chairman, National Committee on the International Union Against Cancer, at the Washington address by Jan. 15, 1954. They should be in letter form giving information concerning age, training, publications in cancer or related fields, and academic or professional status. Applicants not planning to present papers should include five copies of abstracts, as described previously, of major current investigative work. A letter from the laboratory director, or appropriate administrative officer, approving the application is also necessary.

Buffalo Surgical Society

On Feb. 18, 1954, the Buffalo Surgical Society will sponsor the Roswell Park Lecture, this year to be given by Dr. Isador S. Ravdin, John Rhea Barton professor of surgery, University of Pennsylvania Medical School, and Surgeon in Chief at the Hospital of the University of Pennsylvania.

Dr. Ravdin at that time will be awarded the Society's Gold Medal, being given for the seventh time, in honor of Dr. Roswell Park, professor of surgery, University of Buffalo, 1883 to 1914. Previous lecturers and recipients of the Medal are as follows: Dr. Allen C. Whipple (1948), Dr. Evarts A. Graham (1949), Dr. Dallas B. Phemister (1950), Dr. Frederick A. Coller (1951), Dr. Edward D. Churchill (1952), and Dr. Warren H. Cole (1953).

SURGERY

VOL. 35 FEBRUARY, 1954 No. 2

Original Communications

PRIMARY CARCINOMA OF THE LUNG

Results of Surgical Treatment

Mario M. J. Brea, M.D.,* Buenos Aires, Argentina

THE aim of this work is to present the results of our experience with the surgical treatment of bronchiogenic carcinoma. It is based upon a series of 800 cases from our hospital and private practice; 311 were operated upon and in 200 a resection was done.

Table I. Operability (1944 to 1952)

Number of patients observed	880
Number of patients resected	200
Operative index	22.7%

This figure is not quite right in absolute terms, because our cases are surgical and therefore represent a selection; but it is useful for comparative purposes. The operative index depends on the criteria of extension of resection in advanced cases and, mainly, of palliative resections when they are performed. We advocate wide resections in advanced cases and palliative operations only when during thoracotomy the propagation precludes radical resection; in other words, we do not perform deliberate palliative resections.

In 1948,[1] we stated that by taking advantage of all favorable circumstances operability could reach 50 per cent, which is a substantial proportion.

In our series the operative index has increased in these percentages:

1947	13.1 per cent
1949	17.6 per cent
1952	22.7 per cent

It is lower than Ochsner and associates'[2] figures, 35 per cent (1952), but near Churchill and co-workers',[3] 25.1 per cent (1950). Edwards[4] (1946) could resect in only 70 cases out of 1,016, scarcely 7 per cent.

Read before the Inter-American Congress of the American College of Surgeons, São Paulo, Brazil, Feb. 11, 1953.
Received for publication, April 6, 1953.
*Assistant Professor, Thoracic Surgery, University of Buenos Aires Medical School.

Table II. Resectability

Number of patients explored	311
Number of patients resected	200
Resectability index	64.3%

Resectability index reveals the accuracy of operability diagnosis and of handling of advanced cases, in other words, the ability to decide whether a case is resectable or not. It increases with the accuracy of the detection of extension indicating inoperability and with the use of new techniques of radical resection.

In our series the resectability was:

1947	40.7 per cent
1949	56.0 per cent
1952	64.3 per cent

Ochsner's[2] figure is 64.8 per cent and Churchill's[3] 58.0 per cent.

Table III. Mortality (1944 to 1952)

Number of patients resected	200
Number of deaths	37
Gross mortality	18.5%

Thirty-seven patients died immediately or several weeks after operation (18.5 per cent). In order to evaluate the risk of operation we must consider the time the operation was performed, because in later years surgical skill has become greater and antibiotics and a better understanding of prevention of shock have been available. Furthermore, it is essential to consider the extent of resection and, finally, whether the patient is in a private or charity hospital must be considered.

Our series comprises only one period (1944 to 1952).

Table IV. Mortality and Influence of the Type of Operation

Type of operation	Number of cases	Deaths	Per cent
Pneumonectomy	159	35	22.0
Lobectomy	41	2	4.8

Most deaths occurred in the pneumonectomy group, partly because of the greater risk, but chiefly because lesions so treated were more extensive and propagated to the mediastinum as demonstrated by these figures:

	Number of Cases	Deaths	Per Cent
Atypical resections	119	31	26.0
Typical resections	81	6	7.4

We consider reaction atypical when it is carried beyond the borders of the organ, thus altering the standard technique. Details are given in the following figures.

	Number of Cases	Deaths	Per Cent
Mediastinal dissection	33	4	12.1
Parietal and mediastinal dissection	6	2	33.3
Intrapericardiac maneuvers	4	1	25.0
Suture of the auricle	4	2	50.0
Block resection of chest wall	9	6	66.6

TABLE V. MORTALITY AND INFLUENCE OF TYPE OF HOSPITAL

TYPE OF HOSPITAL	NUMBER OF CASES	DEATHS	PER CENT
Charity hospital	104	28	26.9
Private practice	96	9	9.3

Such a remarkable difference depends on the type of patients treated, in that the charity patient generally has a more advanced lesion; also, in private clinics there is better nursing and medical care.

Operation	Hospital	Number of Cases	Deaths	Per Cent
Pneumonectomy	Charity hospital	91	27	29.6
	Private practice	68	8	11.7
Lobectomy	Charity hospital	13	1	7.5
	Private practice	28	1	3.5

In both institutions the mortality in the lobectomy series was low, a consequence of the fewer nursing requirements. Lobectomy was twice as common in private practice as in charity patients, an index confirming the theory that the more favorable cases are predominately those of private patients. Conversely, in the charity series, pneumonectomy, with its higher mortality, was performed more often because the lesions are more advanced.

From the foregoing it is evident that the mortality increases with the extent of the lesion and the type of operation.

We cannot change the extent of the resection except by early diagnosis, which is dependent upon education of the medical profession concerning the frequency of bronchiogenic carcinoma. The extent of resection, which depends on the extent of the growth, rests on a choice between lobectomy and pneumonectomy. In certain cases, with small, peripheral tumors, without glands and with free fissures, we prefer lobectomy because we consider the operation as radical or as palliative as pneumonectomy, with the advantage of its low operative mortality and better functional prognosis. The feasibility of this procedure is still open to question and because of this we cite our results. We do not believe that there is a place for standards in the treatment of a disease such as cancer where we cannot warrant any cure and where we proceed only under the guidance of the gross findings provided by clinical investigation.

Of 200 patients submitted to resection 37 died shortly after operation and, excluding 13 others not traced, there remained 150. Ninety-two of them died postoperatively from recurrence and other causes; 58 are still alive.

Most of the postoperative deaths occurred within two years, the so-called "critical" period. The patients who survive this period without signs of recurrence have a good chance of cure.

TABLE VI. SURVIVALS

	Of 92 Patients Who Died		
Critical period	0 to 6 months	32	81
	6 months to 1 year	31	
	1 to 2 years	18	
	2 to 3 years	8	
	3 to 4 years	3	
	Of 58 Patients Still Alive		
	6 months to 1 year	13	
	1 to 2 years	11	
Over 2 years	2 to 3 years	11	34
	3 to 4 years	8	
	4 to 5 years	8	
	More than 5 years	7	

It is interesting to study the survival rate in relation to the type of resection and to the characteristics of the tumor (histology and spread).

TABLE VII. SURVIVALS OVER TWO YEARS IN RELATION TO TYPE OF RESECTION

TYPE OF OPERATION	NUMBER OF OPERATIONS	NUMBER OF SURVIVALS	PER CENT
Pneumonectomy	104	25	24.0
Lobectomy	21	9	42.8
Total	125	34	27.2

Concerning long-time survivals we can consider only pneumonectomy and lobectomy, as we have not had enough experience with the radical resections because of the small number of such operations performed and the short period of time which has elapsed (under two years). Excluding thirteen cases not traced, 125 resections were performed between 1946 and 1950, with a minimum of two years' postoperative course. Thirty-four patients are still alive (27.2 per cent), a figure very similar to those obtained by Churchill and Ochsner and inferior only to Taylor and associate's.[5] We surmise that our five-year survival rate might be similar to Ochsner's and we believe that the cure rate following surgical treatment of bronchiogenic carcinoma should be 25 per cent.

But the most interesting feature is the comparative study of lobectomy and pneumonectomy to establish their respective curative value. The overall figure is very impressive: 42.8 per cent for lobectomy against 24.0 per cent for the pneumonectomy series. Churchill reports the same results: lobectomy 26 per cent and pneumonectomy 22 per cent survival rate after five years. In Churchill's series the operative mortality was not a significant factor because it was more or less the same for both operations; in our cases mortality was quite different in the two series, thus explaining the great difference between the respective figures.

We do not assume that lobectomy is a more radical operation than pneumonectomy because we know that the tumors treated by partial resection have a better prognosis, but this fact confirms the idea that in selective cases the radicality of the two is equivalent. Therefore, it is advisable not to lose the opportunity to perform a lobectomy with its accompanying advantages, low mortality and excellent immediate and functional results.

TABLE VIII. SURVIVALS. HISTOLOGY AND PROPAGATION OF THE TUMOR

*(A) Histologic classification of 185 resected patients**

TYPE	NUMBER OF CASES	PER CENT
Epidermoid carcinoma	101	55.1
Adenocarcinoma	58	31.3
Undifferentiated	17	9.2
Sarcoma	5	2.7
Alveolar cell tumors	2	1.0
Endothelioma	2	1.0

*Ten cases of bronchial adenoma are not included.

(B) Histologic classification and propagation of 33 resected patients who survived more than two years

TYPE	WITHOUT PROPAGATION	WITH PROPAGATION	TOTAL	PER CENT
Epidermoid	18	2	20	60.6
Adenocarcinoma	11	1	12	36.3
Sarcoma	1	–	1	–
Total	30	3 (9%)	33	–

(C) Histologic classification and propagation of 9 lobectomy patients who survived more than two years

TYPE	WITHOUT	WITH
Epidermoid	3	–
Adenocarcinoma	6	–
Total	9	–

(D) Histologic classification and propagation of 24 pneumonectomy patients who survived more than two years

TYPE	WITHOUT	WITH	TOTAL	PER CENT
Epidermoid	15	2	17	70.8
Adenocarcinoma	5	1	6	25.0
Sarcoma	1	–	1	4.2
Total	21	3	24	–

Of 200 resected cases 15 were not well classified but the remainder, 185, were. Epidermoid carcinoma constituted the majority with 55.1 per cent, followed by adenocarcinoma with 31.3 per cent and undifferentiated 9.2 per cent. These figures are different from those obtained in the pathologic laboratories in which there is a higher proportion of the last grouping. It is recognized that this disparity lies in the smaller degree of malignancy of the epidermoid and adenocarcinoma which offer a greater chance for surgical treatment.

The respective malignancies of these lesions in patients surviving two years is demonstrated in Table VIII, (*b*).

Epidermoid carcinoma was present in 60.6 per cent and adenocarcinoma in 36.3 per cent. Most tumors had no metastases (thirty of thirty-three); only three of the patients, or 9 per cent, who are still alive had metastases. The bad prognosis of carcinoma with lymphatic propagation has been stressed by Ochsner, who considers resection palliative under these circumstances. Although Graham does not subscribe to this opinion, it is prevalent. The poor results obtained in cases with metastases have prompted many surgeons to perform more extensive resections with dissection of the lymphatics of the mediastinum.

It is interesting to consider the relationship of the type of tumor and the type of operation in the patients who survived more than two years [Table VIII, (*c*) and (*d*)]. In the lobectomy group adenocarcinoma was the more prevalent whereas the reverse was true in epidermoid carcinoma. The explanation lies in the fact that adenocarcinoma constitutes most of the peripheral tumors without lymphatic spread which makes lobectomy feasible. In our series many were asymptomatic and were revealed only occasionally by a rheumatoid syndrome of the Bamberger-Marie type. The malignancy of these tumors is not higher than the malignancy of the epidermoid cancers but they have a longer development with a prolonged asymptomatic period.

In the pneumonectomy group, epidermoid carcinomas comprise 70.8 per cent of the cases because of the common localization of these tumors in the hilum of one lung and because of early lymphatic spread which makes it imperative to resect the entire lung.

From the preceding study of the relationships between survivals and the type of excision and the characteristics of the tumor, it is evident that the chief factor in prognosis lies in the extension of the tumor and its actual propagation; the second important factor is histologic type. Conversely, survival is independent of the type of resection. This means that prognosis does not depend as much on histology and extent of resection as on extension of the disease.

SUMMARY AND CONCLUSIONS

1. The operability rate in our series of 880 cases of bronchiogenic carcinoma with 200 resections is 22.7 per cent; it has increased through the years and could reach 50 per cent.

2. Resectability index on 311 thoracotomy cases with 200 resections is 64.3 per cent; it is still increasing, although not as much, because of accuracy of preoperative diagnosis and because of the new field opened by wide resections. There will always be a margin for the exploratory thoracotomy which must not be restricted.

3. Over-all operative mortality is 18.5 per cent. In the pneumonectomy series it was 22 per cent and in lobectomy it was 4.8 per cent. In typical operation, mortality descends to 7.4 per cent, whereas, in atypical operation, it ascends to 26 per cent. The greater risks are in block resections of the chest wall, in patients with suture of the auricle, in combined parietal mediastinal dissection, and in intrapericardial maneuvers. Conversely, mediastinal dissection alone does not add any extra risk. The mortality varies with the type of hospital, 26.9 per cent in charity hospitals and 9.3 per cent in private clinics. This can be explained by major extension and seriousness of disease in charity patients and the better nursing provided by private clinics.

4. Over-all survival includes fifty-eight cases; thirty-four of the patients are living more than two years after the operation, the so-called critical period of recurrences. This represents a 27.2 per cent late-survival rate.

5. Studying the survivals after two years according to the type of resection, it is apparent that lobectomy has advantages over pneumonectomy

because of the different kinds of tumors submitted to each procedure. But at least it is apparent that this operation is as radical as pneumonectomy when strictly circumscribed as to its indications and contraindications.

6. When the relationship between survivals and histology of the tumor is considered, it appears that there is a great prevalence of epidermoid carcinoma in the resected group and that increases in the two-year-survival series are undoubtedly an index of lower malignancy. Late survival in propagated cases was very small, 9 per cent, confirming the opinion that resection in such cases is mostly palliative. This finding is mandatory for more extensive resections, the so-called radicals, with dissection of mediastinal glands.

7. The lobectomy series, which includes less advanced and nonpropagated tumors, shows a sharp predominance of the adenocarcinoma type; this means that its malignancy does not exceed that of the epidermoid group, according to its evolutive degree.

8. General conclusions regarding mortality and survival are:

(a) Operative risk rises with extension of lesions and width of excision.

(b) Prognosis is less dependent on the histologic type of the growth and extension of the excision than it is related to propagation of the disease.

(c) The philosophy of doctors dealing with this problem must be to concentrate their efforts on trying to detect cases earlier than on devising wider operations.

REFERENCES

1. Brea, M. M.: Cáncer de Pulmón, Buenos Aires, 1948, libreria y editorial "El Ateneo."
2. DeBakey, M. E., Ochsner, A., and DeCamp, P. T.: Primary Carcinoma of the Lung, SURGERY **32**: 877, 1952.
3. Churchill, E. D., Sweet, R. H., Soutter, L., and Scannell, J. G.: The Surgical Treatment of Carcinoma of the Lung, J. Thoracic Surg. **20**: 349, 1950.
4. Edwards, A. T.: Carcinoma of the Bronchus, Thorax **1**: 1, 1946.
5. Taylor, A. B., and Waterhouse, J. A. H.: Prognosis for Bronchial Carcinoma, Thorax **5**: 257, 1950.

SHOCK AND THE ADRENOCORTEX

MARK A. HAYES, M.D., PH.D., NEW HAVEN, CONN.

(From the Department of Surgery, Yale University School of Medicine)

SHOCK is a syndrome resulting from depression of many functions, but in which reductions of the effective circulating blood volume and of the blood pressure are of basic importance, and in which impairment of the circulation steadily progresses until it eventuates in a state of irreversible circulatory failure.[25] In any consideration of the shock problem it is necessary to differentiate between the factors which initiate and those which perpetuate the syndrome. The favorable effects of blood-replacement therapy have served to focus attention on the reduction in the effective blood volume and its immediate circulatory consequences to the neglect of other factors. In the past, the concept of decreased effective circulating volume seemed adequate to explain the initiation and the early manifestations of the shock syndrome, such as hypotension and vasoconstriction; it shed no light, however, on either the nature of the compensatory mechanisms involved or the reason for their deterioration as the shock syndrome progressed.

Shorr and his associates, studying the pathophysiology of the terminal vascular bed, provided a clear analysis of the striking contrasts that exist when shock is reversible and when it is irreversible.[19-22] By direct visualization of the peripheral blood vessels in the mesentery, they were able to distinguish two consecutive stages in the shock syndrome. The initial compensatory phase apparently was related to a reduction in blood volume; the decompensatory phase was related to the period of inadequate peripheral blood flow. The compensatory response was characterized by a hyperreactive condition of the peripheral blood vessels, as evidenced by an increasingly enhanced reactivity of the terminal muscular vessels to epinephrine and an increase in the spontaneous vasomotor movements of the smallest arterioles and precapillaries. This type of heightened reactivity persisted even when the blood loss was acute and sufficient to precipitate the collapse of the animal. The resultant capillary ischemia and the restriction of peripheral blood flow into the most direct thoroughfare channels served to maintain an active venous return of blood from the tissues until shortly before death.

On the contrary, with the development of an irreversible type of shock following prolonged hypotension, a new set of vascular changes progressively appeared and disrupted the peripheral circulation. These changes were decompensatory in nature and initially were made evident by a progressive

---

Supported by an Institutional Grant from the American Cancer Society to Yale University.

Presented in part at the Regional meeting of the American College of Surgeons, Los Angeles, Calif., March 31, 1953.

Received for publication, May 11, 1953.

decrease in epinephrine reactivity and a slowing and, finally, complete cessation of spontaneous vasomotor caliber changes in the terminal arterioles. The loss of these compensatory influences on the peripheral circulation resulted in the diversion of increasing amounts of blood into the capillary side channels, from which it failed to return to the active circulation. This, in turn, led to the

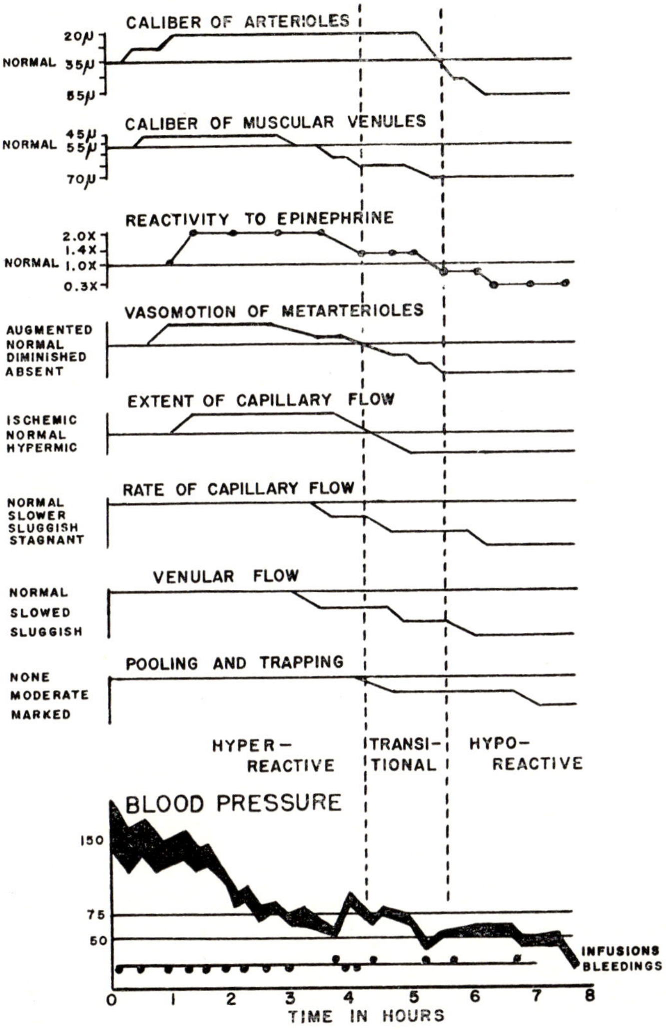

Fig. 1.—Graphic presentation of observations made during shock on the terminal vascular bed contrasting the findings in the hyperreactive or reversible phase and the hyporeactive or irreversible phase of shock. Note the beneficial results on blood pressure from a reinfusion of blood during the reversible state and the failure to improve the hypotension by repeated transfusions in the irreversible state. (From Zweifach.[26])

eventual failure of venous return and to peripheral circulatory collapse. Once this hyporeactive stage had fully developed, transfusions exerted only a transient, if any, benefical effect, a state of irreversibility to replacement therapy having been reached (Fig. 1).[26] In simple contrast, referable to the terminal vascular bed, then, reversible shock is characterized by augmented vasomotion, accentuated response to epinephrine, ischemic capillary blood flow, and slowed venular flow. Irreversible shock is characterized by absent vasomotion, no response to epinephrine, over-all capillary blood flow, and stagnant venular return. In the latter condition, transfused blood is trapped in the stagnant pool of the capacious capillary bed, and results in no improvement in the over-all hemodynamic response.

The immediate readjustments leading to vasoconstriction following hemorrhage are such that an insight into one of the mechanisms perpetuating a shock state may be apparent.[28] Subsequent to a functional reduction in circulating blood volume, there is decreased filling of the right side of the heart and reduced cardiac output. A natural consequence of decreased cardiac output is a fall in blood pressure in the aorta and arteries. As a measure of visceral blood flow, these findings should be correlated with the demonstrated decrease in renal plasma flow,[4, 13, 18] the reduction being greater than the fall in blood pressure, indicating increased renal resistance or vasoconstriction.[11] There is, thus, a decreased minute volume of blood delivered to the kidney and, presumably, to the adrenal gland, with a subsequent possible reduction in the amounts of adrenocortical steroids available in the circulation per unit time for peripheral tissue utilization. This is particularly true as the peripheral vascular bed in general, as well as the vascular bed of the adrenocortex, undergo the changes coincident with the development of irreversible shock. Zweifach,[27] moreover, has reported that the absence of the adrenocortex blunts the adequacy of the compensatory mechanisms in reversible shock and that adrenocortical steroids will restore terminal vascular epinephrine responsivity in decompensated or irreversible shock.

A clinical evaluation of shock occurring in patients who possess an unrecognizedly limited or borderline adrenocortical reserve and of shock in patients who presumably are endocrinologically normal, but who do not respond to blood replacement therapy, seems to be of interest.

Among other changes, it has been well established that the circulating blood level of the C-11, 17-oxygenated adrenocortical steroids is reflected by the number of eosinophils circulating in the blood stream.[3, 5, 8] In man, failure to demonstrate an eosinopenia following the administration of adrenocorticotropic hormone should be considered evidence of adrenocortical insufficiency;[23] if eosinopenia does not follow operation, failure of the adrenocortex should be suspected.[16] Even though many objections have been raised as to the suitability of this measure of adrenocortical activity, it still remains, recognizing its limitations, the simplest and quickest evaluation of adrenocortical function. The demonstration of a high eosinophil count at a time when past experiences indicate it should be low is substantiative evidence of an inadequate supply of adrenocortical steroids.

MATERIALS AND METHODS

The first part of this study demonstrates different patterns of endocrine response in known normal and known abnormal endocrinologic patients. Some of the patients described in this part of the study have been reported previously.[6] Nearly all the patients studied were subjected preoperatively or pretreatment to either the epinephrine-eosinophil response or the ACTH-eosinophil response (Thorn) test, or both. In the former, the test dose of epinephrine was 0.3 c.c. of a 1:1,000 dilution injected subcutaneously. In the latter, the test dose was 25 mg. of ACTH injected intramuscularly. Examinations were made in the postabsorptive state, and the control eosinophil count was taken immediately preceding, and the second count exactly four hours after, the injection of the test material. The cell counts were made in a Levy chamber according to the method recommended by Randolph and Rollins.[14] For the study made during the operative procedure, a control count was taken prior to the induction of anesthesia, and serial counts were made during the course of the operation. The counts were recorded as percentage changes from the control counts in the endocrinologically normal cases and from the pretreatment counts in the adrenocortical-deficient patients. The patients in this part of the study included: normal patients without operative complications, a normal patient with an operative complication, an adrenocortical-deficient patient without preparation, adrenocortical-deficient patients prepared with cortisone, and an adrenocortical-deficient patient prepared with adrenocorticotropic hormone.

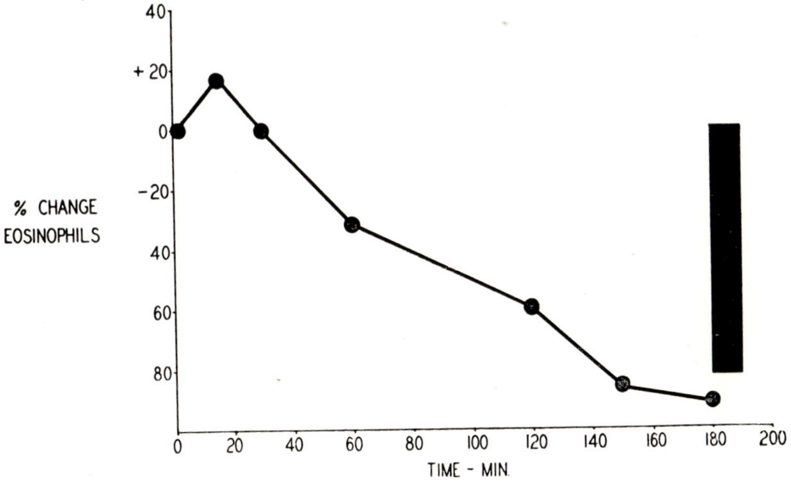

A.

Fig. 2.—Patterns of adrenocortical activity in varying clinical situations depending on severity of stress and type of hormonal preparation as reflected in the eosinophil count.

A, Pattern of normal response. Bar graph indicates means eosinophil fall in the normal cases tested preoperatively by the epinephrine-eosinophil response test. The line graph indicates the average pattern of eosinophil fall during the surgical procedure.

The second part of this study deals with case reports of patients in shock treated with adrenocortical extract, cortisone, adrenocorticotropic hormone, or various combinations of these agents.

RESULTS

Employing the circulating eosinophil level as a measure of adrenocortical function, several characteristic patterns of endocrine response during operative procedures have been obtained (Fig. 2). The type of response depends on the functional integrity of the pituitary-adrenocortical axis, the severity of the stress, and the type of hormone-substitution therapy employed in preparing the deficient patients for operation.

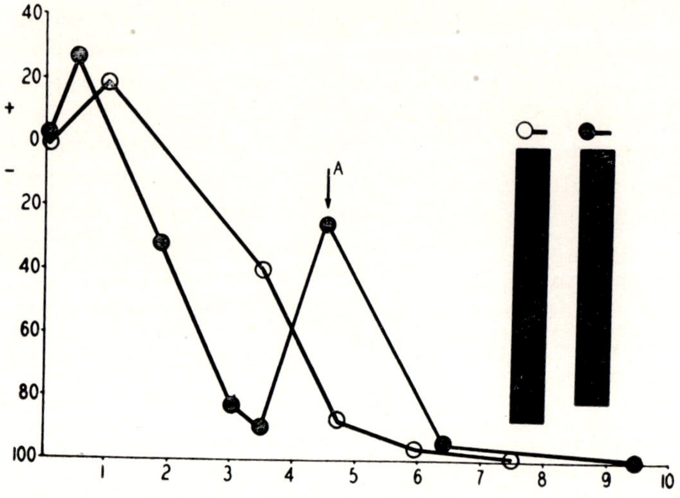

B.

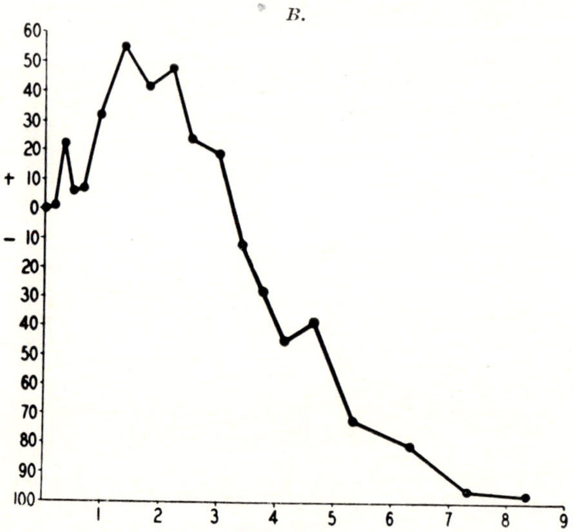

C.

Fig. 2 (*continued*).

B, Pattern of normal response with a superimposed severe stress. Bar graphs show normal preoperative epinephrine-eosinophil tests. These are comparable cases, but the patient represented by the closed circles had a major hemorrhage as a complication at Point *A.*

C, Pattern of mild adrenocortical insufficiency without preoperative preparation. At two and one-half hours adrenocortical extract was given because of severe shock. [From SURGERY 32: 815 (Nov.) 1952.]

Normal Pattern of Response.—Fig. 2, *A* illustrates mean changes in a group of normal patients. The bar graph indicates a satisfactory response to the epinephrine test as a preoperative evaluation. The line graph demonstrates an initial eosinophilia, then a prompt and rapidly progressive activation of the adrenal cortices early in the course of the operative procedure as reflected in the eosinophil count.

Pattern of Severe Stress Superimposed on a Normal Response.—Fig. 2, *B* compares two patients with the same diagnosis of cardioesophageal carcinoma

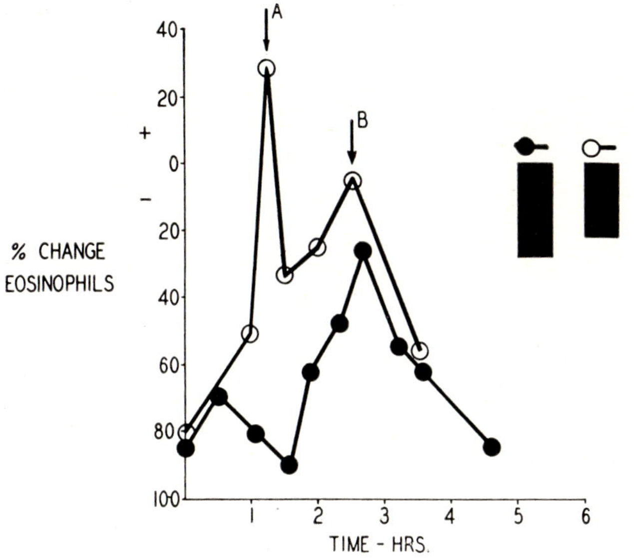

D.

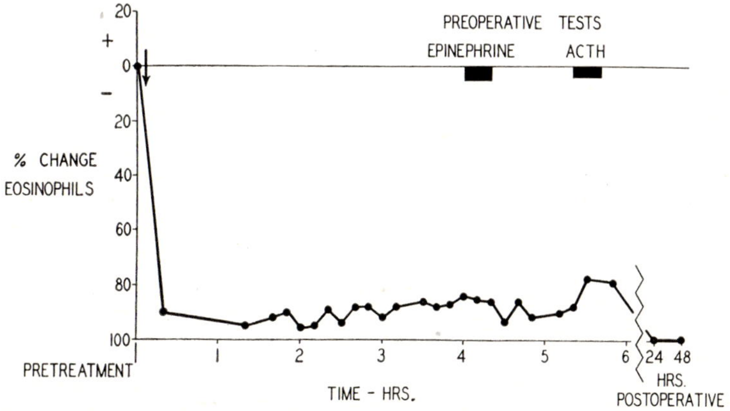

E.

Fig. 2 (*continued*).

D, Pattern of adrenocortical insufficiency in patient prepared for operation with cortisone acetate. The bar graphs are evidence of hypoadrenocorticism. The line graphs compare the minor relative adrenocortical insufficiency of a technically easy operation (closed circles) with the severe insufficiency of a very difficult case (open circles). Both patients required adrenocortical extract during operation. At Points *A* and *B* the patient was without detectable blood pressure but promptly responded to adrenocortical extract in large amounts.

E, Pattern of adrenocortical insufficiency in patient prepared for operation with ACTH. The bar graphs indicate the severe degree of secondary hypoadrenocorticism existing preoperatively. The rate of administration of ACTH during operation was adjusted to the eosinophil counts taken serially throughout the procedure.

subjected to a resection via a thoracoabdominal approach. These patients in all respects were comparable surgical risks and displayed comparable preoperative responses to the epinephrine-eosinophil tests (bar graphs). At Point *A* the patient represented by the closed circles was subjected to a sudden blood loss estimated at 500 c.c. with an immediate rise in eosinophil count and a profound fall in systolic blood pressure to 55 mm. Hg. No drug therapy was given, but overreplacement of 1,500 c.c. of blood was necessary to stabilize the blood pressure and eosinophil count.

Pattern of Mild Adrenocortical Insufficiency Without Hormonal Preparation (Fig. 2, *C*).—This patient had received testosterone propionate 50 mg. daily for one week prior to an exploratory laparotomy of two hours' duration. The preoperative treatment with the androgen had resulted in a progressive loss of the pituitary-adrenocortical response to the same stress of epinephrine. This decreased responsiveness is demonstrated by a change from a 60 per cent fall in eosinophils during the test, prior to the hormone administration, to a 40 per cent fall after hormone administration. This represented a condition of mild pituitary-adrenocortical insufficiency[1, 2] due to a delayed release of pituitary ACTH.[7] During the course of the operative procedure (Fig. 2, *C*), there was strong evidence of adrenocortical insufficiency in the serial eosinophil counts; the operative course was characterized by moderately to severely intractable shock which responded poorly to the continuous use of pressor agents and blood transfusion, although operative blood loss was significantly low. It was necessary at the termination of the operation to give 150 c.c. of aqueous adrenocortical extract, which promptly returned the blood pressure to normal coincidentally with the prompt fall in eosinophils seen after two and one-half hours.

Pattern of Adrenocortical Insufficiency Prepared With Cortisone (Fig. 2, *D*).—The two patients represented in this figure were known to be moderately severe hydroadrenocortical (diagnosis: chromophobe adenoma of the pituitary). The bar graphs indicate the restricted responses to the test dose of epinephrine in each case. Both of these patients were prepared for operation by four daily intramuscular injections of 100 mg. of cortisone acetate. Two hours before operation, each received intramuscular injections of 50 mg. of cortisone acetate at two different sites. The control eosinophil counts just prior to the induction of the anesthesia clearly show that each patient was in a hyperadrenocortical state at that time. Since cortisone acetate has a fixed solubility in tissue fluids, the available synthetic adrenocortical steroid was at a fixed level throughout the operative procedure (craniotomy for optic chiasma decompression). The patient who is represented by the closed circles in Fig. 2, *D* had a primary operation without prior irradiation, which was technically not difficult. In this instance, as evidenced by the rise in the number of eosinophils, temporary very mild adrenocortical insufficiency supervened but was controlled by the prompt administration of aqueous adrenocortical extract. The operative course, as judged from the anesthesia record, was entirely uneventful.

On the other hand, the patient represented by the open circles presented difficulty in management. This was a secondary operation following irradiation and was an extremely difficult procedure technically. It is quite apparent that the degree of adrenocortical insufficiency, as followed by the eosinophil count, was of a much more striking degree. At the points designated *A* and *B*, the patient was without a detectable blood pressure, but the rapid infusion of 100 c.c. of aqueous adrenocortical extract at each instance produced an instantaneous return of blood pressure to 110 mm. Hg. This case presents interesting information concerning the rate of utilization of available adrenocortical hormones (fixed in these cases) as correlated with the severity of the stress and the clinical course; the greater the severity of the stress, the greater is the demand for hormone to effect homeostasis.

Pattern of Adrenocortical Insufficiency Prepared With ACTH (Fig. 2, *E*). —The patient who was the subject of this method of preparation had a recognized case of primary panhypopituitarism with secondary hypoadrenocorticism. Preoperative evaluations by both the epinephrine and ACTH tests are shown by the bar graphs; a very significant degree of hypoadrenocorticism was present. The preoperative preparation consisted of a prolonged course of intramuscular ACTH, to which the metabolic response was sluggish and which required intravenous supplementation (see metabolic data concerning this patient in the Case Reports section of this article).

The patient was carried through the operation (a six-hour pneumonectomy for bronchogenic carcinoma) without adrenocortical extract. A constant intravenous infusion consisting of 40 mg. of ACTH per liter of 5 per cent dextrose in distilled water was maintained. The rate of administration was governed qualitatively by the serial eosinophil counts taken during operation. The course of the surgical procedure as judged by the anesthesia record was completely uneventful. It is of importance to point out how much more physiologic is the control of the patient's response by the varying administration of ACTH, as in this case, than by prior preparation with a fixed level of hormonal activity, as in the preceding cases of patients prepared with cortisone.

CASE REPORTS

CASE 1 (721637).—W. O., a 59-year-old white man, was scheduled for a pneumonectomy for bronchogenic carcinoma. All diagnostic examinations completed prior to operation revealed no stigmata of endocrine dysfunction. Immediately after the induction of anesthesia and the beginning of the skin incision, the patient's blood pressure fell precipitously, and he did not respond adequately to the use of pressor agents or blood transfusion. The operative procedure was discontinued immediately, and the patient was allowed to recover from the anesthesia. No unusual sequelae were apparent. Three days later, on successive days, the patient was tested by the epinephrine and the ACTH tests with remarkably decreased responses (Fig. 2, *E*). Additional examinations made at this time suggested hypogonadism and hypothyroidism. Laboratory examinations revealed a twenty-four hour urinary excretion of pituitary gonadotrophin of 3 M. U. (normal: 6.6 to 53), a serum-protein-bound iodine level of 0.1 gamma per cent, a total serum-cholesterol level of 131 mg. per cent, and a twenty-four hour urinary excretion of 7.6 mg. of 17-ketosteroids. Intravenous pyelograms were normal. The concluded diagnosis was panhypopituitarism with secondary hypoadrenocorticism.

The patient was subsequently placed on a metabolic balance regimen with a constant dietary intake of 125 Gm. of protein (20 Gm. of nitrogen), 350 Gm. of carbohydrate, and total calories of 4,000 per day. This dietary program included 9.3 meq. of sodium and 117.7 meq. of potassium daily. The metabolic data of the entire study are graphically presented according to the method of Reifenstein, Albright, and Wells[15] in Fig. 3. After an equilibration period of six days, intramuscular ACTH therapy was begun at the dosage of 100 mg. per day; the lag in metabolic, eosinophil level and 17-ketosteroid excretion is very apparent and confirms the diagnosis of secondary atrophy of the adrenal cortices. The maximal metabolic responses characteristic of the desired state of hyperadrenocorticism were not attained until an additional daily dose of 10 mg. of ACTH was given intravenously over an eight-hour period. It is noteworthy that water retention was prohibited by the severe sodium restriction and that an additional water load was promptly excreted in the hyperadrenocortical state. At the completion of the metabolic-study period the patient was operated upon under the plan discussed previously, employing ACTH (illustrated in Fig. 2, *E*). The operative course and convalescence were uneventful during the gradual withdrawal of the tropic hormone.

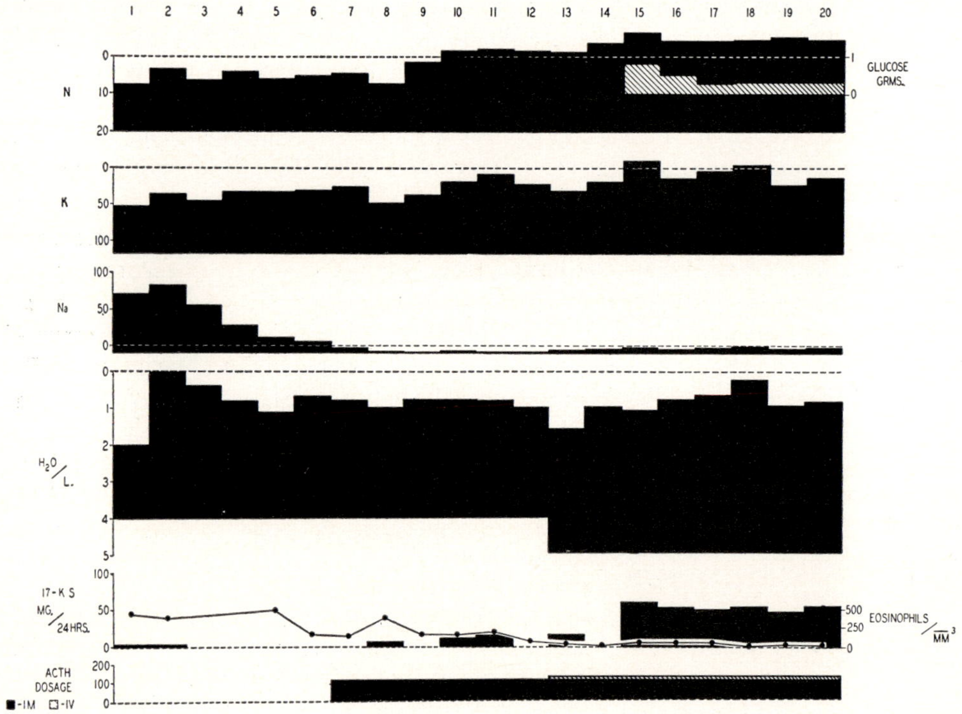

Fig. 3.—Metabolic data on Case 1. (See text for details.)

Case 2 (B58507).—M. H., a 54-year-old white man, was admitted to the hospital with a diagnosis of a residual pulmonary tuberculous cavity under a thoracoplasty; it was planned to perform a left pneumonectomy. Two preoperative ACTH-eosinophil tests are presented graphically in Fig. 4. It is to be emphasized that the patient presented no laboratory or physical evidence of endocrinologic abnormality. This same illustration shows the preoperative preparation of this patient with cortisone. Fig. 5 demonstrates the essential data from this patient's anesthesia record and shows an essentially stable course during the procedure. It is pertinent that aqueous adrenocortical extract was given intravenously during the operative procedure as the quality of the pulse or the surgeon's clinical evaluation of the cardiac action indicated. Fig. 4 shows the plan of withdrawal of the cortisone in the convalescent period and the rising eosinophil count with the withdrawal. The patient's postoperative period was completely uneventful, and he was discharged on the fifteenth postoperative day.

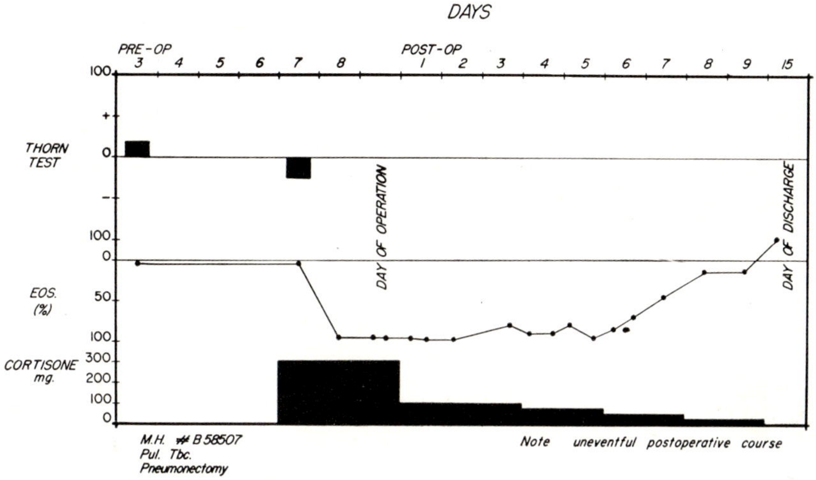

Fig. 4.—Preoperative Thorn tests and essential clinical data on Case 2. (See text for details.)

CASE 3 (38-32-07).—M. C., a 65-year-old white woman, was admitted to the hospital with a diagnosis of carcinoma of the gastric cardia involving the lower esophagus. As a result of the concomitant obstruction, the patient was in a state of severe malnutrition. After what was considered satisfactory preparation for operation, resection was accomplished through a thoracoabdominal incision. The operating surgeon had not been correctly informed of the results of the preoperative Thorn test, which had shown only a 27 per cent fall in eosinophils. Fig. 6 illustrates the important data from the anesthesia record. It is readily apparent that the problem of shock was of great significance. Despite the use of pressor agents and a continuous flow of blood, the situation became precarious about two hours after the induction of the anesthesia. The surgeon by this time was committed to completion of the operation. An eosinophil count taken at this time was 334 cells per cubic millimeter, at a time when it should have been approaching 0. Recalculation of the Thorn test data confirmed the diagnosis of adrenocortical insufficiency. The dramatic response to the first intravenous dose of adrenocortical extract is apparent. The prompt responses of the blood pressure and the general condition of the patient to each administration of the extract were impressive. Because of the rapid utilization of the injected hormone,[24] it was practically impossible to maintain a stable state. At the point indicating cortisone administration, 500 mg. of this synthetic steroid was injected intramuscularly at ten different sites, 50 mg. each to assist maximal absorption.[6] With the continued intensive therapy, the eosinophil count fell progressively, and the operation terminated successfully.

Fig. 7 shows the laboratory data available on this patient. More pertinent to this discussion is the fact that during a period of hypotension on the first postoperative day the patient failed to respond to blood transfusion (there was no blood loss) but promptly responded to intravenous adrenocortical extract; this occurred when serum electrolyte levels would suggest hypoadrenocorticism. The rest of this patient's convalescence was remarkably uneventful, and the method of employing ACTH in withdrawing cortisone is demonstrated in Fig. 7.

CASE 4 (37-74-90).—S. L., a 42-year-old white man, had a diagnosis of carcinoma of the stomach; prior tests showed an intact and responsive pituitary-adrenocortical system. A radical total gastrectomy and total pancreatectomy were performed without event. A

Fig. 5.

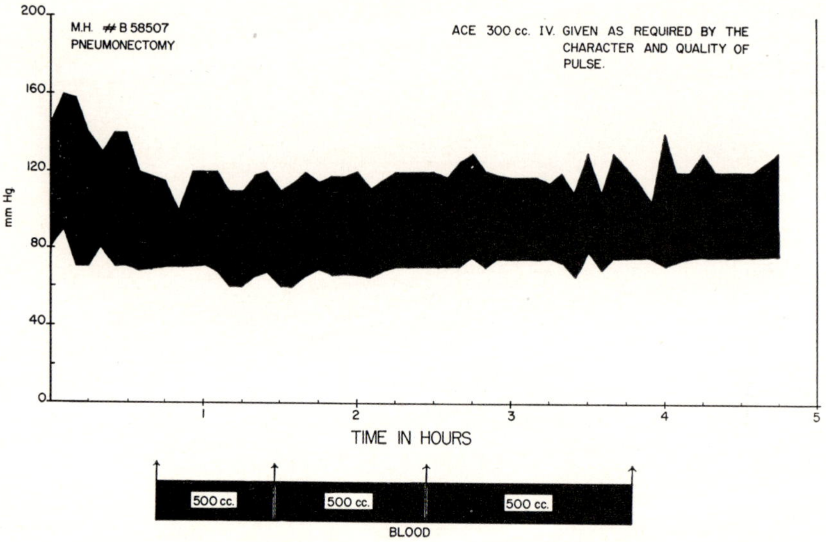

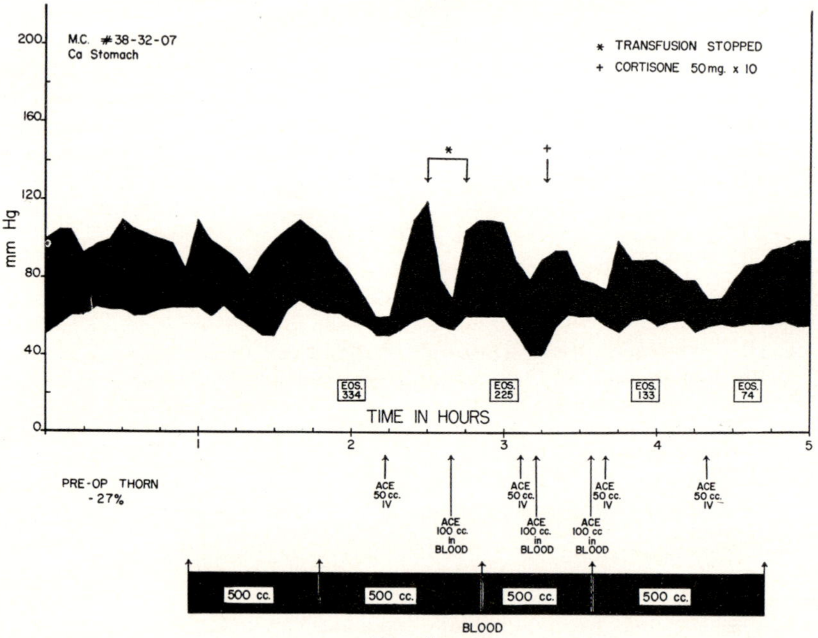

Fig. 6.

Fig. 5.—Pertinent data from the anesthesia record of Case 2. (See text for details.)

Fig. 6.—Pertinent data from the anesthesia record of Case 3. *EOS* represents number of eosinophils per cubic millimeter of blood. *TRANSFUSION STOPPED,* Because of mechanical difficulties, the blood infusion temporarily was interrupted over this period. (See text for details.)

moderately severe degree of hypotension, which did not respond to repeated blood transfusions, appeared on the second postoperative day. It has been demonstrated that an adequate available supply of adrenocortical steroids will prevent ketonemia or ketonuria in a severely diabetic individual.[9, 12] For this reason it is interesting to correlate three evidences of adenocortical insufficiency in this patient: hypotension, high eosinophil count, and ketonuria (Fig. 8). Aqueous adrenocortical extract was given by slow intravenous infusion for a three-day period. It is quite significant that the hypotension was corrected simultaneously with the fall in eosinophils and disappearance of ketonuria, although there had been no change in the fasting blood sugar level and the insulin dosage was essentially constant, but at a low level. The only conclusion to be made from these observations is that the hypotensive state was one manifestation of relative hypoadrenocorticism.

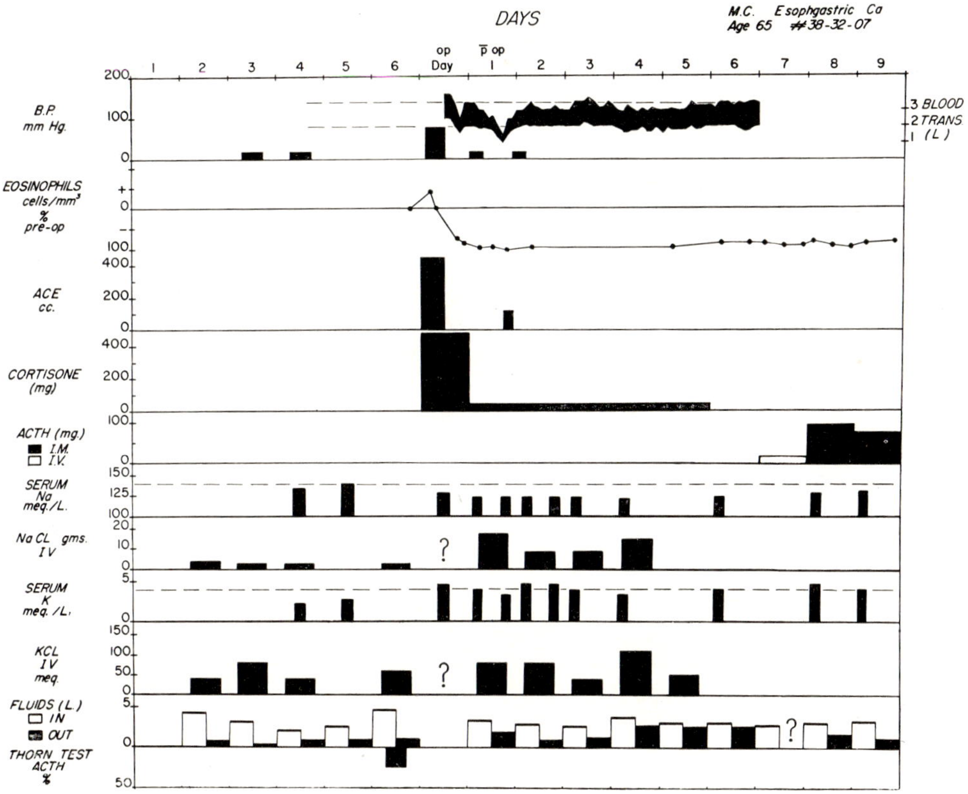

Fig. 7.—Essential clinical data from the record of Case 3, including the preoperative Thorn test. (See text for details.)

CASE 5 (C31696).—F. P., a 63-year-old white man, was first admitted to the hospital twenty-four hours after the perforation of a gastric ulcer, in severe shock and with generalized peritonitis. The left portion of Fig. 9 illustrates pertinent data obtained during the first hospitalization period. Vertical time relationships are portrayed accurately. It is readily apparent that the severe clinical shock did not respond to the administration of 1,500 c.c. of whole blood. An eosinophil count was moderately elevated at a time when it presumably should have been very low. The administration of 150 c.c. of aqueous adrenocortical extract was followed by a prompt rise in blood pressure, clinical improvement, and a fall in eosinophil count. The hemodynamic state began to deteriorate again, and another transfusion was given with no change in the progressing fall in blood pressure

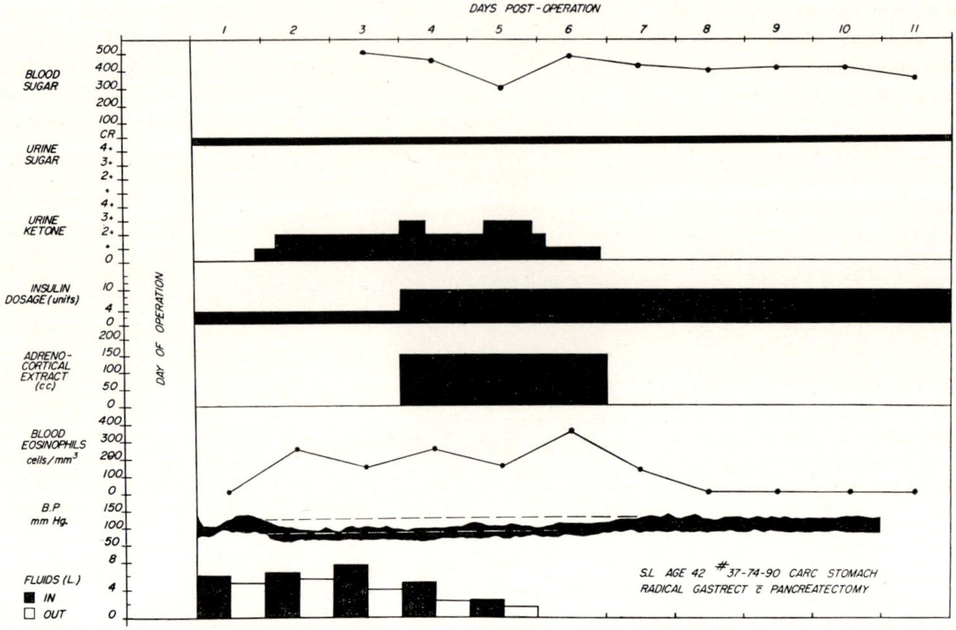

Fig. 8.—Clinical data from Case 4. Note the simultaneous disappearance of three evidences of adrenocortical insufficiency: hypotension, high eosinophil count, and ketonuria. (See text for details.)

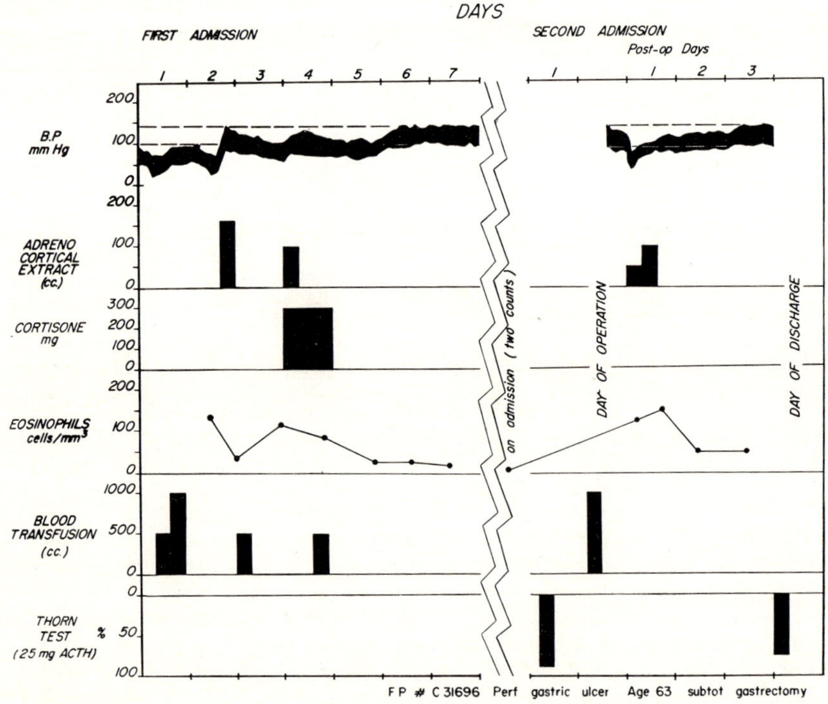

Fig. 9.—Data from the two hospital admissions of Case 5. Note shock, which does not respond to blood transfusions but does respond to adrenocortical extract, occurring during both admissions despite two low normal Thorn tests during the second. (See text for details.)

and rise in eosinophil count. Aqueous adrenocortical extract, 100 c.c., was given with an appropriate rise in blood pressure. Simultaneously, 300 mg. of cortisone acetate was given intramuscularly. Another 500 c.c. of whole blood did not alter the hypotensive state. Approximately thirty-six hours after the cortisone had been given, the eosinophil count had fallen to a satisfactory level, and at that time the blood pressure stabilized. Twenty-four to thirty-six hours is the generally accepted time interval required for a single intramuscular injection of cortisone to produce its maximal therapeutic effect. The subsequent convalescence was uneventful under nonoperative management, and the patient was discharged with a return date six weeks later for a gastric resection.

Forewarned of possible adrenocortical hypofunction, an ACTH-eosinophil (Thorn) test was performed on admission with a 95 per cent fall, a very satisfactory test, as shown in the right half of Fig. 9. The operative procedure was carried on without event. In the immediate postoperative period, shock, which was in no way deterred by 1,000 c.c. of whole blood, supervened, and a high eosinophil count was found. Aqueous adrenocortical extract significantly improved the hypotension and caused a fall in eosinophils. The remainder of the postoperative convalescence was without incident. An ACTH-eosinophil test made the day of discharge again demonstrated a normally responding adrenal cortex by that test.

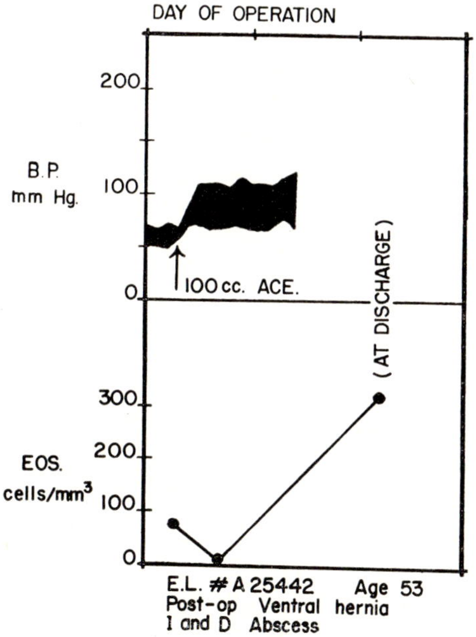

Fig. 10 (Case 6).—(See text for details.)

CASE 6 (A25442).—E. L., a 53-year-old white man, had had a ventral hernia repaired two months prior to the present admission. The current hospitalization was for an incision and drainage of a large wound abscess. No evaluation of pituitary-adrenocortical function was made. In the immediate postoperative period, a state of moderately severe shock occurred. Realizing that this state might have been easily corrected by pressor agents or blood transfusion, we decided to administer a therapeutic trial of adrenocortical extract. The eosinophil count during the shock state was higher than that usually seen in the normal postoperative period. Fig. 10 demonstrates the dramatic blood pressure response to the extract occurring simultaneously with a fall in the eosinophil count.

CASE 7 (38-57-50).—E. S. was a 30-year-old white woman, gravida ii, para i. She was four months pregnant and was admitted because of vaginal bleeding and fever, having passed per vaginam a small bone about twelve hours previously. The final diagnosis was: Rh_0 mother with a dead fetus. A manual extraction of the macerated fetus was performed, and the subsequent severe bleeding required packing. The patient bled through the packs, and a total hysterectomy was performed for a ruptured uterus. At the time of laparotomy it was discovered that the pregnancy had been a cervical implantation, with rupture of the cervix and laceration into the uterine artery on the left. Estimated operative blood loss was 6,000 c.c.; replacement was 7,000 c.c. During operation, the generalized bleeding syndrome characteristic of an incompatible blood transfusion was noted, and whole fresh blood was begun. The hemorrhagic diathesis apparently was brought under control, but the patient's blood pressure remained at 80 mm. Hg systolic and 40 mm. Hg diastolic, irreversible to further transfusion. At this time the patient had received 8,000 c.c. of whole blood. The eosinophil count at this time was 89 cells per cubic millimeter, much higher than had been anticipated. A test dose of 50 c.c. of aqueous adrenocortical extract was given, and the blood pressure immediately but transiently rose to 110 mm. Hg systolic. An immediate infusion was started consisting of 200 c.c. of aqueous adrenocortical extract in 500 c.c. of 5 per cent dextrose in distilled water. The blood pressure rose and stayed within a normal range. A hematocrit taken at this time was 26 per cent. The patient then received two 500 c.c. blood transfusions, each containing 200 c.c. of aqueous adrenocortical extract. The blood pressure stabilized completely at 110 mm. Hg during and following the transfusions, and eosinophil counts were stationary, showing 0 cells per cubic millimeter. No shock state recurred during the remainder of the convalescence.

DISCUSSION

When individuals are subjected to a stress, a rise instead of the anticipated fall in the numbers of eosinophils and lymphocytes can be produced experimentally by maintaining them on a fixed available level of adrenocortical steroids; furthermore, the magnitude of these increases qualitatively parallels the severity of the stress.[10] A clinical counterpart of this phenomenon has been demonstrated amply in the patterns of response in the first part of this study. When the rate of peripheral-tissue utilization of adrenocortical steroids exceeds their availability, the eosinophil count rises. In general, it would appear that the rate of adrenocortical hormone utilization parallels cellular activity and that the hormone is necessary for the mobilization of energy for cellular work. It is quite reasonable that the increased cellular activity which accompanies homeostatic adjustments to stress may be responsible at least in part for the parellel increase in the rate of utilization of adrenocortical hormone[17] and its increased production. At any time of stress during which an elevated eosinophil count can be demonstrated, this fact can be taken as direct evidence for an insufficient supply of adrenocortical hormone.

With the more complete understanding of the pathophysiology of "irreversible" shock and the demonstration that some of the criteria for irreversibility can be improved by the administration of adrenocortical steroids, an avenue for a better evaluation of clinical shock can be found. If a patient is in shock, irreversible to adequate blood replacement, and the eosinophil count is not at the anticipated low level, it is reasonable to assume that an adequate supply of adrenocortical hormone is not available because of hemodynamic failure. In this state, a condition of temporary peripheral adrenocortical insufficiency is present, and a beneficial response in the shock state could well be obtained by therapy with an adrenocortical preparation suitable for rapid intravenous administration. Since there are tremendous demands for adrenocortical hormone in stress, large amounts are necessary for adequate treatment. It may be necessary in some cases to give a test dose of adrenocortical extract (50 c.c.) and to follow the blood pressure; if relative adrenocortical failure is fundamental to the problem, a dramatic and instantaneous, yet transient, response in blood pressure and pulse quality obtains.

It is quite true that several of the patients discussed in this report were endocrinologically abnormal, but the important fact remains that, by ordinary careful histories, physical examinations, and routine laboratory tests, no evidences of endocrinopathic stigmata were revealed. Other patients in this series were endocrinologically normal, at least as far as the tests employed were concerned, yet the stress to which they were subjected exceeded the ability of the adrenal cortex to contend with it. Shock, irreversible by established clinical criteria, supervened.

SUMMARY

Various patterns of adrenocortical response to the trauma of surgical procedures have been presented. The configuration of the pattern depends on the severity of the incurred stress and the availability of endogenous adrenocortical hormone to effect the necessary homeostatic readjustments.

The adrenal cortex incontrovertibly can be implicated in the pathophysiology of irreversible shock when blood replacement is followed by no beneficial response and the level of circulating eosinophils is above a very low level.

The more careful evaluation of the integrity of the pituitary adrenocortical mechanism prior to operation is now required.

In some cases, because of hemodynamic failure in the shock syndrome, a temporary period of relative hypoadrenocorticism may supervene. This complication may be an important contributor to the perpetuation of the shock state with an irreversible outcome.

REFERENCES

1. Albright, F., Parson, W., and Bloomberg, E.: Cushing's Syndrome Interpreted as Hyperadrenocorticism Leading to Hypergluconeogenesis: Results of Treatment With Testosterone Propionate, J. Clin. Endocrinol. **1**: 375-384, 1941.
2. Albright, F.: Cushing's Syndrome, Harvey Lectures, Lancaster, Pa., 1942-1943, Science Press Printing Company, pp. 122-186.
3. Almy, T. P., and Laragh, J. H.: Reduction in Circulating Eosinophils Following Epinephrine, Insulin and Surgical Operation, Am. J. Med. **6**: 507, 1949.
4. Corcoran, A. C., and Page, I. H.: Effects of Hypotension Due to Hemorrhage and of Blood Transfusion on Renal Function in Dogs, J. Med. **78**: 205-224, 1943.
5. Dougherty, T. F., and White, A.: Influence of Hormones on Lymphoid Tissue Structure and Function. The Role of the Pituitary Adrenotropic Hormone in the Regulation of the Lymphocytes and Other Cellular Elements of the Blood, Endocrinology **35**: 1-14, 1944.
6. Hayes, M. A.: Adrenocortical Function During Surgical Procedures, SURGERY **32**: 811-818, 1952.
7. Hayes, M. A., Hodgson, P. E., and Coller, F. A.: The Use of Testosterone in Preventing Postoperative Liver Dysfunction in the Poor Risk Surgical Patient, Ann. Surg. **136**: 643-658, 1952.

8. Hills, A. G., Forsham, P. H., and Finch, C. A.: Changes in Circulating Leucocytes Induced by the Administration of Pituitary Adrenocorticotropic Hormone (ACTH) in Man, Blood **3**: 755-768, 1948.
9. Kinsell, L. W., Margen, S., Michaels, G. D., and Partridge, J.: Hormonal Regulation of Fat Metabolism. I. Effects of ACTH and of Certain Steroid Hormones Upon Fasting Induced Hyperketonemia, Proc. Second Clin. ACTH Conf., J. R. Mote, editor, Philadelphia, 1951, The Blakiston Company, pp. 308-317.
10. Kumagai, L. F.: Stress Induced Lymphocytosis in Adrenalectomized Mice, Fed. Proc. **10**: 76, 1951.
11. Lauson, H. D., Bradley, S. E., and Cournand, A.: The Renal Circulation in Shock, J. Clin. Investigation **23**: 381-402, 1944.
12. Margen, S., Michaels, G. D., Boling, L. A., and Kinsell, L. W.: Hormonal Regulation of Fat Metabolism. II. Effects of ACTH and Certain Steroid Hormones Upon the Utilization of Infused Acetoacetate and Octonoic Acid, Proc. Second Clin. ACTH Conf., J. R. Mote, editor, Philadelphia, 1951, The Blakiston Company, pp. 318-331.
13. Phillips, R. A., Dole, V. P., Hamilton, B. P., Emerson, K., Archibald, R. M., and Van Slyke, D. D.: Effects of Acute Hemorrhage and Traumatic Shock on Renal Function of Dogs, Am. J. Physiol. **145**: 314-336, 1946.
14. Randolph, T. G., and Rollins, J. P.: Eosinophil Observations in Adrenocorticotropic Hormone Therapy, Proc. First Clin. ACTH Conf., J. R. Mote, editor, Philadelphia, 1950, The Blakiston Company, pp. 1-13.
15. Reifenstein, E. C., Jr., Albright, F., and Wells, S.: The Accumulation, Interpretation and Presentation of Data Pertaining to Metabolic Balances, Notably Those of Calcium, Phosphorus and Nitrogen, J. Clin. Endocrinol. **5**: 367-395, 1945.
16. Roche, M., Hills, A. G., and Thorn, G. W.: The Level of Circulating Eosinophils as an Indicator of Adrenal Cortical Adequacy Following Major Surgery, J. Clin. Endocrinol. **9**: 662, 1949.
17. Sayers, G.: The Adrenal Cortex and Homeostasis, Physiol. Rev. **30**: 241-320, 1950.
18. Selkurt, E. E.: Renal Blood Flow and Renal Clearance During Hemorrhagic Shock, Am. J. Physiol. **145**: 699-709, 1946.
19. Shorr, E., Zweifach, B. W., Furchgott, R. F., and Baez, S.: Hepatorenal Vasotropic Factors in Experimental Shock and Renal Hypertension, Tr. A. Am. Physicians **60**: 28-51, 1947.
20. Shorr, E., Zweifach, B. W., and Furchgott, R. F.: Hepatorenal Factors in Circulatory Homeostasis. III. The Influence of Humoral Factors of Hepatorenal Origin and the Vascular Reactions to Hemorrhage, Ann. New York Acad. Sc. **49**: 571-592, 1948.
21. Shorr, E., Zweifach, B. W., Furchgott, R. F., Mazur, A., Baez, S., and Payne, M. A.: Recent Findings Concerning the Role of the Liver and Kidney in Circulatory Homeostasis, Trans. Eighth Conf. Liver Injury, sec. 4, New York, 1949, Josiah Macy, Jr., Foundation, pp. 60-85.
22. Shorr, E., Zweifach, B. W., Furchgott, R. F., and Baez, S.: Hepatorenal Factors in Circulatory Homeostasis. IV. Tissue Origins of the Vasotropic Principles, VEM and VDM, Which Appear During Evolution of Hemorrhagic and Tourniquet Shock, Circulation **3**: 42-79, 1951.
23. Thorn, G. W., Forsham, P. H., Prunty, F. T. G., and Hills, A. G.: Test for Adrenal Cortical Insufficiency; Response to Pituitary Adrenocorticotrophic Hormone, J. A. M. A. **137**: 1005-1009, 1948.
24. Vogt, M.: Output of Cortical Hormone by Mammalian Suprarenal, J. Physiol. **102**: 341-356, 1943.
25. Wiggers, C. J.: The Present Status of the Shock Problem, Physiol. Rev. **22**: 74-123, 1942.
26. Zweifach, B. W., Lee, R. E., Hyman, C., and Chambers, R.: Omental Circulation in Morphinized Dogs Subjected to Graded Hemorrhage, Ann. Surg. **120**: 232-250, 1944.
27. Zweifach, B. W.: Humoral Vasoactive and Other Metabolic Derangements in Shock, Shock, Transactions First Conference, New York, 1951, Josiah Macy, Jr., Foundation, pp. 15-72, p. 224.
28. Zweifach, B. W.: Functional Deterioration of Terminal Vascular Bed in Irreversible Hemorrhagic Shock, Ann. New York Acad. Sc. **55**: 370-380, 1952.

SOME PHYSICAL-CHEMICAL PROPERTIES OF POLYVINYLPYRROLIDONE

LEOPOLD MAY, PH.D., MARGUERITE HINES, M.A., LEONARD WEINTRAUB, M.A., JOHN SCUDDER, M.D., MED.SC.D., AND SAMUEL GRAFF, PH.D., NEW YORK, N. Y.

(From the Departments of Biochemistry and Surgery, Francis Delafield Hospital, and Columbia University)

POLYVINYLPYRROLIDONE (PVP) is a water-soluble, high molecular weight polymer with chemical and physical properties desirable in a plasma extender. It is prepared from acetylene by processes devised by Reppe[2] in 1938. The last stage in the process, polymerization of the monomer, N vinyl pyrrolidone, is carried out in aqueous solution with hydrogen peroxide as catalyst, the concentration of the latter controlling the degree of polymerization.

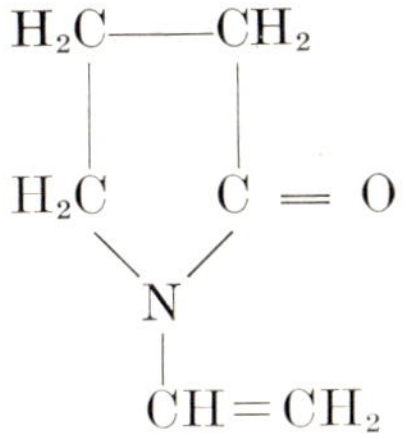

Monomer

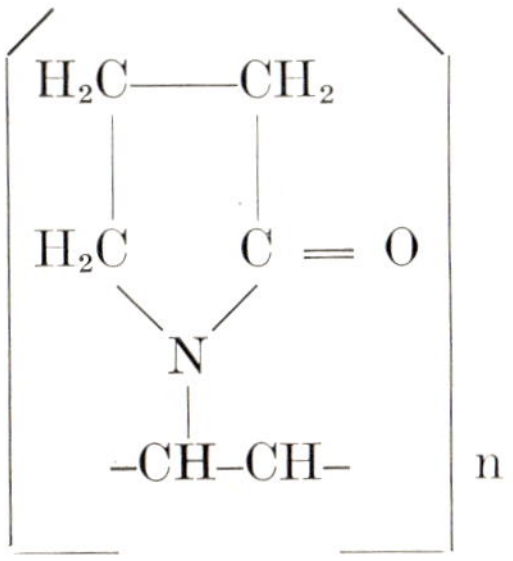

Polymer

Commercial preparations, suitable for use as plasma expanders, are mixtures of the polymer chains, averaging 35,000 to 40,000 molecular weight, with no residual monomer. The latter is appreciably toxic, but is readily identified by virtue of its unsaturation, and is easily extracted with methylene chloride.

The polymer is an undissociated, neutral substance. There is some evidence that the chains of from 150 to 720 units end in acid radicals, which would account for a minimal electrophoretic mobility. The hydrophilic properties are probably assignable to the >N—C=O groups.

Following Starling's dictum that only "colloidal" hydrophilic substances could be efficacious in replacement therapy, Hecht and Weese[1] first evaluated PVP as a plasma expander. Their initial criteria were that the material had to be hydrophilic and chemically indifferent, and a solution of the material should approximate that of the plasma proteins in molecular weight and viscosity.

This study was supported by a grant from Schenley Laboratories, Inc., 350 Fifth Avenue, New York.

Received for publication, May 28, 1953.

Some of the chemical and physical properties of PVP-Macrose* relative to these criteria are included in this report. Clinical experience will appear in other articles.[5]

TITRATION DATA

PVP-Macrose has no groups titrable by either acid or alkali. The pH titration curve (Fig. 1) was determined electrometrically by titration according to standard procedure. PVP exhibits no appreciable buffer capacity, and therefore cannot contribute to, or directly disturb, the acid-base of the recipient. Any electrolyte alterations following PVP administration, if they occur, must then be referable to the saline vehicle employed, or to the physiologic response of the recipient. Numerous serum sodium, potassium, and chloride estimations, before and after PVP, showed that changes in serum electrolytes were within normal limits.

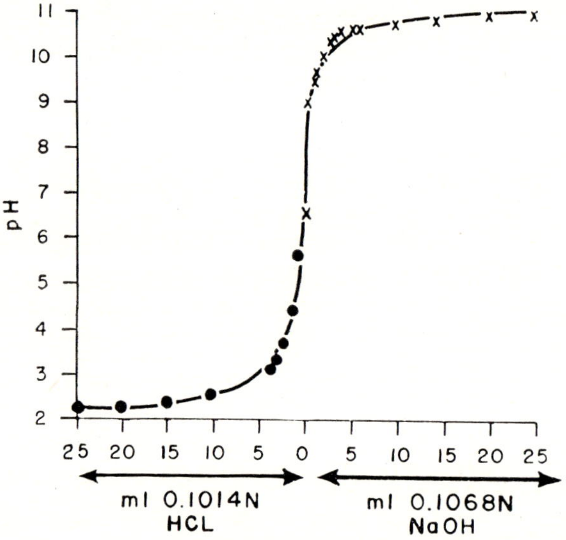

Fig. 1.—Titration curve of PVP-Macrose with standard HCl and NaOH.

ULTRACENTRIFUGAL DATA

The molecular size and size distribution have been determined by industrial procedure in which high polymers are commonly characterized by the K-value, which is a function of viscosity. Solutions with K-values between 28 and 32 are suitable for clinical use. The average molecular weights corresponding to these figures are 30,000 to 40,000 units, no more than 10 per cent of the 15,000-molecular-weight polymer. The distribution had been confirmed by fractionation of the material.

A 3.5 per cent solution of PVP-Macrose in 0.9 per cent NaCl was subjected to centrifugation in the analytic ultracentrifuge.† The pattern obtained (Fig. 2) illustrates the gaussian distribution of the components. The

*PVP-Macrose supplied by Schenley Laboratories, Inc., New York.
†Specialized Instrument Co., Model E.

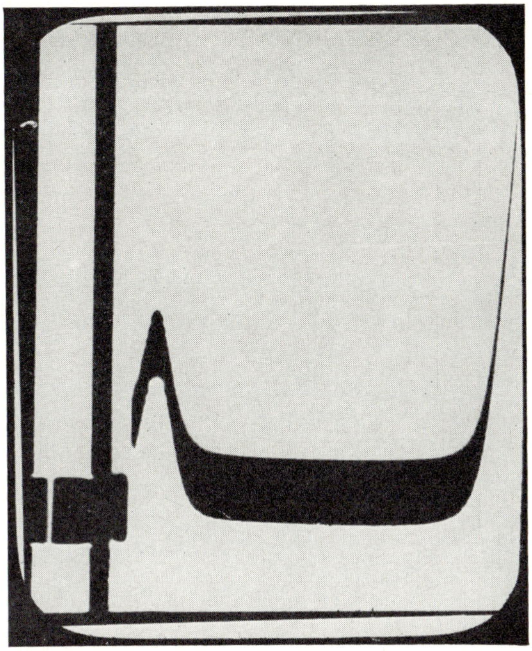

Fig. 2.—Ultracentrifugal pattern of PVP in 0.9 per cent NaCl after forty minutes at 60,000 r.p.m.

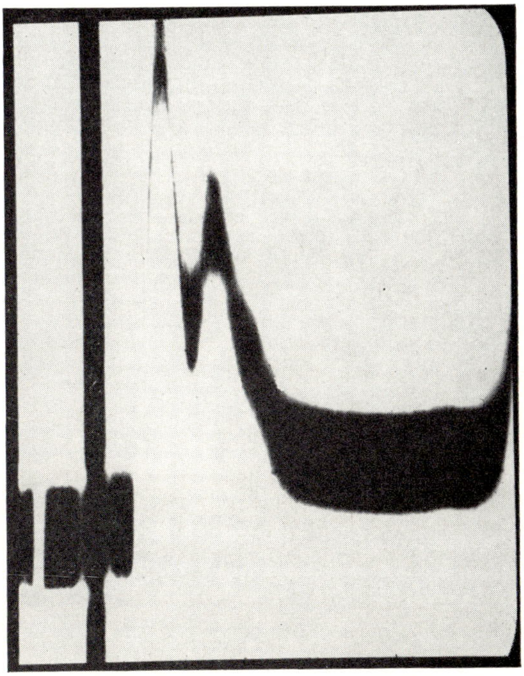

Fig. 3.—Ultracentrifugal pattern of PVP and serum after sixty minutes at 60,000 r.p.m.

average molecular weight, calculated from the sedimentation constant (S_{20} w = 0.9 S) and an assumed diffusion constant of 4 × 10^{-7} cm. per second, is about 40,000. These data are consistent with those obtained by viscosity and light-scattering techniques.

The ultracentrifugal pattern of PVP-Macrose mixture indicates a sharp separation of the apparently undiluted components (Fig. 3). It may be of some significance that PVP does not appear to combine with serum proteins or otherwise affect their distribution.

ELECTROPHORETIC DATA

As expected, PVP exhibits low mobility at pH 8.6 in the Tiselius apparatus.* The serum protein migrated with the characteristic mobilities without apparent interaction between the PVP and the serum proteins. The PVP migrated with the gamma globulin fraction of the serum in all cases examined (Fig. 4). Electrophoretic examination of the serum following PVP administration was carried out at intervals in several cases. The data also indicated that PVP was present in the serum in appreciable amounts up to twenty-four hours after administration. In general, however, PVP can no longer be detected after one week (Table I).

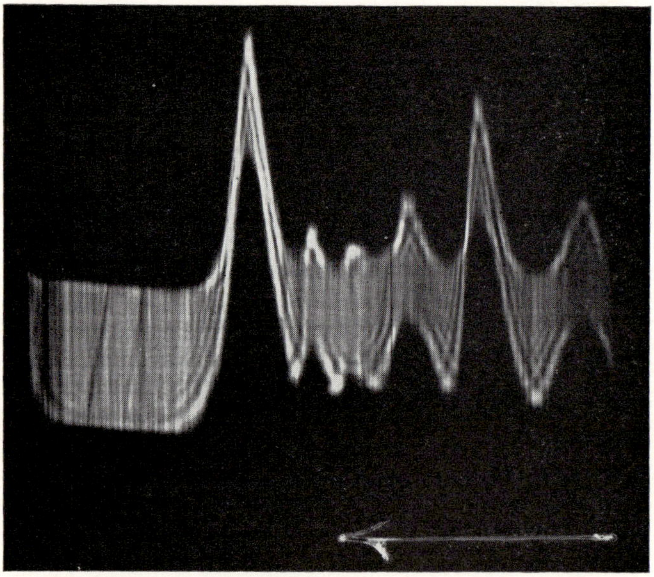

Fig. 4.—Descending electrophoretic pattern of PVP and blood serum in 0.1 ionic strength, diethylbarbiturate buffer of pH 8.6 after sixty minutes at 10.6 volts per centimeter.

ESTIMATION OF PVP IN SERUM AND URINE

PVP in low concentration reacts with I_2 to produce a colored compound absorbing maximally at 5,000 Å and obeying the Beer and Lambert laws. $Zn(OH)_2$ filtrates were employed for serum analysis.

*Perkin-Elmer Corp.

The amount of PVP excreted in the urine was determined by adapting the method of Thrower and Campbell.[4] PVP forms with iodine a colored complex which absorbs maximally at 5,000 Å and follows Beer's law of concentration dependence from 0 to 35 μg per milliliter of PVP. For most samples, urine was diluted 1:1,000 with 0.2 molar citric acid, an aliquot of 10 ml. was withdrawn, and 2 ml. of KI_3 reagent (13.5 Gm. of sublimed iodine dissolved in an aqueous solution containing 24 Gm. of KI and diluted to approximately

TABLE I. SERUM PVP ASSAY BY ELECTROPHORETIC METHODS

PATIENT AND WEIGHT (KG.)	AMOUNT GIVEN	TIME	TOTAL PROTEIN (GRAMS PER 100 C.C.)	COMMENT ON ELECTROPHORETIC PATTERN
C.,	500 c.c.,	Control	7.17	*
55.6	17.5 Gm.	8 days	7.08	*
		17 days	7.06	
R.,	500 c.c.,	Control	6.68	*
63.9	17.5 Gm.	8 days	6.49	
B.,	500 c.c.,	Control	6.86	
80.4	17.5 Gm.	8 days	6.82	*
W.,	500 c.c.,	Control	7.38	
70.6	17.5 Gm.	8 days	6.74	*
H.,	500 c.c.,	Control	6.94	*
78.1	17.5 Gm.	14 days	6.90	
F.,	1,000 c.c.,	Control	6.49	*
57.6	35 Gm.	8 days	6.52	*
	1,000 c.c.,	Control	6.70	
	35 Gm.	24 hr.	5.13	Little PVP detectable
Wh.,	500 c.c.,	Control	7.40	*
54.9	17.5 Gm.	8 days	7.64	*
Re.,	1,000 c.c.,	Control	6.60	
62.5	35 Gm.	24 hr.	5.26	Definite PVP peak
M.,	1,000 c.c.,	Control	5.41	
58.0	35 Gm.	6 days	5.50	Presence of PVP questionable
S.,	1,000 c.c.,	Control	6.20	
64.1	35 Gm.	24 hr.	5.98	*
J.,	1,000 c.c.,	No control		
58.3	35 Gm.	12 hr.	6.57	Presence of PVP questionable
Lu.,	1,000 c.c.,	Control	6.20	
44.6	35 Gm.	24 hr.	5.43	Presence of PVP questionable
Sm.,	2,000 c.c.,	Control	8.15	
70.5	70 Gm.	6 hr.	6.12	Definite PVP
		24 hr.	6.18	Definite PVP
		16 days	6.35	Little PVP
Wi.,	2,500 c.c.,	Control	6.92	
15.6	87.5 Gm.	6 hr.	4.56	Definite PVP
		24 hr.	4.20	Definite PVP
Br.,	3,000 c.c.,	Control	7.07	
83.4	105 Gm.	12 hr.	4.43	Definite PVP
		36 hr.	4.37	Definite PVP
He.,	1,000 c.c.,	Control	5.82	
62.5	35 Gm.	24 hr.	4.96	Definite PVP

*No observable peak or elevation due to presence of PVP.

0.0006 normal) was added. The solution was swirled, a portion was transferred to a 1 cm. cuvette, and the absorption read at 5,000 Å on a Beckman DU spectrophotometer. The readings were compared with those obtained with known concentrations of PVP which were plotted on graph paper.

At this low concentration there is no interference from anything in urine. In serum, however, it is necessary to remove the proteins which would otherwise react with some of the iodine. This was done by the Somogyi zinc hydroxide precipitation.[3] After the proteins had been precipitated, the filtrate was treated in the same way as urine, except that it was only necessary to make a 1:500 dilution to bring it within the correct concentration range.

TABLE II. PVP EXCRETION IN URINE AND DETERMINATION OF PVP IN SERUM: TWENTY-FOUR HOURS POSTINFUSION

PATIENT	AMOUNT OF PVP ADMINISTERED (GM.)	AMOUNT OF PVP EXCRETED IN 24 HOURS (GM.)	AMOUNT OF PVP RETAINED (GM.)	TOTAL PLASMA VOLUME POST-PVP (C.C.)	THEORETICAL CONCENTRATION OF PVP IN SERUM (MG. PER C.C.), RETAINED PLASMA VOLUME (GM.)	OBSERVED CONCENTRATION OF PVP IN SERUM (MG. PER C.C.)
B. F.	35	19.1	15.9	2,325	6.8	4.7
F. L.	35	7.4	27.6	3,435	8.0	3.4
T. W.	35	22.9	12.1	3,226	3.7	3.4
D. R.	35	6.8	28.2	2,948	9.6	4.6
J. F.	35	16.6	18.4	2,516	7.3	3.9
H. L.	35	19.6	15.4	2,490	6.2	4.2
M. H.	35	9.9	25.1	3,319	7.6	3.4
A. B.	35	17.1	17.9	2,802	6.4	4.2

SUMMARY

Polyvinylpyrrolidone is a chemically inert, hydrophilic, water-soluble macromolecule, averaging 35,000 to 40,000 molecular weight. Solutions of PVP have minimal buffer capacity, and electrophoretic and ultracentrifugal analyses indicate no interaction between it and plasma proteins.

Chemical and electrophoretic methods of qualitative and quantitative estimation of PVP in serum and urine have been reviewed.

REFERENCES

1. Hecht, G., and Weese, H.: Periston, ein neuer Blutflüssigkeitsersatz, München. med. Wchnschr. **90**: 11-15, 1943.
2. Reppe, W.: Neue Entwicklungen auf dem Gabret der Chemie des Acetylene und Kohlenoxyds, Berlin, 1949, Springer-Verlag.
3. Somogyi, M.: A Method for the Preparation of Blood Filtrates in Determining Sugar, J. Biol. Chem. **86**: 655, 1930.
4. Thrower, W. R., and Campbell, H.: Plasmosan; A Synthetic Substitute for Plasma, Lancet **1**: 1096-1099, 1951.
5. (a) Posner, A. C., Cordice, J. W. V., Jr., and Scudder, J.: Effect of Polyvinylpyrrolidone in Obstetrical Cases, Surg., Gynec. & Obst. **96**: 581-583, 1953.
   (b) Cordice, J. W. V., Jr., Suess, J. E., and Scudder, J.: Polyvinylpyrrolidone in Severe Burn Shock, Surg., Gynec. & Obst. **97**: 39-44, 1953.
   (c) Cordice, J. W. V., Jr., Suess, J. E., and Scudder, J.: Polyvinylpyrrolidone in Acute Traumatic and Hemorrhagic Shock, Surg., Gynec. & Obst. **97**: 361-367, 1953.

HYPERCHLOREMIC ACIDOSIS FOLLOWING ANTERIOR PARTIAL AND COMPLETE PELVIC EXENTERATION

ALEXANDER BRUNSCHWIG, M.D., NEW YORK, N. Y., AND
MARIE LÜSCHER, M.D.,* ZÜRICH, SWITZERLAND

(From the Memorial Center for Cancer and Allied Diseases, New York)

WITH the increasing frequency of ureterointestinal anastomoses and the formation of wet colostomy in the extended treatment of cancer in the pelvis, attention is drawn to the possibilities of physiologic imbalances resulting from such alterations in the urinary tract. When urine is excreted into the lower colon, a situation foreign to the normal status obtains in that urine, instead of pooling temporarily in the bladder and then being excreted, is pooled in the lower colon and then excreted. The colon itself possesses certain absorptive potencies for substances excreted by the kidneys. The absorption of these substances into the blood stream to be again excreted by the kidney and again poured into the colon conceivably may and does result in certain deviations from normal in regard to chloride levels, acid-base balance, and urea concentration of the circulating plasma.

Clinical experience (A. B.) has shown that, in the large majority of patients subjected to these operations, the subsequent course is clinically asymptomatic in so far as the acid-base balance is concerned, that imbalances detectable by laboratory studies may be present but seem to be asymptomatic, or that a clinical syndrome does supervene in the presence of the imbalance (one patient). Clinically the disturbance, if it occurs, is said to be characterized by (a) fatigability, (b) constant asthenia of varying degree, (c) anorexia, (d) a perverted sense of taste, (e) nausea, sometimes vomiting, (f) loss of weight, and (g) a general feeling of not being well without special emphasis on particular symptoms. Laboratory studies reveal elevated plasma chlorides, lowered carbon dioxide-combining power, and elevated blood urea nitrogen. The syndrome is referred to as "hyperchloremic acidosis," and has been previously discussed in the recent literature.[1-3] Hyperchloremia and depressed plasma carbon dioxide-combining power may obtain in the presence of essentially normal blood urea nitrogen levels.

This report is concerned with two groups of patients, namely, those who received anterior partial exenteration, removal of bladder, vagina, uterus, and pelvic lymph nodes with implantation of the ureters into the intact colon (Fig. 1), and those who received total pelvic exenteration with implantation of ureters into the sigmoid above the end colostomy, a wet colostomy[4, 5] (Fig. 2).

This work was facilitated by a grant from Mr. and Mrs. André Meyer, New York.
Received for publication, May 27, 1953.

*Head of Surgical Service, Swiss Nurses School Hospital, Zürich. Recipient of Travel Grant, American Association of University Women, 1952 to 1953.

In those patients who received anterior partial pelvic exenteration the anal sphincter mechanism is intact, and the urine excretion is under voluntary control. Under these circumstances there is obviously periodic retention of urine in the colon, especially at night, and there is greater opportunity for

Fig. 1.

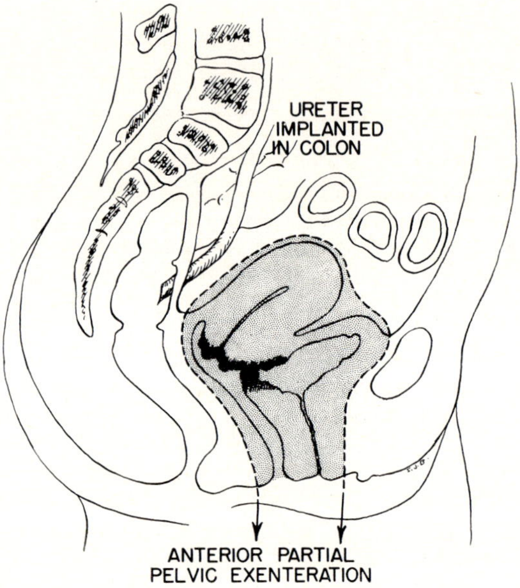

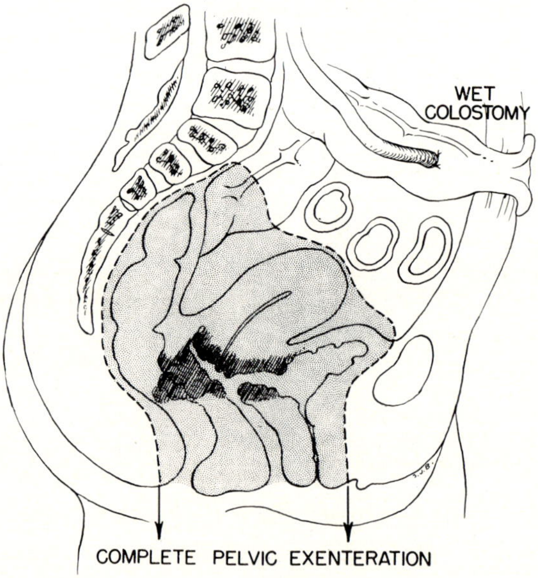

Fig. 2.

Fig. 1.—Diagram of anterior partial pelvic exenteration showing ureters implanted into pelvic colon which is undisturbed.

Fig. 2.—Diagram of total pelvic exenteration showing ureters implanted into sigmoid end colostomy to form a wet colostomy.

absorption of urinary contents into the circulation. As of March 1, 1953, over eighty of these operations had been performed. In Table I a summary is presented of records of seventeen patients selected more or less at random from the survivors ranging from two weeks to five years. It is felt that if significant imbalances are to occur in the absence of other complicating factors, they would develop during these periods. In the patients who died with recurrences or who died during the immediate postoperative period, acid-base imbalance was never observed to be the cause of death.

TABLE I. URETERS IMPLANTED INTO THE COLON (ANTERIOR PELVIC EXENTERATION)

PATIENT	AGE AT OPERATION (YEARS)	PLASMA CHLORIDES (NORMAL: 98-106 MEQ. PER LITER)		CARBON DIOXIDE (23-31 MEQ. PER LITER)	BLOOD UREA NITROGEN (8-15 MG. PER 100 C.C.	INTRVENOUS PYELOGRAMS
1	53	Preop.	97	23	15.0	
		P.O. 2 wk.	102	22	8.5	
2	54	Preop.	97	22	19.8	
		P.O. 2 wk.	105	18	14.0	
3	34	Preop.	106	20	15.7	
		P.O. 6 mo.	113	23	11.1	
4	51	Preop.	107	27	9.1	
		P.O. 10 mo.	101	19	13.8	Moderate bilateral hydronephrosis
5	48	Preop.	112	25	16.4	
		P.O. 11 mo.	120	18	72.0	Slight hydronephrosis, left; marked impaired kidney function, right
6	58	Preop.	110	-	12.2	
		P.O. 1 yr.	106	20	21.8	No hydronephrosis
7	66	Preop.	97	-	13.0	
		P.O. 1 yr., 1 mo.	99.7	22.3	17.2	Marked bilateral hydronephrosis
8	58	Preop.	108	25	11.2	
		P.O. 1 yr.	122	15	20.1	Slight hydronephrosis
9	43	Preop.	110	-	8.8	
		P.O. 1 yr., 4 mo.	98.6	23	8.3	
10	62	Preop.	106	23	12.0	
		P.O. 1 yr., 10 mo.	113	19	19.8	No hydronephrosis
11	71	Preop.	103	22	15.6	Normal right kidney;
		P.O. 1 yr., 6 mo.	107	24	20.6	poor visualization, left kidney
12	48	Preop.	93	27.3	10.0	
		P.O. 2 yr., 6 mo.	100	-	17.2	Slight bilateral hydronephrosis
13	63	Preop.	-	-	-	
		P.O. 3 yr., 9 mo.	119	17	26.1	
14	65	Preop.	-	-	-	
		P.O. 3 yr., 4 mo.	100	22	16.0	No hydronephrosis
15	47	Preop.	94.3	27	16.5	
		P.O. 3 yr., 10 mo.	109	17	37.0	Slight bilateral hydronephrosis
16	44	Preop.	99.5	-	18.0	
		P.O. 4 yr.	107	33	14.8	Slight hydronephrosis
17	54	Preop.	98	-	10.0	Slight bilateral hydro-
		P.O. 5 yr.	105	20	12.0	nephrosis; right nephrolithiasis

In the seventeen patients studied, eight presented at least one abnormal finding among the three chemical determinations (Cases 2-4, 6, 7, 11, 12, 16). In five (Cases 5, 8, 10, 13, 15), the classical chemical features of hyperchloremic acidosis were present, that is, elevated plasma chlorides, depressed carbon dioxide-combining power, and elevated blood urea nitrogen. In four of these the clinical symptoms associated with this syndrome were absent at the time the blood was drawn, and hence no treatment was instituted. Case 15 has moderately severe diabetes which she controls with insulin herself "by the way she feels," since tests upon the urine passed per rectum are not reliable. The excellent clinical status of Case 5 completely belies the blood chemical findings, although she is being carefully observed. On one occasion she complained of a peculiar taste in her mouth, the only symptom ever presented. She was advised to increase her water intake during the day and to take .3 Gm. of sodium bicarbonate four times a day for four days; the symptom disappeared, and the blood urea nitrogen and chlorides returned to nearer normal levels. Case 16 had an attack of food poisoning the day prior to having the blood sample drawn and was taking large doses of sodium bicarbonate by mouth; this probably accounts for the alkalosis observed. Subsequently this has disappeared.

In the wet colostomy the ureters are implanted into the sigmoid colon proximal to the end colostomy. There is no sphincteric mechanism, and the urine is readily discharged more or less at a constant rate or frequently with peristalses. However, in some instances appreciable quantities of urine may pool in the sigmoid and even flow up to the proximal descending or left transverse colon. Under the latter conditions increased opportunity for absorption of urinary products obtains, and there is the possibility of hyperchloremic acidosis.

In Table II are summarized the data in twenty patients selected more or less at random and including some of the three- to five-year survivors with wet colostomy. In five instances (Cases 1, 3, 8, 17, 19) the available data indicated essentially no imbalances. In nine patients (Cases 6, 7, 9, 10, 12-15, 18) one of the factors showed deviation from normal. In none of these was the carbon dioxide-combining power of the plasma altered. In four there was hyperchloremia, and in five there was slight elevation of the blood urea nitrogen. In four patients (Cases 2, 4, 11, 16) there were two abnormal findings in each. One showed hyperchloremia and slight elevation of blood urea nitrogen, while in three there was decrease in carbon dioxide-combining power and slight elevation in blood urea nitrogen. Only two patients showed all the alterations typical of hyperchloremic acidosis (Cases 5 and 20). They are asymptomatic as far as the hyperchloremic acidosis clinical syndrome is concerned, and now survive three and six months to date, respectively, after total pelvic exenteration. The latter patient is working full time as a domestic servant.

DISCUSSION

The plasma chlorides, carbon dioxide-combining power, and blood urea nitrogen in seventeen patients who received anterior pelvic exenteration with implantation of ureters into the intact colon are compared with similar observations made in twenty patients who received total pelvic exenteration with wet colostomy. Among the former there were five instances of the typical chemical abnormalities associated with hyperchloremic acidosis, as compared to two among those with wet colostomies. There were eight patients with partial exenterations who had one abnormal factor, compared to nine among those with wet colostomies. There were four in the partial exenteration group who showed normal findings, compared with five in the wet colostomy series.

TABLE II. WET COLOSTOMY (TOTAL PELVIC EXENTERATION)

PATIENT	AGE AT OPERATION (YEARS)	PLASMA CHLORIDES (NORMAL: 98-106 MEQ. PER LITER)		CARBON DIOXIDE (23-31 MEQ. PER LITER)	BLOOD UREA NITROGEN (8-15 MG. PER 100 C.C.)	INTRAVENOUS PYELOGRAMS
1	48	Preop.	111			
		P.O. 2 mo.	100	21	11.6	
2	32	P.O. 2 mo.	96	19	17.3	
3	48	P.O. 3 mo.	101	26	–	
4	58	Preop.	104	18	9.2	
		P.O. 5 mo.	101	19	22.4	
5	59	Preop.	109	21	15.5	Moderate bilateral hydronephrosis
		P.O. 6 mo.	110	20	18.8	
6	42	P.O. 11 mo.	110	22	11.8	Slight hydronephrosis
7	47	Preop.	112	21	8.0	Moderate hydronephrosis
		P.O. 1 yr.	108	20	12.6	
8	35	Preop.	104	–	14.4	Marked bilateral hydronephrosis
		P.O. 1 yr.	106	–	15.8	
9	48	Preop.	105	–	7.2	
		P.O. 1 yr., 3 mo.	97	22	19.0	
10	41	Preop.	105	–	7.4	
		P.O. 1 yr., 10 mo.	102	22	23.0	
11	50	Preop.	101	–	11.0	
12	61	P.O. 1 yr., 5 mo.	114	–	22.0	Moderate hydronephrosis, left; no function, right
		Preop.	114	24	12.6	
		P.O. 2 yr., 2 mo.	105	–	23.8	Slight bilateral hydronephrosis
13	39	Preop.	101	–	12.0	
		P.O. 3 yr.	99	26	20.0	No hydronephrosis
14	63	Preop.	103	–	9.6	
		P.O. 3 yr., 4 mo.	109	26	28.0	Bilateral moderate hydronephrosis
15	32	P.O. 4 yr.	112	22	–	
16	47	Preop.	98	–	–	
		P.O. 5 yr.	107	17	26.0	Slight bilateral hydronephrosis
17	31	P.O. 1 day	103	–	28.0	
		P.O. 5 yr., 1 mo.	109	24	18.0	No hydronephrosis
18	57	Preop.	98	–	15.0	
		P.O. 5 yr., 6 mo.	113	22	10.0	Slight bilateral hydronephrosis
19	36	Preop.	103	27.6	8.9	
		P.O. 4 yr., 10 mo.	104	27	12.0	Slight hydronephrosis
20	58	Preop.	107	23	17.8	
		P.O. 3 mo.	115	19	24.5	

Thus, the majority of the patients showed some imbalances, and a total of seven among the whole series of thirty-seven patients showed all the alterations associated with hyperchloremic acidosis (nineteen per cent), while a total of nine of the thirty-seven, that is, 24 per cent, showed no changes. Twelve patients (60 per cent) in the total exenteration group showed slight elevations of blood urea nitrogen ranging from 17.3 to 28 mg. per cent. Eight patients (43 per cent) among those with partial exenterations showed the blood urea nitrogen to be slightly elevated, ranging from 17.2 to 37, with one patient showing a blood urea nitrogen of 72 mg. per cent. Of special interest in this group of patients, limited in number, is the fact that there was only one instance of clinical symptoms referable to the imbalance, and this was promptly corrected. Thus, in exenteration operations a certain incidence of acid-base and electrolyte imbalance is to be anticipated and accepted. This certainly does not contraindicate the operations. Table III summarizes the comparative incidence of imbalances. There is greater possibility of hyperchloremic acidosis after partial than complete pelvic exenteration. The reason for this is obviously the intact sphincter mechanism after partial exenteration which results in intermittent retention of urine in the lower colon, whereas this is absent in the wet colostomy where urine excretion occurs more or less uninhibited from the colon.

TABLE III. COMPARISON OF IMBALANCES IN PARTIAL AND TOTAL PELVIC EXENTERATION GROUPS

	PARTIAL EXENTERATION (SEVENTEEN PATIENTS)	TOTAL EXENTERATION (TWENTY PATIENTS)
Normal blood chemical findings	4	5
One abnormal determination	8	9
Two abnormal determinations	0	4
''Typical'' hyperchloremic acidosis:		
Elevated blood chlorides		
Decreased carbon dioxide-combining power		
Elevated blood urea nitrogen	5 (30 per cent of series)	2 (10 per cent of series)

The mechanisms from the production of hyperchloremic acidosis are not clearly understood. According to Mitchell and Valk[2] it is simply a matter of balance between chloride and fluid intake and urinary passage out of the colon, and that when these factors are in proper relationship absorption of chlorine from the colon is such that hyperchloremia does not occur. On the other hand, Lapides'[3] observations are interpreted by him to indicate that renal tubular damage is the prime etiological factor and that intestinal absorption of urinary contituents is of secondary importance. Experimental studies consisting of urine enemas in three patients with poor renal function and, as controls, urine enemas in three patients with normal renal functions showed that electrolyte imbalance occurred in the former and not in the latter. In one patient operated upon by one of us (A. B.) the preoperative blood urea nitrogen was 74.6 mg. per cent (the plasma carbon dioxide-combining power was 19 meq. per liter and chlorides were 106 meq. per liter) because of obstruction. During the period following total pelvic exenteration, the blood urea nitrogen gradually fell to 35 to 40 mg. per cent after a period of one month, the chlorides were 111 meq. per liter with plasma carbon dioxide-combining power at 16 meq. per liter. Thus, a picture of hyperchloremic acidosis evolved following presumable renal damage due to ureteral obstruction for a period before operation. This observation supports Lapides' hypothesis. The patient is not included in the series mentioned previously because of the pre-existing renal obstruction.

In years past, various techniques for the creation of artificial bladders have been described and the operations successfully performed in man. Makkas employed the cecum and ascending colon as a bladder, implanted the ureters into the cecum, and employed the appendix as a "urethra." In 1937 Seiffert detached a segment of jejunum, implanted the ureters into one end, and brought the other open end through the abdominal wall. In recent years, interest in these procedures has again developed, and modifications of them have been devised in connection with total pelvic exenteration. Such attempts are praiseworthy and must be carried out in order to learn what might be the preferred method for dealing with the urinary tract following pelvic exenteration. However, in the experience of one of us (A. B.) the wet colostomy has proved satisfactory under the conditions imposed by the radical pelvic en masse visceral excision; five-year survivals have been achieved, and the patients are in full physical activity and quite well adjusted to the wet colostomy. When sufficient long-range survivals from other methods of dealing with the urinary tract after pelvic exenteration are available for comparison, a more definite orientation in this problem will be possible, based on actual experience and presentation of results.

CONCLUSION

While in the series reported by us there was no serious clinical problem posed by the presence of acid-base and electrolyte imbalance, the latter, as shown, was present in varying degree in the majority of instances. Other methods for dealing with the urinary tract in which chemical imbalances might be avoided altogether and which might afford long survival will be worthy, indeed, of consideration.

REFERENCES

1. Ferris, D. O., and Odel, H. M.: J. A. M. A. **142**: 634, 1950.
2. Mitchell, A. D., and Valk, L. W.: Southcent. Sec. Am. Urol. A. **58**: 29 (Oct.) 1951.
3. Lapides, J.: Surg., Gynec. & Obst. **93**: 691, 1951.
4. Brunschwig, A.: Cancer **1**: 177, 1948.
5. Brunschwig, A.: Tr. Twelfth Brit. Cong. Obst. and Gynec., London, 1949, Austral Press.

THE RELATION OF THE IN VITRO SENSITIVITY TEST TO THE CLINICAL RESPONSE TO AUREOMYCIN THERAPY

Fritz B. Schweinburg, M.D., Elsie M. Sylvester, and
Alexander M. Rutenburg, M.D., Boston, Mass.

(From the Surgical Research Department, Beth Israel Hospital, and the Department of Surgery, Harvard Medical School)

DATA are herewith presented showing that the clinical response to therapy with Aureomycin correlates closely to the results of a properly standardized in vitro sensitivity test to be described in this article.

The test (a modified Rammelkamp-Maxon[1] method).—Aureomycin Hydrochloride, 500 mg., buffered with sodium glycinate is dissolved in 10 c.c. of phosphate-buffered regular broth, pH 7.0. This stock solution is kept at –4° C. Its antibacterial potency does not deteriorate for at least ninety-six hours; it is discarded after this interval.

Immediately prior to making the test, twofold dilutions of the stock solution with phosphate-buffered nutrient broth (Difco), pH 7.0, are prepared, running left to right, from 200 to 0.0125 μg per milliliter. To 1 ml. of each dilution is added 0.1 ml. of an eighteen to twenty-four hour culture diluted so as to contain 500 to 5,000 bacteria per 0.1 ml. A control tube containing 1 c.c. of the buffered broth, to which 0.1 ml. of the diluted culture has been added, is also prepared.

All tubes are then incubated at 37° C. and examined for cloudiness after twenty-four hours.* Reading from left to right, the last macroscopically clear tube is noted. The tubes are incubated for twenty-four hours longer and are again examined. At this time (forty-eight hours) the concentration of the drug in the last macroscopically clear tube is considered to be the minimum bactericidal concentration, because there is no growth on subculture of a large loopful from this tube. The last clear tube after twenty-four hours' incubation, and usually one to three tubes to the left of it, will have become cloudy after forty-eight hours. Although the last clear tube after twenty-four hours does not contain the bactericidal concentration, for purposes of rapid clinical evaluation it may be taken as the measure of the antibacterial effect of the drug on the organism being tested.

The test for each strain was always made twice, the second time two or more days after the first. The results were identical in over 96 per cent of the tests.

From clinical experience with the response to therapeutic doses of Aureomycin (Tables V and VI), strains which are completely inhibited for twenty-

Received for publication, May 4, 1953.

*Because of the slow growth of hemolytic streptococci and pneumococci the control tube may not become cloudy until more than twenty-four hours have elapsed. The test for these organisms is, therefore, first read six hours after the control tube becomes cloudy and again twenty-four hours later.

four hours by concentrations of 50 μg per milliliter or higher can be classified as resistant; strains inhibited by concentrations of 12.5 to 25 μg per milliliter as borderline, and strains inhibited by concentrations of 6.2 μg per milliliter or lower as sensitive. However, as the following studies show, this classification will not apply if the technique described is not followed in every detail, that is, if use is made of a medium of different composition or of a different pH, or if the reading is done at different time intervals.

Factors Influencing the in Vitro Test.—

Period of incubation: Macroscopically visible growth in tubes containing low drug concentrations appears from two to six hours after growth is noted in the control tube. After twenty-four hours, the last clear tube is usually followed by one to three tubes showing less cloudiness than the control tube, but after forty-eight hours these tubes are just as cloudy as the control. As a rule, one or more of the tubes which are clear after twenty-four hours will also have become cloudy at this time. The last clear tube after twenty-four hours remained the same after forty-eight hours in only 6 per cent of 350 strains tested. There are no further changes of significance on incubation beyond forty-eight hours. This, to some extent at least, may be due to the inactivation of Aureomycin in solution at 37° C.

Influence of the size of inoculum: Using sterile nutrient broth (Difco), a series of tenfold dilutions of a twenty-four hour broth culture of the strain to be tested, ranging from 10^1 to 10^7, were prepared. To each tube was added 0.1 ml. of each dilution in seven duplicate sets of tubes each containing the twofold series of dilutions of Aureomycin described previously.

TABLE I. INFLUENCE OF SIZE OF INOCULUM ON RESULT OF TEST

SAMPLE STRAINS	NUMBER OF BACTERIA INOCULATED	CONCENTRATION OF AUREOMYCIN IN THE LAST CLEAR TUBE (MICROGRAMS PER MILLILITER)	
		AFTER TWENTY-FOUR HOURS	AFTER FORTY-EIGHT HOURS
Escherichia coli (sensitive strain)	2×10^1	0.2	1.6
	2×10^2	0.2	1.6
	2×10^3	0.2	1.6
	2×10^4	0.2	1.6
	2×10^5	0.2	1.6
	2×10^6	0.2	1.6
	2×10^7	0.2	1.6
Nonhemolytic *Staphylococcus albus* (refractory strain)	5×10^1	25	200
	5×10^2	25	200
	5×10^3	25	200
	5×10^4	25	200
	5×10^5	25	200
	5×10^6	25	200
	5×10^7	25	200

The twenty-four and forty-eight hour cultures (Table I) showed identical bactericidal and bacteriostatic titers for twenty of twenty-five strains tested, regardless of the size of the inoculum. In five strains (Pseudomonas 2, hemolytic *Staphylococcus aureus* 2, *Bacillus proteus* 1), the last clear tube after twenty-four hours' incubation shifted one tube to the left when the inoculum was in excess of 100,000 bacteria, but in four of these strains the results after forty-eight hours were identical regardless of the size of inoculum. In the fifth (*Bacillus proteus*), this shift of one tube to the left persisted after forty-eight hours.

Comment: With this method, the size of the inoculum, as a rule, does not matter. This finding differs from other reported results.[2-4]

Influence of total dose of Aureomycin (varying volume with the same concentration): Five series of tubes containing the usual twofold dilutions of Aureomycin were set up. The volume of fluid in the five tubes of each concentration was 1, 2, 4, 6, and 10 c.c., respectively.

The last clear tube after twenty-four hours and after forty-eight hours had the same concentration in each series for twenty-one of the twenty-five strains tested (Table II). In the remaining four strains (Proteus 1, Pseudomonas 1, *Escherichia coli* 1, hemolytic *Staphylococcus aureus* 1), the tubes containing 6 and 10 ml. at the various concentrations showed, after twenty-four hours, one more clear tube than those containing 1, 2, and 4 ml. But after forty-eight hours all series read exactly alike. Increasing the size of the inoculum did not change the results.

Table II. Influence of Varying Volumes of Fluid With Equal Concentrations of Aureomycin

	Volume of fluid (milliliters)	Concentration of Aureomycin in the last clear tube (micrograms per milliliter)	
		After twenty-four hours	After forty-eight hours
Example characteristic of 21 strains	1	0.05	0.4
	2	0.05	0.4
	4	0.05	0.4
	6	0.05	0.4
	10	0.05	0.4
Example characteristic of 4 strains	1	12.5	25
	2	12.5	25
	4	12.5	25
	6	6.25	25
	10	6.25	25

Comment: It is evident that the concentration of the drug, not the total amount, is the determining factor.

Influencing of pH: The pH of a stock solution of Aureomycin in unbuffered nutrient broth was adjusted to 6.2, 7.0, and 7.8, respectively, and a series of twofold dilutions of each of these three stock solutions was prepared with broth of the corresponding pH. (The bacterial titer was found to be the same at pH 7.0 in both buffered and unbuffered nutrient broth.) Ten strains, which could grow readily at these various pH's, were tested.

In all instances, the most potent antibacterial action of Aureomycin was exhibited at pH 6.2 (Table III). This is a true pH effect on the drug and is not due to a different rate of bacterial growth at these different pH values, because the controls showed approximately the same number of bacteria after twenty-four hours at all three pH values.

TABLE III. INFLUENCE OF PH ON RESULT OF TEST

SAMPLE STRAINS	PH	CONCENTRATION OF AUREOMYCIN IN LAST CLEAR TUBE (MICROGRAMS PER MILLILITER) AFTER TWENTY-FOUR HOURS	AFTER FORTY-EIGHT HOURS
Hemolytic *Staphylococcus aureus* (sensitive strain)	6.2	0.8	1.6
	7.0	1.6	3.2
	7.8	25.0	100.0
Pseudomonas (resistant strain)	6.2	25.0	100.0
	7.0	50.0	200.0
	7.8	200.0	>200.0

The action of Aureomycin was considerably weaker at pH 7.8 than at pH 7.0 or 6.2, because the drug deteriorates rapidly in an alkaline solution, even if the stock solution is kept at –4° C.

Influence of the medium: Parallel tests were run in nutrient broth (Difco), trypsinized broth, tryptone broth, beef-heart broth, 1 per cent dextrose broth, 5 per cent serum broth, and 10 per cent horse-blood broth, all at pH 7.

The results (Table IV) show that the richer media interfere with the antibacterial action of Aureomycin. The last clear tube after twenty-four hours shifted to the left from one to as many as four tubes. These results confirm similar findings by Bliss and Chandler[2] and by Beigelman.[5]

TABLE IV. BACTERIOSTATIC CONCENTRATION (MICROGRAMS PER MILLILITER) OF AUREOMYCIN IN DIFFERENT MEDIA

SAMPLE STRAINS	NUTRIENT BROTH	TRYPTONE BROTH	BEEF-HEART BROTH (NO PEPTONE)	TRYPSINIZED BEEF-HEART BROTH	1 PER CENT DEXTROSE BROTH	5 PER CENT SERUM (HORSE OR RABBIT) IN NUTRIENT BROTH	10 PER CENT BLOOD BROTH
Hemolytic *Staphylococcus aureus*	0.05-0.1*	0.2-3.2	0.2-6.2	3.2-50	6.25-50	6.25-50	12.5-50
Aerobacter aerogenes	0.8-6.25	1.6-25	3.2-25	12.5-100	12.5-100	25-100	25-200
Proteus vulgaris	3.2-25	6.25-25	12.5-50	50-200	25-100	25-200	50-200
Klebsiella pneumoniae	25-100	50-200	50-200	50-200	100-200	200-200	200-200
Pseudomonas	3.2-6.25	12.5-50	12.5-50	6.25-50	12.5-25	12.5-100	50-200

*The first of each pair of numbers indicates the concentration of Aureomycin in the last clear tube after twenty-four hours; the second, after forty-eight hours.

Tryptose broth interferes least, serum and dextrose broth much more, and blood broth most with the action of Aureomycin. Hence, the sensitivity values obtained by an in vitro test for the effect of Aureomycin on a given strain depends on the medium in which the test is performed. By the method described, the drug is most potent in nutrient broth (Difco).

Correlation Between in Vitro Sensitivity and Clinical Effect of Aureomycin.—

Bacteriologic response: Table V records the findings from a series of 190 patients. The data demonstrate that there is a good correlation between the in vitro sensitivity and the clinical antibacterial effect of Aureomycin. Of 132 strains found sensitive by this method, all but five were eliminated. Of eight borderline strains two were eliminated. None of 124 resistant strains was eliminated. These data are based on cultural data obtained during therapy with Aureomycin and again, in most instances, one to three days after it was discontinued.*

TABLE V. CORRELATION OF IN VITRO SENSITIVITY TEST TO THE CLINICAL BACTERIOLOGIC RESPONSE

		INFECTIONS DUE TO ONE BACTERIAL STRAIN			INFECTIONS DUE TO TWO OR MORE BACTERIAL STRAINS		
DIAGNOSIS	TOTAL NUMBER OF CASES	IN VITRO SENSITIVITY OF RESPONSIBLE STRAIN	NUMBER OF CASES	BACTERIOLOGIC RESPONSE TO AUREOMYCIN	IN VITRO SENSITIVITY OF RESPONSIBLE STRAIN	NUMBER OF CASES	BACTERIOLOGIC RESPONSE TO AUREOMYCIN
Wound infections	62	Sensitive	1	Eliminated	All sensitive	17	All eliminated
		Borderline	1	Not eliminated	Sensitive and resistant mixed	32	31 of 32 sensitive eliminated; all resistant not eliminated
		Resistant	1	Not eliminated	All resistant	10	None eliminated
Urinary tract infections	128	Sensitive	22	21 eliminated; 1 not eliminated	All sensitive	18	17 eliminated
		Borderline	7	2 eliminated; 5 not eliminated	Sensitive and resistant mixed	42	40 of 42 sensitive eliminated; all resistant not eliminated
		Resistant	17	None eliminated	All resistant	22	None eliminated

Clinical response: When there was no complicating pathology, a satisfactory antibacterial effect was followed by rapid disappearance of the clinical evidence of infection. With rare exceptions, the infection did not recur during the patient's hospital stay. When there was complicating pathology, an antibacterial effect either was not secured even with sensitive bacteria or, if secured, was frequently followed by recurrence until complicating pathology was eliminated.

Of 245 patients treated with Aureomycin, 137 were free of complicating pathology before or at the time the antibiotic treatment was started (Table VI). In 53 the infection was due to one or more sensitive strains and in 51 it was rapidly cured. In 5 the infection was due to strains of borderline sensitivity. Only one satisfactory response was achieved by Aureomycin. In

*The dose of Aureomycin, given as the glycinate, varied from 1½ to 3 Gm. daily, averaging 2 Gm. When given intravenously, the dose was 500 mg. twice a day. The route of administration depended principally on presence or absence of nausea or of vomiting. The oral route was always preferred. Treatment was continued for seven to ten days. Cases in which treatment was discontinued earlier are not included in this paper. When treatment for seven to ten days failed, the case was considered and classified as not cured.

23 the infection was due to resistant strains only; none responded to Aureomycin. In 31 the infection was due to a mixture of sensitive and resistant strains; none of these responded to Aureomycin. However, in an additional 25 patients with diffuse peritonitis, caused by a mixture of sensitive and resistant organisms, the cure of the infection was achieved. The sensitive strains were rapidly eliminated. But Pseudomonas or Proteus, or both, which were the resistant strains in all cases, did not disappear in response to Aureomycin. Nevertheless, these strains appeared not to interfere with control of the infection. This observation was also made in experimental peritonitis in the dog.[6]

TABLE VI. CORRELATION OF IN VITRO SENSITIVITY TO THE CLINICAL RESPONSE*

		INFECTIONS DUE TO ONE BACTERIAL STRAIN			INFECTIONS DUE TO TWO OR MORE BACTERIAL STRAINS		
DIAGNOSIS	TOTAL NUMBER OF CASES	IN VITRO SENSITIVITY OF RESPONSIBLE STRAIN	NUMBER OF CASES	RESPONSE	IN VITRO SENSITIVITY OF RESPONSIBLE STRAIN	NUMBER OF CASES	RESPONSE
Wound infections	42	Sensitive	1	Cured	All sensitive	12	11 cured; 1 not cured
		Borderline	1	Not cured	Sensitive and resistant mixed	22	Not cured
		Resistant	1	Not cured	All resistant	5	Not cured
Urinary tract infections	60	Sensitive	18	Cured	All sensitive	12	11 cured; 1 not cured
		Borderline	4	1 cured; 3 not cured	Sensitive and resistant mixed	9	Not cured
		Resistant	10	Not cured	All resistant	7	Not cured
Biliary tract infections	7	Sensitive	2	Cured	All sensitive	5	Cured
		Borderline	–	–	Sensitive and resistant mixed	–	–
		Resistant	–	–	All resistant	–	–
Peritonitis	28	Sensitive	–	–	All sensitive	3	Cured
		Borderline	–	–	Sensitive and resistant mixed	25	Cured†
		Resistant	–	–	All resistant	–	–

*Complicating pathology was absent or had been eradicated in all these patients.

†Peritonitis appears to be the exception to the rule that cure does not result in mixed infections due to resistant as well as sensitive bacteria. The resistant strains were *Bacillus proteus vulgaris* or Pseudomonas or both.

Needless to say, patients with resistant strains who did not respond to Aureomycin frequently improved subsequently because of the effect of other chemotherapeutic agents, surgery, or natural defense mechanism.

DISCUSSION

This study deals exclusively with the relationship of the in vitro sensitivity of the bacteria responsible for the disease to the bacteriologic and clinical response of the patient during and shortly after treatment with the drug. Most patients who responded to the drug were permanently cured. In some cases, especially urinary infections, in which there was a good response to the drug, there was recurrence or reinfection, especially if accompanying pathology had not been dealt with successfully. Others, which were resistant to

Aureomycin, responded to other antibiotics or to surgery, or recovered because of their own defense mechanisms. Since most patients showed some clinical improvement during treatment, even if the bacteria were resistant to Aureomycin,[14] such improvement cannot be attributed to specific drug action, but there are no cases in the series reported here in which bacteria resistant to Aureomycin disappeared during the period of treatment with Aureomycin. That this can and does happen, however, is well known. Even so, the method described provides a reliable index of the clinical response which may be expected from therapy with Aureomycin. A similar method has also proved valid for the sulfonamides.[7] Our data for such a method for penicillin and neomycin, although meager, suggest that the same may prove to be true for these antibiotics as well.

The in vitro titers indicating clinical antibacterial effectiveness are very different for the various drugs. The method described is not the only one that might prove satisfactory.* The clinical validity of this method, or any other, is not established until experience demonstrates a close correspondence between the clinical response and the antibacterial titer.† If such a correspondence is found to hold for a large variety of species, and for many strains within a species, the clinical antibacterial effectiveness of the antibiotic for any given strain will be predictable from the in vitro antibacterial titer alone. For Aureomycin this is 6.2 μg per milliliter or less. Similar data are needed for the other antibacterial agents. A judgment as to the comparative clinical value of different chemotherapeutic agents against a given infecting organism cannot as yet be made by the same test until the correlation between clinical response and in vitro antibacterial concentrations is known for all the agents under consideration.

Jackson and Finland[4] stated that in vitro tests have limited clinical usefulness because of the varying quantitative results of differing techniques. Even with a given technique they obtained a fourfold difference between maximum and minimum values on repeated tests of the same organism. In some 4 per cent of the 350 strains tested with Aureomycin, we found a twofold difference, but the remainder showed no difference on repeat test.

For therapeutic purposes they suggested that it is usually necessary only to identify the causative organism and to dispense with in vitro tests in the case of uniformly sensitive bacteria, that is, Pneumococci or Group A hemolytic Streptococci. In the case of other species, whose susceptibility to the available antibiotics cannot be predicted, they regard the in vitro tests of value. Our data, listed in Table VII, agree with this judgment, for many strains of many species generally considered sensitive to Aureomycin are frequently, in fact, resistant, while some strains of species generally considered resistant are,

*Howe[8] in comparing an agar-plate-disk method with a nutrient-broth method stated that the concentration of Aureomycin required to inhibit growth on the plate is twice as high as that required in broth.

†The disk or tablet method, although very simple, carries a 25 per cent error, according to Spaulding.[9] (This is because the zone of inhibition varies with the medium used, and because the speed of release of the antibiotic to the surface of the plate varies with the surface moisture.) Braude and Dockrill[10] stated in a recent paper that, especially with Aureomycin, the disk method is far inferior to the tube dilution method.

in fact, sensitive. Since a very large percentage of clinical infections are due to strains with unpredictable sensitivity, an in vitro test, such as the one herein reported for Aureomycin, can be used to great advantage in the selection of the appropriate antibiotic. It is obvious that no single test can suffice for all bacteria. Thus the bacilli of tularemia, pertussis, and influenza, as well as other fastidious bacteria, cannot be tested in a simple medium like nutrient broth. Eisenberg and Wagner[11] obtained results similar to ours for a series of antibiotics including Aureomycin in a large series of cases, using a standardized paper-disk method. In a large number of urinary infections, Metzger and associates[12] observed a close correlation between clinical response and antibacterial titer of Aureomycin in vitro. Reiss and co-workers[13] also stated that the in vitro sensitivity test is the most reliable guide for selecting an antibiotic for a given infection.

TABLE VII. SENSITIVITY OF VARIOUS STRAINS WITHIN A BACTERIAL SPECIES TO AUREOMYCIN (LAST CLEAR TUBE AFTER TWENTY-FOUR HOURS)

SPECIES	NUBMER OF STRAINS TESTED	RESISTANT (200 TO 50 μG PER MILLILITER)	BORDERLINE (25 TO 12.5 μG PER MILLILITER)	SENSITIVE (6.25 OR LESS μG PER MILLILITER)
Beta streptococcus Group A	10	–	–	10
Alpha streptococcus	10	3	3	4
Gamma streptococcus	10	2	3	5
Streptococcus faecalis	10	7	1	2
Pneumococcus	10	–	–	10
Hemolytic *Staphylococcus aureus*	20	2	4	14
Nonhemolytic *Staphylococcus aureus*	10	3	3	4
Hemolytic *Staphylococcus albus*	15	8	4	3
Nonhemolytic *Staphylococcus albus*	15	5	5	5
Salmonella typhi	10	–	2	8
Salmonella paratyphi	2	–	–	2
Salmonella schottmuelleri and *Salmonella enteritidis*	8	2	4	2
Various Shigellae	10	1	2	7
Escherichia coli	50	5	5	40
Aerobacter aerogenes	50	13	5	32
Klebsiella pneumoniae	10	5	1	4
Pseudomonas	50	22	16	12
Proteus	50	15	15	20

The method herein described can be simplified for practical clinical purposes by setting up, in place of sixteen tubes, only six, one control tube and five tubes with Aureomycin in concentrations from 50 to 3.2 μg per milliliter.

CONCLUSIONS

1. A standardized twofold serial dilution method for testing sensitivity of bacteria to Aureomycin is described. With this method the clinical antibacterial effectivenes of Aureomycin against the infecting bacteria can be predicted.

2. From the data at hand it appears that if there is no visible growth in vitro after twenty-four hours in an Aureomycin concentration of 6.2 μg per milliliter or less, the bacteria should be eliminated, provided complicating pathology is not present or has been eliminated. If this concentration is between

12.5 or 25.0 μg per milliliter, the clinical affect will probably be a failure. If it is 50 μg per milliliter or higher, the bacteria will almost certainly not be eliminated by Aureomycin.

REFERENCES

1. Rammelkamp, C. H., and Maxon, T.: Resistance of Staphylococcus Aureus to the Action of Penicillin, Proc. Soc. Exper. Biol. & Med. **51**: 386, 1942.
2. Bliss, E. A., and Chandler, C. A.: *In Vitro* Studies of Aureomycin, A New Antibiotic, Proc. Soc. Exper. Biol. & Med. **69**: 467, 1948.
3. Jackson, G. G., and Finland, M.: Turbidimetric Method for Determining Sensitivity of Bacteria to Antibiotics, J. Lab. & Clin. Med. **38**: 289, 1951.
4. Jackson, G. G., and Finland, M.: Comparison of Methods for Determining Sensitivity of Bacteria to Antibiotics *In Vitro*, Arch. Int. Med. **88**: 446, 1951.
5. Beigelman, P. M.: *In Vitro* Determinations of Bacterial Sensitivity to Aureomycin, Proc. Soc. Exper. Biol. & Med. **72**: 89, 1949.
6. Schweinburg, F. B., Rutenburg, A. M., Milrod, S., Glotzer, P., and Fine, J.: The Therapeutic Effect of Aureomycin in Experimental Peritonitis in the Dog, Ann. Surg. **133**: 208, 1951.
7. Schweinburg, F. B., and Rutenburg, A. M.: A Simple Method for Determining Sulfonamide Sensitivity *In Vitro* and Its Clinical Application, J. Lab. & Clin. Med. **34**: 1457, 1949.
8. Howe, C. W.: Studies on the Susceptibility of Bacteria to Various Antibacterial Agents With a Comparison of the Serial Tube Dilution and Filter Paper Disc Methods of Testing, Surg., Gynec. & Obst. **91**: 669, 1950.
9. Spaulding, E. H.: Laboratory Aspects of Antibiotic Therapy, Pediat. **8**: 406, 1951, Spaulding, E. H.: Selection of Antimicrobial Agents by Laboratory Means, J. A. M. A. **147**: 336, 1951.
10. Braude, A. I., and Dockrill, M.: Inaccuracies in the Disc Method for Determining Bacterial Sensitivity to Aureomycin Discovered by Comparison With the Tube-Dilution Method, J. Lab. & Clin. Med. **40**: 149, 1952.
11. Eisenberg, G. M., and Wagner, B. M.: Bacterial Susceptibility to Antibiotics, Am. J. M. Sc. **223**: 600-606, 1952.
12. Metzger, W. I., Wright, L. T., Deluca, F. R., Ford, C. E., and Katske, F.: Aureomycin in Urinary Tract Infections, J. Urol. **67**: 374-389, 1952.
13. Reiss, E., Pulaski, E. J., Amspacher, W. H., and Contreras, A. A.: Penicillin Sensitivity of Staphylococci, New England J. Med. **246**: 611-612, 1952.
14. Rutenburg, A. M., and Schweinburg, F. B.: Oral Administration of Aureomycin in the Treatment of Urinary Infections, New England J. Med. **241**: 698-700, 1949.

THE MANAGEMENT OF PERFORATING INJURIES OF THE COLON AND RECTUM IN CIVILIAN PRACTICE

JAMES W. TUCKER, M.D., AND WILLIAM P. FEY, M.D., SHREVEPORT, LA.

(From the Department of Surgery, Shreveport Charity Hospital)

THIS report is based on an analysis of forty-two cases of penetrating wounds of the colon and rectum treated in the Shreveport Charity Hospital from January, 1948, to January, 1953, inclusive. The structural outline of this report, for purposes of comparison, is very similar to a report by Woodhall and Ochsner,[1] who reviewed fifty-five cases of patients with perforating wounds of the colon and rectum admitted to the Charity Hospital in New Orleans from 1944 to 1948, inclusive.

Prior to their report, Imes[2] was singular in recommending primary suture with enthusiasm. Woodhall and Ochsner's report also pointed out the profound influence that the writings of Ogilvie,[3] Morgan,[4] Mason,[5] Hurt,[6] Hamilton,[7] Colcock,[8] and Taylor and Thompson,[9] dealing with the treatment of colon lesions in combat wounds, had on the treatment of colon and rectal wounds in civilian practice. Woodhall and Ochsner suggested that this influence of the writings of the World War II surgeons may have overemphasized the principle of exteriorization of all wounds of the colon and rectum. With the continuous development of newer and improved antibiotics, better pre- and postoperative care, and early definitive treatment, a critical analysis of the methods of treatment is warranted. This report further suggests that in selected cases with early definitive treatment more wounds can be closed primarily with safety and with the resultant decrease in the number of operations and in economic loss to the patient.

Mortality.—The mortality rates from traumatic injuries of the colon and rectum generally have been high regardless of the type of therapy. Quite consistently, those obtained in civilian practice have been higher than those obtained in battle injury (Table I).

In the present series of 42 patients operated upon, 6 died (14.3 per cent). Although a mortality rate of 14.3 per cent is high, it is considerably lower than those reported both in civilian and military practice (Table I).

TABLE I. MORTALITY RATES IN COLON AND RECTAL WOUNDS

SOURCE	YEAR REPORTED	MORTALITY RATE (PER CENT)	
Present series	1953	14.3	Civilian
Woodhall and Ochsner	1949	20	
Taylor and Thompson	1948	27	Military
Imes	1945	26	
Hurt	1945	33	
Ogilvie	1944	53	
Wilkinson, Hill, and Wright	1946	79.3	Civilian
Elkin and Ward	1943	53	
Rippey	1941	62.5	

Received for publication, April 20, 1953.

Incidence.—

Age: The average age in the present series was 34.8 years, whereas in the fatal cases it was 34.1 years. Generally the prognosis is poorer in the older person because of degenerative conditions.

Sex: Of the 42 patients, 29 (69.1 per cent) were men and 13 (30.9 per cent) were women. The mortality rate for men was 10.34 per cent and for women 23.07 per cent.

Race: Thirty-five patients (83.33 per cent) were Negroes and 7 (16.66 per cent) were white. The mortality rate for Negroes was 14.3 per cent and for whites it was 14.2 per cent.

Mechanism of Injury.—The mechanism by which the injury occurred varies considerably from single gunshot injuries, multiple gunshot injuries, shotgun blasts, stabs, instrumentation, and falls to auto accident (Table II).

TABLE II. INJURING MECHANISM IN FORTY-TWO CASES

CAUSE	NUMBER	DEAD	MORTALITY (PER CENT)
Gunshot	20	0	0
Multiple gunshot	3	0	0
Stab	5	1	20.0
Shotgun	5	4	80.0
Instrumentation	7	1	14.3
Auto accident	1	0	0
Unknown	1	0	0
Total	42	6	

Single gunshot wounds formed almost one-half of the injuries in the present series and were associated with no mortality. Tearing and mangling of the intra-abdominal viscera are less likely with this type of injury.

The mortality rate of stab wounds was 20.0 per cent, and shotgun blasts of the colon carried a mortality of 80.0 per cent in this series, thus illustrating the seriousness of stab wounds and shotgun blasts.

Shock.—The presence of shock in the patient when first seen and its persistence up to the time of operation are of great prognostic value (Table III).

The mortality rate in patients first seen in shock was 23.07 per cent, and in cases when shock persisted up to time of operation it was 75.0 per cent.

TABLE III. SHOCK

	NUMBER	DEAD	PER CENT
Before surgery	13	3	23.07
On arrival at operating room	4	3	75.0

It is likely that more than 13 of these patients were in shock before surgery, since the information was frequently omitted from the admitting record.

Of the 4 patients in whom adequate therapy was employed unsuccessfully and who were sent to the operating room in shock, 3 died (75 per cent).

Time Lag.—The longer the time elapsing from injury to institution of the therapy, the worse the prognosis (Table IV). The mortality rate in the group

TABLE IV. TIME LAG

LAG (HOURS)	NUMBER OF CASES	DEAD	MORTALITY (PER CENT)
0-3	18	1	5.5
3-6	10	2	20.0
6-9	5	1	20.0
9-12	1	0	0.0
12-18	1	0	0.0
18-24	1	1	100.0
24-48	3	0	0.0
48-72	2	1	50.0
10 days	1	0	0.0
Total	42	6	

treated within the first three hours was markedly below the over-all mortality rate. In civilian practice, most patients arrive shortly after injury.

The greater the lag period, the fewer the patients who will survive to reach the hospital. The earlier the casualty is admitted to the hospital, the sooner shock can be treated and the patient prepared for operation. Antibiotics and chemotherapy have reduced much of the danger of delay and resulting peritonitis.

Mortality of Wounds.—Injury to other intra-abdominal viscera in addition to the colon increases the mortality rate considerably (Table V).

TABLE V. WOUNDS

SERIES AND ORGAN INVOLVED	NUMBER OF CASES	DEATHS	MORTALITY (PER CENT)
Present series			
Multiple organs	28	5	17.8
Large intestine alone	14	1	7.1
Woodhall and Ochsner			
Multiple organs	32	9	28.1
Large intestine alone	23	2	8.7
Taylor and Thompson			
Multiple organs	39	12	31.0
Large intestine alone	28	5	18.0

Of the 42 patients in the present series 28 (66.6 per cent) had injuries to other intra-abdominal viscera aside from the colon. The other organs injured were: liver (3 cases), stomach (1 case), kidney (3 cases), spleen (2 cases), small bowel (21 cases), bladder (2 cases), chest and ribs (5 cases), diaphragm (2 cases), urethra (1 case), uterus (1 case), sacral plexus (1 case), external iliac vessels (1 case), spermatic vessel (1 case), bony pelvis (2 cases), gastrocolic ligament (2 cases), suspensory ligament (1 case), buttocks (1 case), and deltoid muscle (1 case).

The low mortality rate in cases when only the colon is injured is indeed striking. This reflects the minor nature of some of the perforations, lack of massive fecal contamination, employment of adequate surgery, and control of peritonitis.

Site of Colon Injury.—Injuries of the right colon and sigmoid and rectosigmoid carried a grave prognosis in this series (Table VI). Injuries of the ascending and descending colon are more likely to be single and therefore associated with a lower mortality rate. Injuries of the transverse colon, because of its relatively central position in the abdomen, generally are accompanied by injuries to other intra-abdominal organs and as a rule cause a high mortality rate; however, this was not reflected in this series. It is of interest that injuries of the extraperitoneal rectum caused no fatalities.

TABLE VI.

SITE OF INJURY	NUMBER OF CASES	DEATHS	
		NUMBER	PER CENT
Right colon	8	3	37.5
Transverse colon	6	0	0
Splenic flexure and descending colon	9	1	11.1
Sigmoid and rectosigmoid	13	2	15.3
Extraperitoneal rectum	6	0	0
Total	42	6	

Methods of Treatment.—In the present series a number of methods were used to treat perforated injuries of the colon and rectum (Table VII).

TABLE VII. METHODS OF TREATMENT

METHOD	NUMBER	DEAD	
		NUMBER	PER CENT
1. Primary suture	17	0	0
2. Primary suture with proximal decompression	6	1	16.6
3. Exteriorization	10	2	20.0
4. Resection with exteriorization	2	1	50.0
5. Resection with primary anastomosis	3	2	66.6
6. Proximal decompression with incision and drainage of perineum (rectum)	4	0	0
Totals	42	6	14.3

1. *Analysis of primary suture:* Of 17 patients there were no deaths. The average hospitalization was 11.8 days. Complications were one wound abscess.

2. *Analysis of primary suture with proximal decompression:* Of 6 patients there was one death (16.6 per cent mortality). The average hospitalization was 65.0 days. Complications were one case of evisceration.

3. *Analysis of exteriorizations:* Of 10 patients there were two deaths (20.0 per cent mortality). The average hospitalization was 48.3 days. Complications were two wound abscesses and one case of evisceration.

4. *Analysis of resection and exteriorization:* Of 2 patients there was one death (50 per cent mortality). The average hospitalization was 144.0 days. Complications were phlebothrombosis with pulmonary embolism. This patient made a complete recovery.

The one death when resection and exteriorization were used occurred in one of the patients taken to the operating room in shock. The traumatic lesions consisted of massive mangling and perforations of the terminal ileum, ascending colon, and hepatic flexture due to a shotgun blast. There was massive hemorrhage from a tear in the superior mesenteric vein and marked retroperitoneal hemorrhage around the right kidney and ureter. An intra-arterial transfusion was necessary using the radial artery. This patient died from irreversible shock and delayed hemorrhage twenty-eight hours after surgery.

5. *Analysis of resection and primary anastomosis:* Of the 42 patients with colon wounds 3 were treated by resection of the traumatized bowel followed by primary anastomosis with two deaths (66.6 per cent mortality). In the patient who survived there was one complication of a fecal fistula of the small bowel, which closed spontaneously in approximately three weeks. The average hospitalization was thirty-one days.

In one of the fatal cases, the patient died on the sixteenth postoperative day from a lower nephron syndrome and peritonitis. This patient received a shotgun blast of the ascending colon and hepatic flexure.

In the second case, the patient died on the sixteenth postoperative day because of delayed hemorrhage from the liver. This patient received a shotgun blast of the right lobe of the liver, terminal ileum, ascending colon, and hepatic flexure. On the seventh day after surgery, the wound of the point of entry broke down, and later massive delayed hemorrhage from the liver occurred on the day of death.

6. *Analysis of extraperitoneal rectal wounds:* There were 6 patients with extraperitoneal rectal wounds, and all recovered. Four patients had sigmoid colostomy with or without drainage of the rectal wound by incision through the perineum. Two patients had primary suture of the rectum performed immediately following laceration of the rectum which inadvertently occurred during colpotomy for a cul-de-sac abscess and a perineal prostatectomy.

TABLE VIII. ANALYSIS OF CASES AND DEATHS BY YEARS

YEAR	NUMBER OF CASES	DEATHS	
		NUMBER	PER CENT
1948	10	1	10.0
1949	1	0	0
1950	11	3	27.2
1951	7	1	14.2
1952	13	1	7.6

Days of Disability.—

1. *Analysis of primary suture:* From the injury to discharge the average hospitalization was 11.8 days (Tables IX).

TABLE IX. DAYS OF DISABILITY

	METHODS OF TREATMENT		
	Primary suture	Resection with primary anastomosis	1. Proximal decompresion with or without primary suture (secondary closure of colostomy) 2. Exteriorizations and colostomies (secondary closure of colostomy) 3. Resection with exteriorization (secondary closure of colostomy)
Time from injury to discharge	11.8 days	31.0 days	58.2 days

2. *Analysis of resection with primary anastomosis:* From the injury to discharge the average hospitalization was 31.0 days.

3. *Analysis of proximal decompression with or without primary suture, exteriorizations and colostomies, resections with exteriorizations, all methods of treatment being followed by closure of colostomy:* From injury to discharge the average period of disability was 58.2 days.

Preoperative Treatment.—The patient is usually brought to the emergency admitting room within six hours of injury (twenty-eight of forty-two cases). Shock is generally the rule, depending on the extent of the injury. If the blood pressure is unobtainable, 0 negative blood is rapidly transfused intravenously and/or intra-arterially. If the shock is not so severe, the patient is typed and matched for blood, nasal oxygen is administered, and portable x-ray pictures of the abdomen and chest are made without moving the patient. Tetanus antitoxin, penicillin, streptomycin, and, in the last two years, intravenous Aureomycin or terramycin are administered.

The majority recover rapidly from shock. Premedication is then given and surgery is performed immediately. A Levin tube is inserted into the stomach and alcohol and food particles are aspirated when present. Four patients in this series did not recover from shock under this management, and it was necessary to perform surgery with the patient in shock with a resultant 75 per cent mortality.

Operative Treatment.—Endotracheal anesthesia with gas-oxygen-ether mixtures is administered. As a rule most of the patients have alcoholic beverages and food particles in the stomach. The anesthetist is instructed to aspirate the Levin tube frequently and allow it to drain throughout the procedure.

A long paramedian incision is employed as a rule. Hemorrhage is first controlled, and perforations of the colon are closed temporarily while a search is made for damage in the small bowel and stomach.

Types of Repair.—Primary closure was employed in seventeen cases with 0 per cent mortality. Primary closure was not employed in any wound in this series which was over six hours old at the time of surgery. This type of closure was employed in single and multiple wounds of the colon and rectum, where it was judged by the operator that a good two-layer closure with viable edges could be obtained without compromising the lumen of the bowel.

Lesions of the extraperitoneal rectum as a rule were not closed. Perineal drainage was employed with a proximal sigmoid colostomy. However, two of six perforations of the extraperitoneal rectum in this series were closed primarily with perineal drainage. One case occurred during a perineal prostatectomy and one occurred during drainage of a cul-de-sac abscess. Both were recognized at the time and were immediately closed in layers.

Shotgun wounds present our most serious problem. Four patients in this series sustained shotgun blasts at close range, which mangled and destroyed the right colon with multiple associated injuries of other abdominal viscera. In three cases the right colon was resected with primary anastomosis of the ileum to the transverse colon. One case of a Mikulicz type ileotransverse colostomy was exteriorized. The shotgun-type lesion carried an 80 per cent mortality.

Many of the twenty-three cases that were exteriorized or closed with proximal decompression were lesions that were small and seen within the first six hours of injury and which could, in retrospect, have been closed primarily without additional risk to the patient.

The abdomen is closed in layers with chromic 0 suture on the peritoneum and interrupted cotton sutures on the fascia and skin. Retention sutures of Dermalon or stainless steel are employed in most cases to help prevent wound dehiscence. Drainage is routinely employed by bringing a rubber drain through a stab wound in the flank.

Postoperative Treatment.—Levin tubes connected to a suction apparatus are routinely employed until bowel sounds are present and flatus is passed per rectum or per colostomy. Streptomycin and penicillin were given routinely from 1948 through 1950, and since 1950 intravenous Aureomycin or terramycin has been employed until the patient is placed on oral feeding, at which time Aureomycin or terramycin is given by mouth.

SUMMARY

A series of forty-two cases of perforating injuries of the colon and rectum with a 14.3 per cent mortality has been reviewed. This comparatively low mortality rate is attributed in part to the increased use of streptomycin, Aureomycin, and terramycin.

Seventeen cases with single or multiple perforations of the colon and rectum were closed primarily with no mortality. This group was comprised, in the greater part, of wounds not over two inches in diameter and which received definitive treatment within six hours of injury. Primary closure in wounds of this type has in this series proved to be a safe procedure.

Primary suture with proximal decompression was employed in six cases with 16.6 per cent mortality. In most of these cases the injuries were in the relatively fixed portion of the colon or rectum.

Exteriorization was employed in ten cases with a 20 per cent mortality. Of this group, those patients who had small wounds and were treated early could have been treated by primary suture with reduction in morbidity and less loss of time.

In two cases, resection with exteriorization was employed with a 50 per cent mortality rate, and in three cases resection with primary anastomosis was performed with 66.6 per cent mortality. The high mortality in this group was primarily the result of severe initial injury with multiple gunshot involving multiple abdominal organs.

In six lesions of the extraperitoneal rectum two were closed primarily without proximal decompression. Four had proximal decompression. All had perineal drainage with no mortality.

So markedly has the use of the more recent antibiotics improved the prognosis of colon wounds that primary closure in selected cases is the preferred procedure.

REFERENCES

1. Woodhall, J. P., and Ochsner, A.: The Management of Perforating Injuries of the Colon and Rectum in Civilian Practice, SURGERY **29**: 305-320, 1951.
2. Imes, P. R.: War Surgery of the Abdomen, Surg., Gynec. & Obst. **81**: 608-616, 1945.
3. Ogilvie, W. H.: Abdominal Wounds in the Western Desert, Surg., Gynec. & Obst. **78**: 225-238, 1944.
4. Morgan, C. N.: Wounds of the Colon, Brit. J. Surg. **32**: 337-345, 1945.
5. Mason, J. M., III: Surgery of the Colon in the Forward Battle Area, SURGERY **18**: 534-541, 1945.
6. Hurt, L. E.: The Surgical Management of Colon and Rectal Injuries in the Forward Areas, Ann. Surg. **122**: 398-407, 1945.
7. Hamilton, J. E.: War Wounds of the Colon and Rectum, New York State J. Med. **44**: 2706-2712, 1944.
8. Colcock, B. P.: Traumatic Perforation of the Colon as Seen in a General Hospital, SURGERY **17**: 1-10, 1945.
9. Taylor, E. R., and Thompson, J. E.: The Early Treatment, and Results Thereof, of Injuries of the Colon and Rectum, With 70 Additional Cases, Internat. Abstr. Surg. **87**: 105-122, 209-228, 1948; in Surg., Gynec. & Obst. Aug.; Sept. 1948.
10. Wilkinson, R. S., Hill, L. M., and Wright, L. T.: Gunshot Wounds of the Abdomen, SURGERY **19**: 415-429, 1946.
11. Elkin, D. C., and Ward, W. C.: Gunshot Wounds of the Abdomen, Ann. Surg. **118**: 780-787, 1943.
12. Rippey, E. L.: The Management of Perforating Gunshot Wounds of the Abdomen, South. Surgeon **10**: 441-450, 1941.

THE ASSOCIATION OF LYMPHOGRANULOMA INGUINALE AND CANCER

Robert Rainey, M.D.,* Chicago, Ill.

(From the Department of Surgery, The Presbyterian Hospital of the City of Chicago and the University of Illinois College of Medicine, Rush)

ELEVEN cases in which lymphogranuloma inguinale apparently predisposed to neoplastic degeneration are reported in this paper. Only in recent years has it been suggested that there may be an association between lymphogranuloma inguinale and cancer. In 1935, Coutts[1] reported a case of round-cell sarcoma developing on a rectal stricture in a 15-year-old boy who had been a passive pederast. The Frei test was positive. Coutts was the first author to suggest that lymphogranuloma inguinale predisposed to malignancy, especially in view of the rarity of sarcoma of the rectum.

Liccione,[2] in 1936, was the first to describe rectal adenocarcinoma complicating lymphogranuloma inguinale. Two cases of adenocarcinoma of the rectum were described. In one, the patient had a rectal stricture with associated fistulas. After two years a Frei test was positive and biopsies of the stricture showed no neoplastic disease. A colostomy was performed, and one year later rectal adenocarcinoma was discovered. The second patient had a rectal stricture with fistulas for fifteen years after which time adenocarcinoma was discovered at the site of the stricture. Although no Frei test had been performed, the chronicity of the anorectal disease and elephantiasis of the vulvar and ischiorectal skin offered presumptive evidence of lymphogranuloma inguinale.

The same year, Lisa[3] described the autopsy findings in a Negro woman who had had a rectal stricture of two years' duration with a positive Frei test. Autopsy findings included: adenocarcinoma of the pelvic colon, squamous-cell carcinoma of the anal canal, and tuberculosis of the femoral, inguinal, and iliac nodes.

David and Loring,[4] in 1939, reported three cases of squamous-cell carcinoma of the rectum, associated with the chronic anorectal manifestation of lymphogranuloma inguinale. Two patients had positive Frei tests and had had operations diverting the fecal stream, one two years and the other twelve years prior to the detection of carcinoma. Although a Frei test was not performed on the third patient, the chronicity and nature of the rectal stricture suggested lymphogranuloma as an etiology.

The tendency for neoplastic degeneration to occur at sites of prolonged chronic inflammation, such as in cutaneous ulcers and scars of burns, is well

---

Presented before the Chicago Surgical Society on May 2, 1952.

Received for publication, April 22, 1953.

*Now serving in Medical Corps, United States Army.

known. Carcinomatous degeneration has been reported to occur in over 5 per cent of cases of chronic idiopathic ulcerative colitis.[28] Although the relationship of lymphogranuloma inguinale to neoplasia is perhaps less apparent, the incidence has been reported as ranging from less than .1 per cent (Guzman)[5] to 8.6 per cent (Barber and Murphy).[6] It remains debatable whether lymphogranuloma inguinale, per se, or its prolonged inflammatory residual, such as rectal strictures, fistulas, sinuses, and esthiomenes, are the factors predisposing to development of carcinoma.

A survey of the literature disclosed ninety-five patients with lymphogranuloma who subsequently developed carcinoma. Only those cases have been included in which either patients had a positive Frei test or the chronic clinical manifestations of lymphongranuloma inguinale were apparent.[1-27] I am reporting eleven additional cases, one from the Presbyterian Hospital and ten from the Cook County Hospital, Chicago, Ill.

These latter cases were found in the records at Cook County Hospital between 1937 and 1950, during which time 220 cases were diagnosed as strictures of the rectum due to lymphogranuloma inguinale. Of this group, ten patients were found in whom carcinoma was associated with lymphogranuloma inguinale. In these latter patients the diagnoses were confirmed by a positive biopsy for carcinoma and a positive Frei test. The incidence of neoplasia was found to be 4.5 per cent. There were twenty additional cases in which either a biopsy for carcinoma or a Frei test had not been performed to support the clinical diagnoses, and therefore they are not included in this series.

An analysis of the ninety-five cases collected from the literature and of the eleven cases in my series reveals that the majority were in Negro women. In some instances in the literature, the information pertaining to sex and race was not available (Fig. 1).

The sites at which these malignancies developed are shown in Fig. 2.

The intradermal Frei test was positive in seventy-three of the cases collected from the literature and in all of the eleven cases which I am reporting. The results of the Frei test were not stated in twenty-two of the cases found in the literature. However, as previously stated, all of these latter patients had the residual manifestations compatible with a diagnosis of lymphogranuloma inguinale. In five instances, two of these cases being in my series, a previously positive Frei test had reverted to negative at the time of carcinomatous degeneration (Fig. 3).[11, 15]

An analysis of the age distribution of these patients at the time of detection of cancer reveals that the majority were in the younger age groups, between the years of 31 and 50. In some instances this information was not available in the literature (Fig. 4).

In twenty-five cases the clear-cut relationship between carcinoma and lymphogranuloma inguinale was complicated by the presence of one or more of the following accompanying diseases: syphilis (20), chancroid (12), granuloma inguinale (6), and rectal tuberculosis (3). Sixteen of the twenty-five patients had two or more of these diseases. Forty-nine patients with lymphogranuloma inguinale subsequently developed anorectal neoplasms. The sex, race, and age distribution of this latter group reveals again that the majority were Negro women between the ages of 31 and 50 years (Figs. 5 and 6). In this group of forty-nine patients with anorectal neoplasms complicating lymphogranuloma inguinale a Frei test was positive in thirty-four instances. In the remaining

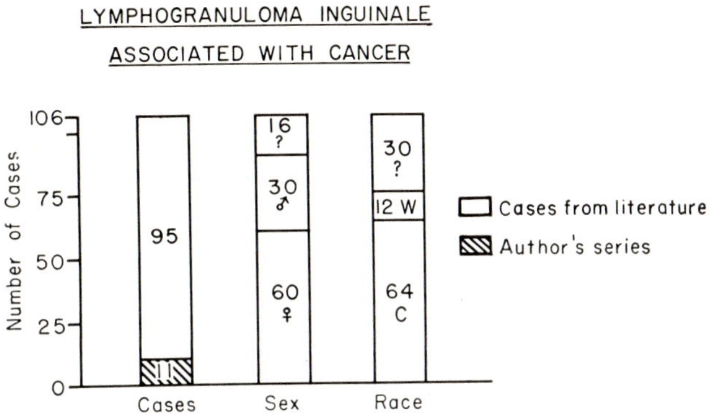

Fig. 1.

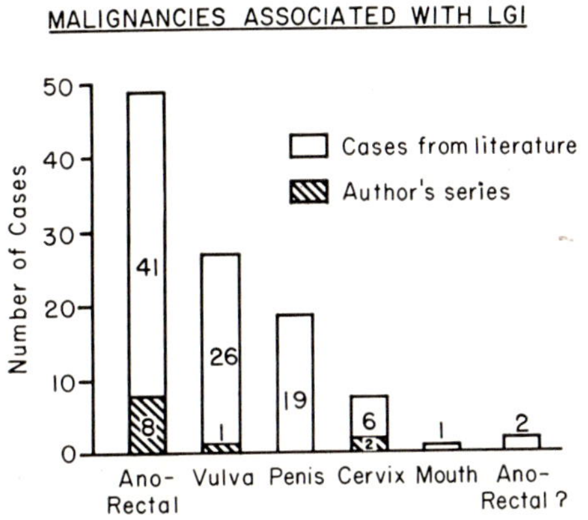

Fig. 2.

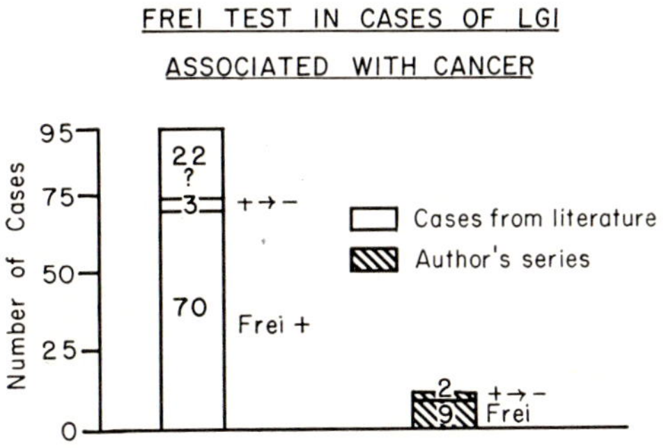

Fig. 3.

Figs. 1-3.

cases these data were not stated in the literature. Anorectal carcinomas were superimposed on a rectal stricture in thirty-one cases; eighteen patients probably had rectal strictures, although this was not stated definitely. Only one of the group definitely did not have a previous rectal stricture.[26] The duration of the lymphogranulomatous process prior to the detection of anorectal neoplasms was in most instances more than ten years. In twenty-five cases reported in the literature, data concerning the duration of the disease were not available (Fig. 7).

The cell type of the anorectal malignancies complicating lymphogranuloma inguinale is shown in Fig. 8. Apparently, rectal adenocarcinoma complicating

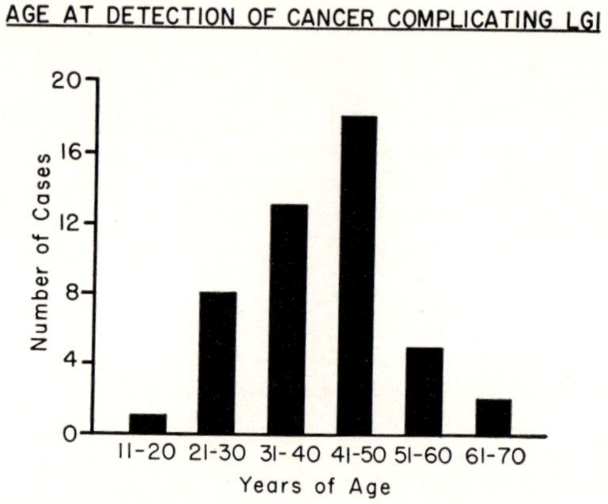

Fig. 4.

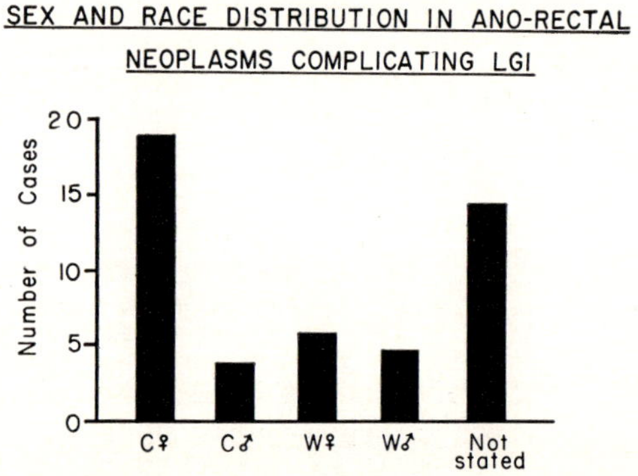

Fig. 5.

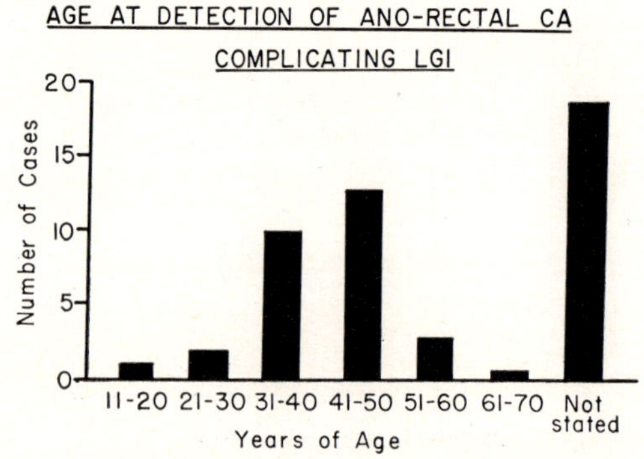

Fig. 6.

Figs. 4-6.

lymphogranuloma inguinale is quite rare, since only seven cases were found in the literature. All these patients had chronic rectal strictures. However, a Frei test was not reported in four of this group.[2, 6, 20] In two other cases, rectal tuberculosis was a complicating factor.[3, 21] In still another case the adenocarcinoma developing in the rectosigmoid may have been coincidental, since the lymphogranulomatous stricture was apparently confined to the rectum.[17]

Fig. 7.

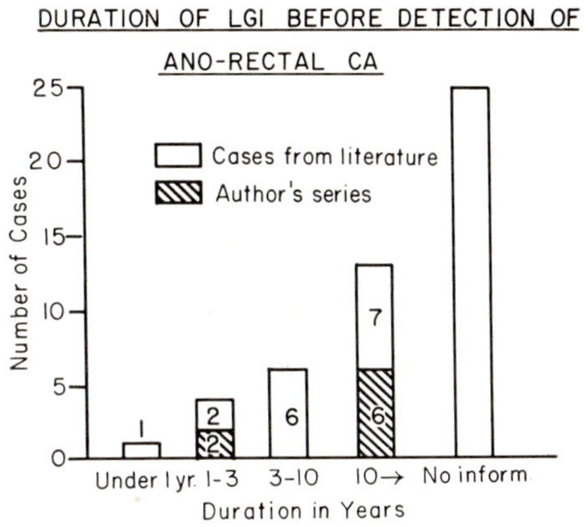

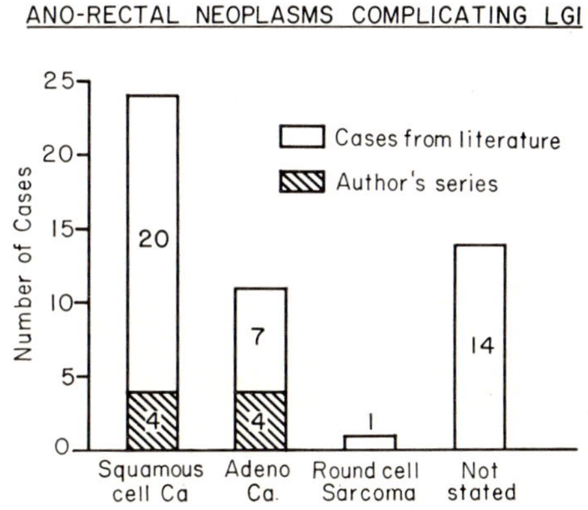

Fig. 8.

I am reporting four additional cases of rectal adenocarcinoma complicating lymphogranuloma inguinale. The following patient, whom I observed at the Presbyterian Hospital of Chicago, is illustrative of this group.

CASE REPORTS

CASE 1.—J. G., a 46-year-old white woman, was first admitted to the Presbyterian Hospital, Chicago, in January, 1939. She then claimed that for the preceding two years she had experienced progressively painful defecation with obstipation and with "pencillike" and frequently blood-streaked stools. In 1938, she had been under the care of a doctor who prescribed mineral oil, cathartics, and enemas, and who dilated the rectum two times a week, with some relief or symptoms. In the week prior to admission she suffered marked rectal distress with progressive difficulty in defecation. Examination on admission revealed the colon to be distended and palpable in its entire extent. A stricture of the rectum admitting the tip of the index finger was located 3 cm. proximal to the anal ring. The mucosa distal to the stricture was rough and granular, and showed changes typical of those seen in lymphogranuloma inguinale. This impression was confirmed by a positive Frei test. The blood Kahn test was negative. A double-barreled sigmoid colostomy in continuity was performed.* A biopsy of the rectal stricture showed no evidence of malignancy (Fig. 9). Postoperatively, the course was uneventful, and the patient received sulfanilamide for the following year.

The second admission was in April, 1940, at which time the patient was apparently in good health. Examination of the rectum under anesthesia revealed a purulent discharge from the rectum. The stricture, which was just above the mucocutaneous line, could not be probed and was felt by vaginal palpation to be like an indurated cord, extending superiorly to the level of the posterior fornix. A catheter passed distally in the colostomy reached this area but would go no further.

The third admission in May, 1940, was preceded by shifting, cramping abdominal pain and obstipation for one week with failure of the colostomy to function for two days prior to admission. Examination revealed the lumen of the colostomy to be markedly stenosed. This was remedied by revising the afferent stoma.

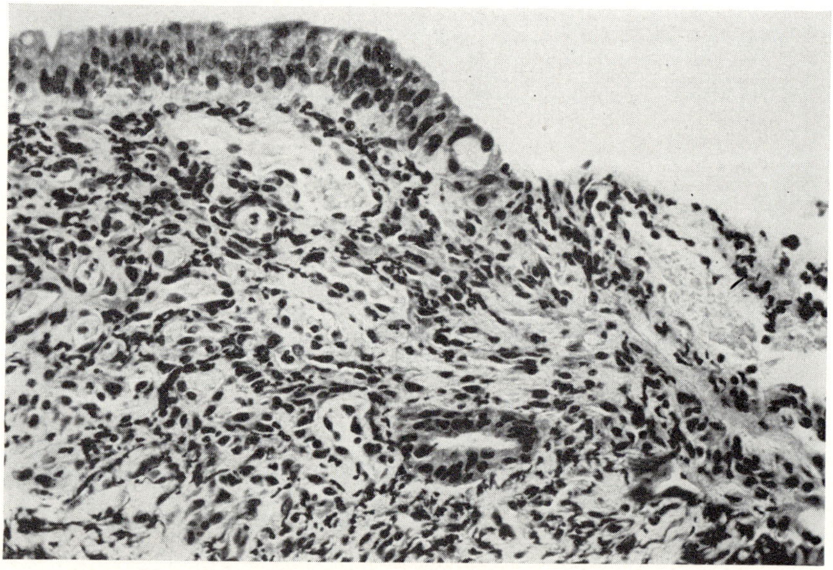

Fig. 9.—Medium-power photomicrograph of a biopsy of the rectal stricture, which was made twelve years before the detection of carcinomatous degeneration. It shows chronic inflammation and fibrosis and an area of mucosal ulceration.

In ensuing years the patient experienced good health and was admitted the fourth time in August, 1944, for consideration of closing the colostomy. However, rectal examination under anesthesia revealed the mucosa at the level of the stricture to be ulcerated and covered with a purulent exudate. Barium-contrast x-ray studies revealed a marked stricture of the rectum involving the distal 10 cm. with an apparently complete obstruction at the proximal end of the stricture (Fig. 10). Consideration of dilating the rectal stricture was therefore abandoned. Examination of the purulent rectal exudate revealed no acid-fast bacilli, and the intradermal Frei test was again positive.

*By Dr. Vernon C. David and Dr. Richard K. Gilchrist, who also performed subsequent operations.

The patient remained in good health until the fifth admission in August, 1950. During the preceding week she had had cramping abdominal pain with poor results from colostomy flushings and had experienced moderate pain in the rectum. This pain was associated with the desire to defecate, and on doing so she would pass bloody purulent material through the anus. Examination on admission revealed a temperature as high as 102.4° F. Vaginal palpation revealed a firm mass, 7 cm. in diameter, in the left perirectal area and about 6 cm. above the anus. The anus would not admit the tip of the little finger, and water from above would barely go through to the anus. The colostomy opening had narrowed. Therefore the colostomy stoma was again revised and the stricture at the anal outlet was dilated, resulting in the evacuation of about 30 c.c. of pus. The mucosa was described as being very red, inflamed, and soft, with nothing that resembled tumor. Ten centimeters above the anus, the rectal stricture was again excessively narrow. A culture of pus from the perirectal abscess revealed predominantly *Streptococcus viridans*, with a minor growth of *Staphylococcus aureus*.

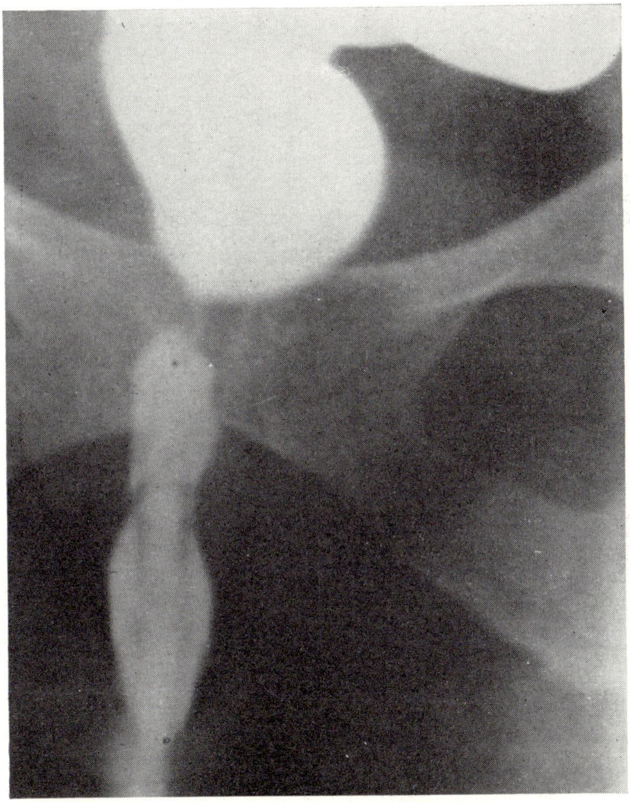

Fig. 10.—Photograph of an x-ray film made of the rectum after a barium enema and introduction of barium into the distal stoma of a sigmoid colostomy. It shows a marked stricture of the distal rectum with an apparent complete obstruction at the proximal end of the stricture. This x-ray picture was made seven years prior to the detection of carcinoma.

Convalescence was uneventful and the patient was able to return to work as a secretary. However, she continued to have an anal discharge of thick yellow pus and small amounts of blood, associated with cramping, lower abdominal pain and night sweats.

In April, 1951, she noted a ten-pound weight loss and progressive malaise, necessitating a sixth admission. Vaginal examination again revealed the rectum to be excessively indurated. Because of the progressively incapacitating course and in view of a suspicion of a superimposed malignancy, an abdominoperineal resection was performed. Abdominal exploration revealed no pathologic changes. The rectum was mobilized with great difficulty, as it was densely adherent to the sacrococcygeal junction and to the base of the bladder and vagina. About 4 cm. from the anus, a small rectovaginal fistula was observed. The postoperative course was uneventful, with the perineal wound granulating and healing at a normal rate. It

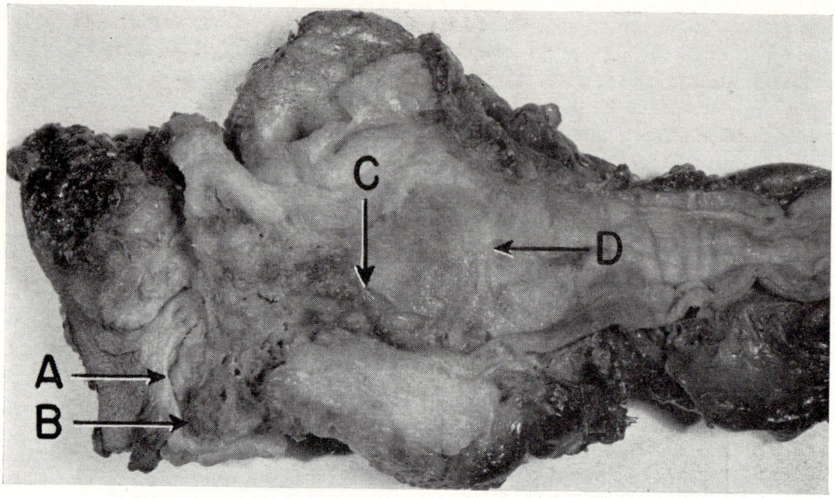

Fig. 11.—Photograph of the surgical specimen from the patient mentioned in the adjoining case report and the preceding two illustrations showing: *A.* squamocolumnar junction, *B,* distal extension of the colloid adenocarcinoma, *C,* proximal extension of the colloid adenocarcinoma, *D,* granular mucosa at the site of the rectal stricture due to lymphogranuloma inguinale.

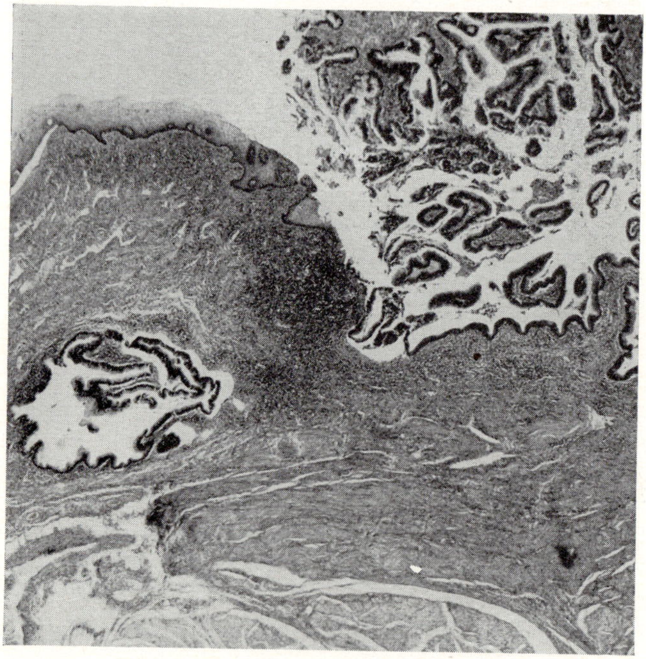

Fig. 12.—Low-power photomicrograph of tissue removed from the previously illustrated surgical specimen showing an adenocarcinoma infiltrating beneath the squamocolumnar junction.

is interesting to note that the intradermal Frei test was repeated preoperatively but resulted in only an area of slight erythema 1.5 cm. in diameter and without induration or elevation. This was interpreted as negative. The Frei test was repeated twice, postoperatively, using

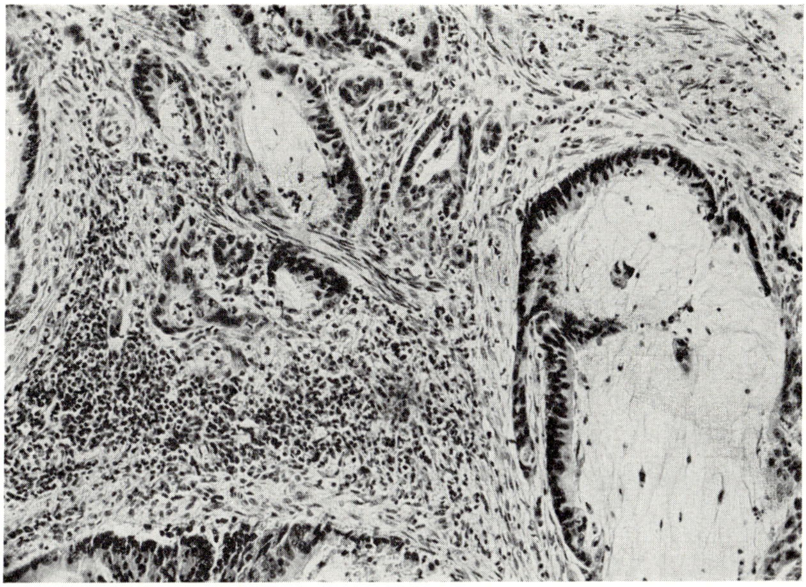

Fig. 13.

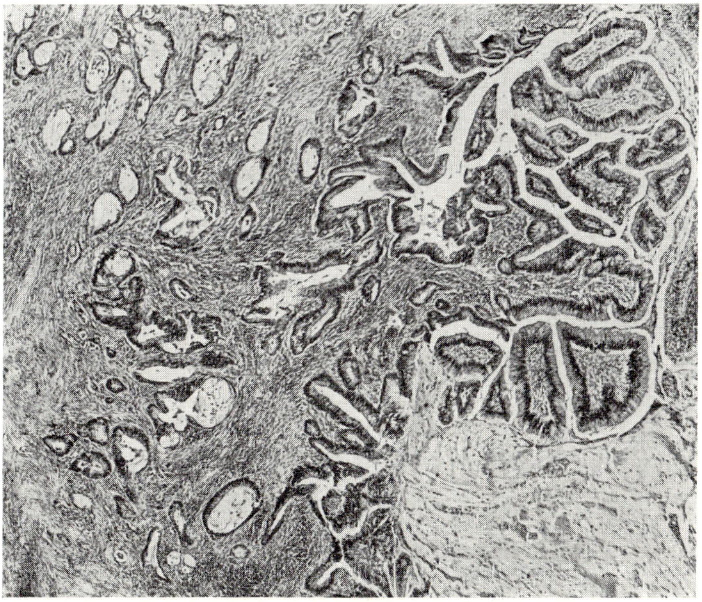

Fig. 14.

Figs. 13 and 14.—High-power photomicrograph of tissue removed from the surgical specimen illustrated in Fig. 11 showing the colloid-producing tendency of this adenocarcinoma with infiltration into the muscular wall of the rectum.

TABLE I*

CASE	SITE	TYPE OF CANCER	CHRONICITY OF LYMPHOGRANULOMA INGUINALE (YEARS)	AGE AT TIME CARCINOMA WAS DETECTED (YEARS)	RACE	SEX	FREI TEST†	BLOOD KAHN TEST†	MISCELLANEOUS DATA
1	Anorectal	Adenocarcinoma	14	45	W	F	P-N		Colostomy 12 yr. prior to detecion of carcinoma
2	Anorectal	Adenocarcinoma	30	50	N	F	P		
3	Anorectal	Adenocarcinoma	14	52	N	F	P		
4	Anorectal	Adenocarcinoma	1	55	N	M	P	P	
5	Anorectal	Squamous-cell carcinoma	24	44	N	F	P	P	Granuloma inguinale
6	Anorectal	Squamous-cell carcinoma	17	48	N	F	P		
7	Anorectal	Squamous-cell carcinoma	12	41	N	M	P	P	Granuloma inguinale (? central nervous system syphilis)
8	Anorectal	Squamous-cell carcinoma	1	45	W	M	P-N		Colostomy 10 mo.
9	Cervix	Squamous-cell carcinoma	18	45	N	F	P		Colostomy 1 yr. prior to detection of carcinoma; pulmonary tuberculosis
10	Cervix	Squamous-cell carcinoma	12	30	W	F	P		Colostomy 4 yr. prior to detection of carcinoma
11	Vulva	Squamous-cell carcinoma	5	32	W	F	P		Vulvar esthiomene; no rectal stricture

*Data from eleven cases of lymphogranuloma inguinale complicated by the development of carcinoma. These previously unreported cases were collected from the Presbyterian Hospital and Cook County Hospital of the City of Chicago.

†P represents positive; P-N represents positive, subsequently becoming negative.

two different commercial antigens and was again negative without erythema or induration. The operative specimen (Fig. 11) was 25 cm. long, with an anal orifice barely admitting the tip of the little finger. One-half centimeter above the pectinate line, a soft, gelatinous, slightly elevated, and polypoid lesion was present, almost completely surrounding the circumference of the bowel and extending proximally for 4 cm. The edges of this lesion in some areas were moderately indurated. The mucosa for 7 cm. proximal to this lesion was rough and granular, the lumen being narrowed to 2 to 3 cm. in diameter. The wall of the rectum in this portion was thickened and surrounded by a moderate amount of excessively indurated perirectal fat. The sigmoid colon and proximal one-third of the rectum were grossly normal. Microscopically (Figs. 12 and 13), the lesion was a colloid adenocarcinoma which had infiltrated deeply in some areas into the musculature of the rectum, but not beyond. The carcinoma extended down to and infiltrated beneath the squamocolumnar junction. In both the carcinoma and the proximal portion of the strictured rectum there were numerous areas of acute and predominantly chronic inflammatory cells. In the entire strictured portion of the rectum, fibroblastic proliferation was excessive and severe perirectal fibrosis was apparent. The mucous membrane over the proximal stenosed portion of the rectum, although not involved by carcinoma, contained atypical glands, the cells of which were well oriented, but larger than normal with hyperchromatic nuclei.

Subsequent examination revealed that in May, 1951, the patient developed a perineal abscess. Biopsy at this site showed recurrent mucus-secreting adenocarcinoma. A local resection of this perineal mass and the posterior vaginal wall was performed in September, 1952. The postoperative course was uneventful.

Information relevant to the remaining ten cases in my series, which were collected from the records at the Cook County Hospital of Chicago, is presented in Table I.

DISCUSSION

A colostomy does not remove the hazard of subsequent carcinomatous degeneration. It is interesting to note that an operation sidetracking the fecal stream, namely, a colostomy, cecostomy, or ileostomy, had been performed in eleven cases at varying intervals prior to the detection of carcinoma (Table II). Nine of these patients subsequently developed anorectal neoplasms; the other two patients had also had colostomies performed, one and four years, respectively, before the discovery of carcinoma of the cervix with infiltration of the rectovaginal septum. There has been little warning in the literature that a colostomy, although relieving the symptoms of a severe rectal stricture and its associated fistulas and abscesses, may not remove the hazard of a complicating carcinoma. In fact, in many of these patients with severe residuals of lymphogranuloma inguinale, a colostomy may temporarily relieve a chronic intestinal obstruction, but fibrobsis, abscesses, and fistulous tracts may persist frequently, with copious amounts of purulent and sometimes sanguineous drainage, in spite of the modern chemotherapeutic agents. In addition, the persistence of the lymphogranulomatous inflammation in some patients is manifested by anemia, amyloid disease, and an extension of the fibrotic granulomatous process, resulting in obliteration of the afferent loop of the colostomy.[29] Therefore, if the inflammatory process persists after proper drug therapy and a defunctioning colostomy, then a combined abdominoperineal resection is indicated. As a result of the latter operation, the greater part of the diseased tissue can be excised and the risk of developing a superimposed anorectal carcinoma is removed. It must be borne in mind, however, that the mortality rate will be higher with this more extensive operation, since these patients are frequently in a severely debilitated condition; also, the extensive inflammation and fibrosis make the perineal dissection considerably more difficult and time-consuming. Therefore, if the patient's health is complicated by severe inflammation, debilitation, or intestinal obstruction, a single-barreled type of sigmoid colostomy may be performed in which the proximal end is brought out through a stab wound and the distal loop is delivered through the laparotomy incision. This maneuver will facilitate the abdominoperineal resection, which should be performed if the inflammatory process persists after adequate conservative therapy.

TABLE II*

PERIOD OF TIME COLOSTOMY OR CECOSTOMY WAS PRESENT BEFORE DETECTION OF CARCINOMA (9 CASES)	AGE, COLOR, AND SEX	TYPE OF ANORECTAL CARCINOMA	REFERENCE
Colostomy, 10 mo.	45, W, M	Squamous-cell carcinoma	Case Report 8†
Colostomy, 1 yr.	35, N, F	Adenocarcinoma	Ref. 2
Colostomy, 2 yr.	29, W, F	Squamous-cell carcinoma	Ref. 4
Colostomy, 3 yr.	Not stated	Squamous-cell carcinoma	Ref. 16
Colostomy, 7 yr.	Not stated	Squamous-cell carcinoma	Ref. 16
Colostomy, 8 yr.	49, N, F	Squamous-cell carcinoma	Ref. 12
Cecostomy, 12 yr.	32, W, F	Squamous-cell carcinoma	Ref. 4
Colostomy, 13 yr.	46, W, F	Adenocarcinoma	Case Report 1†
Colostomy, 18 yr.	Not stated	Adenocarcinoma	Ref. 20
		TYPE OF CARCINOMA OF CERVIX (2 CASES)	
Colostomy, 1 yr.	45, N, F	Squamous-cell carcinoma	Case Report 9†
Colostomy, 4 yr.	30, W, F	Squamous-cell carcinoma	Case Report 10†

*Eleven cases collected from the literature and the present series.
†Present series.

In those patients without severe scarring or extensive fistulous formation, conservative therapy utilizing rectal dilatations, chemotherapy, and supportive measures should be employed. As advocated by David in 1944,[30] a colostomy in conjunction with these conservative measures has in some cases afforded so much improvement as to warrant reanastomosis with apparent cure. It is important, however, to be aware of the persistent hazard of carcinomatous degeneration when such a conservative therapy is utilized. These patients must, therefore, be kept under close observation and, if it is feasible, biopsies must be performed at frequent intervals. In many instances a severely strictured rectum will prevent adequate biopsy examination.

As previously mentioned, the positive Frei test reverted to negative at the time of cancer detection in five cases; two of these were from my series. Further investigation should be made into this possibly anergic phenomenon in which a positive Frei test may revert to negative in the presence of carcinoma, since it is conceivable that such a skin test or a decrease in the complement fixation titer might serve as a diagnostic aid in the detection of latent cancer in these patients.

In my series of cases from Cook County Hospital, there was 4.5 per cent incidence of carcinomatous degeneration in patients whose conditions were previously diagnosed as lymphogranuloma inguinale between the years 1937 and 1950. It is my opinion that had Frei tests and biopsies for carcinoma been performed on all of these 220 patients, a higher incidence of neoplasia might well have been observed.

Binkley and Derrick,[18] in 1945, reported the interesting observation that the average age in their series was lower in those cases of carcinoma of the anus with a positive Frei test, as contrasted with those with negative Frei tests. This observation is verified by my data in which twenty-eight of a total of thirty patients with anorectal neoplasms complicating lymphogranuloma inguinale developed carcinoma prior to 52 years of age, while the average age of onset of anorectal carcinoma in the general population is 54 years.[31] Swink,[24] in 1949, stated that although carcinoma in general is less prominent in Negroes, the incidence of neoplasms of the rectum and anus is considerably less in white than in Negro women at ages under 65 years. In 1951 Pund and Lacy[27] reported that in a group of forty-nine Negro patients with penile, vulvar, or anorectal carcinoma, 63 per cent had a positive Frei test. The incidence of carcinoma of the anus has been reported to comprise 1.7 per cent of anorectal cancer.[32] When the frequency of a positive Frei test in cases of squamous-cell carcinoma in the anorectal, vulvar, and penile areas is considered, these observations are all highly suggestive that lymphogranuloma inguinale predisposes to neoplastic degeneration.

The data collected from the literature and from my series of cases are not extensive enough to prove conclusively that lymphogranuloma inguinale per se predisposes to neoplasia. Rosser[33] maintained that the prolonged chronic inflammation with the fistulous formation present in these patients with lymphogranuloma inguinale is the factor responsible for the carcinomatous degeneration. The incidence of neoplastic degeneration reported in association with fistulas in ano is less than 1 per cent.[4] If my observation is correct, that a minimum of 4.5 per cent of patients with lymphogranuloma inguinale develop superimposed carcinoma over a period of years, then the predisposition of the chronic lymphogranulomatous inflammatory process to carcinomatous degeneration would seem apparent.

SUMMARY

1. In this series of eleven cases there was an apparent association between lymphogranuloma inguinale and carcinomatous degeneration.

2. The incidence of neoplasia in a group of 220 cases of lymphogranuloma inguinale, collected from the records at Cook County Hospital, was found to be 4.5 per cent.

3. In a survey of the literature, ninety-five cases were found in which lymphogranuloma inguinale and carcinoma were associated.

4. A colostomy does not remove the hazard of anorectal neoplastic degeneration in patients with lymphogranuloma inguinale.

5. Patients with less extensive anorectal disease may be treated with more conservative measures but must be followed closely. If the inflammatory process

continues after proper drug therapy and a preliminary colostomy, then more radical surgery is indicated.

6. Five cases are mentioned in which a previously positive Frei test reverted to negative at the time carcinoma was discovered. Further investigation is urged, as it is conceivable that this observation might form the basis of a diagnostic aid in the detection of latent carcinoma in these patients.

7. Evidence is presented from the literature and from my series supporting the hypothesis that lymphogranuloma inguinale may predispose to neoplastic degeneration.

REFERENCES

1. Coutts, W. E.: Sindrome genito-ano-rectal elefantiasico y estenosante de origen linfogranulomatoso, en especial en relacion contrastornos ano-rectales, Bol. Soc. Quir. de Chile **13**: 235-249, 1935.
2. Liccione, W. T.: Venereal Stricture of the Rectum: Adenocarcinoma as a Late Complication of Lymphogranuloma Inguinale, Am. J. Surg. **31**: 551-555, 1936.
3. Lisa, J. R.: Adenocarcinoma of the Rectum, Squamous Cell Carcinoma of the Anal Canal and Chronic Tuberculous Pelvic Adenitis, Arch. Path. **21**: 252, 1936.
4. David, V. C., and Loring, M.: The Relation of Chronic Inflammation and Especially Lymphogranuloma Inguinale to the Development of Squamous Cell Carcinoma of the Rectum, Ann. Surg. **109**: 837-843, 1939.
5. Guzman, L.: Coexistence of Chronic Lymphogranuloma and Cancer, Radiology **41**: 151-156, 1943.
6. Barber, W. H., and Murphy, W. B.: Lymphogranuloma Venereum, Ann. Surg. **113**: 30-40, 1941.
7. Bernstein, P.: Lymphogranuloma Inguinale, Carcinoma, and Syphilis; A Triad of Diseases Occurring in One Patient, Am. J. Obst. & Gynec. **29**: 718-725, 1935.
8. Reaves, J. U.: Granuloma Inguinale Differentiated From Lymphogranuloma Inguinale, J. M. A. Alabama **6**: 317-324, 1937.
9. Smith, T. E.: The Relation of Anorectal Disease to Malignancy, Dallas M. J. **23**: 118-120, 1937.
10. Pund, E. R., Greenblatt, R. B., and Huie, G. B.: The Role of Biopsy in Diagnosis of Venereal Diseases, Am. J. Syph., Gonor. & Ven. Dis. **22**: 495-502, 1938.
11. Weissenbach, R. J., Martineau, J., and Seguin, M.: Esthiomène de la vulve avec rétrécissement du rectum. Epithélioma spino-cellulaire de la région vulvo-vaginale, Bull. Soc. franç. de dermat. et syph. **45**: 1643-1650, 1785-1786, 1938.
12. Cardwell, E. S., and Pund, E. R.: Malignancies Related to Venereal Diseases, J. M. A. Georgia **29**: 60-62, 1940.
13. Taussig, F. J.: Prevention of Cancer of the Vulva, Cancer Research **1**: 901-904, 1941.
14. Deibert, A. V., and Greenblatt, R. B.: Malignancy and Lymphogranuloma Venereum, Am. J. Syph., Gonor. & Ven. Dis. **26**: 330-335, 1942.
15. Fraser, C. K., Kane, H. F., and Parks, J.: Stricture-Forming Lesions of the Female Genitals and Rectum, Am. J. Obst. & Gynec. **43**: 698-703, 1942.
16. Woods, F. M., and Hanlon, C. R.: Inflammatory Stricture of the Rectum, Ann. Surg. **120**: 598-606, 1944.
17. Bacon, H. E., Gass, O. C., and Todhunter, W. D.: The Present Status of the Surgical Treatment of Cancer of the Rectum and Pelvic Colon, Tr. Am. Proct. Soc. 129-150, 1944.
18. Binkley, G. E., and Derrick, W. A.: Association of Squamous Cancer With Anal Manifestations of Lymphogranuloma Venereum, Am. J. Digest Dis. **12**: 46-47, 1945.
19. Wright, L. T., Berg, B. N., Bolden, J. V., and Freeman, W. A.: Rectal Strictures Due to Lymphogranuloma Venereum, Surg., Gynec. & Obst. **82**: 449-462, 1946.
20. Salgado, C.: Retite estenosante e câncer do reto, Rev. brasil. de cir. **15**: 367-370, 1946.
21. Bordon, LaPalle, and Pujosausset: Epithélioma greffe sur une stenose recto-sigmoidienne due à la maladie de Nicholas-favre, J. de méd. de Bordeaux **125**: 49-54, 1948.
22. Costello, M. J., and D'Avanzo, C. S.: Lymphogranuloma Venereum, Arch. Dermat. & Syph. **57**: 112-121, 1948.
23. Kremer, H. U.: Case of Lymphopathia Venereum With Coexistent Carcinoma of the Rectum, Urol. & Cutan. Rev. **52**: 534-535, 1948.
24. Swink, R. L.: Lymphogranuloma Venereum Associated With Squamous Cell Carcinoma, South. M. J. **42**: 217-220, 1949.
25. Lunin, A. B.: Carcinoma of the Vulva, Am. J. Obst. & Gynec. **57**: 742-747, 1949.
26. Schiebel, H. M.: Treatment of Advanced Strictures of the Rectum Due to Lymphogranuloma Venereum, North Carolina M. J. **12**: 49-52, 1951.

27. Pund, E. R., and Lacy, G. R.: Lymphogranuloma Inguinale—A Precipitating Cause of Carcinoma: Statistical Analysis of 135 Cases of Penis, Vulva, and Anorectum, Am. Surgeon **17**: 711-718, 1951.
28. Sloan, W. P., Bargen, J. A., and Baggenstoss, A. H.: Local Complications of Chronic Ulcerative Colitis Based on the Study of 2000 Cases, Proc. Staff Meet., Mayo Clin. **25**: 240-244, 1950.
29. David, V. C., and Loring, M.: Extragenital Lesions of Lymphogranuloma Inguinale, J. A. M. A. **106**: 1875-1879, 1936.
30. David, V. C.: See discussion of Reference 16.
31. Bacon, H. E.: Anus, Rectum, Sigmoid Colon: Diagnosis and Treatment, ed. 3, vol. 2, Philadelphia, 1949, J. B. Lippincott Company, p. 603.
32. Cattell, R. B., and Williams, A. C.: Epidermoid Carcinoma of the Anus and the Rectum, Arch. Surg. **46**: 336-349, 1943.
33. Rosser, C.: See discussion of Reference 4.

CARCINOMA OF THE MAXILLARY ANTRUM

WALTER L. MATTICK, M.D., AND MILTON A. STREUTER, M.D., BUFFALO, N. Y.

(From the Roswell Park Memorial Institute)

THE following is a brief survey of the records of the Roswell Park Memorial Institute, covering epithelial malignancies of primary origin arising in the maxillary antrum in contradistinction to tumors of similar histology occurring in the mucosa of adjacent structures, such as the alveolus, palate, nares, adjoining paranasal sinuses, and/or metastatic tumors secondarily spreading or extending into the antrum. A more recent ten-year period from 1936 through 1946 was chosen so that an over-all evaluation of five-year end results could be ascertained. All cases, even those too far advanced for treatment, are included.

In this particular period, sixty-eight cases of cancer of the antrum, or .14 per cent of all admissions, were noted out of 48,613 patients examined in this clinic where, over the past years, experience has shown that approximately 50 per cent of all patients seen are found to have some form of malignancy. This is an approximate incident of .27 per cent of all cancer, thus being higher than that reported by Perzik,[7] who found that carcinoma of the nasal cavity and paranasal sinuses makes up .2 per cent of all malignancies and 80 per cent of those cases in the antrum.

Of the 68 patients, 67.7 per cent were men and 32.3 per cent were women. Schall,[8] reporting a series of 219 cases of nasal cavity and sinus malignancies seen from 1930 to 1945, found 63 per cent in men and 36 per cent in women, which does not materially differ from our figures of exclusive epithelial malignancy of the antrum. To recapitulate, other types of antral involvement, such as lymphosarcoma, fibrosarcoma, giant-cell tumor, neurinoma, adamantinoma, and so forth, are not included in this study.

All of our patients were of the white or Caucasian race, except 2 who were Negroes. No particular nationality seemed to predominate. In this short series, the greatest incidence was noted in the 56-to-75-year age group, where approximately 58.8 per cent of our cases occurred (Table I). All, incidentally, had a negative serology.

Concerning etiology in this series, little positive information was gained, beyond that known of cancer in general. It is probable, however, as often postulated, that chronic inflammatory hyperplasia, with its tendency to polypoid formation and metaplasia of the mucosa, may play a part. The Cohnheim theory of occurrence in misplaced islands of embryonal squamous cells is also still suggestive.

Primary antral involvement is often difficult to prove as the lesion may have originated in the nose, ethmoid, hard palate, or alveolar mucosa, and

Received for publication, April 21, 1953.

secondarily involved the antrum. More essential from the prognostic point of view is an attempt to ascertain whether the process involves mainly the anterolateral wall and floor, or the posterior wall and roof of the antrum. In this respect, our experience coincides with that generally cited in that the former group, that is, the one involving the anterolateral wall and floor, offers a much better prognosis.

TABLE I. CARCINOMA OF THE ANTRUM (1936 THROUGH 1945, SIXTY-EIGHT CASES): TABULATION OF AGE, SEX,* AND PRESENCE OF METASTATIC NODES

AGE	NO NODES			NODES PRESENT			TOTAL	PER CENT
	MALE	FEMALE	TOTAL	MALE	FEMALE	TOTAL		
35-45	9	1	10	1	1	2	12	17.6
46-55	5	3	8	2	1	3	11	16.1
56-65	13	5	18	4	2	6	24	35.3
66-75	5	5	10	4	2	6	16	23.5
76-85	3	2	5	0	0	0	5	7.3
Totals	35	16	51	11	6	17	68	100.0
Per cent	76.0	72.7	75	24.0	27.3	25	100	

*In the entire group, 67.7 per cent were men, 32.3 per cent were women.

Regional node metastasis, considered a sign of advanced disease, was noted in 25 per cent of our cases on initial examination. Perzik[7] stated that "distant metastasis occurs in over 25 per cent of cases of cancer in the nasal cavity and para-nasal sinus." Watson[12] found metastasis in 29 per cent of 127 cases, and considered lateral pharyngeal node involvement to run high.

Extension of the lesion to the orbit, nose, oral cavity, ethmoids, and cheek muscles is also to be considered as a significant indication of advanced disease, hence offering poor prognosis.

These observations, in addition to x-ray findings of bone destruction, led us to classify fifty-two of our sixty-eight cases in the advanced stage and sixteen in the earlier stages of the disease. These findings will be elaborated later when our results are considered. Age of the patient seemed to bear no essential relationship to prognosis in this series.

On histopathologic examination of the biopsied or autopsied tissues, thirty-eight of our specimens were of the differentiated types of squamous-cell carcinoma, either of the mucous membrane or pearl-cell variety, twenty-five were noted as anaplastic carcinoma, three as papillary, one as glandular epithelial formation, and one as epithelial neoplasm, possibly suggestive of adamantinoma. In twenty-seven cases the lesion occurred in the right antrum and in forty-one it occurred in the left. We believe that this is coincidental because of the small size of our series of cases.

The symptoms encountered were generally those commonly stated, such as swelling and aching of the cheek or teeth, nasal obstruction or bleeding, proptosis of the eye, all on the side of the lesion. In more advanced cases with extension through the infraorbital plate, the eye may be pushed up or proptosed with resulting diplopia, or involvement of the second division of the fifth cranial nerve may be noted causing numbness of the ipsilateral cheek and gums.

On palpation of the oral cavity, a resiliency of the anterolateral wall of the antrum, palate, or alveolus may be noted and is often a diagnostic sign. Extension into the orbit and roughening or destruction of the infraorbital ridge may be felt. The ipsilateral nares may be obstructed by displacement of the naso-antral wall or by extension of the tumor causing bleeding on attempted examination.

X-ray pictures of the chin-nose and lateral projection showed clouding of the antrum in sixty of our cases (88 per cent) and, incidentally, in all seven of our five-year survivals; sclerosis and/or marginal irregularity of outline was noted in twenty-five cases, or 36.8 per cent, and in 4 of the 7 patients surviving five years or more. Bone destruction was noted in twenty-three instances, or 33.8 per cent, but in only 2 patients surviving two years, 1 patient surviving three years, 1 patient surviving four years, and none surviving over five years. Usually, such patients lived less than one to one and one-half years. Thus, we must conclude that this finding is generally of bad prognostic import.

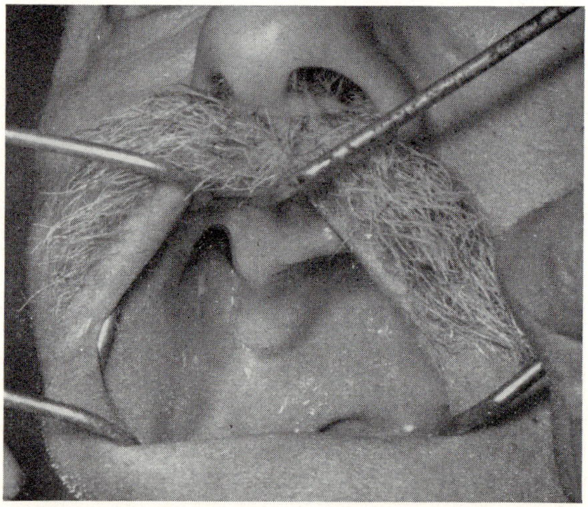

Fig. 1.—A typical seven-year arrest in a case of antral cancer following surgical drainage of antrum and irradiation.

Therapy during these ten years of investigation varied from external x-ray or radium pack to intra-antral radium tube, often supplemented with drainage through the naso-antral window, or modified Caldwell-Luc approach. The intracavitary radium tube was generally placed in the antrum and/or nose for 200 to 400 mg. hr. (100 mg. tube, 1 mm. of platinum for four hours) usually before x-ray therapy. X-ray therapy commonly consisted of one or more fields crossing in the antrum on 200 to 400 kv. modality with dosage up to tissue tolerance (Fig. 1). In a few of the cases, the palate was removed, the antral tumor tissue curetted out, and a radium mold applied with dosage to tissue tolerance supplemented by x-ray.

In more recent cases not included in this series, we have attempted to follow the principle of more radical surgery, that is, superior maxillary resection with or without exenteration of orbit and ethmoids where necessary, or a modified excision with electrocoagulation followed by intracavitary radium buried in gauge for dosages of 1,000 to 1,500 mg. her. (Fig. 2, *A* and *B*). This is followed later by external x-ray. This sequence of surgical drainage, radium, and x-ray in the present series of sixty-eight cases was often reversed as reflected in the results herein reported. We now believe that radical surgery and/or electrocoagulation followed by heavy dosage of gamma radiation up to 1,500 or more mg. hr. and these followed by x-ray to be the procedure of present choice, as is well shown by the results of Schall,[8] and as advocated by Weaver,[13] Schuknecht,[9] New,[6] Ward and Hendrick,[11] and others.

Results.—We divided the sixty-eight cases into sixteen early ones and fifty-three advanced cases as seen on admission and, as noted previously, we found that 7 of 16 patients with early cases survived from three to thirteen years (40 per cent). Six of these have been free of disease (Fig. 1) from seven to thirteen years (35 per cent arrests); 9 survived from two and one-half to thirteen years.

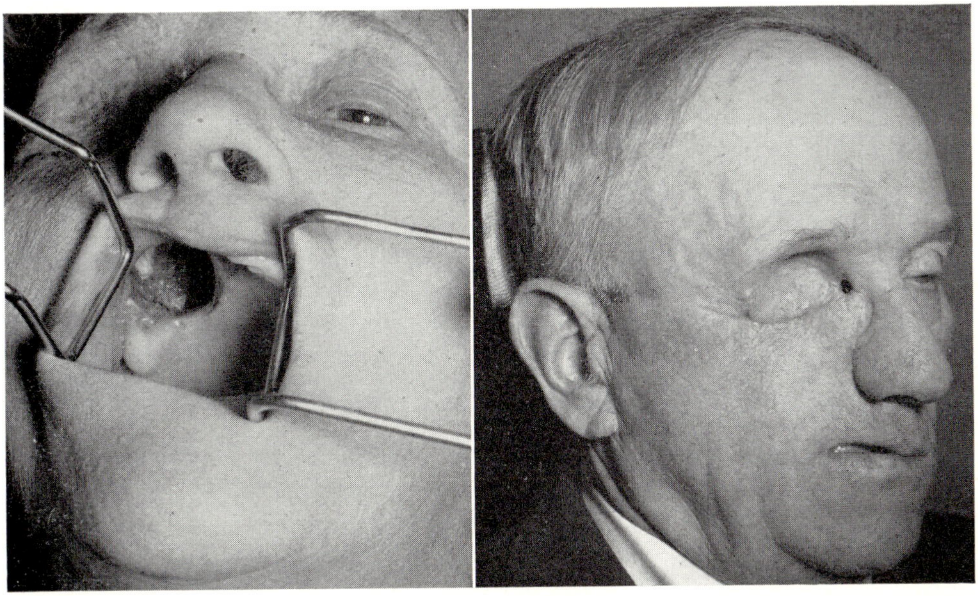

A. B.

Fig. 2, *A* and *B*.—Final results three months after exenteration of orbit and maxillary resection for antral cancer with invasion of orbit and skin of infraorbital cheek region.

Only 5 of 53 patients with advanced cases survived over two years under treatment of any kind. The longest survivals of patients with demonstrable bone destruction were three years, ten months and three years, three months, respectively. The average survival of such patients was seven months. The absolute survival rate of the 68 patients was 10.3 per cent in this series.

When the ten-year period from 1936 to 1946 is broken down into two five-year periods we note that the absolute five-year survival rate for the 1936-through-1940 period is approximately 6 per cent and that of the 1941-through-1945 period is 15 per cent. This is probably the result of more adequate surgical exposure and drainage in addition to the radiation in the later five-year period.

In the three-year period from 1943 to 1945 there were 18 patients with 7 living over five years, in fact, seven years or more, which constitutes 16.7 per cent of all patients as calculated on an absolute survival basis (Table II).

TABLE II. CARCINOMA OF THE ANTRUM (1936 THROUGH 1945, SIXTY-EIGHT CASES): TABULATION OF CASES BY YEARS

YEAR	DEAD	NOW ALIVE	TOTAL
1936	7	0	7
1937	8	0	8
1938	5	1	6
1939	7	1	8
1940	5	0	5
1941	6	1	7
1942	8	1	9
1943	6	1	7
1944	4	2	6
1945	5	0	5
Totals	61	7	68

Discussion.—Considerable literature has accumulated on cancer of the paranasal sinus and a lesser amount concerning the specific entity of cancer of the antrum. This is quite conceivable due to the difficulty in many cases, when the patient is first seen, of determining the site of primary origin.

Also, there has been considerable change in the methods of management from the earlier periods when radiation therapy was the mainstay, then through the period of less radical surgical procedures, such as electrocoagulation and drainage supplemented by irradiation, up to the present epoch when radical surgery with or without supplemental electrocoagulation and radiation is being advocated.

As the material presented here is concerned mainly with the first and second of these periods, we feel that the results herein stated may serve in a way as average end results achieved in a small series under such management.

Our 35 per cent five-year arrests in the earlier cases and 15 per cent absolute results in all cases for five years seem to be a fair average and fairly consistent with those quoted from other sources. For example, Holt Radium Institute[4] in Manchester, in a series of seventy-five cases, reported five-year survivals in 41 per cent of early cases, 14 per cent in more advanced cases, and a 25 per cent over-all survival rate.

Todd[10] in 100 cases and Windeyer[14] of Middlesex Hospital reported end results for five years as 26 and 25 per cent, respectively. Del Regato,[3] in a series of 10 patients treated exclusively by x-ray, noted a five-year salvage rate of 40 per cent and Lenz at Presbyterian Hospital noted 11 per cent.

Berven,[1] also using x-ray, achieved only 6 per cent five-year end results in 220 patients. It seems thus quite apparent that a greater number of cases under similar types of therapy must be collected before a stable base line of results by the various methods can be evaluated.

Schall[8] made a very substantial contribution to methods of management of these lesions when he showed in a good-sized series of 219 cases a 27 per cent five-year survival rate when surgery supplemented by radiation was used, 17.6 per cent when this sequence was reversed, and no lasting results from radium alone. Berven[2] at Radiumhemmet reported 38.4 per cent five-year survivals in 112 cases from electrocoagulation alone; New with 30 five-year survivals of 75 patients also reported a 40 per cent rate from electrocoagulation followed by radium and/or x-ray.

The future trend in therapy of these tumors seems, therefore, quite obvious, that is, radical surgery and/or electrocoagulation supplemented by irradiation (Fig. 2). Our later impression here would seem to bear out this conclusion.

SUMMARY

1. Sixty-eight cases of cancer of the antrum from 1935 to 1946 comprised .27 per cent of all cancer seen at the Roswell Park Memorial Institute. The prevalence in men was about twice that in women, with the greatest incidence between the fifty-sixth and seventy-fifth years.

2. The usual histopathology was squamous-cell carcinoma with a scattering of papillary carcinoma and adenocarcinoma.

3. The diagnosis was commonly made on symptomatology, physical findings, x-ray picture, and biopsy.

4. X-ray findings of cloudiness in the involved antrum were commonly noted. The finding of bone destruction carried a bad prognosis, as did also involvement of the orbital plate and posterior wall.

5. Treatment in this series was mainly by radiation often combined with conservative surgery, that is, surgical drainage, radium installation, and x-ray, with an absolute over-all five-year cure rate of 15 per cent in all cases and a relative rate of 35 per cent in early cases.

REFERENCES

1. Berven, E.: Carcinoma of the Antrum, Proc. 30th Annual Meeting, Amer. Radiol. Soc., Chicago, June, 1948.
2. Berven, E.: Report of Cancer Society, Stockholm, 1949, p. 112.
3. Del Regato, J. A.: Roentgenology in Epithelioma of the Maxillary Sinus, Surg., Gynec. & Obst. **65**: 657-665 (Nov.), 1937.
4. Holt Radium Institute, Manchester: Results of Radium and X-ray Therapy in Malignant Disease. Second Statistical Report, 1934-1938. Compiled 1945.
5. Lenz, M.: Malignant Neoplasms of Nose, Naso-Pharynx and Paranasal Sinuses. Evaluation of Radiation Therapy, Tr. Am. Acad. Ophth. **55**: 214, 1951.
6. New, G. B.: Malignant Tumors of the Paranasal Sinuses, Am. J. Surg. **42**: 170-173 (Oct.), 1938.
7. Perzik, S. L.: Management of Cancer of the Nasal Cavity and Paranasal Sinuses, California Med. **74**: 374-376 (May), 1951.

8. Schall, L. A.: Malignant Neoplasms of the Nose, Paranasal Sinuses and Nasopharynx. Evaluation of Surgical Treatment, Tr. Am. Acad. Ophth. **55**: 209-213 (Jan.-Feb.), 1951.
9. Schuknecht, H. F.: The Surgical Management of Cancer of the Paranasal Sinuses, Laryngoscope **61**: 874-890 (Sept.), 1951.
10. Todd, M. C.: The Treatment of Cancer of the Maxillary Antrum by Radium, Brit. J. Radiol. **21**: 270-275 (June), 1948.
11. Ward, G. E., and Hendrick, J. W.: The Diagnosis and Treatment of Tumors of the Head and Neck, Baltimore, 1950, Williams & Wilkins Company.
12. Watson, W. L.: Cancer of the Paranasal Sinuses, Laryngoscope **52**: 22-42 (Jan.), 1942.
13. Weaver, D. F.: Tumors of the Maxillary Antrum, Laryngoscope **62**: 139-159 (Feb.), 1952.
14. Windeyer, B. W.: Carcinoma of the Antrum, Proc. 30th Annual Meeting, Amer. Radiol. Soc., Chicago, June, 1948.

LONG-ACTING DRUGS FOR AVOIDANCE OF POSTHEMORRHOIDECTOMY PAIN: A NEGATIVE REPORT

ROBERT TURELL, M.D., NEW YORK, N. Y.

RECENTLY a repository injection of d-tubocurarine chloride[1] and a "new" anesthetic solution[2, 3] have been advocated for the control of pain following hemorrhoidectomy,[1-3] as well as pain following other anorectal operations.[3] I have received a large number of inquiries concerning the merits of these agents, particularly the anesthetic solution, from general surgeons, anesthesiologists, gynecologists, and general practitioners. It is, therefore, timely to report the results of the following study concerning the pain-relieving features of these agents, especially since the virtues of prolonged local anesthesia have even been communicated to the layman, who is demanding it (Galton, L.: Cosmopolitan, May, 1953, p. 22).

MATERIALS AND METHODS

One cubic centimeter of a suspension containing 25 mg. of d-tubocurarine chloride pentahydrate and chlorobutanol 0.5 per cent in a menstruum of peanut oil, oxycholesterol derivatives, and 2 per cent of beeswax, marketed as Tubadil, was injected into one of the deltoid muscles prior to the commencement of hemorrhoidectomy in 11 alternate patients. Another eleven alternate hemorrhoidectomies served as controls. All patients were operated upon under regional, saddle-block spinal, or caudal anesthesia.

A solution containing 1 per cent procaine, 0.25 per cent procaine hydrochloride, and 5 per cent butyl p-aminobenzoate in a solvent composed of 2 per cent polyethylene glycol-300, 78 per cent propylene glycol, and water, marketed as Efocaine, was injected into the perianal tissues in a dosage varying from 5 to 10 c.c., by the methods employed either by Tucker[2] or Gross,[3] at the conclusion of thirty-nine alternate open-type hemorrhoidectomies.[4] Another thirty-nine alternate open techniques of hemorrhoidectomy served as immediate controls; these in turn were fortified by a recent study of 535 personally performed hemorrhoidectomies.[4] Low or saddle-block spinal or caudal anesthesia was employed.

The nurses, who knew nothing about this clinical experiment, had been instructed to give the patients pain-relieving drugs such as morphine or Demerol by injection on the complaint of pain only (morphine was more desirable than Demerol). In addition, orders for the oral administration of hypnotic drugs and/or pain-relieving coal-tar derivatives were left to be used at the discretion of the nurses in attendance, particularly for sedation against apprehension and restlessness.

Received for publication, May 11, 1953.

About eight hours after the operation, when the effects of spinal anesthesia were dissipated, most of the patients were made ambulatory. During that eight-hour period the patients received abundant amounts of fluid given primarily as an aid for the prevention of postspinal headache. Those patients who could not void while in the lying position were permitted to stand out of bed whenever they developed the urge to urinate. The day following the operation, all patients were given regular house diets, and hot hip baths were begun. Those patients who had been operated upon under caudal anesthesia were served food immediately after operation, and most of them were ambulatory almost from the outset.

Originally it was planned to extend these studies to at least 100 cases in each series. However, as this investigation progressed and the results revealed themselves, I could not justify the continuation of this clinical experiment.

RESULTS

Seven of the 11 patients who had received the d-tubocurarine required one to two doses of either morphine or Demerol for the relief of pain. Two of the 4 patients who did not require narcotics exhibited some general muscular relaxation but without respiratory embarrassment. Another patient (the eleventh of this series) could not talk for almost ten hours, appeared flaccid, and had sufficient difficulty in breathing so as to alert the anesthesiologist for fear that artificial respiration might become necessary.

Of the controls, 3 patients did not require narcotic drugs for the relief of postoperative pain.

Postoperative pain requiring one to two doses of morphine or Demerol was complained of by 27 patients following the injection of the anesthetic solution; 2 additional patients required three doses of narcotics because of a combination of pain and a peculiar burning sensation, the latter lasting in various degrees of intensity for more than five days. Thus, 29 patients had postoperative pain requiring an analgesic narcotic drug for its control. Burning sensation was complained of by 2 patients without direct questioning and by 5 more patients who registered this complaint on direct interrogation. Pain during the first act of defecation was mild in 8 patients and only moderate, although erratic, in severity in the remaining patients. Edema, hyperemia, and occasional bleeding were noted in the wounds of nine patients; the burning sensation already alluded to was present in 4 of these 9 patients. Some delay in the healing of the anorectal wounds was present in 7 of these 9 patients and in 3 other patients of this series. The wounds of 4 patients had failed to heal completely until the end of the fifth postoperative week, and did not heal until the end of seven weeks in 6 other patients. However, once healed the wounds remained well healed and were indistinguishable from those of the controls. Garson[5] independently has obtained somewhat similar results in fifty-four anorectal operations, including many hemorrhoidectomies.

Fecal incontinence lasting for from sixteen to thirty days was observed in 3 patients, all of whom exhibited the peculiar burning sensation and delay in the healing of the wounds. In two instances, the patients had some warning so that they could "hurry" to the lavatory, while the third patient had to be confined to her house for about one month.

Twelve of the control patients required no morphine; 23 had received one to two injections, and 4 patients were given three injections of narcotic drugs. All patients had experienced somewhat more pain during the postoperative first act of defecation; this pain was, however, always relieved promptly by a hot hip bath and has never constituted a problem in either the control or the injected cases. None of the other complications was noted in the controls.

Additional Data.—To this absolutely personal experience may be added the occurrence of a localized suppuration in a patient on one of my services several days posthemorrhoidectomy, which was performed by a competent associate (Garson) who has had a much wider experience with the use of this drug than I have had. Similar experiences have been reported to me by other surgeons.[5] I have also seen similar suppurations and/or areas of necrosis following the injection of this anesthetic solution for the "conservative" treatment of anal fissures.* Squire and Weiner,[5] as well as other obstetricians, have observed necrosis in episiotomy wounds. Intractable paresthesias, similar in character to those observed following injections of procaine hydrochloride or its derivatives,[6] occurred in 2 patients approximately three weeks after this solution was injected deeply subcutaneously for the control of anal pruritus. As in the case of other long-acting "anesthetics," complications following Efocaine such as "postinjectional suppurations are unreported for various obvious reasons."[6]

DISCUSSION

Using personal experience and a recent comparative study of the open versus the closed methods of hemorrhoidectomy[4] as a background for this investigation, I believe that pain following hemorrhoidectomy has to a large degree a direct relationship to the type of technique employed. It was shown that following the open technique, which consisted of a sharp dissection of the hemorrhoidal mass well beyond the mucocutaneous or dentate line without suturing of the wound except for the mucosal pedicle (which in principle is a Milligan-Morgan procedure), the patient seldom required more than two doses (usually 0.01 Gm. or 1/6 gr.) of morphine postoperatively for relief of pain; narcotic drugs were unnecessary for the control of restlessness or apprehension. Significantly, about 40 per cent of these patients required no morphine at all; coal-tar derivatives and/or barbiturates sufficed for sedation in these patients. However, following a semiclosed method of hemorrhoidectomy, which was essentially the same as the open type except that the subcutaneous structures of the hemorrhoidal bed were approximated but without suturing of the skin, all patients required morphine for postoperative sedation, and more than two doses had to be used in a considerable number of these patients. Importantly, following the closed type of hemorrhoidectomy in

*M. H. Adelman, an anesthesiologist who has participated in parts of this work, has encountered two instances of chronic, slowly healing ulcers on the chest wall following the injection of this solution into the "trigger zones" for relief of pain.

which the wounds, including the skin, are closed by suture following the excision of the hemorrhoidal mass, about four times more morphine was required for the control of postoperative pain than after the open operation.

The competence and gentleness of the surgeon also enter into this picture. In 1941, referring to the pitfalls and hazards of the then heralded slowly absorbable, oil- or water-soluble anesthetic agents which have since fallen into considerable disrepute, I stated that "numerous competent proctologists have questioned the wisdom and need for the employment of the anesthetic agents when clean-cut and gentle surgery and meticulous preoperative and postoperative care are utilized. Following a well-performed surgical anorectal procedure there should be no need for these anesthetic agents; at best these drugs are poor substitutes for good surgery. I have never found a need for the employment of these drugs for the avoidance of postoperative pain"[7]; this still holds true.

Gross,[3] in a study of sixty-five cases including some forty-five hemorrhoidectomies, stated that "35 patients required no postoperative medication, 28 received one or two doses, and 2 patients received three doses of postoperative medication." He, however, summarized his studies thus: "Efficient pain control was achieved in 96 per cent of anorectal surgery series in which patients required one or two doses of postoperative medication." Tucker[2] reported that 32 (80 per cent) of his 40 patients had received no doses or one dose of postoperative medication, while 4 (10 per cent) had received two doses and another 4 patients (10 per cent) had been given more than two (varying between four and six) doses. To me "efficient pain control" means no pain and, consequently, no need for any drugs, neither of which was accomplished in all cases by Gross or Tucker, who are the present proponents of injectional proctologic postoperative anesthesia. Their figures, therefore, do not seem to entitle this drug to the designation of anesthetic, as absolute postoperative anesthesia had not been produced.

The lesson I have learned is clear: considering that about one-third of patients who undergo the open type of hemorrhoidectomy do not ordinarily require morphine for postoperative sedation[4] and that the pain in the remainder of the patients can be easily controlled on the average by two doses of morphine, I find little, if any, need or justification for taking even the slightest risk by injecting any of the slow-absorbing "anesthetic" agents. Garson[5] has also indicated a dissatisfaction with such drugs. This also applies with equal force to repository injections of d-tubocurarine, as I was not impressed with the alleged "abolition of painful spasm of the sphincters—practically the only source of pain following hemorrhoidectomy."[1]

Parenthetically, if it is desired, pain following a properly executed open type of hemorrhoidectomy can be safely and effectively prevented by the employment of the simple classic or modified sphincterotomy as described for the treatment of chronic anal fissure.[8] I employ this maneuver at the conclusion of hemorrhoidectomy only when preoperative spasm of the anal sphincter muscles of undetermined origin accompanies hemorrhoids. However, there seems to be little or no justification for the routine employment of sphincterotomy following hemorrhoidectomy.

Edema and hyperemia with some delay in the healing of the anorectal wounds were observed in ten patients although, once healed, the wounds were indistinguishable from those of the controls. In these cases, complete healing failed to take place within the usual three- to four-week interval observed in the control cases as well as in the hundreds of other patients operated upon by the identical technique.[4, 6] It is possible that these phenomena may be caused by the adverse, although temporary, degenerative effect exerted by the injected anesthetic solution on the innervation of the anorectum. Experimentally, using guinea pigs, rats, and rabbits, Weinberg[9] has noted a fibroelastic proliferation about injected nerves during the early postinjectional stages which, however, disappeared in time; concerning this he stated that "one is dealing with a benign process which is apparently reversible." He has also observed macroscopic "necrosis in the line of injections" of the muscles as well as microscopic "necrosis and partial disappearance of muscle fibers with a replacement by a moderately cellular, loose connective tissue" with "little or no inflammatory reaction" in those experimental animals that had been submitted to autopsy up to thirteen days after the injection of the anesthetic solution. Neither "a foreign body giant cell reaction" nor "significant permanent damage" was observed, except in one instance in which a "small focal area of fibrous replacement of muscle fibers" was noted at necropsy performed some time between eighty-nine and ninety-eight days following the injection of the solution. The clinical and histopathologic aspects of this problem need much more urgent investigation, particularly as they apply to the tissues of the human anorectum, one of the most potentially, if not actually, grossly infected areas in the body.

Fecal incontinence, although temporary, carries an undesirable psychologic import and is quite annoying.

SUMMARY AND CONCLUSIONS

1. Repository injection of d-tubocurarine does not appear to control posthemorrhoidectomy pain. The generalized muscular relaxation observed in three cases, which was alarmingly pronounced in one patient, constitutes a potential respiratory danger.

2. The failure of an anesthetic solution, injected into the perianal tissues at the conclusion of thirty-nine hemorrhoidectomies, to eliminate postoperative pain completely in a significant number of cases (which is also reported by the proponents of postoperative injectional anesthesia) plus the occurrence of complications such as temporary fecal incontinence, frank suppuration, and/or necrosis, noted by others, lead me to believe that postoperative injectional anesthesia is not a procedure to be used.*

*Since submission of this paper for publication, the neurological complications[10] and even death[11] following the use of Efocaine have been reported. Efocaine is now regarded by some former users as an unsatisfactory medicament because of complications noted in late postoperative examinations.[12]

3. In my experience, severe pain after operation or during the first act of defecation does not follow a well-performed open type of hemorrhoidectomy. The pain observed following the open type of hemorrhoidectomy performed upon a non-neurotic person can be controlled safely and effectively with ease by sedatives or analgesic drugs. These drugs also effectively allay preoperative and postoperative apprehension and are given freely, as a matter of sound practical therapeutics, to all patients who have a natural fear of any operation.

ADDENDUM

Since submission of this paper for publication, Mannheimer, Pizzolato, and Adrian[13] have stated that, like alcohol and phenol, Efocaine and the vehicle in Efocaine ''cause anesthesia by nerve destruction rather than by blockade due to their anesthetic effects.''

REFERENCES

1. Fuller, J. D.: Advantages of Preoperative Use of Slowly-Absorbed d-Tubocurarine, Anesthesiology **13**: 370 (July) 1952.
2. Tucker, C. C.: Control of Postoperative Pain in Anorectal Surgery, J. Kansas M. Soc. **53**: 230 (May) 1952.
3. Gross, J. M., and Shaftel, H. E.: Role of Efocaine in Anorectal Anesthesia and Analgesia, New York State J. Med. **52**: 1413 (June 1) 1952.
4. Turell, R.: Hemorrhoidectomy, With Special Reference to Open Versus Closed Technics, S. Clin. North America **32**: 677 (April) 1952.
5. Alexander, R. M., Feitel, A., Garson, B. J., Peskin, H., Rhodes, M. P., Squire, J. J., and Weiner, I.: Personal communication.
6. Turell, R.: Treatment in Proctology, Baltimore, 1949, Williams & Wilkins Company.
7. Turell, R.: Disease of Colon and Rectum, Am. J. M. Sc. **202**: 282 (Aug.) 1941.
8. Turell, R.: Surgical Treatment of Chronic Anal Fissure, Surg., Gynec. & Obst. **86**: 434 (April) 1948.
9. Weinberg, T.: Study of Effects of Efocaine Upon Nerves, Muscle, Skin and Subcutaneous Tissue, Sinai Hosp. J., Baltimore **1**: 21 (Nov.) 1952.
10. Shapiro, S. K., and Norman, D. D.: Neurological Complications Following Use of "Efocaine," J. A. M. A. **152**: 608 (June 13) 1953.
11. Angerer, A. L., Su, H. H., and Head, J. R.: Death Following Use of Efocaine, J. A. M. A. **153**: 550 (Oct. 6) 1953.
12. Eastwood, D. W., and Bartlett, R. W.: Correspondence, J. A. M. A. **152**: 1067 (July 11) 1953.
13. Mannheimer, W., Pizzolato, P., and Adrian, I.: Mode of Action and Effects on Tissues of Long-acting Local Anesthetics, J. A. M. A. **154**: 29, 1954.

MECHANISM OF OMENTAL MIGRATION

A Review of the Literature and Experimental Study*

M. Shannon Allen, Jr., M.D.,** Kingsport, Tenn.

(From the Department of Surgery, University of Virginia School of Medicine, Charlottesville, Va.)

INTRODUCTION

THE presence of the omentum at sites of inflammation throughout the abdominal cavity, with its attempts to wall off and protect against infection, has been recognized since ancient times. The mode of travel of the omentum from its normal position to the site of inflammation is not so definitely understood. If the most important function of the omentum is considered to be its ability to limit or wall off peritoneal insults by the formation of adhesions, it is necessary to assume that, in order to be efficient at its job, it must travel or migrate into contact with the offending agent or to the site of inflammation. It is the object of this work to attempt to explain the migration of the omentum.

Historically, there has been much speculation on the function and mode of travel of the omentum. Hippocrates (460 to 385 B.C.)[2] associated the omentum in some way with the formation and absorption of intraperitoneal fluid. Aristotle (384 to 322 B.C.)[3] regarded the omentum as a fatty apron designed to protect the intestines against cold. Vesalius (1514 to 1564)[3] thought of it as a fixation ligament or supportive ligament for the transverse colon. Ross[16] in 1893 assumed that the omentum protected the intestines against injury by assisting them in gliding away from the point of greatest pressure. He observed the way the omentum seemed to hasten to prevent the invasion of the general peritoneum by some intraperitoneal poison, gluing itself to the site of inflammation and thus preventing dangerous invasion of the general peritoneal cavity. "It is like a man-of-war ready to sail to any port in which there is impending trouble."[16]

Durham[8] in 1897 cited the omentum as the seat of selection for the cells being removed from the peritoneal fluid after bacterial contamination.

Buxton and Torrey (1906)[4] described the omentum as a battleground or area of support for phagocytosis by the macrophages and the polymorphonuclear leukocytes of inert particles and microorganisms in the peritoneal cavity.

Rutherford Morison (1906)[12] was the first to recognize the importance of the omentum in arresting the spread of inflammation by forming adhesions around its borders. Fisher[9] in 1906, Ruben[19] in 1911, Schutz[20] in 1930, and Rothenberg and Rosenblatt[18] in 1943 made similar observations regarding the

Received for publication, April 25, 1953.

*Abridgment of a thesis submitted in partial requirement of the degree of Master of Science, awarded June, 1951.

**Formerly Clinical Trainee of the American Cancer Society.

part played by the omentum in intraperitoneal inflammation, namely, that the most important function of the omentum is the part that it plays in limiting intraperitoneal inflammation.

Other functions, such as neutralization of toxins,[6, 14] plugging of peritoneal openings to prevent herniation,[12] providing a blood supply to a tissue or organ not adequately nourished,[3] providing a vascular bed for the relief of arterial tension,[7] providing a direct avenue from the peritoneal cavity into the vascular system,[15] and causing leukogenesis,[21] have all been ascribed to the omentum.

Finding the omentum frequently at the site of inflammation, at the operating table and in the post-mortem room, has led surgeons and pathologists alike to speculate concerning the motion of the omentum. Many theories of motion have evolved.

Ross,[16] in 1893, wrote that the omentum was endowed with some vermicular-like action and that it was able to move itself from place to place. Durham (1897)[8] noted that the omenta of animals dead of peritoneal infection became rolled and folded up because of the peristalsis of the intestines. Adami (1898)[1] thought that the omentum was endowed with the power of active locomotion. He thought of it as rolling up and down to the right and left and in effect, covering the entire abdominal cavity. Morison (1906)[12] believed that the omentum was attracted to the point of injury by some sort of information. He likened its movement to that of a jellyfish.

Theodore Fisher (1906),[9] Norris (1908),[13] Wilkie (1911),[23] and Adams (1913)[2] believed that the movement of the omentum was dependent on peristalsis of the intestines. Fisher postulated that if the peristalsis affected all areas of the intestines, the omentum was spread out over the intestines; however, if there were paresis of one segment of the intestines, the active, moving segments propelled the omentum to the area of stasis.

Dickinson (1906)[7] postulated that the position of the omentum in the abdomen was determined by (1) pumping action of the diaphragm, (2) intra-abdominal pressure, and (3) peristaltic movement of the intestines.

Rubin (1911)[19] denied spontaneous motility of the omentum. Like Wilkie and Adams, he denied the theory of a positive or negative chemotaxis of the omentum as advocated by Milian.[19] His theory of motion was similar to that of Dickinson.[7]

Hertzler (1935)[11] stated that if there were no leukocytic-cell infiltration into the omentum, there would be no migration. He explained the motion as similar to the influence that draws any leukocyte to an area of infection or inflammation. He did not believe that the position of the normal omentum was influenced by a change in the position of the individual or animal, or that peristalsis influenced the advance of the omentum to the site of injury. ''If we are to speak of the 'intelligence' of the omentum, we may safely add that an individual's omentum is as smart as his leukocytes.''[11]

Schutz[20] in 1930 approached the mechanism controlling migration of the omentum from an entirely different point of view and one not previously presented. He likened the motion of stretching out of the omentum to the uncoiling of a curled-up garden hose when an increased pressure of water is caused to flow through it. Similarly in the omentum, he postulated that the arteries become hyperemic, the intra-arterial blood supply is increased, the arteries straighten out, and the omentum loosely attached to the arteries is pulled by them to their advanced position. He noted a resemblance between the omentum and erectile tissue.

Cantacuzène and Soru (1931)[5] stated that the migration of the omentum to a lesion of the intestines was strictly a function of the difference of electric potential that existed between these two points. They determined that the electric potential between the omentum and the intestines was usually 8 or less millivolts. After an injury to the peritoneal surface, the electric potential between the two areas was immediately elevated to 53 millivolts. The omentum, which was electronegative under normal conditions, became electropositive; thus, the omentum was attracted to the injured area.

Rothenberg and Rosenblatt (1942)[17] by means of omental-marking agents and fluoroscopic studies concluded that omental migration depended on the motion of the underlying bowel.

Thomas, Greene, and Rhoads (1950)[22] studied the process of adhesion formation through abdominal windows made of methyl merhacrylate or Lucite in animal experiments. In the course of their observation they stated that, in respect to an area of injury, the omentum seems to be pushed or attracted to the sticky coagulum to which it adheres.

In summary, it is seen that, in the literature, omental migration has been attributed to (1) an inner intelligence, (2) peristalsis, (3) action of the diaphragm, (4) intra-abdominal pressure, (5) positive or negative chemotaxis, (6) leukocytic-cell infiltration, (7) arterial hyperemia, and (8) change in electric potential.

It is the object of this experimental work to study the mechanism of omental migration and thereby make steps toward an accurate, simple, and scientific explanation for the migration of the omentum.

Experimental Data.—An omental-marking agent for radiographic recording was selected. Studies were made of the normal omental pattern, omental pattern response to food and starvation, omental pattern response to peristalsis, omental pattern response to experimental appendicitis, omental pattern response to sterile gauze in right lower quadrant of abdomen, omental migration in response to inaccessible inflammation (1. sterile gauze sutured to undersurface of diaphragm and 2. experimental liver abscess), omental migration in response to increase in omental blood volume flow, dilation of the omental bed with maintenance of systemic pressure, and the omentum in an isolated fluid medium.

Dogs were used in all animal experiments. They were healthy adult mongrel dogs weighing five to fifty pounds, both male and female. All dogs were fed standard basic diet for laboratory dogs and were kept in cages throughout the experiments.

All operative procedures were performed on anesthetized dogs which were given veterinary Nembutal in the jugular vein in the amount of 1 gr.

for each five pounds of weight. Subsequent maintenance doses were given throughout the procedure as indicated, and all operations were performed using aseptic technique. All the dogs used in the experiment were studied for movement of the omentum uninfluenced by intraperitoneal procedures.

X-ray pictures were obtained on all dogs immediately after the operation while the dog was still anesthetized and at two subsequent intervals, making a total of three sets of films. Anteroposterior and left-lateral abdominal films, size twelve by fourteen inches, were obtained. A Bucky diaphragm was used with a time of one-fifth second and a distance of thirty-six inches. Three hundred milliamperes were routinely employed, and the kilovoltage depended on the size of the dog.

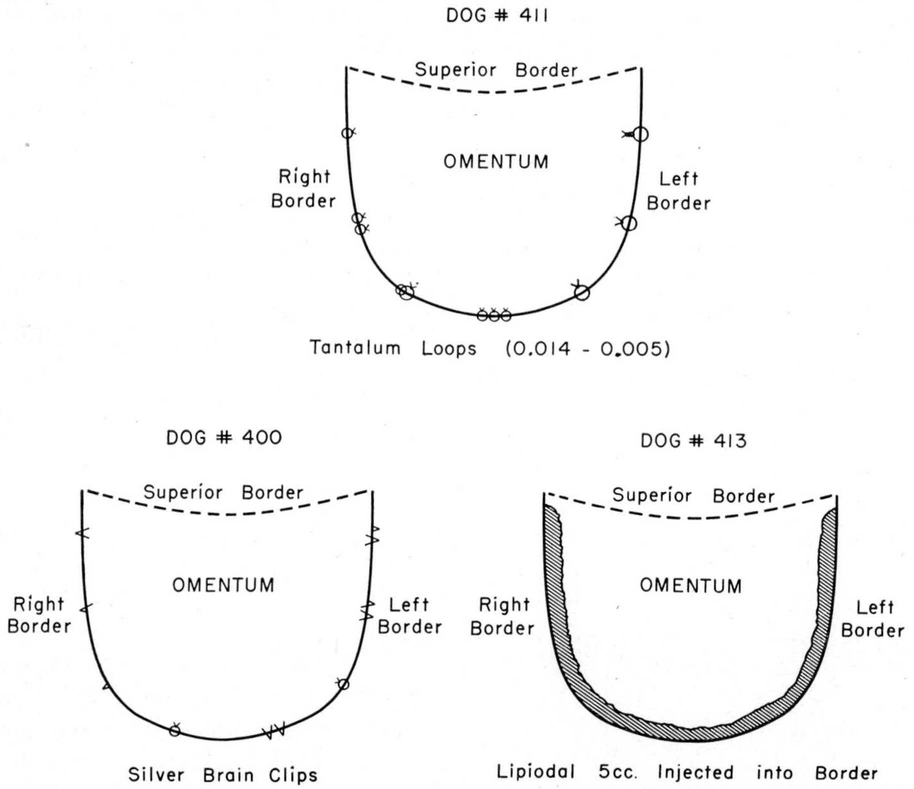

Fig. 1.—Diagram of omental-marking agents and their sequence in the omental edge.

Selection of a Marking Agent.—As a preliminary experiment it was necessary to determine an agent that would mark the omentum in such a fashion that its position could be determined roentgenographically. Four requirements had to be met in order for the agent to be used: (1) it had to be radiopaque; (2) it had to cause minimal tissue reaction; (3) it had to be light in weight, thus eliminating a static effect; and (4) it had to retain its position as originally placed in the omentum.

Three agents were chosen for testing: (1) tantalum wire loops (ethicon tantalum surgical wire sutures, Size 0.005 and 0.014), (2) silver brain clips, and (3) Lipiodol Lafay (E. Fougera and Company, Inc., New York, N. Y.).

In each experiment, the abdominal cavity of an anesthetized dog was entered through a short midline epigastric incision. The omentum was gently drawn out of the abdominal cavity and carefully inspected for adhesions. The omentum was kept moist with physiologic saline solution throughout the procedures. The marking agents were placed in the omental edge as atraumatically as possible, and the omentum was then returned to the abdominal cavity and the abdominal wound was closed in layers. Diagrams of the omentum containing the marking agents are seen in Fig. 1.

Results.—

Dog 411 (omentum marked with tantalum wire): In each film the tantalum loop could be identified as such; however, some of the loops were superimposed, and identification as to the actual site of the loop in the original sequence was often impossible. A second difficulty proved to be chance profile of an occasional loop on edge so that its character could not be identified. In an area of the loop, there was no evidence that the loop exerted a drag effect on the omentum and, in each instance, the loops had maintained their original position in the omentum.

Dog 400 (omentum marked with silver brain clips): The clips were very difficult to interpret. Although they were radiopaque, they were set at various angles, thereby making their identification in the sequence impossible without multiple oblique films. At time of operation, it was difficult to secure the clips in the omental borders, and at post-mortem one clip had been dislodged (possibly while returning the omentum into the abdominal cavity) from its original setting. As with tantalum loops no gross tissue reaction to the silver brain clips could be determined at autopsy.

Dog 413 (omentum marked with Lipiodol): X-ray pictures of this dog were obtained immediately following operation, twenty-four hours following operation, and fifteen days following operation. The first two sets of x-ray pictures showed an irregular opaque mass approximately 6 by 6 cm. in the anteroposterior view. Fifteen days following injection there was still faint evidence of the presence of the opaque oil in its original position; however, its outlines could not be determined, and the shadow it cast was not unlike that of fecal matter in the intestines. The Lipiodol gradually shifted away from the omental border toward the greater curvature of the stomach. Here again there was little gross evidence of tissue reaction in the Lipiodol.

Results: It was concluded that tantalum wire was by far the best marking agent of the three agents studied; therefore, it was used exclusively in subsequent experiments. Because of the complicated sequence originally used and the difficulty in the interpretation when loops became superimposed, it was decided to mark the right border of the omentum with three single tantalum loops appropriately placed and the left border with three double loops, one small and one large, similarly placed (Fig. 2).

Normal Omental Pattern.—Since it had been suggested that the omentum under normal circumstances traveled to different parts of the abdominal cavity,[7, 23] it was thought necessary to determine the position of the marked omentum under physiologic conditions at various time intervals. If the omentum routinely migrates to different parts of the abdominal cavity, this should be demonstrated by a change in the position of the tantalum loops and an over-all change in omental pattern. It was presumed that there were no omental adhesions after placing the loops, and this was proved in all instances at later operation.

Ten dogs with marked omenta which had been x-rayed immediately following operation were then x-rayed each week for a period of three weeks. In one of these animals, x-ray pictures were obtained at weekly intervals for eight weeks following operation. All dogs were maintained on ordinary laboratory diets and were allowed freedom of their cages for the entire period. Both anteroposterior and left lateral films were obtained. Although a complete outline of the omentum is not expected, a general picture of the change in omental pattern can be obtained from the displacement of various loops. At time of obtaining the x-ray pictures the dogs were not sedated; however, they were centered on a crossbar on the x-ray table in an effort to have each film taken from the same position as the previous one.

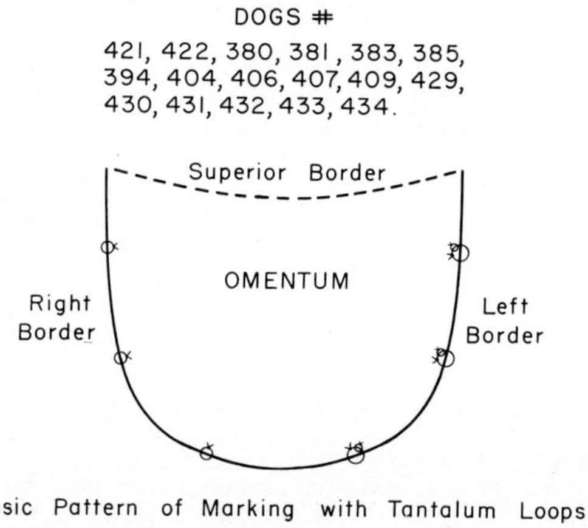

Fig. 2.—Diagram of omental outline with tantalum loops as marking agent. Pattern used in later experiments.

Results: A diagram of the omental pattern from one of the ten dogs presenting the apparent position of the omentum on successive weeks is shown in Fig. 3. The single loops represent the right border and the double loops represent the left border. The remaining nine dogs present similar patterns.

From the diagram it is seen that although the general pattern of the edge of the omentum changes considerably in most instances during ordinary unrestrained existence of the dog, the omentum, however much its border varies, lies in approximately the normal relationship to the upper abdominal organs and does not appear to fold on itself or migrate cephalad to its normal line of attachment.

Omental Pattern Response to Food and Starvation.—Since the omentum is so closely related both in position and blood supply to the stomach it was decided to study the effects of feeding and starvation on the motion of the omentum. Three marked dogs were used. (1) Dog 421 was starved for twelve hours prior to the first film and was allowed no food whatsoever for the duration of the experiment; (2) Dog 404 was starved for twelve hours prior to the first film

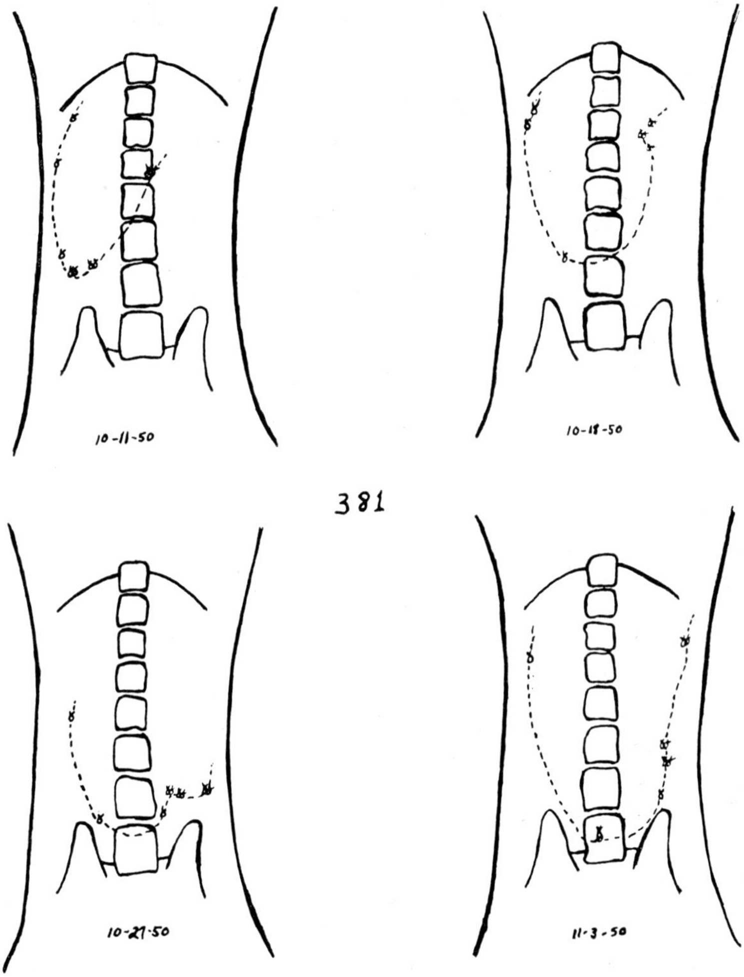

Fig. 3.—Normal omental pattern. Single loops in right omental edge; double loops in left omental edge. Seven-day, nine-day, and seven-day interval.

but was given food as desired for twenty minutes before each x-ray exposure. In the interim he was given no food; (3) Dog 409 was maintained on normal laboratory routine with no change in feeding habits, that is, with available food in the cage at all times.

Films were taken initially and at six, eighteen, and forty-two hours. The total period of starvation was fifty-four hours.

The diagram of each film is presented (Figs. 4 through 6).

Results: The most marked pattern change is seen in Dog 404 (dog given food as desired for twenty minutes before each film). Although this change is not marked, it is unmistakable and is thought to be explained by the increased peristalsis initiated by feeding.

The pattern of the starved dog and the control dog remain fairly constant and are not outside the range of ordinary movement as seen in the second experiment.

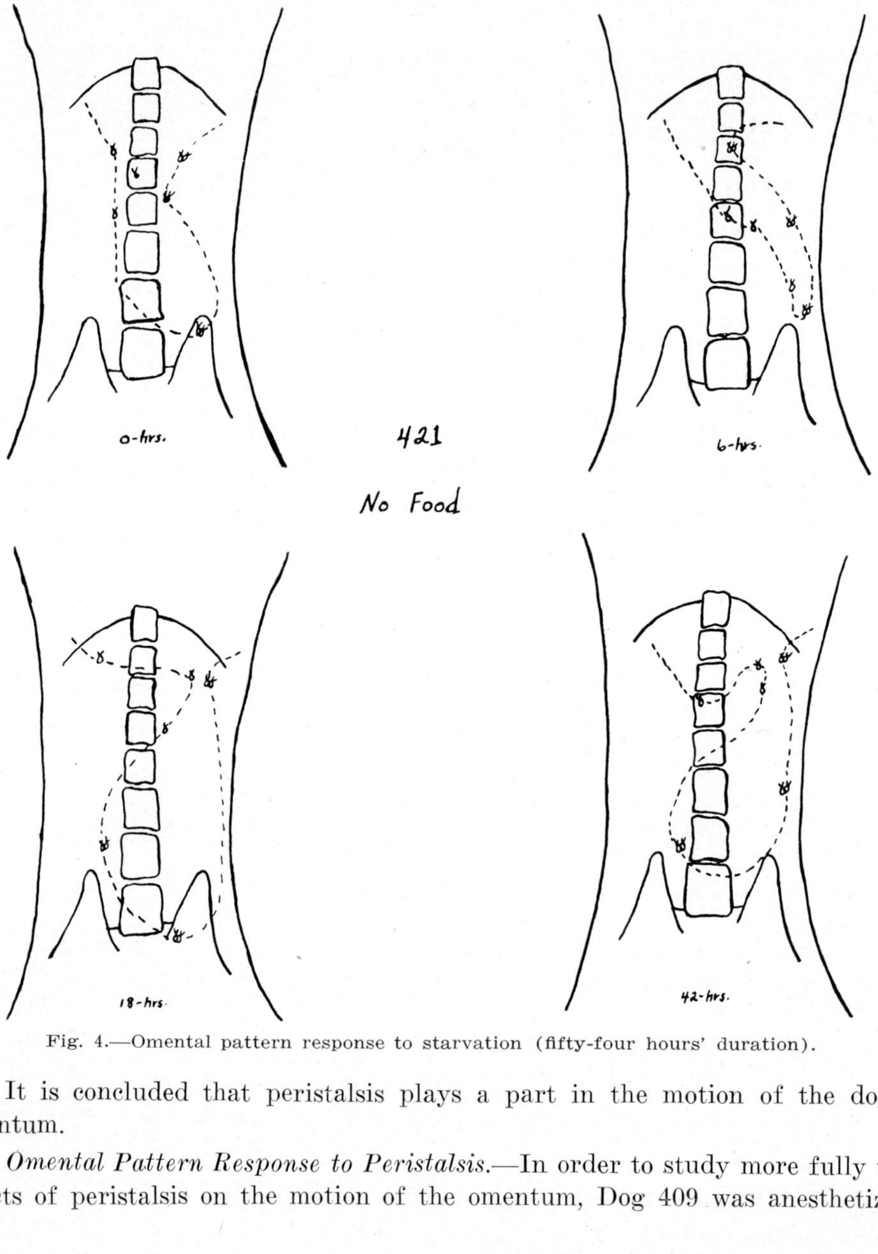

Fig. 4.—Omental pattern response to starvation (fifty-four hours' duration).

It is concluded that peristalsis plays a part in the motion of the dog's omentum.

Omental Pattern Response to Peristalsis.—In order to study more fully the effects of peristalsis on the motion of the omentum, Dog 409 was anesthetized with intravenous veterinary Nembutal and tied to a frame, in the dorsal supine position. The dog had been allowed food for twenty-eight hours.

Dog 409: Twenty-five cubic centimeters of castor oil was given per os, and films were obtained at one-half hour, one and one-half hours, two and one-half hours, and three and one-half hours. During this time the anesthesia was

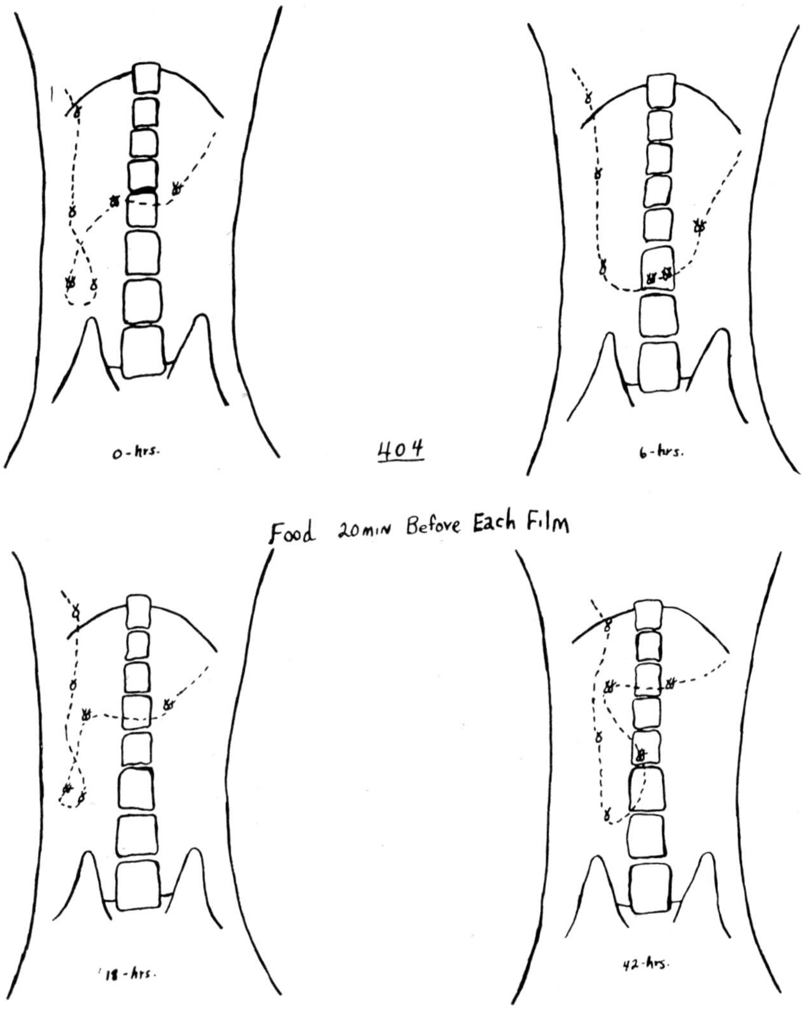

Fig. 5.—Omental pattern response. Dog given food as desired for twenty minutes prior to film, starved in interim.

continued and the dog was constantly observed. There was no visible peristalsis, and peristaltic sounds were heard with auscultation of the abdomen. The pattern of the dog's omentum during a period of three and one-half hours is diagramed (Fig. 7).

Since there was no visible or audible stimulation of peristalsis and since the pattern diagrams showed no appreciable motion of the omentum, the dog was then given 2 c.c. of 1:2,000 Prostigmine intravenously. Within five minutes, marked waves of peristalsis could be seen through the abdominal wall. The dog defecated and passed flatus. Films were taken fifteen and thirty minutes after the injection; diagrams of the omental pattern are presented (Fig. 8).

Results: Castor oil fails to initiate peristalsis in the anesthetized dog over a period of three and one-half hours and fails to change the omental pattern. Prostigmine given intravenously is followed by marked peristalsis and a definite movement of the omental edge.

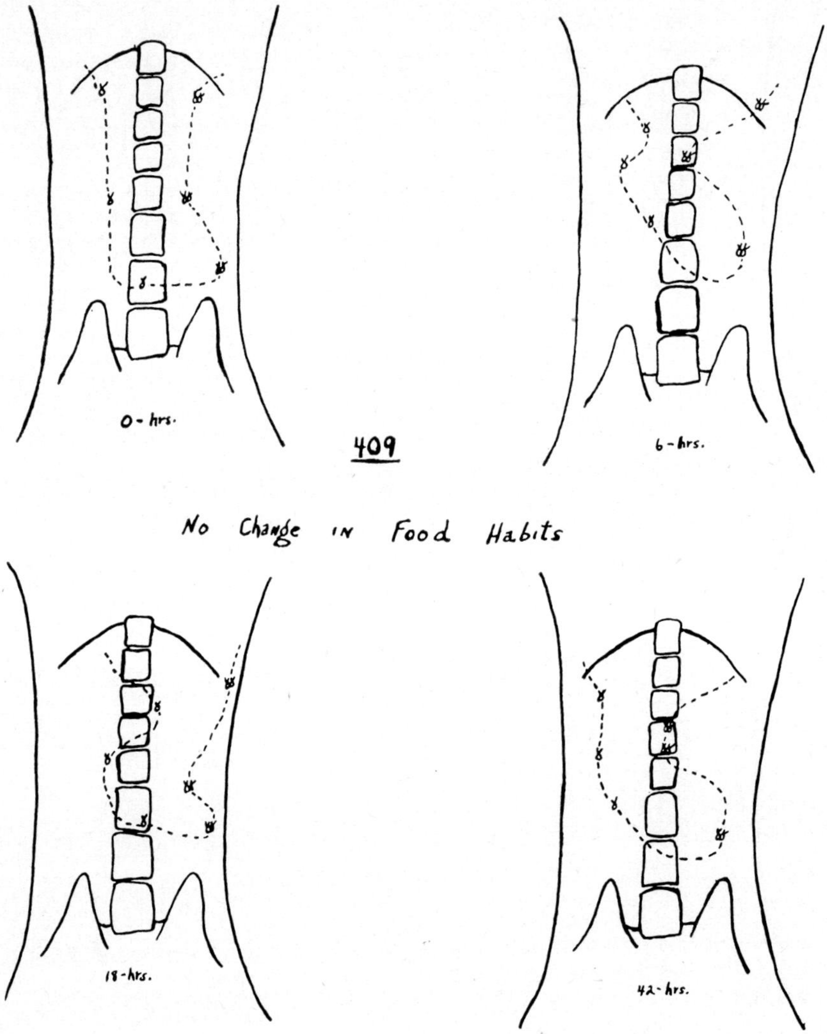

Fig. 6.—Omental pattern response. No change in food habits; control for this experiment.

It is concluded that peristalsis in the underlying intestines causes migration of the omental edge.

Omental Pattern Response to Change of Position.—Since there was shown to be considerable variation in the position of the omentum in day-to-day observation it seemed of interest to determine whether gravity as well as peristalsis played a part in this movement.

A dog with a marked omentum was anesthetized and securely fastened in the dorsal supine position to a wooden frame, and a film was obtained. The dog was then placed in a vertical position with the head down for fifteen minutes and at the end of this time another film was obtained. Again

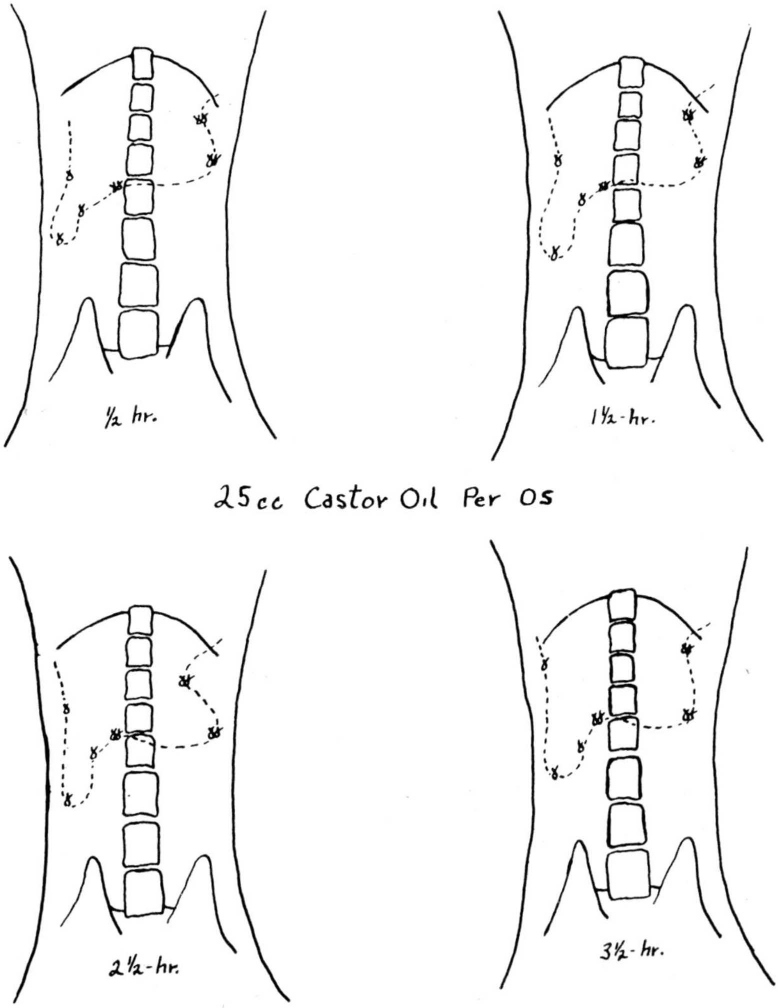

Fig. 7.—Omental pattern response to castor oil. (No visible or audible peristalsis produced by the castor oil.)

after being horizontal for fifteen minutes, the dog was placed in a vertical position for fifteen minutes with the head up, and a third film was obtained. Diagrams of the omental pattern are presented (Fig. 9).

Results: It is seen that there is a marked shift in the omental pattern corresponding to the change in position of the animal. The omentum seems to move as a unit rather than to fold on itself. It is concluded that gravity is a factor in omental movement.

Omental Pattern Response to Experimental Appendicitis.—Five dogs (Nos. 433, 385, 383, 404, and 381) with marked omenta were used in a study of omental migration in response to experimental appendicitis.

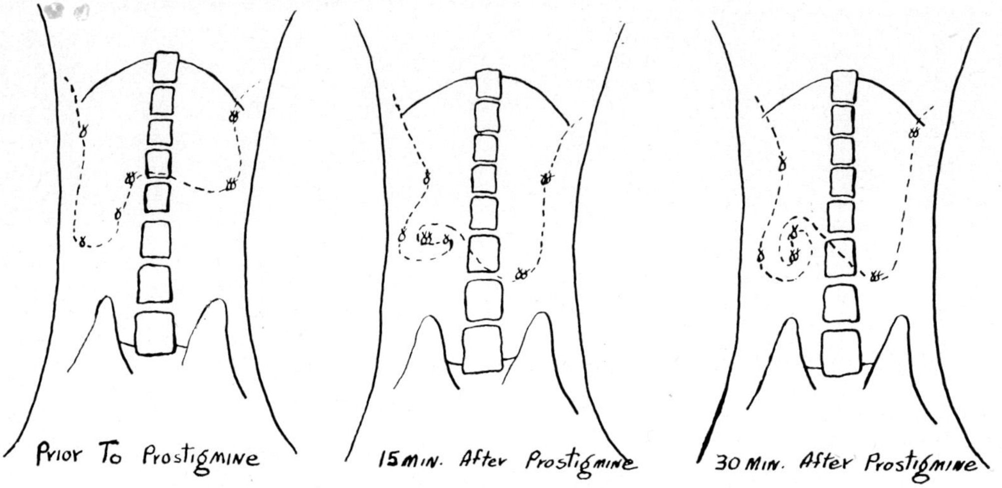

Fig. 8 (Dog 409).—Omental response to intravenous Prostigmine. Anesthetized dog secured to frame. This dog was given castor oil previously (see Fig. 7).

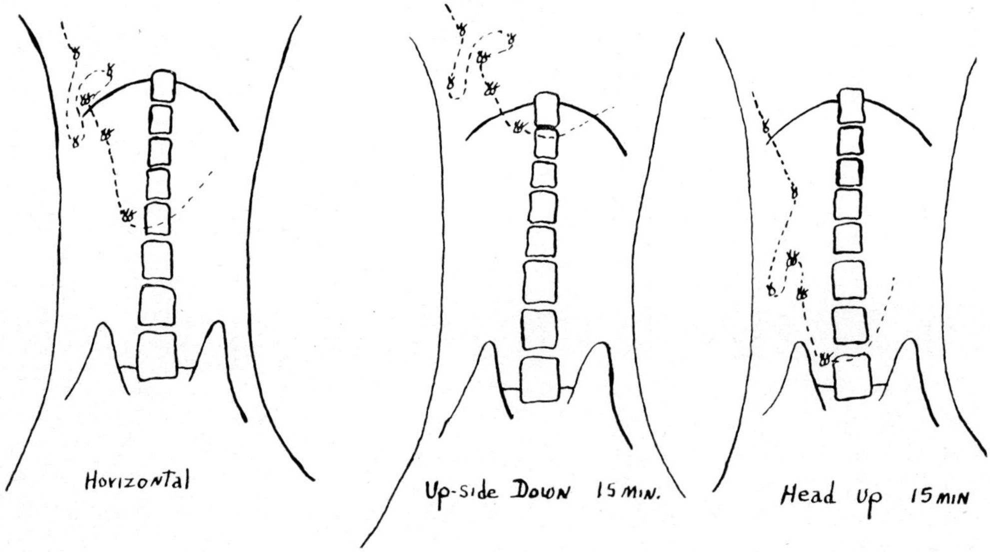

Fig. 9.—Omental pattern response to change in position. Anesthetized dog secured to frame.

The appendix of the dog is situated high in the abdominal cavity, approximately 4 cm. from the greater curvature of the stomach, in easy reach of the great omentum. In the human being at operation and at post-mortem, the omentum is often observed in the right lower quadrant adherent to an acutely inflamed appendix or a periappendiceal mass. If the omentum were inherently "interested" in "policing the abdominal cavity"[12] and in isolating infection by forming adhesions and thus walling off the inflammatory process, it seems logical to expect a large part of its entire free border to migrate to the area of injury and enter into the protective process.

In these experiments, after anesthesia the abdomen was explored through a right lower quadrant incision. It was first ascertained that there were no omental adhesions from the previous operation. A ligature was then placed around the base of the appendix and tied sufficiently tight to obstruct the venous return. Care was taken to prevent cutting into the appendiceal wall. A No. 1 catgut ligature was used in the first three dogs and a No. 0.004 tantalum ligature was used in the latter two dogs. The abdominal wound was closed in three layers with continuous fine cotton.

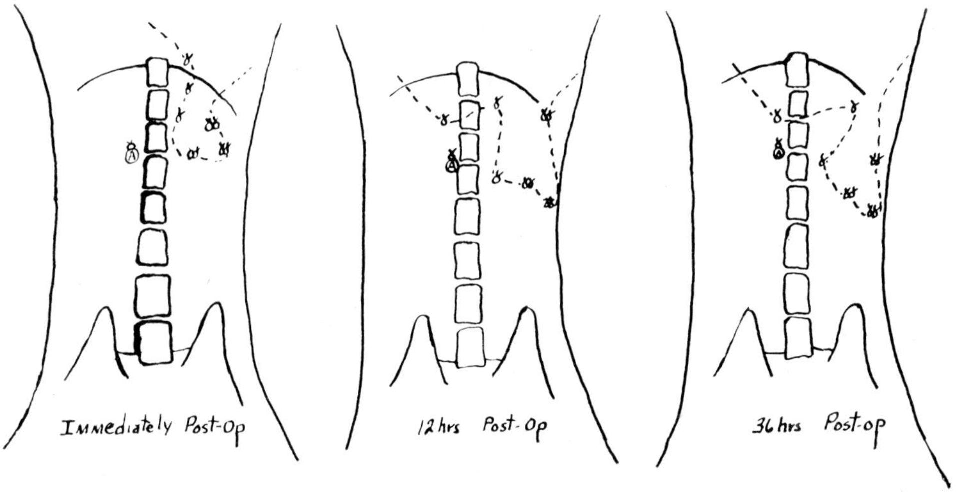

Fig. 10 (Dog 433).—Omental pattern response to experimental appendicitis. Tantalum as a ligature shows position of appendiceal base of x-ray picture. Dog died thirty-six hours postoperatively of generalized peritonitis.

Films were obtained at intervals following the surgical procedure. An autopsy was performed on all dogs. The omental pattern of Dog 433 is shown in Fig. 10. The autopsy findings in Dog 433 are shown in Fig. 11.

Results: In each dog at the time of experimental production of appendicitis, the right border of the omentum was in the same general area as the appendix. During the operative procedure there was a tendency to push the omentum up and to the left. This is reflected in the omental patterns. Roentgenographic observation of the omental pattern revealed no mass migration of the omentum to the site of injury, but the free border nearest the offending agent becomes adherent to that agent by the process of inflammation with resultant firm fibrous adhesions.

If loops of small bowel completely surround the offending agent, the omentum may become adherent to the inflammatory mass rather than to the actual offending agent, in this case a necrotic appendix. Other peritoneal surfaces such as the mesentery of the small bowel or the mesentery of the fallopian tube may, if physically capable (being limited by their attachments), become adherent to the inflammatory mass just as readily as the omentum, and may perform a similar function in prevention of generalized peritonitis.

The failure of the omentum to become widely attached to the area of inflammation strongly suggests that any attachment which does occur is due to chance proximity of a portion of the omentum to the inflammatory process during its normal excursion already demonstrated.

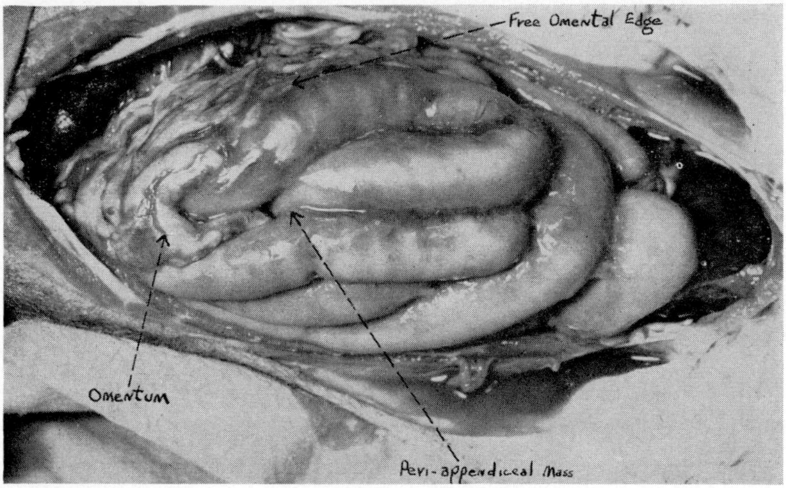

Fig. 11.—Autopsy Dog 433. Dog died thirty-six hours after ligation of appendiceal base (generalized peritonitis). Omentum in left upper quadrant of abdomen except for one small omental stalk.

Omental Pattern Response to Sterile Gauze in Right Lower Quadrant of the Abdomen.—The possibility of omental migration in response to a fixed sterile foreign body was also studied.

Five dogs with marked omenta, No. 421, 409, 407, 406, and 422, were anesthetized, and the abdominal cavities were explored through a short right lower quadrant incision. No omental adhesions were found. A small Raytex gauze sponge was sutured to the parietal peritoneum of the right lower quadrant of the abdomen, and the abdominal wound was closed. X-ray pictures were obtained at intervals. One omental pattern is presented in Fig. 12.

At autopsy there was no evidence of acute peritonitis. The gauze sponge had in each case been peritonealized in its entirety. In three dogs, this was accomplished by the parietal peritoneum, small bowel, and omentum. In Dog 421, the medial aspect of the gauze sponge had been covered by the mesentery of the right fallopian tube, and the omentum had become adherent over a small area to the medial surface of the fallopian tube mesentery. In Dog 407 the gauze sponge was covered by a loop of small bowel, including the mesentery of this loop. The omentum was attached to the resultant mass over an area of small intestine of approximately 1 by 1 by 1½ cm.

Results: Fixed, sterile foreign bodies (gauze sponges) in the abdominal cavity may be covered by intestine, mesentery of intestine, mesentery of fallopian tube, or omentum, singularly or in any combination. Mobility and position determine the part that forms the new peritoneal surface over the

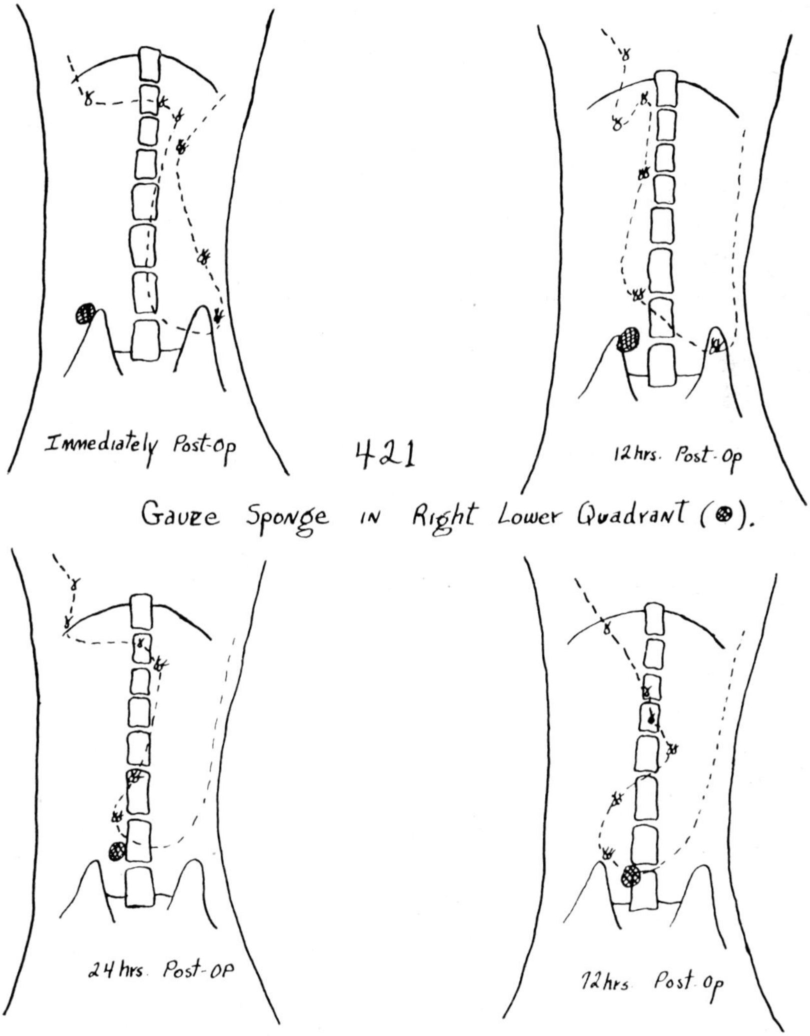

Fig. 12.—Omenta pattern response to marked gauze fixed in right lower quadrant of abdomen. Shift in position of gauze indicates shift in dog's position on x-ray table.

foreign body. Since the omentum is very mobile and since it offers an excellent surface for peritonealization purposes, it is most often involved in this reaction. However, if another part, such as a loop of small intestine with its mesentery or the mesentery of the fallopian tube, happens to make contact with the foreign body first, it too will just as readily attach itself to the foreign body and isolate it from the general peritoneal cavity.

The omental patterns reveal no massive migration of the omentum toward the foreign body; however, once the omentum comes in contact with the foreign body, its excursion away from this area is limited, as shown by the constancy of relation of one marker to the radiopaque foreign body at twelve hours and later (Fig. 12). In no instance was the entire free edge of the omentum adherent to the foreign body; in each case the edge nearest the foreign body made the initial contact and became involved in the isolation process. These results lead to the same conclusion as the observation made concerning experimental appendicitis.

Omental Migration in Response to Inaccessible Inflammation: (A) Sterile Gauze Sutured to Undersurface of the Diaphragm and (B) An Experimental Liver Abscess.—

(a) Sterile gauze sutured to undersurface of the diaphragm: In each dog in which a sponge was placed in the right lower quadrant of the abdominal cavity it was necessary to push the omentum away while the gauze was being sutured to the parietal peritoneum. In one dog, the omentum was "stuck" to the sponge before the abdominal incision was closed. This task seemed too easy for the omentum, and it was therefore decided to place the same type of foreign body in a part of the abdominal cavity that was not readily accessible to the omentum in its normal position, but which was within easy reach of the trailing omental edge if it chose to migrate in the right direction. The undersurface of the diaphragm was selected as the site.

Three unmarked dogs without previous laparotomies (Nos. 439, 440, and 441) were anesthetized, and the abdominal cavity was entered through a short epigastric midline incision. A small sterile gauze roll was sutured to the undersurface of the diaphragm above the left lobe of the liver. The abdomen was closed in layers, and each dog was returned to his cage and permitted the customary freedom of activity, food, and water. Seven days later the dogs were autopsied.

Autopsy findings: The findings were similar for all dogs and they will be described together. There was no evidence of acute peritonitis. In each case the sponge had been "walled off" or surrounded by the diaphragm, the left lobe of the liver, and the falciform ligament. In one of the three dogs (Dog 439), the sponge protruded slightly below the liver edge, and the resultant free margin was covered with fibrin. The omentum in each case was spread out over the loops of small intestine, showing no attachment to, or evidence of, an attempt to migrate toward the foreign body.

(b) An experimental liver abscess: To simulate more closely an inflammatory process, it was decided to produce an abscess in the upper surface of the left lobe of the liver and to study the omental migration response.

Two unmarked dogs (No. 422 and 443) had abdominal explorations as in the previous cases. A small stab wound was made in the upper surface of the left lobe of the liver. (This was facilitated by rotating the liver anteriorly and inferiorly from beneath the diaphragm.) A cotton pledget was soaked in a warm fresh culture of *Staphylococcus albus* and sutured in the stab wound. The abdominal wound was closed in layers; the dogs were sacrificed on the fifth postoperative day.

Autopsy findings: There was no generalized peritonitis. The left lobe of the liver was adherent to the undersurface of the diaphragm and to the falciform ligament. The omentum was in its normal position, covering the loops of small bowel and had obviously made no attempt to migrate to the upper surface of the liver. Adhesions about the superior surface of the left lobe of the liver were separated, and an abscess cavity containing thick, white pus was encountered.

Results: An inflammatory lesion created either by the introduction of a sterile foreign body or by an experimental infectious process is walled off by the structure normally nearest it. When the area of inflammation is created at a point outside the normal range of motion of the omentum, it takes no part in the walling-off process. These experiments again indicate the chance nature of omental participation in peritoneal inflammations.

Omental Migration in Response to Occlusion of Omental Venous Return.—As noted earlier, Schutz[20] postulated that the omentum migrated in response to hyperemia or distention of its vessels as a reflex response of the omentum to peritoneal irritation. He observed a similar response experimentally after obstructing the venous return from the omentum in a normal dog.

This experiment was repeated as follows:

Three normal dogs were anesthetized, and the abdominal cavities were explored through a midline incision. The intestines and omentum were kept moist with warm saline solution throughout the procedure. All venous return from the omentum was obstructed by fine cotton ligatures. Care was taken not to injure the right and left gastroepiploic arteries and the splenic artery. The anesthesia was continued and the omentum was observed for a period of approximately two and one-half hours.

Results: There was no visible motion of the omentum other than that observed with movements of the diaphragm and peristalsis of the intestines. At the conclusion of each experiment, the omentum was slightly edematous, thickened, and congested and had occasional scattered petechial hemorrhages over its surface; however, it maintained its relative position.

It is concluded that hyperemia or distention of the omental vessels does not cause migration of the omentum.

Omental Migration in Response to Increase in Omental Arterial Pressure, Increase in Omental Blood Volume, and Dilation of the Omental Vascular Bed With Maintenance of Systemic Pressure.—Schutz[20] stated that when pressure in the omental arteries is increased, the omentum migrates. The abdominal cavities of three anesthetized dogs were explored through a midline incision. The observations were uniform in all three animals. It was observed that the omentum lay free over the loops of small bowel with no adhesions whatsoever. After heparinization, a glass cannula was placed in each femoral artery, one to record the systemic blood pressure and the other for blood donation. A similar, smaller glass cannula was placed in the right gastroepiploic artery approximately 3 cm. from the pylorus along the greater curvature of the stomach. The small arteries and veins between the stomach and the gastroepiploic vessels were ligated with fine cotton ligatures. All cannulas contained a solution of heparin and saline to prevent clot formation. The arterial pressures in the gastroepiploic artery and in the left femoral artery were 100 mm. Hg and 120 mm. Hg, respectively. Three hundred cubic centimeters of blood was withdrawn from the right femoral artery into 50 c.c. of a heparin and saline solution. Both arterial pressure recordings dropped 30 mm. Hg but returned to normal with partial replacement of the blood volume with 150 c.c. of saline solution. By means of a T-tube connection to the gastroepiploic cannula, the 300 c.c. of blood plus the 50 c.c. of saline and heparin solution was perfused through the omental vascular tree at a known pressure of 250 mm. Hg over a period of sixteen minutes. During this time there was no recognizable migration of the omentum whatsoever. This part of the experiment was repeated three times with no change in the results. A period of stabilization was allowed before each venesection and perfusion.

Since a primary increase in pressure limited to the omental vessels created, as demonstrated, no change in the omentum, it remained to be determined whether general changes in the systemic blood pressure, which would be expected to be reflected also in the omental blood pressure, would create alteration in the omentum. For this purpose, three drugs were used, namely, (1) histamine, (2) ephedrine, and (3) amyl nitrite.

After a period of stabilization, 1 c.c. of a histamine solution on 5 c.c. of saline solution was injected into the right gastroepiploic artery. Thirty seconds later, a blood pressure fall amounting to 20 mm. Hg was recorded in both the femoral and gastroepiploic arteries. This fall gradually leveled off and the pressure returned to normal. The blood pressure curves could be superimposed. Observation of the omentum revealed no change in the gross physical appearance, and there was no indication whatsoever of a migration in its trailing edge.

Another period of stabilization was allowed, after which 1 c.c. of ephedrine sulfate solution was injected intravenously. There was an immediate parallel rise in both recorded pressures; the pressure in the gastroepiploic artery was recorded at 200 mm. Hg and the pressure in the femoral artery was recorded at 220 mm. Hg. Observation of the omentum revealed the arterial pulsation to be of greater volume, but with close observation there was no visible migration of the omental edge.

Observation of the Omentum in an Isolated Fluid Medium.—The preceding observations were confirmed by a study of the omentum in an isolated fluid medium.

In three dogs, glass cannulas were placed in both femoral arteries and in the left femoral and left jugular vein. The abdominal cavity was entered through a long midline incision, and all vessels leading to and away from the omentum were carefully ligated with the exception of the splenic artery and vein. Care was taken to ligate the vessels near the greater curvature of the stomach to avoid injury to the gastroepiploic vessels. The latter were ligated on the right and left individually. All vessels to the spleen were ligated near the splenic capsule, and the spleen was removed. At this point the omental circulation was maintained by the relatively large splenic artery and vein.* All omental arterial pulsations appeared normal and there was no discoloration of the tissue.

After heparinization, glass cannulas were placed in the omental artery and vein (in the direction of the omentum) and were connected by means of heparinized rubber tubing to similar cannulas in the femoral artery and vein. The vessels were then severed proximal to the cannulas so that with an active circulation the entire omentum could be delivered from the abdomen and submerged in a large glass bowl containing Ringer's solution at a constant temperature of 99° F. Pressures were recorded from a T connection in the tubing between the femoral artery and the omental artery and between the femoral vein and the omental vein. The abdominal wound was closed in order to minimize exposure and shock. The circulation from the femoral vessels was adequately maintained in the transplanted omentum. Its color remained good, and arterial pulsation could be observed in the most distal omental margin.

In an effort to study the effect of omental blood flow on omental migration in the excised specimen maintained as far as possible under physiologic conditions, the following five experiments were performed:

1. Obstruction to venous return.
2. Rapid intra-arterial transfusion.
3. Perfusion of blood through the omental vascular system under a known increased pressure.
4. Dilation of the omental vascular system with maintenance of systemic blood pressure.
5. Increase in systemic blood pressure by a vasoconstrictor drug.

1. *Obstruction to Venous Return.*—This was accomplished very readily by compressing the rubber tubing connecting the omental vein with the femoral vein. The venous pressure was recorded at 80 mm. of water and it rose gradually to 200 mm. of water. The tubing was released and venous return re-established. This was repeated three times in each animal.

The omental vein near the cannula became distended as venous pressure was elevated, and the entire omental specimen moved approximately ½ cm., but in no instance was there evidence of migration of the omental edge.

2. *Rapid Intra-Arterial Transfusion.*—Rapid intra-arterial transfusion elevates the blood pressure by rapidly increasing the circulating blood volume. It was thought advisable to see if an increase in omental blood pressure and in omental circulating blood volume has any effect on omental migration.

The experimental dog was given 500 c.c. of whole blood, in a solution of heparin and saline from a donor dog, through the femoral artery not supplying

*Hereafter to be referred to as the omental artery and vein.

the omentum over a period of approximately five minutes. The arterial pressure in the omentum rose 80 mm. Hg above the normal line, with a rise in venous pressure of approximately 30 mm. of water. There was no evidence of omental migration.

3. *Perfusion of Whole Blood Through the Omental System Under a Given Pressure Increase.*—From the right femoral artery was removed 250 c.c. of whole blood, and the blood pressure was allowed to stabilize. The blood was then perfused through the omental arterial system under a pressure of 250 mm. Hg. This produced a rise in omental venous pressure to 210 mm. of water. Observation of the omentum revealed no evidence of omental migration.

4. *Dilation of Omental Vascular System With Maintenance of Systemic Blood Pressure.*—Dilation of the omental vascular system with maintenance of the systemic blood pressure was accomplished by the injection of 1 c.c. of histamine in 5 c.c. of saline solution directly into the omental arterial tree. Histamine produces capillary dilation by direct action and arterial dilation indirectly through the axon reflex.[10] This was evidenced first by a slight fall in venous pressure followed by a very slight transitory fall in arterial pressure.

There was no omental response following the intra-arterial injection of histamine.

5. *Increase in Systemic Blood Pressure by a Vasoconstrictor Drug.*—Increase in systemic arterial pressure by intravenous ephedrine sulfate is paralleled by an increase in omental arterial pressure. This pressure increase was readily recorded with the present preparation, and its influence on omental migration was observed. Following the injection of 1 c.c. of ephedrine sulfate intravenously, there was a rise in arterial pressure to the omentum to 200 mm. Hg. The pressure gradually returned to normal and the injection was repeated with a second similar rise in omental arterial pressure. Observation of the omentum throughout the experiment revealed no movement or migration of its edge.

The entire experiment produced identical results in the three dogs.

It is concluded that (1) elevation of omental venous pressure, (2) increase in omental arterial pressure and volume flow, (3) omental perfusion with whole blood under a pressure of 250 mm. Hg, (4) maintenance of systemic blood pressure with dilation of the omental vascular tree, and (5) increase in systemic blood pressure with resulting increase in omental blood pressure have no effect whatsoever on omental migration.

SUMMARY AND CONCLUSIONS

1. Tantalum wire is an excellent radiopaque, nonirritating, stable marking agent for the omentum.

2. The normal omental pattern, as shown in x-ray films after its edge had been marked with tantalum, undergoes variations of considerable degree.

3. These variations have been shown to be dependent in varying degrees on: (a) peristalsis, (b) gravity, and (c) diaphragmatic movement.

4. Migration of the omentum has no relationship to: (a) hyperemia of the omentum, (b) elevation of mental arterial pressure, (c) increase in omental volume flow, or (d) any combination of these factors.

5. The omentum is involved only in those intra-abdominal inflammatory processes which are situated within its normal range of excursion and with which therefore it might by chance come into contact.

6. The omentum reacts as other peritoneal surfaces when in contact with intra-abdominal inflammations.

REFERENCES

1. Adami, J. G.: The Great Omentum, Phila. M. J. **1**: 373, 1898.
2. Adams, J. E.: Peritoneal Adhesions (The Omentum and Its Functions), Lancet **1**: 663, 1913.
3. Bloomhardt, S. L., Andrews, C. F., and Heatherington, B. R.: Surgical Research of the Great Omentum, Surg., Gynec. & Obst. **24**: 474-479, 1917.
4. Buxton, B. H., and Torrey, J. C.: Absorption of Particles From the Peritoneal Cavity. V. The Function of the Omentum, J. Med. Research **15**: 73-87, 1906.
5. Cantacuzène, J., and Soru, E.: Recherches sur le mécanisme de l'accolement de l'épiploon aux portions lésées de la cavité peritonéale; intervention de phénomènes d'ordre électrostatique, Arch. roumaines de path. expér. et de microbiol. **4**: 173, 1931.
6. De Renzie, and Boeri, G.: Das Netz als Schutzorgan, Berl. klin. Wchnschr. **40**: 773-775, 1903.
7. Dickinson, G. K.: The Omentum and Its Functions, Ann. Surg. **45**: 652, 1906.
8. Durham, H. E.: The Mechanism of Reaction to Peritoneal Infection, J. Path. & Bact. **4**: 338, 1897.
9. Fisher, T.: Some Functions of the Omentum, Brit. M. J. **1**: 235, 1906.
10. Fulton, J. F.: Howell's Textbook of Physiology, ed. 16, Philadelphia, 1950, W. B. Saunders Company.
11. Hertzler, A. E.: Surgical Pathology of the Peritoneum, XIX; Philadelphia, 1935, J. B. Lippincott Company.
12. Morison, R.: Functions of the Omentum, Brit. M. J. **1**: 76, 1906.
13. Norris, C. C.: The Omentum, Its Anatomy, Histology, and Physiology in Health and Disease, Univ. Penn. M. Bull. **21**: 119-127, 1908.
14. Pirone, R.: Sulla Furzione difensiva del grande epiloon, Riforma med. **19**: 768-770, 1903.
15. Poynter, C. W.: Concerning the Great Omentum, M. Clin. North America **12**: 499, 1928.
16. Ross, J. F. W.: The Omentum and the Role It Plays in Operative Work Upon the Abdomen, Jour. of Obst. **28**: 763, 1893.
17. Rothenberg, R. E., and Rosenblatt, P.: Motility and Response of the Great Omentum, Arch. Surg. **44**: 764, 1942.
18. Rothenberg, R. E., and Rosenblatt, P.: Omental Response (Observations in 160 Consecutive Autopsied Cases), Am. J. Surg. **62**: 200, 1943.
19. Rubin, I. C.: The Functions of the Great Omentum: A Pathological and Experimental Study, Surg., Gynec. & Obst. **12**: 117, 1911.
20. Schutz, C. B.: Mechanism Controlling Migration of the Omentum, Surg., Gynec. & Obst. **50**: 544, 1930.
21. Seifert, E.: Peritoneum einschiesslich Netz, Möllendorff: Handbuch der Mikroskopischen Anatomie des Menschen, Bd. 5, Berlin, 1927, pp. 337-360.
22. Thomas, J. W., Green, J. W., Jr., and Rhoads, J. E.: An Experimental Study of Factors Affecting the Development and Persistence of Intra-peritoneal Adhesions, Proc. Surg. Forum, Clin. Congress Am. Coll. Surgeons, Philadelphia, 1950, W. B. Saunders Company, pp. 125-128.
23. Wilkie, D. P. D.: Some Functions and Surgical Uses of the Omentum, Brit. M. J. **2**: 1103, 1911.

Case Reports

APPENDICITIS IN THE NEWBORN INFANT

Case Report in a Premature Infant

Douglas H. Riddell, M.D., and David M. Mullins, M.D., Nashville, Tenn.

(From the Department of Pediatrics and the Department of Surgery, Vanderbilt University School of Medicine)

ABT,[1] in 1917, published a review of eighty cases of acute appendicitis in infants under 24 months of age, thirty-seven of whom were less than 12 months old. In 1950, however, the rarity of this disease in infancy was emphasized by Abel and Allen[2] in a collection of 1,165 patients under 12 years of age, among whom only two, or 0.17 per cent, were less than 12 months old. Acute appendicitis in infants under 3 months of age is extremely rare,[3] and in the neonatal period it is seldom diagnosed before laparotomy or necropsy.[4-10] The frequency with which acute appendicitis in the newborn infant is associated with strangulated inguinal hernia has been emphasized.[5, 11-13]

Few instances of acute appendicitis have been recognized in the premature infant. Lilenthal[5] operated upon an infant 3 weeks of age, weighing 5 pounds, who was found to have acute appendicitis within a strangulated inguinal hernia sac. The patient survived. John[7] reported a premature twin weighing 2 pounds, 15 ounces who expired at the age of 20 days. Autopsy revealed acute appendicitis.

The following case report is of interest because of the patient's prematurity, weight, and survival.

CASE REPORT

G. K. (Vanderbilt University Hospital 196179), a 15-day-old premature white male twin, was admitted to the Vanderbilt University Hospital on Jan. 23, 1951, with a chief complaint of "not doing well."

Family history was not remarkable.

Past History.—The twins had a seven-month gestation and an uncomplicated delivery. The patient's birth weight was 3 pounds, 12.25 ounces; the twin's birth weight was 4 pounds, 8.5 ounces. The early condition was not known, but the patient was referred to this hospital because of his debilitated state.

Physical examination on admission revealed a small, ashen, and dehydrated white male infant who appeared critically ill. Weight was 3 pounds, 12 ounces; temperature 97.6° F.; head circumference 29.5 cm.; chest circumference 24 cm.; length 41.5 cm. The abdomen was firm and moderately distended, and the umbilicus was dry with minimal surrounding erythema. There were no palpable masses. Soft fluctuant accumulations of fluid were present on the lateral aspects of the thighs, presumably due to hypodermoclysis. The remainder of the examination was not remarkable. Prematurity and probable septicemia were the initial diagnoses.

Received for publication, Feb. 5, 1953.

Laboratory Data on Admission.—Hemoglobin was 16 Gm. per cent; white blood count was 25,400. Urine was not remarkable. Blood culture revealed a light growth of *Staphylococcus aureus.*

Course and Treatment.—The patient was given constant oxygen, nothing by mouth, 20,000 units of aqueous penicillin every four hours intramuscularly, and an injection of 2.5 mg. of vitamin K (Hykinone).

On the following day, the patient's condition was unchanged. It was thought that he had cellulitis of the abdominal wall and thrombophlebitis of the lower extremities. Dihydrostreptomycin, 75 mg. every four hours, was administered intramuscularly.

The patient appeared improved during the next two or three days, and was given small amounts of skimmed milk formula through a polyethylene tube introduced into the stomach. There was no vomiting, but the abdomen remained quite firm, distended, and red. Abdominal peristalsis was audible. The stools were normal. He was afebrile.

On the fifth hospital day, he passed some bright red blood with mucus in the stools; however, the general condition seemed improved, and he was slowly gaining weight.

On the sixth day, roentgenograms of the abdomen were made because of continued abdominal distention. There was no x-ray evidence of obstruction. Dihydrostreptomycin was discontinued, and chloromycetin, 50 mg. every eight hours, was started by mouth. The accumulations of fluid in the thighs were aspirated of serosanguineous, sterile fluid.

Oral feedings were discontinued on the seventh hospital day because of occasional vomiting and abdominal distention. Hydration was maintained with parenteral fluids. The patient's general appearance, however, continued to improve.

The next day another abdominal x-ray film was obtained which revealed distention of the stomach and upper small intestines. A barium enema revealed very slow filling of the cecum and terminal ileum. The patient's general appearance was not good. His weight was 3 pounds, 12.75 ounces. Surgical consultation was obtained, and laparotomy was advised.

Through a right rectus incision, the abdomen was opened, revealing slight distention of the small bowel and a small amount of free peritoneal fluid. A peritoneal band was found stretching over the terminal ileum, and the appendix was edematous, red, and gangrenous in one area. The peritoneal band was divided, and the appendix and meso-appendix were ligated and amputated at the base without inversion of the stump. The abdominal wound was closed with through-and-through sutures of braided silk because the infant's condition was extremely poor throughout the operation.

Following operation, therapy included constant Wangensteen suction, oxygen, intravenous fluids, and whole blood. Terramycin hydrochloride,* 20 mg. per kilogram per day, was given in the intravenous drip; cortisone, 25 mg., was given, immediately followed by 10 mg. daily intramuscularly.

During the next five days, the patient was maintained on parenteral fluids. Steady improvement ensued. The abdomen became soft, and he began to pass small yellow stools. On the fifth postoperative day small amounts of electrolyte mixture† were started by gastric polyethylene tube. Parenteral fluid supplements and intravenous terramycin were continued until the seventh postoperative day. On the eighth postoperative day, the patient was able to take formula from a nipple. Cortisone dosage was diminished at the end of the second week postoperatively.

The postoperative course was complicated by *Staphylococcus aureus* septicemia on two occasions; these occurred during the sixth and tenth postoperative weeks. The patient was treated with penicillin, terramycin, and chloromycetin, and received several small whole blood transfusions. He also developed bilateral inguinal hernias and small herniations along the line of abdominal incision.

He continued to thrive and gain weight, and was discharged from the hospital weighing 7 pounds, 4 ounces. The total length of hospitalization was sixteen weeks.

*Manufactured by Chas. Pfizer and Co., Inc.
†Meade's No. 297.

Since discharge he has been followed in the outpatient department, and was gaining weight and doing well when last seen at the age of seven months.

COMMENT

Treatment of acute appendicitis in the neonatal and infancy periods requires the combined cooperation of the pediatrician and surgeon, for the disease in this period presents problems which are extremely formidable. These problems result from the following facts:

1. Perforation of the appendix is likely to occur early because of the infant's poor response to the infection.
2. Generalized peritonitis is common, for the role of the greater omentum in localizing the infection is not adequate.
3. Clinical signs and symptoms may be misleading because of the rarity of the condition in this age group.
4. The operative procedure requires meticulous handling of delicate and diseased tissue.
5. Postoperative management necessitates almost constant observation of the patient and an exacting regulation of the patient's fluid balance and nutrition.

SUMMARY AND CONCLUSIONS

1. Acute appendicitis in the neonatal period is extremely rare, but must be considered in differential diagnoses of intra-abdominal disease, particularly when vomiting and abdominal distention are present.
2. Adequate treatment of these patients requires the combined care of the pediatrician and the surgeon.
3. An instance of acute appendicitis is presented in a premature infant who survived.

REFERENCES

1. Abt, Isaac A.: Appendicitis in Infants, Arch. Pediat. **34**: 641, 1917.
2. Abel, William G., III, and Allen, P. D.: Acute Appendicitis in Children, Ann. Surg. **132**: 1093, 1950.
3. Emerson, A. H.: Acute Appendicitis in Infancy, Am. J. Surg. **59**: 563, 1943.
4. Jackson, W. F.: A Case of Prenatal Appendicitis, Am. J. M. Sc. **127**: 710, 1904.
5. Lilenthal, H.: Strangulated Hernia and Gangrenous Appendicitis in a Premature Infant, J. Mt. Sinai Hosp. **5**: 607, 1939.
6. Engstrom, C. G.: Akute Appendicitis bei Einem 3 Wochen Alten, Frühgeborenen Kinde, Acta Pediat. **37**: 355, 1949.
7. John, R. W.: Acute Perforative Appendicitis in an Infant of Twenty Days, Lancet **2**: 1907, 1936.
8. Hill, W. B., and Mason, C. C.: Prenatal Appendicitis With Rupture and Death, Am. J. Dis. Child. **29**: 86, 1925.
9. Reed, E. N.: Infant Disemboweled at Birth—Appendectomy Successful, J. A. M. A. **61**: 199, 1913.
10. Corcoran, W. J.: Prenatal Rupture of the Appendix, Am. J. Dis. Child. **39**: 277, 1930.
11. Black, B. M., and Waugh, J. M.: Hernial Appendicitis: Report of Two Cases, Proc. Staff Meet., Mayo Clin. **17**: 328, 1942.
12. Dixon, C. H.: Gangrene of Appendix in a Three-Week-Old Infant, Ann. Surg. **47**: 57, 1908.
13. Remsen, C. M.: Appendicitis in an Infant Sixteen Days Old With Appendix in an Inguinal Sac, Ann. Surg. **56**: 911, 1912.

LARYNGOCELE: AN UNUSUAL TUMOR OF THE NECK

Case Report

Malcolm R. Hill, Jr., M.D., and Charles S. Kipen, M.D.,
Los Angeles, Calif.

(From the Surgical Service of the Wadsworth Hospital, Veterans Administration Center, and the Department of Surgery, School of Medicine, University of California at Los Angeles)

IN 1947, McLaurin[10] found approximately forty cases of laryngocele reported in the literature. However, most of the reports concerning this unusual tumor of the neck appeared in the specialized literature of otorhinolaryngology,[6, 8-10, 12, 14] and a review of the literature revealed that this lesion was rarely included in the differential diagnosis of tumors and cysts of the neck.[1-5, 7, 11, 13]

CASE REPORT

A 29-year-old white male brewmaster's apprentice was referred to the Surgical Service in December, 1951, for investigation of a mass in the left side of the neck. He stated that he had first noted a swelling in the neck in 1947 and concurrently had begun to have recurrent episodes of sore throat and dysphagia. There was no hoarseness or dyspnea. The patient had been told that the swelling was caused by recurrent tonsillitis and a tonsillectomy was performed, but without relief of symptoms. The patient received no further treatment prior to our consultation. During the intervening period, the swelling gradually increased and the episodes of dysphagia and sore throat occurred more frequently. The patient noted that when he sang loudly, the mass became more prominent or increased in size. External pressure on the mass was not painful and had never caused a hissing sound in the throat. There was no history of external drainage from the neck.

Examination revealed a soft, movable, nontender, cystic mass lying in the anteromedial border of the sternocleidomastoid muscle in the upper third of the neck. The mass measured 5 cm. in its greatest diameter. There was no surrounding induration, enlargement of the thyroid gland, or cervical adenopathy. The mass did not move with swallowing. All laboratory studies were within normal limits.

A diagnosis of left branchial cleft cyst was made, and on March 19, 1952, exploration was carried out under endotracheal anesthesia through a transverse incision across the mass. The mass was exposed by retracting the sternocleidomastoid muscle laterally and the strap muscles medially. It appeared to be a unilocular cyst about 5 cm. in diameter, with a thin, rubbery, translucent wall. A narrow stalk was found posteromedially which extended behind the strap muscles and entered the lateral thyrohyoid membrane. The cyst was aspirated, and air, but no fluid, was recovered. The stalk was transected at the base and a probe inserted through its lumen into the larynx. The base of the stalk was inverted with interrupted fine chromic sutures, and the small defect in the thyrohyoid membrane was reapproximated over the inverted stalk. A small Penrose drain was placed down to the thyrohyoid membrane and was brought out through the lateral end of the incision. The remainder of the wound was closed in layers with interrupted sutures of fine cotton. Microscopic examination of the sac revealed a lining of ciliated pseudostratified columnar epithelium (Fig. 1).

Received for publication, March 2, 1953.

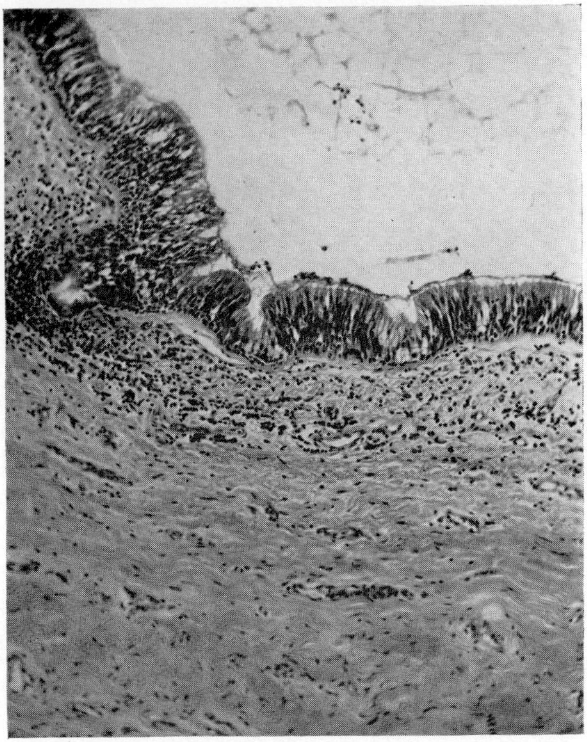

Fig. 1.—Microscopic section of laryngocele, showing ciliated pseudostratified columnar epithelium.

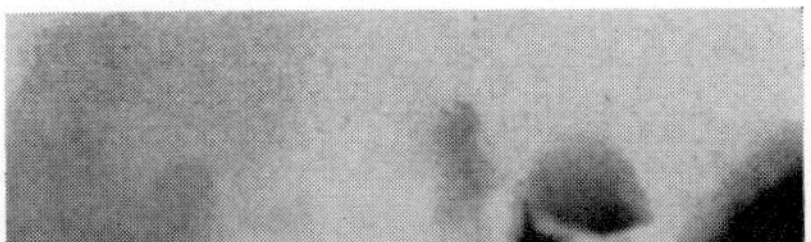

Fig. 2.—Lateral cervical film showing air-filled sac. (From Taylor.[14])

The drain was removed twenty-four hours after operation. Penicillin and streptomycin were given parenterally for four days. The patient recovered uneventfully and was discharged seven days after operation. Three months after operation he was asymptomatic, and direct laryngoscopy and roentgenograms of the neck revealed no abnormalities.

DISCUSSION

The differential diagnosis of tumors and cysts of the neck, as considered by most authors,[1-5, 7, 11, 13] has not included laryngocele. In 1947, Jackson[6] briefly reviewed the history and incidence of laryngocele. He defined the lesion as a "hernia of the larynx" and reiterated that the air sac connected with the larynx usually arises in the laryngeal ventricle. Most authors[6, 9] mention two or three types of laryngocele. The internal type is contained within the thyroid cartilage. The external type pierces the thyrohyoid membrane and presents itself externally as a tumor of the neck. Jackson[6] quoted Leborgne as stating that the laryngocele may be associated with laryngeal carcinoma in 10 to 15 per cent of the cases. Lathrop[8] reported purulent inflammation complicating two cases of laryngocele (laryngopyocele). Lindsay[9] observed changes in the size of the sac with intralaryngeal pressure change by the use of planograms. He discussed increased intralaryngeal pressure as the generally accepted etiology of this lesion.

Hoarseness is the most common symptom,[6, 10] but it was not noted by this patient. Often, patients note that pressure over the mass elicits a hissing sound in the larynx.[6] Again, this patient was an exception. Dyspnea occurs only if an intraglottic (internal) component causes obstruction. Coughing, singing, or any rise in intraglottic pressure usually enlarges the external mass.[9] Examination should include direct laryngoscopy to note the presence and size of any intraglottic component and to rule out associated papilloma or carcinoma of the larynx.[12] The importance of routine neck films for examination of neck tumors is emphasized by this lesion, for an x-ray picture usually establishes the diagnosis by demonstrating an air-filled sac (Fig. 2). Diagnostic aspiration of the cyst or tumor, with its risk of introducing infection, is thus avoided.

Treatment is by excision.[6, 10] Attention should be paid to careful inversion of the base of the transected laryngocele stalk. Whenever possible, the defect in the thyrohyoid membrane should be reapproximated, in an attempt to prevent recurrence.

SUMMARY

A case of superior external laryngocele is presented. Diagnosis and treatment are discussed, and a brief review of the literature is included. It is recommended that differential diagnosis of neck cysts and tumors include this unusual lesion.

REFERENCES

1. Baumgartner, C. J.: Differential Diagnosis Between Thymic Duct and Branchial Cleft Fistulas, Am. J. Surg. **59**: 99, 1933.
2. Baumgartner, C. J.: Congenital Lesions of the Neck, J. A. M. A. **113**: 1860, 1939.
3. Baumgartner, C. J.: Surgery of Congenital Lesions of the Neck, Post-grad. M. J. **1**: 181, 1947.

4. Baumgartner, C. J.: Lateral Cysts and Fistulas of the Neck, California Med. **73**: 466, 1950.
5. Gross, R. E., and Ladd, W. E.: Congenital Branchiogenic Anomalies, Am. J. Surg. **39**: 234, 1938.
6. Jackson, C. L.: Laryngocele, Laryngoscope **57**: 788, 1947.
7. Lahey, F. H., and Nelson, H. S.: Branchial Cysts and Sinuses, Ann. Surg. **113**: 508, 1941.
8. Lathrop, O. A.: Laryngopyocele, New England J. Med. **229**: 681, 1947.
9. Lindsay, J. R.: Laryngocele Ventricularis, Ann. Otol., Rhin. & Laryng. **49**: 661, 1940.
10. McLaurin, J. W.: Laryngocele, Laryngoscope **57**: 616, 1947.
11. Meyer, H. W.: Congenital Cysts and Fistulas of the Neck, Ann. Surg. **95**: 1, 226, 1932.
12. Moore, I.: The So-Called Prolapse of the Laryngeal Ventricle and Eversion of the Sacculus, J. Laryngol. & Otol. **37**: 265, 333, 381, 1922.
13. Neal, H. D., and Pemberton, J.: Branchial Cysts and Fistulas, SURGERY **18**: 281, 1945.
14. Taylor, H. M.: Ventricular Laryngocele, Ann. Otol., Rhin. & Laryng. **53**: 536, 1944.

MESENCHYMOMA

Report of a Case

George T. Pack, M.D.,* and James R. Lisa, M.D.,**
New York, N. Y.

THE mesenchymoma has been recognized and described as a tumor entity by Arthur Purdy Stout who referred to it as a "neoplasm composed of an admixture of two or more nonepithelial mesenchymal derivatives that ordinarily are not found together in a single tumor." To quote Stout again in this connection, he stated that "mesenchyme is an extremely versatile tissue, which in ordinary development produces the normal prototypes of all of the tissues of which these malignant cells are the grotesque caricatures."

The primitive mesenchymal cell endowed with amazing growth energies is the ultimate ancestor of the various tumors of the soft somatic tissues, both benign and malignant. In the ordinary course of differentiation these mesenchymal cells finally emerge into specific functional tissues such as fat, muscle, fascia, nerve, synovia, and so forth, but seldom in pure form because of the variable proportions of stromal elements which are present. The connective or fibrous tissue component of the somatic tumors may constitute a relatively small proportion of the neoplasm as in some liposarcomas or a major part of the bulk as in some malignant synoviomas. The preponderance of connective tissue in some sarcomas has led to the erroneous appellation of "fibrosarcoma" without due consideration of the histogenesis of the more differentiated type cell, which is present but less conspicuous. The term mesenchymoma as employed by Stout excludes from the classification any tumor in which one of the two elements is fibroblastic, and rightly so because fibroblasts can be elaborated by synovial cells and others. Also excluded are tissues of metaplastic change, such as the occurrence of bone in a liposarcoma or the development of sarcoma in myositis ossificans.

The mixed mesenchymal tumors are comprised of two or more somatic tissues of different histogenesis in addition to the variable proportions of fibrous stroma present. Theoretically, the mesenchymomas should be frequent instead of rare. The neoplasm may contain adipose, angiomatous, osseous, cartilaginous, hematopoietic, myxomatous, and smooth muscle tissues, but such multiple admixtures are seldom found. Each of the component tissues may be as fully malignant as any sarcoma of pure histogenetic type. The potpourri of tissues varies widely in composition and in degree of malignancy. In lieu of the term mesenchymoma, implying a malignant tumor, compound terms have found some usage in medical literature, but Stout's identification of them in the single category is a definite titling which should be adopted. Some of the sarcomatous elements are in greater proportion than others; therefore, there is no set pattern of composition.

Received for publication, March 9, 1953.

*Pack Medical Group.
**Doctors Hospital.

Although Stout admitted that metaplasia may play a role in the genesis of these tumors, he was inclined to consider them largely as dysontogenetic neoplasms, originating as developmental aberrations. An argument in favor of metaplasia, he pointed out, is the possible occurrence of heterotopic bone and cartilage, whereas in substantiation of the dysontogenetic theory is the occurrence of mesenchymomas in regions where congenital abnormalities are found.

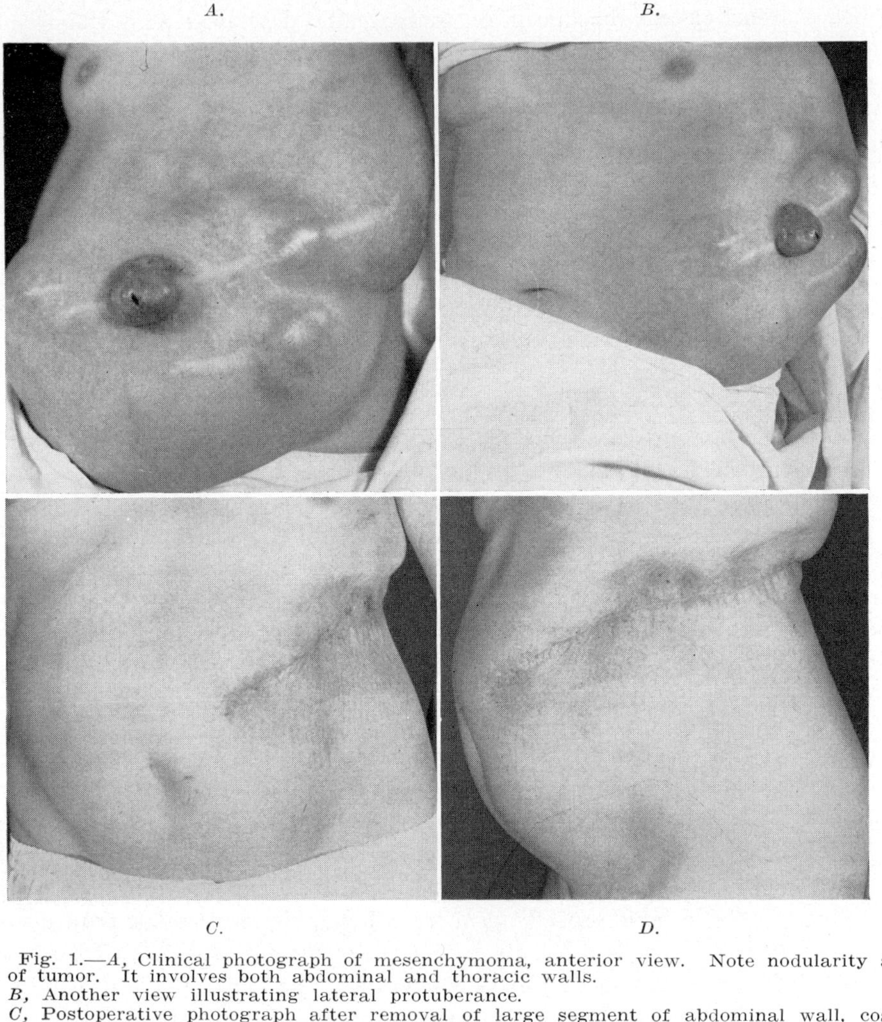

Fig. 1.—*A*, Clinical photograph of mesenchymoma, anterior view. Note nodularity and bulk of tumor. It involves both abdominal and thoracic walls.

B, Another view illustrating lateral protuberance.

C, Postoperative photograph after removal of large segment of abdominal wall, costal margins, portions of diaphragm, and pericardium.

D, Photograph showing defect after it was closed by tantalum mesh and skin.

The proper treatment is radical surgical excision with ruthless sacrifice of the containing tissues, viscus, or extremity. Radiation therapy may secure a palliative end result of variable duration, but cure by such treatment would not be anticipated.

CASE REPORT

C. K., a 54-year-old white man, was first seen on Oct. 14, 1949. In May, 1949, he had observed a lump in the left upper anterolateral abdominal wall, which tumor was resected at St. Joseph's Hospital, Paterson, N. J. on May 19, 1949. At that time, portions of the ninth and tenth ribs were removed. Within two months, a recurrence had developed in the medial aspect of the incision involving the abdominal wall. X-ray therapy had been given without apparent effect. Weight was maintained at 208 pounds.

A.

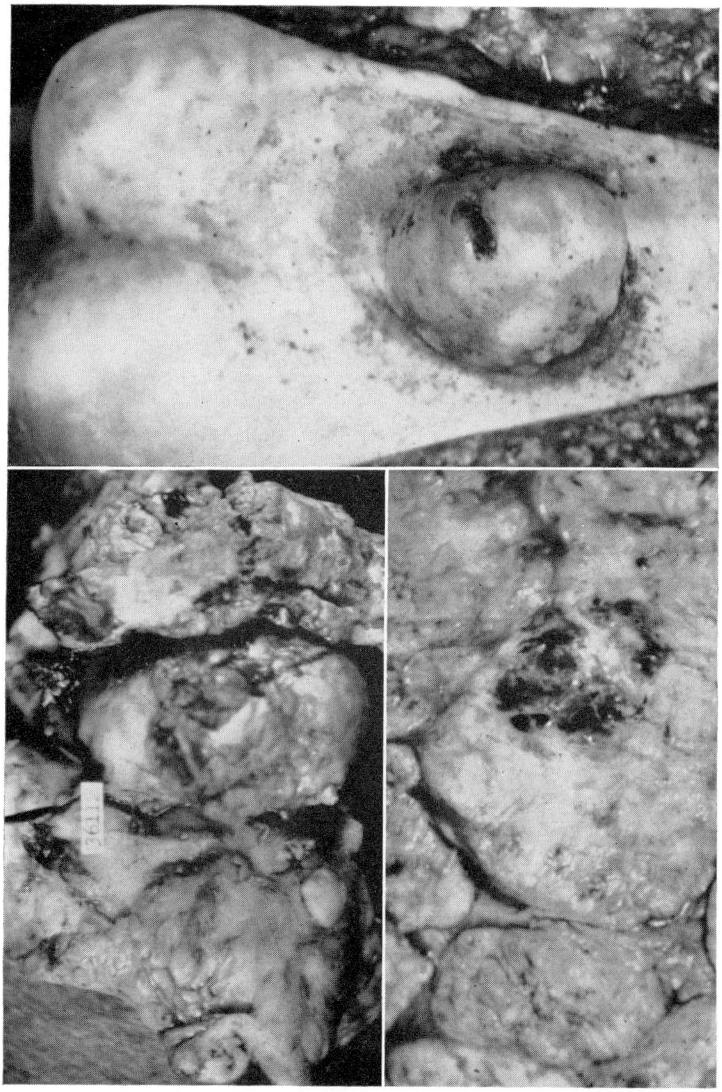

B. *C.*

Fig 2.—Photographs of mesenchymoma showing the external nodular appearance of the skin (upper), the nodular appearance of the undersurface (lower left), and the cut surface (lower right).

At the time of our first examination, a fungating recurrent sarcoma was seen to involve the left lower anterolateral chest wall adherent to and involving the ribs. It was fixed and immovable. A roentgenogram of the chest revealed evidences of pulmonary metastases. Posterior-anterior and left lateral x-ray films of the chest showed densities in the lower portion of the right lung field in the posterior gutter. There were no axillary or lymph nodes palpable at the time. On fluoroscopy, the diaphragm moved well, and on physical examination, ventilatory excursion was adequate and the patient had good respiratory reserve.

The patient refused surgical intervention and went to a tumor hospital in Philadelphia. While there, he received fractionated treatments with polysaccharides at monthly

A.

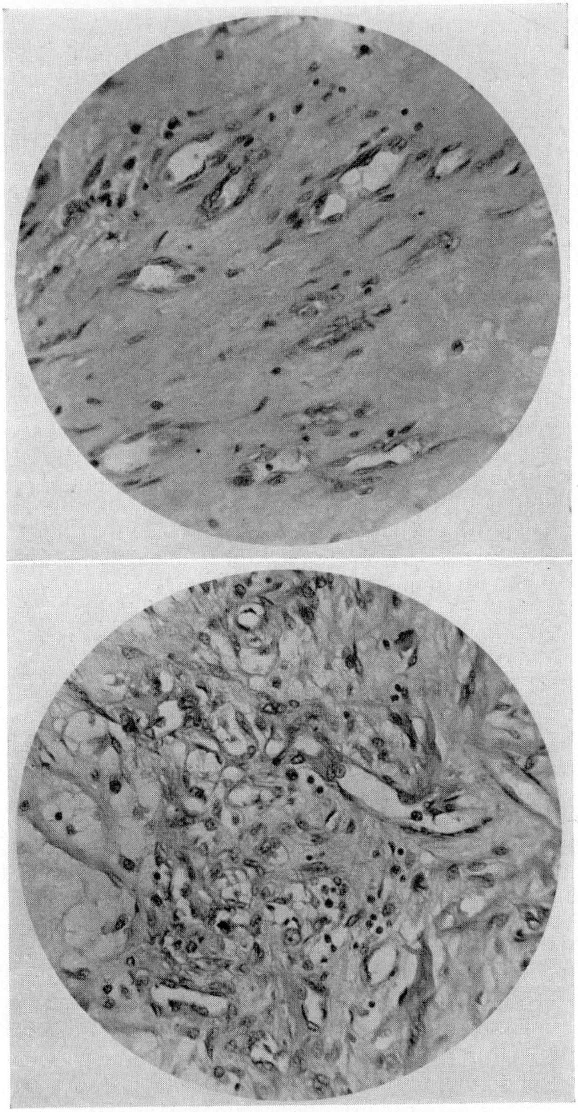

B.

Fig. 3.—*A*, Photomicrograph of the vascular channels which are lined by endothelial cells showing moderate anisocytosis and hyperchromia. They merge into the surrounding tissue which has a few cells of similar nature. There are foci of necrobiosis. (×200, reduced ⅓.)

B, Photomicrograph showing more marked vascularity. The endothelial cells display a greater degree of anisocytosis and the surrounding tissue is richer in neoplastic elements. (×300, reduced ⅓.)

intervals, starting on Nov. 30, 1949, and continuing until April 16, 1951. During this time, the recurrent tumor of the chest wall tripled in size; when he returned in May, 1951, the huge fungating tumor was as shown in Fig. 1. In the meantime, the patient had lost considerable weight. The roentgenograms of the chest now showed the pulmonary metastases to be much larger than at previous times.

C.

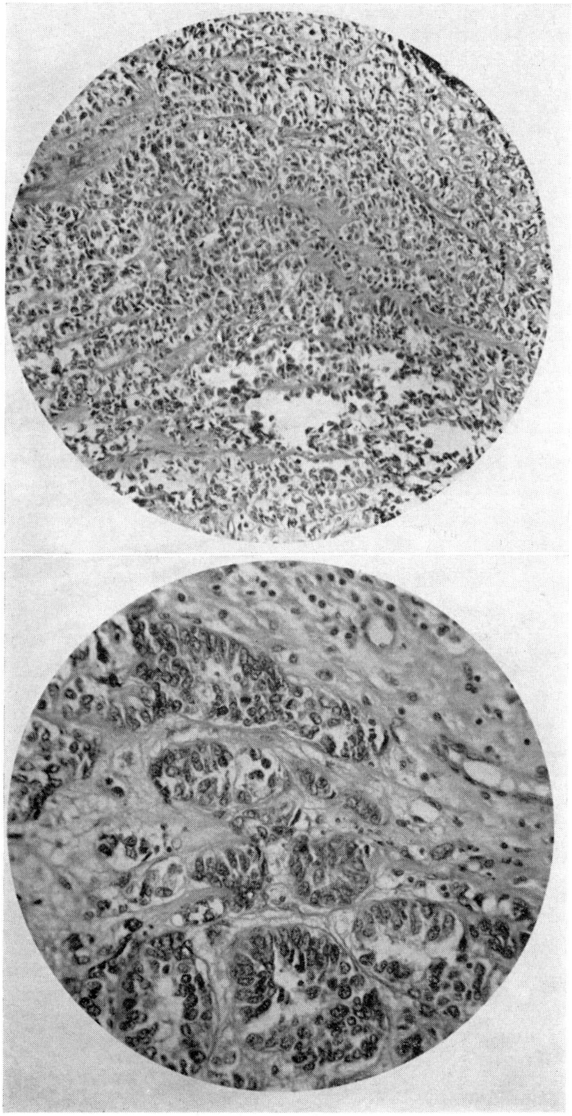

D.

Fig. 3 (*continued*).

C, Photomicrograph showing how the richly cellular area closely simulates epithelial structures. Other foci reveal primitive chondroblasts. (×70, reduced ⅓.)

D, Photomicrograph showing the neoplastic cells arising directly from the wall and producing solid nests which fill the channels. There is marked anisocytosis and hyperchromia. Mitoses are present in moderate numbers. There are a few inflammatory cells. (×300, reduced ⅓.)

On June 11, an operation was performed by making an incision along the course of the twelfth rib with extension inferiorly and medially toward the midportion of the abdominal wall. The skin was then dissected away from the mass and, by encompassing the contours of the tumor, the musculature of the abdominal wall which had become extremely frayed was dissected away from the mass. The external oblique, transversalis, internal oblique, and left rectus muscles were transected, and in one portion of the abdominal wall, where the tumor had infiltrated these muscles and the peritoneum, it was necessary to excise all of these structures, leaving a huge defect in the abdominal wall. As the dissection progressed superiorly, it was necessary to resect the lower three ribs, after which the intrathoracic portion of the mass was excised by removing a portion of the pericardium and a large segment of the left leaf of the diaphragm. Numerous implants of the tumor were noted within the substance of the lung, on the diaphragm, and on the parietal pleura.

After the huge tumor mass had been dissected free from the body wall and removed, the resultant defect was repaired by suturing the diaphragm to the chest wall at the level of the ninth rib. The chest wall was then closed with interrupted silk sutures, and a drain placed under water. The abdominal cavity was closed by suturing the peritoneum and the remaining abdominal musculature in the four quadrants of the defect to each other, leaving a central defect 10 cm. square, which was repaired by suturing a tantalum mesh in place, over which the skin was approximated. The tantalum mesh was in direct contact with the viscera and was the only structure intervening between the subcutaneous fat and the viscera.

Convalescence was completely uneventful. The wound healed well. The patient gained twenty pounds in weight after the operation, and the metastases in the lungs remained relatively quiescent. Six months later, pleural effusion developed requiring thoracentesis. He died ten months after the date of operation. The period of complete palliative relief was approximately six months.

Gross Pathologic Anatomy.—The tumor was a huge, grossly nodular mass measuring 34 by 23.5 by 11.8 cm. and covered by a triangular segment of skin with a healed central surgical scar. The mass was divided into lobules of milky-white or yellow-white firm tissue with occasional hemorrhagic foci. It was tightly adherent to the periosteum of the rib segments (Fig. 2).

Histologic Features of the Tumor.—The neoplasm was extremely vascular. Within the tumor could be seen thin-walled blood vessels lined by neoplastic endothelial cells lying in a relatively loose tissue which had a few necrobiotic foci (Fig. 3, *A*). Other portions were much richer in blood vessels and lay in tissue which had the same type of cell as that which lined the vessels. Other segments of the neoplasm (Fig. 3, *C*) were much more cellular, and some foci resembled primitive cartilage. These channels were lined by malignant cells similar in character to those of the other areas but displayed more anaplasia and anisocytosis. A moderate infiltration by inflammatory cells was present.

Diagnosis.—Diagnosis was mesenchymoma of thoracoabdominal wall.

REFERENCES

1. Alston, E. F., and Paulson, D.: Mesenchymoma of the Pleura, J. Thoracic Surg. **18**: 518-525 (Aug.) 1949.
2. Bowen, J. A.: Mesenchymoma, Secondary Invasion of the Urinary bladder, J. Urol. **64**: 311-317 (Aug.) 1950.
3. Hyde, W. R., White, J. E., and Stout, A. P.: Mesenchymoma of the Mesentery, Cancer **3**: 653-656 (July) 1950.
4. Huneman, M. W., and Lehman, M. L.: Mediastinal Mesenchymoma Masquerading as Liposarcoma, Cancer **4**: 692-696 (July) 1951.
5. Scarrow, G. D., and Ainsworth, J.: Calcification in Retroperitoneal Mesenchymoma, Brit. J. Radiol. **24**: 167-169 (March) 1951.
6. Stout, A. P.: Mesenchymoma, the Mixed Tumor of Mesenchymal Derivatives, Ann. Surg. **127**: 278-290, 1948.
7. Symmers, W. St. C., and Nangle, E. J.: An Unusual Recurring Tumor Formed of Connective Tissue of Embryonic Type, So-called Mesenchymoma, J. Path. & Bact. **63**: 419-428 (July) 1951.

CONGENITAL DUPLICATION OF THE GALL BLADDER

Review of the Literature and Report of an Unusual Symptomatic Case

Thomas C. Moore, M.D., and Anson G. Hurley, M.D., Muncie, Ind.

(From the Surgical Service, Ball Memorial Hospital, Muncie, and the Department of Surgery, Indiana University School of Medicine, Indianapolis)

CONGENITAL duplication of the gall bladder is quite rare. From a review of this and other types of gall bladder malformation, it would appear that the incidence of gall bladder anomalies is considerably less than that of other segments of the extrahepatic biliary system.[21] Furthermore, gall bladder anomalies, when symptomatic, do not become so until adult life in contrast to the frequency of neonatal symptoms, generally obstructive jaundice, accompanying anomalies of the hepatic and common bile ducts.

Because of the wide range of variations in size, shape, and location encountered in the recorded cases of gall bladder duplication,[10, 20] it is desirable to classify these malformations only within rather broad limits. Accordingly, a duplication may be regarded as either a complete or a partial one. In the cases of complete duplication, the "vesica fellea duplex" group of Boyden,[5] the two gall bladders do not communicate and may or may not have separate serosal coverings. Furthermore, in these cases the cystic ducts may be completely duplicated, entering the common duct each with its own orifice, or they may be only partially duplicated, joining at a "Y" junction with a single opening into the common duct.

The gall bladder may be bilobed or partially septate in cases of incomplete duplication, Boyden's "vesica fellea divisa" classification. Only a very few instances, approximately eight in number, of incomplete duplication have been reported,[20] and it is with the occurrence of complete duplication that this study will be largely concerned.

Thirty-five cases of complete duplication of the gall bladder, proved either by operative or necropsy examination, have been reported up to the present time.[2-4, 5-15, 17-20, 22-39] Unconfirmed cases in which the diagnosis was based solely on roentgen interpretation have been excluded. The first case of complete duplication to be discovered on post-mortem examination was described in 1674 by Blasius.[4] Yet, it was not until 1911 that Sherren[31] reported the first discovery of this singular malformation at operation.

Because of the rarity of gall bladder duplication, it has seemed desirable to report an unusual symptomatic case in which there was complete duplication of both the gall bladder and cystic duct, each gall bladder having a separate serosal covering, and in which one gall bladder was normal and the other acutely inflamed.

Aided in part by a grant from the James Whitcomb Riley Memorial Association.
Received for publication, March 19, 1953.

CASE REPORT

The patient, a 30-year-old white woman, was admitted to the hospital on May 9, 1951, because of severe right upper quadrant abdominal pain of twelve hours' duration. The pain was referred to the tip of the right shoulder and was associated with nausea and vomiting. She had had five similar attacks during the two years prior to admission, and complained of intolerance to fatty foods. There was no history of jaundice.

Physical examination revealed epigastric and right upper quadrant tenderness. The findings otherwise were within normal limits. The red blood count was 4.2 million and the hemoglobin 13 Gm. The serology was negative and the urine normal. White blood count was 16,200 with 83 per cent neutrophils. The serum amylase level was 94 Somogyi units. On May 11, cholecystography demonstrated a normal functioning gall bladder (Fig. 1). The symptoms subsided and the patient was discharged from the hospital May 12.

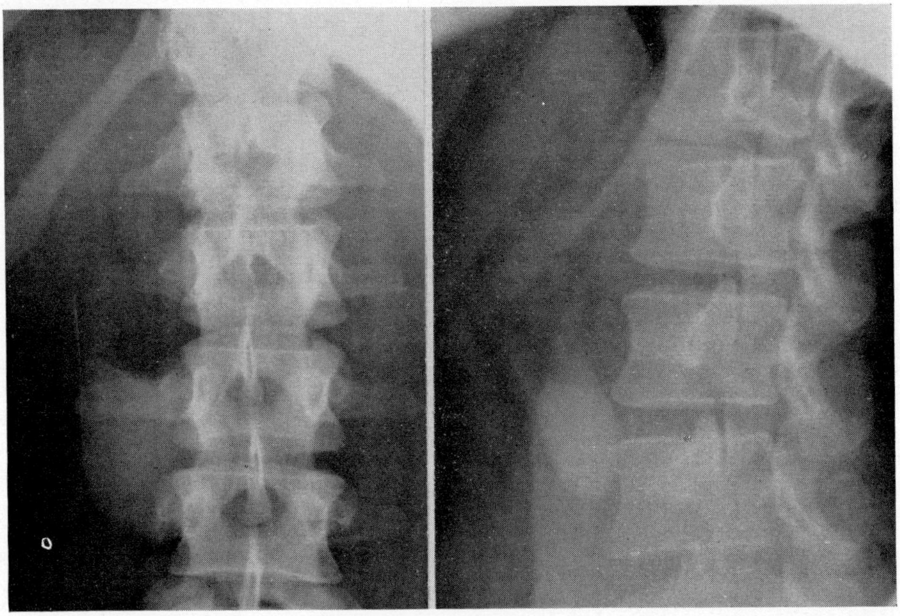

Fig. 1.—Anterior-posterior and lateral films showing cholecystographic evidence of normal function of one of the gall bladders, presumably the normal-appearing distal one.

She remained relatively asymptomatic until she was readmitted to the hospital on Jan. 20, 1952, with a recurrence of the severe right upper quadrant abdominal pain of three days' duration. The pain was again associated with nausea and vomiting, and she had not been jaundiced. In addition to right upper quadrant tenderness, a mass was palpated just below the right costal border. The red blood count was 4.4 million, the hemoglobin 14.5 Gm., and the white blood count 8,800. The Bromsulphalein test demonstrated normal excretion of the dye. The fasting amylase was 133 units and the Prostigmine amylase test levels were within normal limits. Cholecystography again revealed a normally functioning gall bladder. Despite roentgen evidence of an apparently normal gall bladder, it was felt that a right upper quadrant exploration should be carried out.

On Jan. 23, under cyclopropane anesthesia, the peritoneal cavity was opened through a right subcostal Kocher-type incision. On examination of the extrahepatic biliary system, two well-developed and separate gall bladders were found (Fig. 2). Each gall bladder had its own serosal covering, and the cystic ducts were completely duplicated. The distal gall bladder had a smooth, glistening serosal covering and appeared to be normal in every way. The proximal gall bladder, on the other hand, was red, tense, and edematous, and its serosa had a dull, granular appearance. Stones could not be palpated within either structure or within the hepatic or common bile ducts. Because of the normal appearance and the apparently normal functional capacities roentgenologically of the distal gall bladder, it was decided to leave this organ intact and to remove only the acutely inflamed proximal gall bladder. This was accomplished by dissection of the proximal gall bladder from above down. The cystic duct was ligated and divided near its junction with the common duct, and a Penrose drain was placed down to the site of removal. The wound was closed in layers. No stones were found when the excised gall bladder was opened. Nevertheless, evidence of acute inflammation was found on microscopic study.

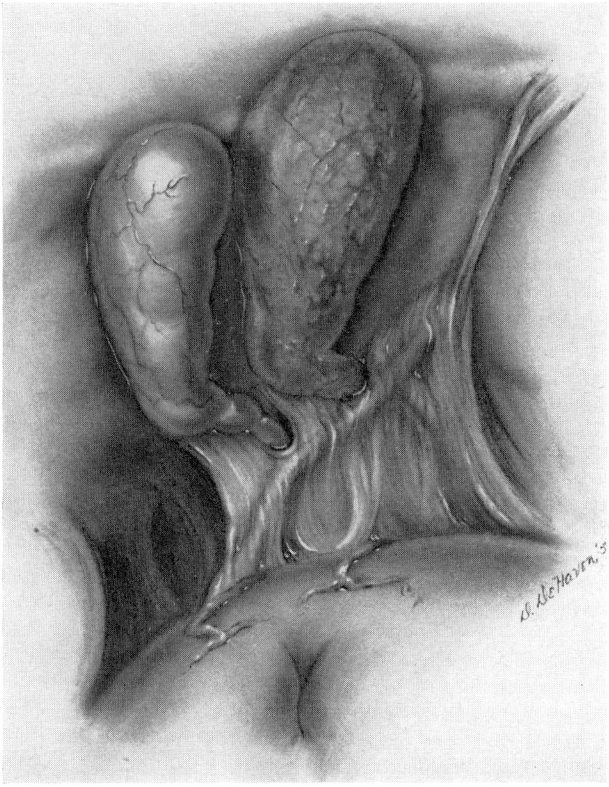

Fig. 2.—Drawing of the appearance, at operation, of the two gall bladders and their cystic ducts.

The postoperative course was uneventful, and the patient was discharged from the hospital on Jan. 26. Since her release from the hospital, she has had no recurrence of abdominal pain and has been otherwise free of symptoms.

DISCUSSION

Although gall bladder duplications are exceedingly rare in human beings, there is a rather high incidence of them in other animals. This fact accounts for a considerable historical interest in gall bladder anomalies which can be traced to ancient times. This interest, to be sure, derives principally from the frequent discovery of these anomalies in sacrificial animals.

Jastrow,[16] in a comprehensive study of the religion of the Babylonians and Assyrians, cited some forty cuneiform texts dealing with gall bladder malformations. A similar interest is to be found in Hebrew literature pertaining to the certification of kosher meats.[5] The finding of gall bladder anomalies also was regarded by the ancients as being of some prophetic significance. In this regard, Pliny considered worthy of mention the finding of a double gall bladder in a sacrificial animal on the day of the great naval victory of Octavianus Caesar over the combined forces of Anthony and Cleopatra at Actium (31 B.C.).

Because of his apparently significant incidence of gall bladder duplications in some animals, Boyden attempted to determine the incidence of this abnormality in certain animals by examining large numbers of them. He found that partial or complete gall bladder duplication occurred once in every eight cats examined and in a ratio of 1:28 in calves, 1:85 in sheep, and 1:198 in pigs. Only 7 per cent of the duplications in cats were complete, whereas 52 per cent of those in calves were. In a few animals, multiple duplications were encountered.

In human beings, on the other hand, complete duplication of the gall bladder is quite uncommon, only thirty-six instances, including the one herein recorded, having been reported up to the present time. The anomaly was encountered as an incidental necropsy finding in nine of the cases, and in twenty-seven, the discovery was made at the time of operation, generally for symptoms suggesting gall bladder disease. As pointed out by Gross,[10] this finding might appear to suggest that the majority of gall bladder duplications ultimately become symptomatic.

The ages of the patients with symptomatic duplications ranged from 19 to 69 years, and averaged 43 years. Eighteen of the patients were women and six were men. Information was available concerning the cystic ducts in twenty-nine cases. In twenty-two cases, they were completely duplicated, entering the common duct at separate orifices, while in seven cases, they were found to join at a Y junction with a single opening into the common duct.

Although considerable variation in the size and location of the two gall bladders has been described, the commonest single form of the malformation appears to be side-by-side occurrence, with a common serosal covering. For this reason, the existence of the duplication in a few cases was not established until the surgical specimen was examined. Occasionally, the gall bladders may be more widely separated, as they were in the case reported by Wischnewsky,[37] in which one gall bladder was located to the right and one to the left of the falciform ligament. In the interesting case reported by Croudace,[7] the cystic duct from one gall bladder entered the common bile duct, whereas the duct from the accessory gall bladder passed directly into the liver.

Symptoms accompanying gall bladder duplication are, as a rule, those of cholecystitis, generally secondary to cholelithiasis involving one or both of the gall bladders. Cholecystitis has been discovered in a few instances in the absence of cholelithiasis. In one case, the inflammation was due to parasites[2] and in another, obstructive cholecystitis was found to be due to hypertrophied tissues, resembling Brunner's glands, at the ampulla of one of the gall bladders.[31] In the case reported here, no clear cause of the acute cholecystitis was demonstrated. In the case reported by Recht,[27] symptoms resulted from volvulus and gangrene of one of the two gall bladders. The cystic ducts joined at a Y junction in this case.

Although roentgenographic demonstration of gall bladder duplication is possible either from the identification of two separate areas containing gallstones or the visualization of two functioning gall bladders on cholecystography, the findings may also prove misleading.[1] The establishment of this diagnosis depends, to be sure, on operative or necropsy identification of the duplication.

The surgical management of symptomatic cases of gall bladder duplication is, in essence, the management of cholecystitis and cholelithiasis. The diseased organ or organs should be removed. Since both gall bladders are generally diseased, and since they are often rather intimately attached to one another, it is seldom possible to excise an abnormal gall bladder and leave a normal one. The case reported here is unusual in that separation of the two gall bladders made it possible to remove the acutely inflamed proximal one and leave undisturbed the normal-appearing distal one which had previously been shown to function normally on cholecystography. This approach has been possible in only two other reported cases of this malformation. In the case reported by Wischnewsky,[37] the acutely inflamed gall bladder to the left of the falciform ligament was excised and the normal one to the right of the ligament was left intact. Recht's[27] case of a volvulus of an accessory gall bladder with gangrene was treated by removal of only the accessory organ. Although the experience with this anomaly is, as yet, too small to permit any rigid conclusions, there seems to be no impelling reason to excise the normal one of duplicated gall bladders when it can be left behind with apparent safety. Furthermore, there does not seem to be any clear indication for operating upon patients with asymptomatic gall bladder duplication, even though initial impressions might be interpreted as suggesting that there may be a greater tendency for duplicated gall bladders to be affected by cholelithiasis and cholecystitis than nonduplicated ones.

SUMMARY

1. The literature pertaining to congenital duplications of the gall bladder is reviewed, and the classification of these malformations into complete and incomplete duplications is discussed.

2. A symptomatic case of complete duplication of both the gall bladder and cystic duct is reported. Each gall bladder had a separate serosal covering. The proximal gall bladder was acutely inflamed and was removed. The distal one was normal in appearance and had been shown to function normally

by cholecystography. It was left behind. Neither gall bladder contained stones.

3. Thirty-six cases of complete duplication, including the one herein recorded, have been reported up to the present time. Of this number, nine were discovered at post-mortem examination and twenty-seven at operation.

4. In the vast majority of cases, the symptoms have been those of cholecystitis and cholelithiasis. Seventy-five per cent of the patients have been women, and the age of onset of symptoms has ranged from 19 to 69 years, with an average age at onset of 43 years.

5. In approximately 75 per cent of the cases of complete duplication of the gall bladder, the cystic duct has also been completely duplicated. In the remaining cases, the cystic ducts have joined at a Y junction and have entered the common duct with a single opening.

6. Although it has occasionally been possible to remove a pathologic gall bladder and leave a normal one, the surgical management in the majority of symptomatic duplications has involved the removal of both gall bladders, either because both were diseased or because their relatively intimate approximation prevented selective removal.

REFERENCES

1. Alexander, R. E.: Roentgen Appearance of Double Gallbladder Simulated by Gallbladder With Congenitally Folded Fundus, Am. J. Roentgenol. **58:** 112, 1947.
2. Alfredo, J.: Ascaridiose e anomalia anatomica das vias biliares extrahepaticas, Rev. med. de Pernambuco **10:** 317, 1940.
3. Andreon, E.: Vesícula doble, Arch. urug. de med., cir. y especialid. **31:** 375, 1947.
4. Blasius, G.: Observata anatomica in Homine, variisque animalibus aliis, Amstelod. p.: 128, Tab. XV, Fig. XIII, 1674.
5. Boyden, E. A.: The Accessory Gall Bladder—An Embryological and Comparative Study of Aberrant Biliary Vesicles Occurring in Man and the Domestic Animals, Am. J. Anat. **38:** 177, 1926.
6. Braun, A.: Doppelbildung der Gallenblase, Zentralbl. f. Chir. **53:** 1055, 1926.
7. Croudace, W. H. H.: A Case of Double Gall-Bladder, Brit. M. J. **1:** 707, 1931.
8. Erdmann: Personal communication to Boyden, E. A., Am. J. Anat. **38:** 177, 1926.
9. Garofalo, F.: Un caso di cistifellea doppia, Bull. d. sc. med. **5:** 380, 1927.
10. Gross, R. E.: Congenital Anomalies of the Gallbladder; A Review of One Hundred and Forty-eight Cases With Report of a Double Gallbladder, Arch. Surg. **32:** 131, 1936.
11. Haberer, H.: Ueber Doppelung der Gallenblase, Arch. f. klin. Chir. **126:** 25, 1923.
12. Hermann, S. F., Hicks, G. S., and Martin, D. L.: Double Gallbladder, Arch. Surg. **27:** 905, 1933.
13. Holderman, H. H.: Double Gall-Bladder, Ann. Surg. **91:** 475, 1930.
14. Huber, J. J.: Acta Phys. Med Ac. Caes. **9:** 382, 1752.
15. Ingegno, A. P., and D'Albora, J. B.: Double Gallbladder, Am. J. Roentgenol. **61:** 671, 1949.
16. Jastrow, M., Jr., quoted by Boyden, E. A., Am. J. Anat. **38:** 177, 1926.
17. Kennon, R.: A Double Gall Bladder Opening by Two Cystic Ducts Into the Common Bile Duct, Brit. J. Surg. **20:** 522, 1933.
18. Lambert: Personal communication to Boyden, E. A., Am. J. Anat. **38:** 177, 1926.
19. Lamprecht, W.: Dopplungen der Gallenblase, Chirurg. **21:** 105, 1950.
20. Millbourn, E.: Ueber die doppelte Gallenblase, im Anschluss an zwei beobachtete Fälle, Acta. chir. Scandinav. **84:** 97, 1940.
21. Moore, T. C.: Congenital Atresia of the Extrahepatic Bile Ducts, Surg., Gynec. & Obst. **96:** 215, 1953.
22. Priesel, A.: Verdoppelung der Gallenblase beim Menschen, Virchows Arch. f. path. Anat. **265:** 76, 1927.
23. Purser: Liver With Two Gall-Bladders, Brit. M. J. **2:** 1102, 1886.
24. Nichols, B. H.: Double Gall-Bladder, Radiology **6:** 255, 1926.
25. Oldfield, M. C., and Wright, C. J. E.: Double Gallbladder, Brit. J. Surg. **38:** 116, 1950.

26. Petrina, E.: Un caso raro di duplice cistifellea, con doppio cistico, in uno dei quali trovasi un calcolo, Policlinico (sez. prat.) **37**: 1416, 1930.
27. Recht, W.: Torsion of a Double Gall-Bladder, Brit. J. Surg. **39**: 342, 1952.
28. Schachner, A.: Anomalies of the Gall Bladder and Bile Passages, Ann. Surg. **64**: 419, 1916.
29. Schulz, J.: Ein Beitrag zur Gallenstein chirurgie, Beitr. z. klin. Chir. **92**: 359, 1914.
30. Scott, W. R., Sanes, S., and Smith, H. A.: Cholecystographic Diagnosis of Double Gallbladder With Pathologic Verification, Radiology **37**: 492, 1941.
31. Sherren, J.: A Double Gall-Bladder Removed by Operation, Ann. Surg. **54**: 204, 1911.
32. Slaughter, F. G., and Trout, H. H.: Duplication of the Gall Bladder, Am. J. Surg. **19**: 124, 1933.
33. Strukow, A. J.: Zwei Gallenblasen beim Menschen, Centralbl. f. allg. Path. u. path. Anat. **50**: 420, 1931.
34. Wakeley, C. P. G.: A Double Gall-Bladder Removed by Operation, Brit. J. Surg. **15**: 334, 1927.
35. Weiss, S.: Diseases of the Liver, Gall-Bladder, Ducts and Pancreas, New York, 1935, Paul B. Hoeber, Inc.
36. Wilson, C. L.: Double Gallbladder With Two Cystic Ducts and Two Cystic Arteries, Ann. Surg. **110**: 60, 1939.
37. Wischnewsky, A. W.: Doppelgallenblase während der Operation aufgedeckt (Ektomie der erkrankten supplementären Blase), Arch. f. klin. Chir. **135**: 779, 1925.
38. Wittie: An Anatomical Observation Respecting a Stone in the Kidney, Philosophical Transactions (No. 207, p. 30, 1693-1694), Roy. Soc. London, vol. 3 (1683-1694), London, 1809, C. and R. Baldwin.
39. Wolfson, W. L.: Supernumerary Gall-Bladder, Am. J. Surg. **6**: 88, 1929.

Editorials

The Research and Development Board

ON JUNE 30, 1953, the Research and Development Board ceased to exist. Instead, its functions are now under an Assistant Secretary of Defense in charge of Research and Development. This announcement probably meant very little to the vast majority of persons in the medical profession, yet since 1948 this Board has advised the armed services in their research programs and has endorsed, increased, or decreased vast amounts of money for this purpose. Several of the committees of the Board had intimate association with medical affairs: atomic energy, biologic warfare, chemical warfare, human resources, and medical sciences, for example, and others somewhat more remotely.

"The committees function in broad technical fields to assist the Board in providing constructive guidance for the research and development activities of the Department of Defense."

The committees in turn appointed numerous panels: "Panels function in specific technical fields to assist committees in carrying out their responsibilities."

How the new organization will operate has not yet been officially determined. As one who has been intimately associated with the Panel on Military and Feld Medicine and also with the Committee on Medical Sciences since 1948, I want to take this opportunity to point out how this civilian group works with the services. True, the Committee on Medical Sciences overlapped other committees, made contact with the Armed Forces Medical Policy Council, and stretched out into the development of engineering devices and matériel, into the Quartermaster Department concerning clothing and its protective cooling effects in cold and hot climates, into the food laboratory in Chicago under the Quartermaster Department, and into the entomologic laboratory in Orlando, Fla., under the Department of Agriculture, with its important role in preventive medicine and public health.

The machines invented by man have now become so complicated and fearsome that some are well ahead of man's ability to cope with them. Therefore, we have a real interest in human engineering. These problems are being studied both from research and practical application at the Special Devices Center of the Navy and in the laboratories of the Air Force and the Naval Air Arm. In particular, the research of the Marine and Army laboratories has brought about revolutionary changes in the types and proportions of serious chest and abdominal wounds by the development of lightweight protective armor, which has met with such notable success in Korea concerning both protective and morale factors. The results have been a marked decrease in serious chest and abdominal wounds and a corresponding increase in multiple extremity wounds with the saving of lives. Building on these foundations and the report by the Board for the Study of the Severely Wounded in the North African Mediterranean theater of operation, surgical research teams are at work both in the field and laboratories of Korea and Japan and in the larger hospitals in this country, carefully studying and recording the altered physiology of the wounded, various and improved techniques in vascular repair and plasma expanders, the use of whole blood as carried forward by helicopters, and extensive studies in the treatment of burns.

These are but a few of the problems that are now the active concern of the medical departments of our armed forces, and all are of prime interest to the surgeon. Each year, members of the Committee have made a short tour of some of the laboratories and facilities where this work is being carried out, and some have also visited the battlefields of Korea and the hospitals and laboratories of Japan. It is essential that the armed forces maintain this program of research and that their work be expanded by further studies in their own hospitals and also through contracts with various medical schools and hospitals throughout the country. This research in human engineering and in many of the problems associated with trauma, mass casualties, and evacuation can only be performed by the services. They are our representatives and, as such, need the cooperation and help of each and all of us. What impresses one when traveling about, however, is the difficulty they operate under in the sense of continuity of personnel in problems of research. Except for the purely laboratory workers, a career pattern in research is difficult to assure, but this is necessary if worth-while and constructive research is to be performed, otherwise there will be mere repetition. This was evident in a recent tour of various facilities by members of the Committee on Medical Sciences. We found almost universal satisfaction with the assignments of personnel and considerable enthusiasm. On the other hand, it was evident that some ground was being replowed that had been tilled before.

Since the creation of the Board in 1948, there has been a steady increase in coordination, sharing of information, and joint participation in and sharing of benefits derived from the various research projects. Each service knows what the other is doing, and unnecessary duplication is gradually being eliminated. We on the civilian side can be of real assistance by scrutinizing closely and evaluating carefully our own research programs so as to be sure that they are not mere schemes to obtain easy money from the services.

Whether we like it or not, we are apparently in a state of expanded military activity on a semipermanent basis, so we had best make the most of it and use the opportunities afforded for the training of interns and residents during their tour of duty in the armed services. There is no reason why the various boards, for example, should not allow basic science, research, or laboratory credit for at least part of the time spent by the group of young men who are on these assignments. Many are doing just as good work with equally good leadership and as ample opportunities as they have in our own civilian hospitals for a similar period in their training. Furthermore, those in the armed services who are responsible for and in charge of the research programs will welcome sincere interest and suggestions from the civilian profession in helping carry forward this program so that it may bring true progress and not just change.

—*Frank B. Berry*

Cardiac Arrhythmia as a Predictable Surgical Risk

IT IS rather generally believed that heart disease is less certainly an insurmountable contraindication to surgical operations than disease of the liver or kidneys. This has become increasingly true as the understanding and treatment of congestive failure has improved. Indeed, there seems to be a trend to reduce the preoperative evaluation of the heart to the recognition of congestive failure. Evidence for this opinion is the often repeated assertion that cardiac reserve is adequate when the patient can sleep lying down and walk up a flight of stairs without dyspnea or pain. This eminently practical approach to the problem of heart disease was one of the first postulates of Sir Thomas Lewis, but it should be remembered that it was designed to evaluate heart function during the course of usual living. Recently it has been recognized that there is an increasing incidence of sudden failure or arrest of the heart during surgical operations. For the most part, these catastrophes have occurred in individuals without prior evidence of diminished tolerance to exercise.

The recognition of impending sudden failure or arrest of the heart has become a pressing obligation. Special problems arise with two classes of patients: those with aortic stenosis and those with first degree heart block.

Aortic stenosis predisposes to sudden death during surgical procedures. The lesion precludes effective cardiac support of the peripheral circulation when blood volume is reduced by surgical blood loss. Furthermore, alarming hypotension and ineffective coronary circulation may result from the diminished peripheral resistance of general anesthesia or anoxia. The clinical recognition of aortic stenosis fortunately presents few difficulties.

First degree heart block can be recognized only by measurement of the P-R interval on an electrocardiographic record. It is an ominous finding because of the hazard of complete auriculoventricular dissociation and ventricular standstill during surgical or anesthetic stress. Digitalis, quinidine, and Novocain increase the likelihood of these complications. Ephedrine-like compounds offer considerable promise in the treatment of delayed conduction time, but their most effective utilization requires further study. It is not uncommon for patients to present coexisting first degree heart block, congestive failure, and severe anemia. Under such circumstances, careful digitalization with short-acting glucosides may be necessary to permit correction of the anemia with concentrated red cells. Withdrawal of digitalis is often possible after anemia is corrected and is an indicated preoperative safeguard. It is also helpful to have established the response to Adrenalin before operation.

There remains for consideration a group of patients destined to develop cardiac arrhythmia during operation in spite of a normal exercise tolerance, no aortic stenosis, and no heart block. Prophylactic quinidine has fallen from favor because of undesirable side effects and because of a growing conviction that cardiac arrest in a quinidinized patient is especially refractory to restoration of cardiac rhythm by massage. The logical approach to this problem is the more careful scrutiny of cardiac function throughout the period of anesthetic and surgical stress. The cathode-ray oscillograph and the pulse tachometer have proved helpful to us for this purpose. It is surprising how frequently in elderly patients, during induction and intubation, there occurs a series of ventricular premature beats comparable to those seen regularly during manipulation of the mitral valve. Such evidence of cardiac irritability seems likely to have prognostic import, aside from its sobering influence on the anesthetist.

A further virtue in the constantly visualized electrocardiographic record is the sound basis for selection of drugs for specific arrhythmias: Cedilanid for supraventricular tachycardias, Novocain compounds for ventricular premature beats, and ephedrine compounds for prolonged conduction defects. Such precise therapy, with immediate observation of its effectiveness, has obvious advantages over blind therapy and renders questionable the use of a combination of Novocain and Adrenalin. The oscillograph not only provides immediate and certain evidence of cardiac arrest, but also defines impending and established ventricular fibrillation with great clarity.

It seems reasonable to conclude that evaluation of the cardiac risk during surgery should include, in addition to the exercise tolerance test, some consideration of the vulnerability of the heart to arrhythmia. It is suggested that a continuous electrocardiographic record during anesthetic induction may permit recognition of an irritable heart with postponement of the operation and more careful preparation. It also seems likely that early recognition and appropriate treatment of incipient irregularities may reduce the incidence of ultimate cardiac arrests.

—*Champ Lyons*

Recent Advances in Surgery

CONDUCTED BY ALFRED BLALOCK, M.D.

RIB FRACTURES FROM MUSCULAR EFFORT WITH PARTICULAR REFERENCE TO COUGH

VINCENT J. DERBES, M.D., AND THOMAS HARAN, M.S. IN C. E.,
NEW ORLEANS, LA.

(From the Department of Medicine, Tulane University, School of Medicine, and the Ochsner Clinic)

THE appearance of pleural pain following cough may be the result of fracture of one or more ribs. Although such fractures are not extremely common, they are certainly not rare, and the possibility of their occurence is especially to be considered in the presence of otherwise unexplained pleural pain. Some idea of the incidence of these fractures may be obtained from several investigators. In an interesting study of 500 patients with atypical pneumonia in an Army station hospital made by Harvey[72] in 1942-1943, 19 had recent rib fractures; excluding one with a history of trauma, there remained an incidence of 3.6 per cent. Many of these had been overlooked at the original examination. The serial studies made during the course of the pneumonia would often reveal a callus, and review of the earlier films showed fracture lines at the same site. In several cases reviewed, these fractures were quite apparent, but the attention of the examiner was centered on the more obvious inflammatory process in the lungs. In an analysis[116] of 1,194 incipient cases of tuberculosis, there was one patient with a rib fracture (0.08 per cent); among 601 moderately advanced cases, there were 12 patients with rib fractures (2 per cent); and among 108 far-advanced cases, there were 7 with rib fractures (6.5 per cent). Oechsli,[105] who routinely examined patients for rib fractures, found 22 (0.7 per cent) with such fractures in 3,000 admissions to Olive View Sanatorium. A careful search for fractures of the rib following cough among 64 patients with pleural pain in whom no other cause was apparent was made by Mitchell; of these, 14 (21.9 per cent) had fractured ribs.

HISTORY

The first instance of rib fracture produced by coughing that could be found in the literature is the one reported by Gooch[61] in 1773. His patient suffered from necrosis of a rib caused by a kick. When nearly recovered, he fractured a rib on the opposite side during a paroxysm of coughing. Monteggia[100] in 1802 reported seing a man of about 50 years of age who had fractured a rib while coughing. The sound produced at the moment of fracture was heard by all in the room.

Received for publication, June 30, 1953.

In 1834, R. J. Graves[63] of Dublin reported in excellent detail what he considered to be the first case of this nature.

A 47 year old woman, tall and unusually strong and muscular for a female, had a violent fit of coughing 5 days previous during which she suddenly felt a stitch in the left side, with a sensation of something snapped or given way. The pain was so severe and so affected her breath she sought professional advice when some leeches and afterwards a blister were applied without relief. Inspiration was painful and pain radiated down to the left kidney and up to the right shoulder. The central point of tenderness was at the midpoint of the 9th or 10th rib and that from which the pain radiated was situated not between the ribs but on one of them. Pressure made at exactly this spot could scarcely be tolerated. She had observed that she was much easier during the days when her stays were on, than at night when she had unlaced and taken them off. A compress and roller over the part affected afforded immediate relief. Altogether the case is instructive not merely for its singularity, but because it affords a useful lesson with regard to the extreme importance of making an accurate examination of every disease before we hazard an opinion concerning its nature.

The following year at Val-de-Grace at the examination of a patient suffering from chronic pneumonia, Broussais[26] found a painless tumor, the size of a pigeon's egg, on the fourth rib; crepitus was elicited and a fracture was diagnosed.

In 1838, the scholarly and erudite surgeon Malgaigne[89] published a most impressive survey of the medieval and ancient medical literature on fractured ribs; he had been able to collect 7 cases. Early case reports were also published by Nankivell (1836),[103] Bérard (1841),[15] Hilton (1852),[74] Denonvillier (1853),[39] and Hérard (1855).[73]

In 1860, Gurlt[67] recorded 14 instances of rib fracture from muscular action; 10 of these were from coughing, 1 from a repressed sneeze, and 1 each from turning in bed, mounting a restless horse, and through an effort to maintain bodily equilibrium.

In 1882, Mazeillé[94] published a series of 24 cases including one previously unreported. In 1890, the list was extended by Tunis[132] to a total of 40 rib fractures from muscular action. In more recent times Wahl[134] (1926) collected 66 cases (including 3 personal cases). Oechsli[105] (1936) reported 22 personal cases and Mitchell[99] (1951), 14 personal instances.

ETIOLOGY

Rib fractures from muscular effort occur as the result of the most varied circumstances but especially following a violent paroxysm of coughing. The most frequently identified cause of the cough in the reported cases has been tuberculosis, but it is likely that the frequency of roentgenographic examination of tuberculous persons accounts for this apparent excess. Thus, Cohen[36] reported 7 such instances, Richardson[116] 30, Oechsli[105] 22, and Webb[135] 3. Richardson[116] stated that there were ten times as many such fractures in patients with advanced as in those with incipient tuberculosis. It is true that as the disease worsens the cough becomes of greater severity and frequency; prolonged bed rest predisposes to osteoporosis.

Mazeillé[94] considered bronchitis the chief cause of rib fractures; certainly a large number of isolated instances have been ascribed to acute or chronic bronchitis, influenza, coryza, infections of the upper respiratory tract, and the like. Bronchial asthma is not infrequently mentioned. Laryngeal irritation from aspirated foreign matter has been the cause of rib fractures in 2 or 3 reported cases. In one young woman, both eleventh ribs were fractured during a paroxysm of whooping cough.

Sneezing has been blamed for the broken rib in several reports in the literature. One concerned the patient of Castella[31] (1861), a powerful 39-year-old Swiss hotelkeeper. Although he did not use snuff, on one occasion he took a pinch of it from a guest. After sneezing repeatedly, he attempted unsuccessfully to suppress the act by expanding his thorax with his mouth closed. A powerful exhalation followed, after which there was a definite crack accompanied by pain and difficulty in breathing. In explaining his case, Wyman[138] (1885) remarked that in the act of sneezing two powerful sets of muscles may be brought into antagonism in such a way as to expend their opposed forces on the ribs, making the fracture simply a mechanical matter. Podrazki[112] reported the case of a strong healthy lady ''of some thirty years'' who fractured the tenth costal cartilage while sneezing.

It is well known that coughing often follows vigorous laughter. Speed[126] and Palfrey[106] as well as Breslin[23] have called attention to rib fracture under such circumstances. Muscle strain incident to straining at stool or vomiting has also resulted in this accident.

Bones have been broken as a result of intervention of muscles not primarily concerned with respiration; these may act alone or in conjunction with those involved in such physiologic acts as are discussed in the preceding paragraphs. Thus, the patient of Atkinson[10] fractured a rib after coughing while in the act of hanging up his coat; Somerset[124] reported the case of a patient who fractured a rib after coughing while removing her stays; in Seilin's[121] report, the rib fracture followed cough while the patient was attempting to close a window. The patient of Fisk[54] after a sudden violent cough felt a rib break while sitting sidewise on a chair, with his legs crossed, his right arm and his hands clasped on the back of the chair. Groninger's[64] patient made an effort to right himself to prevent falling while walking home, with immediate pain and dyspnea resulting. Aitken and Lincoln[4] reported the instance of a well-developed and -nourished white man aged 29 years who with a cardboard box on his head was climbing a ladder; the box slipped, and to maintain balance he jerked his head suddenly to the right, thereby fracturing the left first rib. Analogous perhaps are those accidents induced by suddenly turning in bed or attempting to mount a restless horse. Rectification of asymmetrical posture seemed operative in the instance of Michael-Phillip's[97] young woman who had been out earlier with her young man. On arising from the bank on which they had been sitting, she felt something snap "like a twig"; a rib fracture was demonstrated roentgenographically.

A frequent complaint of occasional golfers is soreness or tenderness over the lower left ribs and upper abdomen. These might well be symptoms of fractured ribs. Two medical colleagues fractured ribs on the golf links, and a similar accident was at first thought to be due to coronary artery disease (Case 2). Fractured ribs are also said to be common among scullers; Arnold[9] reported a broken rib from a medicine ball workout, and Mandl[91] one from the Telemarkschwung in skiing.

When one is set to perform some action requiring heightened muscular activity which does not eventuate, rib fractures may occur. Chenery's[34] old but active farmer broke three ribs when a root which he was pulling up gave way, causing him to sit suddenly on a rock behind him. Kevin Byrne[28] described a case in which muscular effort alone accounted for six badly fractured ribs, three on each side. His patient was tossing cabbages with a pitchfork, and a particularly heavy forkful slipped off as he started to toss; the anticipated exertion was used on the lightened load. Perhaps the case of Nancrede[102] is parallel. The patient was a healthy vigorous laborer who fractured the second rib while trying to straighten a scythe blade; he was holding it down with one hand while lifting the free end with a monkey wrench held in the other hand when the accident took place.

SEX

There is no doubt that in instances in which these fractures are due to violent muscular action other that that involved in coughing or sneezing, men are definitely more prone to these injuries. Also, men are more often exposed to physical trauma, and fractures of all sorts from external violence predominate in men. This is not the case when the responsible forces derive from physiologic or quasiphysiologic activities (coughing, sneezing, vomiting, straining at stool, parturition). In 140 such instances in which the sex was noted, there were 85 women and only 55 men.

AGE

On a priori grounds, it might be anticipated that increasing age would incline to a heightened incidence of rib fractures. In addition to their greater dependence and helplessness, as a rule there is in aged individuals progressive atrophy of bones resulting from senile osteoporosis. Increasing calcification of the costal cartilages and the tendency to ankylotic fusion of the ribs with the vertebral column lead to reduced elasticity of the thoracic cage. Moreover, the wasting with senescence of muscles which formerly protected the ribs exposes them especially to indirect as well as to direct violence. The fact seems to be, however, that this very decrease in muscularity precludes the development of stresses adequate to break the now more predisposed ribs.

On the other hand, in youthful individuals the elasticity of the ribs affords a significant measure of protection. In quite young people, rib fractures from muscular action alone must be extraordinarily rare. One exception must be made. Cough develops in patients with progressive rickets, and this cough may occur in paroxysms. In a study of 32 children, ranging in age from 8 months to 4½ years, who suffered from severe rickets, Park and Howland[109] found rib fractures almost regularly present. In one case, 20 were counted. Although these fractures were often not apparent on physical examination, the roentgenograms of the patients studied by Park and Howland characteristically showed remarkably slender porous-appearing ribs. Pospischill[114] described a "dozen" instances of fractured ribs in autopsies of children who died from whooping cough; perhaps they also had rickets. In the 113 reported cases in which the age was specified, the youngest was a 16-year-old girl; 3 were 18-year-old and two 19-year-old women. The majority of the remainder occurred in patients in the third to sixth decade. Thus, the likelihood of rib fracture from muscular action is greatest from 20 to 50 years of life, that is, when the resiliency of extreme youth is lost but the feebleness of advanced years is not yet apparent (Table I).

TABLE I. DISTRIBUTION OF RIB FRACTURES BY AGE AND SEX

	AGE (YEARS)							
	10-19	20-29	30-39	40-49	50-59	60-69	70-79	TOTAL
Men	2	5	8	12	6	4	4	41
Women	6	18	16	14	10	6	2	72
Totals	8	23	24	26	16	10	6	113

PREGNANCY

In the literature there are reports of 24 rib fractures during pregnancy, all of which occurred in the last trimester, but only two during labor. Ahern's (1894)[3] patient, a strong, healthy woman in labor with her third child, sustained a fracture of the left sixth rib a little in front of the anterior axillary line when she was seized with a violent fit of coughing during a severe pain accompanied by powerful expulsive efforts. Freeland's (1895)[57] case, which seems to have escaped general attention, is quoted because of its interesting features: "A black woman of Herculean frame, who in a long pain during parturition fractured the eighth and ninth ribs on the left side. I was present when the accident occurred, and the loud report I heard when the bones gave away proves, I think, that although the ribs were large, solid, and fixed they were not strong enough to resist the powerful action that was being exerted by this unusually muscular woman."

Reference to Table II will show, as noted by Paulley and co-workers,[111] that in these cases the fractures occur late in pregnancy, tend to be left-sided, and affect chiefly the lower ribs. Paulley and co-workers also pointed out that multiple fractures are exceptional under such circumstances, but this observation is not confirmed in the present series.

Cazeau[32] asserted that there is an increase of fragility of the ribs in pregnancy because of fetal demands on maternal calcium. This idea has been alluded to repeatedly by later writers on the subject, but it was first studied critically by Paulley and co-workers. Their comparisons of bone density with controls of the same sex and age revealed slight osteoporosis in only one case; blood calcium and phosphorus estimations were within normal limits. Barr (1949)[13] is of the opinion that some degree of decalcification may be present late in pregnancy although it is not revealed by roentgenographic or blood chemistry studies. Lachmann and Whelan[82] experimentally removed calcium by acid and studied roentgenographically the bones before and afterward. It is clear from their results that normal roentgenograms do not exclude osteoporosis, for only under favorable circumstances can decalcification of less than 20 per cent be diagnosed roentgenologically. In most bones, including the ribs, the calcium loss, in order to be visible, must be in the vicinity of 20 to 40 per cent.

TABLE II. SUMMARY OF REPORTED RIB FRACTURES DURING PREGNANCY

SOURCE	AGE (YR.) AND PARITY	DURATION OF PREGNANCY	SITE OF FRACTURE (RIB)	EXCITING CAUSE
Adkins (1949)	36	1 week before confinement	Left 7th and 8th	Cough
Ahern (1894)	Multipara	In labor	Left 6th	Coughing paroxysm
Barr (1949)	26	36 weeks	Left 11th	Coughed while rising from bed
Benoît		9th month	Left 9th	Coughing fit from chronic bronchitis
Blanc (1908)	37	End of pregnancy	Multiple	Cough
Brookhouse (1879)	36	Late pregnancy	Left 6th	Coughed while sitting sideways
Chenery (1878)	23			Coughing fit
Dogadkin (1885)	27; multipara	10th month	Left 8th	Bronchitis
Evans (1949)	Late 20's; multipara	8th month	Left 8th and 9th	
Freeland (1895)		In labor	Left 8th and 9th	Straining with hard pain
Hérard (1855)	22	7th month	Mid ⅓ of left 11th	Violent cough from chronic bronchitis
Inglima (1938)	29	Last of pregnancy	Left 9th	Coughing fit (acute bronchitis)
Miall (1871)	29	7th month	10th	Violent paroxysm of coughing
Paulley, Lees, and Pearson (1949)	21; primipara	36 weeks	Left 10th	Coughing fit (chronic bronchitis)
	25; multipara	38 weeks	Left 9th and 10th	Coughing mildly
	36; multipara	40 weeks	Left 11th	Lifting and coughing
	25; multipara	29 weeks	Left 11th	Coughing after previous choking
Telhouni (1937)	40; multipara	8 months	Left 11th	Asthmatic attack
Trillat and Pizzera (1932)	34; primipara	8 months	Left 10th	
	27; multipara	8 months	Right 11th and 12th	Bronchitis
	32; multipara	4 days before delivery	Right 11th and left 7th	Bronchitis
	35; primipara		Left 11th	
Vidal (1894)	32; multipara	7th month	Left 10th	Bronchitis
Wynn-Williams (1951)	28	6 months	Right 6th	Coughing from respiratory tract infection

In any case, gestation does not retard consolidation in spite of the classic conception to the contrary; in the case reports in which comment was made, healing was noted to progress normally even before delivery.

The presence or absence of increased fragility of bones in late pregnancy would in no way explain the left-sided preponderance of these fractures. It has been suggested that the position of the liver seems to protect the right ribs, the net effect of the blow being delivered against the lower left ribs. Paulley and co-workers considered that the laterality was favored by the bulky uterus being driven violently upward and backward with forceful contractions of the abdominal muscles in coughing or sneezing. They further called attention to the posteral alterations in the pregnant state: compensatory to the backward thrust of the head and shoulders is a lordosis with increased tone of the sacrospinalis. In their view, incoordinate action in association with depression of the lower ribs by the iliocostalis could provide conditions for a shearing stress sufficient to fracture a lower rib. Telhouni[128] commented on the exaggerated distension of the abdomen in advanced pregnancy and on the derangements provoked thereby in the last ribs; thus the direction of forces generally applied by the ribs is modified, at times deleteriously. None of these speculations is satisfactory, and it may well be that the explanation can be found in a combination of these with as yet unappreciated factors.

SITE AND NUMBER OF THE FRACTURES

Fractures resulting from cough have been reported in every rib, but rarely occur in the uppermost and lowermost ribs. The first rib is, however, frequently the site of fracture from muscle stress unrelated to cough. Most fractures are found in the fifth through the tenth ribs (Table III). As a rule (102 of 142 instances), a single rib is involved. In 15 patients, two ribs were broken; in 12 patients, three ribs; four and six were broken in four instances each; and eight were broken in one person. There are a number of reports in which it is clear that in multiple rib fractures not all of the ribs break simultaneously. Edgecombe's[49] patient sustained a fracture on the left side; one week later a second break took place on the right. The second fracture in Halliwell's[68] case occurred sixteen days after the first. Evans'[51] patient felt the second rib crack with a subsequent bout of coughing about twenty minutes after the first. In the case reported by Swineford and McKinnon[127] there were eight independent rib fractures during one single bout of upper respiratory tract infection.

TABLE III. DISTRIBUTION OF RIB FRACTURES BY SITE INVOLVED

LOCATION	RIB												TOTALS
	1	2	3	4	5	6	7	8	9	10	11	12	
Right side	0	0	1	2	9	15	19	10	9	4	5	1	75
Left side	1	1	0	2	7	21	18	16	14	8	6	0	94
Totals	1	1	1	4	16	36	37	26	23	12	11	1	169

Analysis of the location of fractures in the cases reported in the literature suggests that those in the first rib seem conditioned by the attachment of the scalene muscles as well as by the subclavian groove. There were too few fractures in the second, third, and fourth ribs to elaborate on this point. There was a definite increase in incidence of fractures between the anterior and posterior axillary lines from the fifth through the ninth ribs.

They were less commonly found mesiad to this area and were definitely rare adjacent to the cartilages and vertebral column.

Reference to Table III shows that in those instances in which the side involved was noted, there was a moderate preference for the left. In the 134 case reports in which this point was recorded, 7 patients had bilateral fractures, the remainder (approximately 93 per cent) having but one side involved. The discrepancies in the various totals stem from the lack of detail in many instances.

PSYCHOSOMATIC FACTORS

The old-fashioned fault of carelessness and its counterpart carefulness have been replaced in more modern circles by accident proneness and compulsive behavior. Much has been written on accident proneness as a cause of fractures.[30, 45, 46] Only one reference was found to emotional or psychosomatic factors in the reported cases of rib fracture. In a letter to the editor of the *British Medical Journal,* Harold[70] wrote: "A young female, after some months estrangement from her boy friend met him again, was lovingly embraced, and soon after experienced what she described as a sharp pleuritic pain in the chest. Medical opinion was nonplussed for three days when an x-ray revealed a fractured lower rib. Could this, sir, be etiologically ascribed to emotional trauma?"

THEORIES

It is generally agreed that muscular contraction can fracture healthy ribs, but there is no unanimity either as to the precise muscles involved or to their method of action. In general, it is supposed that the accident takes place by virtue of opposed forces. Seilin[121] invoked the simultaneous contraction of the diaphragm and the upward pull of the latissimus dorsi. Tunis also believed that the diaphragm was a major factor, together with the other powerful muscles attached to the ribs. Oechsli,[105] whose views are most widely accepted, excluded the diaphragm from consideration because the attachments of this muscle do not correspond to the location of the fractures. In his cases, these fractures were found in a line extending from a point 4 cm. from the costochondral articulation of the fourth rib obliquely caudad and laterally to the ninth rib in midaxillary line. This line, he stated, corresponds to the interdigitations of the external oblique and the serratus anterior. The contrasting contractions of these muscles, in his view, produce the fractures.

Malgaigne[89] invoked torque: "in powerful inspiration preceding cough, slight torsion which the elevation of the sternum produces on ribs is not completely executed because of ossification of cartilages; bones are ruptured because they cannot yield." Telhouni[128] also favored the concept of torsion. Parenti[108] thought that the site of the fractures was conditioned by the moment of curvature which is greatest posteriorly near the region of the angle, and anteriorly near the costochondral junction.

Sustained tetanic contractions are quite capable of breaking bones; such fractures may appear in 35 per cent of patients subjected to electric shock therapy,[95] or in 23 per cent of those treated with Metrazol.[47] Fractures have also been reported in tetanus: in the ribs and vertebral column,[84, 117] elbow,[125] femoral neck,[12] and forearm.[137]

Moreover, it is by now well established that repeated subminimal trauma may produce fracture, particularly of weight-bearing bones. Large numbers of such fractures have been reported under various names (March fracture, March foot, Deutschländer's disease, Pied forcé, fracture de recrue) ever since World War I, although they were known earlier.[22] This mechanism has been called on to explain rib fracture from coughing, a view which has been championed especially by Zur.[140] He doubts that such fractures come about from a particularly strong cough, feeling it more likely that they are instances of "schleichende Frakturen" (creeping fractures). Alderson,[6] too, considered stress from repeated contraction of the scalenes to be a plausible explanation of breaks of the first rib appearing after strenuous physical training. The constant location of the fracture line in relation to the insertion of the scalene muscle is invoked as the explanation of rib fractures following thoracoplasty in the report of Guggenheim and Cohn.[65] They analyzed 208 cases of thoracoplasty in which fractures of the first or second rib or both occurred on the contralateral side in eight patients. After operation, the pull of the muscles on the first and second ribs is unopposed by similar muscles on the side operated on. The fractures did not take place during or immediately after the operation. The authors commented that it was noteworthy that all fractures with one exception occurred in the area of greatest muscular stress and where the bone structure was thinnest due to the subclavian grooves. Further reference to these points is made in the structural analysis section.

STRUCTURAL ANALYSIS OF RIB FRACTURES FROM MUSCULAR CONTRACTION

Before the structural analysis is discussed, it is considered best to define, from an engineering standpoint, those terms which may be used differently in other fields. When a force is applied to an object, the object is subjected to *stress;* the fundamental stresses may act singly or in combination. The diagrams in Fig. 1 illustrate these stresses, which are called *tension, compression* (direct stresses), *shear,* and *bending.* As a result of these stresses the object undergoes *deformation;* this deformation is called *strain. Enlongation* is the strain which results from tensile stresses; under compression the body is shortened; as a result of shearing stress, one part of the body tends to slide past the other. When one prunes a branch in his garden, he is subjecting the branch to a shearing stress.

In order to facilitate and simplify the engineering analysis, an object is isolated from its surroundings by means of a *free body diagram* which permits the application of vectors to those points at which forces are acting. This principle is shown in Fig. 2.

A moment, mathematically defined, is $\int(x\text{-}a)^k dm$, where dm is the differential of measure over the appropriate portion of space. In engineering it is customary for k to be 1 or 2, that is, for the first and second moments only to be used. The first moment is the moment of a force; the second is the moment of inertia.

The *moment of a force* ("moment") with respect to a point is the tendency of the force to turn or rotate about the given point. This tendency to rotate is expressed as the force times the perpendicular distance from the line of action of the force, as illustrated in Fig. 3. In this analysis, three basic

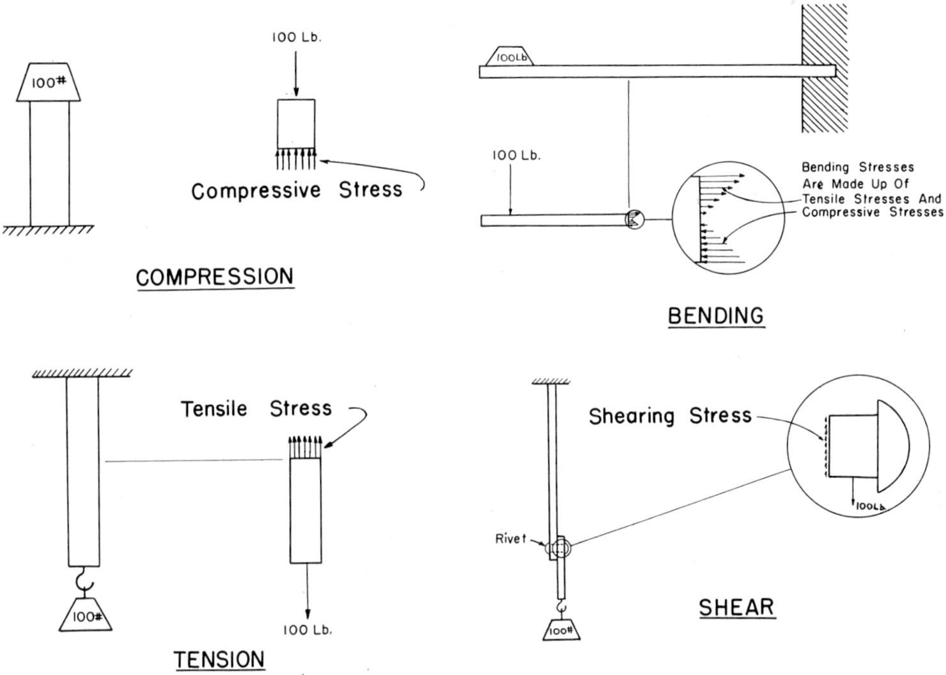

Fig. 1.—The fundamental stresses.

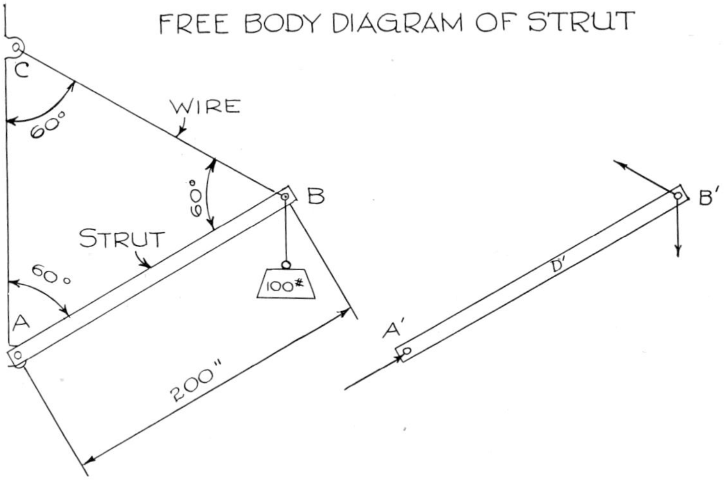

Fig. 2.—Free body diagram of strut.

laws of static equilibrium have been used: (1) summation of horizontal forces acting on a free body equals zero, $\Sigma F_x = 0$; (2) summation of vertical forces acting on a free body equals zero, $\Sigma F_y = 0$; (3) summation of moments of forces acting on a free body about any point in the free body equals zero, $\Sigma M = 0$. In the free body diagram of the strut, which represents a condition of static equilibrium, these principles can be applied to solve for the unknown forces acting on the body as shown in Fig. 4.

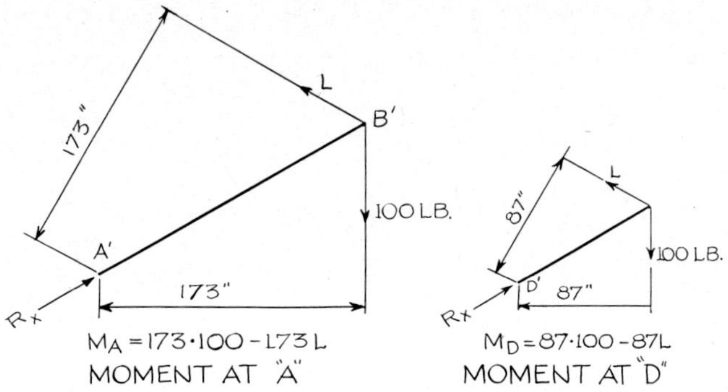

Fig. 3.—Example of computations of moment of a force with respect to points "*A*" and "*D*."

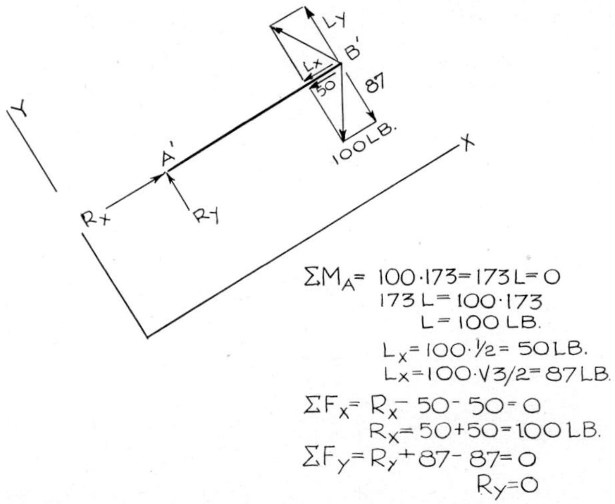

Fig. 4.—Computation of unknown forces. R_X and R_Y are reactions with respect to the *x* and *y* axes; L_X and L_Y are components of *L* with respect to the *x* and *y* axes; F_X and F_Y are the resultant forces on the *x* and *y* axes.

Of the reported rib fractures from muscular action, the sixth rib was involved the greatest number of times and, therefore, this one was selected for the structural analysis. The first step was to draw a free body diagram of this rib and solve for the reactions. (See Fig. 5.) *Reactions* in this sense are resultant forces at the supports of the ribs, that is, the costochondral junction and vertebral column due to muscular action. At various points along the rib, imaginary cross sections were established and stresses were computed at these points. These stresses consisted of shearing stresses, tensile stresses, compressive stresses, and bending stresses. For example, in order to compute the stress in Section 4, a free body diagram was established for the portion of the rib extending from the vertebral column to Section 4. The free body diagram and computations of stresses at Section 4 are shown in Fig. 6. Bending stress was computed from the formula $f = \frac{M}{S}$ in which S is the *section modulus,* M the moment at the section, and f the extreme bending stress. The section modulus is the *moment of inertia* divided by ½d. For

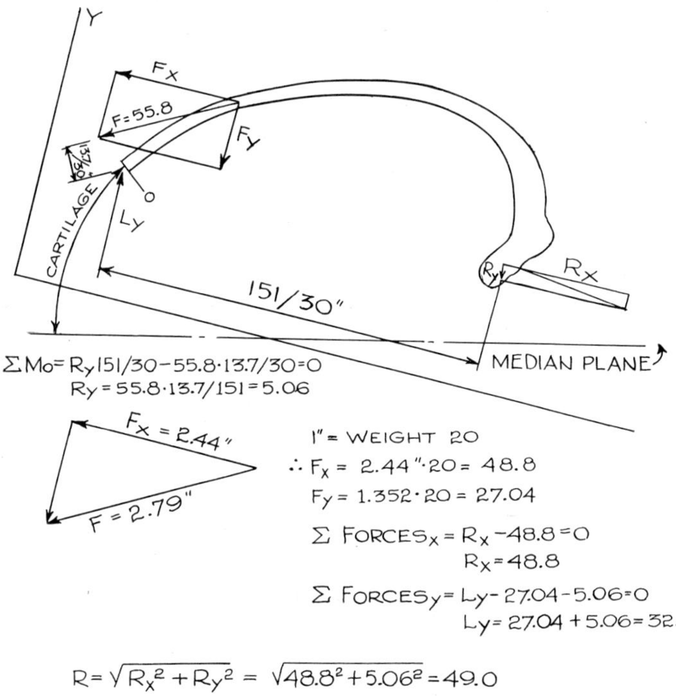

Fig. 5.—Free body diagram of sixth rib with calculations of reactions at costochondral and costovertebral junctions.

the purposes of calculating stresses, the rib sections were assumed to possess properties of equivalent ellipses. Table IV summarizes the values obtained from computations at the various sections indicated. It should be noted that direct stresses and bending stresses at the same section are additive. In Fig. 7 is shown the variation of the combined direct and bending stresses along the rib. The variation of shear stresses is shown in Fig. 8. In each case the relative magnitude of the stresses at the various sections is represented by the distance from the center line of the rib to the curve. Sites of reported fractures are indicated on the ribs themselves. The incidence of fractures in each zone is indicated by encircled numbers. Fractures are of greatest frequency in those areas where bending stress is greatest; they are of least frequency where shearing stress is maximal. Torsion is not believed to be present, but if there were any torsion present it would be in the portion

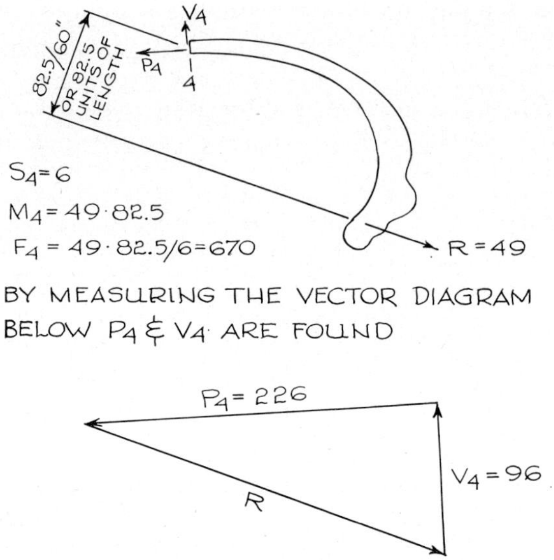

Fig. 6.—Free body diagram with computations of stresses at Section 4.

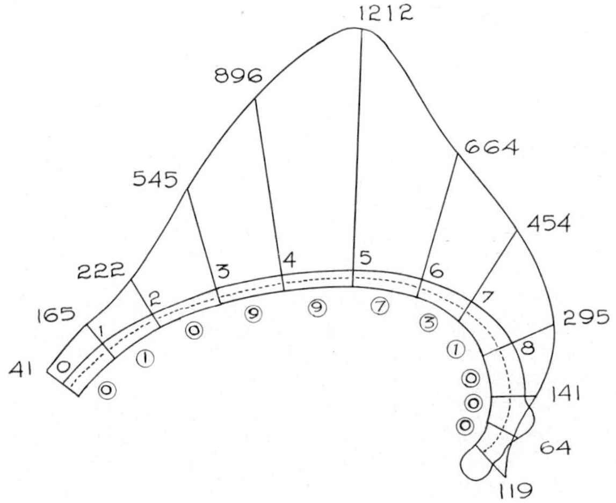

Fig. 7.—Variation of combined direct and bending stresses along the rib. See text.

of the rib extending from Section 7 posteriorly; fracture produced by torsion in this portion would tend to assume a helical path.

The actual fracture may be the result of a gradual failure of the rib due to a progressive cracking across a given section. Even though the stress at this section may be computed to be below the *elastic limit,* stress concentrations in minute regions occasionally exceed the elastic limit. The elastic limit is the maximum stress to which a material can be subjected without any permanent deformation. Prior to the development of a crack, there is a period of inelastic deformation which is graphically illustrated in Fig. 9. Cracks are

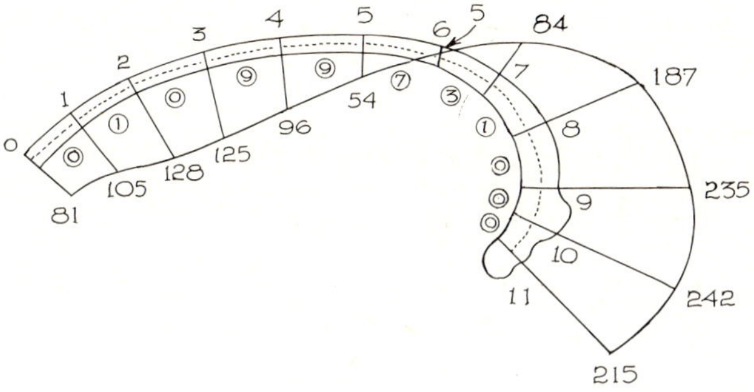

Fig. 8.—Variation of shear stresses. See text.

thus started which reduce the cross-sectional area resulting in an increase in maximum stress, as illustrated in Fig. 10. This cycle is repeated with progressive reduction in area of intact bone, which may suddenly snap. Throughout the failure, the region of high stress has always been so small that the deformation does not extend sufficiently to become apparent. This mechanism is illustrated by those patients in whom a definite localized area of tenderness persists for several days prior to audible fracture at this site.

TABLE IV. VALUES OBTAINED FROM STRESS COMPUTATIONS AT DESIGNATED SECTIONS OF SIXTH RIB

SECTION	S*	y*	M*	f*	P*	A*	p*	f + p*	V*	v*
0	18	0	0	0	141	1	141	141	81	81
1	18	22.5	735	40.9	124	1	124	165	105	105
2	14	52.5	1710	122	100	1	100	222	128	128
3	9	61.5	3000	333	212	1	212	545	125	125
4	6	82.5	4020	670	226	1	226	896	96	96
5	5	98.6	4860	972	240	1	240	1212	54	54
6	12	103.0	5030	419	245	1	245	664	5	5
7	21	96.5	4710	224	230	1	230	454	84	84
8	27	76.0	3710	137	158	1	158	295	187	187
9	30	44.0	2150	72	69	1	69	141	235	235
10	30	20.5	1000	33.3	31	1	31	64	242	242
11	30	0	0	0	119	1	119	119	215	215

*Symbol notation:
S = Section modulus,
y = Perpendicular distance from center of section to the line of action of the reaction at support,
M = Bending moment at section,
f = Maximum bending stress at section,
P = Direct force on section,
p = Direct stress on section (p = P/A),
A = Cross-sectional area of rib, which is taken as 1 since it is practically constant at all sections,
V = Shearing force on section,
v = Shearing stress on section.

In the foregoing analysis, certain assumptions were made initially.

1. The weight of the rib was assumed to be negligible. This would not have altered the location of the maximum stress.
2. The support of the rib at the vertebral column was assumed to act as a hinge joint.

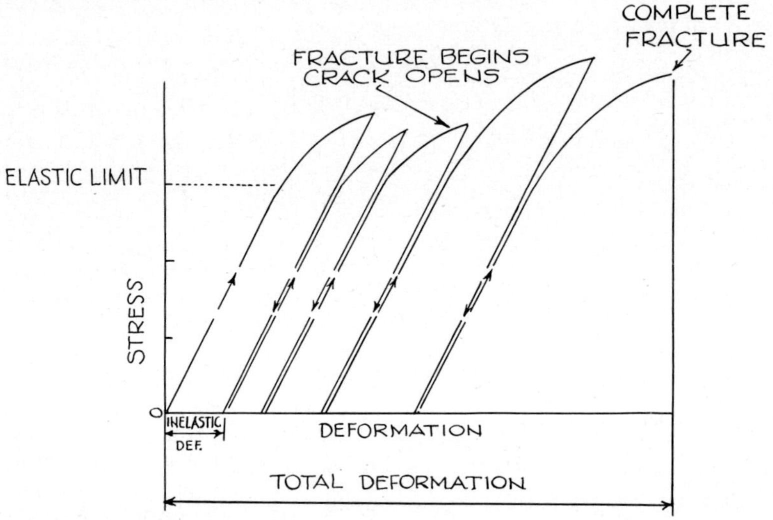

Fig. 9.—Stress-strain diagram. In coughing, the rib returns to its initial dimensions, the zero position, as long as the elastic limit is not exceeded. When the elastic limit is exceeded, it no longer returns to the zero position but a certain small amount of permanent set takes place which is indicated by *inelastic deformation.* Each time the elastic limit is exceeded, the inelastic deformation is increased. Ultimately the rib breaks.

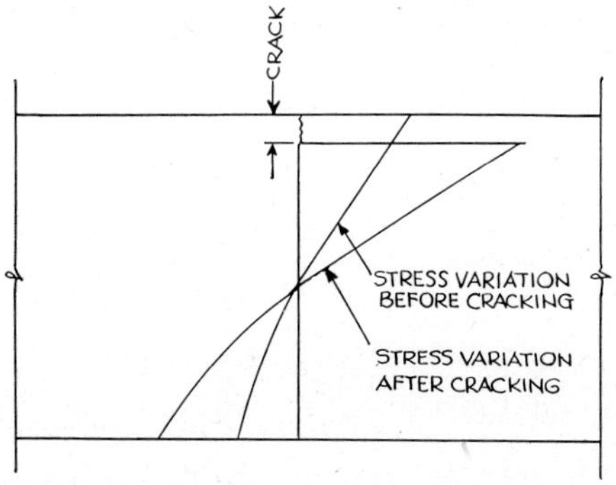

Fig. 10.—Example of change in stress variation caused by small crack in rib. The parallel horizontal lines represent the upper and lower margins of the much enlarged rib. It will be seen that prior to the crack the displacement of the stress line from the vertical is considerably less than after the cracking has begun. As the depth of the crack increases, the maximum stress in the remaining intact bone is progressively increased. Finally, complete fracture results.

3. The anterior support was taken to be at the costochondral junction; the moment induced by the cartilage was considered to be negligible.
4. It was assumed that the rib was supported only at its extremities.
5. It was assumed that there was no chance of failure in a vertical plane because of the uniform action of the intercostals and also because of the ratio of the depth of the vertical plane to the depth of the horizontal plane of the rib. Strength varies directly with the cube of the depth.

6. It was assumed that the section modulus was proportional to the outside dimension of the rib, that is, that the ratio of the cross-sectional areas of the compact bone to the cross-sectional areas of the cancellous bone did not vary and that the cancellous bone trabeculae were uniformly distributed. Consequently, stress units are of arbitrary dimension.
7. It was considered that muscle force is directly proportional to its effective cross section,[50] and that in addition the Muskelkrafteinheit of Fick[53] (10 kg. per square centimeter) is valid in so far as it permits contractile forces of various muscles to be compared. This force has been estimated by Franke[55] to be 11 kg. per square centimeter.
8. It is clear that a number of variables are also involved in the area of cross section of the respiratory muscles, variations not alone from age, sex, and muscularity of the individual, but also from the effect of the incident disease. As a standard, the *Cross-Section Anatomy* of Eycleshymer and Shoemaker[52] was employed.
9. A mean position of the rib was assumed. A series of roentgenograms was taken on full inspiration and expiration in the hope of deriving information useful to this analysis. Extent of thoracic expansion and degree of costal or diaphragmatic breathing varied not only from person to person but also in the same person at different times.
10. Other stresses, such as radial stresses, have not been discussed, as they are negligible.
11. Bending stresses were assumed to vary along a straight line instead of hyperbolically as they actually vary. It is realized that this assumption yields inaccurate stress calculations, but since the ratios of the radii of curvature to their corresponding depths are not of great magnitude, the variation of maximum stresses along the rib would be similar to that obtained by virtue of this assumption.

The criticism might be offered that an analysis based on so many assumptions could not produce valid results. Rashevsky[115] pointed out that the study of such nonreal idealized systems does lead to practical results, at least within certain limits; within these limits the real things have common properties with the fictitious idealized ones. "Only a superman could at once grasp mathematically all the complexities of a real thing. We ordinary mortals must be more modest and approach reality asymptotically, by gradual approximation."[115] Finally, there is a close correspondence of the predicted and actual zones of greatest likelihood of fracture.

THEORY OF RIB FRACTURES DUE TO VIBRATION

Whereas many rib fractures are probably the result of stress concentrations and progressive cracking, as has already been explained, some fractures may be caused by a sudden muscular contraction that is repeated at a frequency which corresponds to the natural frequency of vibration of the rib. Under such a condition, the stresses and strains are tremendously increased. This can best be seen by inspecting the equation of motion of a spring under forced vibration,

$$\frac{W}{g}\frac{d^2x}{dt^2} = W - (W + kx) + P \sin t,$$

together with the magnification factor curve in Fig. 11. W is the weight acting on a spring, g is the acceleration of gravity, k is a physical property of the spring called the spring constant, x is the deflection of the spring at time t, and the term P sin t is known as the disturbing force and is related to the magnification factor.*

Of course, the preceding equation pertaining to a spring is not directly applicable to the action of ribs, but the magnification curve for rib vibrations would take a similar form, and even though the vibration of a rib would be subjected to some damping, due to contiguous tissues, stresses and strains in excess of the elastic limit (and sometimes in excess of the ultimate strength) would be reached. This is due to the fact that the magnification factor approaches a limit of infinity at $\omega/p = 1.0$.

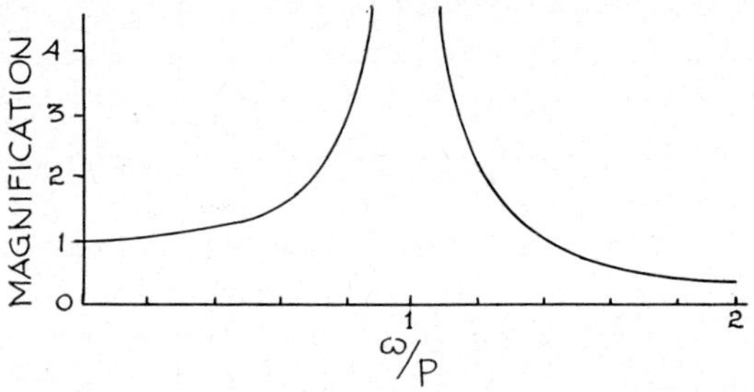

Fig. 11.—Magnification of forces results when coughing occurs at the natural frequency of vibration of the rib. At the time when $\omega/p = 1$, the force approaches infinity.

It should be pointed out that the probability of rib vibrations occurring at the natural frequency of a rib is extremely low; however, such a condition must have occurred, when one considers the periodic function of a coughing seizure and the billions of people who have had many coughs during their lifetimes.

PATHOLOGY

In those instances in which fractures produced by muscular action have been examined pathologically, essentially normal features have been revealed grossly and histologically. Hérard[73] reported a case of fracture of the eleventh rib on the left side which at autopsy showed rich callus at the fracture site; the tissues of this rib and of the other bones as well were normal. Matthes and Thelen[93] excised two such fractures which were initially thought to be malignancies; biopsy showed new formation of bone and cartilage and no tumor but "reactive changes in the sense of callus formation." In the third case of this paper, the biopsied fracture disclosed essentially normal rib including bone marrow. Finally, Bodenheimer's[19] case showed little beyond osteoid formation with low-grade perichondritis.

It may be relevant to cite here the results of post-mortem examinations of vertebrae fractured during convulsions of tetanus. Eberstadt's[48] patient was a 29-year-old soldier. The autopsy disclosed in the third and fourth thoracic vertebral bodies numerous shattered, broken, and collapsed bone trabecu-

*For a complete explanation of this equation and graph see S. Timoshenko's Vibration Problems in Engineering, Chapter 1, D. Van Nostrand Company, Inc.

lae, which comprised a rather disordered group. In many places, the medullary cavity was replaced by an edematous vascular fibrillar marrow, which contained some plasma cells and round cells with much protoplasm. There was limited new bone formation with irregular calcification. There was no evidence of pre-existing bone disease.

Autopsy of a powerful boy, 15 years of age, in whom tetanus developed following a foot injury showed the fifth thoracic vertebra to be compressed and to project into the spinal canal. The fourth intervertebral disc was infiltrated with blood. Aside from the mechanical disorder, microscopic examination revealed completely intact bone.[11]

CLINICAL PICTURE

The symptomatology of rib fractures produced by muscular action does not differ from that produced by trauma. At the moment of the accident, many patients have felt something break or give way in the side; certain of these fractures have been accompanied by noises which at times could be heard across the room.[3, 7, 8, 38, 40] The noise is generally likened to that produced by breaking a stick, fagot, or twig. Pain is not an invariable symptom, especially in breaks of the uppermost ribs; thus, of Alderson's[6] 35 patients with fracture of the first rib, only 5 volunteered significant symptoms or history. The patient of Brewster[24] felt something snap in the chest but experienced no pain; three days later a small tender swelling was noted at the fracture site. The onset of pain may be sudden; 3 of Wynn-Williams'[139] 9 patients and 5 of Mitchell's[99] 14 reported development of abrupt pain. Patients stated, for example, that for days they had had aches in the side which suddenly became stabbing pains. Once present, the pain is usually intense and sticking or cutting in nature. All movements of the thorax, especially coughing, sneezing, or deep breathing, intensify the pain. Movement of the arm of the affected side, contracting the serratus magnus, or moving the trunk may similarly worsen the discomfort. The pain is accompanied by an instinctive restriction of respiratory motion and often by a splinting of the ipsilateral muscles of the thorax, particularly in instances of multiple fracture. If coughing continues, the pain will ordinarily interfere greatly with sleep. Severe pain persists from two days to two weeks. Some degree of discomfort probably persists for about three months. In a number of the reported cases, pain was present after six months. Just as with traumatic fractures, immobilization affords relief; Graves'[63] patient felt better in her stays and Mitchell's[99] patient was more comfortable when lying with the painful place pressed against a hard pillow.

The pain usually is localized in the area contiguous to the fracture site, but not infrequently it is referred along the distribution of the involved intercostal nerve. Particularly in fractures of the lower ribs, pain may extend to the hypochondrium, mediated through the anterior cutaneous branches of the sixth through the eleventh intercostal nerves. Pain may extend above as well as below the fracture site because of the superior and inferior branches of these nerves. Two instances of paradoxical referred pain have been reported. Ginsburg's[60] patient complained of an aching pain in the right side of the neck; roentgenogram showed a recent fracture of the left first rib. Because the pain was on the wrong side, another roentgenogram was made and it confirmed the fracture site. Webb's[135] patient felt no pain at the termination of the ninth intercostal over the abdomen on the same side as the fracture, but had severe pain on the opposite side in this area of distribution.

Moderate to exquisite tenderness may be elicited by finger point pressure over the fracture site. Pressure on the rib at some distance from the site of injury causes pain in patients with rib fracture but not in those with contusions or muscular injury.

Innumerable instances of crepitus, at times audible at a considerable distance, are reported after rib fractures produced by coughing. Crepitation naturally is to be expected only in complete fracture; it is ordinarily not elicited in infractions or in insignificant separation of the fragments from one another. When present it is usually quite clear and may be felt with the palpating hand during ordinary respiration or heard with the ear or stethoscope applied to the chest. It is often apparent to the patient.[38, 104, 135] Gurlt[67] noted that crepitation could at times be elicited by applying pressure with the fingers of both hands placed on either side of the suspected fracture site. In order to appreciate the sound with the stethoscope or feel it with the applied palm, pressure might be exerted on the rib at a greater distance or the patient might be asked to cough.

At times, palpation immediately after the fracture might reveal a deformity produced by overriding of the displaced fragments.[7, 8, 10, 37] Later the callus may be palpable as a somewhat indistinct ridge; gradations from this finally include definite tumors as large perhaps as 2.5 by 2 cm. The discovery of crepitation, abnormal mobility, or callus is difficult when the broken ribs are covered with unusually thick soft parts, as in significant obesity or location under a large breast or under powerful muscles such as the pectoralis major and sacrospinalis. The patient should be in the optimum position for examination, that is, standing erect or in the dorsal decubitus. The seated position, especially in fat people, is the most disadvantageous.

The similarity between the pain of pleurisy and that caused by rib fracture has led to the diagnosis of many rib fractures as pleurisy. There are several reported cases, however, in which rib fracture led to pleural friction rub either from the fragments irritating the pleura or from localized hemorrhage. Hilton[74] reported the first such case. Wahl[134] reported 2 cases in which pleurisy developed at the fracture site. There was a suggillation the size of a Viennese thaler in Podrazki's[112] patient. The hemorrhage may be extensive as in the patient of Bodenheimer,[19] a man 67 years old, in whom the hemorrhagic spot over the fracture site was the size of the palm of the hand. The hemorrhage continued to spread until it involved the entire surface of the left half of the thigh. There was otherwise no bleeding tendency and the excised fracture site showed only perichondritis. Browning[27] reported the case of a patient with advanced tuberculosis who suffered from generalized emphysema secondary to two rib fractures with displacement of the fragments following severe coughing. This seems to be quite rare after cough fractures but is well known to occur after trauma to the chest.[62, 88]

Roentgenography.—Occasionally, the roentgenogram shows definitely less density than normal, but usually there is no radiographic evidence of decrease of bone density. The ease with which early rib fractures might be overlooked in roentgenograms has been commented on repeatedly. The initial line of fracture is quite delicate, and because of the tendency for crowding of the ribs laterally, fractures in this zone may be missed. At times when callus has formed, reviewing of the earlier films may disclose the initially undiscovered break.

The need for oblique views was stressed by Mitchell[99]: of 14 fractures, 8 were seen only in the oblique views. However, Wynn-Williams[139] was unable to find fractures in lateral or oblique views which were not obvious in the anteroposterior position. It is our belief that not only should oblique views be taken but the film should also be exposed for bone detail (including use of Bucky diaphragm) rather than for soft tissue information, as is usually done in views of the chest.

CASE REPORTS

CASE 1 (Rib fracture simulating pleurisy).—Mrs. W. R., white, 55 years of age, had suffered from bronchial asthma since childhood. Within three or four days after development of an infection of the upper respiratory tract, moderately severe asthma associated with a persistent nonproductive cough appeared. Several days later she complained of intense pain over the right hemithorax anteriorly in the region of the seventh and eighth ribs which was aggravated by deep inspiration and particularly by coughing. Physical examination disclosed sibilant râles but no friction rub. It was thought that the patient had pleurisy, but a roentgenogram revealed definite linear fractures in the eighth and ninth ribs in the anterior axillary line on the right side.

CASE 2 (Rib fracture simulating angina).—D. G. R., a white attorney, 54 years of age, had suffered from "asthma" for the past two years. The asthma never awakened him at night. He had an intermittent nonproductive cough and exertional dyspnea which was worse shortly after arising. While playing golf one afternoon he had a paroxysm of coughing almost simultaneously with teeing off the ball. This was followed by severe precordial pain, radiating to the left shoulder and left hypochondrium, and severe dyspnea. He was barely able, with the help of friends, to return to the clubhouse. The pain persisted and was accompanied by some nausea. His physician had him hospitalized for the exclusion of a myocardial infarction. Numerous electrocardiograms were within normal bounds, and after two weeks' observation he was discharged. Roentgenogram of the chest had not been made. One week later, examination at the Ochsner Clinic disclosed obstructive emphysema plus callous formation over the fifth left rib near the costochondral junction.

CASE 3 (Rib fractures confused with metastatic carcinoma fractures).—Mrs. W. M. Y., a white housewife 43 years old, had had a left mammectomy elsewhere because of possible carcinoma of the breast. She had an attack of unrelieved coughing followed by generalized thoracic pain. A roentgenogram of the chest revealed slight accentuation of the pulmonary markings at the right base and multiple fractures involving the sixth and eleventh right ribs and the sixth through the eleventh on the left side with faint rarefaction of the bone on the region of several of these. In view of the multiplicity of the fractures with slight rarefaction and absence of trauma, these were considered to represent pathologic fractures secondary to metastases. Rib marrow aspiration disclosed no abnormality. Rib biopsy was performed. The periosteum over the ninth rib was incised after palpation had failed to disclose the fracture site. A rather fresh fracture was found; the rib was cleaned off and this segment excised. Microscopic examination revealed essentially normal rib, marrow, and early callus. No metastatic tumor was present.

DIAGNOSIS

The diagnosis of rib fracture may be obvious, or not even suspected. Rarely does one think of a fractured rib if there has been no fall or blow to the chest or if the patient has heard no sound of fracture or felt anything give way. Sudden pain in a circumscribed region of the thoracic wall following cough is a daily occurrence; it is frequently a sign of minimal muscle damage or pleural irritation, and therefore one may easily pass over a fracture and attribute the pain to much more frequent occurrences of this sort. The ease of dismissing these lesions is illustrated by Tunis'[132] (1890) patient, who felt something snap in her side following a cough. "Not believing it possible she could have fractured a rib in this fashion, I gave her a sedative cough mixture and told her to apply a turpentine stupe. The next day she was complaining bitterly so *she was then examined* and a definite fracture discovered." (Italics mine.)

The clinical manifestations of rib fracture may be indistinguishable from pleurisy, in which case the diagnosis must be established roentgenologically. At times intermittent thoracic pain, often diagnosed pleurodynia, may precede the onset of pleural effusion by three to six months; in such cases the radiograph is usually normal. This was true in 10 per cent of 200 cases of tuberculous pleurisy with effusion studied by Sibley.[122] In epidemic pleurodynia there is usually no difficulty in making the diagnosis, for the triad of pain, fever, and headache is pathognomonic. According to Locke and Farnsworth,[86] the pain varies from mild pressure or discomfort to the extreme degree described as having an intense cutting or knifelike quality; in its severe form it may be paroxysmal and quite overwhelming. Locke and Farnsworth added other characterisitc features of the pain: (1) It is directly related to sneezing, laughing, coughing, deep breathing, and especially exercise. (2) Commonly the victim is leaning over a table or chair in a fixed position, or sitting or lying in a relaxed state. If relieved in this manner, motion of any sort is likely to precipitate a paroxysm of pain. (3) The patient walks slowly and deliberately, bent over with the body held rigidly. (4) Referred pain may be located anywhere on the trunk but the commonest sites are along the lower or lateral portion of the abdomen or chest in areas about three inches in diameter. (5) In the epidemic studied by Locke and Farnsworth the onset of fever was coincident with the pain and showed a sharp rise to a maximum of 104° or 105° in very severe cases. Prostration is at times extreme, but most cases subside promptly.

Pre-eruptive herpes zoster of one of the intercostal nerves may also present a clinical picture indistinguishable from pleurisy or rib fracture. With the appearance of vesicles, the differentiation becomes obvious.

Bone changes not produced by muscle action but rather by systemic disease must also be borne in mind when rib fractures are discovered on roentgenography. There is a large number of conditions in which pseudofractures mimic true breaks in bone. Camp and McCullough[29] listed the following conditions in which transverse zones of rarefaction may appear in various bones including the ribs: osteomalacia, rickets and late rickets, renal rickets, celiac disease, chronic idiopathic steatorrhea, Gee's disease, nontropical sprue, sprue, early and late osteogenesis imperfecta, fragilitas ossium, hyperparathyroidism, hyperthroidism, osteitis deformans or Paget's disease, adrenal-pituitary bone dystrophy, severe chronic acidosis or hyperglycemia, congenital syphilis, osteomyelitis, osteopetrosis (marble bones, osteosclerosis fragilis generalisata), states of overloading of bone (march fracture, insufficiency fracture), and certain blood dyscrasias. In referring to this list Albright, Burnett, Parson, Reifenstein, and Roos[5] pointed out that the bone disturbance in the first eight of these conditions is rickets or osteomalacia, depending on the age of the patient, and that the disturbance in the next two may be osteomalacia or rickets. They believed that "the ribbon-like zones of decalcification which occur in otherwise normal appearing bone, which last for months or years without regressing, and which exhibit a marked tendency to be symmetrical, occur only in osteomalacia or rickets." Looser[87] first described these under the term "Umbauzonen" (zones of transformation) in an extensive essay which appeared in 1920.

Milkman's syndrome derives from a carefully studied case first reported under the title "Pseudofractures" (1930); a second report entitled "Multiple Spontaneous Idiopathic Symmetrical Fractures" appeared in 1934 after the death of the patient. This patient exhibited "fractures" of the ribs as well as other bones. Although Albright and co-workers[5] established the identity of this condition as a variant of osteomalacia, they believed it should be retained as a separate entity because of the coexistence of pseudofractures and a skeleton which otherwise is not definitely abnormal as judged by roentgenograms. LeMay and Blunt[85] demonstrated that one factor determining the location of pseudofractures in osteomalacia is the position of the main arteries which lie on the bones. In their patients with rib lesions, it is surmised that these were at the site of branches of the intercostals; vessels were found in these areas in one of three cadavers examined by them.

Another "new" syndrome closely related, in the opinion of its discoverers Guichard and Lehmann,[66] to Milkman-Looser syndrome, has recently (1952) been reported under the name of costal fissures in chronic pulmonary disease. The reproduced roentgenograms certainly resemble those of rib fractures produced by cough; no indication is given of the status of the blood calcium, phosphorus, or alkaline serum phosphatase which would be useful in differentiating osteomalacia, osteoporosis, and osteitis fibrosa generalisata. Since there were no other bone anomalies than those noted in the ribs, it is believed that there is no validity for considering this syndrome as a separate entity.

Rib fractures have been considered to be malignancies either from the roentgenographic appearance or on physical examination. Wynn-Williams[139] remarked that if the rounded area of callus lies over the pulmonary field, it may be taken for an intrapulmonary shadow more easily than is generally realized. He saw two instances in which a callus around a rib fracture was temporarily diagnosed disease in the lung. I know of a patient who narrowly escaped operation for a cough fracture initially diagnosed malignancy. Case 3 (Mrs. W. M. Y.) had had a breast removed for suspected carcinoma. Because of slowly growing, slightly painful masses over the osteochondral junction of the second or third ribs, four patients were referred to Matthes and Thelen[93] with diagnosis of chondroma, sarcoma, osteochondritis, or tuberculosis. They were men between 20 and 35 years of age in good health with rather delicate bony structure but powerfully built musculature. Physical examination revealed a clearly visible mass ranging from the size of a pigeon's egg to that of a plum, and extending perhaps 0.5 cm. above the surface of the chest; it was in firm union with the rib, of the consistency of cartilage, and unattached to the overlying skin. On palpation the masses were slightly painful. Biopsy in 2 patients disclosed callous formation. In all 4 patients, questioning revealed that the fractures were probably caused by excessive physical exertion.

PROGNOSIS

The outlook in rib fractures is favorable for complete recovery with rich callus binding the rib ends together. In many cases the callus appears exuberant, especially with anterior or lateral fractures, probably because of the greater movement of this portion of the costal arch and hence the greater irritative stimulus exercised on the periosteum.[119] These fractures are rarely followed by any of the numerous complications of traumatic fractures of the ribs.[16] There are isolated reports of pseudoarthrosis (Wahl's[134] patient had pseudoarthrosis involving four ribs), of hemoptysis,[33] of extensive emphysema,[27] and of subcutaneous hemorrhage.[19, 112]

TREATMENT

The standard treatment for fractured ribs is strapping with adhesive. Blades[17] advised encirclement of the lower costal margin with a single four-inch strip of adhesive plaster regardless of the level of the fracture. The strapping should remain in place for at least three weeks. Christopher[35] recommended application of a tight circular muslin bandage around the entire chest; it gives much relief, does not irritate the skin, and can be changed easily and painlessly. Harmon[69] found that the use of a local anesthetic with prolonged action (eucupine hydrochloride) eliminated the necessity of strapping the thoracic wall and of excessive use of sedatives.

SUMMARY AND CONCLUSIONS

Rib fractures due to muscular action are not uncommon; in patients with infections of the respiratory tract the incidence of such fractures ranged between 0.08 and 6.5 per cent. The first instance of rib fracture from coughing was reported by Gooch[61] in 1773.

Muscular effort induced by coughing, sneezing, laughter, vomiting, straining at stool, or parturition may lead to broken ribs. Women are somewhat more prone to such accidents than men, approximately in a 3:2 ratio. Although these fractures occur at all ages, they occur most commonly in persons between 20 and 50 years of age. There are reports of 24 of these accidents in pregnancy; all occurred in the last trimester but only two occurred during labor.

Cough fractures have been reported in every rib but are quite rare in the uppermost and lowermost ribs. The first rib is, however, frequently the site of fracture from muscle stress unrelated to cough. Most fractures are found in the fifth through the tenth ribs, with a moderate preference for the left side. Ninety-three per cent of the reported cases were unilateral, and in 102 of the 142 reported instances only a single rib was involved.

The symptomatology or rib fractures produced by muscular action does not differ from that produced by trauma. At the moment of the accident, patients may feel something break or give way in the side; some fractures have been accompanied by a cracking sound. Pain is often intense and worsened by movements of the thorax.

Crepitation is common, and at times deformity may be palpated. The fractures are easily overlooked in the roentgenograms, especially if these are made before callus has formed.

The diagnosis may be simple, or not even suspected. The clinical manifestations may be indistinguishable from pleurisy; epidemic pleurodynia and preeruptive herpes zoster also have features in common. Rib fractures should also be distinguished from the pseudofractures seen in osteomalacia and other states. Rib fractures have at times been considered malignancies.

In those instances in which fractures produced by muscular action have been examined pathologically, essentially normal features have been revealed.

A structural analysis was made of the sixth rib using engineering principles to study the relative importance of various stresses. It was concluded that the incidence of fractures is greatest where bending stresses are greatest and shearing stresses least, and contrariwise, fractures occur least often where shearing stresses are greatest. Many rib fractures are probably the result of stress concentration and progressive cracking. Fractures may rarely be produced by sudden muscular contractions that are repeated at a frequency which corresponds to the natural frequency of vibration of the rib.

The outlook is favorable for complete recovery. Treatment consists in immobilization and/or local anesthesia.

REFERENCES

1. Adkins, G. E.: Cough Fracture in Pregnancy, Brit. M. J. **1**: 681-682, 1949.
2. Adler, A.: Eine seltene Fraktur der ersten Rippe durch Muskelzug, Zentralbl. f. Chir. **59**: 518-521, 1932.
3. Ahern, M. J.: Fractured Rib and Dislocated Clavicle as a Result of Fits of Violent Coughing, N. York M. J. **59**: 503, 1894.

4. Aitken, A. P., and Lincoln, R. E.: Fracture of the First Rib Due to Muscle Pull; Report of a Case, New England J. Med. 220: 1063-1064, 1939.
5. Albright, F., Burnett, C. H., Parson, W., Reifenstein, E. C., Jr., and Roos, A.: Osteomalacia and Late Rickets, Medicine 25: 399-479, 1946.
6. Alderson, B. R.: Stress Fractures of the First Rib, Brit. J. Radiol. 17: 323-326, 1944.
7. Alexander, J.: Spontaneous Fracture of a Rib in Coughing, Brit. M. J. 1: 61, 1871.
8. Antony: Fracture de côte indépendente de tout traumatisme extérieur, Bull. et mém. Soc. méd. d. hôp. de Par., 3rd ser. 3: 247-248, 1886.
9. Arnold, A.: Rippenfraktur durch Muskelzug als Sportverletzung, München. med. Wchnschr. 75: 1918-1920, 1928.
10. Atkinson, A. M. B.: Fracture of the Rib During Cough, Brit. M. J. 1: 490, 1898.
11. Bäcker, W.: Wirbelfraktur bei Tetanus, Beitr. z. klin. Chir. 138: 555-558, 1926.
12. Baisch, K.: Ueber chronischer Tetanus, München. med. Wchnschr. 65: 127-129, 1918.
13. Barr, J. S.: Cough Fracture During Pregnancy: Report of a Case, Glasgow M. J. 30: 410-411, 1949.
14. Benoît, cited by Paulley.[111]
15. Bérard: Gaz. d. Hôp. 1841, cited by Mazeillé.[94]
16. Bistolfi, S.: Sulle complicanze pleuro-polmonari delle fratture costali, Radiol. med. 17: 1255-1308, 1930.
17. Blades, B.: Emergency Treatment of Traumatic Chest Injuries, S. Clin. North America 20: 1473-1483, 1940.
18. Blanc, L. C.: Ein Fall von Spontanfraktur mehrerer Rippen im Verlaufe der Schwangerschaft, Zentralbl. f. Gynäk. 32: 1153, 1908; Un cas de fractures spontanées de plusieurs côtes au cours de la grossesse, Bull. Soc. d'obst. de Par. 11: 152-155, 1908.
19. Bodenheimer, J. M.: Fractured Ribs From Coughing, New Orleans M. & S. J. 100: 474-475, 1948.
20. Bond, T. B.: Spontaneous Fractures of the Ribs in Healthy Individuals, Texas J. Med. 40: 642-643, 1945.
21. Breck, L. W., in discussion of article by Bond.[20]
22. Breithaupt: Zur Pathologie des menschlichen Fusses. Medicin. Zeitung 24: 169, 175, 1855, cited by Kirchner, A.: Die Aetiologie der indirecten Metatarsalfracturen, Arch. f. klin. Chir. 77: 241-265, 1905.
23. Breslin, F. J.: Fractures of the First Ribs Unassociated With Fractures of Other Ribs, Am. J. Surg. 38: 384-389, 1937.
24. Brewster, E. S.: An Unusual Case of Fracture of the Rib Due to Paroxysmal Cough Following Laryngeal Aspiration of Foreign Body, M. Rec. 150: 159-160, 1939.
25. Brookhouse, C. T.: Curious Case of Fracture of a Rib, Lancet 1: 503, 1879.
26. Broussais, C.: Journal Hebdon (Oct.), 1835, p. 107, cited by Mazeillé.[94]
27. Browning, C. C.: Generalized Subcutaneous Emphysema Secondary to Pathologic Fracture of Rib in Advanced Pulmonary Tuberculosis, Am. Rev. Tuberc. 25: 571-575, 1932.
28. Byrne, K.: Letters to Editor on Rib Fracture, Brit. M. J. 1: 832, 1949.
29. Camp, J. D., and McCullough, J. A. L.: Pseudofractures in Diseases Affecting the Skeletal System, Radiology 36: 651-663, 1941.
30. Cappon, D.: Some Psychosomatic Aspects of Injuries, Canad. M. A. J. 65: 321-325, 1951.
31. Castella, F.: Fracture de côte produite par un éternument, Gaz. d. Hôp. 34: 599, 1861, cited by Mazeillé.[94]
32. Cazeau, cited by Mazeillé.[94]
33. Chelmonski, A.: (Abstr. from Gaz. lek., 1901, No. 21) Ueber spontane night traumatische Rippenfrakturen bei Phthisikern und kakektischen Individuen, Centralbl. f. Chir. 28: 1188, 1901.
34. Chenery, E.: A Rib Fractured by Cough, Boston M. & S. J. 98: 673-674, 1878.
35. Christopher, F.: Minor Surgery, ed. 6, Philadelphia and London, 1950, W. B. Saunders Company.
36. Cohen, R. S.: Cough Fracture of Ribs, Brit. M. J. 1: 133-134, 1949.
37. Daukes, S. H.: Fracture of a Rib Due to Muscular Action, Lancet 1: 1691, 1906.
38. de Coquet: Fracture de côte par contraction musculaire, J. de méd. de Bordeaux 92: 78, 1921.
39. Denonvillier: Union méd., 1853, cited by Mazeillé.[94]
40. Desnos, L.: Des fractures de côtes independentes du traumatisme, Gaz. hebd. de méd., Par. 22: 691-693, 1885.
41. Després: Fractures de côtes par contraction Musculaire, Gaz. d. Hôp. 55: 193-194, 1882.
42. Dogadkin: Rippenbruch bei einer Schwangeren ohne äussere Veranlassung, Zentralbl. f. Gynäk. 9: 535-536, 1885.
43. Douthwaite, A. H.: Cough Fracture of Ribs, Brit. M. J. 1: 241, 1949.

44. Dubs, J.: Rippenfraktur durch Muskelzug, Deutsche Ztschr. f. Chir. **135**: 380-387, 1916.
45. Dunbar, H. F., Wolfe, T. P., and Rioch, J. M.: Psychiatric Aspects of Medical Problems; the Psychic Component of the Disease Process (Including Convalescence), in Cardiac, Diabetic and Fracture Patients, Am. J. Psychiat. **93**: 649-679, 1936.
46. Dunbar, H. F., Wolfe, T. P., Tauber, E. S., and Brush, A. L.: The Psychic Component of the Disease Process (Including Convalescence) in Cardiac, Diabetic, and Fracture Patients. Part 2, Am. J. Psychiat. **95**: 1319-1342, 1939.
47. Easton, N. L., and Sommers, J.: The Significance of Vertebral Fractures as a Complication of Metrazol Therapy, Am. J. Psychiat. **98**: 538-543, 1942.
48. Eberstadt: Ueber Gibbusbildung bei Tetanus, München. med. Wchnschr. **65**: 1318-1319, 1918.
49. Edgecombe, W.: Fracture of the Ribs in Whooping Cough, Lancet **2**: 374, 1935.
50. Elftman, H.: Skeletal and Muscular Systems: Structure and Function, Glasser, O.: Medical Physics, Chicago, 1944, The Year Book Publishers, Inc.
51. Evans, F. A.: Letter to Editor on Rib Fracture, Brit. M. J. **1**: 241, 1949.
52. Eycleshymer, A. C., and Shoemaker, D. M.: A Cross-Section Anatomy, New York and London, 1911, D. Appleton-Century Company, Inc.
53. Fick, R.: Handbuch der Anatomie und Mechanik der Gelenke. Zweiter Teil: Allegemeine Gelenk-und Muskelmechanik, Jena, 1910, Gustav Fischer, p. 297.
54. Fisk, S. A.: Spontaneous Fracture of a Rib, Boston M. & S. J. **99**: 325-326, 1888.
55. Franke, F.: Kraftkurve menschlicher Muskeln, Arch. f. d. ges. Physiol. **184**: 300, 1920.
56. Frank-Pittowa, H.: Zwei Fälle von isolierten Spontanfraktur der ersten Rippe, Röntgenpraxis **4**: 1011-1013, 1932.
57. Freeland, J.: Spontaneous Fracture of Ribs, Brit. M. J. **1**: 362, 1895.
58. Garber, R. L.: Isolated Fracture of the First Rib Produced by Muscular Traction, Radiology **42**: 395-396, 1944.
59. Gelfand, M. L.: Spontaneous Rib Fracture in Bronchial Asthma, Ann. Allergy **7**: 217-218, 296, 1949.
60. Ginsburg, M.: Spontaneous Fracture of the First Rib as a Complication of Status Asthmaticus. Ann. Allergy **5**: 488-489, 1947.
61. Gooch, B.: Medical and Chirurgical Observations, London, 1773, 8°, appendix, p. 53.
62. Goodliffe, R. V.: Spreading Subcutaneous Emphysema After Fracture of Rib, Brit. M. J. **1**: 153, 1929.
63. Graves, R. J.: Fracture of a Rib Produced by a Violent Fit of Coughing, Dublin J. M. and Chem. Sc. **3**: 353-355, 1833; Am. J. M. Sc. **13**: 553-554, 1834.
64. Groninger, L.: Ueber einen Fall von spontaner Rippenfractur durch Muskelaction, Archiv der Heilkunde **1**: 473-474, 1860.
65. Guggenheim, A., and Cohn, B. N. E.: Contralateral Fracture of First and Second Ribs Following Thoracoplasty, J. Thoracic Surg. **17**: 366-373, 1948.
66. Guichard, A., and Lehmann, M.: Contribution à l'étude des ostéoses respiratoires (ostéopathies d'ordre pneumique). L'ostéose fissuraire costale de l'insuffisance respiratoire chronique, Lyon méd. **185**: 429-539, 1951; **186**: 2-10, 1952.
67. Gurlt, E.: Handbuch der Lehre von den Knochenbruchen vol. 2 Chapter 2: Bruch der Rippen und Rippenknorpel, Hamm, 1862-1864, G. Grote, pp. 191-263.
68. Halliwell, B. T.: Fracture of Ribs Caused by Coughing, Brit. M. J. **2**: 1056, 1929.
69. Harmon, P. H., Baker, D. E., and Kornegay, R. D.: Uncomplicated Fractures of Ribs and Major Injuries of the Chest Wall, J. A. M. A. **118**: 30-34, 1942.
70. Harold, J. T.: Letter to Editor on Rib Fracture, Brit. M. J. **1**: 241, 1949.
71. Hartley, J. B.: "Stress" or "Fatigue" Fractures of Bone, Brit. J. Radiol. **16**: 255-262, 1943.
72. Harvey, R. M.: Rib Fractures in Atypical Pneumonia, Am. J. Roentgenol. **52**: 487-493, 1944.
73. Hérard: Union méd. **9**: 447, 1855; Soc. méd. d. hôp. Juillet, 1855, cited by Mazeillé.[94]
74. Hilton, J.: Clinical Lectures Delivered at Guys Hospital, Lancet **1**: 141-144, 1852.
75. Howson, C. R.: Rib Fracture by Cough, Am. Rev. Tuberc. **30**: 566-567, 1934.
76. Inclán, A.: Fracturas raras que merecen publicarse; Fractura aislada de la primera costilla por contracción muscular, Cir. ortop. y traumatol., Habana **11**: 3-7, 1943.
77. Inglima, A.: Frattura di costola da colpo di tosse, Policlinico **45**: 824-825, 1938.
78. Jones, H. E.: Rib Fractured by Coughing, Glasgow M. J. **61**: 168, 1904.
79. Kleiner, S. B.: Fracture of Ribs by Muscular Action, Boston M. & S. J. **190**: 1034-1035, 1924.
80. Knopp, L. F.: Fractures of the Ribs, A Review of 386 Cases, Am. J. Surg. **52**: 405-414, 1941.
81. Kohlbach, W.: Verschiedenartige Kontinuitätstrennungen der I. Rippe, Röntgenpraxis **11**: 626-629, 1939.

82. Lachmann, E., and Whelan, M.: The Roentgen Diagnosis of Osteoporosis and Its Limitations, Radiology **26**: 165-177, 1936.
83. Ladroitte: Fracture de côte par contraction musculaire, France méd. **2**: 1133-1135, 1886.
84. Lehndorff, H.: Deformitäten der Wirbelsäule und der Rippen im Verlaufe eines schweren Tetanus, Wien. med. Wchnschr. **67**: 2477-2789, 1907.
85. LeMay, M., and Blunt, J. W.: A Factor Determining the Location of Pseudofractures in Osteomalacia, J. Clin. Investigation **28**: 521-525, 1949.
86. Locke, E. A., and Farnsworth, D. L.: The Clinical Characteristics of Epidemic Pleurodynia, Tr. A. Am. Physicians **51**: 399-406, 1936.
87. Looser, E.: Ueber Spätrachitis und Osteomalacie. Klinische, roentgenologische und pathologisch-anatomische Untersuchungen, Deutsche Ztschr. f. Chir. **152**: 210-357, 1920.
88. Macewen, J. A. C.: Extreme Emphysema Involving the Greater Part of the Body: Report of 2 Cases, Brit. M. J. **2**: 892-893, 1928.
89. Malgaigne, J. F.: Recherches sur les variétés et le traitement des fractures des côtes, Archives gén. de méd. IIIe Série, Tome II, pp. 256-277; 415-454, Paris, 1838.
90. Malgaigne, J. F.: A Treatise on Fractures, Translated by John H. Packard, Philadelphia, 1859, J. B. Lippincott Company, chap. VI, p. 347.
91. Mandl, F.: Chirurgie der Sportunfälle, 1925, cited by Arnold.[9]
92. Masser, E. C.: Fracture of a Rib From Coughing in a Patient With Chronic Brights Disease, Brit. M. J. **1**: 953, 1890.
93. Matthes, H. G., and Thelen, A.: Ermüdungsbrüche der Rippen mit typischer Lokalisation, Chirurg. **11**: 537-542, 1939.
94. Mazeillé, T.: Des fractures de côtes par action musculaire, Thèse de Paris, No. 263, 1882.
95. Meschan, I., Scruggs, J. B., Jr., and Calhoun, J. D.: Convulsive Fractures of the Dorsal Spine Following Electric Shock Therapy, Radiology **54**: 180-193, 1950.
96. Miall, P.: Fracture of a Rib From Coughing, Brit. M. J. **1**: 8, 1871.
97. Michael-Phillips, A. H.: Letter to Editor on Rib Fracture, Brit. M. J. **1**: 414, 1949.
98. Milkman, L. A.: Pseudofractures (Hunger Osteopathy, Late Rickets, Osteomalacia), Am. J. Roentgenol. **24**: 29-37, 1930; Multiple Spontaneous Idiopathic Symmetrical Fractures, **32**: 622-634, 1934.
99. Mitchell, J. B.: Cough Fracture, Brit. M. J. **2**: 1492-1493, 1951.
100. Monteggia, G. B.: Institutioni Chirurgiche, Milano, 1802-03, Pirotta and Maspero.
101. Nadler, F.: Beitrag zur isolierten Fraktur der ersten Rippe, Zentralbl. f. Chir. **62**: 2790, 1935.
102. Nancrede, C. B.: Three Rare Surgical Cases, Phil. Medical Times **4**: 535-536, 1874.
103. Nankivell, C. B.: Two Cases of Fracture of the Ribs by Muscular Action, Am. J. M. Sc. **17**: 519-520, 1836.
104. Nash, J. T. C.: Fracture of Rib Due to Cough, Lancet **1**: 245, 1893.
105. Oechsli, W. R.: Rib Fracture From Cough, Report of 12 Cases, J. Thoracic Surg. **5**: 530-534, 1936.
106. Palfrey, F. W.: Fracture of Ribs by Muscular Action, Boston M. & S. J. **191**: 498-499, 1924.
107. Palmer, P. E. S.: Cough Fractures, Brit. M. J. **2**: 732, 1953.
108. Parenti, O.: Doppia frattura costale da colpo di tosse, Arch. di radiol. **14**: 318-323, 1938.
109. Park, E. A., and Howland, J.: The Dangers to Life of Severe Involvement of the Thorax in Rickets, Bull. Johns Hopkins Hosp. **32**: 101-109, 1921.
110. Parker, R. W.: Rickety Deformity of the Thorax With Spontaneous Fractures of Several of the Ribs, Tr. Path. Soc. Lond. **33**: 257-258, 1882.
111. Paulley, J. W., Lees, D. H., and Pearson, A. C.: Cough Fracture in Late Pregnancy, Brit. M. J. **1**: 135-137, 1949.
112. Podrazki: Frakturen der 10 Rippe durch Muskelaction. Oester. Ztschr. f. prakt. Heilk. **18**: 201-205, 1872; Fraktur des x. Rippenknorpels durch Niesen, **19**: 677-678, 1873.
113. Porzelt, W.: Ein Fall von isoliertem Bruch der ersten Rippe durch Muskelzug, Zentralbl. f. Chir. **58**: 1264-1267, 1931.
114. Pospischill, D.: Ueber Klinik und Epidemiologie der Pertussis, Berlin, 1921, S. Karger.
115. Rashevsky, N.: Mathematical Biophysics, Chicago, 1948, University of Chicago Press.
116. Richardson, E. C.: Indirect Fracture of the Rib in Pulmonary Tuberculosis, J. A. M. A. **106**: 1543-1544, 1936.
117. Roberg, O. T.: Spinal Deformity Following Tetanus and Its Relation to Juvenile Kyphosis, J. Bone & Joint Surg. **19**: 603-629, 1937.
118. Rodman, H. D.: Spontaneous Fracture of the Ribs, With Report of Case, Am. Pract. & News **38**: 611-614, 1904.

119. Sabbione, C.: Studio radiologico delle fratture spontanee delle coste in soggetti affetti da tubercolosi polmonare, Radiol. med. **25**: 528-541, 1938.
York M. J. **59**: 434, 1894.
120. Scherck, H. J.: A Case of Fractured Rib as a Result of Fit of Violent Coughing, N. York M. J. **59**: 434, 1894.
121. Seilin, J.: Fracture of the 11th Rib by Muscular Action; Résumé of Reported Cases, M. Rec. **91**: 281-283, 1917.
122. Sibley, J. C.: A Study of 200 Cases of Tuberculous Pleurisy With Effusion, Am. Rev. Tuberc. **62**: 314-323, 1950.
123. Skyrme, H. E.: Fracture of a Rib Six Days After Injury to the Side, Brit. M. J. **2**: 733, 1890.
124. Somerset, E.: Fracture of Rib From Coughing, Brit. M. J. **1**: 408, 1894.
125. Sonntag, E.: Die bisherigen Erfahrungen ueber den Wundstorrkrampf in dem jetzigen Kriege, Ergebn. d. Chir. u. Orthop. **10**: 1-6, 1918.
126. Speed, K.: A Textbook of Fractures and Dislocations, Philadelphia and New York, 1916, Lea & Febiger, pp. 331-333.
127. Swineford, O., and McKinnon, J.: Multiple Fractures of Ribs by Cough: Report of a Case, Ann. Int. Med. **23**: 442-444, 1945.
128. Telhouni, T.: Des fractures des côtes dites spontanées au cours de la grossesse, Thèse de Lyon, 1937, No. 440.
129. Tisné, C.: Note sur les fractures de côtes par contraction musculaire, Ann. méd.-chir. française et étrangère **2**: 289-293, 1886.
130. Trifan, I.: Fractura cóstei a 7-a strângă, printr'un acces de tusă, Spitalul, Bucuresci **17**: 604-605, 1897.
131. Trillat and Pizzéra: Fractures spontanées des côtes pendant la gestation, Bull. Soc. d'obst. et de gynéc. **21**: 275-278, 1932.
132. Tunis, J. P.: Rib Fracture From Muscular Action With 40 Collected Cases, Univ. M. Mag. **3**: 57-65, 1890.
133. Vidal, E.: Des fractures dites spontanées pendant la grossesse et l'accouchement, Thèse de Paris, 1894, No. 330.
134. Wahl, E.: Ueber Spontanfrakturen der Rippen insbesondere Hustenfrakturen, Wien. klin. Wchnschr. **39**: 1213-1217, 1926.
135. Webb, G. B., and Gilbert, G. B.: Ribs Fractured by Cough, J. A. M. A. **81**: 25, 1923.
136. Werthmann, H., and Scholz, W.: Der Ueberlastungsschaden der I. Rippe, Röntgenpraxis **11**: 322-325, 1939.
137. Wilhelm, T.: La cyphose tétanique, J. de chir. **22**: 295, 1923.
138. Wyman, H. C.: Fracture of the Rib Caused by Sneezing, J. A. M. A. **5**: 512, 1885.
139. Wynn-Williams, N.: Cough Fracture of the Ribs Unassociated With Pulmonary Tuberculosis, Brit. M. J. **2**: 1494-1496, 1951.
140. Zur, G.: Osteoporotische Hustenfrakturen der Rippen, Fortschr. Geb. Röntgenstrahlen **72**: 144-153, 1949.

Surgical History

CONDUCTED BY JOHN R. PAINE, M.D.

EPONYMIC FRACTURES: ABRAHAM COLLES AND COLLES' FRACTURE

LEONARD F. PELTIER, M.D., MINNEAPOLIS, MINN.

(From the Department of Surgery, Division of Orthopedic Surgery, University of Minnesota Medical School)

. . . for be assured, that no man can know his own profession perfectly who knows nothing else.[4]

ABRAHAM COLLES (1773-1843) was the greatest of the Irish surgeons. He excelled as a clinician, as a teacher, and as an anatomist. His eponym is attached to a fascia, a space, a ligament, a law, and to a fracture. These suffice to keep his name alive, but in no way illuminate his great contribution to the surgical art.

THE FRACTURE

Colles had the good fortune to describe the most common fracture occurring in practice. As a result, his eponym is one of the most widely known and used. Although he himself was unaware of their reports, the French surgeons Pouteau (1725-1775)[8] and Desault (1744-1795)[6] had made previous mention of this fracture of the distal end of the radius. Colles' description appeared in 1814, and it has been recognized as a classic of brevity and clarity.[2] Unfortunately, this description is unaccompanied by an illustration, and surprisingly enough in view of Colles' reputation as an anatomist, there was no description of the dissection of such an injury. Perhaps this accounts for the fact that Colles placed the fracture so far proximally.

> This fracture takes place at about an inch and a half above the carpal extremity of the radius, and exhibits the following appearances.
>
> The posterior surface of the limb presents a considerable deformity; for a depression is seen in the forearm, about an inch and a half above the end of this bone, while a considerable swelling occupies the wrist and the metacarpus. Indeed the carpus and base of the metacarpus appear to be thrown backward so much as on first view to excite a suspicion that the carpus has been dislocated forward.
>
> On viewing the anterior surface of the limb, we observe a considerable fulness, as if caused by the flexor tendons being thrown forwards. The fulness extends upwards to about one-third of the length of the forearm, and terminates below at the upper edge of the annular ligament of the wrist. The extremity of the ulna is seen projecting towards the palm and inner edge of the limb; the degree, however, in which this projection takes place, is different in different instances.

Received for publication, July 22, 1953.

> The hard swelling which appears on the back of the hand, is caused by the carpal surface of the radius being directed slightly backwards instead of looking directly downwards. The broken extremity of the radius being thus drawn backwards, causes the ulna to appear prominent toward the palmar surface, while it is possibly thrown more towards the inner or ulnar side of the limb, by the upper end of the fragment of the radius pressing against it in that direction.[2]

Dissections of these fractures, such as those illustrated by Malgaigne,[8] and the use of x-ray pictures have resulted in a clearer concept of these fractures.

A Colles' fracture is a transverse fracture of the distal end of the radius, usually occurring within one inch of the articular surface. The articular surface of the distal fragment is tipped dorsally with the loss of its normal slightly volar inclination. The fracture may be accompanied by an avulsion of the styloid process of the ulna. There may be some comminution of the distal fragment with longitudinal fissures extending to the joint surface. These are rarely displaced. Such cases should not be confused with Barton's fracture-

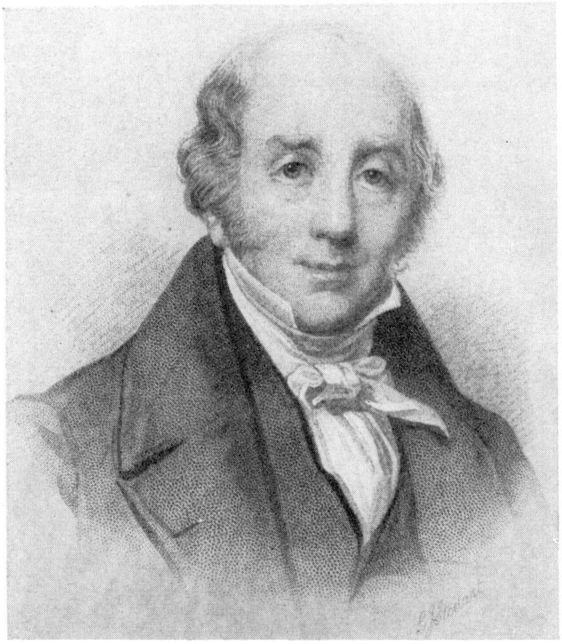

Fig. 1.—Abraham Colles (1773-1843).

dislocation of the wrist.[11] Regardless of the methods of treatment employed, the functional end result following Colles' fracture are generally good, a fact recognized by Colles himself.[9]

THE MAN

Colles was born in Kilkenny, Ireland, in 1773. His father died when Abraham was 6 years old, and he was raised by his mother, who saw to his early education. In 1790, accompanied by his older brother, he entered Trinity College, Dublin. One biographer remarks that while the older brother took the academic laurels, Abraham aimed at success in life rather than success in college.[10] During this period, Colles was apprenticed to Dr. Woodroffe, resident surgeon at Steevens' Hospital. Having gained his license from the Royal College of Surgeons in Ireland in 1795, he proceeded directly to Edinburgh for further study. Always an indefatigable worker, he notes in a letter home:

> As for my landlady, Mrs. Williams, she is positively afraid I shall read myself into a coffin, and actually comes to keep me idle at different times, out of her desire to keep me in health.[10]

After two years of further training, he was granted the degree of Doctor of Medicine.

Colles then set off for London, a distance of 400 miles, which he covered in only eight days. He had not been in London long before he fell under the spell of Astley Cooper. Cooper enlisted his aid in the preparation of some of the dissections for Cooper's monumental work on hernia, then in preparation. Plates of some of these dissections have recently been republished.[1] Colles' ligament, a portion of the aponeurosis of the external oblique muscle extending from Poupart's ligament to the linea alba, attests to his early interest in anatomy.

On his return to Dublin in 1797, while waiting for his practice to become established, Colles attached himself to a free dispensary maintained by the Quakers, and had an appointment as District Visitor to the Sick and Indigent Roomkeepers' Society. Two years later he succeeded his former chief, Dr. Woodroffe, as Resident Surgeon at Steevens' Hospital. At the age of 26 years, he had complete charge of one-third of the surgical beds in one of Ireland's leading hospitals.[7] Abraham Colles had arrived on the surgical scene. In 1802, he was elected President of the Royal College of Surgeons in Ireland, and two years later became Professor of Surgery, a post he filled with distinction for thirty-two years.

Toward the end of his career, he was passed over because of his life-long political views when the British Government sought to honor the leading figure in Irish medicine, a distinction uniquely Colles'. Public indignation over the slight caused the government to reconsider, and Colles was offered a baronetcy. He firmly, but modestly, declined.

> Mr. Colles won his way to eminence by means which are, to some extent, within the reach of all. He may be said to have wrested success from the hands of adverse fortune by his energy and indomitable perseverance. His family and decendants may point with pride to the unadorned name of Abraham Colles, and boast that they are sprung from one who merited a title, but declined it.[10]

THE ANATOMIST

> The subject of anatomy too generally ends at that point where it begins to be useful.[4]

Anatomy at the beginning of the Nineteenth Century was still taught on the basis of systems. The bones, the muscles, the nervous system, the vascular system were all taken up in succession and dissected individually without any attempt to correlate them with the human fabric as a whole. As a result, the student might know the structures which cross the antecubital space but be totally unaware of their relationship to one another. It can be readily appreciated that such incomplete understanding had no value in the practical application of anatomy at the operating table. Colles was one of the first to recognize the need for the study of topographic anatomy with emphasis on the relationship between important structures in an area. His *Treatise on Surgical Anatomy*[4] published in 1811 introduced a new era in the teaching of anatomy.

> . . . while systems of anatomy are multiplied beyond number, we have scarcely any elementary treatises, the sole object of which is, to describe the relative position of the parts, or to point out the subserviency of anatomical knowledge to surgical practice. To supply that defect for the pupils of this school, is the design of the present work.
>
> The plans for the dissections have been laid down in such a manner as will enable the student to enjoy, from the dissection of each part of a single subject, a connected and comprehensive view of the structure: so that he may have it in his power to form an accurate idea of the various relations which the structure of this part bears to the phenomena of its diseases, and the modes of operation recommended for their removal.[4]

The book is literally a dissecting manual with a commentary on the surgical application of the anatomic relationships exposed. Its character is best illustrated by the perusal of Colles' description of what is now known as Colles' fascia.

> Now proceed to dissect the perinaeum. Raise the skin of the perinaeum, extending the dissection beyond the tubera ischii to the thighs. This exposes to view a strong fascia, which, on dissection, will be found to cover the entire of the perinaeum, and to blend itself with the structure of the scrotum. This fascia, although on a superficial view it appears continuous with the fascia of the muscles of the thigh, will yet be found, on closer examination, to attach itself very firmly to the rami of the ischium and pubes. The texture and connections of this fascia will serve to explain many of those phenomena attendant on the effusion of urine into the perinaeum, by rupture or ulceration of the posterior part of the canal of the urethra.
>
> First, then, you will find that this fluid, when so effused, although it forms a tumor in perinaeo, rarely terminates by suppuration and ulceration in this spot; being here resisted by the dense and unyielding texture of the fascia, diffusion laterally towards the thighs is prevented by the close attachment of this fascia to the rami of the pubes and ischium; while its progress forwards if favoured by a quantity of cellular substance, interposed between the surface of the perinaeal muscles and this fascia. In general, then, we find that the urine having caused some tumefaction in perinaeo, passes on into the scrotum. Here meeting with only a very feeble resistance from the lax texture of this part, it quickly distends it to a very considerable size. In some instances the mischief does not extend further, for suppuration takes place in the scrotum, and a quantity of very foetid fluid, composed of urine and pus, is discharged as soon as the abscess spontaneously bursts, or is opened by the surgeon. In other cases, the effused urine continues its progress until it arrives at the pubes.[4]

THE TEACHER

Among his contemporaries Colles was widely known for his ability as a teacher and lecturer.[12] His lectures on surgery were attended by as many as 300 students. He spoke fluently and relieved the tedium of his subject with the interspersion of practical anecdotes, sharply contrasting figures of speech, and an occasional *double entendre*. He was the outstanding attraction on the teaching staff, and largely as a result of his teaching the College attained the highest enrollment of any medical school in Britain during his tenure as Professor of Surgery. At the time of his retirement in 1836, the Royal College of Surgeons in Ireland passed a resolution stating:

> . . . it was the unanimous feeling of the College that the exemplary and efficient manner in which he had fulfilled the chair of the Theory and Practice of Surgery, for thirty-two years, had been the principal cause of the success and consequent high character of the school of Surgery in this Country.[12]

Colles had advanced ideas on medical education. His address to the pupils of the Royal College of Surgeons in Ireland, "On the Preparatory Education Necessary for the Surgical Student,"[4] should be required reading for deans and medical educators. He begins with a strong endorsement of a classical education and emphasizes the need for a knowledge of foreign languages.

> [Mathematics] No science tends so effectually to strengthen the understanding, and to improve the reasoning faculties, as that of mathematics; for it requires that complete retirement of the mind within itself, that straight-forward, unbroken progress of thought, which can alone enable us to follow up a long chain of arguments, and arrive at a remote conclusion. But besides the important benefits which are thus derived from the cultivation of this science, it is also in a great degree the key to most of the other sciences.
>
> [Natural philosophy] Natural philosophy will be found of great use to explain some of the functions of the animal body, and the laws to which they are subject. Thus it is impossible that any person unacquainted with the general principles of optics can form an accurate idea of the manner in which vision is performed in the natural state of the eye, and he consequently cannot clearly comprehend why distinct vision is in some persons confined to objects close to the organ while in others, those objects only which are placed at a distance can be seen distinctly.
>
> [Chemistry] Chemistry, Gentlemen, affords such a luminous explanation of the great phenomena of nature, and leads to such important improvements in the various arts subservient to human life that mankind at large must regard it as a science at once most highly pleasing, and most eminently useful. *To the surgical student in particular,* it is of indispensable importance. [Italics mine.]
>
> [Physiology] Physiology, which comprises a knowledge of the living actions of individual parts, and of the various functions of the animal system in a state of health, must obviously strike you, as being of essential importance to the surgeon. For without a knowledge of the healthy actions and functions, how can he know which of them are disturbed by disease? How can he undertake to regulate them when out of order? *Study them not in books, but in nature.* [Italics mine.]
>
> [Anatomy: To Colles, the study of anatomy was the foundation stone of the surgical education. He spent all of his life increasing the effectiveness of the teaching of this, his favorite subject.]

The stress on the basic sciences in the education of surgeons, which we like to think of as a recent trend, was nothing new to Colles, who justified it as follows:

> You may think, that if the time required for those general studies were devoted solely to the pursuits of your own particular profession, it would be more wisely and profitably employed. But his opinion is equally narrow and unfounded: for be assured, that no man can know his own profession perfectly who knows nothing else; and that he who aspires to eminence in any particular science, must first acquire the habit of philosophizing on matters of science in general.

Although limiting himself to a surgical practice, Colles had decided feelings in regard to the general medical education of the specialist.

> Since then it is absolutely necessary for the benefit and security of the patient, that the physician and surgeon should each be acquainted with both medical and surgical diseases, that surgeon must be inexcusable who is found to want this combined knowledge . . . Let it not be supposed that I would inculcate the idea of unnecessarily uniting the *practice* of both physic and surgery in the same person; on the contrary, I am decidedly of opinion, that in great cities the surgeon should never undertake the cure of a case purely medical, nor the physician of a case purely surgical. All I mean to assert is, that the *study* of both professions should be combined by the man who wished to practice either to the greatest advantage.[4]

In addition to writing about medical education, Colles took an active part in its reform and improvement. In 1828 he was responsible for establishing the chair of chemistry in the College, the first in any nonuniversity medical school.[12] The institution of chairs in medical jurisprudence, comparative anatomy, and botany also received his active support.

THE CLINICIAN

In 1837, late in his career, Colles published what he believed was his most important work, *Practical Observations on Venereal Disease and on the Use of Mercury.*[5] The dedication was to Sir Astley Cooper, his friend for over thirty-five years. In this work, Colles pitted his clinical acumen against that of John Hunter himself, and came off with the laurels. From the observation of cases in his practice, Colles demonstrated that, contrary to Hunter's opinion, the secondary lesions of syphilis can spread the contagion. Since they read the tragic case reports of women infected with syphilis by the examining fingers of their physicians, it is surprising that these clear-cut examples of disease transmission escaped the notice of both Semmelweis and Holmes in their search for evidence to support the theory of the contagiousness of puerperal sepsis.

Some of Colles' comments on the venereal diseases demonstrate his understanding of the human factor in disease, and also his sense of humor.

> I may be told by some that men may contract syphilis by sitting in a public privy; to this I can only answer that I have never witnessed a single instance; nor did the late Mr. Obre, who had been for many years most extensively engaged in treating the venereal disease; for on asking him if he believed that the disease was propagated in this manner, he shrewdly answered, that it sometimes was the manner in which *married* men contracted it, but *unmarried* men never caught it in this manner.[10]

In a masterful description of congenital syphilis, Colles traced the course of the disease from the child to the wet nurse, and then to the nurse's family. These observations form the basis of what is known as Colles' law, which is best stated in his own words.

> One fact well deserving our attention is this: that a child born of a mother who is without any obvious venereal symptoms, and which, without being exposed to any infection subsequent to its birth, shows this disease when a few weeks old; this child will infect the most healthy nurse, whether she suckle it or merely handle and dress it; and yet this child is never known to infect its own mother, even though she suckle it while it has venereal ulcers of the lip and tongue.[10]

It was observations such as this, based on a careful appraisal of a wide experience, which established Colles' reputation as a clinician.

CONCLUSION

In closing, Colles' ability as a surgeon should be mentioned. His description of the ligation of the subclavian artery is evidence enough of this.[3] His conception of the procedure was based on knowledge of the pathologic process; its execution was aided by his anatomic studies; the assessment of the end results was candid and critical. Here was a master surgeon who excelled as a teacher and writer. The ubiquity of his eponym is well deserved.

REFERENCES

1. Brock, R. C.: The Life and Work of Astley Cooper, Edinburgh, 1952, E. & S. Livingstone.
2. Colles, A.: On the Fracture of the Carpal Extremity of the Radius, Edinb. M. & Surg. J. **10**: 182-186, 1814; M. Classics **4**: 1038-1042, 1939-40.
3. Colles, A.: On the Operation of Typing the Subclavian Artery, Edinb. M. & Surg. J. **11**: 1-25, 1815; M. Classics **4**: 1043-1072, 1939-40.
4. Colles, A.: Treatise on Surgical Anatomy, 2nd American ed. With Notes by J. P. Hopkinson, Philadelphia, 1831, Carey and Lea.
5. Colles, A.: Practical Observations on Venereal Disease and on the Use of Mercury, London, 1837, Sherwood.
6. Desault, P. J.: A Treatise on Fractures, Luxations and Other Affections of the Bones, Edited by Xav. Bichat, Translated by Charles Caldwell, ed. 3, Philadelphia, 1817, Kimber and Sharpless.
7. Jones, A. R.: Abraham Colles, J. Bone & Joint Surg. **32B**: 126-130, 1950.
8. Malgaigne, J. F.: A Treatise on Fractures, Translated by John H. Packard, Philadelphia, 1859, J. B. Lippincott Company.
9. Mason, M. L.: Colles' Fracture, A Survey of End Results, Brit. J. Surg. **40**: 340-346, 1953.
10. McDonnell, R.: Selections From the Works of Abraham Colles, London, 1881, The New Sydenham Society.
11. Peltier, L. F.: John Rhea Barton and Barton's Fracture, Surgery, **34**: 960, 1953.
12. Widdess, J. D. H.: An Account of the Schools of Surgery Royal College of Surgeons, Dublin, Edinburgh, 1949, E. & S. Livingstone.

Book Reviews

Pathology of the Fetus and the Newborn. By Edith L. Potter, M.D., Ph.D. Chicago, Ill., 1953, The Year Book Publishers, Inc.

The volume is not a functional pathology but a complete description of the normal variations in growth and development of the fetus and newborn infant, as well as the relation of the more extreme variations considered pathologic. The book is well organized into twenty-eight chapters, including weight and length tables for calculating the rate of antenatal growth and tables with the initial appearance of centers of ossification. There are 601 illustrations included and an important number of photomicrographs.

This book is a valuable addition to the library of the gynecologist and as a reference source for students and teachers.

The Principles of Neurological Surgery. By Loyal Davis, M.S., M.D., Ph.D., D.Sc. (Hon.), Professor of Surgery and Chairman of the Division of Surgery, Northwestern University Medical School, Chicago, Ill. Pp. 544, with 186 engravings, containing 354 illustrations and 5 plates, 4 in color. Philadelphia, 1953, Lea & Febiger.

The purpose of this book is to present the general principles of neurological surgery as applied to general diagnosis, therapy, and prognosis. A determined effort has been made by Dr. Davis to offer the material from the clinical viewpoint, and he has written it so that it may be a valuable book for referral by physicians engaged in general practice as well as those in special fields. It is comprehensive and includes a discussion of all the important neurological lesions. He has included the necessary neuroanatomic and neurophysiologic data required to understand properly the clinical development of the various lesions and methods of therapy. The first chapters include a thorough discussion of the techniques and significance of the neurological examination. Following this fundamental material, the various lesions of the nervous system are discussed. These include injuries, neoplasms, and inflammatory lesions of the skull, brain, spinal cord, and peripheral nerves. The remainder of the book includes material on the treatment of intractable pain, sympathetic nerve surgery, surgery of convulsive disorders, vascular malformations, anomalies, psychoses, and abnormal involuntary movements.

This fourth edition differs from the preceding editions in that many important additions and rearrangements have been made in the text. The material on peripheral nerve surgery has been entirely revised and rewritten to incorporate experiences obtained in World War II. The new diagnostic procedures, such as angiography for intracranial aneurysms and tumors, and radioactive isotope studies for localization of intracranial tumors, have been included. This greatly enhances the book as far as the majority of physicians are concerned.

This book has never been a particular reference work for specialists in neurological surgery, but has been directed more at those men in general practice, or in allied fields, who encounter neurological cases in the course of their practice. The emphasis has been on fundamental methods of diagnosis and prognosis, rather than on the outlining of specific operative procedures. The book is written, at times, with a confusing editorial style. This detracts from its usefulness but, in general, it is felt that it will be found to be a relatively authoritative source of ready information for most physicians. There are 354 illustrations, all of which seem to be well selected to demonstrate the desired data. The volume itself is on high-grade paper, and is excellently bound.

Clinical Orthopaedics, Vol. I and II. Edited by Anthony F. DePalma. Philadelphia, 1953, J. B. Lippincott Company.

The first two volumes of this new publication are now available, and from their contents the value of this series to the orthopedic scene can be fairly evaluated. In the prospectus, we read that this series will not be a ''rehash'' of material published elsewhere. but will provide an outlet for valuable orthopedic investigations, material of scientific, practical, and academic value. Alas, this is not the case.

In Volume I, the first sentence of the first article, ''Rheumatism is the leading cause of death in children,'' is obviously untrue. The second article describes the treatment of a normal anatomic variation with corrective braces and exercises. Fig. 73 illustrates an improper treatment for femoral shaft fractures mislabeled Bryant's traction. In this same section on femoral fractures, the writer states his preference for the Hansen-Street intramedullary nail rather than the Küntscher nail, ''which bends or breaks in a great percentage of cases.'' This is not true. With incredible naïveté, the author of an article on ''Trigger Thumb in Infants,'' after describing this operation in fourteen such cases, says, ''The author, however, is at a loss to explain what happens to these youngsters if no treatment is given. . . . The inference is that some infants must have this condition and recover without benefit of treatment. . . .'' Meddlesome surgery?

Volume II, devoted in a large part to the intramedullary nailing operation developed and popularized by Küntscher, fails even to mention his name in the historical introduction, a damnable omission. Of the remaining material on intramedullary nailing, hardly any is appearing for the first time. Indeed, a great deal of it has been published by the American Academy of Orthopaedic Surgeons.

The material in these volumes is not scientific, for there is not one article on the investigation of a basic problem of an orthopedic nature; it is not practical, unless overtreatment and meddlesome surgery can be considered practical; and it is hardly academic, as a glance at the bibliographic references will quickly reveal.

Morris' Human Anatomy. A Complete Systematic Treatise. Edited by J. P. Schaeffer. Ed. 11. Pp. 1718, with 1220 illustrations. New York and Toronto, 1953, The Blakiston Company.

The eleventh edition of *Morris' Anatomy* appears for the second time under the editorship of Dr. Schaeffer. All the contributors are Americans. The first edition appeared under the editorship of Sir Henry Morris, an English surgeon and anatomist. This reviewer came to know this anatomic text best under the editorship of the late distinguished anatomist, Dr. C. M. Jackson, who continued as editor of the fifth (1914) through the ninth editions (1933).

The present volume is a very readable book. The illustrations, many of which are in color, are considerably better than those in the earlier editions. And this consideration is one of great importance, not only to undergraduate students of medicine, but also to physicians and especially to surgeons, whose eyes, of necessity, must pore often and at frequent intervals over anatomic texts. It is to be hoped that medical students may some time enjoy the great privilege of studying anatomic texts profusely illustrated in color, as in some of the well-known German texts of an earlier day.

This volume should find favor with medical students as well as surgeons who want a ready, readable anatomic text with superior illustrations by well-known American anatomists.

The Year Book of General Surgery (1953-1954 Year Book Series). Edited by Evarts A. Graham, with a Section on Anesthesia edited by Stuart C. Cullen. Pp. 590. Chicago, 1953, The Year Book Publishers, Inc. $6.00.

The Year Book of Surgery, edited by the distinguished American surgeon Evarts A. Graham, continues to be a very interesting and instructive monograph. Some of the best readings in the text are the mature comments made by the author. The tone of the volume is set in the Introduction written by Dr. Graham, which suggests very forcefully the nature of the change in surgery which has occurred in this country during the past three decades. That interesting foreword to the volume indicates the editor's attitude toward what constitutes modern surgery, and is reprinted here in full. The volume can be recommended enthusiastically as interesting reading which will hold the reader's attention.

"At the meeting of the International Surgical Society in New Orleans in 1949 one of the prominent older European members criticized the program to your editor. His chief complaint was, as he put it, there was too much chemistry and not enough surgery. The remark led to my query, what is surgery anyway? His answer revealed the fact that to him the surgery of today is very little different from that in the early days of this century. That is to say, surgery is an art dependent upon the application of anatomy and pathology to the job at hand. To him the advances made in the last half-century or so and those still to be made consist chiefly of new operations. He completely overlooked the great improvements in diagnosis, in postoperative care and in surgical mortalities which have occurred.

"This astonishing concept of our profession raised several questions in my mind. Does he not realize that there is a science as well as an art of surgery? Must we still think of it in the etymologic sense as the work of the hand? Does the surgeon not require also a brain? Surely we have advanced beyond the stage of being practitioners of external medicine as contrasted with those who practice internal medicine.

"To one who during his life has seen a change from a glorification of the art of surgery to a recognition of the importance of the scientific aspects, the criticism by my European friend came as an unbelievable expression of an opinion supposedly obsolete for many a year. During the period of glorification of the art of surgery, manual dexterity and rapidity of operating were criteria used in gauging the excellence of the surgeon. He who performed a greater number of operations per year was ordinarily considered a better surgeon than he who perhaps sought to be less busy in the operating room but to have more time for meditation, reading, research, of either a clinical or a laboratory nature, and, yes, even perhaps to learn something of a science that might contribute to the solution of some of his daily problems. The one-thousand-laparotomies-a-year man was the big shot, and on him most of the young surgeons looked with envy.

"The teaching of surgery in this country in those days was carried out by herding together in an amphitheater a crowd of medical students to watch the professor gallop through a string of operations with occasional remarks about what he was doing. That was about the only information which the students got, because they could see practically nothing of the field of operation. A big list of operations meant a big surgeon. Aspiring young surgeons learned their profession by acting as assistants to established surgeons if they were lucky enough to know men with whom they could work or, as more often occurred, they learned to operate by using the experimental method on such unsuspecting patients as were willing to allow the tyros to operate on them. It was a sort of catch-as-catch-can procedure. Catch the patient and learn operative technic on him.

"Now how different the whole situation is! Standards of judging surgeons have changed. Much of the glamor has gone. Facilities for obtaining a good training in surgery are abundant. The amphitheater operating clinics as a method of teaching surgery have become obsolete.

"My friend who was critical because he thought there was too much chemistry and not enough surgery on the program failed to recognize one of the most important contributions to surgery which Lister made. Of course, everybody knows that the introduction of the antiseptic method revolutionized the practice of surgery and greatly extended its field of application. But perhaps a greater revolution was a philosophic one which has never received the emphasis it deserves. Here was a young surgeon well versed in, but dissatisfied with, the current art of practice who saw the possibility of applying to surgery the work of a young chemist by the name of Pasteur who was working in a foreign land and publishing his results in a foreign language. Could anything at that time have seemed less applicable to the practical art of surgery than a chemist's contributions to the philosophic problems of spontaneous generation, fermentation and putrefaction?

"Nowadays it is true that more and more young surgeons are calling upon chemistry and physics to assist in the study of surgical problems. This is as it should be. More power to them! Every cell is a chemical laboratory. Even as practical a matter as the healing of a wound is fundamentally a chemical phenomenon. Some day a new young Lister will come along and by applying chemistry to his studies will learn how to shorten the period of wound healing from a week or 10 days to 2 or 3 days. In the meantime, let the programs of the surgical societies and the surgical journals contain more rather than fewer papers dealing with the application of chemistry to surgical problems! Anyway, the Year Book is glad to publish abstracts of many of the papers of that kind, because they represent the surgery of 1953 and not that of 1900."

Conduction Anesthesia. By George P. Pitkin, M.D., edited by James L. Southworth, M.D., Robert A. Hingson, M.D., and Winifred M. Pitkin, M.D. Ed. 2. Pp. 1005, with 36 tables and 585 illustrations. Philadelphia, 1953, J. B. Lippincott Company.

A comprehensive and thorough revision and modernization of the original "encyclopedia" of regional anesthesia is offered in the second edition of *Conduction Anesthesia.*

The basic neuroanatomy section of the book has been enlarged by the inclusion of a chapter on the vertebral canal. Modern techniques such as transtracheal cocainization appear in the new chapter on topical anesthesia agents. Similarly, a chapter on the complications of conduction anesthesia, including their causes, preventions, and specific treatments, has been added.

Of even greater interest in the revision of the section on the pharmacology of local anesthetics, which places major emphasis on hypotension, the principal untoward action of these agents. Many obsolete compounds have been deleted, and such popular new compounds as Xylocaine have been added. The use of vasopressor drugs in conjunction with anesthetic agents is dealt with much more fully. Furthermore, the addition of new equipment (polyethylene and vinoplastic catheters) to the surgeons' and anesthesiologists' armamentarium is included.

The recent popularity of extradural anesthesia has necessitated the revision of the chapter on this subject. Alterations have been made in the section on spinal anesthesia so that it now contains the most modern spinal anesthetic techniques and agents. In addition, there is a topographic table of the relationships of the spinal nerves and attachments to the spinal cord and their vertebrae. An important supplement to the chapter on the anatomy of the spinal nerves concerns the dermatomes, myotomes, and scleratomes, with numerous diagrammatic illustrations. The anatomic section on the autonomic nervous system has been rewritten, and emphasis placed largely on various reflex arcs which are more fully described and illustrated. Included also are diagrammatic illustrations of the afferent and efferent innervation of the various organs by both the parasympathetic and sympathetic pathways. Another important addition is the section dealing with anatomic innervation of the adrenal glands. Moreover the section on local anesthesia now includes specific nerve block techniques for cesarean section and labor, and there has been much revision and enlargement of the section on therapeutic and diagnostic conduction anesthesia.

As in the first edition, this volume represents a complete encyclopedic treatment of nerve block anesthesia. The various sections dealing with specific nerve blocks are individually approached from an anatomic standpoint, even though this necessitates much repetition of the pertinent neuroanatomy involved. The techniques of the specific blocks themselves are described from every practical anatomic approach. This in itself makes the book unique since many patients have pathologic restrictions to what is perhaps the best approach, and it becomes necessary for the surgeon or anesthesiologist to choose some alternative approach.

Although this text is specifically intended for the anesthesiologist and the surgeon, it will prove of immeasurable benefit as a reference guide to the neurologist, the obstetrician and gynecologist, the ophthalmologist, and the dentist, as well.

Pathologie vasculaire, medicale et chirurgicale (Vascular Pathology, Medical and Surgical). By Marceau Servelle. Paris, 1952, Masson & Cie.

This book is essentially a text for the surgeon interested in clinical applied vascular surgery. It includes the practical approach to the various arterial, venous, and lymphatic problems and also includes the surgical treatment of the congenital cardiac anomalies, as well as those of the acquired type.

Written in French, it reads very easily, and the author presents reasonable arguments for his particular approach to the various vascular lesions. There are adequate illustrations to emphasize his statements. While the reference form is not that which the American medical reader is used to, the author does include some references in his historical accounts and discussions of the subject. However, no formal bibliography is presented.

In some areas, the author has gone a little further than the average vascular surgeon's interests, for example, in discussion of intracranial aneurysms and their treatment. In other areas, the discussion is usually brief, as in his short section on thoracic and abdominal aortic aneurysms. There are many errors that would have been picked up by more careful proofreading. (As examples of this, one can cite the misspelling of Raynaud which appears on page 38 as Reynaud. Also such errors as the author's reference on page 61 to Dr. E. Allen of the Mayo Clinic as a vascular surgeon.)

The advances being made in the field of vascular surgery are so rapid that a text such as this is outdated much more than the average textbook by the time it goes to print. The loose paper binding does not stand up well. A table of contents is given at the end of the book which is of some value, but it would seem that a text of this sort would deserve an index as well as a table of contents.

In summary, this French text presents in a fairly clear fashion some worth-while material for the clinical surgeon interested in vascular disorders of various types. The rapid advances which have been made recently in the field of vascular surgery make the author's experiences which are presented here somewhat more out of date than in the usual textbook.

Prostatectomy: A Method and Its Management. By Charles Wells, professor of surgery, University of Liverpool. Pp. 103, with 72 figures, 17 tables, and 65 references. Cloth. Chapters on history, pathology, sequellae, clinical features, indications for treatment, anesthesia, surgical technique, postoperative care, severe chronic urinary retention; fluids, electrolytes, and proteins; analysis of 205 consecutive admissions to hospital for prostatism, and late results. Edinburgh and London, 1952, E. & S. Livingstone.

Of the 205 patients in the series, 47 had acute and 56 high-grade chronic retention. The blood urea was normal in 84 and elevated in the remainder. Ninety were past 70 years of age. Ten had stones in the bladder, 10 had vesical diverticula, and 4 had papillomata. The surgical mortality was 3 per cent. While the catheter was removed on the fifth day, only 27 patients were discharged before the fourteenth day; the others stayed longer, many up to three or four weeks. Penicillin and a triple sulfonamide were used before operation, and Mandelamine afterward.

Follow-up was carried out for one to three years in 194 patients. None was incontinent of urine, and none had obstructive symptoms.

This book is a forthright discussion of the experience of the author and his associates with their version of the ''aseptic'' suprapubic enucleation of Wilson Hey. The novel aspects of this technique include avoidance of catheterization before operation, and the retrograde passage and fixation of a urethral catheter at its conclusion. Otherwise, the operation itself is a conventional suprapubic enucleation with careful hemostasis with diathermy, Oxycel, and Gelfoam.

The urinary tract is investigated beforehand only by excretory urography. Urinalysis and culture are carried out before operation only if the patient is able to void. Impaired renal function is not regarded as a contraindication to operation; indeed, 121 of the 205 patients had elevated blood ureas, some as high as 150 mg. per cent. In many instances, operation is performed as an emergency in patients with acute retention. Drainage with a catheter is employed only when serious extraurogenital lesions require treatment in patients with complete or nearly complete retention.

While this attitude toward preliminary drainage contravenes one of the most firmly established principles of modern urology, the author's results suggest that the old principles may be wrong. He states that no patient was refused operation; yet, the mortality was but 3 per cent in 205 consecutive cases! This leads one to wonder what could be achieved by applying the same principles to transurethral resection.

The reviewer does not share Mr. Wells's grim attitude toward catheterization, and has achieved a mortality in transurethral resection considerably lower than the author's in "aseptic prostatectomy," despite free use of the catheter. It is necessary to point out, too, that a mortality of 3 per cent in 205 cases does not mean that it would be the same in 1,000 such cases. That there may have been a certain element of luck in a surgical mortality of 3 per cent with this operation is suggested by Aiken's report (Brit. J. Urol. **25:** 20 [March] 1953) of fifteen deaths in 150 cases.

This book should be read by every surgeon who has occasion to operate upon the prostate gland. One who does so, and then reads the treatises of Millin on retropubic, of Nesbit and of Barnes on transurethral, and of Young on perineal prostatectomy will be very well informed about prostatectomy.

ANNOUNCEMENT

1953-1954 SCHOLARSHIPS IN PLASTIC AND RECONSTRUCTIVE SURGERY

The Foundation of the American Society of Plastic and Reconstructive Surgery announces the regulations of the Fifth Annual Scholarship Contest:

1. The contest in *Junior* Classification is restricted to residents in training and to plastic surgeons who have been in practice *no longer than five years.*
2. Two main prizes are offered, each consisting of a *three-month plastic surgery scholarship* with full maintenance in a number of selected leading services, in the United States and abroad.
3. The subject matter of the essay must be the result of some *original* research (either clinical or experimental) in the field of plastic and reconstructive surgery. The thesis should be of about 5,000 words, and written in English.
4. Work previously published wholly or in part is not acceptable.
5. Expenses of travel between the services will be allotted.
6. A silver plaque or a certificate of honorable mention is also offered for a winning essay in *Senior* Classification to contestants active in practice of plastic and reconstructive surgery for *more than five years.*
7. Manuscripts will not be accepted by the Award Committee *after July 1, 1954.*
8. The winning essays will be presented in person at a formal program of the Foundation of the A. S. of P. and R. S. to be held in the fall of 1954.

The 1953 Scholarships were awarded to Robert M. McCormack, M.D., Rochester, N. Y., for an essay, "Simultaneous Chordee Repair and Urethral Reconstruction for Hypospadias," and to James Calnan, F.R.C.S., Oxford, England, for an essay, "The Error of Gustav Passavant," subtitle: "A Refutation of the Recognized Velo-Pharyngeal Mechanism in Speech."

For further information, write to the Award Committe, c/o Jacques W. Maliniac, M.D., Chairman, 30 Central Park South, New York, N. Y.

SURGERY

Vol. 35 March, 1954 No. 3

Original Communications

OCCULT CARCINOMA OF THE MAJOR BRONCHI*

William H. Wierman, M.D.,** John R. McDonald, M.D.,*** and
O. Theron Clagett, M.D.,**** Rochester, Minn.

THE purpose of this study is to describe five cases of surgically resected squamous cell carcinoma of the major bronchi in which there was no readily apparent gross tumor formation. One of the lesions was a carcinoma in situ, while the others were small, superfically invasive malignant growths with surrounding areas of in situ carcinoma.

These lesions exhibited a growth pattern in which the malignant epithelium grew in a rather centrifugal manner, often over wide areas, rather than in a centripetal fashion where growth was concentrated in one region with a resultant gross tumor formation. Such lesions may be overlooked rather easily, but we believe that with proper correlation of cytologic studies of sputum and bronchoscopic examination, they may be recognized.

These cases have important clinical and surgical implications because of the difficulties encountered in detecting and localizing the carcinoma, the decision as to the extent of the resection, and, last, the surgical and pathologic recognition of such occult lesions.

REVIEW OF LITERATURE

Since 1932 when Broders[1] first used the term "carcinoma in situ," much has been written about it. Most of the discussion has concerned the cervix,[2, 3] but carcinoma in situ has been reported as occurring in the breast,[4] larynx,[5] endometrium,[6] kidney,[7] stomach,[8] skin,[9] appendix,[10] and even pharyngeal diverticula.[11]

Much of the knowledge of preinvasive carcinoma has been obtained from studies of carcinoma in situ of the cervix uteri, from which the following features have been determined:

Received for publication, July 6, 1953.

*Abridgment of thesis submitted by Dr. Wierman to the Faculty of the Graduate School of the University of Minnesota in partial fulfillment of the requirements for the degree of Master of Science in Surgery.

**Fellow in surgery, Mayo Foundation.

***Division of Surgical Pathology, Mayo Clinic.

****Division of Surgery, Mayo Clinic.

1. By definition there must be no invasion. The malignant epithelium is separated from the underlying stroma by an intact basement membrane.

2. A malignant epithelium growing on a free surface exfoliates its cells, which may then be recognized as such when the appropriate secretions are studied cytologically.

3. The results of cytologic study are more often positive when there is involvement of the mucous glands than when there is only surface epithelial involvement. Younge, Hertig, and Armstrong[3] have shown that when only the surface epithelium of the cervix is carcinomatous, the results of cytologic study are positive in 53 per cent of cases, whereas with mucous glandular involvement, malignant cells are found in 93 per cent.

4. There are no gross characteristics of carcinoma in situ of the cervix. This has been emphasized by many.

5. Appropriate biopsies of a cervix when the results of cytologic study are positive will reveal the carcinomatous area in a high percentage of cases. Foote and Stewart[2] found that biopsies of such cervices at the twelve, three, six, and nine o'clock positions at the squamous-columnar epithelial juncture revealed the carcinoma in 90 per cent of cases.

6. All carcinomas in situ eventually invade the underlying stroma. The time factor generally accepted for the cervical variety is approximately ten years.

7. Complete eradication of the affected epithelium effects a cure.

These findings may then possibly be applied to carcinoma of the bronchial tree. Thus, probably all bronchogenic carcinomas begin as in situ lesions. If they could then be recognized and treated adequately, the survival rate might be expected to equal that of persons with cervical lesions of this nature.

However, the bronchial tree, with its anatomic pairing, large surface area, vital nature, and relative inaccessibility, presents a much more complex problem in the detection and treatment of an early carcinoma than does the cervix. The sputum may be positive for malignant cells, but if the roentgenogram of the chest does not reveal any abnormality, the question then arises as to which side should be operated on.

Our interest in bronchogenic carcinoma in situ was stimulated by a case encountered in 1951, and since then we have studied the literature on this variety of lesion. Papanicolaou and Koprowska[12] reported a case of squamous cell bronchogenic carcinoma initially diagnosed by means of cytologic examination of sputum. Pneumonia and pulmonary edema developed, and the patient died, with the carcinomatous focus being undetected. At necrospy, no grossly visible tumor of the lungs could be found. However, a minute area of roughening of the bronchial mucosa of the right lower lobe proved, on sectioning, to contain an epidermoid carcinoma in situ. Papanicolaou and Koprowska stressed the importance of cytologic studies in making an early diagnosis of carcinoma of the lung, and mentioned the confusing dilemma of being confronted with positive sputum findings and a normal-appearing roentgenogram of the chest, a situation we have experienced several times.

Umiker and Storey[13] later reported a case of epidermoid bronchogenic carcinoma in situ detected at bronchoscopy when a "small, slightly granular and thickened area" was noted in the bronchus of the right lower lobe. Biopsy revealed the nature of the lesion. A right lower lobectomy for "a grossly invisible lesion" was then performed.

Recently, Black and Ackerman[14] and Williams[15] separately have written of the importance of carinoma in situ in the histogenesis of bronchogenic carcinoma. Black and Ackerman stated that 22 per cent of their invasive epidermoid and undifferentiated carcinomas were associated with adjacent areas of malignant change in situ.

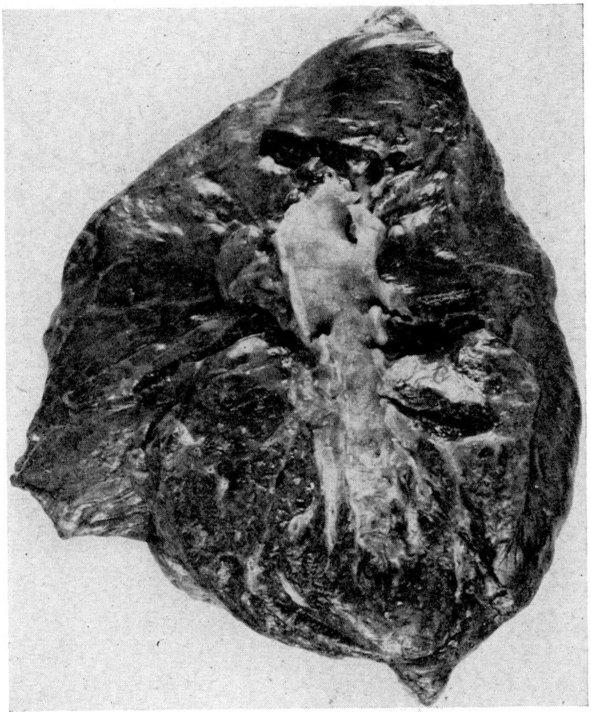

Fig. 1 (Case 1).—Right lung removed because of extensive epidermoid carcinoma in situ. There is practically complete obliteration of the mucosal longitudinal furrows. No gross tumor was present, yet microscopic examination revealed that the carcinoma in situ involved most of the bronchial epithelium.

Previously, Carlisle, McDonald, and Harrington[16] reported that carcinoma in situ frequently surrounds an invasive epidermoid tumor.

Griess, McDonald, and Clagett[17] have demonstrated that approximately 43 per cent of excised bronchogenic carcinomas have a proximal extension of the tumor beyond grossly recognizable limits. Squamous cell epitheliomas comprised 80 per cent of the group, and one-fifth of these showed in situ extension over an average area of 5 mm.

In the literature, there are numerous reports of minute peripheral pulmonary tumors believed by some to represent early bronchogenic carcinoma. Prior and Jones[18] collected reports of twelve such cases from the literature and added eight of their own. They reviewed the data on these cases and found the following to be true: the majority of the lesions were found incidentally in necropsy or surgical material; most occurred in a subpleural location, and approximately 70 per cent were in women; 20 per cent of the patients were less than 40 years of age; 70 per cent had an associated bronchiectasis. These findings cast serious doubt on the possibility that these foci represent early bronchogenic carcinoma.

A.

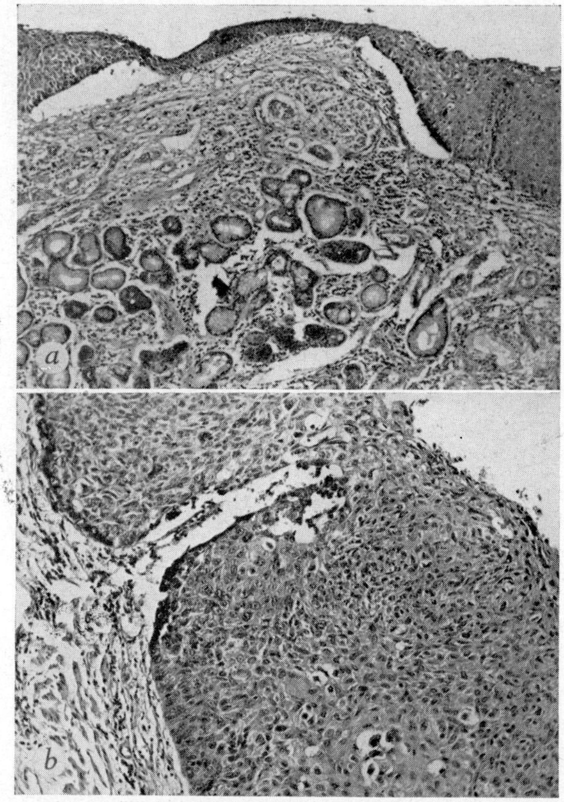

B.

Fig. 2 (Case 1).—*a*, Section of an epidermoid carcinoma in situ of the middle lobe bronchus. The epithelial proliferation extended into the mucosal invaginations and obliterated the longitudinal furrows (hematoxylin and eosin; ×75, reduced ¼). *b*, Section of an epidermoid carcinoma in situ involving the right lower lobe bronchus (hematoxylin and eosin; ×150 reduced ¼).

CASE 1.—The first case to stimulate our interest in this subject was that of a 50-year-old white plumber. He reported that three weeks previously he had experienced an acute respiratory infection characterized by a productive cough and a temperature of 104° F., which had persisted for three days and had then responded to penicillin therapy. Since that time, he had complained of an aching pain in the right lower anterior part of the chest and a cough productive of small amounts of mucoid sputum. There was no history of hemoptysis. A roentgenogram of the chest three months before admission was said to have disclosed no abnormality.

The initial roentgenograms of the chest taken at the clinic revealed a diffuse infiltration with linear fibrosis in the right base, and the patient was admitted to the hospital with the diagnosis of bronchopneumonia of the right lower lobe. He received penicillin both as an aerosol and as an intramuscular injection, and ten days later the pulmonary infiltration had greatly subsided. While he was under study at the hopsital, a cytologic examination of sputum disclosed malignant cells.

Bronchoscopy was performed. Although the bronchoscopist could see no tumor, he described a roughening of the mucosa on the medial wall of the right bronchus intermedius. Biopsy of this area revealed a Grade 3 squamous cell carcinoma in situ.

A right thoracotomy was performed. The surgeon found the middle lobe and the anterior portion of the lower lobe to be quite indurated, and he performed a right pneumonectomy. The patient made an uneventful convalescence, and was doing well twenty months after operation.

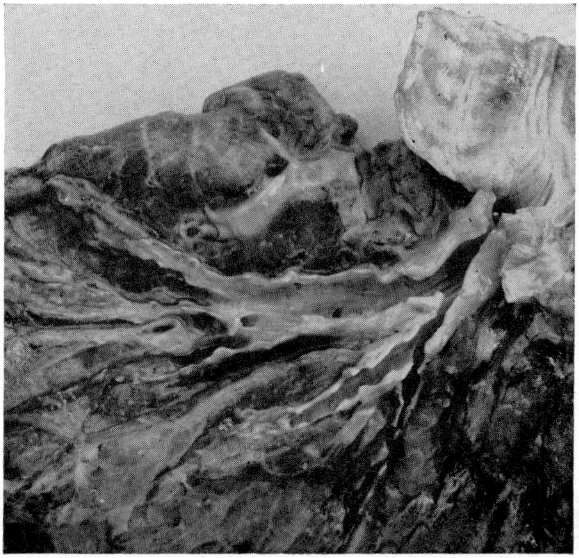

Fig. 3.—Specimen showing the normal pattern of the bronchial mucosa. Note the longitudinal furrows that are present in the main bronchus and extend into the secondary and tertiary divisions as well.

When the surgically removed lung was examined in the pathology laboratory, a group of physicians who were present were told that the patient's sputum was positive for malignant cells, and they were asked to identify ''the tumor.'' None was able to do so. Several mentioned that the bronchial mucosa appeared to be peculiarly roughened, but the consensus was that no carcinoma was present and that the results of cytologic examination had been falsely positive.

Numerous microscopic sections at various levels of the right main bronchus, bronchus intermedius, upper middle, and lower lobe bronchi, and to a varying degree their secondary branches revealed a diffuse, Grade 3 squamous cell carcinoma in situ. The involved epithelium was irregularly thickened, and exhibited a ''heaping action'' extending into the mucosal invaginations and obliterating them. The mucous glands were involved with carcinoma, but no invasion of the stroma in any of the sections examined could be demonstrated.

Although the epithelial involvement with carcinoma was widespread, there were numerous ''skip areas'' measuring up to 1 cm. in diameter where the bronchial mucosa was devoid of carcinomatous changes. At one point, the cancer was seen to extend as close as 2 mm. to the line of resection of the right main bronchus.

The gross appearance of the right bronchial tree (Fig. 1) was found to parallel the microscopic appearance (Fig. 2), namely, that of a shaggy proliferation of the bronchial epithelium with carcinoma which imparted a diffuse gross roughening of the mucous membrane. The photograph of the surgical specimen when compared to a normal one (Fig. 3) showed granular obliteration of the mucosal invaginations by carcinoma and loss of the typical sheen.

No evidence of involvement of the lymph nodes was found.

The typical pathologic appearance of obstructive pneumonitis was found in the middle lobe and the anterior portion of the lower lobe. This correlated with the preoperative roentgenologic appearance. It might well be asked why an obstructive pattern is present when no ''obstruction'' of the corresponding bronchi can be found. We believe that the obstruction in such a case is physiologic rather than organic. The normal ciliated epithelium has been replaced by a carcinomatous squamous epithelium, and the lack of cilia, along with the bronchial splinting caused by the epithelial proliferation, results in inability to propel secretions. The cough reflex is apparently adequate to keep the mainstem bronchus clear.

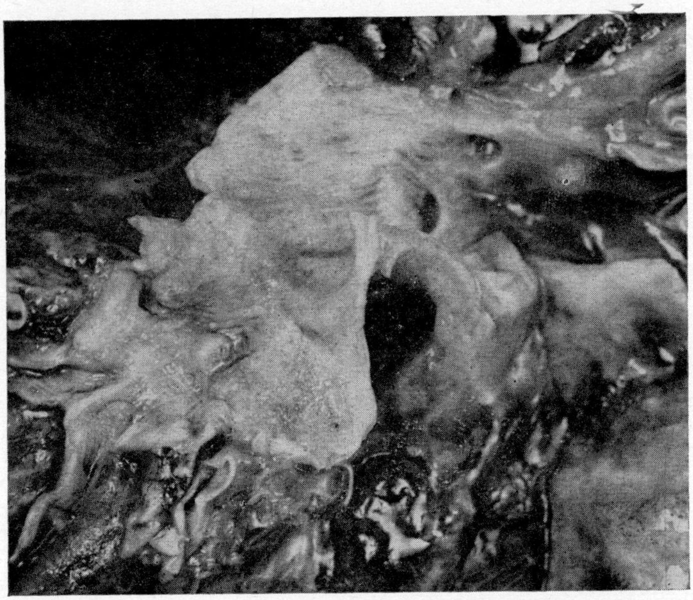

Fig. 4 (Case 2).—Surgically removed lung showing a hidden epidermoid carcinoma in the right upper lobe bronchus. The lesion has obliterated the bronchial striae over an area of 3 cm., and the mucosa has a granular appearance. Bronchial striations are present in the uninvolved portions of the bronchial tree.

Case 2.—A 62-year-old white man gave a history that one year previously he had had virus pneumonia followed by a productive cough and intermittent hemoptysis. Roentgenographic examination of the chest gave negative results, but cytologic examination of the sputum disclosed the presence of malignant cells. Bronchoscopy revealed an area of roughening of the mucosa of the right upper lobe bronchus, but no tumor was visible. Biopsy of this area disclosed a Grade 3 squamous cell carcinoma. At the time of bronchoscopy, both sides of the bronchial tree were aspirated and the secretions studied cytologically. Malignant cells were found in each specimen. The patient underwent a right thoracotomy, and the lung was described as being normal to palpation. A right pneumonectomy was performed. Pathologic examination revealed a superficially invasive epidermoid carcinoma, 2 mm. in diameter, in the orifice of the right upper lobe bronchus (Fig. 4). Extending from the right main bronchus into the right upper lobe bronchus for a distance of 3 cm., and completely surrounding the invasive tumor, was a carcinoma in situ. This area exhibited grossly a granular obliteration of the mucosal invaginations. None of the lymph nodes was found to be involved with carcinoma.

CASE 3.—A 67-year-old white man had been seen at this clinic eight years before, at which time a diagnosis of squamous cell carcinoma in situ of both vocal cords was made. Thyrotomy was performed, and the cords were electrocoagulated. Subsequent examinations revealed no recurrence. On the present visit, he complained that a recent upper respiratory infection had left him with a residual cough slightly productive of mucoid sputum. X-ray examination of the chest revealed an obstructive pneumonitis of the right upper lobe. He was immediately examined bronchoscopically, but no cytologic examination of the sputum was made. Bronchoscopy revealed an area of nodularity in the depth of the right upper lobe bronchus, but no tumor per se was visualized. Biopsy of the region disclosed a Grade 4 epidermoid carcinoma. Bronchial aspiration for cytologic study gave negative results. A right pneumonectomy was performed, and because of carinal involvement it was necessary to resect a portion of the trachea as well. On pathologic examination a superficially invasive Grade 4 epidermoid carcinoma, 3 mm. in diameter, was found in the orifice of the right upper lobe bronchus, and extending proximally for a distance of 3 cm. into the main-stem bronchus and distally into all three subdivisions of the upper lobe was a carcinoma in situ. No lymph nodes were found to be involved with carcinoma.

The original laryngeal carcinoma was compared to the present one, and although the two lesions were similar, it was felt that they undoubtedly represented separate primary lesions.

CASE 4.—A 63-year-old white man stated on admission that seven months previously he had contracted a severe cold, and that since then he had had pain in the left side of the chest and a nonproductive cough. One week before admission he had had hemoptysis. Roentgenograms of the chest disclosed a poorly defined infiltration in the left upper lobe. Initial cytologic examination of the sputum revealed malignant cells. At bronchoscopy, although an excellent view of the left upper lobe bronchus was obtained, nothing abnormal could be seen, and the results of examination were interpreted as being negative. However, examination of aspirated secretions from the left upper lobe at the time revealed malignant cells. A left pneumonectomy was performed. A Grade 3 infiltrating squamous cell epithelioma, 3 mm. in diameter, was found in the left upper lobe bronchus at the bifurcation of the apical posterior and anterior divisions. Extending proximally for a distance of 1.5 cm. was an epidermoid carcinoma in situ. None of the examined lymph nodes were positive for carcinoma.

CASE 5.—A 64-year-old white man stated that six weeks previously he had experienced pleurisy in the left anterior part of the chest and a productive cough which had persisted to the time of admission. X-ray examination of the chest disclosed obstructive pneumonitis of the lingula. Examination of the sputum revealed the presence of malignant cells. Bronchoscopy gave negative results, but atypical cells were found in aspirated secretions. A left pneumonectomy was performed. At the orifice of the lingular bronchus and extending distally for 1.2 cm. was a superficially invasive, Grade 3 epidermoid carcinoma which formed no definite gross tumor. No lymph nodes were found to be involved with carcinoma.

The following case, although characterized by the eventual development of a readily recognizable gross tumor, is reported merely to illustrate how "hidden" a bronchogenic carcinoma can be.

A 58-year-old white man had complained, for many years, of a chronic cough which had increased following a cold approximately one month previously. On admission, he was raising about one tablespoon of mucoid sputum daily. There was no history of hemoptysis. Examination of the chest revealed numerous rhonchi bilaterally, but they were more numerous on the left. The results of roentgenographic examination of the chest were negative. Cytologic examination of the sputum disclosed the presence of malignant cells. In the hope of isolating the lesion, bronchoscopic examination was performed. An area of reddening within the orifice of the left upper lobe bronchus was detected, and biopsy of this region was attempted, but it was felt by the bronchoscopist that representative tissue was not obtained; only inflammation of the mucosa was observed on microscopic examination of the biopsy specimen. Bronchial secretions aspirated from the left upper lobe bronchus contained malignant cells. Because of the unreliability of bronchial aspirations alone in the localization of an intrabronchial neoplasm, it was with considerable reluctance that the patient was submitted to a left exploratory thoracotomy. When the chest was opened, no pulmonary abnormality could be found by either inspection or palpation; consequently, a left upper lobectomy was performed. No bronchial lesion could be found on pathologic examination. Two weeks postoperatively, cytologic examination of the sputum again disclosed the presence of malignant cells. The patient was sent home for convalescence and returned in two and one-half months, at which time the sputum was again positive for malignant cells. Bronchoscopy then revealed a gross tumor in the stump of the left upper lobe bronchus. A left pneumonectomy was performed. A Grade 4 epidermoid carcinoma measuring 1.8 by 1.5 by 1.5 cm. was found in the stump of the left upper lobe bronchus. It extended through the bronchial wall into the surrounding lung and directly invaded one lymph node.

Woolner and McDonald[19, 20] have stated that the obvious shortcoming of examination of the sputum for malignant cells is that it does not localize the source. Carcinoma cells found in the sputum may originate from a lesion situated anywhere in the respiratory tract, pharynx, esophagus, or possibly stomach. They reported a case of an esophageal carcinoma developing in the region of an old lye stricture. Subsequently, a treacheo-esophageal fistula resulted and malignant cells were recovered in the sputum.

As Papanicolaou and Koprowska[12] have indicated, the cytologic examination of the sputum and bronchial washings may reveal an early bronchogenic carcinoma. But the lesion must be localized before effective treatment can be instituted. When obstruction is present, a roentgenogram of the chest permits such localization, but when the results of roentgenographic examination are negative, the situation can be trying. Because of the ease with which ''contamination'' can occur, bronchial washings and aspirated material taken from selected sites for cytologic study in an attempt to isolate the involved lobe do not appear to offer a reliable basis for localization of the lesion.

COMMENT

In an attempt to determine whether there is a gross change, however slight, in the bronchial mucosa of these ''hidden'' bronchogenic carcinomas, the surgically removed specimens in Cases 1 to 5 were carefully studied. Normally the main, secondary, and, for a variable distance, the teritiary bronchi have an invaginated mucosal pattern. This pattern grossly appears as a series of longtitudinal furrows or grooves (Fig. 3). The corresponding ridges of the furrows are due to irregularly placed submucosal smooth-muscle bundles (Fig. 5). Just as a carcinoma may destroy this topography by invasion, likewise a carcinoma in situ may alter it by proliferation of the carcinomatous epithelium, and by a ''heaping'' action it may extend into the sulci and obliterate them. Thus, the typical undulating mucosal pattern is destroyed even though no grossly protruding tumor is present. We have found no specific mention of this phenomenon in the literature, although Papanicolaou and Koprowska,[12] in describing their case, mentioned that the bronchial mucosal invaginations became completely lined by neoplastic epithelium and finally were transformed into short, thick neoplastic cords or nests which occupied the entire thickness of the epithelium. Likewise, Umiker and Storey,[13] in the description of their case, spoke of replacement of the invaginated mucosal folds with neoplastic epithelium.

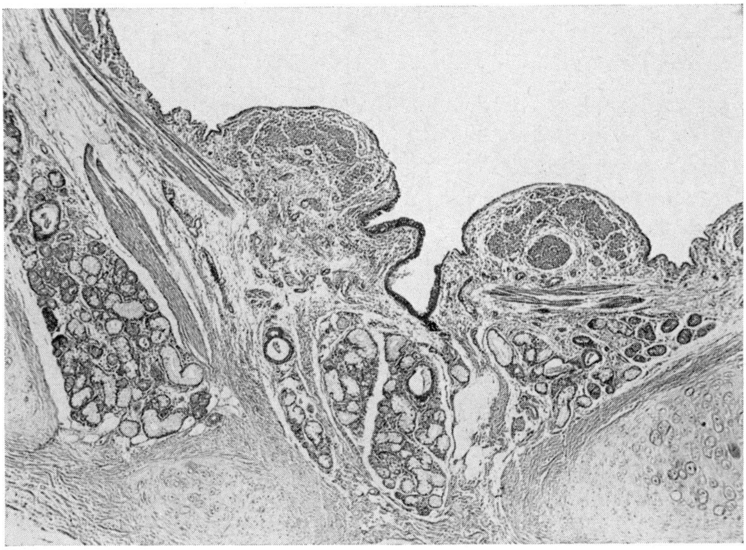

Fig. 5.—Cross section of a normal secondary bronchus showing the longitudinal furrows and corresponding ridges of the bronchial mucosa (hematoxylin and eosin; ×30). This normal topography may be destroyed by proiferation of malignant epithelium, yet no grossly recognizable tumor may be formed.

We believe that an appreciation of this mucosal pattern can aid significantly in the bronchoscopic detection of bronchogenic carcinoma even though no tumor per se is seen. From the study of our own cases plus the few appearing in the literature, it seems that it is advisable to subject to biopsy any area of the bronchial mucosa in which the longitudinal furrows have become obliterated. The obliterative process may be associated with a wrinkling, thickening, granular, or nodular appearance of the mucosa which should call attention to the correct area to be examined by biopsy or smear. If such areas are routinely subjected to biopsy, early bronchogenic carcinoma will be detected more often than at present.

The scope of surgical treatment of superficially invasive and in situ bronchogenic carcinoma should be considered. One might think that such an early lesion as a carcinoma in situ could be treated adequately by lobectomy. However, when the tendency toward widespread involvement is considered, pneumonectomy would appear to be the procedure of choice. Moreover, one should be aware of the possibility that the process may involve the opposite side.

Aufses and Neuhof[21] have reported two cases of bronchoscopic removal of carcinoma and subsequent resection, in which no residual tumor could be found. The first patient was treated by pneumonectomy and was well some six years later. The second was treated by a right middle lobectomy. Subsequently, the carcinoma involved the right main bronchus and extended to the trachea. Aufses and Neuhof stated that if an unequivocal diagnosis of carcinoma is made by a pathologist from biopsy tissue removed from a major bronchus, a pneumonectomy should be performed even though no gross evidence of a malignant lesion is found at operation.

Black and Ackerman[14] have stated that the finding of an in situ bronchogenic carcinoma usually implies an associated invasive tumor. Our study would seem to substantiate this. Further, since these tumors have a central origin, pneumonectomy would appear to be the procedure of choice.

SUMMARY AND CONCLUSIONS

Our study of five cases of occult bronchogenic carcinoma disclosed the following pertinent facts:

1. Surgical resection was performed in all cases.
2. Squamous cell carcinoma was the lesion in each case.
3. The major bronchi were involved in all cases.
4. The lesions were not readily apparent. One was in situ and four were grossly minute lesions with a rather wide area of in situ carcinoma surrounding the invasive portion.
5. In four of the cases, cytologic examination of the sputum disclosed the presence of malignant cells. This examination was not made in the remaining case.
6. In none of the cases were lymph nodes found to be involved with carcinoma.
7. In two of the cases, grave surgical implications were presented. In Case 1, although the carcinoma was in situ, the process was widespread, involving most of the right bronchial tree, and it extended to within 2 mm. of the line of resection. Furthermore, there were multiple skip areas where the epithelium was devoid of carcinoma. This further raises the possibility of carcinomatous involvement of the opposite bronchial tree. In Case 3, an in situ epidermoid carcinoma of the vocal cords had been treated eight years previously, and there were no signs of recurrence. The bronchogenic focus had extended from the right upper lobe bronchus proximally to the carina, and resection of a portion of trachea was necessary.

We wish to stress the fact that an epidermoid bronchogenic carcinoma can appear as a superficial nonprojecting tumor. The malignant epithelium grows in a somewhat centrifugal manner, and by its epithelial proliferation it obliterates the normal longitudinal furrows of the bronchial mucosa, imparting a granular or roughened appearance. Such an area of morphologic change can be detected bronchoscopically, and it should be subjected to biopsy. When biopsy is performed in conjunction with cytologic studies of the sputum, bronchogenic carcinoma may be detected early, when treatment is more likely to be effective.

REFERENCES

1. Broders, A. C.: Carcinoma in Situ Contrasted With Benign Penetrating Epithelium, J. A. M. A. **99**: 1670-1674, 1932.
2. Foote, F. W., and Stewart, F. W.: Anatomical Distribution of Intraepithelial Epidermoid Carcinomas of Cervix, Cancer **1**: 431-440, 1948.
3. Younge, P. A., Hertig, A. T., and Armstrong, D.: A Study of 135 Cases of Carcinoma in Situ of the Cervix at the Free Hospital for Women, Am. J. Obst. & Gynec. **58**: 867-892, 1949.
4. Foote, F. W., Jr., and Stewart, F. W.: Lobular Carcinoma in Situ; Rare Form of Mammary Cancer, Am. J. Path. **17**: 491-496, 1941.
5. Gordon, G. R.: Keratosis of Larynx. Report of Case With Underlying Carcinoma in Situ, Laryngoscope **60**: 1201-1209, 1950.
6. Hertig, A. T., Sommers, S. C., and Bengloff, H.: Genesis of Endometrial Carcinoma. III. Carcinoma in Situ, Cancer **2**: 964, 1949.
7. Foot, N. C., and Papanicolaou, G. H.: Early Renal Carcinoma in Situ: Detected by Means of Smears of Fixed Urinary Sediment, J. A. M. A. **139**: 356-358, 1949.
8. Mallory, T. B.: Carcinoma in Situ of the Stomach and Its Bearing on the Histogenesis of Malignant Ulcers, Arch. Path. **30**: 348-362, 1940.
9. Montgomery, H.: Precancerous Dermatosis and Epithelioma in Situ, Arch. Dermat. & Syph. **39**: 387-408, 1939.
10. McCollum, W., and Pund, E. R.: Preinvasive Adenocarcinoma of the Appendix: Report of Sixteen Cases, Cancer **4**: 261-264, 1951.
11. Bullock, W. K., and Snyder, E. N., Jr.: Carcinoma in Situ Occurring in a Pharyngeal Diverticulum, Cancer **5**: 737-739, 1952.
12. Papanicolaou, G. N., and Koprowska, I.: Carcinoma in Situ of the Right Lower Bronchus: A Case Report, Cancer **4**: 141-146, 1951.
13. Umiker, W., and Storey, C.: Bronchogenic Carcinoma in Situ: Report of a Case With Positive Biopsy, Cytological Examination, and Lobectomy, Cancer **5**: 369-374, 1952.
14. Black, H., and Ackerman, L. V.: The Importance of Epidermoid Carcinoma *in Situ* in the Histogenesis of Carcinoma of the Lung, Ann. Surg. **136**: 44-55, 1952.
15. Williams, M. J.: Extensive Carcinoma in Situ in the Bronchial Mucosa Associated With Two Invasive Bronchogenic Carcinomas: Report of Case, Cancer **5**: 740-747, 1952.
16. Carlisle, J. C., McDonald, J. R., and Harrington, S. W.: Bronchogenic Squamous-cell Carcinoma, J. Thoracic Surg. **22**: 74-82, 1951.
17. Griess, D. F., McDonald, J. R., and Clagett, O. T.: The Proximal Extension of Carcinoma of the Lung in the Bronchial Wall, J. Thoracic Surg. **14**: 362-368, 1945.
18. Prior, J. T., and Jones, D. B.: Minute Peripheral Pulmonary Tumors: A Study of Eight Cases, J. Thoracic Surg. **23**: 224-236, 1952.
19. Woolner, L. B., and McDonald, J. R.: Bronchogenic Carcinoma: Diagnosis by Microscopic Examination of Sputum and Bronchial Secretions; Preliminary Report, Proc. Staff Meet., Mayo Clin. **22**: 369-381, 1947.
20. Woolner, L. B., and McDonald, J. R.: Carcinoma Cells in Sputum and Bronchial Secretions: A Study of 150 Consecutive Cases in Which Results Were Positive, Surg., Gynec. & Obst. **88**: 273-290, 1949.
21. Aufses, A. H., and Neuhof, Harold: Minute Carcinoma of the Major Bronchi: A Follow-up Report, J. Thoracic Surg. **23**: 219-223, 1952.

INTRACRANIAL METASTASIS FROM CARCINOMA OF THE LUNG

BÉLA HALPERT, M.D., WILLIAM S. FIELDS, M.D., AND MICHAEL E. DE BAKEY, M.D.
HOUSTON, TEXAS

(From the Departments of Pathology, Psychiatry and Neurology, and Surgery, Baylor University College of Medicine, and the Veterans Administration Hospital)

METASTASIS to the brain from carcinoma of the lung occurs frequently.[1-3] While this is generally conceded, information is not available as to how often it occurs in a substantial number of consecutive patients.[4] The reasons are that authorization for necropsy may not be obtainable and the brain may not be included in the examination. During the past three and one-half years (July 21, 1949, to Jan. 20, 1953) in this Veterans Administration Hospital the authorization for post-mortem examination was consistently 90 per cent or over, and in nearly 95 per cent of these cases the brain was included in the examination. Furthermore, the patients were almost exclusively men in the third through the ninth decades of life, yielding a large percentage of patients with carcinoma. During this period, among 891 necropsies there were exactly 100 performed on patients with carcinoma of the lung, and in 92 of these the brain was included in the examination.

An analysis of the 100 cases was undertaken to determine the frequency of metastatic involvement of the brain from carcinoma of the lung and to provide information as to which cell type is most likely to do so. An attempt was also made to determine from clinical data the time relation between the appearance of the neoplasm in the lung and the metastasis in the brain.

Material and Method.—For the purpose of this study the clinical histories and findings at necropsy were reviewed in the 100 patients. A photograph of the gross specimen of the lung and of the brain, when involved, was usually available, as well as the gross specimen and microscopic preparations from the primary site and from all other locations listed in the anatomic diagnosis. All brains were fixed in formalin (10 per cent) for periods of at least three weeks prior to examination.

Incidence.—All of the patients were men (85 white, 15 Negro), 3 were in the third, 7 in the fourth, 14 (3 Negro) in the fifth, 50 (8 Negro) in the sixth, 19 (4 Negro) in the seventh, and 7 in the eighth decade of life. The youngest patient was 23 and the oldest 76 years. Thus, 76 per cent of the patients were in the sixth decade of life or older.

Among the 92 patients in whom the brain was examined, intracranial metastasis occurred in 30 (32.6 per cent). Of these, 2 were in the third decade, 3 in the fourth, 4 in the fifth, 14 in the sixth, 7 in the seventh, and none in the eighth decade of life (Table I).

Cellular Structure.—Among the 92 patients with carcinoma of the lung in whom the brain was included in the examination, 55 had squamous cell

Received for publication, May 25, 1953.

carcinoma, 23 reserve cell[5] (undifferentiated, oat cell), 6 columnar cell, and 8 mixed columnar and squamous cell carcinomas. Intracranial metastasis occurred in 19 of the squamous cell (34.5 per cent), in 8 of the reserve cell (34.7 per cent), in 2 of the columnar cell (33.3 per cent), and in 1 of the mixed squamous and columnar cell carcinomas (12.5 per cent). Thus, the frequency of intracranial metastasis from carcinoma of the lung seemed to bear no relationship to the cell type (Table II).

TABLE I. FREQUENCY OF INTRACRANIAL METASTASIS FROM CARCINOMA OF THE LUNG

AGE	WHITE MEN	NEGRO MEN	TOTAL	BRAIN EXAMINED	INTRACRANIAL METASTASIS
21-30	3	0	3	3	2
31-40	7	0	7	7	3
41-50	11	3	14	12	4
51-60	42	8	50	46	14
61-70	15	4	19	18	7
71-80	7	0	7	6	0
Totals	85	15	100	92	30 (32.6%)

TABLE II. RELATIONSHIP OF CELLULAR STRUCTURE TO INTRACRANIAL METASTASIS

TYPE OF CARCINOMA	METASTASIS TO BRAIN	NUMBER OF CASES	PER CENT
Squamous cell	19	55	34.5
Reserve cell (oat cell, small cell, undifferentiated)	8	23	34.7
Columnar cell (adenocarcinoma)	2	6	33.3
Mixed squamous and columnar cell	1	8	12.5
Total	30	92	32.6

Spread.—Local extension of the carcinoma with involvement of regional lymph nodes occurred in 83 of the 100 patients. Metastatic foci were encountered in the liver 43 times, in the suprarenal glands 37 times, in the skeleton 29 times, in the pancreas 19 times, in the kidneys 18 times, in the spleen 10 times, in the heart 7 times, in the skin and prostate 3 times each, and in the eye and thyroid gland once each. Thus intracranial metastasis from carcinoma of the lung was exceeded in frequency only by involvement of the regional lymph nodes, liver, and suprarenal glands. It occurred more often in the brain than in the skeleton, pancreas, and kidneys (Table III).

TABLE III. FREQUENCY OF INTRACRANIAL METASTASIS FROM CARCINOMA OF THE LUNG IN RELATIONSHIP TO METASTASIS ELSEWHERE

REGION	SPREAD (PER CENT)
Regional lymph nodes	83
Liver	43
Suprarenal glands	37 (unilateral 9)
BRAIN	32.6
Skeleton	29
Pancreas	19
Kidneys	18

Sites of Intracranial Involvement.—A single focus in the brain was observed in 12 patients, and multiple foci were observed in the remaining 18 patients. In the cerebral hemispheres the involvement was bilateral in 12 patients; the right hemisphere alone was involved in 3, and the left alone in 7. The cerebellar hemispheres were involved by a solitary lesion in 3 patients, and in 1 the brain stem was the only site of intracranial involvement. Metastasis was encountered in the hypophysis three times and in the pineal body once.

Methods of Diagnosis.—The diagnosis of carcinoma of the lung was established during life by bronchoscopic biopsy in 16, by lymph node biopsy in 20, by skeletal biopsy in 6, and by other biopsy in 5 of the patients. Exploratory thoracotomy was performed in 10 and craniotomy in 2 of the patients. Pneumonectomy was performed in 14 patients and lobectomy in 4. The clinical diagnosis was made by roentgenographic study alone in 9; the diagnosis of carcinoma of the lung was not made in 14 of the patients.

Clinical Manifestations.—Among the 30 patients with intracranial metastasis, 10 had clinical manifestations of central nervous system involvement as the presenting complaint. The diagnosis of carcinoma of the lung was eventually established during life in 7 of these patients: by x-ray film alone in 4, by biopsy of the lymph node in 1, and by craniotomy in 2. The diagnosis of carcinoma of the lung was not made at all in three patients, and they were thought to have encephalomalacia, pontine glioma, and cerebellar degeneration, respectively.

Of the 20 remaining patients, 11 had no clinically recognized involvement of the central nervous system, while 9 had neurologic symptoms for six weeks or less prior to death. In only these 9 patients was it possible to estimate the time between the probable appearance of the neoplasm in the lung and that of the metastasis in the brain. The shortest time interval between the onset of pulmonary symptoms and neurological symptoms was one month and the longest was fourteen months.

Among the patients in whom the brain was included in the post-mortem examination, 13 had been treated by pneumonectomy and 4 by lobectomy. Of the 13, 1 already had, and 2 subsequently developed, intracranial metastasis. Of the 4 treated by lobectomy, 2 subsequently developed intracranial metastasis.

COMMENT

These studies provide tentative answers to some basic questions. The data indicate that metastasis to the brain may be expected in one of three patients with carcinoma of the lung. Metastasis to the brain is exceeded in frequency only by metastasis to regional lymph nodes, liver, and suprarenal glands.[6, 7]

The cell type of carcinoma of the lung bears no relationship to the frequency of intracranial metastasis.

It is of particular significance that 10 of the 30 patients with intracranial metastasis had clinical manifestations of central nervous system involvement as the presenting complaint and 11 had no clinical manifestations of central nervous system involvement. The time relationship between the appearance of the neoplasm in the lung and the metastasis in the brain could be estimated only in the 9 remaining patients.

SUMMARY

The clinical histories and findings at necropsy were reviewed in 100 consecutive patients with carcinoma of the lung, in 92 of whom the brain was included in the post-mortem examination.

All patients were men (85 white and 15 Negro), and 76 per cent were in the sixth decade of life or older.

Intracranial metastasis occurred in 30 of the 92 patients, that is, one in three. Metastasis to the brain was exceeded in frequency only by metastasis to regional lymph nodes, liver, and suprarenal glands, and occurred more often in the brain than in the skeleton, pancreas, and kidneys.

The frequency of intracranial metastasis from carcinoma of the lung bore no relationship to the cell type.

Among the 30 patients with intracranial metastasis, 10 had clinical manifestations of central nervous system involvement as the presenting complaint, 9 had neurological symptoms for six weeks or less prior to death, and 11 had no symptoms indicative of central nervous system involvement.

REFERENCES

1. Dosquet: Ueber die Metastasenbildung bei primären Lungen- und Bronchial-Krebsen, Arch. f. path. Anat. **234:** 481-484, 1922.
2. Grant, F. C.: Concerning Intracranial Malignant Metastases, Ann. Surg. **84:** 635-646, 1926.
3. Koletsky, S.: Primary Carcinoma of the Lung; a Clinical and Pathologic Study of One Hundred Cases, Arch. Int. Med. **62:** 636-651, 1938.
4. King, A. B., and Ford, F. R.: A Clinical and Anatomical Study of Neurological Conditions Resulting From Metastases in the Central Nervous System Due to Carcinoma of the Lung, Bull. Johns Hopkins Hosp. **70:** 124-156, 1942.
5. Halpert, B., and Pearson, B.: The Cellular Structure of Carcinoma of the Lung, Am. J. Cancer **40:** 213-218, 1940.
6. Halpert, B.: Morphologic Aspects of Carcinoma of the Lung, SURGERY **8:** 903-909, 1940.
7. Ochsner, A., and De Bakey, M.: Carcinoma of the Lung, Arch. Surg. **42:** 209-258, 1941.

PRINCIPLES IN MANAGEMENT OF SOFT TISSUE SARCOMAS

A Clinical and Pathologic Review of One Hundred Cases

Zelig Lieberman, M.D., and Lauren V. Ackerman, M.D., St. Louis, Mo.

(From the Departments of Surgery and Surgical Pathology, Barnes Hospital and Washington University School of Medicine)

IN RECENT years a more exact classification of soft tissue sarcomas has evolved (Stout). The principles of diagnosis and treatment have not been so well defined. One hundred cases of sarcoma were reviewed from Barnes Hospital, Jefferson Barracks Veterans Hospital, St. Louis, Mo., and Ellis Fischel State Cancer Hospital, Columbia, Mo. The clinical history, the gross findings, and the microscopic pathology were evaluated. Follow-up was obtained in all cases with the exception of seven, each of the seven patients presenting initially with either a locally inoperable lesion or evidence of pulmonary metastases. Nineteen cases were clinically inoperable locally or had distant metastasis at the time of first examination. This study does not include sarcomas arising in the soft tissues of the viscera, in the retroperitoneal area, or in the mediastinum. Sarcomas of the retroperitoneal and mediastinal regions are practically never cured because the anatomic conditions prevent adequate excision (Ackerman, DeWeerd). We excluded sarcomas with origin in the skin, nerves, bone, and cartilaginous tissue.

The tumors in this study have been classified into five main groups: liposarcoma, fibrosarcoma, rhabdomyosarcoma, synovial sarcoma, and desmoid tumors (Table I). The average age of patients in our total series was 52 years, with an equal sex ratio (49 men, 51 women).

In thorough reviews of synovial sarcomas and rhabdomyosarcomas, Haagensen and Stout have demonstrated that these tumors have an unfavorable clinical course, are difficult to control locally, and have a high incidence of pulmonary metastases. Most of these tumors are completely refractory to all forms of therapy. Pack has reported the best results. There are three cases of patients with synovial sarcoma in this series, and two are dead, six and seven months, respectively, after therapy. The surviving patient had an 8 cm. forearm lesion widely excised, and is now thirty-nine months postoperative without evidence of persistent disease. There were eight cases of rhabdomyosarcoma. All patients but one are dead, this patient being only seven months postoperative following wide excision of an upper arm lesion; thus her prognosis is still uncertain. With this single exception, attempts at local excision were followed in all cases by rapid local recurrence of the tumor. The clinical course typically was rapid, lung metastases being demonstrable clinically in five cases an average of ten months after the onset of symptoms. The average duration of symptoms to death in the seven patients who died was 31.0 months.

Received for publication, May 30, 1953

TABLE I. SOFT TISSUE SARCOMA, TOTAL CASES

Liposarcoma	31
Fibrosarcoma	27
Desmoid	10
Rhabdomyosarcoma	8
Synovial sarcoma	3
Malignant granular cell myoblastoma	2
Leiomyosarcoma	2
Angiosarcoma	1
Sarcoma, unclassified	16
Total	100

There were sixteen cases classified as undifferentiated sarcomas. Ten of these patients presented with either a far-advanced locally inoperable lesion or clinically demonstrable lung metastases. Most of these undifferentiated lesions ran a rapid course and did not respond to treatment. In highly undifferentiated, rapidly growing tumors it is doubtful whether any therapy, no matter how well planned, will be successful except in rare instances.

DESMOID TUMORS

Desmoid tumors are fibrous lesions which arise from musculo-aponeurotic structures throughout the body, and are most frequently seen in the abdominal muscles of women most of whom have a history of severe labor during one or more pregnancies. The desmoid tumors have the peculiar property of locally replacing and engulfing surrounding skeletal muscle tissue, yet having no tendency to metastasize (Fig. 1). Because of this locally infiltrating characteristic, frequently these tumors are clinically considered to be highly malignant lesions, and excessively radical procedures are unnecessarily performed (Case 4) (Table II).

TABLE II. DESMOID TUMORS

Total cases	10
Age, average	35.4 years
Sex	
Women	9
Men	1
Size, average	9.1 cm.
Location	
Abdomen	5
Shoulder	2
Upper extremity	1
Lower extremity	1
Chest	1

TABLE III. FIBROSARCOMA

	NUMBER OF CASES	LOCAL RECURRENCES	LUNG METASTASIS	SYMPTOMS TO DEATH
Well differentiated	16	10 (62 %)	3 (18%)	7 yr., 6 mo.
Intermediate	6	6 (100 %)	2 (33%)	6 yr.
Undifferentiated	4		3 (75%)	2 yr., 7 mo.
Mixed	1		1	1 yr., 6 mo.

The microscopic pattern of this tumor is that of mature fibrous connective tissue which engulfs surrounding striated muscle (Fig. 2). Individual cells are uniform, with only rare mitotic figures and abundant intercellular collagen. In the abdominal wall the lesion may become so extensive that fixation occurs to pelvic bones and the lesion is therefore erroneously considered

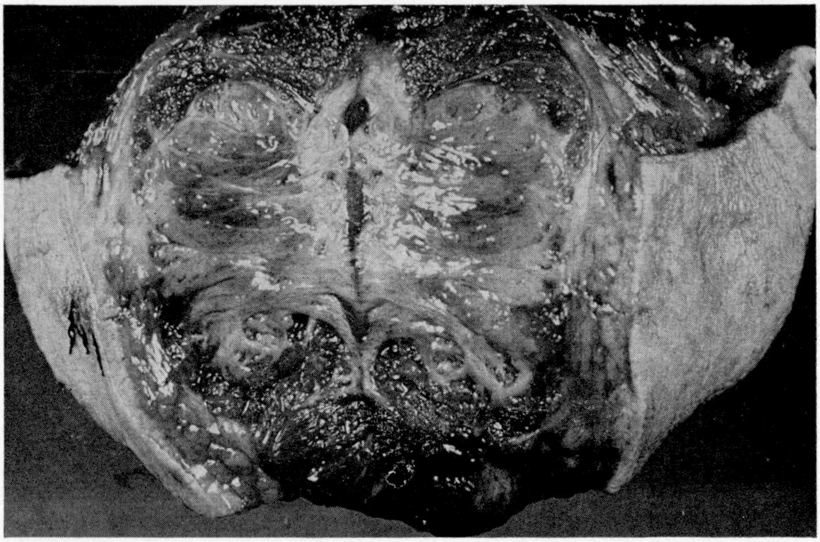

Fig. 1.—Gross photograph of a desmoid tumor of the shoulder showing the typical replacement and inclusion of muscle bundles at the periphery of the tumor (Case 5, W.U. 48-3924).

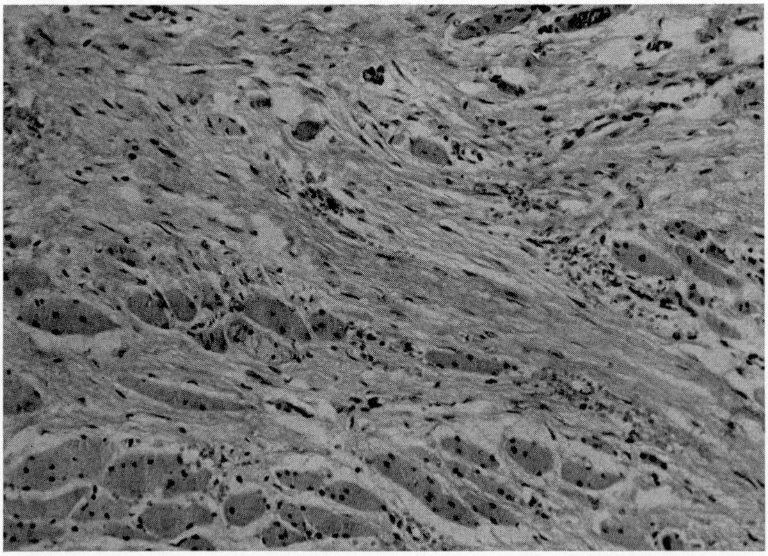

Fig. 2.—Photomicrograph of the same tumor shown in Fig. 1. The striated muscle is engulfed by this mature fibrous connective tissue tumor (W.U, 53-2995).

malignant. We know of cases where hemipelvectomy has even been performed. It is not so generally realized that identical microscopic lesions, often with a history of trauma, appear in regions other than the abdominal wall (Musgrove). In our group, these lesions have been located in soft tissues of leg, popliteal space, and upper arm. In these areas, the lesions often feel firm, are fixed to deep structures, and are clinically diagnosed as malignant. In children, these lesions are more cellular and appear to have a greater tendency for local recurrence (Booher).

FIBROSARCOMA

Twenty-seven cases of fibrosarcoma were reviewed. The average age of the patients was 49.5 years, with a mean age of 35 years. There were thirteen men and fourteen women. These tumors were classified into three groups according to microscopic degree of differentiation (Table III). The typical gross appearance of a well-differentiated fibrosarcoma is that of an apparently well-circumscribed neoplasm. This tumor is pseudoencapsulated, and on cut section it appears as a grayish white homogenous mass (Fig. 3). The undifferentiated fibrosarcoma, having a faster growth, is less well encapsulated and more invasive, and scattered areas of cellular necrosis and hemorrhage are prominent (Fig. 4).

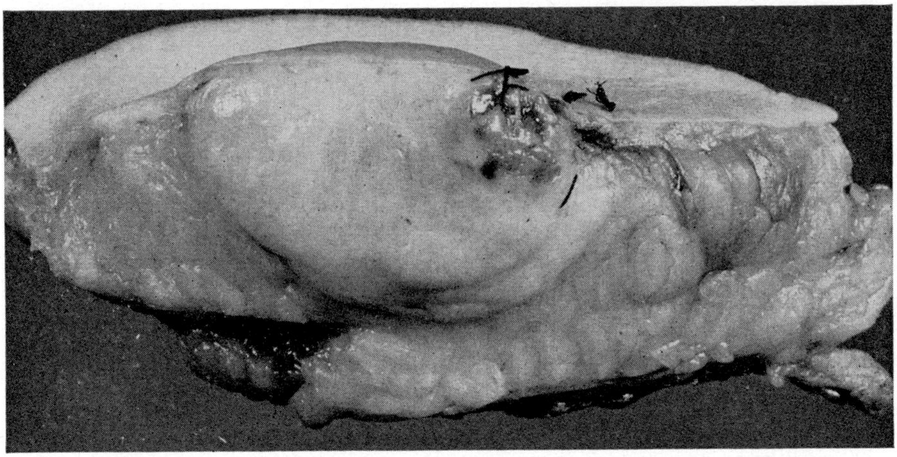

Fig. 3.—Gross photograph of a well-differentiated fibrosarcoma of the abdominal wall illustrating the typical pseudoencapsulation of these tumors (W.U. 52-7320).

Microscopically the well-differentiated lesions are composed of relatively uniform cells with abundant intercellular substance, and have few mitoses (Fig. 5). As the tumor becomes more malignant, there is an increase in the cellularity, the nuclei become more prominent, there is decreased intercellular substance, and mitoses are more frequent (Fig. 6). The majority (59 per cent) of our tumors were well differentiated. These well-differentiated tumors typically have a slow local growth rate, with infrequent tendency to distantly metastasize. These tumors, without treatment or with inadequate local control of the tumor, will in time metastasize and cause the death of the patient. The following case is an excellent illustration of the potentialities of these well-differentiated tumors to metastasize if repeated local recurrences are allowed to occur.

Case 1.—P. S., a 44-year-old man, was admitted with a 9 cm. cicatrix on the infrascapular area of the back, with multiple surrounding persistent tumor nodules. The initial tumor had been present fifteen years, and in the previous six years there had been seventeen unsuccessful attempts to excise the tumor locally. A wide local excision was performed with a split-thickness graft to cover the area. Three years later, a lung metastasis appeared radiographically, and death occurred 5.5 years postoperatively, a total of twenty years after the onset of symptoms and eleven years after first treatment. Microscopically the tumor was an extremely well-differentiated fibrosarcoma (Fig. 5).

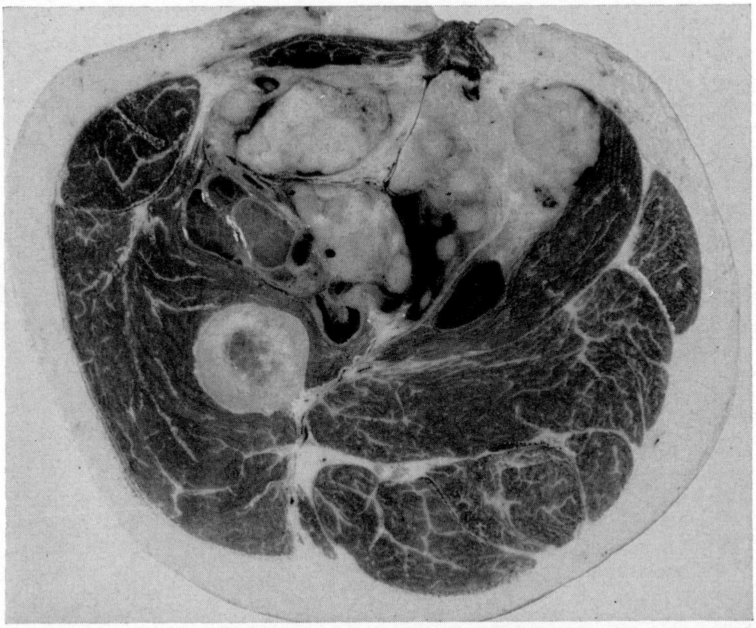

Fig. 4.—Gross photograph of an undifferentiated fibrosarcoma of the thigh. The tumor extends deeply into the thigh and cellular necrosis is prominent (Case 2, W.U. 50-505).

The finding that lung metastases are most frequently found in patients presenting postsurgical persistent lesions emphasizes the importance of adequate primary treatment of the local tumor (Warren).

The highly undifferentiated fibrosarcomas typically have a rapid growth rate and are often refractory to all therapeutic efforts, as illustrated in the following case.

Case 2.—L. P., a 44-year-old man, was admitted with a five-month history of an upper thigh tumor. On physical examination there was a 20 by 15 cm. tumor of the upper medial thigh, extending deeply into the thigh muscles. The lesion was biopsied, and then an immediate hemipelvectomy was performed. Follow-up revealed lung metastases two years postoperatively. Pathology examination revealed the tumor to be an undifferentiated fibrosarcoma (Figs. 4 and 6).

Comment.—In the total group of fibrosarcomas, there were fifteen which locally recurred (55 per cent), and lung metastases appeared in eight cases (29 per cent).

Fig. 5.

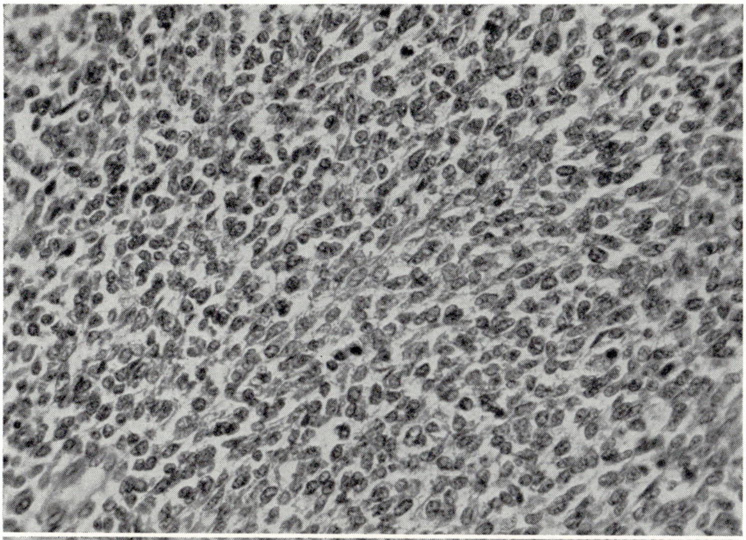

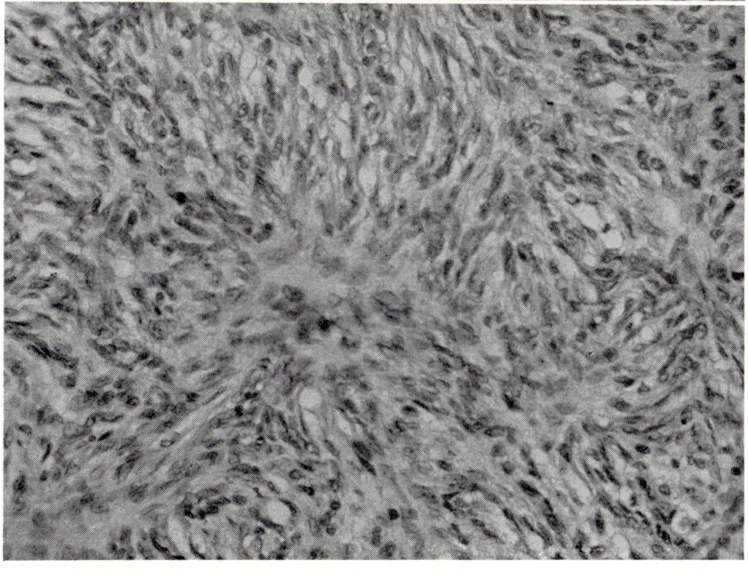

Fig. 6.

Fig. 5.—Photomicrograph of a well-differentiated fibrosarcoma showing the uniform pattern and well-developed intercellular substance. The patient developed multiple locally persistent tumors and a fatal lung metastasis (Case 1, W.U. 53-1686).

Fig. 6.—Photomicrograph of an undifferentiated fibrosarcoma showing the high cellularity of the tumor with frequent mitosis and poorly developed intercellular substance (Case 2, W.U. 53-80).

LIPOSARCOMA

Thirty-one cases of liposarcoma were included in our series. The average mean age was 54 years. There were 14 women and 17 men.

These tumors were classified into two main groups according to degree of differentiation (Table IV). The gross appearance of these well-differentiated liposarcomas is varied, but in general these tumors form large, bulky, nodular masses of apparently encapsulated tumor which is firmer than

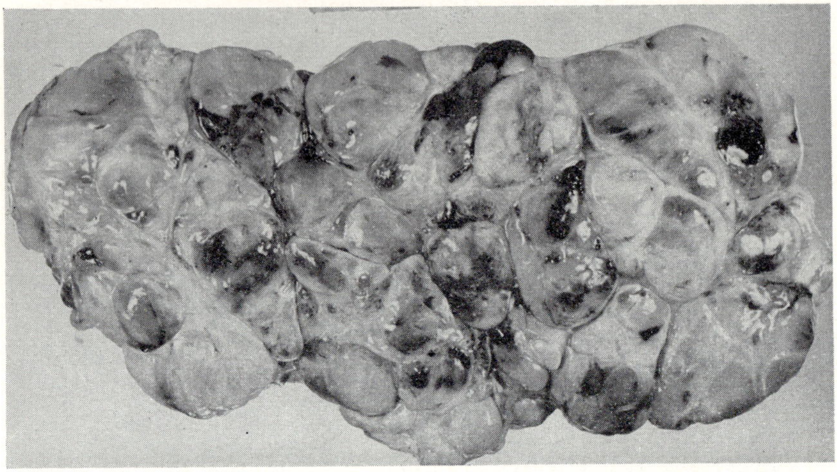

Fig. 7.—Gross photograph of a well-differentiated liposarcoma of the thigh illustrating the typical pseudoencapsulation of this bulky, nodular tumor (W.U. 49-608).

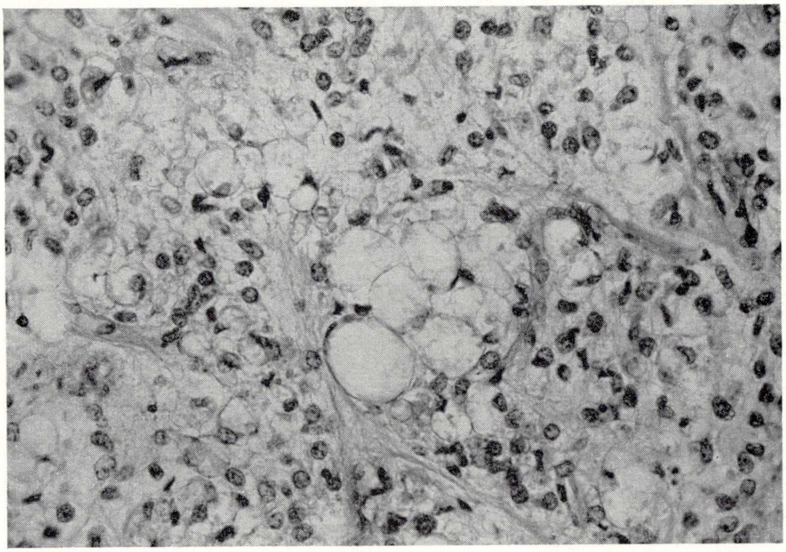

Fig. 8.—Photomicrograph of a well-differentiated liposarcoma showing the characteristic signet-ring cells in which the nuclei are compressed by cytoplasmic fat (W.U. 53-83).

the adipose tissue of simple lipomas. A majority of these neoplasms are slimy and mucoid in consistency. The microscopic picture is also variable, and within a given tumor there is often an admixture of histologic types. The well-differentiated liposarcoma classically shows signet-ring cells in which the nuclei are compressed by stainable cytoplasmic fat (Figs. 7 and 8). The undifferentiated liposarcomas are typically less well encapsulated and have more tendency to invade the surrounding tissues. Microscopically, these undifferentiated lesions are usually difficult to recognize and are commonly

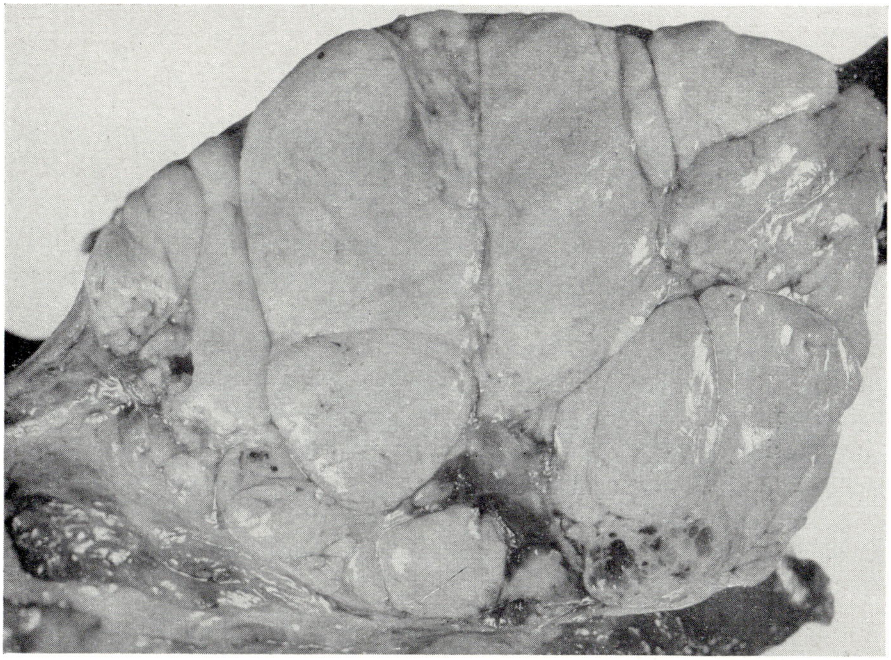

Fig. 9.—Gross photograph of an undifferentiated liposarcoma. There is infiltration of the surrounding tissues as well as cellular necrosis within the tumor (W.U. 49-1801).

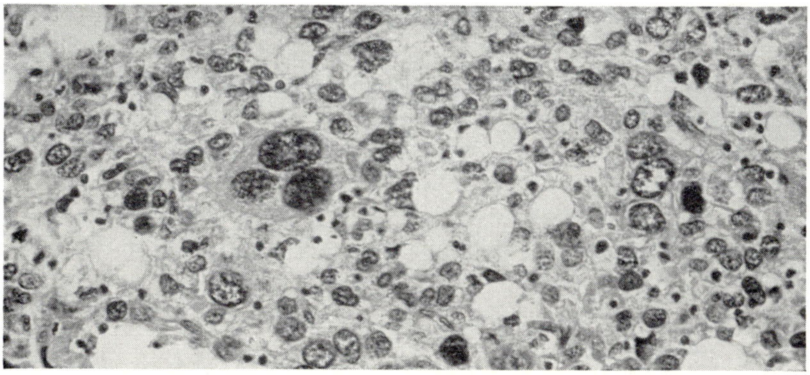

Fig. 10.—Photomicrograph of an undifferentiated liposarcoma. The large bizarre lipoblasts are thought by most pathologists to represent degenerated nuclear forms (W.U. 53-79).

mistaken for rhabdomyosarcoma because of the bizarre tumor giant cells present (Figs. 9 and 10).

Clinically, these lesions have capacities of local recurrence and lung metastases similar to those of the fibrosarcomas, with the additional ability to have multicentric foci, as demonstrated in six of our cases (Ackerman, Starkloff). Local recurrence occurred in fifteen cases (48 per cent), and lung metastases were clinically identifiable in four cases (12.8 per cent).

TABLE IV. LIPOSARCOMA

	CASES	LOCAL RECURRENCE	LUNG METASTASIS	SYMPTOMS TO DEATH
Well differentiated	14	6 (43%)	1 (7.1%)	4 yr., 9 mo.
Undifferentiated	11	6 (55%)	3 (30%)	2 yr., 8 mo.
Multicentric	6			6 yr., 4 mo.

PRELIMINARY BIOPSY

It is important to stress the necessity of the preliminary biopsy of soft tissue tumors before instituting definitive therapeutic measures. The presence of a soft tissue tumor does not necessarily indicate that it is a sarcoma, for it may be a Baker's cyst, inflammatory mass, a bursal sac, a lipoma, or other benign neoplasm. If it is a sarcoma, it is important to the surgeon to know the histologic type of tumor and its degree of differentiation. Benign lesions must be identified to prevent needless radical therapeutic measures.

Unfortunately, the sarcomas, in general, have a gross appearance at the operating table of encapsulation, and if the surgeon operates without the benefit of previous biopsy, he often believes he is dealing with a benign neoplasm. Tissue planes are easily developed, and tumor can often be apparently enucleated.

Microscopic examination reveals this encapsulation to be completely false, as tumor is seen in all cases to extend to the edge of the enucleated mass and penetrate beyond the limits of this false capsule in fine fibrils of tumor (Fig. 11). This procedure results in contamination of the entire field and often forces, at a later time interval, a much more radical procedure. In soft tissue tumors, needle biopsy with paraffin sectioning of the material obtained may at times be diagnostic. We have also not hesitated to use frozen section. However, in both the needle biopsy and the frozen section, we may not be able to make a definite diagnosis, and whenever there is doubt, the paraffin section is awaited. This conservative attitude is justified because of the serious important therapeutic decisions which depend on the interpretation of this biopsy.

TABLE V. CLINICAL EVALUATION OF PRELIMINARY BIOPSY

	NUMBER OF CASES	LOCAL RECURRENCES
Without biopsy	27	21 (78.8%)
With biopsy	12	2 (16.6%)
Totals	39	23 (59.9%)

Clinical cases also bear out this concept of false enucleation. Thirty-nine cases of fibrosarcoma and liposarcoma, which were followed for over ten months, were analyzed in this respect (Table V). Of twenty-seven cases of enucleation without biopsy, twenty-one recurred (78.8 per cent). In twelve patients in whom preliminary biopsy was performed, there were only two cases of local recurrence. These two local recurrences appeared when tumor was situated in such a location (upper arm, back) where even the most radical local excision could not circumscribe the tumor.

The following cases indicate the necessity of preliminary biopsy prior to performing definitive surgical treatment.

CASE 3.—H. G., a 32-year-old woman, was admitted with a mass, 3 cm. in diameter, in the popliteal fossa which had been present for one month. The preoperative impression was Baker's cyst. At surgery, the lesion was thought to be encapsulated and was easily enucleated without the benefit of previous biopsy. Pathology examination revealed this to be a well-differentiated fibrosarcoma, and thus reoperation with wide dissection of popliteal fossa was performed. The pathology examination of the specimen from the second operation revealed tumor nodules to be scattered throughout the removed specimen. (Fig. 11 is taken from the original specimen of this case.)

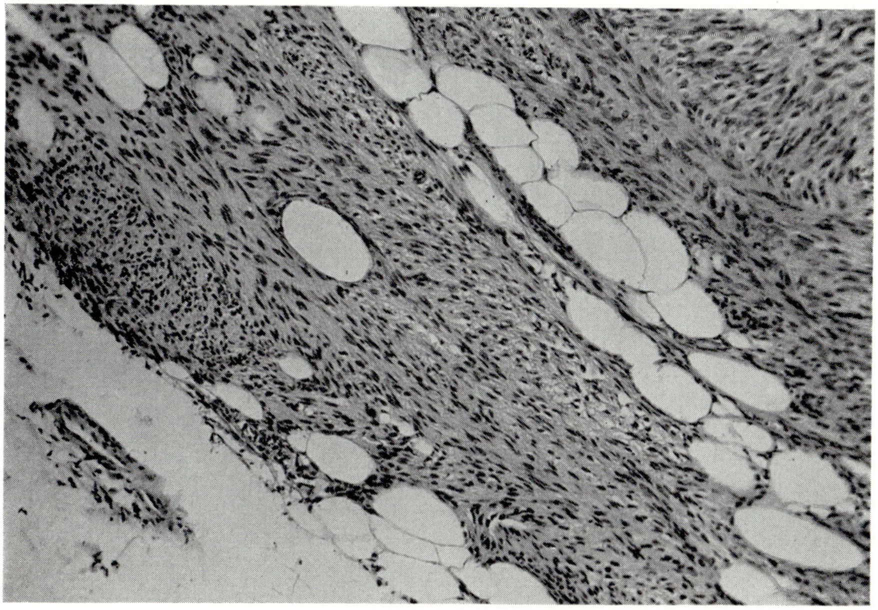

Fig. 11.—Photomicrograph of the periphery of a well-differentiated fibrosarcoma. Surgically, false cleavage planes may be developed, with tumor being on both sides of the line of dissection (Case 3, W.U. 53-85).

Comment.—This case demonstrates that primary enucleation of a sarcoma does not eradicate the local disease, and reoperation is mandatory. If this is not done, local recurrence is inevitable. This method of enucleation followed by subsequent wide excision has many disadvantages: (1) the absence of the palpable tumor at the second operation does not allow the surgeon to determine as accurately the adequacy of the excision during the operation; (2) the initial enucleation, as in the previous case, spreads tumor cells over the exposed operative area, and this, of course, makes subsequent removal of all the tumor more difficult and much more radical.

Case 4.—L. Y., a 23-year-old woman, was admitted with a 10 by 5 cm. soft circumscribed mass in popliteal fossa of two months' duration. The preoperative impression was Baker's cyst. At the time of surgery, the tumor grossly infiltrated the surrounding tissues and was considered to be malignant. Without biopsy of the lesion, radical dissection of popliteal fossa was performed with transection of popliteal artery and tibial and common peroneal nerves. Postoperatively the lower leg became gangrenous, requiring an above-the-knee amputation on the tenth postoperative day. Microscopic examination of the tumor revealed it to be a desmoid.

Comment.—If an initial biopsy of this lesion had been performed, this catastrophe could have been prevented. In the desmoid tumors, if radical excision implies amputation or gross disturbance of function, we feel that conservative removal is permissible even if this implies an inadequate excision. We have never experienced trouble from this method of handling. The worst thing that can happen is local recurrence.

Case 5.—B. P., a 61-year-old woman, was admitted with a 10 by 4 by 3 cm. tumor infiltrating the left trapezius muscle. Preoperatively, this was thought to be an infiltrating malignant soft tissue tumor. A preliminary biopsy was performed. The biopsy was reported as a desmoid tumor, and therefore a wide local excision was performed. The patient is living without evidence of persistent disease 4.5 years postoperatively.

Comment.—If a preliminary biopsy had not been performed and if the lesion had been treated as a malignant sarcoma, an interscapulothoracic amputation would have been needlessly performed.

Case 6.—H. C., a 45-year-old man, was admitted with a lesion, 3 cm. in diameter, on the sole of the foot, which had been biopsied and diagnosed by another pathologist as sarcoma. An amputation had been advised. Examination of the specimen in our laboratory revealed the lesion to be composed of mature fibroblastic tissue having an abundance of collagen matrix (Fig. 12). Further review of the patient's history revealed that he had had, in the previous five years, excisions of bilateral Dupuytren's contractures of the hand. The clinical history with the microscopic pattern suggested the diagnosis of plantar fibromatosis, and thus simple excision was all that was advised for this benign process (Fig. 13). Pickren has previously reviewed plantar fibromatosis, emphasizing the importance of recognizing this lesion as benign.

LOCATION OF THE SOFT TISSUE TUMOR

The specific surgical management of soft tissue sarcomas is modified by the anatomic location of the tumor. The limitations of local surgical procedures in many areas of the body must be recognized, and radical surgical therapy may be indicated as the initial therapeutic procedure. Therapy must be well conceived when a tumor is located in an area in which radical surgery is anatomically restricted. If a preliminary incisional biopsy is obtained without disturbing the tumor bed, frequently a wide local excision will adequately circumscribe the neoplasm. However, if the tumor is primarily enucleated without a preliminary biopsy, the confines of the tumor area are destroyed, and tumor is spread throughout the operative field, perhaps forcing an amputation or even making complete removal impossible.

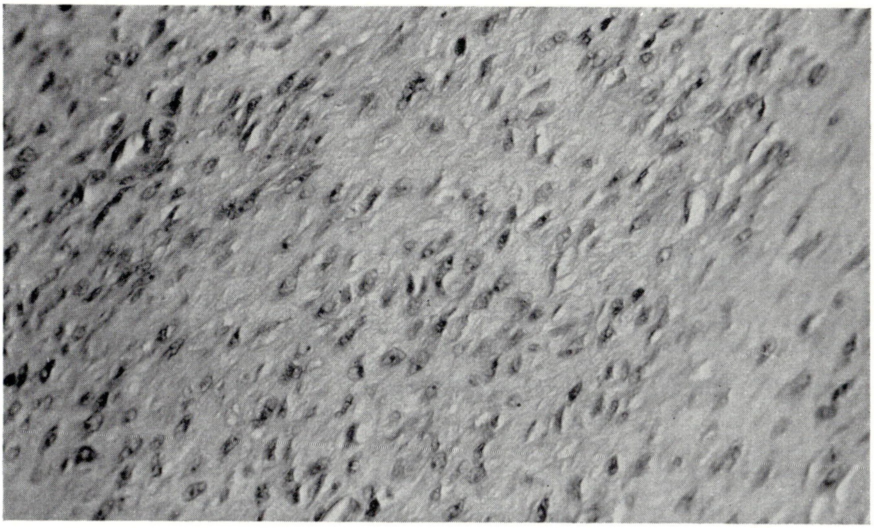

Fig. 12.—Photomicrograph of plantar fibromatosis showing proliferation of mature fibroblastic tissue which infiltrates the plantar fascia (Case 6, W.U. 53-82).

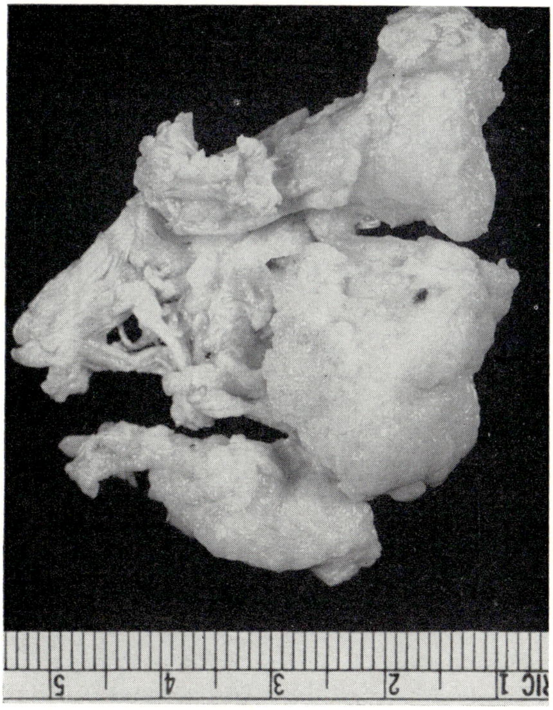

Fig. 13.—Gross photograph of specimen shown in Fig. 12 which was excised from plantar fascia. These small hard nodules may simulate a fibrosarcoma (W.U. 52-7310).

The location of tumors in this series (Table VI) reveals that the tumors are diffusely scattered throughout the body; however, the greatest incidence is in the lower extremity (32 per cent).

TABLE VI. SOFT TISSUE SARCOMAS: LOCATION

Lower extremity	35
Upper extremity	15
Chest, shoulder, back	15
Abdomen	12
Head, neck	11
Buttocks	6
Multicentric	6
Total	100 cases

The popliteal fossa poses many surgical obstacles, for the anatomic structure is such that wide surgical dissection is limited by the important nerves and vessels which traverse the space. The popliteal artery, lying deep in the fossa, cannot be safely ligated with the assured preservation of viability of the lower leg (Case 4). The terminal branches of the sciatic nerve (common peroneal, tibial) traverse this space superficially, just deep to the deep fascia. In addition, the bulk of the fossa is composed of adipose tissue, and thus accurate surgical dissection within the fossa itself is impossible. These factors necessitate a carefully planned therapeutic regimen if successful results are to be obtained. Of the lesions in the popliteal space on which attempts at local excision were made, all of the six cases which have been followed over eighteen months have recurred.

The medial aspect of the thigh, a common site for sarcomas, also presents the problem of adequate local excision because of proximity of the femoral vessels and nerves, whereas lesions on the anterior, lateral, and posterior aspects of the thigh lend themselves well to wide excisions because of the bulk of underlying muscle and the absence of adjacent vital structures. Of the eight lesions on the medial aspect of the thigh which were locally excised, all but one has recurred, this being a well-differentiated liposarcoma which is now only two years postoperative. Microscopic sections of this case reveal the original tumor to extend to the edge of the excision; thus local recurrence can be anticipated.

Lesions of the abdominal and chest walls usually lend themselves well to wide local excision (Fig. 3). The following case report illustrates both the value of preliminary biopsy of tumors and the advisability of radical wide excisions of chest wall lesions.

CASE 7.—B. C., a 53-year-old woman, was admitted with a four months' history of a progressively enlarging 8 by 6 cm. tumor in the fifth intercostal space, anterior axillary line. X-ray picture revealed the lesion to be invading the rib cage (Fig. 14). A preliminary biopsy was performed, and the lesion was reported as liposarcoma, highly undifferentiated, following which a wide local excision of the chest wall was performed, including the underlying rib cage and pleura (Fig. 15). The patient is now thirty-nine months postoperative with no evidence of persistent disease.

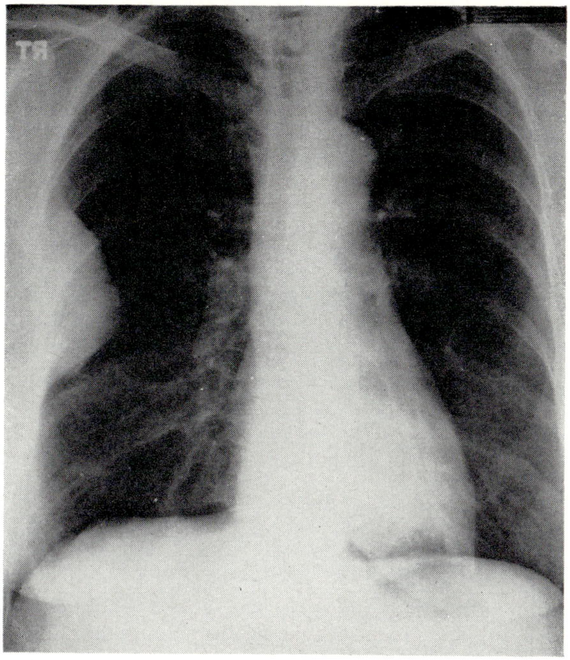

Fig. 14.—Chest x-ray picture of large liposarcoma of chest wall invading the rib cage (Case 7, W.U. 49-6224).

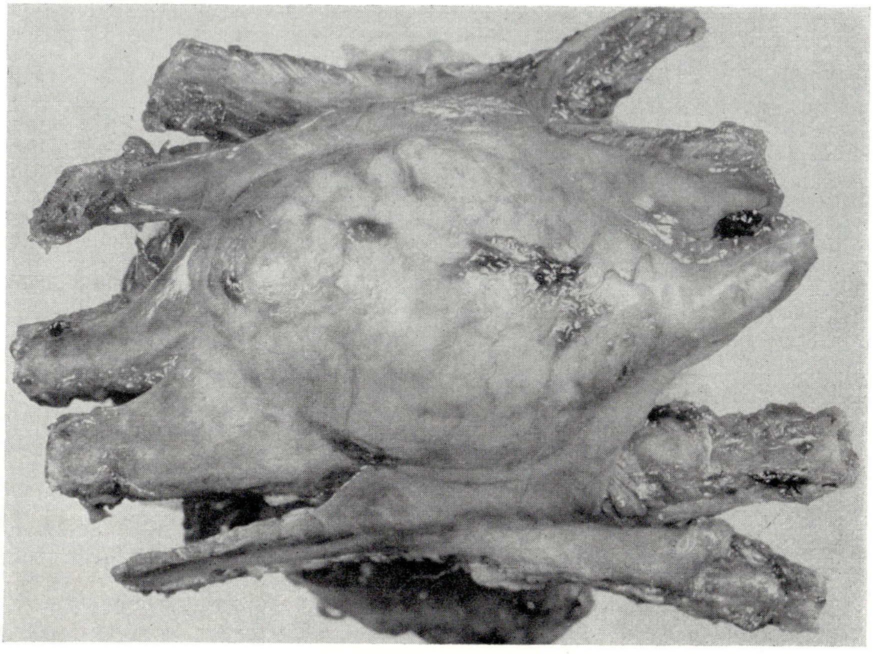

Fig. 15.—Gross photograph of surgical specimen following wide excision of the undifferentiated liposarcoma of chest wall shown in Fig. 14 (W.U. 49-1800).

Most lesions of the back and buttocks in this series were found to be locally far advanced, and the depth of the tumor extension made local excision ineffective in most of the cases as exemplified by Case 8. Radical resection of some sarcomas of the buttock is possible. However, if the tumor has invaded underlying periosteum, bone, or sciatic nerve, hemipelvectomy is necessary (Bowden). In the undifferentiated group, practically none will be cured, no matter how radical the procedure.

CASE 8.—J. B., a 71-year-old man, was admitted with a 15 by 10 cm. tumor of the back, just above the sacrum, which had been slowly enlarging for the past seven months. A biopsy was performed and the lesion was reported as fibrosarcoma, well differentiated. An attempt to excise the tumor radically was made, the excision including ribs and transverse process of lumbar vertebrae; however, the tumor extended through the vertebral foramina to lie adjacent to the spinal cord, and thus a total excision of tumor could not be performed. A lung metastasis was noted nine months postoperatively, and local recurrence became clinically detectable seventeen months postoperatively, the patient dying five months later.

Adequate local excisions of large lesions of the upper extremity are frequently impossible because of its narrow circumference and the wide dispersal of vital vessels and nerves throughout the arm. This is especially true of lesions located in the region of the elbow and medial aspect of the upper arm. The depth of penetration also affects the prognosis, both in inability to excise the tumor locally (Case 8) and in the high incidence of lung metastases (Case 2). Eleven cases were noted to extend deeply into muscles of the back, buttocks, or thigh. Extensive local recurrence and/or lung metastases occurred in all cases. Of the seven cases noted specifically to be superficial in extent, local recurrences occurred in those cases which were inadequately excised; however, there were no instances of lung metastases.

IRRADIATION

The use of irradiation in this series is limited, and it was used either as an adjunct to surgical excision or in several locally inoperable cases. Of the ten liposarcoma lesions on which irradiation alone was used, clinical regression of the local tumor occurred in five cases, and in the other five cases no appreciable effect was noted. The two inoperable fibrosarcoma lesions receiving irradiation had no beneficial response. Nine cases of liposarcoma were treated with a combination of irradiation and local excision, and there has been local recurrence in one of these cases. No valid conclusion can be drawn from this small group of cases. However, irradiation seems definitely indicated in those cases of liposarcoma which are locally inoperable and in those cases of multicentric foci in which radical surgery seems contraindicated.

CONCLUSIONS

1. The microscopic pattern of soft tissue sarcomas gives a fair index of the clinical growth rate of the tumor. Certain types such as rhabdomyosarcoma and synovial sarcoma have a poor outlook.

2. Highly undifferentiated sarcomas usually have a rapid clinical course, and prognosis is poor, no matter what treatment is given.

3. Incisional biopsy of soft tissue tumors is essential to diagnose and classify the lesions accurately prior to the institution of specific therapy.

4. Primary enucleation of a soft tissue tumor may result in contamination of the entire operative field by tumor.

5. Primary surgery without biopsy may result in unnecessary sacrifice of vital structures.

6. The decision of the extent of surgical therapy must depend on consideration of the histologic pattern of the tumor and its anatomic location.

7. Consideration of primary amputation must be given to deeply seated sarcomas of the inner thigh and popliteal fossa.

REFERENCES

1. Ackerman, L. V.: Multiple Primary Liposarcoma, Am. J. Path. **20**: 789-798, 1944.
2. Ackerman, L. V., and Taylor, F. H.: Neurogenous Tumors Within the Thorax, Cancer **4**: 669-691, 1951.
3. Booher, R. J., and Pack, G. T.: Desmomas of the Abdominal Wall in Children, Cancer **4**: 1052-1065, 1951.
4. Bowden, L., and Booher, R. J.: Surgical Considerations in the Treatment of Sarcoma of the Buttock, Cancer **6**: 89-99, 1953.
5. Cade, S.: Soft Tissue Tumors: Their Natural History and Treatment, Proc. Roy. Soc. Med. **44**: 19-36, 1951.
6. Coley, B.: Treatment of Soft Tissue Tumors, Am. J. Surg. **85**: 259, 1952.
7. DeWeerd, J. H., and Dockerty, M. B.: Lipomatous Retroperitoneal Tumors, Am. J. Surg. **84**: 397-407, 1952.
8. Haagensen, C. D., and Stout, A. P.: Synovial Sarcoma, Ann. Surg. **120**: 826-842, 1944.
9. Ivins, J. C., Dockerty, M. B., and Ghormley, R. K.: Fibrosarcoma of the Soft Tissues of the Extremities, SURGERY **28**: 495-508, 1950.
10. Musgrove, J. E., and McDonald, J. R.: Extra-Abdominal Desmoid Tumors, Arch. Path. **45**: 513-540, 1948.
11. Pack, G. T., and Ariel, I. M.: Synovial Sarcoma (Malignant Synovioma); A Report of 60 Cases, SURGERY **28**: 1047-1084, 1950.
12. Pickren, J. W., Smith, A. G., Stevenson, T. W., and Stout, A. P.: Fibromatosis of the Plantar Fascia, Cancer **4**: 847, 1951.
13. Starkloff, G. B., Saxton, J. A., and Johnson, R. E.: Liposarcoma of an Extremity Associated With Multiple Subcutaneous Lipomas, Ann. Surg. **133**: 261-266, 1951.
14. Stout, A. P.: Liposarcoma—The Malignant Tumor of Lipoblasts, Ann. Surg. **119**: 86, 1944.
15. Stout, A. P.: Rhabdomyosarcoma of the Skeletal Muscle, Ann. Surg. **123**: 447-472, 1946.
16. Stout, A. P.: Fibrosarcoma, Cancer **1**: 30-63, 1948.
17. Warren, S., and Sommers, G. N. J.: Fibrosarcoma of the Soft Parts, Arch. Surg. **33**: 425-450, 1936.

COMPARATIVE STUDIES, IN NORMOTENSIVE MAN, OF THE EFFECTIVENESS, RETENTION, AND ELIMINATION OF VARIOUS PLASMA EXPANDERS

RICHARD A. BADER, M.D.,* MORTIMER E. BADER, M.D.,* SOON WON KIM, B.A., AND ANDRE COURNAND, M.D., NEW YORK, N. Y.

(From the Department of Medicine, Columbia University, College of Physicians and Surgeons, and the Cardio-Pulmonary Laboratory of the First Medical and Chest Services [Columbia University Division], Bellevue Hospital)

INTRODUCTION

THE need for an effective plasma expander which is easily stored, inexpensive, nontoxic, and not indefinitely retained in the body has stimulated investigation of three major types of preparations: (1) dextran, a polysaccharide, (2) polyvinylpyrrolidone (PVP), a "plastic" polymer, and (3) oxypolygelatin (OPG), a gelatin polymer. The characteristics of these agents have been extensively studied, and a variety of preparations of each, varying in osmotic activity, have been prepared and evaluated.

The purpose of this report is to present the observations on the effectiveness of a number of preparations of these three agents as plasma expanders in fifty-three patients, as well as data on the time course of their distribution and excretion. During these studies, observations were also made on the validity of the blue dye plasma volume determination in the presence of PVP and OPG.

MATERIAL AND METHODS

General.—All studies were made on patients who were convalescent from either surgery or medical illness, none of whom were in shock or had cardiovascular or renal disease. They were studied in a fasting state. All blood samples for hematocrit and blood volume determination were obtained via an indwelling arterial needle. Plasma volume was measured in all cases by the Evans blue dye technique (T 1824), the dye being introduced in a vein in the opposite arm. After control observations, 1 L. of plasma expander (all of which are made up in normal saline solution) was infused at a rate of 1,000 c.c. in forty minutes. Hematocrit determinations were made after 500 c.c. of the infusion (twenty minutes), after the full liter had been given (forty minutes), and one hour after the completion of the infusion. Repeat blue dye plasma volume and hematocrit determinations were made at six hours and twelve hours and/or twenty-four hours after the completion of the infusion.

Urine was collected at one, six, twelve, twenty-four, and forty-eight hours following the infusion, and blood for plasma levels of the agent infused was collected at the same time periods. In some instances, seventy-two hour blood

---

This work was done under Contract DA-49-007-MD-127, issued by the Medical Research and Development Boards, Office of the Surgeon General, Department of the Army.

Received for publication, July 30, 1953.

*Fellow of the Dazian Foundation.

and urine collections were made. Data on excretion and storage of the expander were not collected in all cases.

Plasma Expanders Used.—The agents used and the number of patients receiving them are tabulated as follows:

Material	*Number of Patients*
PVP, Lot GA 111 (3½%)	12
PVP, Lot GA 148 (3½%)	3
OPG, Lot Baxter S 152 AY (5%)	5
OPG, Lot Baxter S 153 BY (5%)	4
OPG, Lot Baxter S 230 XA (5%)	6
OPG, Lot Baxter S 233 XA (5%)	5
Dextran, Lot CSC 255 F4 (6%)	6
Dextran, Lot CSC 258 L6 (6%)	8
Dextran, Lot Baker 256 R8 (6%)	4

Determinations in Blood and Urine.—Dextran levels in blood and urine were carried out by the method of Bloom and Willcox.[1] OPG was determined by Kjehldahl measurement of OPG nitrogen,[2] and PVP by the method suggested by Cannan.[3] Measurement of the K value, a coefficient of viscosity, which is a useful indicator of average molecular weight, for PVP excreted in the urine was determined in Dr. R. Keith Cannan's laboratory.

Validity of the Blue Dye Technique for Plasma Volume Determination in the Presence of PVP or OPG.—Since Cannan, Allen, and Gregersen[4] have pointed out that PVP and plasma protein separately produce characteristic changes in the spectral absorption of T 1824, the validity of the determination of the plasma volume by the blue dye (T 1824) technique in the presence of PVP and OPG was investigated at the outset of the study. These authors have indicated that the maximum absorption of T 1824 in plasma is at 620 mμ as compared to a peak of 640 mμ for T 1824 in PVP. This observation was confirmed in our studies. Fig. 1 illustrates the spectral absorption curves for T 1824 in plasma and in a 3.5 per cent solution of PVP in normal saline solution, and demonstrates a definite shift of the latter curve to the right. The possibility existed that in spite of this shift due to PVP, there was a minimal alteration of the spectral transmission characteristics of blue dye in the presence of concentrations of PVP which are actually encountered in the plasma of the patients studied. Studies were carried out to evaluate this possibility.

Various dilutions of PVP in plasma were prepared. In Fig. 2 the spectral absorption of T 1824 in 1.0 per cent and 0.35 per cent PVP in plasma is shown. It may be seen that the point of maximal optical density is at 620 mμ. Furthermore, this curve is, for practical purposes, similar to that of dye in plasma alone, especially in the critical range. Since the first dye plasma volume determination performed in the presence of PVP was at six hours, it is important that at that time, as will be seen in Table VI, the average plasma level was about 4 mg. per cubic centimeter (a figure well within the range of dilutions illustrated in Fig. 2). Additional evidence for the validity of the blue dye method in the presence of PVP in low concentrations in plasma is the fact that at 620 mμ various dilutions of plasma and PVP containing the same amount of dye have similar optical densities when the corresponding mixture is used as the blank. Comparison was made of the optical density of 0.001 c.c. of T 1824 for 1.1 c.c. of solution, using as solvent plasma alone, 3.5 per cent PVP in saline solution, and 1.0, 0.7, and 0.35 per cent solutions of PVP in plasma. In each case, the blank contained the corresponding mixture except that a corresponding amount

Fig. 1.

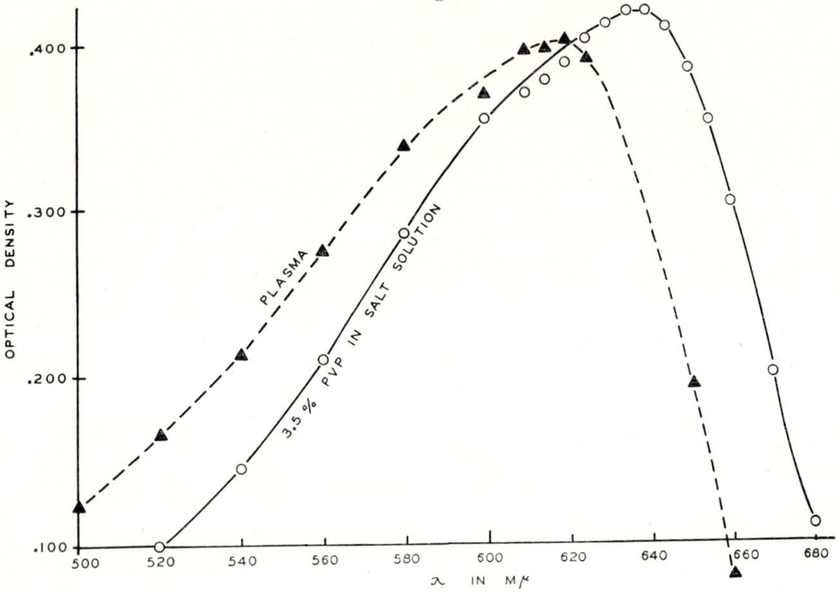

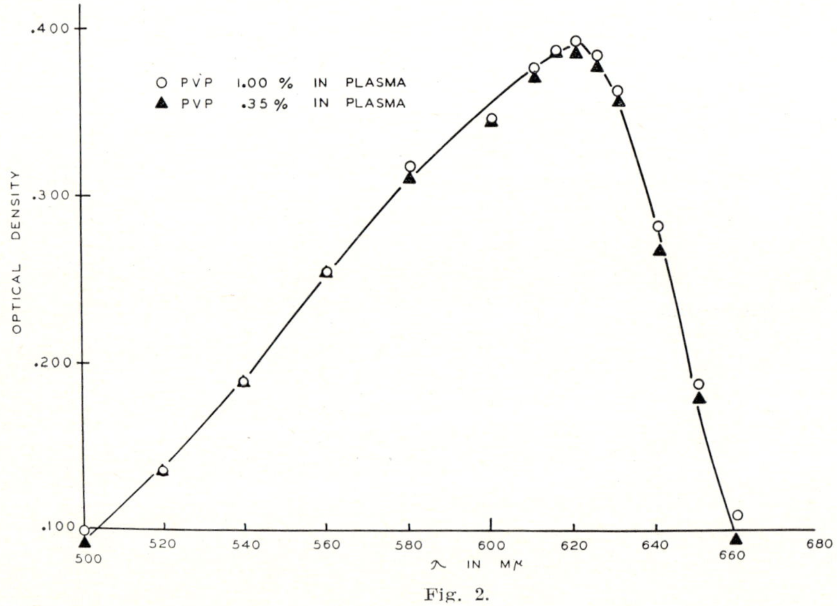

Fig. 2.

Fig. 1.—Spectral-optical density curve for blue dye (T 1824) in plasma and a 3.5 per cent solution of PVP (in solution of electrolyte).

Fig. 2.—Spectral-optical density curve for blue dye (T 1824) in various mixtures of PVP and plasma.

of distilled water was used in place of dye. In Table I, the results of two such series of studies revealed that the optical density was approximately the same in all the solutions tested. It may, then, be concluded that for the range of concentration of PVP encountered in this group of patients, there was no significant interference with the plasma volume determination by the blue dye method.

TABLE I. EFFECTS OF VARIOUS CONCENTRATIONS OF PVP ON THE OPTICAL DENSITY OF BLUE DYE (T 1824)

SOLUTION TESTED	OPTICAL DENSITY*	
	STUDY I	STUDY II
Dye in plasma	0.320	0.338
Dye in 3.5% PVP in saline solution	0.325	0.330
Dye in 1.0% PVP in plasma	0.320	0.329
Dye in 0.7% PVP in plasma	0.328	0.333
Dye in 0.35% PVP in plasma	0.319	0.334

*Optical density of 0.001 c.c. of T 1824 per 1.1 c.c. of solution made up in vitro (spectrophotometer set at 620 mμ).

TABLE II. AVERAGE PLASMA VOLUME INCREMENT IN CUBIC CENTIMETERS FOLLOWING THE INFUSION OF 1 L. OF PLASMA EXPANDER

MATERIAL	NUMBER OF PATIENTS	PLASMA VOLUME BEFORE INFUSION (C.C.)	PLASMA VOLUME INCREMENT AFTER INFUSION* (C.C.)		
			1 HR.	6 HR.	24 HR.
PVP 3½%					
GA PVP 111 } GA PVP 148 }	15	3,000		406 ± 229	212 ± 158
Dextran 6%					
CSC 255 F4	6	2,926		668 ± 85	
CSC 258 L6	8	2,699		492 ± 310	349 ± 218
Baker 256 R8	4	2,569		463 ± 132	
OPG 5% Baxter					
S 152 AY } S 153 BY }	9	3,156		519 ± 237	340 ± 142
S 230 XA	6	2,770		398 ± 162	285 ± 199
S 233 XA	5	2,442	123 ± 147		

*All values expressed as mean and standard deviation in cubic centimeters.

TABLE III. AVERAGE ARTERIAL HEMATOCRIT CHANGES DURING AND FOLLOWING INFUSION OF 1 L. OF PLASMA EXPANDER

MATERIAL	NUMBER OF PATIENTS	CONTROL VALUE (PER CENT)	PERCENTAGE OF DECREMENT FOLLOWING INFUSION*			
			1 HR.	6 HR.	12 HR.	24 HR.
PVP 3½%						
GA PVP 111 } GA PVP 148 }	15	40.8	14.5 ± 1.9	10.1 ± 4.8	–	8.4 ± 3.4
Dextran 6%						
CSC 255 F4	6	43.1	13.4 ± 3.9	10.6 ± 3.0	7.2 ± 1.6	6.8 ± 1.0
CSC 258 L6	8	44.7	16.4 ± 2.2	13.4 ± 2.6	13.0 ± 1.6	11.2 ± 2.8
Baker 256 R8	4	42.2	17.5 ± 2.4	17.8 ± 5.2	11.3 ± 3.4	–
OPG 5% Baxter						
S 152 AY } S 153 BY }	9	43.6	8.4 ± 2.4	7.5 ± 2.0	–	4.6 ± 3.5
S 230 XA	6	44.5	10.5 ± 1.0	8.2 ± 3.3	6.1 ± 2.4	–
S 233 XA	5	45.8	7.3 ± 2.4	5.4 ± 3.2	5.8 ± 3.6	–

*Expressed as percentage of decrement from initial control value. Values given are mean and standard deviation.

TABLE IV. URINE EXCRETION FOLLOWING INFUSION OF 1 L. OF VARIOUS PLASMA EXPANDERS

MATERIAL	NUMBER OF PATIENTS	TOTAL AMOUNT OF INFUSION (GM.)	AVERAGE EXCRETION FOLLOWING INFUSION* (GM.)					
			1 HR.	6 HR.	12 HR.	24 HR.	48 HR.	72 HR.
PVP 3½%								
GA PVP 111 } GA PVP 148 }	11	35	8.00 ± 1.69	4.60 ± 1.65	-	3.17 ± 0.71	1.13 ± 0.42	0.58 ± 0.29
Dextran 6%								
CSC 258 L6	5	60	13.71 ± 2.38	7.19 ± 2.41	4.35 ± 0.49	3.83 ± 1.04	1.98 ± 0.24	–
Baker 256 R8	5	60	12.46 ± 2.58	9.57 ± 1.30	3.94 ± 1.52	3.25 ± 0.72	2.18 ± 0.92	-
OPG 5% Baxter								
S 230 XA	5	50	10.73 ± 3.66	6.24 ± 1.21	2.15 ± 0.35	1.18 ± 0.99	0.41 ± 0.26	-
S 233 XA	5	50	16.98 ± 5.64	8.22 ± 2.17	–	2.51 ± 1.67	0.33 ± 0.45	-

*All values expressed as mean and standard deviation in grams.

RESULTS

Plasma Volume Changes.—Plasma volume increments following the infusion of the various plasma expanders are listed in Table II, and the average hematocrit values in Tables III.

At six hours following the infusion, the material which afforded the largest increase in plasma volume was a dextran preparation (Lot CSC 255 F4), which produced an average increment of 668 c.c., compared to values between 450 and 500 c.c. with the other lots of dextran, 406 c.c. with PVP, 519 c.c. with two OPG preparations (S 152 AY and S 152 BY), and 398 c.c. with a third (S 230 XA). The least effective agent was OPG (Lot S 233 XA), which produced an increment of only 123 c.c. one hour following the infusion. At twenty-four hours following the infusion, dextran still produced the largest increment in plasma volume of 349 c.c. The other preparations tested at this time produced increments ranging from 340 c.c. to 212 c.c.

In all cases, the hematocrit changes reflected the increments in plasma volume. Indeed, in the case of OPG Lot S 233 XA, which produced the smallest increment of all, there was only a 4.7 per cent decrement in hematocrit at one hour following the infusion, compared to values ranging from 8 to 17 per cent for the other expanders at this time period.

Urine Excretion of Plasma Expanders.—The data on the urine excretion of the various plasma expanders are listed in Table IV. The general pattern for all the agents was a rapid early excretion followed by a prolonged excretion at a slower rate.

TABLE V. RELATIVE VISCOSITY AND K VALUE OF PVP IN SPECIMEN OF URINE AT DIFFERENT TIME INTERVALS AFTER INFUSION*

PATIENT	HOURS	RELATIVE VISCOSITY	K
W. L.†	24-48	1.229	29.0
	48-72	1.232	29.4
C. M.†	24-48	1.220	28.3
	48-72	1.219	28.3
S. G.†	24-48	1.212	27.8
	48-72	1.229	29.0
J. W.†	24-48	1.197	26.8
	48-72	1.237	29.5
J. D.‡	1	1.115	19.5
	1-6	1.124	20.4
	6-24	1.159	23.8
	24-48	1.196	26.7

*Measurements obtained in Dr. R. K. Cannan's laboratory.
†Lot number GA PVP 111.
‡Lot number GA PVP 148.

In the case of PVP, 23 per cent was lost in the urine in the first hour, 36 per cent at six hours, 45 per cent at twenty-four hours, and 50 per cent by seventy-two hours. In order to assess the influence of molecular size on the loss of the PVP at the various time periods, the K value of the PVP in the various urine fractions was measured. Determinations were carried out* on urine specimens collected at the twenty-four to forty-eight hour periods, and forty-

*In the labtoratory of Dr. R. Keith Cannan.

TABLE VI. PLASMA LEVELS FOLLOWING INFUSION OF 1 L. OF VARIOUS PLASMA EXPANDERS

MATERIAL	NUMBER OF PATIENTS	AVERAGE PLASMA LEVEL AT END, AND FOLLOWING INFUSION* (MG./C.C.)						
		0 HR.	1 HR.	6 HR.	12 HR.	24 HR.	48 HR.	72 HR.
PVP 3½%								
GA PVP 111 / GA PVP 148	15	7.46 ± 1.44	6.41 ± 1.24	4.89 ± 0.88	–	3.40 ± 0.70	2.84 ± 1.44†	2.52 ± 0.02‡
Dextran 6%								
CSC 258 L6	5	13.33 ± 1.81	11.38 ± 1.46	7.81 ± 0.94	6.54 ± 0.84	4.82 ± 0.62	3.48 ± 0.51	–
Baker 256 R8	5	15.48 ± 1.57	13.76 ± 1.25	9.57 ± 1.61	7.05 ± 1.22	–	3.36 ± 0.17	–
OPG 5% Baxter								
S 230 XA	5	–	4.24 ± 0.77	1.97 ± 0.75	–	0.32 ± 0.55	0.06 ± 0.10	–
S 233 XA	5	10.49 ± 0.79	6.87 ± 0.45	4.79 ± 0.82	–	2.35 ± 0.56	1.05 ± 0.47	–

*All values expressed as mean and standard deviation.
†Mean and standard deviation of seven patients.
‡Mean and standard deviation of four patients.

eight to seventy-two hour periods, as seen in Table V. The K values for these time periods were of the order of 27 to 29, figures greater than those found by Welt and Cannan[5] for the first twenty-four hours for the same lot of PVP. The excretion of a urine with PVP of a low K value early and of higher K values later is seen in Case J. D., where the figures increased from 19.5 to 26.7. These data indicate an early rapid urinary loss of osmotically active smaller-sized molecules.

In the case of dextran, there was an excretion of about 20 per cent in the first hour, 35 per cent by twelve hours, and about 50 per cent in forty-eight hours, figures of the same order as those for PVP excretion.

In the case of OPG, there was a considerable difference in the urinary excretion of both lots tested. Lot S 230 XA was excreted at a rate of 32 per cent in six hours, with only 7 per cent more lost in the urine up to the forty-eight hour period, while 33 per cent of the other lot (S 233 XA) was excreted in one hour, 50 per cent by six hours, and 56 per cent by forty-eight hours.

TABLE VII. TOTAL PLASMA EXPANDER IN CIRCULATION FOLLOWING INFUSION OF 1 L.

MATERIAL	TOTAL AMOUNT INFUSED (GM.)	AMOUNT OF SUBSTANCE IN CIRCULATION AFTER INFUSION					
		1 HR.		6 HR.		24 HR.	
		GM.	%*	GM.	%*	GM.	%*
PVP 3½%							
GA PVP 111							
GA PVP 148	35			16.46	47.0	10.89	31.2
Dextran 6%							
CSC 258 L6	60			24.92	41.6	14.67	24.4
Baker 256 R8	60			29.00	48.4	–	–
OPG 5% Baxter							
S 230 XA	50			6.24	12.5	0.98	2.0
S 233 XA	50	17.6	35.2				

*Per cent of total amount of expander administered.

Plasma Levels.—The plasma levels of the various plasma expanders are listed in Table VI. Comparison of the levels in terms of milligrams per cubic centimeter cannot give an index of osmotic activity, since the material present may vary in molecular size. A high early level is achieved, which then rapidly falls off, so that very small ineffective levels are present at forty-eight hours. In general, with all material tested one hour after the competion of the infusion of the plasma expander, the plasma levels were 80 to 90 per cent of the level immediately following the infusion; by six hours, the level had fallen to 50 per cent of the peak value, it further decreased to about 30 to 35 per cent at twenty-four hours, and in the twenty-four to forty-eight hour period it fell only 10 per cent. This uniform pattern reflects in part the early urinary loss of the small osmotically active molecules. In Table VII, the data are given on the total amount of plasma expanders still in the circulation at one, six, and twenty-four hours after the infusion. It will be seen that after twenty-four hours, from 25 to 30 per cent of the administered dextran and PVP were present. In the case of PVP, despite the rapid disappearance of the bulk of the administered expander, small amounts remain in the body for some time. In one patient

(J. D.) who had received 35 Gm. of PVP, plasma levels were measured intermittently as late as seventy-one days following the infusion. At six days the level was 2.16 mg. per cubic centimeter, at twenty-one days 1.59 mg. per cubic centimeter, and at seventy-one days there was still 0.27 mg. per cubic centimeter of PVP present in the patient's plasma.

Unaccounted-for Fraction of Plasma Expander.—At any time in the course of the study, the total urinary loss of plasma expander plus the total amount of expander in the plasma (the product of plasma volume and plasma concentration) gives the total amount of expander which can be accounted for. The difference between this figure and the total amount of expander administered is the unaccounted-for moiety of the agent. Such calculations were carried out for the PVP, two lots of dextran, and two lots of OPG.

TABLE VIII. QUANTITY OF PLASMA EXPANDERS NOT ACCOUNTED FOR IN URINE AND PLASMA AFTER INFUSION OF 1 L. OF THE EXPANDER

MATERIAL	AVERAGE UNACCOUNTED-FOR PLASMA EXPANDER FOLLOWING INFUSION							
	1 HR		6 HR.		24 HR.		48 HR.	
	GM.	%*	GM.	%*	GM.	%*	GM.	%*
PVP 3½%								
GA PVP 111								
GA PVP 148			5.92	16.9	8.31	23.8	9.58	27.4
Dextran 6%								
CSC 258 L6			14.18	23.6	–	–	20.55	34.2
Baker 256 R8			8.97	14.9	–	–	19.97	33.3
OPG 5% Baxter								
S 230 XA			27.70	55.4	–	–	30.40	60.8
S 233 XA	15.52	30.0	–	–	–	–	19.39	38.8

*Per cent of total amount of expander administered.

At six hours following the infusion, about 17 per cent of the administered PVP could not be accounted for, and by forty-eight hours, this figure had increased to 27 per cent. The loss of dextran (Baker 256 R8) to the unaccounted-for moiety was approximately the same as PVP. In the case of the other dextran lot (CSC 258 L6), the early loss to the unaccounted-for fraction was greater (27 per cent), but at forty-eight hours, the figure was about the same as the previously mentioned expanders, being approximately 34 per cent.

There was a considerable difference in the two lots of OPG studied. Lot S 230 XA had the largest early unaccountable expander loss, 55 per cent in six hours, reaching a total of 61 per cent in forty-eight hours. OPG Lot S 233 XA contrasted sharply with a 30 per cent unaccounted-for fraction at one hour and about 39 per cent in forty-eight hours.

Miscellaneous.—

Blood pressure: No significant changes were noted in the blood pressure of the patients receiving these various types and lots of plasma expanders. It should be remembered, however, that only normotensive persons without evidence of cardiovascular or renal disease and not in shock were used as subjects.

Toxicity: No untoward reactions of allergic or other nature were noted in these patients.

DISCUSSION

From these studies in normotensive men, dextran appears to be the most effective plasma expander, while one lot of OPG was the least effective, the other substances tested ranging in between. In general, these findings are in agreement with those of Fine,[6] who also found dextran to be the most effective plasma expander in normotensive dogs. According to him, it was somewhat superior to OPG and modified fluid gelatin, and considerably more effective than a PVP preparation of small molecular size (average K value of 28). However, a PVP preparation of higher molecular size (K value of 70) was approximately as effective as dextran. Fine also noted, in normotensive human subjects, that the increment in plasma volume with the same lots of dextran used in this study was of similar order of magnitude as we have observed. With a different lot of dextran, not studied by us, Ebert[7] has found even larger increments in plasma volume in unbled human subjects. The relatively poor plasma-expanding properties of OPG and certain lots of PVP confirm the findings of Myers and Taylor[8] and of Higgins.[9]

While the present study was concerned solely with normotensive men, data from investigations in which dog or man was bled also offer evidence of the superior effectiveness of dextran as a plasma expander. Vars,[10] using his "Bleeding Volume Index" as a standard of effectiveness of a given agent as a plasma expander in bled dogs, reported dextran to be superior to OPG, saline solution, and dog plasma, and almost as good as human albumin, although slightly inferior to whole blood. In bled human subjects, Ebert[7] observed that dextran produced increments in plasma volume which were greater and more sustained than in the unbled group, although the rate of disappearance of the dextran was about the same for both groups.

Our studies also provide some information concerning the factors accounting for the extent and duration of the plasma expansion. Theoretically these factors are: (1) the amount of material administered, (2) its osmotic properties, and (3) the rate of disappearance of the expander from the circulation, the two latter factors being dependent on the molecular size of the polymer. Early urinary excretion of all the plasma expanders studied was large, followed by a much slower rate of excretion. These observations are comparable with the findings of Bloom,[11] Ebert,[7] Higgins,[9] and Vars[12] in studies using various preparations of dextran and OPG. Our observations, in addition, revealed that the early rapid urinary loss of PVP consists largely of the smaller more osmotically active molecules, a finding which agrees with that of Welt and Cannan[5] and with the general concept summarized by Gropper and associates,[13] which states that there is an inverse relationship between urinary excretion and molecular weight. With rapid urinary and probable extraurinary loss of the most osmotically effective molecules of plasma expander, it is not surprising that even with the best material, not more than 25 to 30 per cent of an administered amount is retained in the plasma at the end of twenty-four hours. Some of the material, however, may remain in the circulation for a considerable length of time. This is illustrated by the finding noted previously, of PVP in plasma seventy-one days following the infusion, and is consistent with Hellman's[14] observations that 0.6 per cent of an injected dose remains in the circulation thirty days following the infusion. On the other hand, Hecht and associates[15] have reported complete disappearance of a PVP preparation from the circulation in fifteen to twenty days.

In the present study, the quantity of expander not present in the urine or plasma was regarded as "unaccounted for." This fraction, in general, appeared rapidly, and was largest in the case of the two lots of OPG. The magnitude of this fraction confirms the finding of Higgins.[9] Large urinary and unaccounted-for loss of OPG is the obvious reason for its limited plasma-expanding ability. Unaccounted-for PVP and dextran were smaller in amount, and about equal for the two materials. No study was made by us of the metabolic outcome of these materials. However, the work of Hellman indicates a 40 to 50 per cent storage of PVP, which is then eliminated at a rate of 0.02 per cent daily. Since only 1 per cent appears in stool and a negligible amount in expired air, storage rather than metabolic degradation is the most likely outcome of this material.[16] On the other hand, dextran, according to Hellman,[17] is metabolized to a greater extent and is not stored in the same degree as PVP.

In conclusion, it would appear that dextran Lot CSC 255 F4 was the best of the expanders which we studied in terms of plasma-expanding properties, persistence in the circulation, and lack of storage in the body. Preparation of PVP with a uniform K value, which limits too rapid an excretion, is not stored indefinitely, and exerts a satisfactory osmotic effect, would appear to be a desirable step if another plasma expander, as good or even better than dextran, is needed.

SUMMARY AND CONCLUSIONS

1. Comparison of the effectiveness of a variety of preparations of plasma expanders (dextran, OPG, and PVP) was made in fifty-three normotensive men. The time course of distribution and excretion was also studied.

2. The most effective preparation in terms of plasma-expanding properties was one lot of dextran (CSC 255 F4), while the poorest was one lot of OPG (Baxter S 233 XA). The remaining lots of dextran, OPG, and PVP were intermediate in effectiveness.

3. All the materials had an early rapid excretion followed by a slower rate of loss. In the case of PVP, this early loss was demonstrated to consist of the more osmotically active smaller molecules.

4. The urinary and extraurinary loss of expanders accounts for the limited extent and duration of activity of these agents.

REFERENCES

1. Bloom, W. L., and Willcox, M. L.: Determination of Dextran in Blood and Urine, Proc. Soc. Exper. Biol. & Med. **76**: 3, 1951.
2. Vars, H. M.: Estimation of Modified Fluid Gelatin in Plasma and Urine by Nitrogen Analyses. Report to the Subcommittee on Shock, National Research Council, July 3, 1952.
3. Cannan, R. K.: The Estimation of Polyvinylpyrrolidone by Iodometry. Report to National Research Council, March 12, 1951.

4. Allen, T. H.: Memorandum to National Research Council, March 14, 1951.
5. Welt, L., and Cannan, R. K.: Examination of Samples of PVP Recovered From Urines of Human Subjects. Progress Report, National Research Council, June, 1951.
6. Fine, J.: Progress Report No. 8. Subcommittee on Shock, National Research Council, September, 1952.
7. Hammarsten, J. F., Heller, B. I., and Ebert, R. V.: The Effects of Dextran in Normovolemic and Oligemic Subjects, J. Clin. Investigation **32**: 340, 1953.
8. Myers, J. D., and Taylor, W. J.: Progress Report, National Research Council, Novermber, 1951.
9. Higgins, A. R., Hayes, A., Kimmel, J. R., Burns, T. W., Jones, R. E., Jr., Smith, T. W. D., and Klein, C. L.: Oxypolygelatin, a Plasma Expander. Preliminary Report. National Research Council, September, 1951.
10. Vars, H. M.: Tests of Clinical Evaluation and Results of Clinical Studies. Working Conference on Dextran. Peoria, Ill., July 9, 1951. National Research Council, Subcommittee on Shock.
11. Bloom, W. L.: Carbohydrate Changes in the Blood and Urine Following Dextran Administration. Plasma Substitutes Program, Progress Report, National Research Council, August, 1951.
12. Vars, H. M.: Progress Report, National Research Council, September, 1952.
13. Gropper, A. L., Raisz, L. G., and Anspacher, W. H.: Plasma Expanders, Surg., Gynec. & Obst. **95**: 521, 1952.
14. Hellman, L.: Preliminary Report on the Metabolism of C^{14} Labelled PVP and Dextran. Plasma Volume Expander Program, Progress Report, National Research Council, October, 1951.
15. Hecht, G., Joppich, G., and Weese, H.: Peristonwirkung und Nachweiss bei exsiccatischen Saeuglingen, Monatschr. Kinderheilkunde **96**: 145, 1948.
16. Hellman, L.: A Study of C^{14} Labelled Plasma Substitute. Report to Subcommittee on Shock. National Research Council, October 31, 1952.
17. Hellman, L.: A Study of C^{14} Labelled Plasma Substitutes. Progress Report, National Research Council, April 30, 1952.

URINARY LOSS OF AMINO ACIDS AFTER SURGERY

GEORGE L. NARDI, M.D., BOSTON, MASS.

(From the Department of Surgery of the Harvard Medical School at the Massachusetts General Hospital)

INTRODUCTION

IT IS well known that patients who have undergone surgery lose large amounts of nitrogen in the urine in the immediate postoperative period.[1, 2] However, it is not known in what proportions these nitrogen-containing constituents are excreted during this negative nitrogen phase. Since urine normally contains only traces of free amino acids amounting to 1 or 2 per cent of the total urinary nitrogen,[3] it was thought of interest to study the amino acids present in the urine of patients undergoing surgery of varying degrees of magnitude.

METHODS

Twenty-four hour urine collections were obtained from patients on the surgical wards of the Massachusetts General Hospital; aliquots were analyzed for nitrogen (Kjeldahl method), and volumes containing equal amounts of nitrogen were chromatographed two dimensionally on paper, using the technique of Dent.[4] Phenol and water were used as the first solvent, and butanol-propionic acid-water as the second.[5] The amino acids were developed by spraying with 0.1 per cent Ninhydrin in ethanol. Using this technique, urine of normal persons contains mainly glycine and alanine and occasional small quantities of serine, glutamic acid, and threonine.[6-8] In general, only the lower molecular weight, nonessential amino acids are to be found in urine. Fig. 1 represents a typical daily normal excretion pattern of one of our laboratory personnel.

Five patients were studied. The operations represented are: excision of anal fissure, hemorrhoidectomy, inguinal herniorrhaphy, total hysterectomy and perineorrhaphy, and subtotal gastrectomy.

RESULTS

Fig. 2 represents the effects of the minimal anesthesia and surgery which are required for excision of a small anal fissure. As can be seen, there is little deviation from normal.

Hemorrhoidectomy, a procedure of somewhat greater magnitude, produced a slight but definite increase in amino acid excretion (Fig. 3).

Figs. 4 and 5 represent the aminoaciduria occurring after herniorrhaphy and hysterectomy, respectively. The greater loss of amino acids as compared to the two previous lesser procedures is obvious.

The work described in this paper was done under contract between the Office of Naval Research and Harvard University.

Received for publication, June 18, 1953.

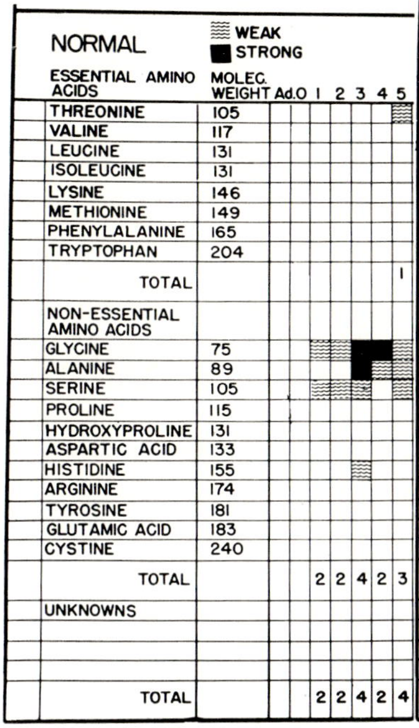

Fig. 1.

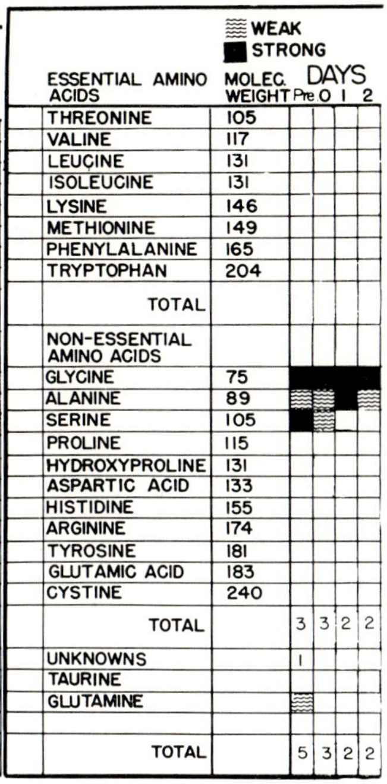

Fig. 2.

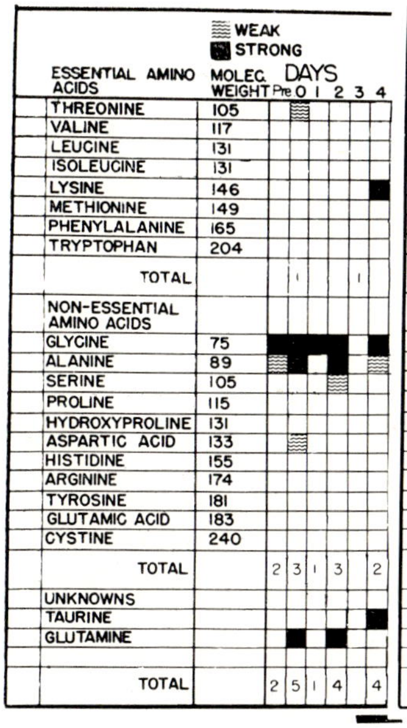

Fig. 3.

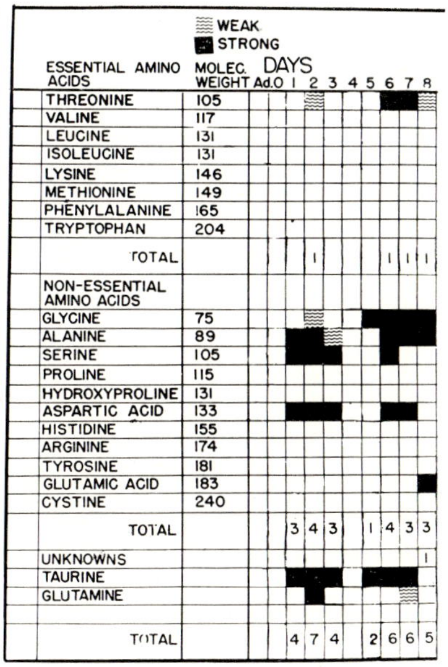

Fig. 4.

The marked aminoaciduria produced in a patient undergoing subtotal gastrectomy is illustrated in Fig. 6.

Aminoaciduria accompanies the increase in urinary nitrogen loss which follows surgical trauma. This aminoaciduria consists of an increase in both the lower molecular weight, nonessential amino acids normally found in urine and the higher molecular weight, essential amino acids not usually present. The degree of aminoaciduria seems proportional to the magnitude of the surgical trauma.

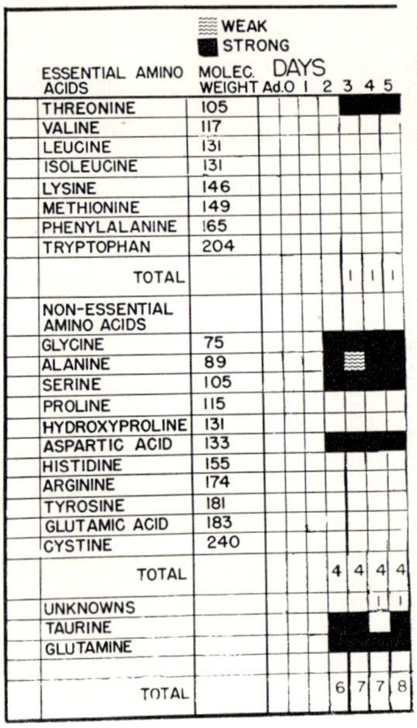

Fig. 5.

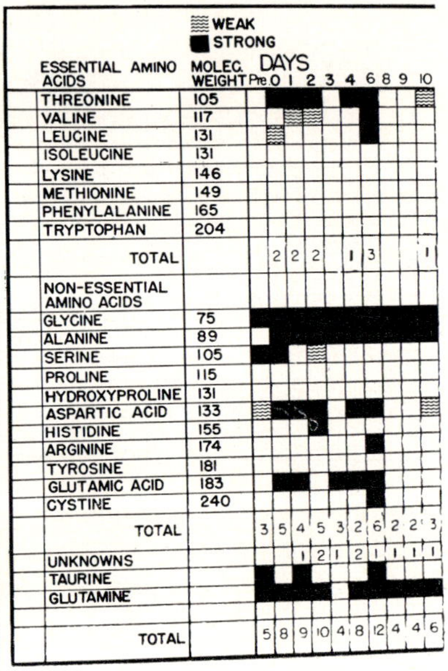

Fig. 6.

DISCUSSION

There are three causes of aminoaciduria.[7] It may result if blood amino acid levels exceed the renal threshold. Another cause with normal amino acid blood levels is renal damage or failure of tubular reabsorption. A third mechanism is the aminoaciduria occurring with normal blood levels of amino acids and normal renal function—the primary aminoaciduria of various metabolic diseases. The latter need not concern us.

Everson and Fritschel[9] have shown no rise in plasma amino nitrogen subsequent to anesthesia and surgery. Man[10] has found a postoperative fall in these levels. It would seem then that the aminoaciduria seen after surgery is primarily a failure of tubular resorption. A possible explanation for this failure of resorption may be the finding of Nathanson and Wilson[11] that after trauma, increased amounts of creatine are excreted. Pitts[12] has shown a competitive tubular reabsorption for creatine and glycine. It is possible that an increased excretion of other urinary constituents may overload the tubular reabsorption mechanism and result in this aminoaciduria.

SUMMARY

An abnormal aminoaciduria consisting of excretion of essential and non-essential amino acids not normally present is to be found in the urine of the postoperative surgical patient.

The qualitative and quantitative aspects of this aminoaciduria are proportional to the magnitude of the surgery.

This loss of amino acids is probably the result of failure of tubular reabsorption.

Acknowledgment.—I wish to express my thanks for help and encouragement to Dr. Oliver Cope, and to Miss Anne Poulos for invaluable aid in making and interpreting the chromatograms.

REFERENCES

1. Moore, F. D., and Ball, M. R.: The Metabolic Response to Surgery, Springfield, 1952, Charles C Thomas, Publisher.
2. Moore, F. D.: Bodily Changes in Surgical Convalescence. I—The Normal Sequence—Observations and Interpretations, Ann. Surg. **137**: 289, 1953.
3. Peters, J. P., and Van Slyke, D. D.: Quantitative Clinical Chemistry Interpretations, vol. 1, Baltimore, 1946, Williams & Wilkins Company.
4. Dent, C. E.: A Study of the Behaviour of Some Sixty Amino-acids and Other Ninhydrin-reacting Substances on Phenol-''Collidine'' Filter-paper Chromatograms, With Notes as to the Occurrence of Some of Them in Biological Fluids, Biochem. J. **43**: 169, 1948.
5. Calvin, M., and Benson, A. A.: The Path of Carbon in Photosynthesis: IV. The Identity and Sequence of the Intermediates in Sucrose Synthesis, Science **109**: 140, 1949.
6. Dent, C. E.: Applications to Study of Amino Acid and Protein Metabolism. Partition Chromatography, Biochem. Soc. Symposia No. 3, Cambridge, 1950, Cambridge University Press.
7. Brick, I. B.: The Clinical Significance of Amino Aciduria, New England J. Med. **247**: 635, 1952.
8. Individual Metabolic Patterns and Human Disease. An Exploratory Study Utilizing Predominantly Paper Chromatographic Methods. (No. 5109), Austin, Texas, 1951, The University of Texas.
9. Everson, T. C., and Fritschel, M. J.: The Effect of Surgery on the Plasma Levels of the Individual Essential Amino Acids, SURGERY **31**: 226, 1952.
10. Man, E. B., quoted by Peters and Van Slyke.[3]
11. Nathanson, I. T., and Wilson, H.: Personal communication.
12. Pitts, R. F.: A Renal Reabsorption Mechanism in the Dog Common to Glycine and Creatine, Am. J. Physiol. **140**: 156, 1943-44.

CIRCULATORY CHANGES IN THE LOWER LIMB FOLLOWING LUMBAR SYMPATHECTOMY

DAVID MESSENT, F.R.C.S., AND PETER BEACONSFIELD, M.D., LONDON, ENGLAND

(From the Department of Surgery, Postgraduate Medical School of London)

RETURN of tone in the peripheral blood vessels following sympathectomy, first demonstrated by Lewis and Landis (1929), has been recorded by several investigators (Freeman and associates, 1934; Barcroft and Walker, 1949; Grant and Pearson, 1938; Hoobler and co-workers, 1949). Lynn and Barcroft (1950) carried out day-to-day studies of the changes in the blood flow in the feet following lumbar sympathectomy, and Duff (1951) investigated the blood flow in the forearm and hand of the same limb in similar circumstances. We have studied the circulatory changes in the calf and foot during anesthesia, during the operation of lumbar sympathectomy, at hourly intervals for the first seven hours immediately following operation, and on the first and second postoperative days. Changes in calf flow have also been studied on the first, second, fourth, fifth, sixth, eighth, eleventh, and fourteenth days, and again four, six, and twelve weeks after sympathectomy.

METHODS

The investigations were carried out in either the wards, the anesthetic room, the operating theater, or the laboratory, and the maximum temperature variation was never more than 3° C. The patients were left at rest with the limbs covered until just before the commencement of each test.

Calf and foot flows were measured by venous occlusion plethysmography (Barcroft and Edholm, 1945, 1946). In the case of the calf, occlusion cuffs were used above and below the plethysmograph. An occlusion pressure of about 60 mm. Hg was used in both cuffs, the pressure being adjusted to give the maximal flow. It is our opinion after varying the pressure in the lower cuff that the use of arterial occlusion in this cuff is not of significance.

We found that it was technically unsatisfactory to take simultaneous tracings of foot and calf flows in the same limb. Our observations on foot and calf flows were therefore made in two separate series of patients.

Whenever possible, resting calf and foot flows were measured over a period of one-half hour on two separate days prior to operation: on the day of operation, recordings were made immediately prior to the induction of anesthesia, at approximately five-minute intervals throughout the operation, and at hourly intervals for the first seven hours following operation.

RESULTS

(The flows in both calf and foot were recorded in milliliters of blood per 100 ml. of tissue per minute.)

Received for publication, June 28, 1953.

Changes in Calf and Foot Flows During Operation and in the Immediate Postoperative Period (Fig. 1, Tables I and II).—In this group of patients (seven calves and six feet studied), the average preoperative resting flow was 1.4 ml. per 100 ml. of tissue per minute in the calf and 0.9 ml. in the foot. In the immediate preanesthetic phase, the average values were 1.5 ml. and 1.3 ml., respectively. With the induction of anesthesia, the calf flow increased to 5.4 ml. and the foot flow to 4.1 ml. In the time between the resection of the sympathetic chain and the end of the operation there was a further slight increase to 5.9 ml. in the calf and to 4.7 ml. in the foot. Over the first seven hours, at the twenty-fourth, and at the forty-eighth hour after operation, the average calf and foot flows were as follows:

Hour	*Calf Flow (Milliliters)*	*Foot Flow (Milliliters)*
1	8.7	5.8
2	8.1	7.0
3	7.5	5.8
4	6.0	7.4
5	7.3	7.3
6	7.2	8.0
7	7.5	
24	5.8	6.7
48	5.5	6.4

Changes in Calf Flow From the First Postoperative Day, at Intervals up to Two Months (Fig. 2, Table III).—The average preoperative resting calf flow in the group (thirteen calves studied) was 1.7 ml. On the first postoperative day after lumbar sympathectomy, an average flow of 8.6 ml. was recorded. On the second, fourth, and fifth days, the calf flows were 6.2 ml., 5.0 ml., and 4.1 ml., respectively. After the fifth day, the decline in flow was more gradual, and the average readings for the sixth, eighth, eleventh, and fourteenth days were 4.0 ml., 4.3 ml., 3.4 ml., and 2.9 ml., respectively. At the fourth postoperative week, an increase to 4.3 ml. was recorded, but this had fallen again to 4.1 ml. at the sixth week, and at twelve weeks the calf flow was 3.1 ml., still nearly double the average preoperative resting flow.

It will be noticed that in the first group of patients studied (that is, during operation) the calf flow twenty-four hours after operation was 5.8 ml., whereas in the present group at the same postoperative period the calf flow was 8.6 ml. This is accounted for by including in the latter group "normal" limbs (without organic arterial disease) with a higher response in calf flow to lumbar sympathectomy.

COMMENTS

Previous investigators (Barcroft and Walker, 1949; Lynn and Barcroft, 1950; Duff, 1951) have drawn attention to the presence of a delayed development of maximal flow in both the hand and foot following sympathetic section as compared to development in forearm and calf. Our results suggest that this delay is more apparent than real and that the peak flow following sympathectomy occurs in the first seven hours in both the calf and the foot.

Table I. Resting Calf Blood Flows Before, During, and Immediately After Operation
(Milliliters per 100 Ml. of Tissue per Minute)

Case No. and Patient	Age (Yr.)	Sex	Limb	Diagnosis	Resting Calf Flow (Perop.) 1	Resting Calf Flow (Perop.) 2	Preanesthesia Phase	Maximum Before Removal of Chain	End of Operation	Postoperative Calf Flows, Hour 1	2	3	4	5	6	7	24	48
1. E. C.	30	F	R	Erythrocyanosis	1.2	1.2	1.2	6.5	100	**18.7**	16.6	14.4	9.9	15.2	11.1	10.4	8.3	5.7
3. C. M.	44	F	R	Postoperative thrombosis of popliteal artery	1.0	1.6	1.5	5.3	5.0	**9.3**	8.6	8.6	6.4				4.5	
4. H. B.	51	M	R	Diffuse obliterative arteritis	3.0	1.5	1.5	6.6	5.8	6.0	6.0	6.4	5.4	6.8	**9.3**	8.8	6.2	7.2
5. W. B.	61	M	R	Diffuse obliterative arteritis	1.1		1.1	4.4	5.0		6.5	4.7	6.0	6.6			**7.5**	6.6
6. A. H.	60	M	L	Diffuse obliterative arteritis	1.1	1.2	1.1	5.6	**8.7**	8.0	8.0	4.0	5.1	6.0	6.8	6.5	4.6	
7. L. S.	37	F	R	Thromboangiitis obliterans		1.3	1.3	2.5	2.0	3.6	4.2	**4.6**	4.6	4.0	3.7	4.3	2.2	
8. M. C.		F	L	Erythrocyanosis		1.8	3.1	7.0	5.2	6.5	6.8	5.9	5.0	5.2	5.2		**7.3**	2.8
				Averages		1.4	1.5	5.4	5.9	8.7	8.1	7.5	6.0	7.3	7.2	7.5	5.8	5.5

Table II. Resting Foot Blood Flows Before, During, and Immediately After Operation
(Milliliters per 100 Ml. of Tissue per Minute)

Case No. and Patient	Age (Yr.)	Sex	Limb	Diagnosis	Resting Foot Flow (Preop.)	Preanesthetic	Maximum Before Removal of Chain	End of Operation	Postoperative Resting Flows, Hour 1	2	3	4	5	6	24	48
1. M. C.	25	F	R	Erythrocyanosis	1.3	2.0	4.2	6.0	4.1	3.7	3.5	5.0	5.2	**6.7**	5.2	6.5
2. V. C.	17	F	L	Erythrocyanosis	2.4	2.8		4.1	10.2	10.4	8.7	10.5	10.8	**12.6**	9.9	11.2
3. J. D.	24	F	R	Erythrocyanosis	0.9	0.8	4.2	4.2	5.1	11.8	11.8	**12.7**	12.3	8.8	7.4	6.2
4. O. B.	50	M	R	Diffuse obliterative arteritis	0.5	0.6	3.2	3.9	4.3	3.4	2.3	4.3	3.2	3.7	**9.9**	6.3
5. R. D.	54	M	L	Diffuse obliterative arteritis	1.0	1.0	7.3	7.3	6.3	5.9	3.3	7.5	7.9	**8.2**	5.9	
6. J. E.	63	F	R	Peripheral senile arteritis	0.7	0.6	2.2	2.8	4.7		**5.2**	4.6	4.7		1.9	2.1
				Averages	0.9	1.3	4.1	4.7	5.8	7.6	5.8	7.4	7.3	8.0	6.7	6.4

TABLE III. RESTING CALF BLOOD FLOWS UP TO THREE MONTHS POSTOPERATIVELY (MILLILITERS PER 100 ML. OF TISSUE PER MINUTE)

CASE NO. AND PATIENT	AGE (YR.)	SEX	LIMB	DIAGNOSIS	FLOWS (PREOP.)		POSTOPERATIVE CALF FLOWS										
							DAYS										
					1	2	1	2	4	5	6	8	11	14	28	42	3 MO.
1. E. C.	30	F	R	Erythrocyanosis	1.2	1.2	8.3	5.7	7.1	4.1	4.0	5.3	3.4		5.3	4.7	3.9
			L		3.5	2.5	19.3	6.3	7.7	5.6	4.3	6.5	4.1	2.5	3.1	3.7	3.5
2. G. G.	41	F	R	Idiopathic Raynaud's phenomenon	1.5		17.5	10.8	6.0	4.3	3.4	4.3		2.7	2.9	3.0	2.5
			L		0.9		12.5	8.7	4.6	3.8	3.3	4.4		2.7	1.9	2.2	2.5
3. L. N.	39	F	L	Postphlebitic leg	1.6	2.7	12.0	9.5	7.8	8.0	5.8	5.5			4.6	4.6	4.3
4. C. M.	44	F	R	Postoperative popliteal artery thrombosis	1.0	1.6	4.5		2.8	2.8	2.9	4.7	5.0	3.7	2.1	5.0	2.9
5. S. H.	61	M	R	Diffuse obliterative arteritis	2.1		6.0	4.2	3.5	2.3	4.2	4.0	2.6	4.0	6.5	5.8	2.2
			L		3.1		6.6	4.5	3.9	2.6	4.4	4.3	2.3	3.7	7.3	6.3	2.7
6. W. B.	61	M	R	Diffuse obliterative arteritis	1.2	1.1	7.5	6.6	4.3		3.6	3.1		3.2	4.6	4.0	3.4
			L		1.0	0.8	3.2	4.5	4.1		2.4	2.1		2.1	3.7	3.7	2.2
7. C. H.	52	M	R	Diffuse obliterative arteritis	1.2		3.0	2.9	2.6	2.6	2.7	2.0	1.9	2.3	1.8	1.6	2.1
8. H. B.	51	M	R	Diffuse obliterative arteritis	3.0	1.5	6.2	7.3	6.9	5.3	5.6	4.8	5.2		5.4	5.2	3.7
			L		1.7	1.4	5.8	3.6	3.8	4.1	4.9	5.6	4.8		6.6	5.3	4.0
				Averages	1.7		8.6	6.2	5.0	4.1	4.0	4.3	3.4	2.9	4.3	4.1	3.1

We have not studied the calf and foot flows in the same limb concurrently and therefore are not in a position to offer evidence as to the exact time relationship between the development of the peak calf and foot flows in any specific limb following lumbar sympathectomy. However, from our results it can be seen that the average peak flow occurs in the foot some three hours

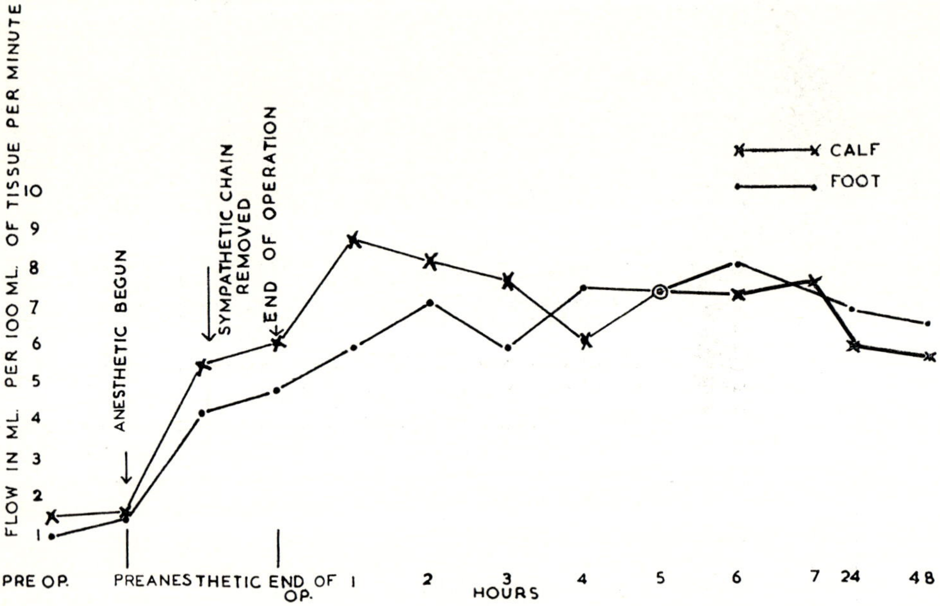

Fig. 1.—Average calf and foot flows during operation of lumbar sympathectomy and from one to forty-eight hours after operation.

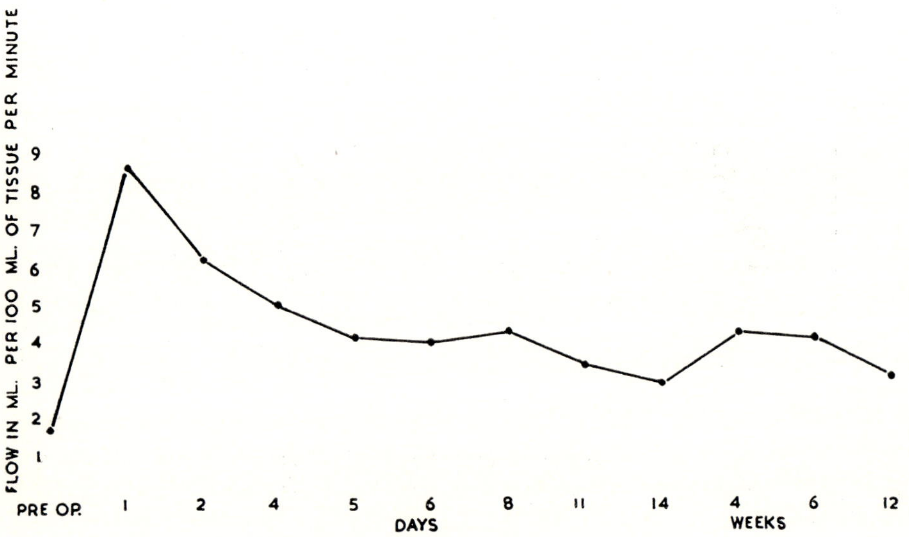

Fig. 2.—Average calf flow following lumbar sympathectomy from first day to twelve weeks.

after it does in the calf. We would suggest that this may be explained by the "current of injury" (Best and Taylor, 1950), which always follows nerve section. This exists for some hours after division of a nerve while chemical changes in the distal portion of the cut nerve continue to produce a flow of impulses in that portion. Such impulses could maintain some degree of vasoconstriction in the area of distribution of the cut nerve, and full vasomotor release following sympathectomy would not take place until this "current" ceased.

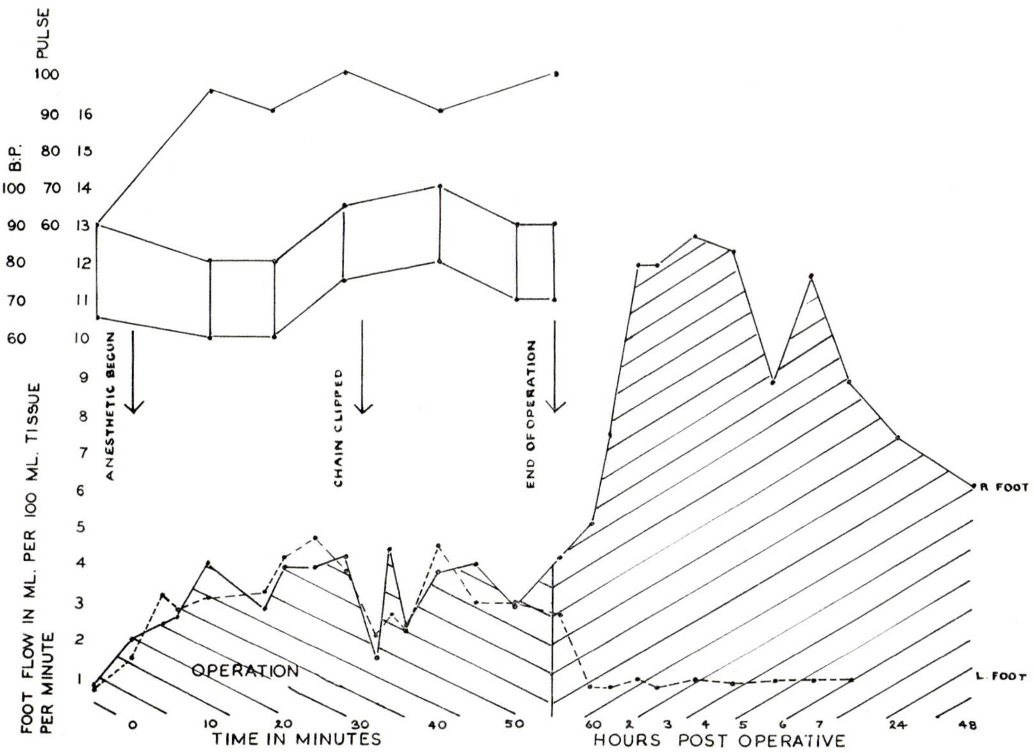

Fig. 3.—Right and left foot flows. Average foot flows during operation and from one to forty-eight hours after operation of right lumbar sympathectomy.

Three exceptions (two calves and one foot) to the general rule occurred in our series; in these the peak flow occurred twenty-four hours after operation; it is difficult to explain them with certainty. It is our practice normally to remove the second, third, and fourth lumbar sympathetic ganglia. On occasion, however, it is possible that the removal has been more extensive, and variation in the behavior of the circulation following sympathectomy may be associated with this variation of operative technique. Similarly, the presence of sympathetic ganglia in and behind the psoas muscle (Boyd and Monro, 1949), with numerous connections with the lumbar sympathetic chain, could account for, through their varying anatomic arrangements, exceptional vasomotor responses in the lower limb following lumbar sympathectomy.

It may be argued that the rise in foot or calf flow immediately following operation is due to the continued effects of anesthesia. We have shown (Fig. 3), however, that the foot flow in the contralateral unsympathectomized limb falls to the preanesthetic resting level during this period.

A secondary rise in blood flow, although less than the peak flows, often occurs in both foot and calf on the second or third postoperative day. This may be associated with the resumption of activity by the patient, although we have no evidence to substantiate this.

Duff (1951) showed that in the forearm the return of tone was almost complete in three to four days. Barcroft and Walker (1949) concluded that in the calf this process took some weeks. In our series we have found that, in general, the preoperative resting level of calf flow was not regained in the first three months. We have also noticed that after its initial rapid fall over the first few postoperative days, the resting calf flow is subject to considerable variation. We are at a loss to explain these variations. Grant and Pearson (1938) suggested that high resting flows in muscle might be associated with muscle tremors. Muscle tremor is common in obliterative arterial disease, but we did not find the variations confined to patients with that type of disease, nor is there evidence to suggest that muscle tremor is any more marked in sympathectomized limbs. Possibly the vessels of the sympathectomized limb are unable to adjust themselves rapidly to the varying influences of posture.

In conclusion, it should be noted that that when sympathectomy is being considered as an adjuvant to some other operative procedure, for example, plastic surgery or arterial grafting, it should be performed at the same time if the maximum benefit is to be obtained.

SUMMARY

1. Changes in blood flow in the foot and calf have been studied by plethysmography during anesthesia, during the operation of lumbar sympathectomy, at hourly intervals for the first seven hours, and at twenty-four and forty-eight hours following the operation.

2. The blood flow in the calf has been studied on the first, second, fourth, fifth, sixth, eighth, eleventh, and fourteenth postoperative days, and again at four, six, and twelve weeks after operation.

3. Both in the foot and the calf, flows become maximal within one to seven hours following operation.

4. Calf flows declined rapidly in the three days after operation; thereafter the fall was slower, but they still remained greater than the preoperative resting flow for at least as long as three months.

REFERENCES

1. Barcroft, H., and Edholm, O. G. J. Physiol. **104:** 161, 1945.
2. Barcroft, H., and Edholm, O. G.: J. Physiol. **104:** 366, 1946.
3. Barcroft, H., and Walker, A. J.: Lancet **1:** 1035, 1949.

4. Best, C. H., and Taylor, N. B.: Physiological Basis of Medical Practice, ed. 5, London, 1950, Baillière, Tindall & Cox.
5. Boyd, J. D., and Monro, P. A. G.: Lancet **2:** 892, 1949.
6. Duff, R. S.: Clin. Sc. **10:** 529, 1951.
7. Freeman, N. E., Smithwick, R. H., and White, J. C.: Am. J. Physiol. **107:** 529, 1934.
8. Grant, R. T., and Pearson, R. S. B.: Clin. Sc. **3:** 119, 1938.
9. Hoobler, J. W., Avera, J. W., Little, W. J., Peet, M. M., and Bassett, R. C.: Fed. Proc. **8:** 77, 1949.
10. Lewis, T., and Landis, E. M.: Heart **15:** 151, 1929.
11. Lynn, R. B., and Barcroft, H.: Lancet **1:** 1105, 1950.

EVALUATION OF A METHOD FOR THE STUDY OF BURN HEALING

RODERICK E. JENSEN, B.A.,* CAMP LEJEUNE, N. C.

INTRODUCTION

THE healing of wounds is a process in which many variable factors are involved. As a consequence, there is much disagreement and confusion concerning the efficacy of therapy designed to accelerate healing. A quantitative method of controlling the injury and measuring the subsequent healing is unquestionably necessary if reproducible results are to be obtained. Carrel[1] and DuNouy[2] in 1916 proposed a quantitative method in which the area of the unhealed surface was measured and described mathematically. Rhode, Morales, and Lozner[3] proposed in 1944 a quantitative method in which the wound-healing curve may be described by a single constant which is the slope of a straight-line function of the healing curve. A modification of the latter method has been used in this study to ascertain the variability in the healing of standard untreated burns, and the purpose of this report is to evaluate this method concerning its suitability for studying the wound-healing process.

EXPERIMENTAL PROCEDURE

Three New Zealand white rabbits, nine months old and weighing two to three kilograms, and five black and white Dutch rabbits, six months old and weighing one and one-half to two kilograms, were given eight paired burns on the back (Fig. 1). All burns were produced with a modification of the burning iron described by Leach, Peters, and Rossiter[4, 5] (Fig. 2) through which hot water is circulated by means of a centrifugal pump. The burning surface of the iron was 3.6 cm. in diameter. Since pressure probably is not a critical factor,[6] the iron was held firmly against the animal by hand for one minute.

This method of burning gives a relatively slight transcutaneous thermal gradient,[6] which gives rise to a larger sublethally injured region than is commonly seen in accidental burns. In spite of this possible disadvantage, it has been used by a number of investigators[3, 5-7] because of its simplicity and the ease of obtaining the necessary temperatures. Rabbits were prepared for burning by removing the hair from the back with electric clippers and shaving, using warm water and soap. Intraperitoneal pentobarbital sodium was used to anesthetize the rabbits for all burns.

Subcutaneous temperatures reached during exposure were determined in forty burns on the black and white rabbits, by means of a 30 gauge copper-constantan thermocouple threaded beneath the skin with the aid of a 22 gauge

This work is not to be construed as necessarily reflecting the views of the Department of the Navy.

Received for publication, May 25, 1953.

*Lt. (JG), Medical Service Corps, United States Naval Reserve, Department of Physiology, Naval Medical Field Research Laboratory.

needle which was removed prior to burning. Following the burn, the position of the thermocouple was noted with respect to the center of the burn.

Four different temperatures were used in producing burns. The two burns at each temperature were bilaterally paired. Progressing cephalad along the back they were 55°, 60°, 65°, and 70° C., respectively, for one-minute exposure (Fig. 1). Temperatures were measured by a thermometer in the burning iron (Fig. 2). These temperatures were selected to give burns of both second and third degree. (From previous experience it has been learned that an exposure of 50° for one minute produces no measurable damage.)

The edema formation in these burns was determined by measuring the thickness of a double fold of burned skin with a vernier caliper and comparing the thickness to a double fold of normal skin. Measurements were taken every thirty minutes for six hours postburn.

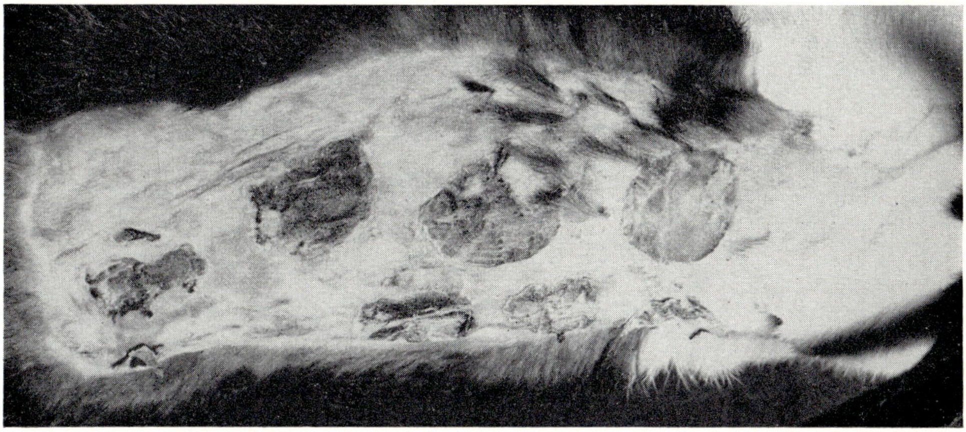

Fig. 1.—Types of burns inflicted. See text.

Healing rate was determined by daily estimates of the unhealed area of the burn which were made by measuring the length and breadth of the area with a vernier caliper. The areas approximated an ellipse, and the formula for the area of an ellipse was used to compute the area of unhealed tissue. ($A = \pi ab$ where a and b are the semimajor and semiminor axes.)

None of the burns received topical treatment. The New Zealand white rabbits reecived 100,000 units of procaine penicillin G in peanut oil, intramuscularly, weekly for four weeks. The burns of one New Zealand white rabbit were excised ninety minutes postburn, fixed in 10 per cent formalin, and stained with hematoxylin and eosin for histologic study.

THEORETICAL CONSIDERATIONS

The growth and migration of the cell population in a regenerating wound follows a typical curve which may be applied to many types of growth processes. Numerous attempts have been made to define growth in the terms of the physical chemist in order to find a "master reaction" which controls it. The growth curve, in general, is the same as that of a monomolecular or first-order reaction where one substance is transformed to another: A → B.

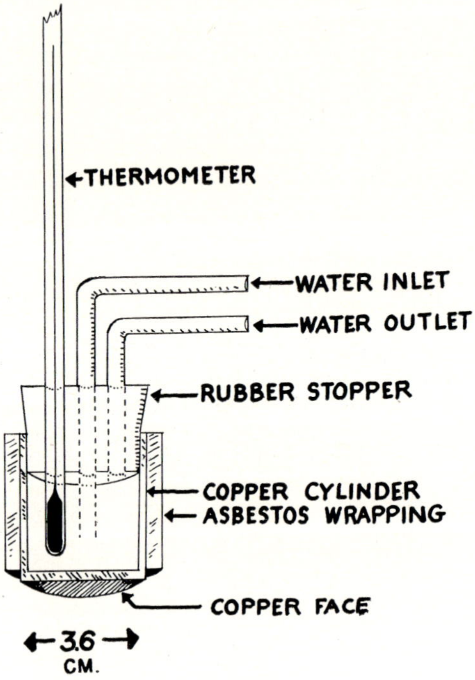

FIO 2 BURNING IRON

Fig. 2.

Brody[8] has divided the general curve of growth into two components, an initial, self-accelerating phase where growth is proportional to amount already grown (W):

$$\frac{dW}{dt} = k_1W, \qquad (1)$$

and a final self-inhibiting phase where growth is proportional to amount of growth remaining to be made before a limit is reached:

$$\frac{dW}{dt} = k_2(A - W) \qquad (2)$$

In this study, W has been used to represent the healed area of the burn, proportional to the number of new cells in the regenerating epithelium constant thickness, or other population parameters of the healing burn. A represents the limiting size or, in the case of wound healing, the original size of the wound. The symbols k_1 and k_2 are rate constants, and t is time.

To describe a growth curve, these exponential equations may be used separately or combined in a number of ways together with the use of additional constants necessary to fit the curve to the experimental data. Some investigators have attempted to link the constants with specific growth processes; however, the mathematical treatment used in this study is not designed to interpret the healing curve but only to describe it.

Equation 1 and Equation 2 may be combined[8]:

$$\frac{dW}{dt} = kW(A - W) \qquad (3)$$

or

$$\frac{dW}{dt} = kWA - kW^2.$$

In this formulation, by one possible rationale both intrinsic proliferation (W) and cellular interaction (W^2) may be taken into account.[3] The rationale for the use of Equation 3 has been established elsewhere,[3, 19, 20] and will not be discussed in detail here. This is the "autocatalytic" curve of the physical chemists which has been used with modifications by Crozier[9] and Robertson.[10] The integral form of (3), which when plotted forms a sigmoid curve, is:

$$W = \frac{A}{1 + e^{k(t + c)}}$$

where c is the constant of integration.

After rearrangement and by taking the logarithm of each term, this becomes the linear equation used as the working formula for analyzing the data from these experiments.

$$\ln \frac{A - W}{W} = -k\left(t - \frac{t^*}{2}\right), \qquad (4)$$

A is selected close to the original wound size. Unhealed area (A − W) has been measured daily, from which W, healed area, is determined by subtraction. Equation 4 describes by means of the constant k and the 99 per cent healing time intercept, t*, the curve represented by the data for each burn. The symbol k represents the rate of change of the ratio of unhealed to healed surface. Deviations from the basic curve may be analyzed by more formal mathematical treatments if desired.

The use of the k term here is not in the sense of a reaction rate constant but has a number which, when known, permits the reconstruction of the sigmoid curve representing the experimental data. In order to do this with precision, the 99 per cent healing time intercept, t*, is also necessary. Thus, by means of two constants a complete description of the healing curve is obtained. How well this description fits the data is discussed in later sections.

RESULTS

Temperatures, edema, and healed characteristics of the fifty-six burns of the four severities studied are summarized in Table I. No effects on healing rate that could be attributed specifically to edema, age, weight, strain, or sex of rabbit could be demonstrated in these experiments. The mean subcutaneous temperature prior to burning was 35° ± 1° C.

TABLE I. SUMMARY OF EFFECTS OF BURNS RESULTING FROM FOUR INCIDENT TEMPERATURES

Exposure	Temperature Time	55° C.	60° C. One minute	65° C.	70° C.
Average subcutaneous temperature	Central 50%	48° C.	50° C.	52° C.	56° C.
	Peripheral 50%	44° C.	45° C.	47° C.	52° C.
Degree of burn		Second	Second-third	Third	Third
Number of burns		14	14	14	14
Edema	Range	1-4 mm.	2-4 mm.	1-4 mm.	2-5 mm.
	Average	2.3 mm.	2.7 mm.	2.7 mm.	3.1 mm.
	Time of maximum	3.2 hr.	2.2 hr.	3.5 hr.	3.7 hr.
Healing rate (k) (average)		0.46 ± 0.08	0.32 ± 0.11	0.23 ± 0.04	0.25 ± 0.04
Healing time (average)		18 days ± 2.2	29 days ± 5.7	37 days ± 3.7	33.5 days ± 3.2

All burns were covered by a tough eschar in one week. The eschar, although curled and cracked, remained in place on the more severe burns for an average of three weeks. The appearance of the burned areas changed little during this period except for a reduction in size. After twelve days, the 70° C. burns were still the pale yellow of ischemic burned skin while the others were red-brown (Fig. 1). There was no infection in the penicillin-treated white rabbits. However, two of the 65° burns in the black and white rabbits became grossly infected early in healing. The infection spontaneously disappeared without treatment. (These burns were not included when computing averages.)

When the natural logarithm of the unhealed area divided by the healed area, equal to a constant X time, is plotted against time, a straight line is approximated. The slope k of this line plotted for each burn is used as the criterion of the healing rate. When the k's of the individual burns are set equal to each other and the data are plotted, the closeness of fit is shown (Fig. 3).

All burns studied could be classified into two significantly different groups on the basis of their healing rates. There was no significant difference between the 70° C. and 65° C. burns, and eight of the 60° C. burns. Six of the 60° C. burns on the New Zealand white rabbits were significantly different from the other eight 60° C. burns; however, they were not significantly different from the healing rates of the 55° C. burns. This is due to the fact that the 60° C. burn represents the threshold between second and third degree burns. The thirty-four burns in the third degree group presented an average k of 0.24 ± 0.04, and healed in 35 days, ± 3.5 days. The twenty burns in the second degree burn group presented an average k of 0.46 ± 0.08, and healed in 20 days, ± 3.3 days. The plot of the mean data of the second and third degree burn groups given in Table II is shown in Fig. 4.

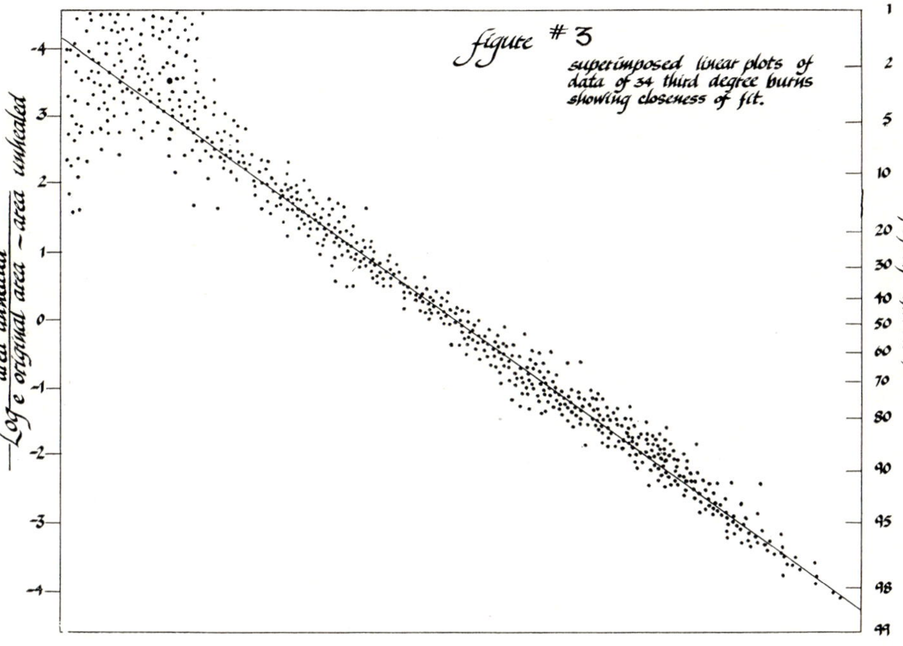
figure # 3
superimposed linear plots of data of 34 third degree burns showing closeness of fit.
-Log e area unhealed / original area - area unhealed
percent healed

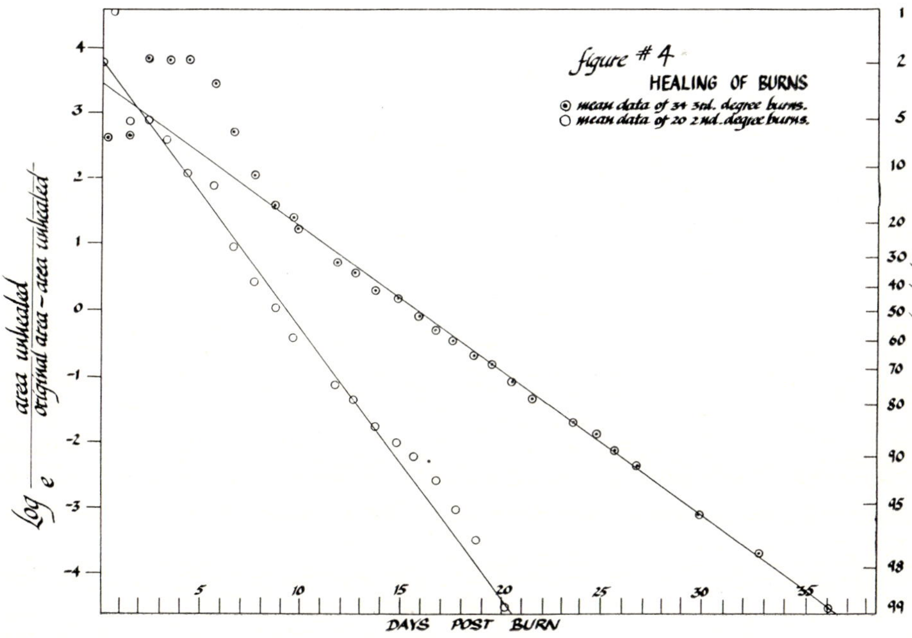
figure # 4
HEALING OF BURNS
mean data of 34 3rd. degree burns.
mean data of 20 2nd. degree burns.
Log e area unhealed / original area - area unhealed
percent healed
DAYS POST BURN

TABLE II

DAYS POSTBURN	SECOND DEGREE BURNS (20 BURNS)			THIRD DEGREE BURNS (34 BURNS)		
	UNHEALED AREA (SQ. CM.)	PER CENT HEALED (W)	$\log_e \frac{100-W}{W}$	UNHEALED AREA (SQ. CM.)	PER CENT HEALED (W)	$\log_e \frac{100-W}{W}$
0	8.0	2	3.9	8.2	7	2.6
1	8.1	1	4.6	8.2	7	2.6
2	7.8	5	2.9	8.6	2	3.9
3	7.8	5	2.9	8.8	0	–
4	7.6	7	2.6	8.6	2	3.9
5	7.3	11	2.1	8.5	3	3.5
6	7.1	13	1.9	8.2	7	2.6
7	5.8	29	0.9	7.7	12	2.0
8	5.0	39	0.4	7.3	17	1.6
9	4.1	50	0	7.1	19	1.4
10	3.3	60	–0.4	6.6	25	1.2
11	–	–	–	–	–	–
12	2.1	74	–1.1	5.9	33	0.7
13	1.7	79	–1.3	5.6	36	0.6
14	1.3	84	–1.7	5.0	43	0.3
15	1.0	88	–2.0	4.8	45	0.2
16	0.8	90	–2.2	4.2	52	–0.1
17	0.6	93	–2.6	3.7	58	–0.3
18	0.4	95	–3.0	3.3	63	–0.5
19	0.2	97	–3.5	2.8	68	–0.7
20	0.1	99	–4.6	2.6	70	–0.8
21	–	–	–	2.2	75	–1.1
22	–	–	–	1.8	79	–1.3
23	–	–	–	–	–	–
24	–	–	–	1.4	84	–1.7
25	–	–	–	1.2	87	–1.9
26	–	–	–	0.9	89	–2.1
27	–	–	–	0.8	91	–2.3
28	–	–	–	–	–	–
29	–	–	–	–	–	–
30	–	–	–	0.4	96	–3.2
31	–	–	–	–	–	–
32	–	–	–	–	–	–
33	–	–	–	0.2	97	–3.5
34	–	–	–	–	–	–
35	–	–	–	–	–	–
36	–	–	–	0.8	99	–4.9
37	–	–	–	–	–	–

DISCUSSION

Wound healing may be followed histologically by excising the wound at various intervals during healing, as has been done recently by McCleery, Schaffarzick, and Light.[11] A method using the tensile strength of the wound was introduced by Howes and Harvey in 1929[12] and has been used in a number of investigations since, including one reported in a recent paper by Sandblom.[13] The tensile strength method is used with wounds that can be sutured or which heal by primary intention. This may be a measure of some other process than rate of epithelization. Both methods have the disadvantage of interfering in the healing process because a wound may be used only once. For repeated measurements, the most widely used method is that used by Carrel[1] and DuNouy[2] in their early attempts to quantitate the wound-healing process. This consists of tracing the perimeter of the wound on cellophane and then measuring the area with a planimeter,[14] or transferring the tracing to heavier material and determining the area gravimetrically. Electrometric measurements as criteria of wound healing have been used by Burr and associates[15] and Barnes.[16] Radioactive tracer techniques are also being used.[17, 18] Healing time alone, as determined by inspection, has been used by a number of investigators. This method is subject to considerable error, since the healed area approaches 100 per cent healed asymptotically, and there is no clear-cut end point.

The method of estimating area from its length and breadth employed in this study is a modification of the method used by Rhode, Morales, and Lozner.[3] Measurements are rapid and the area may be determined in thirty seconds. In addition, this method has the distinct advantage of delimiting the unhealed area as it recedes beneath the covering eschar by the sliding of the caliper beneath the eschar to the wound's edge. It is a common occurrence in burns for a large eschar to remain as the area diminishes in size and in some cases until it is almost healed. The repeatability of this method of measurement was determined from ten measurements on each of thirty unhealed areas (1.5 to 6 square centimeters) in one day of routine measurement. The standard deviation was 0.2 square centimeter (6 per cent). As an added check, the caliper method was compared with the gravimetric tracing method described previously, which is the more accurate method of area estimate. Burn areas were traced on cellophane, and the area was computed from caliper measurements and by weighing a cardboard template of the area. The gravimetric tracing method gave a larger estimate of area than the caliper method used in these experiments. The difference was 0.3 ± 0.3 square centimeter (8 per cent).

The advantages of treating the data so that they will fit a linear function are readily apparent. A line is obtained which can describe the average slope of scattered points in the terms of a single constant. The line forms sharp intercepts with the percentage of healed values. The use of the slope of the line as an index of the healing rate, in addition to having certain theoretical implications,[19-21] has the advantage of accounting for deviations in healing rate due to differences in the initial latent period, which would contribute an error to the average healing rate as determined by other methods.

The data will also fit the self-inhibitory equation (2)[8] alone without the necessity of using Equation 3, in which case the points for the initial phase are disregarded. The estimated initial wound size, A, has more of an effect on k in Equation 2 than in Equation 3. In addition, deviation from linearity in a treatment by Equation 2 indicates that there may be some interaction between initial and final phases. Since the inflection point of the sigmoid curve of healing occurs close to the 50 per cent healed point in the majority of the burns studied, the use of Equation 3, which would include both phases, was felt to be justified.

In these experiments, deviations from the theoretical healing curve during the first week are attributed to relaxation and contraction of the wound prior to the formation of an eschar. This relaxation and contraction is caused in part by skin tensions. For example, the positional effect of the 70° C. burns was such as to close the wound while the 60° C. and 65° C. burns were stretched. The 70° C. burns also showed contraction due probably to the coagulation of the skin at time of burning.

During the first phase of healing, contraction of another sort is important in wound closure. This contraction may be attributed to dermal fibroblastic regeneration and may account for a large percentage of the reduction in size of third degree wounds. It has been previously shown that large- and medium-sized wounds will contract to a size of 1 to 1.5 cm. across when epithelization will take over as the dominant healing factor.[1] Arey[22] discussed these problems in detail in his review of the literature on wound healing. Some investigators[23, 24] have attempted to eliminate contraction in the study of wound healing in order to study only epithelization and its response to therapy. However, since contraction probably forms an important component of most clinically observed healing, this may be an unnecessary refinement.

The pairing of burns in these experiments offered no advantage in analysis. The average difference in k between pairs was 0.036 ± 0.023, while the standard deviation of the mean k of the paired burns of each rabbit was 0.022.

The optimal positions for the burns is considered to be that occupied by the 60° C. and 65° C. burns in the mid-lumbar region of the animal. The temperature used to produce a third degree burn is not critical and may be between 65° and 70° C. for a one-minute exposure. A reproducible second degree burn is produced at 55° C. However, healing is not as reliably followed in second degree burns as in the third degree burns where all healing takes place from the edges. A temperature close to 60° C. for one minute could theoretically be used to determine whether treatment will make this threshold burn heal in the manner of a second or third degree burn.

The accelerated healing in two infected burns and a wide difference between pairs as noted in these experiments warrant further study.

Rhode, Morales, and Lozner[3] have used a similar method of burn production and k (healing rate constant) determination in the evaluation of several types of therapy. It is of interest to note that for twenty untreated burns produced at from 75° C. to 82° C. for one-minute exposure, they found a mean k of 0.26 ± .07. In the experiments reported here, the mean k for 70° C. burns is 0.25 ± .04.

CONCLUSIONS

An attempt has been made to evaluate the method used in this study, in all its aspects, with regard to its applicability to the study of wound healing. In addition, pertinent descriptive information concerning the method used and the burns produced has been presented. It is considered that the method for producing burns is standard with the exception of the 60° C. one-minute threshold burn. This conclusion is based on the fact that the 65° to 70° C. change does not materially affect the healing rate of the burn. The second degree burns produced at 55° C. are more sensitive to small temperature variations. The edema formation was not found to be reproducible; however, this is considered a property of the animal burned and not of the burn source. Subcutaneous temperatures and histology of the burn were not found to be reliable enough to serve as criteria for the reproducibility of the burn. The caliper technique for measuring the diminishing unhealed area is considered superior to other methods because of its speed and simplicity. In addition, it makes it possible to follow the wound's edge as it recedes beneath the covering eschar. The mathematical treatment employed has been shown to describe the data observed during all except the first week of healing, the fit being fair to good depending on the precision required. This method is considered preferable to other widely used mathematical treatments because of its ease of application together with the minimal use of arbitrary constants. A clear rationale is considered established for its use which takes into account the simultaneous action of both an initial and final phase of healing. It is estimated that thirty treated third degree burns would be required in order to show a decrease in healing time of two days at a .02 level of significance when compared to the control group in this study. The agreement with previous experiments of this type[3] is excellent, and indicates that this is a reproducible method which may be useful as an indicator of the physiologic and therapeutic variations attendant upon wound healing.

SUMMARY

1. Sixty-four burns were produced on eight rabbits using a standard method. None of the burns was given topical therapy.

2. Burns were produced at four temperatures for one-minute exposure. The temperatures were 55°, 60°, 65°, and 70° C., respectively.

3. Methods for describing the burn and its subsequent healing are discussed. An equation which may represent the healing curve is given.

4. Subcutaneous temperature, edema, histology, healing rate, and healing time of the four types of burns are compared.

5. Burns studied may be divided into two significantly different groups by means of their healing rate. They are second degree burns (twenty days to heal) and third degree burns (thirty-five days to heal).

6. Standard deviation of the healing-rate constant for third degree burns is 16 per cent; of the healing time, 10 per cent. The contribution of the method error is a small component, and it is considered that the large deviations from the mean have a physiologic basis which can be studied by this method of analysis.

REFERENCES

1. Carrel, A., and Hartmann, J.: Cicatrization of Wounds. I. Relationship Between Size of Wound and Its Rate of Cicatrization, J. Exper. Med. **25**: 429, 1916.
2. DuNouy, P. L.: Cicatrization of Wounds. III. Relationship Between Age of Patient, Area of Wound, and Index of Cicatrization, J. Exper. Med. **24**: 461, 1916.
3. Rhode, C. M., Morales, M. F., and Lozner, F. L.: Quantitative Evaluation of Certain Treatments in the Healing of Third Degree Burns, Naval Medical Research Institute Report No. 82, National Naval Medical Center, Bethesda, Md., 1944, J. Clin. Investigation **24**: 372-379, 1945.

4. Leach, E. H., Rossiter, R. J., and Peters, R. A.: Observations on Thermal Burns, Medical Research Council, War Wounds Committee, Subcommittee on Burns. BS 14, Report No. 2—British.
5. Leach, E. H., Peters, R. A., and Rossiter, R. J.: Experimental Thermal Burns, Especially the Moderate Temperature Burn, Quart. J. Exper. Physiol. **32**: 67, 1943.
6. Moritz, A. R., and Henriques, F. C.: Studies of Thermal Injury. II. The Relative Importance of Time and Surface Temperature in the Causation of Cutaneous Burns, Am. J. Path. **23**: 695, 1947.
7. Brooks, J. W., Robinette, P. W., and Evans, E. I.: A Standard Burn. Method of Production and Observations on the Blood Picture Following Its Production in Dogs, Surg., Gynec. & Obst. **93**: 543, 1951.
8. Brody, S.: Bioenergetics and Growth, Chap. 116, New York, 1945, Reinhold Publishing Corporation.
9. Crozier, W. J.: On Curves of Growth, Especially in Relation to Temperature, J. General Physiol. **10**: 53, 1926.
10. Robertson, T. B.: The Analysis of the Growth of the Normal White Mouse Into Its Constituent Processes, J. General Physiol. **8**: 463, 1926.
11. McCleery, R. S., Schaffarzick, W. R., and Light, R. A.: The Experimental Study of the Effect of Heparin on the Local Pathology of Burns, SURGERY **26**: 548, 1949.
12. Howes, E. L., Sooy, J., and Harvey, S. C.: Healing of Wounds as Determined by Their Tensile Strength, J. A. M. A. **92**: 42, 1929.
13. Sandblom, P. H.: The Effect of Injury on Wound Healing, Ann. Surg. **129**: 305, 1949.
14. Brush, B. F., and Lam, C. R.: The Effect of Topical Application of Several Substances on the Healing of Experimental Cutaneous Wounds, SURGERY **12**: 353, 1942.
15. Burr, H. S., Taffel, M., and Harvey, S. C.: The Electrometric Study of the Healing Wound in Man, Yale J. Biol. & Med. **12**: 483, 1940.
16. Barnes, T. C.: Electrical Measurement of the Healing Rate of Human Skin, Hahneman Monthly **81**: 8, 1946.
17. Neil, C. M.: Thermal Radiation Burns in Rabbits. II. Quantitative Studies Relating P^{32} Uptake to Healing Rates, Naval Medical Research Institute, Project NM 007 081. 03. 04. In preparation.
18. Williamson, W. B., and Fromm, H. J.: Distribution of Methionine S^{35} During Healing of Experimental Burns, Fed. Proc. **12**: 291, 1953.
19. Morales, M. F., and Kreutzer, F. L.: Some Nutritional and Excretional Interactions and the Growth of an Organ or Colony, Bull. Math. Biophysics **7**: 15, 1945.
20. Shock, N., and Morales, M.: A Fundamental Form for the Differential Equation of Colonial and Organismal Growth, Bull. Math. Biophysics **2**: 63, 1942.
21. Rashevsky, N.: Mathematical Biophysics, Chicago, 1948, University of Chicago Press, p. 224.
22. Arey, L. B.: Wound Healing, Physiol. Rev. **16**: 327-406, 1936.
23. Howes, E. L.: Recent Advances in Studying the Problems of Healing and Their Effect on the Treatment of Wounds and Burns, New York State J. Med. **44**: 2006, 1944.
24. Scheinberg, S., Bralow, S. P., and Necheles, H.: Experimental Study of Wound Healing, SURGERY **24**: 972, 1948.

A CONTROLLED PRESSURE PLASTIC DRESSING FOR SKIN GRAFTING, BURNS, AND THROMBOPHLEBITIS

ARNOLD L. LEHMANN, M.D., SPOKANE, WASH., AND
LYLE J. HAY, M.D., MINNEAPOLIS, MINN.

(From the Department of Surgery of the Veterans Administration Hospital)*

WE HAVE searched for a surgical dressing which exerts uniform pressure and is easily applied; a polyvinyl plastic sheath has been developed as a simple pressure dressing. Although extensive investigation of this method will be necessary, we wish to present a preliminary report of our findings.

Numerous useful techniques for applying pressure to wounds have been described. Douglas[1] has reported a pressure jacket for the treatment of burns and other extensive wounds. He utilized a single layer of transparent jacket demanding a seal to the proximal portion of the extremity; this requires moderate time and skill. Bunyan[2] used a similar envelope about the extremity for the irrigation of burns and wounds, thus avoiding painful changes of dressings. Curry[3] described a pneumatic leg splint for the emergency treatment of lower extremities; he suggested the application of this principle in treating compound fractures and burns. Scott[4] developed an inelastic legging with an inflatable rubber bladder for the treatment of venous and lymphatic stasis of the legs. Blair[5] discussed the salutary effect of mechanical pressure on wound healing. Allen and Koch[6] utilized the surgical principle of compression in the treatment of burns of the extremities. Glenn, Gilbert, and Drinker[7] have considered the physiologic implications of this method of therapy. Rossiter and Peters[9] found that external pressures of the order of 10 mm. of mercury applied with an air cuff greatly reduced edema formation in burned guinea pig skin; this pressure was most effective if applied immediately after the thermal insult. Similar pressures applied with an air cuff greatly reduced edema formation in the burned ear of a rabbit. They searched for a method by which unskilled hands could apply pressures of this order.

METHOD

A polyvinyl plastic sheath for the arm and leg has been developed. It consists of a cylinder within a cylinder, sealed along a longitudinal line and at both ends. The extremity is inserted into the sheath. The longitudinal seam is lifted away from the extremity, and the pressure dressing is inflated. The longitudinal seam and inner dressing enclose the extremity much like mesentery and serosa envelop the small bowel. Thus a uniform pressure is exerted

Received for publication July 9, 1953.

*Published with the approval of the Chief Medical Director. The statements and conclusions published by the authors are the result of their own study and do not necessarily reflect the opinion or policy of the Veterans Administration.

on the extremity. To regulate the level of pressure within the sheath, the tube used for inflation is submerged 15 to 20 cm. in a column of water; when bubbles of air cease to escape, the tube is clamped (Figs. 1 through 5).

Prior to use, we have soaked the plastic dressing in an aqueous Zephiran solution at least twenty-four hours for sterilization; the plastic dressing withstands autoclaving poorly.

Fig. 1.

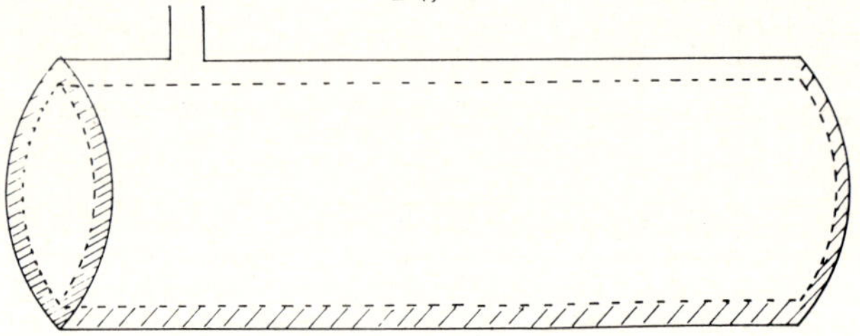

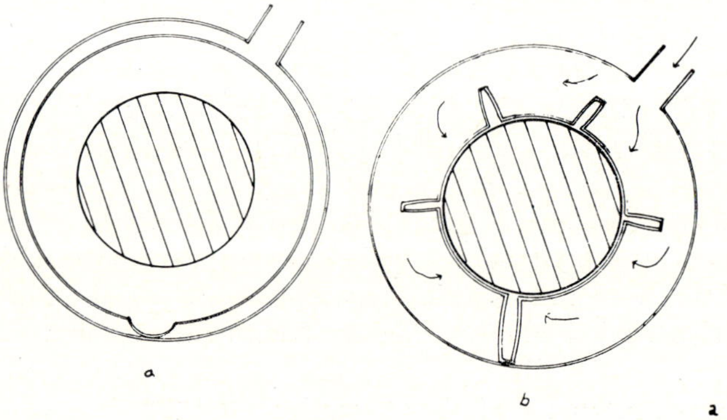

Fig. 2.

Fig. 1.—Diagram of arm sheath. Solid lines represent outer layer of sheath; dotted lines represent inner layer of sheath; at the shaded lines the outer layer is sealed to the inner layer.

Fig. 2.—Cross section of sheath: (*a*) diagram of sheath uninflated; cross-hatched area represents arm, (*b*) sheath is inflated; note how inner layer of sheath is compressed against arm.

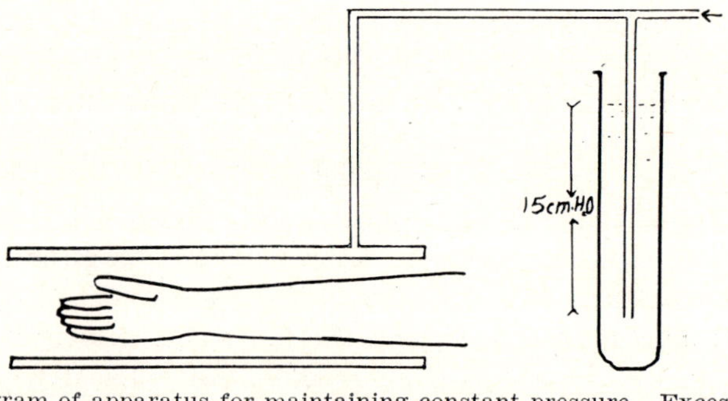

Fig. 3.—Diagram of apparatus for maintaining constant pressure. Excess air escapes from a T tube submerged in water to a distance of 15 cm., while an inflow of air from a pump maintains a constant pressure.

We have measured the changes in the volume of mouse tails following a standard ischemic insult. Pressures from 10 to 30 mm. of mercury effectively decreased the amount of swelling following ischemia of the tail; pressures above 30 mm. of mercury produced necrosis of the tip of tail, adequate evidence of a noxious effect. Like Rossiter, we found that the bulk of fluid accumulated in the tail within one hour following injury.[9-11]

Theoretical considerations appear to favor the rapid application of controlled uniform pressure to an injured part such as a burn. Intense hemoconcentration follows a burn because protein and fluid is lost at the site of the burn. It is hoped that pressure dressings may prevent the shift of fluid from the blood stream to the injured tissue.

CASE REPORTS

CASE 1 (No. 112631).—C. S., a 24-year-old white man, was pinned beneath a jeep, resulting in avulsion of skin and subcutaneous tissue from the left elbow and distally for several inches, with fracture of the radius and ulna. Extensive skin grafting was necessary at that time. Three years later he complained of a burning sensation radiating to the fourth and fifth fingers. A neuroma of the left ulnar nerve was excised. Postoperatively, the skin over the operative site sloughed.

Fig. 4.

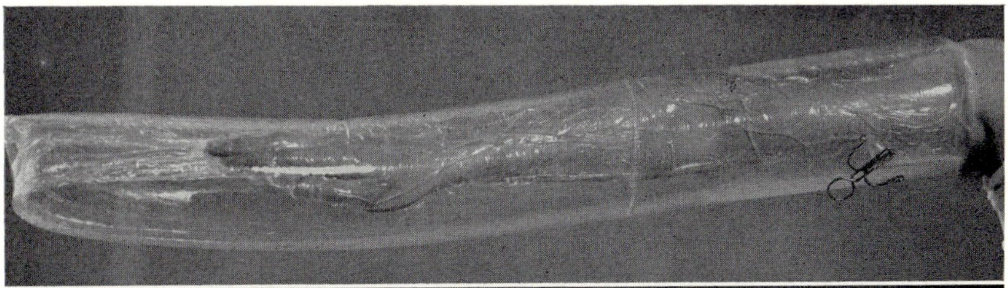

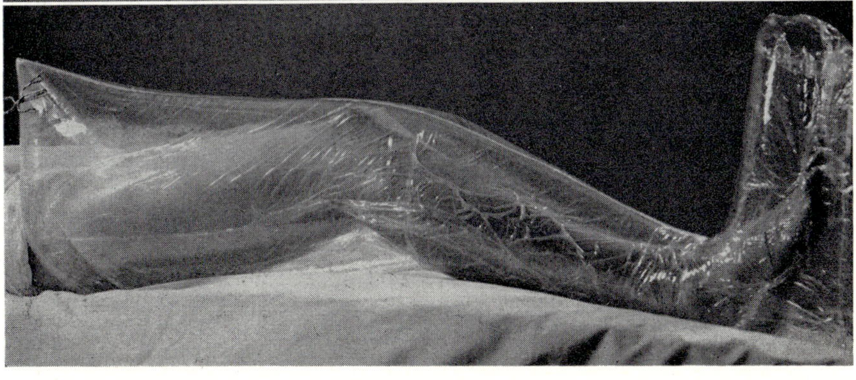

Fig. 5.

Fig. 4.—Plastic pressure dressing applied to arm.
Fig. 5.—Plastic pressure dressing applied to leg.

A split thickness graft was obtained with the Padgett dermatome, and sewed into place. A pneumatic plastic sheath was applied directly to the skin using 15 cm. of water pressure. The postoperative course was afebrile, and six days later, on removal of the dressing on May 16, 1951, the arm was moist but there was a 100 per cent take of the graft.

CASE 2 (No. 115302).—E. Z., a 55-year-old man, had a duodenal ulcer with a choledochoduodenal fistula for which a gastric resection and choledochostomy were carried out. On the sixth postoperative day he developed a thrombophlebitis of the left lower extremity with marked swelling. He was treated with heparin and the pneumatic pressure dressing. There was a dramatic reponse. The patient felt subjective relief, and the leg rapidly decreased to normal size following the application of the pneumatic boot. It was felt that the pressure dressing contributed to the rapid recovery.

CASE 3 (No. 120184).—C. N., a middle-aged white man, sustained second and third degree burns of the left thigh one week prior to admission. Twenty-six days after the injury, on Nov. 21, 1951, a split thickness graft was applied. A pneumatic pressure dressing was applied for six days, and on removal a 95 per cent take of the graft was revealed.

COMMENT

This method provides a simple means of applying uniform pressure. The transparent dressings make possible constant observation of the wound. However, there is collection of considerable moisture when the plastic sheath is applied directly to the skin. There may be an occasional sensitivity reaction to the polyvinyl plastic, and other plastics may eventually be found to be more satisfactory. In hot weather, an increased loss of body heat due to this insulating jacket may add to the patient's discomfort. Nevertheless, we believe that this pneumatic pressure dressing may be satisfactory for many wounds of the body. Pressures of 10 to 30 mm. of mercury are desirable and can be attained easily by this method, whereas practice and skill are needed for the proper pressure application with various other bandages.

SUMMARY

A pneumatic plastic pressure sheath has been found to be an efficacious dressing for many surgical wounds.

Acknowledgment.—We are indebted to Dr. C. R. Arnold of Doughboy Industries, Inc., of New Richmond, Wis., for the aid in designing and fabricating of test samples of the pneumatic dressing.

REFERENCES

1. Douglas, B.: The Treatment of Burns and Other Wounds With Special Emphasis on the Transparent Jacket System, SURGERY **15**: 96, 1944.
2. Bunyan, J.: The Treatment of Burns and Wounds by the Envelope Method, Brit. M. J. **2**: 4200, 1941.
3. Curry, G. J.: A Pneumatic Leg Splint, J. A. M. A. **125**: 966, 1944.
4. Scott, W. J. M., and Radakovick, M.: Venous and Lymphatic Stasis in the Lower Extremities, SURGERY **26**: 970, 1949.
5. Blair, V. P.: The Influence of Mechanical Pressure on Wound Healing, Illinois M. J. **46**: 249, 1924.
6. Allen, H. S., and Koch, S. L.: The Treatment of Patients With Severe Burns, Surg., Gynec. & Obst. **74**: 914, 1924.
7. Glenn, W. W. L., Gilbert, H. H., and Drinker, C. K.: The Treatment of Burns by the Closed-plaster Method, With Certain Physiological Considerations Implicit in the Success of This Technique, J. Clin. Investigation **22**: 609, 1943.
8. Duncan, G. W., and Blalock, A.: The Uniform Production of Experimental Shock by Crush Injury: Possible Relationship to Clinical Crush Syndrome, Ann. Surg. **115**: 684, 1942.
9. Rossiter, R. J., and Peters, R. A.: Controlled External Pressure and Oedema Formation, Lancet **246**: 9, 1944.
10. Lehmann, A. L., and Reinecke, R. M.: Effects of Graded Pressures on the Tail of the Mouse, Am. J. Physiol. **158**: 113, 1949.
11. Lehmann, A. L., and Reinecke, R. M.: Measurement of Increase in Volume of Tail of Mouse Following Ischemia, Am. J. Physiol. **162**: 226, 1950.

THE EFFECT OF SPLENECTOMY ON THE SURVIVAL RATE OF HOMOLOGOUS SKIN GRAFTS IN C.F.W. MICE

ALVAR A. WERDER, PH.D., AND CREIGHTON A. HARDIN, M.D.,
KANSAS CITY, KAN.

(From the Departments of Microbiology and Surgery, University of Kansas Medical Center)

IT HAS been postulated[1, 2] that immunologic mechanisms may play an important role in the transplantability of homologous tissues. The exact site of antibody formation is unknown although the reticuloendothelial system is thought to be involved.[3] Lymphocytes[4] and plasma cells[5, 6] are reported to play an important role in antibody response. The lymphocytes act as the transporters of the already formed antibody, while the plasma cells actually are involved in their production. Reports in the literature tend to show that antigens localize in the spleen and that antibodies may be detected here before appearing in the peripheral blood stream. Splenectomy has also been reported as reducing the animal's ability to produce antibodies.[7-9] Since the reticuloendothelial system, particularly the splenic portion, appears to be related to the immune response, attempts to alter this reaction might allow a homologous graft to survive. The following experiments were carried out on C.F.W. mice in an attempt to prolong the survival time of skin homografts.

Methods.—A study of 129 homologous and autologous skin transplants was made using a random selection of 6-week-old heterozygous C.F.W. mice. Their average weight was about twenty grams. Anesthesia consisted of 0.6 to 0.8 c.c. of a 5 per cent solution of Nembutal Sodium injected intraperitoneally. Splenectomy was performed through a left oblique subcostal incision. The wound was closed with two interrupted through-and-through 0000 black silk sutures. Two control series of mice were subjected to laparotomy. In one series the spleen was delivered through the abdominal incision and then returned intact to the peritoneal cavity. This will be referred to as "mock splenectomy."

In the other series a left nephrectomy was performed. The mice were put in individual cages, and two to three weeks was allowed for complete healing.

In the homologous skin-grafted groups two mice were closely shaved over the dorsal area; a full thickness skin graft was removed from each mouse and then transplanted to the other animal. These grafts were approximately 2.5 cm. in area and weighed, on the average, 150 mg. Fixation of the skin grafts was accomplished by means of interrupted and continuous running 0000 black silk suture. A thin layer of collodion was applied over the graft and the surrounding skin of the mouse to minimize contamination. The grafted mice were then placed in individual cages.

This investigation was supported in part by a grant from the National Cancer Institute, National Institutes of Health.

Received for publication, June 18, 1953.

Recording of Results.—To insure consistency, one observer recorded the daily appearance of the skin grafts. The outcome of the autografts and homografts was recorded by photography, biopsy, and observation, and they were placed into one of four categories according to the following criteria:

1. *Survival:* No color changes, lack of necrosis at the edges, healing without contracture, and regrowth of hair in the graft (Fig. 1).
2. *Necrosis:* Dark discoloration and disintegration (Fig. 2).
3. *Sloughing:* Varying degrees of separation of the graft from the contiguous skin edges of the recipient (Fig. 3).
4. *Contractile healing:* Spontaneous healing of the defect by cicatrix (Fig. 4).

Fig. 1.

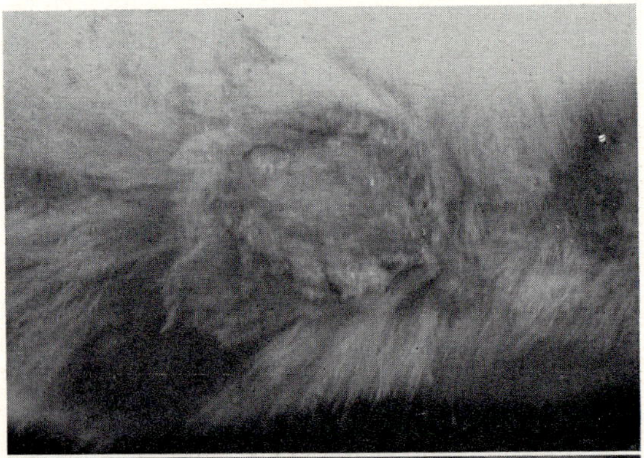

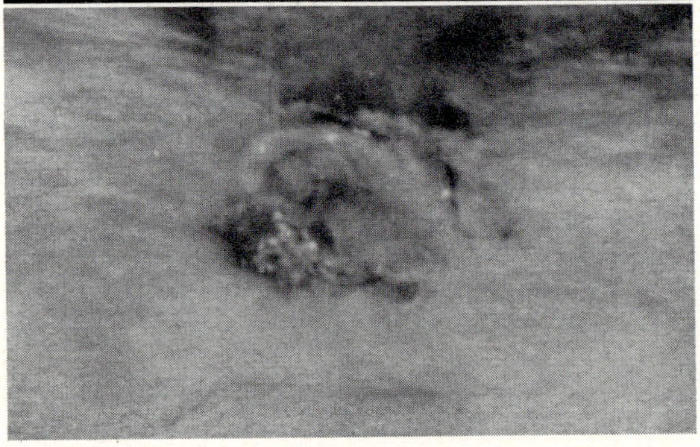

Fig. 2.

Fig. 1.—Appearance of surviving homologous skin graft.
Fig. 2.—Beginning necrosis of homologous skin graft.

Each final recording was correlated with microscopic findings. The pathologic processes of necrosis, sloughing, and contractile healing are continuous and simultaneous. These arbitrary groupings were utilized as an aid in recording the fate of the homografts.

RESULTS

Survival Rate of Autologous Skin on Normal and Splenectomized C.F.W. Mice (see Table I).—Seventeen autografts were made on normal mice for control purposes. By the ninth postoperative day, fifteen of the seventeen autografts were viable. The remainder were permanently viable at the end of a sixty-day observation period (Fig. 5).

There were eighteen autografts performed on previously splenectomized mice. By the fourth postoperative day, fifteen of the eighteen autografts were alive, and remained so at the end of a sixty-day period.

The survival rate of autologous skin grafts was not enhanced by splenectomy. Hemorrhage and infection were the causes of failure in the autografts which did not survive permanently.

Fig. 3.

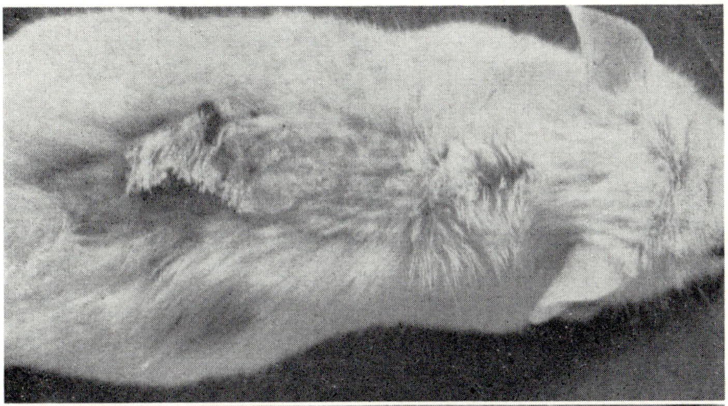

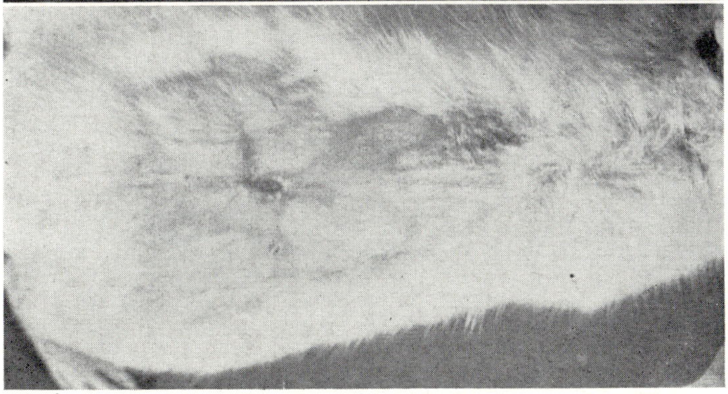

Fig. 4.

Fig. 3.—Sloughing of necrotic skin graft.
Fig. 4.—Contractile healing of defect previously occupied by homologous graft.

Survival Rates of Homologous Skin on Normal and Splenectomized C.F.W. Mice (see Table II).—Forty homologous skin grafts were transplanted to nonsplenectomized mice. Forty per cent of the homografts were viable by the fifth day, but by the tenth postoperative day all of the skin grafts were necrotic. This series includes the mice which were subjected to mock splenectomy. There were thirty-one homologous skin grafts made on previously splenectomized mice. By the fifth postoperative day, 61 per cent of the homografts were viable, but by the nineteenth day, all of the grafts were necrotic.

Survival Rates of Homologous Skin on Nephrectomized C.F.W. Mice.—Nephrectomy was selected as a control procedure to determine whether the operative trauma incident to organ removal influenced the survival rate of homologous skin grafts. Twenty-three homologous skin grafts were transplanted to previously nephrectomized mice. The rate of necrosis paralleled that of the homologous skin grafts transferred to normal animals. Ten days after homotransplantation all of the grafts were nonviable.

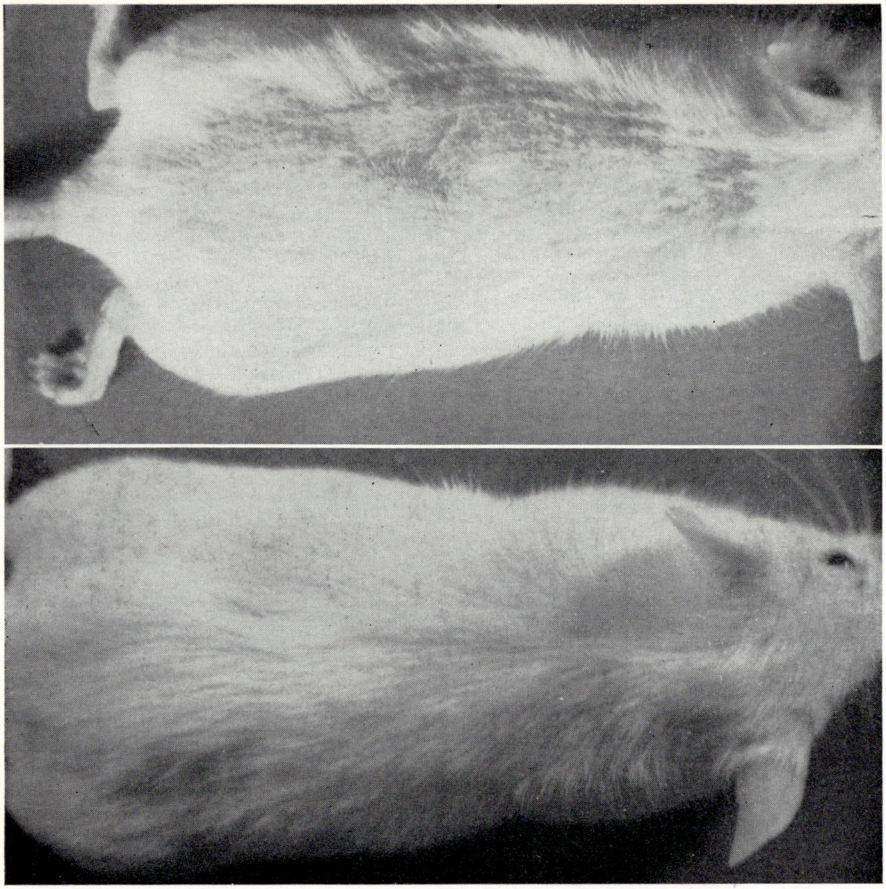

Fig. 5.—Autologous skin graft showing permanent viability.

DISCUSSION

Splenectomy resulted in an extended survival time of the homologous skin grafts. This observation could possibly be explained by a quantitative decrease of a significant part of the reticuloendothelial system. The prolonged survival of a homograft on such an animal could then be explained by a depressed antibody response.

Another possibility to be considered is the concept of "immunological paralysis."[10, 11] It is postulated that the immune mechanism of an animal could be "paralyzed" by large quantities of antigen. With a reduced amount of reticuloendothelial tissue present due to splenectomy, the amount of skin antigen could be sufficient to hold the immune response in abeyance.

It would, therefore, seem to follow that the necrosis of the fixed amount of homografted skin is due to: (1) the immune response of the remaining reticuloendothelial cells, or (2) the fact that the dosage of the homograft antigen was not sufficient to permit continuous paralysis of the reticuloendothelial system.

TABLE I. SURVIVAL RATES OF AUTOLOGOUS SKIN GRAFTS ON NORMAL AND SPLENECTOMIZED CFW MICE

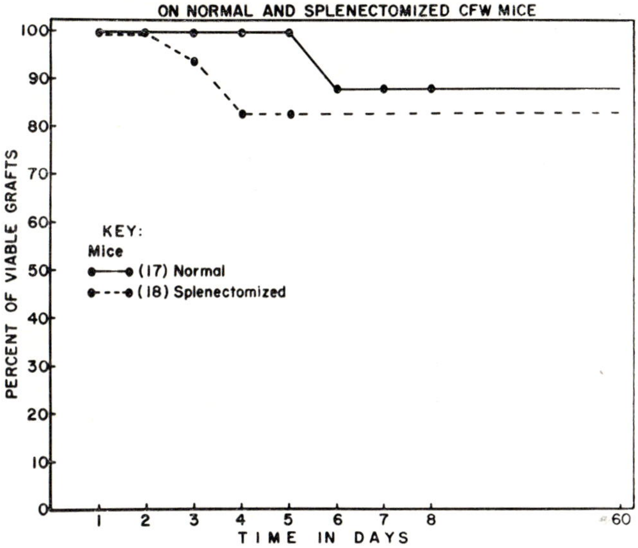

TABLE II. SURVIVAL RATES OF HOMOLOGOUS SKIN GRAFTS ON NORMAL AND SPLENECTOMIZED CFW MICE

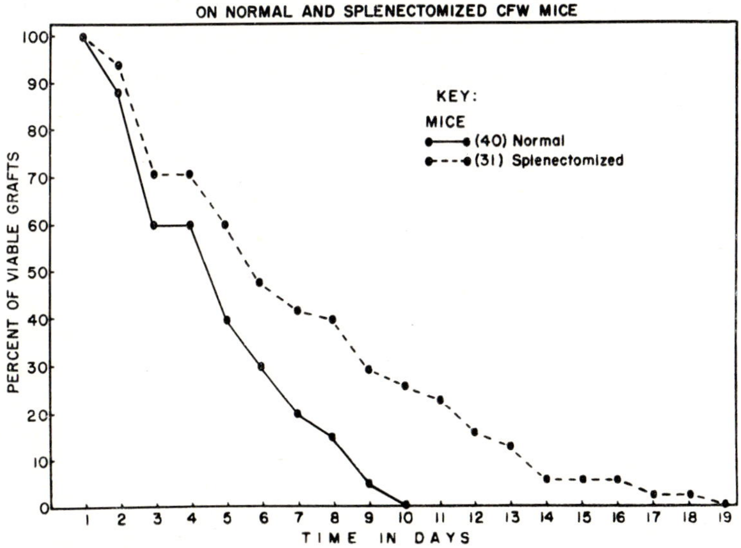

SUMMARY

Splenectomy has been used in an attempt to lower the resistance of the recipient animal to homotransplants of skin.[12] This procedure has been reported as being unsuccessful in prolonging the survival of the homografts. The species of animals used previously in this work was not specifically stated.

We have found that homologous skin grafts transplanted to splenectomized C.F.W. mice have a prolonged survival time. The exact mechanism and site of the immune response are still not definitely known. The results of these animal experiments would seem to add further data to the premise that immunologic factors play an important role in the transplantability of homologous skin grafts.

REFERENCES

1. Dempster, W. J.: Problems Involved in the Homotransplantation of Tissues With Particular Reference to Skin, Brit. M. J. **2**: 1041, 1951.
2. Medawar, P. B.: Immunity to Homologous Grafted Skin: III. Fate of Skin Homografts Transplanted to the Brain, to Subcutaneous Tissue and to the Anterior Chamber of the Eye, Brit. J. Exper. Path. **29**: 58, 1948.
3. Metchnikoff, E.: Immunity in Infective Diseases, London, 1907, Cambridge University Press.
4. Harris, T. N., Grim, E., Mertens, E., and Ehrich, W. E.: The Role of the Lymphocyte in Antibody Formation, J. Exper. Med. **81**: 73, 1945.
5. Ehrich, W. E., Drabkin, D. L., and Forman, C.: Nucleic Acids and the Production of Plasma Cells, J. Exper. Med. **90**: 157, 1949.
6. Fagreaeus, A.: The Plasma Cellular Reaction and Its Relation to the Formation of Antibodies, J. Exper. Med. **58**: 1, 1948.
7. Motohashi, S.: Fixed-tissue Phagocytosis, J. M. Research **43**: 419, 1922.
8. Rowley, D. A.: The Effect of Splenectomy on the Formation of Circulating Antibody in the Adult Male Albino Rat, J. Immunol. **64**: 289, 1950.
9. Woolridge, R. L., Crawford, Y. E., Cretzinger, J. E., Rossner, G. G., and Parpart, R. D.: The Effect of Splenectomy Upon Serum and Tissue Antibody Formation, Naval Medical Research Unit #4, Project Report NM 005 051.06. 01, November, 1950.
10. Felton, L. D.: The Significance of Antigen in Animal Tissues, J. Immunol. **61**: 107, 1949.
11. Morgan, P., Watson, D. W., and Cromartie, W. J.: Type Specificity of "Immunological Paralysis" Induced in Mice With Pneumococcal Type II Polysaccharide, J. Bact. **65**: 224, 1953.
12. Rodhe, C.: Veber Versuche Zur Ueberwindung der Anheilungsschwierigkeiten Homoplasticher Transplantate, Beitr. z. klin. Chir. **134**: 111. 1925.

THE MIXING OF MATERIAL INJECTED INTO PULSATILE AND NONPULSATILE STREAMS: APPLICATION TO REGIONAL HEPARINIZATION

W. R. Cate, Jr., M.D., and T. S. Culley,* Nashville, Tenn.

(From the Department of Surgery, Vanderbilt University School of Medicine)

"REGIONAL heparinization is the term used to describe the administration of heparin in such a way that the coagulation time of the blood of one limb, for example, is increased without materially affecting the blood in other parts of the body. Thus, with an infusion of heparin into the femoral artery of one limb, blood samples from the veins of the same leg show a longer clotting time than those secured at the same time from other parts of the body. This is true, however, only when small doses of heparin are administered."[1]

Since this original description of regional heparinization by Murray and associates in 1937, other investigators[2-5] have been attracted by the possibility of rendering blood relatively incoagulable locally without the attendant dangers of systemic heparinization. They too have been concerned with the comparison of clotting times of blood samples drawn regionally and those obtained from some distant site.[2, 5] We are not aware of any previous studies directed at another factor which would appear to be of importance, that of adequate local mixing of the injected heparin.

The experiments reported in this communication were designed to determine the degree of mixing of materials injected into both pulsatile and nonpulsatile streams under controlled conditions. They were therefore conducted primarily in models. They have demonstrated a marked lack of mixing with pressures and rates of injections ordinarily utilized for regional heparinization. They have pointed to the need for much higher pressures of injection if uniform distribution of the injected material at a reasonable distance from the site of injection is to be achieved.

Materials and Methods.—Fig. 1 illustrates the method of injection of dye into a nonpulsatile stream. Water flowed from a hydrant (*A*) through plastic hosing of 12.5 mm. internal diameter. The pressure in the system was controlled by rubber tubing and attached screw clamp (*I*). The water was ejected into a drain in order to provide a constantly clear stream proximal to the point of injection, and the volume flow was checked by intermittent sampling. Dye was injected with a 50 c.c. syringe (*C*) with a centering device on the plunger for the shaft of the injection pump (*B*). It was necessary to operate the drive shaft of the injection pump manually for high-pressure injections. The syringe was connected to fine polyethylene catheters (*F*) by means of a converted three-way stopcock, so as to form a T connector (*D*), and a 24 gauge needle.

Read before the Society of Clinical Surgery, May 1, 1953.
Received for publication, May 29, 1953.
*Senior medical student.

The other arm of the connector was utilized for the measurement of injection pressures with a Bourdon tube gauge (*E*). Pressures in the stream were recorded by a U-tube mercury manometer (*G*). The sampling needles (*H*) were used for the withdrawing of samples at varying distances from the site of injection. The polyethylene injection catheters were inserted into the hose through 18 gauge needles and sealed there with Du Pont cement; they were pointed in an upstream direction. A catheter length of twelve inches was employed in all experiments.

Fig. 2 illustrates the method of obtaining a pulsatile stream. It is a diagrammatic sketch of a component part of a modified Joengblood heart-lung apparatus isolated from the remainder of the apparatus by clamps. The rubber diaphragm is activated by an eccentric cam, and the stroke volume is adjustable. Water was constantly supplied to the reservoir through a separate hose; the stream was again ejected into a drain, and volume flow was determined by intermittent sampling as with the nonpulsatile stream.

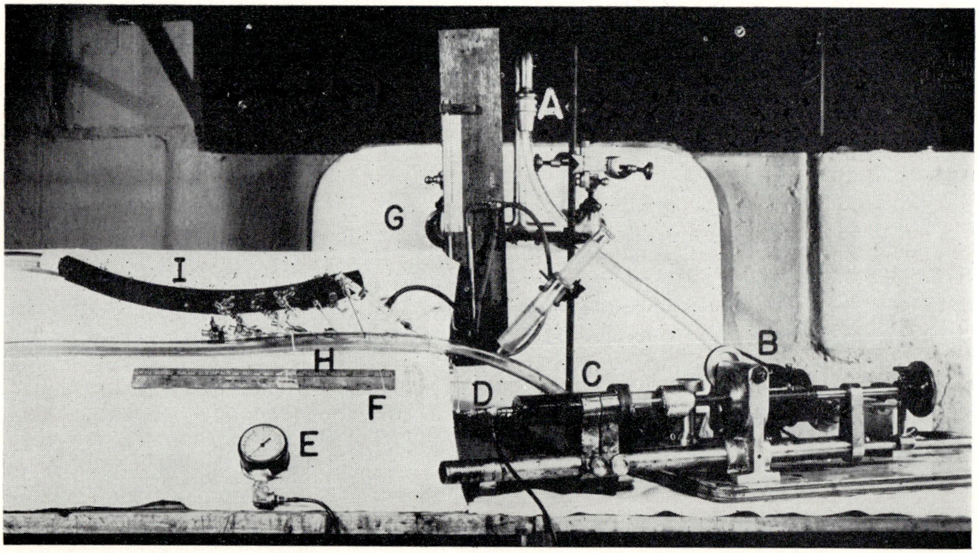

Fig. 1.—Photograph illustrating nonpulsatile stream and injection apparatus. Description in text.

The diameter of the polyethylene injection catheters was decreased for high-pressure injections by melting them about tantalum wire of the desired diameter. The wire was then extracted. Heat of low intensity was obtained for this purpose by placing a glass chimney over a Bunsen burner. The injected dye was methylene blue, 1.6 per cent, in all experiments. Dye concentrations (in terms of optical density) were recorded on a Coleman Junior Spectrophotometer at a wave length of 460 mμ. Samples were withdrawn through previously placed needles at intervals of one inch from the site of injection; the samples were withdrawn either from the periphery or from the center of the stream. Each point on the graphs in Fig. 5 represents an average of six determinations.

Five experiments, as diagrammatically represented in Fig. 6, were performed utilizing mongrel dogs. Following anesthetization with veterinary Nembutal, the abdominal aorta and the trifurcation were exposed through long midline incisions. Polyethylene injection catheters were inserted through 18 gauge needles into the aorta at varying distances from the trifurcation ranging from three to five inches; the catheters were pointed in an upstream direction in all cases. Bleeding about the catheters was prevented by purse-string ligatures (Fig. 6, *A*). Dye was injected in the same manner as in the model experiments. Cournand needles were placed in the femoral arteries (Fig. 6, *B* and *D*)

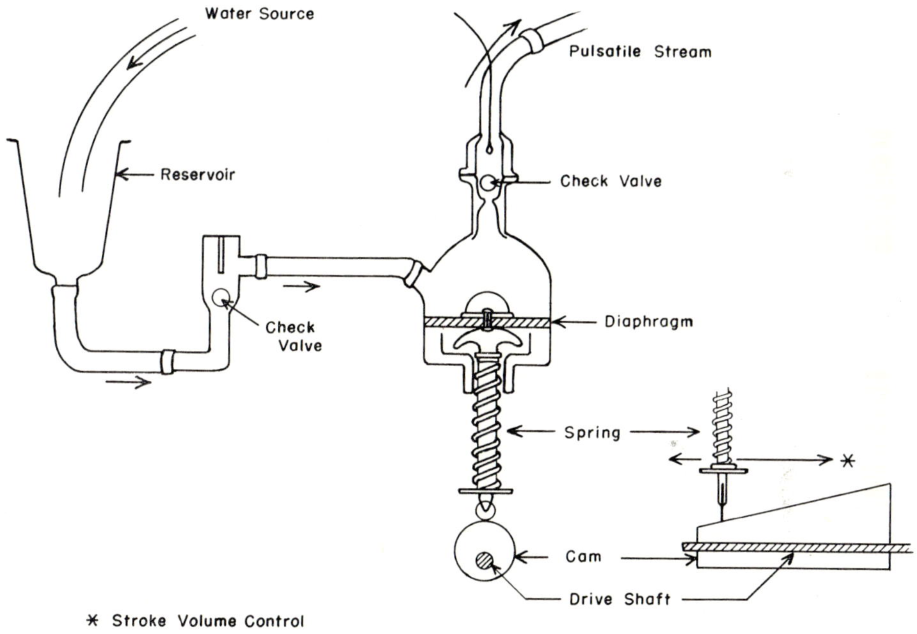

Fig. 2.—Diagram of method of obtaining a pulsatile stream. Description in text.

through separate groin incisions and a large polyethylene catheter in a branch of the common hypogastric artery (Fig. 6, *C*) for the obtaining of blood samples. A separate catheter was secured either in the external jugular vein or in the carotid artery (Fig. 6, *E*). With a team of four, samples were then drawn from these four sites as nearly simultaneously as possible during the intra-aortic injection of dye, either 1.6 per cent methylene blue or 0.18 per cent Evans blue. Dye concentrations were again recorded on the Coleman Junior Spectrophotometer at a wave length of 600 mμ. These determinations were made on supernatant plasma after centrifugation of the oxalated specimens and were compared with plasma blanks.

Results.—Marked streaming of dye injected into nonpulsatile streams of water flowing through clear plastic hose was observed. Fig. 3 records this streaming effect photographically. The mean velocity of flow in the stream is somewhat less than that in the human aorta (0.27 M. per second as compared to 0.4 M. per second).[12] It is to be noted that complete mixing of the dye is not present at a distance of twelve inches from the site of injection, even though an injection pressure of sixty-eight pounds per square inch was employed (Fig. 3, *b*). Streaming can be observed in these models for a distance of two, three, and more feet from the site of injection.

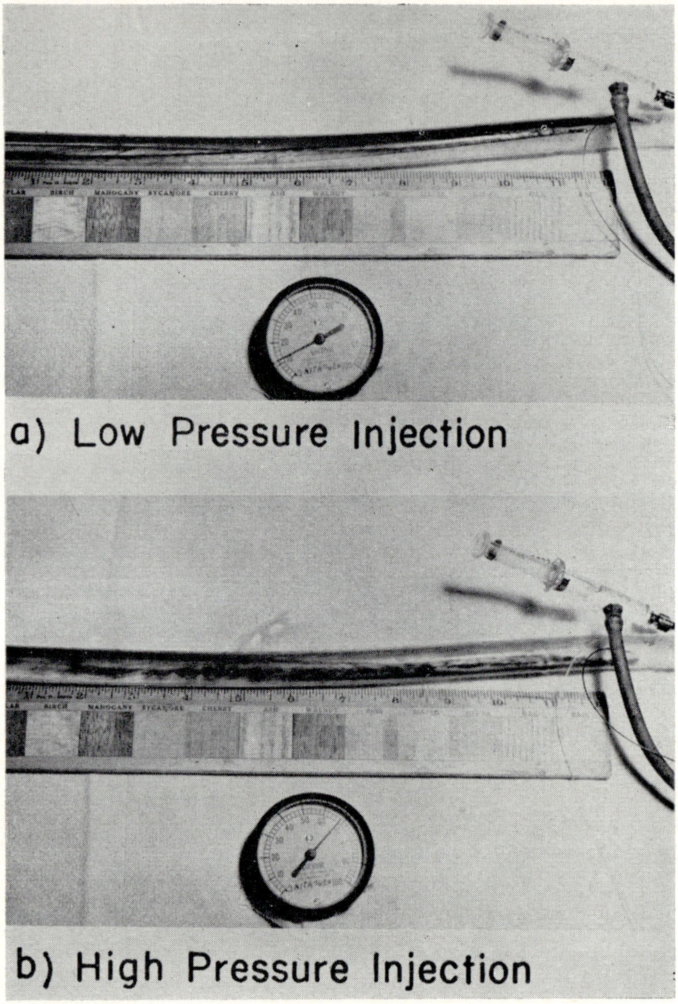

Fig. 3.—Nonpulsatile stream. *a,* Stream: pressure, 30 mm, Hg; flow, 30 c.c. per second; velocity, 0.27 M. per second. Injection: pressure, twelve pounds per square inch; rate, approximately 2.5 c.c. per minute; orifice, 0.011 cm. internal diameter. *b,* Stream: same. Injection: pressure, sixty-eight pounds per square inch; rate, approximately 2.5 c.c. per minute; orifice, 0.0044 cm. internal diameter.

The internal diameter of the injection catheter used in the experiment shown in Fig. 3, *a* was 0.011 cm. It can be inserted through an 18 gauge needle and is of the size frequently used clinically for regional heparinization. The injection pressure recorded on the gauge (twelve pounds per square inch) delivers approximately 2.5 c.c. per minute through a twelve-inch catheter. This rate of injection was chosen since, for purposes of comparison with methods of regional heparinization, it represents a twenty-four hour volume of approximately 3,600 c.c. Significantly greater rates of injection at higher pressures would improve mixing but would result in twenty-four hour volumes beyond the range of practical consideration. The upper graph in Fig. 5 corresponds with the experiment shown in Fig. 3, *a* in that velocity of flow and pressures are the same both for the stream and for the injection. Concentrations of dye in samples drawn from the center of the stream (upper line) and the periphery (lower line) are plotted in terms of optical density against the distance in inches from the site of injection. The shaded area in effect, then, depicts streaming. It should be pointed out that manipulations attendant upon withdrawing the samples alter the concentrations in the direction of apparently better mixing than is actually present.

Fig. 3, *b* represents an experiment with the same factors as in Fig. 3, *a* with the exception of a much higher pressure of injection (sixty-eight pounds per square inch) through a catheter with a smaller injection diameter (0.0044 cm.). Streaming persists, but there is some tendency toward turbulence and better mixing. This is further borne out by the lower graph in Fig. 5 in terms of dye concentrations. Streaming, as depicted by the shaded area, is considerably less than with the low-pressure injection.

Reynold's number is a constant for liquids flowing through tubes of circular cross section. When the value for the constant is reached, normal streamline or laminar flow gives way to turbulent flow. The factors involved in this constant are depicted in Fig. 7. Reynold's number varies for blood flowing under different conditions due to the anomalous character of the suspension and variations in apparent viscosity. Since density is a factor in the numerator and viscosity in the denominator, it is obvious that turbulent flow is approximately two to five times more likely to occur with water than with blood flowing under the same conditions.

When injections of dye were made in a pulsatile stream of water, marked variations in concentration of the dye occurred in the long axis of the stream, as is represented photographically in Fig. 4. The pressures and velocities of the stream are comparable to those observed physiologically. Increasing the pressure of injection (Fig. 4, *b*) did not significantly improve the situation. The model obviously cannot be compared without reservation to the vascular system. It is inelastic except at the rubber diaphragm (Fig. 2) and the rubber tube used for pressure control (Fig. 1, *I*). In addition, a significant backflow component was present. Backflow components have been demonstrated in the arteries of both experimental animals and human beings.[11] As will be pointed out subsequently, however, we are inclined to doubt the importance of this axial variation in concentration as applied to regional heparinization.

The results of five animal experiments are diagrammatically demonstrated in Fig. 6. These experiments consisted of the simultaneous withdrawal of samples of blood from primary branches of the trifurcation of the aorta in dogs with continuous intra-aortic injection of Evans blue (0.18 per cent) or methylene blue (1.6 per cent). The site of injection was three to five inches above the trifurcation. Another sample was also drawn simultaneously either from a carotid artery (*C*) or external jugular (*J*) vein.

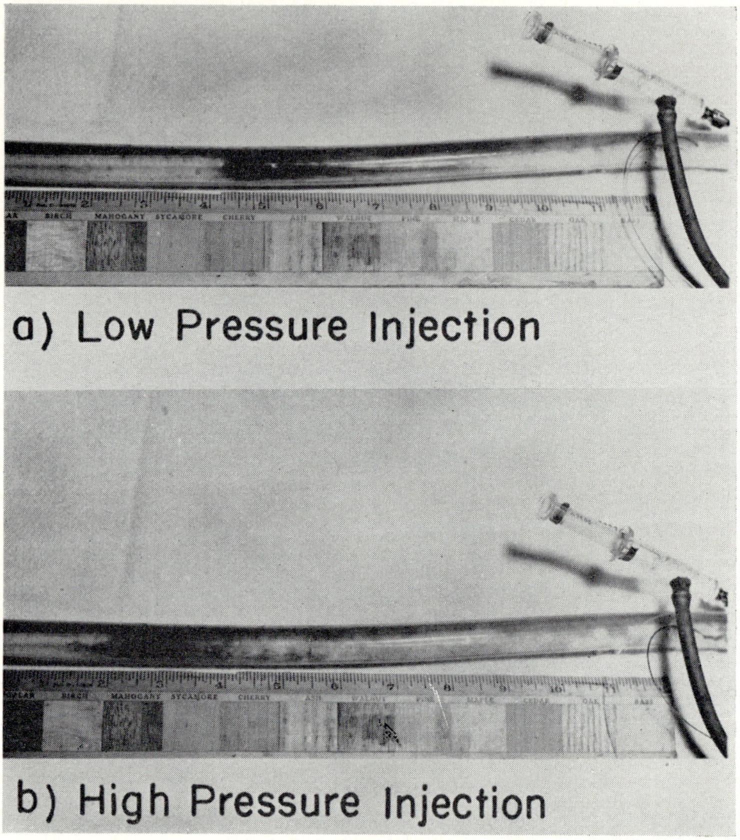

Fig. 4.—Pulsatile stream. *a*, Stream: pressure 120/80; pulse, 128; mean flow, 40 c.c. per second; mean velocity, 0.33 M. per second. Injection: pressure, twelve pounds per square inch; rate, approximately 2.5 c.c. per minute; orifice, 0.011 cm. internal diameter. *b*, Stream: same. Injection: pressure, seventy pounds per square inch; rate, approximately 2.5 c.c. per minute; orifice, 0.0044 cm. internal diameter.

The differences in concentration of dye, expressed as optical density, are apparent. They vary from no difference to a factor of 9.4 times for samples drawn below the site of injection. No vessel consistently contained the greatest concentration of dye. These findings can only be explained on the basis of streaming of the injected dye. The main stream of dye is entirely capricious in its choice of a branch of the trifurcation, and probably depends on such factors as the position of the injection catheter in the aorta. Similar findings have been recorded by Ralston and associates[8, 9] using India ink. These workers removed blood samples from a mesenteric artery, a renal artery, and the aorta below the renal arteries with injection of the ink into the thoracic aorta or the left ventricle. Their injections were made through No. 27 gauge needles. In addition, using brightly illuminated glass tubes, they directly observed streamlined filaments of India ink as far distal as the lower abdominal aorta and the femoral arteries. They made no mention of variations in axial concentration of the India ink. They did, however, observe distinct backflow components to the pulse cycle. Model experiments using water flowing through glass tubes and India ink were also recorded.

A.

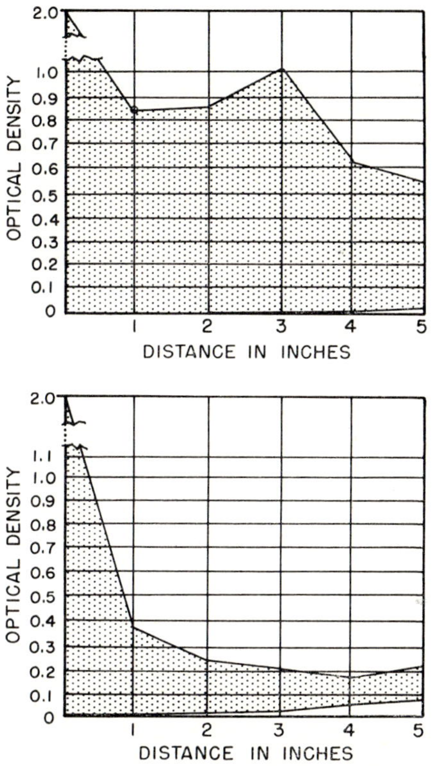

B.

Fig. 5.—Comparison of optical densities of samples drawn centrally (upper line) and peripherally (lower line) at varying distances from site of injection of 1.6 per cent methylene blue (optical density, 2.0). The stream is nonpulsatile. Graph *A* corresponds with Fig. 3, *a* and Graph *B* with Fig. 3, *b*. Each point on the graph represents an average of six determinations.

The differences in concentration of dye in samples drawn from below the site of injection and from the general circulation were greater with methylene blue than with Evans blue. This is due to the rapidity with which the former leaves the blood stream. The differential of 0.9 for a sample from the left femoral artery as compared to one from the external jugular vein in the Evans blue series can only be explained on the basis of some discrepancy in timing.

DISCUSSION

Regional heparinization is a term coined by Murray in 1937[1] to describe the production of a local heparin effect without systemic prolongation of coagulation time. Its achievement would appear to be dependent on two factors: first, the administration of heparin at such a rate that it does not produce a cumulative systemic effect; second, adequate mixing.

Previous investigations have demonstrated that it is possible to achieve the first of these objectives provided the rate of injection is rigidly controlled.[1-5] The experiments reported in this communication have demonstrated the difficulty in achieving the second, that of adequate local mixing.

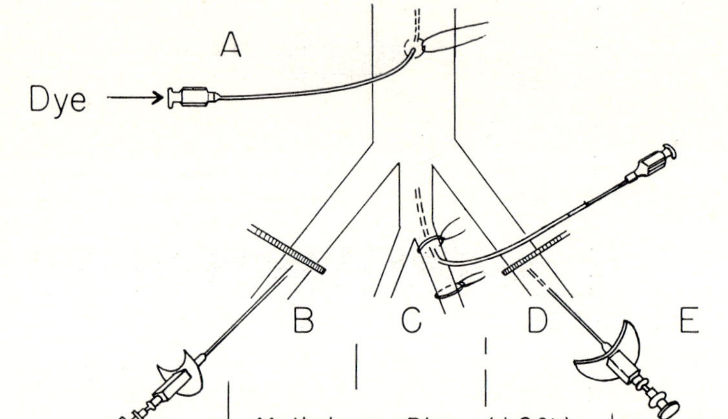

	B	C	D	E
	Methylene Blue (1.6%)			
Max. Dif. x 5.2	0.220		1.152	Systemic
Min. Dif. x 1.05	1.000	0.950		
Max. Dif. x 37.5			1.500	0.040 (J)
Min. Dif. x 5.5			0.220	0.040 (J)
	Evans Blue (0.18%)			
Max. Dif. x 9.4		0.770	0.082	
Min. Dif. x 1.0	0.125		0.125	
Max. Dif. x 7.3			0.320	0.044 (C)
Min. Dif. x 0.9			0.228	0.25 (J)

Fig. 6.—Diagram of animal experiments. At the left are maximum and minimum differentials in dye concentrations of simultaneously drawn samples from right and left common femoral (*B* and *D*), common hypogastric (*C*), general circulation ([*E*], external jugular [*J*], carotid [*C*]). There is continuous injection of dye at *A* at twelve pounds per square inch, approximately 2.5 c.c. per minute, at distances of three to five inches from trifurcation. Internal diameter of injection catheter is 0.011 cm. The figures represent optical densities.

Dye was injected into both pulsatile and nonpulsatile streams of water flowing through clear plastic tubing. Streaming of the injected dye was noted. Mixing was incomplete at considerable distances from the sites of injection. This is illustrated photographically in Fig. 3 and in terms of dye concentrations in Fig. 5. Streaming persisted even though high injection pressures (up to seventy pounds per square inch) were utilized.

In addition, a marked variation in the axial concentration of injected dye was observed in pulsatile streams. The backflow component to the pulse cycle in these model experiments was rather marked. Although backflow components to the pulse cycle in the arteries of both experimental animals and the human being have been demonstrated,[11] we are inclined to question the importance of this axial variation in concentration under more physiologic conditions. It was not recorded by Ralston and co-workers[8, 9] in experiments on cats and dogs in which the streaming of injected India ink was directly observed by the use of brightly illuminated glass tubes.

Five experiments were performed on mongrel dogs. Blood samples were withdrawn simultaneously from the right and left femoral arteries and a branch of the common hypogastric artery with continuous intra-aortic injection of either methylene blue or Evans blue at distances of three to five inches above the trifurcation. Marked variations in the concentration of dye in these simultaneously drawn samples were observed which can only be explained on the basis of streaming (Fig. 6).

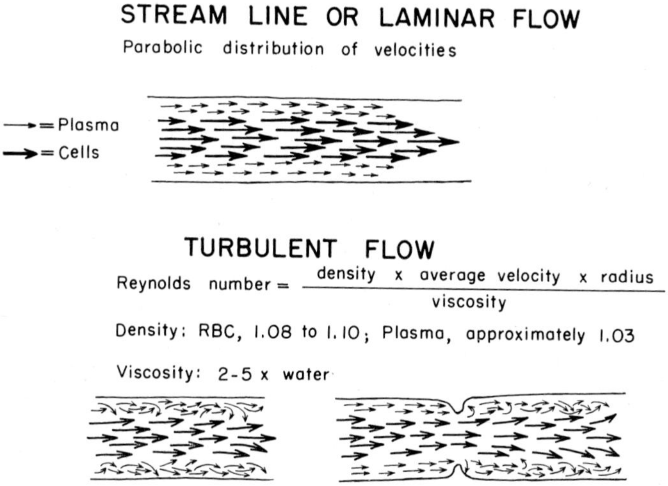

Fig. 7.—Diagrammatic representation of some of the characteristics of the flow of blood. The upper figure depicts normal flow with an axial concentration of cells. The velocity is greatest in the center of the stream and decreases toward the periphery. The lower figures illustrate the tendency for turbulence to occur primarily at the periphery of the stream. The appearance of turbulent flow is dependent upon the factors represented by Reynold's number.

The flow of blood is normally streamline or laminar, as depicted in Fig. 7. Turbulence rarely occurs. Its appearance is dependent on a constant, Reynold's number. This constant varies for blood flowing under different conditions since blood is an "anomalous" suspension.[6] The important consideration to the problem at hand is that, as indicated in Fig. 7, turbulence when it does occur is present primarily only in the peripheral plasma sleeve.[7]

Ralston and co-workers,[8, 9] in studies on the streamline flow of blood in the dog and cat, have demonstrated the lack of mixing of India ink injected into the aortas of these animals. Hahn and associates[10] have detected a lack of mixing of various components of the portal circulation in the dog by the determination of tagged phosphoric acid in the liver after injection into either a mesenteric vein or the splenic vein. Bayliss[6] in referring to studies of this type has stated that ". . . turbulence would, in any case, occur only in the thin peripheral zone of plasma, so that in no circumstance would one expect the injected dye to mix completely with the blood."

These considerations, as applied to regional heparinization, lead to the conclusion that in order to achieve a uniform local effect, completely turbulent flow must be produced. Otherwise, prolongation of the coagulation time of much of the blood in contact with the damaged area will be dependent upon recirculating heparin. Greater pressures than were utilized in these experiments, administered through catheters with smaller lumina, could theoretically produce the desired results. The determination of the practicality of such measures awaits further investigation.

SUMMARY

Streaming of dye injected into streams of water flowing under conditions simulating those observed physiologically has been demonstrated photographically and in terms of dye concentrations. This streaming effect was not overcome by injection pressures of seventy pounds per square inch. The streaming of dye injected into the aorta of the dog has also been demonstrated indirectly by variations in concentration of injected dye in simultaneously withdrawn samples from branches of the trifurcation. The application of these findings to regional heparinization is discussed.

REFERENCES

1. Murray, G. W., Jacques, L. B., Perrett, T. S., and Best, C. H.: Heparin and the Thrombosis of Veins Following Injury, SURGERY **2:** 163-187, 1937.
2. Wylie, E. J., Gardner, R. E., Johansen, R., and McCorkle, H. J.: An Experimental Study of Regional Heparinization, SURGERY **28:** 29-36 (July) 1950.
3. Freeman, N. E., Wylie, E. J., and Gilfillan, R. S.: Regional Heparinization in Vascular Surgery, Surg., Gynec. & Obst. **90:** 406-412, 1950.
4. Freeman, N. E., and Gilfillan, R. S.: Regional Heparinization After Thromboendarterectomy in the Treatment of Obliterative Arterial Disease, SURGERY **31:** 115-131 (Jan.) 1952.
5. Blakemore, A. H., and Fitzpatrick, H. F.: The Surgical Management of the Post-Splenectomy Bleeder With Extra-Hepatic Portal Hypertension, Ann. Surg. **134:** 420-432 (Sept.) 1951.
6. Bayliss, L. E.: Rheology of Blood and Lymph, Chap. VI in Frey-Wyslling, A.: Deformation and Flow in Biological Systems, Amsterdam, 1952, North Holland Publishing Company.
7. Coulter, N. A., and Pappenheimer, J. R.: Development of Turbulence in Flowing Blood, Am. J. Physiol. **159:** 401, 1949.
8. Ralston, H. J., and Taylor, A. N.: Streamline Flow in the Arteries of the Dog and Cat, Am. J. Physiol. **144:** 706, 1945.
9. Ralston, H. J., Taylor, A. N., and Elliott, H. W.: Further Studies on Streamline Blood Flow in the Arteries of the Cat, Am. J. Physiol. **150:** 52, 1947.
10. Hahn, P. F., Donald, W. D., and Grier, R. C., Jr.: The Physiological Bilaterality of the Portal Circulation, Am. J. Physiol. **143:** 105, 1945.
11. Shipley, R. E., Gregg, D. E., and Schroeder, E. F.: An Experimental Study of Flow Patterns in Various Peripheral Arteries, Am. J. Physiol. **138:** 718, 1942-43.
12. Best, C. H., and Taylor, N. B.: The Physiological Basis of Medical Practice, ed. 5, Baltimore, 1950, Williams & Wilkins Company, p. 178.

MAJOR VESSEL DAMAGE IN LUMBAR DISC OPERATION

BRIGADIER GENERAL SAM F. SEELEY, MEDICAL CORPS, UNITED STATES ARMY, LIEUTENANT COLONEL CARL W. HUGHES, MEDICAL CORPS, UNITED STATES ARMY, AND MAJOR EDWARD J. JAHNKE, JR., MEDICAL CORPS, UNITED STATES ARMY, WASHINGTON, D. C.

(From the Vascular Surgery Section, Walter Reed Army Hospital, Walter Reed Army Medical Center)

THE operative removal of herniated nucleus pulposus is an established procedure in selected cases. As is true following any major operation, a certain percentage of complications can be anticipated. One such complication, probably occurring more often than is recorded in the literature, is accidental injury of the common iliac artery. This might be anticipated, considering the relatively contiguous position of the anterior surface of the lumbar vertebrae, especially at the intervertebral space between the fourth and fifth lumbar vertebrae and between the fifth lumbar vertebra and the first sacral vertebra, and the vessels surrounding the aortic bifurcation. Another anatomic relationship of significance is the relative stability of the great vessels in the retroperitoneal space. This prevents their displacement, without potential injury, by instruments passing through the intervertebral space.

Simple awareness of this potential danger is not sufficient. Holscher[4] reported perforation of the common iliac artery and vein while cognizant of the possibility and making a determined effort to avoid it. He cited four other such cases with vascular damage, the outcome, in the majority, being fatal. We are aware of three unreported incidences of common iliac artery injury and one of inferior vena caval injury attending operation for herniated lumbar disc. Two such vascular complications have been treated by us within the last two years and are being reported. Our object is to present and discuss the interesting vascular problems created and to re-emphasize the ever-present danger of this complication.

CASE 1.—A young soldier was transferred to Walter Reed Army Hospital on Sept. 26, 1949, because of low back pain, the result of having jumped from a crane seven months previously. Five months following the initial injury, the pain recurred with radiation to the left leg. Examination was suggestive of a herniated nucleus pulposus at the level of the fourth and fifth lumbar vertebrae. This was confirmed by myelography. Operation for removal of the offending disc was performed. Postoperatively, the symptoms were not altered. Repeat myelography demonstrated persistence of the initial defect. Five months following the original procedure, the intervertebral spaces between the fourth and fifth lumbar vertebrae and between the fifth lumbar and first sacral vertebrae were re-explored under spinal anesthesia. During removal of a segment of disc material from the intervertebral space between the fourth and fifth lumbar vertebrae with an angled pituitary rongeur, a sudden gush of bright red blood obscured the operative field. Immediately the patient complained of nausea. The disc space was packed with gelatin sponge, and pressure was applied for

Received for publication, July 6, 1953.

several minutes. After release of the pressure, the wound was irrigated without evidence of further bleeding. The possibility of aortic or left common iliac artery damage was considered but believed improbable since bleeding was so readily controlled with Gelfoam. The blood pressure and pulse rate remained stable, and the patient's general condition appeared satisfactory. The fifth lumbar-first sacral intervertebral space was explored, and a necrotic disc was removed.

The operation was performed with the patient in the prone position, a supporting pillow under the abdomen. Following the procedure he was placed in the supine position. Apparently the abdominal compression caused by the pillow retarded hemorrhage, for he immediately complained of nausea associated with pain in the back and chest. Perspiration became profuse and there was a sudden drop in blood pressure to 60 mm. Hg systolic and 40 mm. Hg diastolic. At once the patient was taken to the operating room and ether anesthesia was administered. While the abdomen was being prepared and draped, intra-arterial transfusions of whole blood were given under pressure in both radial arteries. Through a left transverse skin incision, the abdominal muscles were opened in the direction of their fibers, and the left common iliac artery was approached retroperitoneally. A clot of 500 to 700 c.c. of blood was evacuated, exposing active bleeding from the artery. Hemorrhage was minimized by manual pressure on the aorta near the bifurcation. The intra-arterial transfusion through the radial arteries was discontinued and replaced by transfusion directly into the aorta above the area of digital compression. The iliac artery was isolated and the retrograde blood flow was controlled by umbilical tapes above and below the injured area. A 3 mm. longitudinal defect was identified on the posterolateral wall of the left common iliac artery approximately 2 cm. distal to the aortic bifurcation. The defect was repaired with interrupted everting mattress sutures of fine arterial silk. The blood pressure, unobtainable prior to intra-arterial transfusion, returned to normal. Following closure of the abdomen, good arterial pulsations were palpable at the left ankle.

Postoperatively, the arterial supply to both lower extremities were functionally adequate, but recovery of the patient was delayed by the development of acute hepatitis. At the time of discharge, the patient's only complaint was slight residual back pain.

CASE 2.—A 20-year-old airman gave a history of having been operated upon for symptoms of herniated nucleus pulposus at the fourth-fifth lumbar intervertebral space one month prior to admission. The operation was uneventful, with no evidence of vascular complication. Postoperatively, however, the patient complained of back pain, and vomited intermittently. This was followed by vascular collapse with a blood pressure of 84 mm. Hg systolic and 50 mm. Hg diastolic, pulse rate of 130 per minute, erythrocyte count of 3,000,000 cells per cubic millimeter, hematocrit of 33, and hemoglobin of 10 Gm. (Fig. 1). Vigorous blood replacement therapy was instituted. Signs of bleeding continued and, to localize the hemorrhage, a transverse exploratory incision was made in the right upper quadrant of the abdomen. A massive retroperitoneal hematoma was discovered. Without further ado, the wound was closed and supportive treatment continued. The general condition of the patient improved, but on the fifth postoperative day he complained of back pain with "spasm" in the lower abdomen and testes. Auscultation revealed a systolic bruit over the right common iliac artery, and a thrill was palpable. When the patient's condition stabilized, transfer to this hospital was initiated for management of the right common iliac aneurysm.

While on the ward, the patient refused to move, and remained in bed with the knees drawn up against the abdomen. He continually complained of severe pain in the lower abdomen radiating to the right flank.

On physical examination, a diffuse mass was palpable in the lower quadrants of the abdomen, but no pulsations were evident. On auscultation, however, a systolic bruit was heard. Operation was delayed one week while a homologous artery graft was being obtained. During this time, the patient developed intense pain in the back of the legs, hypesthesia, weakness, and some loss of deep tendon reflexes. Urinary incontinence also developed.

At operation, six weeks after the initial disc operation, exposure was obtained through a transverse transperitoneal lower abdominal incision (Figs. 2 and 3). An enormous false sac, containing at least 1,000 c.c. of blood, was encountered. After tedious dissection, during which the aorta and both iliac arteries were controlled with umbilical tapes, the defect

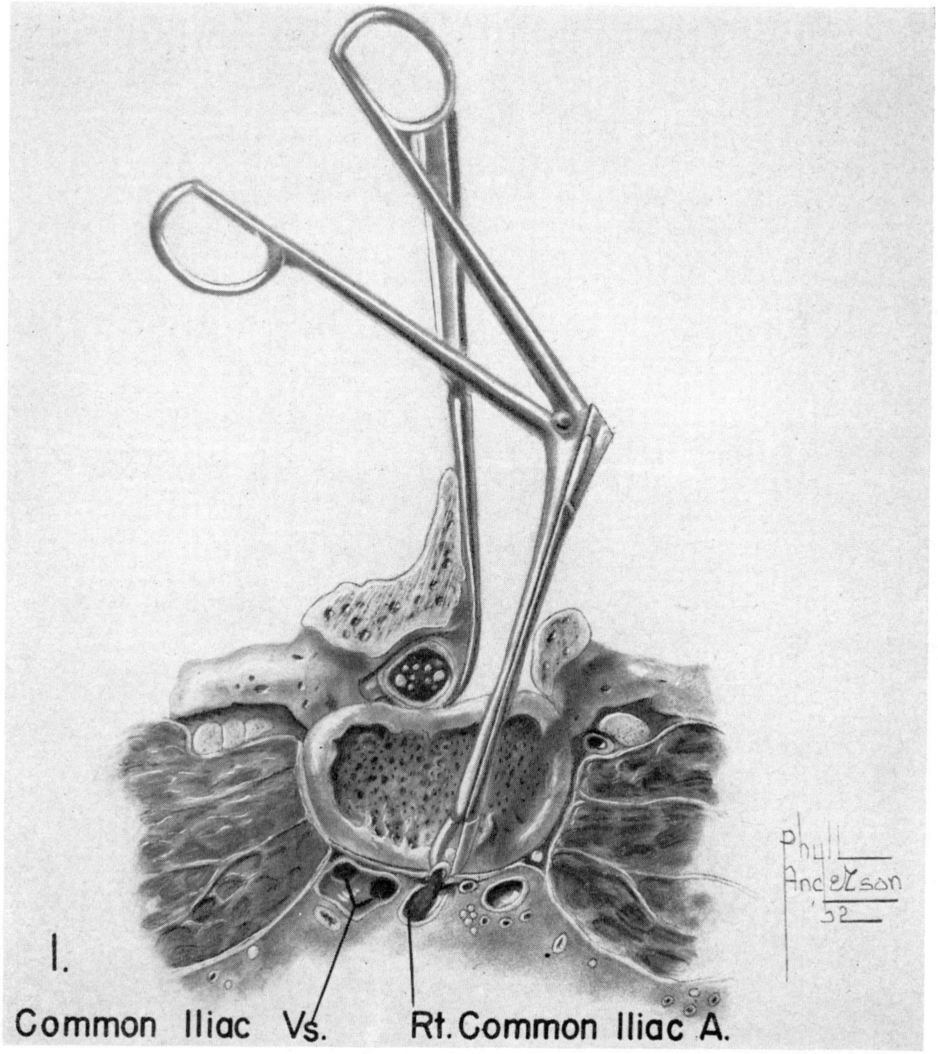

Fig. 1.—Diagrammatic representation of the manner in which the common iliac artery was injured while using an angled pituitary ronguer at the fourth-fifth lumbar intervertebral space.

in the right common iliac artery was isolated approximately 3 cm. from the aortic bifurcation. It was impossible to remove the false sac, which had enmeshed ureter, femoral nerve, and sympathetic chain bilaterally in addition to the hypogastric plexus. The wall of the sac was approximately 2.5 cm. thick and quite rigid, and did not collapse when the clotted contents were removed. Débridement of the involved vessel necessitated ligation of the internal iliac artery. This made the defect too extensive to permit direct end-to-end suture anastomosis (Figs. 4, 5, and 6). Therefore, arterial continuity between the common and external iliac artery was restored by insertion of a 2 cm. homologous arterial graft preserved in Hank's modificant of Tyrode's solution.[2] The medial and lateral surfaces of the graft were covered by the wall of the sac, and the anterior surface by the intestines and mesentery. Posteriorly it was impossible to cover the graft, since it stretched above the cavity of the aneurysmal sac. Prior to abdominal closure, a rubber tissue drain was placed in the remnants of the sac and brought out through the lateral part of the incision.

Postoperatively, the right femoral arterial pulse was stronger than the left. The severe pain which the patient had experienced completely disappeared, and urinary continence returned. His course was uneventful until the fifteenth postoperative day. While he was sitting in bed, approximately 200 c.c. of old and new blood exuded from the apparently healed drain site. The drainage tract was explored in the operating room, and a loculated pocket was identified in the abdominal wall. This suggested that the bloody drainage had accumulated there from a small uncontrolled bleeder. The graft site was approached and found covered with dense adhesions from the bowel, mesentery, and wall of the unremoved sac. These adhesions were not disturbed since there was no evidence of bleeding in that area.

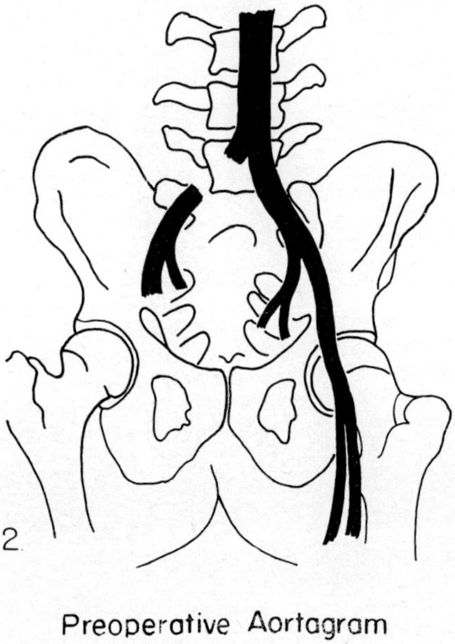

Fig. 2.—Line drawing of the aortagram obtained in Case 2 prior to vascular repair. The defects in the artery on the right caused by pressure of the false aneurysmal sac.

The patient became ambulatory, and recovery progressed until the thirtieth postoperative day, when he again began to complain of leg and back pain. The blood pressure, pulse, and hemogram revealed no evidence of hemorrhage, but were checked frequently. The pain gradually became more intense, and laboratory studies revealed a slow progressive blood loss. This deficit was meticulously replaced by whole blood in the hope that bleeding was confined to the old sac and might be self-contained. However, pain became more intense and blood loss more evident, and a progressively enlarging mass was palpable at the site of the previous aneurysm. Again, in the right leg the tendon reflexes were depressed and femoral hypesthesia developed. When the healed transverse abdominal incision was opened under general anesthesia, the extensiveness of the hemorrhage was immediately apparent.

Digital pressure from within the aneurysmal sac, deep to the common iliac artery, was necessary to occlude the bleeding site. The aorta was manually compressed just above its bifurcation as additional control. When all blood had been aspirated from the wound and the false sac, it was noted that the retroperitoneal dissection by the recurrent hemorrhage was more extensive than that caused by the initial aneurysm. Further attempts at arterial repair were believed inadvisable. Before digital control of the common iliac artery and aorta was released, the artery and vein were ligated proximally and distally to the bleeding point. The graft was not dissected to determine the exact area from which the hemorrhage occurred because of the poor condition of the patient and the dense adhesions encountered. It was believed, however, that the breakdown occurred in the posterior uncovered surface of the homologous arterial graft.

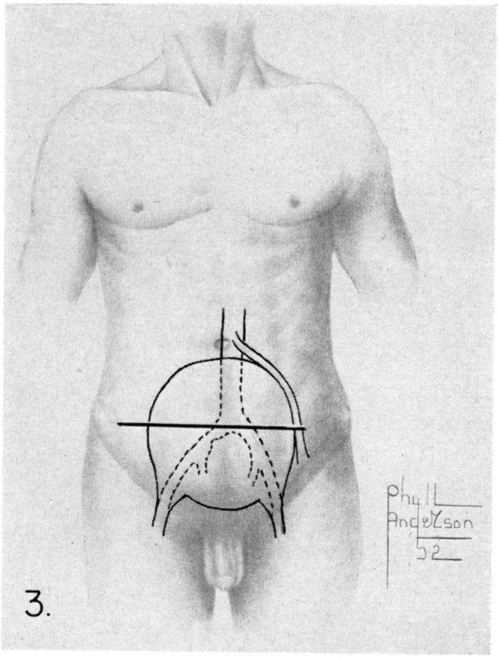

Fig. 3.—Sketch of the estimated size of the aneurysm filling the lower abdomen and the transverse incision employed to expose the sac and the vessels seen in dotted lines.

Postoperatively, careful observations were made frequently for evidence of loss of viability of the right lower extremity. Such was not the case and, on the contrary, the blood flow steadily improved. The right femoral nerve, which sustained stretch injury secondary to the expanding aneurysmal sac, slowly improved, as evidenced by return of sensation and motor function. The only remaining symptom was intermittent recurrent back pain, probably a residual of the initial pathologic process and its operative correction.

DISCUSSION

Although accurate data are available on only three patients sustaining major vascular damage as a result of lumbar disc operation, several important observations can be made. The validity of these observations is enhanced in view of the known relational anatomy of the lumbar vertebrae, terminal aorta, inferior vena cava, and iliac vessels.

In the majority of adults, the bifurcation of the aorta is located anterior to the body of the fourth lumbar vertebra or occasionally at the level of the fourth-fifth lumbar fibrocartilage. It usually lies approximately 2 cm. to the left of the midline. The inferior vena caval relations are similar except that its bifurcation is slightly lower than that of the aorta and to the right of the midline.

The common iliac arteries are approximately 5 cm. in length. On the right, the iliac artery diverges from the aorta at a slightly more acute angle

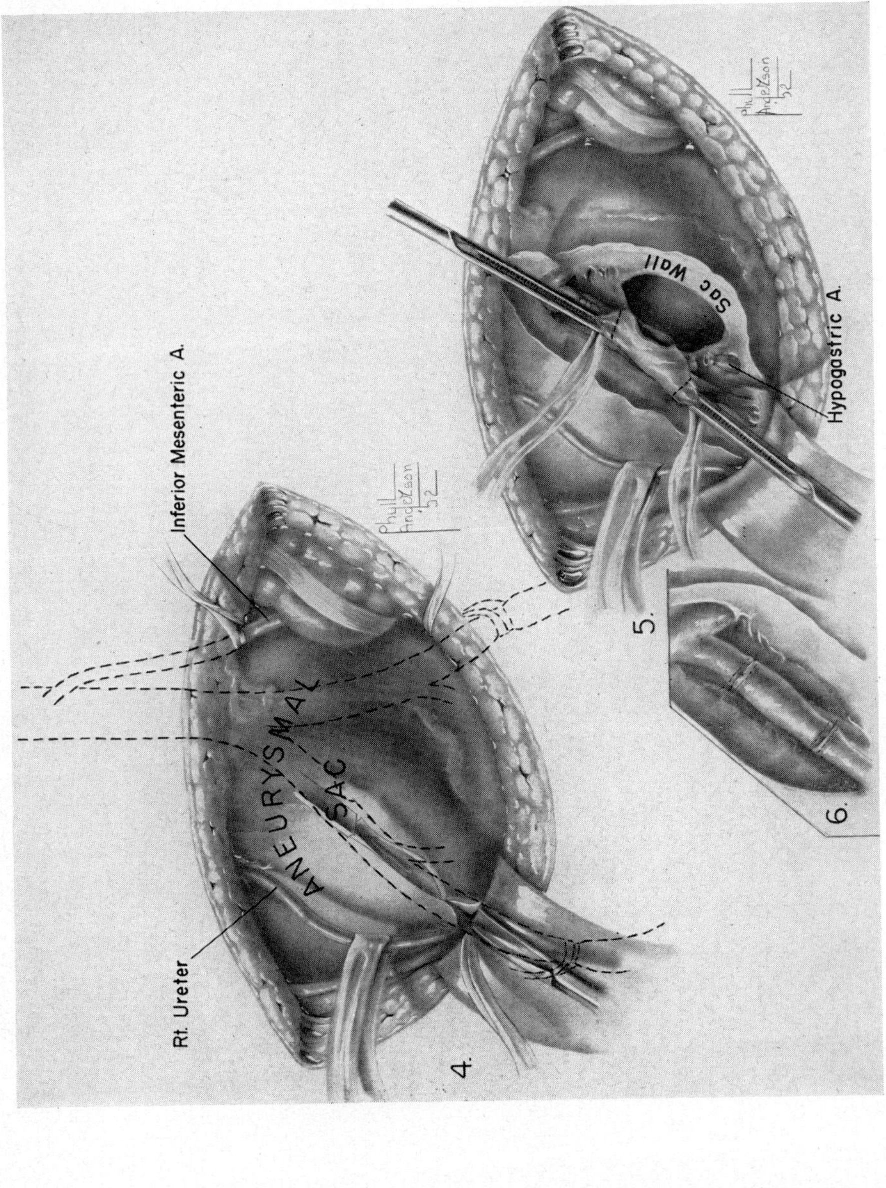

Figs. 4, 5, and 6.—*4*, The aneurysm as it appeared with the abdomen open. The right ureter was displaced laterally. Umbilical tape controls were placed on the iliac arteries bilaterally with manual occlusion of the proximal aorta. *5*, The opened sac with the defect in the posterior wall of the common iliac artery. The hypogastric artery was ligated and Potts coarctation clamps were applied to the artery for local vascular control. Note the thick wall of the sac which prevented its collapse after evacuation of the contents. *6*, The 2 cm. homologous arterial graft used to bridge the defect which was created.

than on the left, and also may be slightly longer. The junction of the external iliac and hypogastric arteries is usually at the level of, but just lateral to, the fifth lumbar-first sacral fibrocartilage. The relationships of the common iliac veins vary significantly. On the right, this vessal lies behind the artery and against the fourth and fifth lumbar vertebrae, its course being slightly oblique from right to left. The left common iliac vein lies medial to the proximal portions of the right and left iliac arteries and posteromedial to the distal portion of this artery on the left.[1, 3]

Correlating the relational anatomy with the level of intervertebral space exploration permits speculation as to the possibility and type of vascular complication which may ensue. Since the position of the major vascular channels is anterior to, or in close anterolateral apposition with, the fourth-fifth lumbar fibrocartilage, operation at this intervertebral space is unquestionably the more potentially dangerous. In contradistinction, the farther removed, lateral position of the iliac vessels in relation to the fifth lumbar-first sacral intervertebral space would make arterial injury at this level unlikely. These suppositions are substantiated, since the vascular complications in the three patients on whom detailed information is available occurred during operation at this fourth-fifth lumbar level.

It is possible to localize further the type of injury occurring at the fourth-fifth lumbar fibrocartilage. Since the right common iliac vein lies behind the artery and passes from right to left in its distal course, and since the left common iliac vein lies medial to the proximal portions of both right and left iliac arteries and posteromedial to the distal part of the artery on the left, several possibilities become apparent. (1) While operating on the extreme right lateral portion of the intervertebral space, vascular damage is probably limited to the terminal vena cava or iliac vein. (2) More medial to this, one can conceivably damage the right iliac artery and vein or damage the artery alone. (3) Removal of disc material in the midline is rarely followed by vascular damage. (4) Just to the left of the midline, the left iliac vein is most likely to be damaged. (5) Slightly more lateral to this, the damage can involve both artery and vein. (6) Finally, on the extreme left side of the fourth-fifth lumbar intervertebral space, only the iliac artery can be damaged.

These suppositions are borne out in clinical practice. An arteriovenous fistula of the right common iliac vessels developed in the case reported by Holscher. Our cases, described herein, differed in location and type of lesion. In the first case, the left common iliac artery was lacerated. In the second, an aneurysm developed on the right common iliac artery. Both were of special interest in that the lesions were within 2 to 3 cm. of the aortic bifurcation. All three lesions were produced by the use of pituitary rongeurs, which understandably would be more dangerous than the spoon curette, especially when visibility is poor. Holscher also cited four cases of vascular damage, with fatal outcome in the majority. Obviously these patients were not fortunate enough to develop a fistula or aneurysm.

It seems plausible that, in some unsuspected cases, damage may be confined to the major veins. This is probably seldom recognized as such, since it may be manifested only by excessive bleeding during the operation, which is adequately controlled by pressure or local hemostatic agents. Only those cases with obvious arterial bleeding under great pressure may be diagnosed. Even the gravity and significance in these instances may be masked, as in our first reported case.

Although recognition of vascular complications cannot be overemphasized, proper management is also of paramount importance. When such a lesion is suspected and confirmed by evidence of impending vascular collapse and continued retroperitoneal bleeding, immediate operation is indicated. The location of the damaged segment can usually be anticipated in the iliac artery several centimeters from the aortic bifurcation. Further isolation as to the involved side may be more difficult. Therefore, a low transverse transabdominal approach should be employed to secure adequate exposure. Restoration of blood volume can be rapidly performed by intra-arterial transfusion of whole blood directly into the aorta[5] (Case 1). Blood flow through the damaged segment of vessel can be prevented by controls with umbilical tape above and below the injured area. Every attempt should be made to restore the arterial continuity. Since the arterial tear is usually quite small, simple repair can be performed using either a continuous or interrupted everting mattress suture of 00000 arterial silk.

Immediate operation with vascular repair in Case 1 was not only lifesaving, but resulted in a functionally viable limb. Delayed operation in Case 2 resulted in prolonged hospitalization, repeated surgical procedures, and permanent nerve damage, the result of aneurysmal pressure.

SUMMARY

Reference to major arterial damage resulting from lumbar intervertebral disc operation is uncommon. Two such cases treated by us on the vascular surgery service are reported. In both, the common iliac artery was injured by capable and careful neurosurgeons fully aware of the possibility of such injury. The lesions were located within 2 to 3 cm. of the aortic bifurcation and followed exploration of the fourth-fifth lumbar intervertebral space. Both patients were salvaged by heroic surgery, but not without partial disability, one with residuals of hepatitis following multiple blood transfusions, and one with femoral nerve palsy and arterial insufficiency as a result of false aneurysmal formation and what was believed to be a breakdown in the homologous arterial graft.

The relational anatomy of the lumbar vertebrae and contiguous major vessels is described and correlated with the potential types of vascular complications. Operation at the fourth-fifth lumbar intervertebral space and use of the pituitary rongeur are emphasized as being most commonly associated with these lesions.

Immediate transabdominal exploration and arterial repair are recommended when this condition is confirmed or seriously suspected.

REFERENCES

1. Callender, C. L.: Surgical Anatomy, Philadelphia and London, 1941, W. B. Saunders Company.
2. Cooke, F. N., Hughes, C. W., Jahnke, E. J., Jr., and Seeley, S. F.: Homologous Arterial Grafts and Autogenous Vein Grafts Used to Bridge Large Arterial Defects in Man, SURGERY **33**: 183, 1953.
3. Gray, H.: Anatomy, Philadelphia and New York, 1913, Lea & Febiger.
4. Holscher, E. C.: Vascular Complications of Disc Surgery, J. Bone & Joint Surg. **30-A**: 968, 1948.
5. Seeley, S. F., and Nelson, R. M.: Intra-arterial Transfusion, Surg., Gynec. & Obst. **94**: 209, 1952.

A METHOD FOR EXPOSURE OF MIDLINE LESIONS OF THE BRAIN: CRANIOTOMY ON THE "DOWN SIDE"

CAPTAIN KEASLEY WELCH, MEDICAL CORPS, UNITED STATES ARMY RESERVE,*
SAN FRANCISCO, CALIF.

(From the Neurosurgical Service, Letterman Army Hospital)

IN ORDER to approach the medial aspect of the brain, a portion of the cerebral hemisphere must be retracted from the falx, or resected. More often than not, the cortex thus treated is innocent of any disease process. Simple elevation of the brain from the falx for a short time is harmless. However, the damage caused by retraction for more than a few minutes can ordinarily be seen before the operation is completed.

Several years ago, during the course of experiments involving the midline surface of the brain in monkeys, it was learned that wide exposure was available, without retraction, when the animal was positioned so that the exposed hemisphere was lowermost. When this was done, the hemisphere settled away from the midline under the influence of gravity.

More recently this technique has been applied in the treatment of four patients. Three of these harbored arteriovenous malformations at the midline, and the fourth, a colloid cyst of the third ventricle.

CASE REPORT

A young Negro woman of 22 years developed a common cold on Oct. 20, 1952. Four days later, while sneezing, she experienced a strange sensation in the head which she likened to a "pop." She immediately experienced severe, sharp pain between the eyes. Before eight hours had passed, the neck was stiff, and during the ensuing days headache persisted and there was anorexia and vomiting. On Oct. 27 she was admitted to Letterman Army Hospital.

Physical examination showed: temperature 100° F., pulse 90, blood pressure 125/80. The patient was in distress because of headache. The pharynx was injected. There was rigidity of the neck and limitation of straight leg raising to forty-five degrees. On the left, there was mild weakness of the hand and wrist and questionable weakness of dorsiflexion of the foot. The biceps, radial, and finger flexion reflexes were slightly less active on the left side than those on the right. The superficial abdominal reflexes were preserved, and there was no Babinski response.

The spinal fluid was pink and contained 19,000 red cells per cubic millimeter.

The symtoms subsided, and by Nov. 5, 1952, she felt completely well and was discharged from the hospital.

On Nov. 24 she was readmitted for study. The physical examination was normal. Right common carotid arteriography, Nov. 25, outlined an arteriovenous angioma at the midline in the frontal region (Fig. 1). Pneumoencephalogram Nov. 28 revealed a small filling defect in the right ventricular roof at the place where the angioma was known to exist.

Received for publication, July 13, 1953.
*Present address: University of Colorado, Department of Medicine, Denver, Colo.

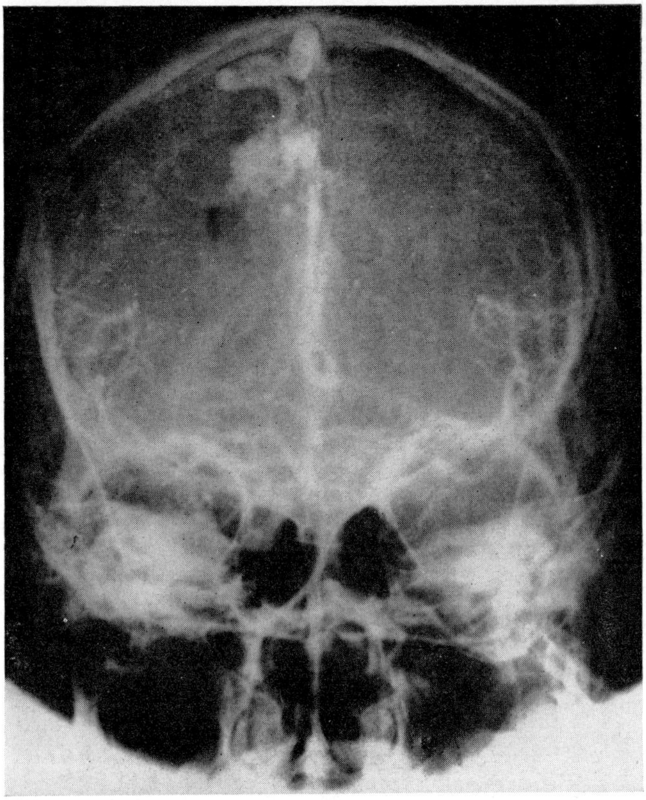

A.

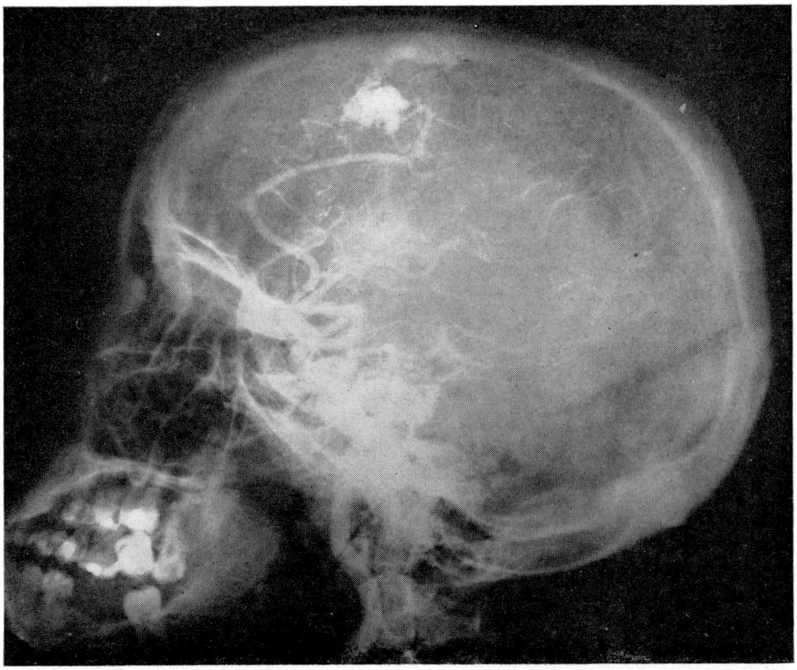

B.

Fig. 1.—Right common cartotid arteriogram. The left carotid was compressed during the injection for the anteroposterior film.

On Dec. 9, surgical excision of this lesion was carried out (Fig. 2). The patient was placed on the operating table in a semirecumbent position. The head was resting with the right side lowermost and with the vertex protruding well above the headrest. A craniotomy was made on the right or lowermost side, and the medial extent of the bony opening uncovered a portion of the sagittal sinus. Ninety cubic centimeters of spinal fluid was removed from the lumbar subarachnoid space while the dura was opened and hinged at the midline. Under the influence of gravity, the hemisphere settled nicely from the falx. A bridging vein from hemisphere to sinus required ligation. The large vein which drained the lesion came up onto the convexity of the brain and described a loop before joining the sinus. There was a small communication between the interhemispheral portion of this vein and the sinus, however, and this also required ligation. In dealing with this lesion, gentle retraction of the medial surface was required from time to time.

On the seventh day a subgaleal hematoma was evacuated. The recovery was smooth. At no time were there any unusual neurological signs postoperatively.

Because of the position, the opening and closure were made at a disadvantage, and required more time than usual.

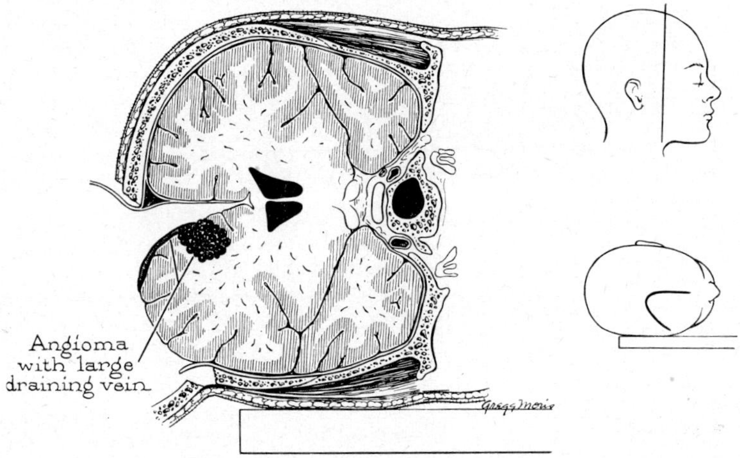

Fig. 2.—Diagrammatic representation of the exposure of the lesion at operation.

DISCUSSION

It does not appear to be of importance whether the craniotomy is actually made on the down side of the head or whether the head is later turned so that the opening is on the undermost side. There is inconvenience either way, and either way this inconvenience is compensated for at a more important stage of the operation.

Retraction of the medial surface is not entirely obviated even with this exposure. However, it is minimized, and need never be forceful. It is more of a molding of the shape of the lobe which is necessary, and the position of the spatula may be changed frequently without losing sight of the lesion.

The extent to which the hemisphere falls from the falx is determined by the size of the dural opening and the amount of displacement allowed by evacuation of spinal fluid or cyst contents. These factors must be governed carefully lest bridging veins, which are not meant to be interrupted, undergo excessive stretch.

SUMMARY

A method of surgical approach to midline supratentorial lesions is presented. This involves positioning of the patient so that the craniotomy is on the lowermost side. The hemisphere then settles away from the falx because of its own weight. Exposure is improved and retraction is minimized.

PREOPERATIVE PREPARATION OF THE BOWEL WITH NEOMYCIN

CAPTAIN JOHN H. DAVIS, MEDICAL CORPS, UNITED STATES ARMY, LIEUTENANT COLONEL LUDWIG R. KUHN, MEDICAL SERVICE CORPS, UNITED STATES ARMY, COLONEL JOSEPH R. SHAFFER, MEDICAL CORPS, UNITED STATES ARMY, AND COLONEL WILLIAM H. AMSPACHER, MEDICAL CORPS, UNITED STATES ARMY, FORT SAM HOUSTON, TEXAS

(From the Surgical Research Unit, Brooke Army Medical Center)

IN A letter to the editor published in the August, 1950, *Annals of Surgery,* Dr. John Lockwood[1] asked three fundamental questions concerning preparation of the bowel preoperatively. The three questions asked were: ''Is it worthwhile?" "Is it sound professional judgment?" "How is intestinal preparation best accomplished?'' There is little doubt that, since the introduction of sulfaguanidine by Poth in 1940, there has been a marked reduction in the morbidity and mortality rates after operations on the colon. The percentage of this reduction in the morbidity and mortality rates which can be attributed to bowel preparation with various antibiotics is very difficult to evaluate. Many other advances have been instituted in this same twelve-year period, such as the administration of large amounts of whole blood, more adequate parenteral therapy in preparing the patient who is debilitated, and an increased understanding of the pathologic physiology of distended bowel. It is certain that all of these measures have been important in the reduction of complications which occur after intestinal operations.

The first question, ''Is it worthwhile?'' can be adequately answered by examining the experimental work of Poth,[2] who has demonstrated in the laboratory these advantages to preoperative preparation of the bowel: (1) There is a 60 to 80 per cent reduction in the distance that edema extends along the bowel from the anastomotic line. (2) Prepared bowel shows clean edges which heal primarily. (3) There is an extensive fibroplasia which occurs to promote healing. (4) There is a marked ingrowth of capillaries at the anastomotic site in the prepared bowel.

To answer the second question, ''Is it reasonable to use intestinal antisepsis?'' we are forced to rely on logic. Certainly, some contamination of the peritoneal cavity can occur during intestinal operations, even under ideal circumstances. It would appear sensible, therefore, to limit contamination to a minimum by having the smallest number of organisms possible in the intestinal tract at the time of operation.

The answer to the third question, ''How is intestinal preparation best accomplished?'' has, as yet, probably not been found. The answer varies as new antibiotics and chemotherapeutic agents become available for clinical trial.

In order to determine the value of neomycin in bowel preparation, fifty patients were prepared for operation with the use of this antibiotic agent.

Received for publication, May 29, 1953.

Neomycin was isolated from *Streptomyces fradiae* in 1949 by Waksman and Lechevalier.[3] It is water-soluble and nontoxic when given orally, although it does cause liquid stools. It has a wide spectrum of bactericidal activity against gram-positive and gram-negative organisms, and it does not favor the development of resistance, as does the closely related antibiotic streptomycin. There is practically no absorption of this antibiotic through the gastrointestinal tract, and the 3 per cent which is absorbed is rapidly excreted by the kidneys.

MATERIALS AND METHODS

The following plan of study was adopted and used in all cases, the only variable being the dosage of neomycin that was given. In the first twenty-five cases, 1 Gm. of neomycin was given every four hours, starting twenty-four hours before operation. None of the patients received the drug postoperatively. Seventy-two hours before operation, a stool specimen was obtained, a warm saline enema was given, and the patient received one ounce of Fleet's phosphate of soda. From this time on, a liquid diet was given, since elimination of solid material in the intestine is one of the most important factors in proper preparation of the bowel. Forty-eight hours before surgical treatment, another stool specimen was obtained, and the same procedure with the enema was repeated. Twenty-four hours before operation, the dose of Fleet's phosphate of soda was repeated and, after this, the neomycin was given. A stool specimen was obtained approximately twelve hours after the first dose of neomycin. Another stool was obtained just before surgery was performed. Whenever possible, stool specimens were obtained for three days after the operation. In some cases, of course, a stool was not passed for two to three days after operation, and the first stool that was passed had to be used as a follow-up specimen.

In the second group of twenty-five cases, a single dose of 4 Gm. of neomycin was administered twenty-four hours before operation. Otherwise, the preparation was the same as outlined.

RESULTS

The effect on the fecal flora of mechanical cleansing of the bowel by means of saline catharsis and enemas together with a low-residue diet had been studied previously in this laboratory by Pulaski and Connell,[4] Baker and Pulaski.[5] They had shown that although some reduction in bacterial counts of some organisms may occur, the total bacterial count is not sufficiently suppressed by mechanical cleansing alone.

Six patients were studied as controls at this time. These patients received the standard preoperative routine except for the neomycin, which was omitted. The results, which showed no consistent diminution of the fecal flora, were as expected. The value of good mechanical cleansing lies in its removal of formed material, thus permitting the antibiotic to work. It has no bactericidal effect in itself.

The results in twenty-five cases of patients treated with neomycin 1 Gm. every four hours for twenty-four hours preoperatively are shown in Table I.

This regimen of drug administration had been established as the most satisfactory method by Poth in his work with neomycin. Tests showed complete disappearance of the coliform group of organisms twenty-four hours after the administration of the drug. Suppression of this group of organisms was affected for forty-eight to seventy-two hours after the last dose of neomycin. Both Pseudomonas and Proteus were markedly suppressed in most of the cases. There was one case, however, in which Pseudomonas was unaffected. The drug did not affect the yeast forms that were present before therapy, but there was no evidence of overgrowth of these organisms during the period of depression of the more common fecal flora. The hemolytic and nonhemolytic streptococci were effectively suppressed during the first forty-eight hours after therapy.

Poth[6] had originally shown a rather effective suppression of the fecal flora after a single 1 Gm. dose of neomycin, and it was decided to use a single 4 Gm. dose in an equal series of cases to test the effectiveness of single-dose therapy.

TABLE I. TWENTY-FIVE PATIENTS TREATED WITH NEOMYCIN, 1 GM. EVERY FOUR HOURS FOR TWENTY-FOUR HOURS PREOPERATIVELY

ORGANISM	PRE-DRUG	TWENTY-FOUR HOURS POSTDRUG: COMPLETE DISAPPEARANCE	MODERATE DISAPPEARANCE	UNAFFECTED	ORGANISMS PRESENT FORTY-EIGHT HOURS POSTOPERATIVELY	ORGANISMS PRESENT SEVENTY-TWO HOURS POSTOPERATIVELY
Micrococci including hemolytic Staphylococcus	23	18	5	0	0	0
Nonhemolytic Streptococcus	25	23	2	0	0	1
Hemolytic Streptococcus	18	18	0	0	0	0
Pseudomonas	10	8	1	1	1	1
Proteus	13	10	2	1	1	1
Coliforms	25	25	0	0	2	5
Yeasts	2	0	0	2	2	0

TABLE II. TWENTY-FIVE PATIENTS TREATED WITH NEOMYCIN, ONE 4 GM. DOSE PREOPERATIVELY*

ORGANISM	PRE-DRUG	18 TO 24 HOURS POSTDRUG: COMPLETE DISAPPEARANCE	MODERATE DISAPPEARANCE	UNAFFECTED	ORGANISMS PRESENT 24 TO 48 HOURS POSTDRUG
Aerobic					
Hemolytic staphylococci	9	8	1	0	0
Hemolytic streptococci	3	3	0	0	1
Other micrococci	13	10	3	0	0
Other streptococci	6	6	0	0	1
Gram-positive bacilli	18	17	0	1	0
Coliforms	25	22	3	0	0
Proteus	2	2	0	0	0
Pseudomonas	13	13	0	0	1
Yeast and fungi	13	3	7	3	3
Anaerobic					
Micrococci	7	7	0	0	1
Streptococcus	2	1	1	0	2
Gram-positive bacilli	13	9	3	1	2
Gram-negative bacilli	11	9	2	0	1

*Types of cases: normal volunteer subjects, 11; closure of colostomy, 8; colostomy, 4; resection of colon, 2.

It was deemed necessary to use 4 Gm. as a single dose in place of 1 Gm. in order to establish adequate stool levels of neomycin. The results in twenty-five cases in which one 4 Gm. dose of neomycin was given before operation are shown in Table II. As can be seen in this table, a more thorough differentiation was attempted in order to establish which organisms might be resistant to a single 4 Gm. dose of neomycin. Coliform organisms, present in all cases, were completely suppressed in twenty-two of the cases, but in 3 cases only a moderate suppression was shown on the single dose in the first twenty-four hours after administration of the drug. However, it can be seen that these organisms were further suppressed and had completely disappeared thirty-six to forty-eight

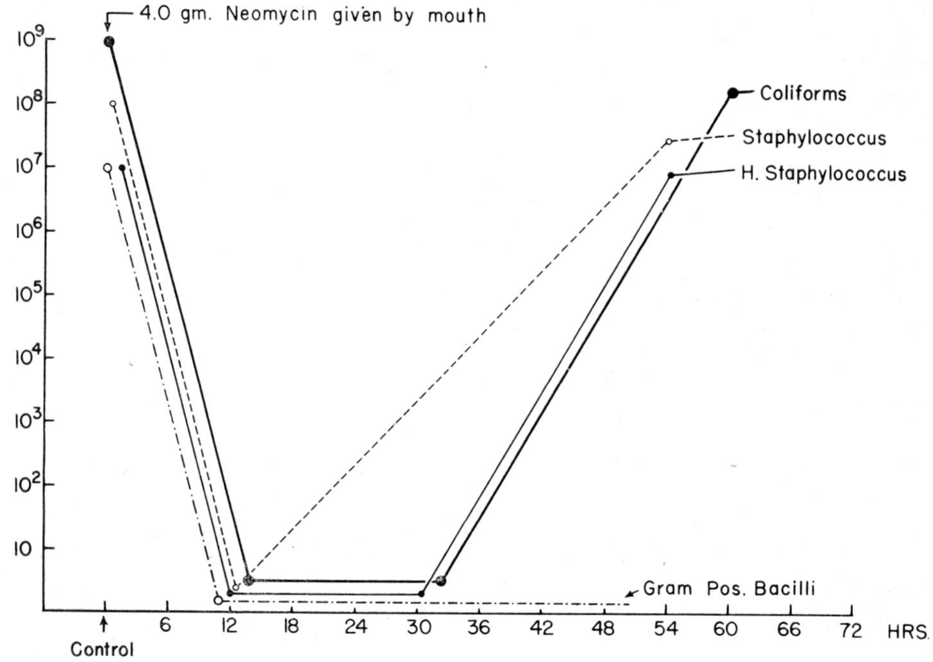

Fig. 1.—Case E. R. Suppression of fecal flora following single 4 Gm. dose of neomycin in a healthy adult.

hours after the drug was administered. Proteus and Pseudomonas, two organisms which are usually resistant to most intestinal antiseptics, were completely eliminated at the end of the twenty-four hour period by this single dose of neomycin. There was some suppression of the yeast and fungi in the fecal flora; however, except in three cases, they were not completely eliminated, but there was no overgrowth of these organisms while the bacteria of the intestinal flora was suppressed. There is no evidence in this series of twenty-five cases to indicate that more than a single dose of the antibiotic is necessary if the bowel has been adequately prepared before the administration of the drug. Baker and Pulaski, as well as Poth, have shown that any of the intestinal antiseptics are much more effective if the solid, formed material has been adequately removed from the colon by proper predrug cleansing of the intestinal tract with catharsis and enemas.

In Fig. 1, the data on E. R., a patient with a typical case of suppression of the fecal flora after a single 4 Gm. dose of neomycin in a normal healthy adult, are shown. Predrug preparation of the bowel was the same as that discussed earlier in the paper. It can be noted that after a single 4 Gm. dose of neomycin all organisms were suppressed by the end of the twelve-hour period. All but the staphylococci remained suppressed for twenty-four hours more, and then all returned toward normal in the next twenty-four to forty-eight hours.

DISCUSSION

Since the effectiveness of Sulfasuxidine and Sulfathalidine was first demonstrated by Poth in 1941, preoperative preparation of the bowel with an antibiotic or chemotherapeutic agent has become a routine preoperative preparatory measure. However, the use of sulfa drugs has several disadvantages. Perhaps the most important of these is the length of time required for adequate preparation, which is usually seven to nine days before operation. Since, in many instances, it means that the patient must be hospitalized during this period of time, the expense involved is a serious problem.

The sulfa drugs also tend to make the stool tenacious and ropy in character and, thus, it clings to the wall of the colon. This is a decided disadvantage, as one of the most important functions of the preparation routine is to remove from the colon all of the formed material in which the bacteria are residing.

The sulfa drugs are rather ineffectual against Proteus and Pseudomonas organisms and although these bacteria are not usually pathogenic in man, they can, under certain circumstances, become a serious problem in the operative treatment of the colon.

For these reasons, the search has continued for a more effective agent to suppress fecal flora. Nearly all of the antibiotics that have been developed in the last twelve years have been tried, but most of them show a specific action against several strains of bacteria without reduction of the total number of aerobes or anaerobes. Combinations of several of the antibiotics have been tried in an attempt to cover the spectrum of bacteria that is found in the colon, but none have proved much more effectual than the sulfa drugs.

Neomycin, a new antibiotic, has been studied in recent months as an intestinal antiseptic. It has been found to be very effective against nearly all of the fecal flora, and the development of resistant strains is most uncommon. Poth has reported the development of resistance of *Aerobacter aerogenes,* but the incidence of resistance is rather low. There is some indication that the drug is not effective against the Shigella organisms; however, these bacteria are not commonly found in the intestinal tract of most Americans. The use of neomycin has several advantages in that it causes the formation of a liquid or semiliquid stool, thus aiding in the elimination of solid material from the colon. In addition, it can be given in a single- or a multiple-dose regimen which requires only twenty-four hours after the administration of the last dose of the drug. It has a very low rate of absorption, less than 3 per cent being absorbed from the gastro-intestinal tract. The small amount absorbed is excreted in the urine and, as a result, toxicity is practically nonexistent when neomycin is given by the oral route. There is no evidence that the bleeding, clotting, and prothrombin times have been prolonged by the suppression of the intestinal bacteria with neomycin, even when therapy is extended over a period of weeks.

SUMMARY AND CONCLUSIONS

Fifty cases of preoperative preparation of the bowel with neomycin have been presented. (1) In twenty-five cases, 1 Gm. every four hours was given for twenty-four hours before operation. In an additional twenty-five cases, a single 4 Gm. dose of neomycin was given twenty-four hours before operation. (2) In all cases, the patients were prepared on a low-residue diet and saline catharsis for three days before surgery. During preoperative preparation, enemas were given in those cases when indicated. (3) Neomycin effectively suppressed all intestinal bacteria in this series without evidence of the development of resistant forms. (4) Overgrowth of yeast or fungi was not evident. (5) Toxicity from absorption of the drug did not occur. Neomycin appears to be the most effective antibiotic available for intestinal preparation, but it must stand the test of time as final proof of its effectiveness.

Acknowledgment.—We wish to acknowledge the technical assistance of Rudolph J. Massari and Anthony A. Contreras of the Bacteriology Section of the Surgical Research Unit.

We are indebted to Dr. Harold R. Reames, of The Upjohn Company, for the neomycin used in this investigation.

REFERENCES

1. Lockwood, J. S.: Letter to the Editor, Ann. Surg. **132**: 319-320 (Aug.) 1950.
2. Poth, E. J.: Sulfasuxidine and Sulfathalidine in Surgery of Colon, South. M. J. **40**: 369-375 (May) 1947.
3. Waksman, S. A., and Lechevalier, H. A.: Neomycin, a New Antibiotic Active Against Streptomycin-resistant Bacteria, Including Tuberculosis Organisms, Science **109**: 305-307 (March) 1949.
4. Pulaski, E. J., Connell, J. F., and Seeley, S. F.: Sterilization of Intestinal Tract by Antibiotics and Supplemental Agents, Ann. Surg. **132**: 225-234 (Aug.) 1950.
5. Baker, H. J., and Pulaski, E. J.: Effects of Terramycin on Fecal Flora, Ann. New York Acad. Sc. **53**: 324-331 (Sept.) 1950.
6. Poth, E. J., et. al.: A Critical Analysis of Neomycin as an Intestinal Antiseptic, Texas Rep. Biol. & Med. **9**: 631-644, 1951.

THE MIDLINE INCISION FOR SURGERY OF THE GALL BLADDER AND COMMON BILE DUCT

HORACE G. MOORE, JR., M.D.,* SEATTLE, WASH.

(From the Department of Surgery of the University of Washington School of Medicine and the King County Hospital)

THE upper midline incision has been used for gastric resection in the South Surgical Service of the King County Hospital, Seattle, for the past five years. Occasionally, cholecystectomy has been performed for coincidental disease of the gall bladder at the time of gastric resection. It was noted that exposure of the cystic duct, cystic artery, and common bile duct was excellent through the midline incision.

With this experience in mind, on April 30, 1952, a policy was deliberately instituted of using the upper midline incision for cholecystectomy and for exploration of the common bile duct. Usually the incision was started in the right xiphocostal angle and extended down to the level of the umbilicus. On occasion, either the umbilicus was excised or the incision was extended slightly below that structure when increased exposure seemed desirable. In most instances the peritoneum has been opened to the left of the round ligament, but in some cases the opening has been made to the right of this structure. No great difference in ease of exposure was noted between these two approaches. Since we began to use this incision, neither I nor the Chief of the Surgical Service (H. N. H.) has used any other type of incision for gall bladder or common duct surgery. We have been pleased with the exposure in all instances, regardless of the patient's degree of obesity or the size of the costal angle.

Between April 30, 1952, and Feb. 12, 1953, the midline incision was used on the South Surgical Service forty-eight times for cholecystectomy. In eighteen of these patients, an exploration of the common bile duct was carried out. In one of the forty-eight patients, repair of a hiatal hernia was performed in addition to the cholecystectomy. During this same period, five common bile duct explorations were performed through the midline incision in patients who had had previous cholecystectomy. In addition, three cholecystostomies were performed, using the midline incision for exploration.

Summers (1952) sent questionnaires to 1,000 diplomates of the American Board of Surgery to obtain information concerning types of preferred abdominal incisions. It is of interest that none of the surgeons who replied used the midline incision. Their preference of incisions for cholecystectomy in instances of chronic cholecystitis was as follows: (1) 34.8 per cent used Kocher's subcostal incision, (2) 34 per cent used a vertical right upper quadrant incision, (3) 18 per cent used a transverse right upper quadrant incision, and (4) 13.2 per cent used a right rectus incision when the subcostal angle is narrow,

Received for publication, July 13, 1953.

*Formerly instructor in surgery. Present address: Wilmington, N. C.

and a transverse or subcostal incision when the subcostal angle is wide. Approximately the same preference distribution obtained in cholecystectomy for acute cholecystitis.

Kocher (1895), after whom one of the oblique incisions was named, stated: "An anterior *mesial incision* gives access to the viscera of the abdomen with least injury." It is only fair to point out, however, that this advice pertained to abdominal surgery as a whole. For gall bladder surgery, Kocher specifically advised the oblique subcostal incision at that time.

The following advantages have been noted in using the midline incision for surgery of the biliary tract: (1) It is faster and easier to make and to close. (2) No muscles or nerves are incised or damaged. This is not true of the transverse, subcostal, or right rectus incision. In the case of the muscle-splitting right rectus incision, the medial portion of the rectus muscle is denervated, thus predisposing to incisional hernia. (3) Neuralgia of the intercostal nerves is avoided. Several patients with this symptom have been observed following transverse or subcostal incisions. (4) Exposure is usually as good or better than that from other types of incisions. In transverse or subcostal incisions retraction of the wound is limited somewhat by the immobility of the costal margin. The anatomic fact should be considered that the cystic duct, cystic vessels, and common bile duct are only 2 to 3 cm. to the right of the midline and are therefore readily accessible through a midline incision. It is doubtful that a right paramedian incision, which is only about 2 cm. from the midline incision, would give enough added exposure to justify the extra difficulty in its use.

Rienhoff (1945) stated: "In the upper abdomen the midline incision traverses the linea alba which is the most avascular portion of the abdominal wall. Obviously, there is no interference with the nerve supply to the rectus muscle or further weakening of that structure from direct trauma in splitting its fibers. The round, or falciform ligament of the liver lies immediately beneath the linea alba, but under the right lip of the incision, the reflection of the peritoneum to cover the ligament may be incised and the entire body, i.e., ligament, fat and peritoneum, reflected laterally. When the peritoneum is incised somewhat to the right of the reflection of the round ligament, it is not necessary to suture the edges of the former when closure of the abdomen is made. The round ligament falls into its normal position covering the posterior surface of the wound as a peritoneal flap, when the linea alba and thus the abdominal wall is closed."

Interrupted sutures of No. 30 stainless steel wire through the linea alba are routinely used for closure. As Rienhoff has suggested, the peritoneum is not closed separately. At the present time I do not know of any instance of incisional hernia in the patients in this series.

SUMMARY

Complete satisfaction has been experienced in the use of the upper midline incision for surgery of the biliary tree. Ease and speed of performance and excellent exposure are its main advantages. Others are urged to utilize this incision for cholecystectomy and for surgery of the common bile duct.

REFERENCES

1. Kocher, T.: Textbook of Operative Surgery, Translation From the Second German Edition by Harold J. Stiles, London, 1895, A. & C. Black, Ltd., p. 126.
2. Rienhoff, W. F., Jr.: An Analysis of the Results of the Surgical Treatment of 260 Consecutive Cases of Chronic Peptic Ulcer of the Duodenum, Ann. Surg. **121**: 583-599 (May) 1945.
3. Summers, J. E.: Abdominal Incisions: Present Status in the United States, Am. J. Surg. **84**: 177-181 (Aug.) 1952.

HYALURONIDASE AND EXPERIMENTAL EXOPHTHALMOS

K. Aterman, M.D., M.R.C.P., D.C.H., Birmingham, England

(From the Department of Anatomy, University of Birmingham)

IN A recent issue of the Journal, Nuzum[1] described the effects of the retrobulbar injection of hyaluronidase on the eyes of normal and of exophthalmic guinea pigs. He observed an immediate mechanical protrusion which, in the exophthalmic animals, was followed by a relative sinking-in of the eyeball. Enophthalmos could not be seen in a normal guinea pig after the injection of hyaluronidase. Some of his conclusions do not agree with those from similar experiments undertaken independently in this laboratory, and briefly reported here.

METHODS

Thirty-four normal, three intact, and three thyroidectomized exophthalmic male and female guinea pigs, ranging in weight from 180 to 450 grams, were lightly anesthetized with ether; retrobulbar injections of 0.1 to 0.8 ml. of physiologic saline solution only, or of hyaluronidase freshly dissolved in 0.1 to 0.15 ml. of saline solution, were then made. The other eye served either as the normal control or as an injection control by being treated either with fresh or with inactivated hyaluronidase solution or saline solution. In most animals the experiments were repeated after the lapse of several days, saline solution being injected into the eye which previously had been treated with hyaluronidase, and vice versa. The hyaluronidase used was either Diffusin (Ortho brand of hyaluronidase, 70 to 900 turbidity reducing units in 0.1 to 0.15 ml.; T.R.U.) or Hyalase (Benger, 330 to 3,000 Benger units in 0.1 to 0.15 ml.; B.U.).

RESULTS

1. The retrobulbar injection of small volumes of saline solution only (0.1 to 0.2 ml.) either had no effect or produced a varying degree of "ballooning" of the conjunctiva. Protrusion of the eyeball was either absent (Fig. 1) or very slight, but became progressively more pronounced if the volume of the injection was gradually increased (0.4 to 0.8 ml.). A characteristic feature of this mechanical protrusion was that it set in almost immediately, reaching its maximum at the end of the injection.

2. The retrobulbar injection of hyaluronidase (70 to 150 T.R.U., or 330 to 500 B.U.) in 0.1 to 0.15 ml. of saline solution produced definite ocular protrusion of varying degree, frequently, but not always, accompanied by a rapidly spreading ballooning of the conjunctival sac. The proptosed eyeball was then surrounded by a rim of prolapsed, edematous tissue which somewhat obscured, but could not obliterate, the appearance of ocular protrusion (Fig. 1). The impression was gained that the conjunctival edema was more marked in eyes

Received for publication, July 16, 1953.

treated with hyaluronidase than in the controls injected with saline solution only, but that the severity of the edema was not dependent on the degree of ocular protrusion. The nature of this edema is not clear. It pitted on pressure, but an incision of the conjunctival sac did not lead to its disappearance; only a small amount of seemingly viscous material escaped.

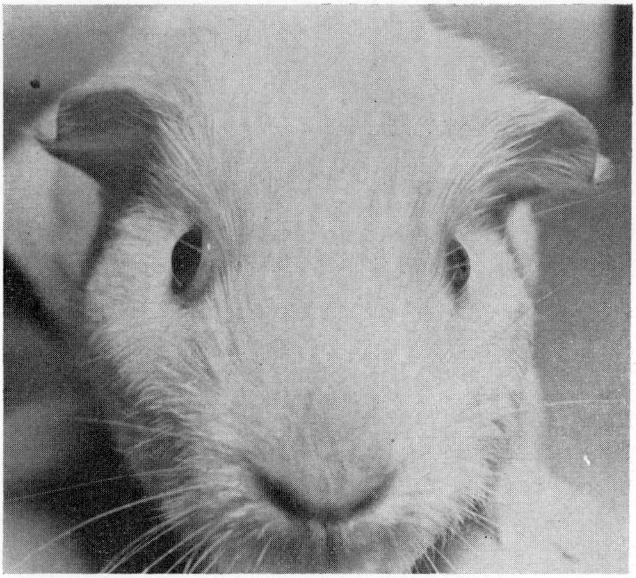

Fig. 1.—The effect of hyaluronidase on the retrobulbar tissues of the normal guinea pig. Five minutes after the injection of 500 Benger units of hyaluronidase in 0.1 ml. of saline solution, protrusion of the eyeball and conjunctival edema have developed in the right eye. A simultaneous control injection of 0.1 ml. of saline solution only, given into the left eye, had no obvious effect.

3. The course of the ocular protrusion produced by hyaluronidase was of interest. It could best be observed when the volume of the injection was kept small (0.1 to 0.15 ml.), since the mechanical protrusion caused by larger volumes tended to obscure the specific enzymic effect. Ocular protrusion could first be seen after a latent interval of four to five minutes after the injection; it rapidly reached its maximum and then slowly declined. Measurements of the intercorneal distance by a method to be described elsewhere[2] supported this observation (Fig. 2). On pressure against the proptosed eyeball, the resistance was felt to be much greater in the eye treated with hyaluronidase than in the control eye. A second injection of the same amount of hyaluronidase into the same eye after the intercorneal distance had returned to its preinjection value produced a similar, but this time much smaller, effect (Fig. 2). The ocular protrusion was frequently followed after a varying interval of time by a definite sinking-in of the eyeball. This enophthalmos persisted for some time, but was never permanent, since twenty-four to thirty-six hours later no obvious difference between the injected eye and its control could be seen. Of interest was the fact that on occasion the conjunctival edema was still present when enophthalmos had already become unmistakable.

4. The injection of larger amounts of hyaluronidase (600 to 900 T.R.U., or 3,000 B.U.) in 0.1 to 0.25 ml. of saline solution was not followed by obvious ocular protrusion, but produced a rapidly spreading conjunctival edema and, somewhat later, definite enophthalmos (Fig. 3). This sinking-in of the eyeball could be seen even when the volume of the injection was increased to 0.4 ml. Both signs disappeared slowly.

5. None of these effects was observed after the injection of hyaluronidase preparations which had been inactivated by heating.

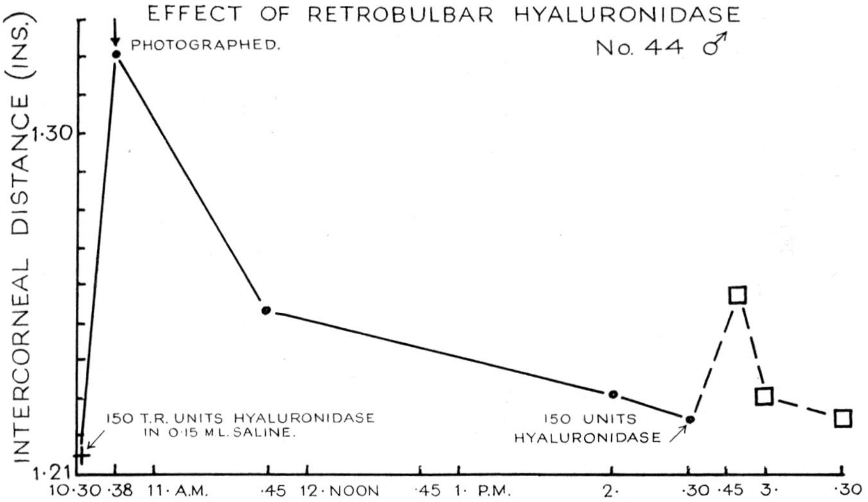

Fig. 2.—Measurements of the changes in the intercorneal distance after the retrobulbar injection of hyaluronidase in a normal guinea pig. The first injection of 150 T.R.U. in 0.1 ml. of saline solution produced a marked ocular protrusion which gradually subsided. A second injection of hyaluronidase into the same eye after the intercorneal distance had reached its preinjection level produced a similar, but less marked, effect.

6. Three intact and three thyroidectomized guinea pigs in which exophthalmos had been produced by treatment with thyrotropin and cortisone[2, 3] responded to the injection of hyaluronidase (70 to 150 T.R.U. in 0.15 ml. of saline solution) in the same manner as normal guinea pigs. A rapid, transient ocular protrusion was followed by a definite sinking-in of the eyeball which, because of the previously established endocrine exophthalmos, could be seen more easily than in the normal animal. Since a quantitative comparison has not been attempted, no statement can be made concerning possible differences in the speed or the degree of the reaction in exophthalmic animals as compared with normal animals.

7. A notable feature of these experiments was the marked individual variation in the response to hyaluronidase.

COMMENT

The protrusion of the eyeball after the injection of hyaluronidase was attributed by Nuzum[1] to a "mechanical proptosis due to the volume of fluid introduced into the retrobulbar space.'' The experiments presented here do not support this view, since the retrobulbar injection of small volumes of fluid produced proptosis only when they contained active hyaluronidase. The mechanical protrusion of the eyeball caused by the injection of larger volumes of saline solution could be distinguished from the proptosis due to hyaluronidase by the rapidity with which it reached its maximum at the end of the injection. In addition, the latent interval, which lapsed before the effects of hyaluronidase could be observed, was missing. That the protrusion after the injection of hyaluronidase was not caused by the bulk of the injection only is borne out by the experience of Kadin,[4] who noted little or no change in a case of endocrine exophthalmos immediately after hyaluronidase had been injected, but observed a definite increase in the degree of swelling and proptosis within twenty minutes, which became pronounced within one hour. The observations of Atkinson[5] and of Key and Key,[6] on the other hand, whom Nuzum[1] quoted as having noted a ''mechanical proptosis'' after the injection of hyaluronidase, have no bearing on the issue in question since these workers merely referred in their papers to ballooning of the tissues, but not to ocular protrusion.

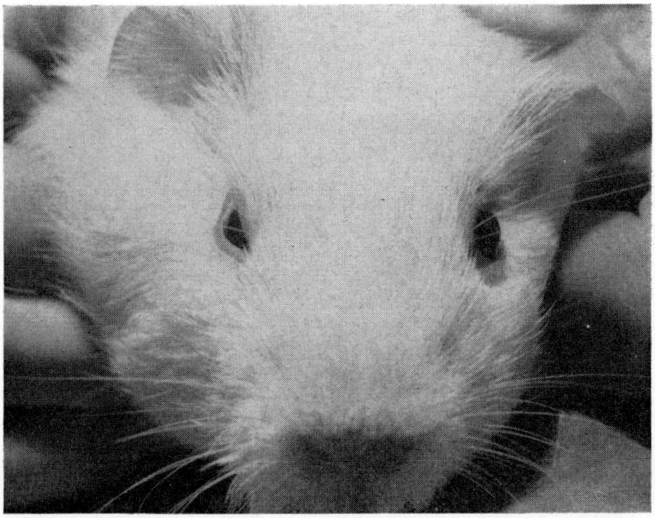

Fig. 3.—Enophthalmos in a normal guinea pig photographed about twenty minutes after the retrobulbar injection of 3,000 Benger units in 0.1 ml. of saline solution into the right eye.

The fact that Nuzum[1] did not observe in a normal animal the enophthalmos noted after the injection of hyaluronidase in guinea pigs treated with thyrotropin led him to postulate that the ''retrobulbar tissue of the normal animal is different from the thyrotropin-treated pigs with respect to its water content and water-binding properties.'' Although it is known from the work of Smelser,[7] and of Ludwig, Boas, and Soffer,[8] that there are differences in the composition, notably in the water content, of the retrobulbar tissues of normal and of exophthalmic guinea pigs, it is questionable whether such differences can be deduced from the response of these tissues to hyaluronidase, especially since in the experiments reported here a definite sinking-in of the eyeball could be seen in normal as well as in exophthalmic animals. It is, of course, possible that detailed measurements of the degree and of the speed with which changes in the position of the eyeball take place after the injection of hyaluronidase will confirm Nuzum's assumption.

The seemingly biphasic effect of hyaluronidase reported here is of interest. In view of the depolymerizing action of this enzyme, it is probable that the initial protrusion, followed by the sinking-in of the eyeball, merely represents different phases of the enzymatic degradation of hyaluronic acid, a component of the connective tissues, and/or similar mucopolysaccharides. The splitting up of the large molecules of hyaluronic acid into smaller units presumably leads to an increase in the content of water and, in view of the findings of Yielding and Rosano,[9] also of electrolytes in the retrobulbar tissues which would cause a swelling of these structures. In the closed space of the orbit, an increase in the volume of its contents would exert a pistonlike action on the eyeball, which therefore becomes more prominent. As the depolymerization of the hyaluronic acid molecule continues, however, the decreasing size of the particles, aided possibly by changes in the permeability of the capillaries, could lead to a diffusion of these particles into the blood stream and therefore to a decrease of the water-binding capacity of the retrobulbar connective tissues; this would then manifest itself as enophthalmos. The normal position of the eyeball would be restored by the resynthesis of highly polymerized polysaccharides after the injected enzyme had been inactivated.

These considerations imply that there is at present little to be gained by the use of hyaluronidase in the management of most cases of endocrine exophthalmos, since in an assessment of the benefit of the unfortunately transient sinking-in of the eyeball, the risk of the temporary increase of the ocular protrusion may have to be taken into account.

Attention should finally be drawn to an erroneous statement by Nuzum[1] which, if left uncorrected, may tend to confuse views on the nature of endocrine exophthalmos. Smelser[10, 11] has not "produced exophthalmos in guinea-pigs by removal of the left cervical ganglia," but has, on the contrary, demonstrated that hormonally induced exophthalmos "was not dependent on a nervous mechanism." His observations were confirmed by me in a guinea pig in which accidental damage to the cervical sympathetic in the course of thyroidectomy had produced unmistakable enophthalmos with narrowing of the palpebral fissure. Measurements of the intercorneal distance showed that the appropriate treatment with thyrotropin and cortisone nevertheless produced definite exophthalmos, which disappeared again when the endocrine treatment was discontinued.

SUMMARY

The retrobulbar injection of active preparations of hyaluronidase in small volumes of saline solution produces in normal and in exophthalmic guinea pigs a protrusion, followed by a sinking-in of the eyeball. The initial bulging of the eyeball is not caused by the volume of fluid introduced, but represents a specific enzymic effect. Changes in the position of the eyeball could be accounted for by changes in the degree of polymerization of hyaluronic acid, the degradation of which at first leads to an increase in the water content of the retrobulbar tissues, and therefore to exophthalmos. Enophthalmos would be the result of the continuation of this process, since the decreasing size of the particles would finally lead to their diffusion into the blood stream, and therefore to a decrease of the water-binding capacity of the orbital structures.

Thanks are due to the Ortho-Pharmaceutical Corporation and to Benger Laboratories Ltd. for the supply of their brands of hyaluronidase.

REFERENCES

1. Nuzum, J. W.: The Effect of Hyaluronidase on Experimental Exophthalmos, SURGERY **33**: 550, 1953.
2. Aterman, K.: Exophthalmos. In preparation.
3. Aterman, K.: Cortisone and Experimental Exophthalmos, Lancet **1**: 1143, 1952.
4. Kadin, M.: Hyaluronidase in Thyrotropic Exophthalmos, Am. J. Ophth. **33**: 962, 1950.
5. Atkinson, W. S.: Use of Hyaluronidase With Local Anaesthesia in Ophthalmology; Preliminary Report, Arch. Ophth. **42**: 628, 1949.
6. Key, S. N., Jr., and Key, S. N.: Use of Hyaluronidase in Ophthalmology, Texas State J. Med. **46**: 31, 1950.
7. Smelser, J. K.: Water and Fat Content of Orbital Tissues of Guinea-Pigs With Experimental Exophthalmos Produced by Extracts of the Anterior Pituitary Gland, Am. J. Physiol. **140**: 308, 1943.
8. Ludwig, A. W., Boas, N. F., and Soffer, L. J.: Rôle of Mucopolysaccharides in Pathogenesis of Experimental Exophthalmos, Proc. Soc. Exper. Biol. & Med. **73**: 137, 1950.
9. Yielding, K. L., and Rosano, C. L.: Effects of Hyaluronidase on Electrolytes (Sodium and Potassium) of Dog Synovial Fluid, Proc. Soc. Exper. Biol. & Med. **78**: 54, 1951.
10. Smelser, J. K.: Experimental Production of Exophthalmos Resembling That Found in Graves' Disease, Proc. Soc. Exper. Biol. & Med. **35**: 128, 1936.
11. Smelser, J. K.: Comparative Study of Experimental and Clinical Exophthalmos, Am. J. Ophth. **20**: 1189, 1937.

A NEW APPROACH TO THE TREATMENT OF ELECTROLYTE DISTURBANCES IN SHOCK AND SEVERE STRESS*

JØRGEN U. SCHLEGEL, M.D., ROCHESTER, N. Y.

(From the University of Rochester, School of Medicine and Dentistry, and the Department of Surgery, Buswell Urological Research Laboratory)

RETENTION of sodium as seen following burns, crush injuries, major operations, and so forth, even where shock is not manifest, is a serious complication in the treatment of these conditions. If sodium is retained, a concomitant amount of water is held back with it, and this makes treatment difficult, since overhydration with resulting edema is easily encountered.

According to the present-day handling of such conditions, the salt retention following shock and severe stress is accepted as an unavoidable complication beyond acute treatment.[1] Consequently, sodium and water are restricted to an absolute minimum. In cases where only small amounts of fluid are needed, complications are rare, but where large quantities of fluid have to be given, as in severe burns, hemorrhage, and so forth, the problem of fluid replacement therapy becomes complex, and overhydration is common.

For the purpose of clarifying the matter we are dealing with, a definition of what we mean by sodium retention may be justified. In this presentation we will consider two types of sodium retention: (1) physiologic and (2) pathologic.

Physiologic salt retention represents a condition of a limited maximum sodium reabsorption in the renal tubules, usually as a result of an acute loss of sodium. When the amount of sodium lost has been replaced, the retention ceases, and thus the process is limited. The validity of labeling such a condition physiologic salt retention may be questionable, since it is understood that sodium is not retained in excess of the amount originally present. However, on an hour-to-hour or day-to-day basis, sodium is retained in excess of the intake.

Whether loss of sodium is to the outside through the intestines, kidneys, or the skin, or to the inside to localized edema, as in burns or damaged cells, the end result is the same, a drop in available sodium. When the loss is to the outside, it is often accompanied by a concomitant loss of water, and therefore the serum sodium stays normal and a status of dehydration is evident. If water without salt is administered faster than the kidneys can excrete it, serum sodium will drop and a condition of water intoxication and oliguria will result. In certain conditions where a great number of cells are traumatized, as in burns, crush injuries, and so forth, serum sodium may drop as a result of a migration of sodium into the damaged cells in exchange for potassium. The depression of serum sodium in such conditions is thus not necessarily a result of water intoxication, although this naturally will aggravate it. Administration of sodium to

Received for publication, July 16, 1953.

*This investigation was supported with funds from the Dr. Henry C. Buswell Memorial and the Office of Naval Research.

a person who has been subjected to an acute sodium loss will usually result in a retention, since the excretion will be less than the intake.

A physiologic salt retention will then be the condition in which a sodium retention is seen until the original loss is made up for. A salt load in excess of the loss should result in a sodium excretion maintaining balance.

A pathologic salt retention is seen when administration of sodium will lead only to a positive balance, irrespective of the dosage, concentration, or route. This syndrome is always accompanied by a lack of ability to handle water and is therefore a feared complication in several types of shock where fluid replacement is needed.

A person who is on a low sodium intake will after a few days excrete practically no sodium in the urine. If such a person is subjected to a sodium load, he will be able to excrete sodium as well as would a person who has had a normal salt intake.

If, however, the restriction in salt intake lasts for more than a few days, even intravenous administration of hypertonic salt solutions will not increase the excretion of sodium in the urine.[2]

The reason for the lack of response to a salt load in a person who has had maximum salt retention for several days is not clear. It seems as if some adaptation has taken place, perhaps mediated through the adrenal cortex. In a normal person who has been on a salt-poor diet for several days, the serum sodium is usually normal, and therefore the retention of sodium does not seem to reflect any drop in serum sodium. It is also reported difficult to induce water diuresis in normal persons who have been on a low sodium intake for five days.[2]

Since the amount of sodium given apparently was in great excess of the total loss, we will define such a retention as pathologic. These experiments then seem to indicate that a physiologic salt retention can develop into a pathologic one if allowed to persist uncorrected for a number of days.

It seems quite important to determine whether the sodium retention seen following stress and shock is physiologic or pathologic in nature. If it is physiologic in nature, administration of sodium in proper amounts should lead to urinary excretion of sodium. Fluid replacement therapy should then be relatively simple, since water and salt retention would not have to be feared and overhydration would thus be difficult to achieve. If, however, the salt retention is of the pathologic type, no improvement in our present-day therapy can be accomplished before we learn how to reverse this process. It may well be that carbonic anhydrase inhibitors will prove of value in such conditions.

It has been shown by several investigators that all major surgery, as well as other types of stress, causes a drop in serum sodium and an increase in excretion of potassium.[3-8] The more extensive the surgery, the more pronounced is the fall in serum sodium.[5] This drop in serum sodium need not be caused by an actual loss of sodium from the organism but instead is usually caused by a shift in the normal distribution. Normally the cells contain a high concentration of potassium and a low concentration of sodium. In the plasma and extracellular space, the conditions are reversed. Following a condition of severe stress, more sodium goes into the cells at the expense of potassium, which would be excreted provided the kidneys were functioning. Damaged cells, and especially damaged muscle cells, take up large amounts of sodium,[3] which will further aggravate such a condition, resulting in an increasing hyponatremia. The urine from such patients contains practically no sodium.

The important question is whether the maximum sodium reabsorption in such cases reflects a physiologic or a pathologic sodium retention. If administration of sodium to such a patient results in a corresponding sodium excretion in the urine, it means that we are dealing with a physiologic salt retention, and consequently no water intoxication should result from a water load. The situation, however, is different from that seen in persons who have been deprived of salt for a short period. The patient who has been subjected to a severe stress has lost sodium into the intracellular space, and in order to evaluate whether or not he can handle sodium as a normal individual, it would first be necessary to restore the serum sodium to normal levels. The sodium which has gone into the cells must be considered temporarily lost for the extracellular fluid. Consequently, sodium must be administered to bring the serum sodium up to the level it was at prior to the stress. The amount of sodium needed for this should not be considered a pathologic retention, but rather a physiologic replacement. If the patient can then excrete salt following a salt load, it would probably be justifiable to consider the condition a physiologic salt retention.

Since an acute drop in serum sodium very often is accompanied by oliguria or even anuria,[4, 5, 9-14] restoration of serum sodium to normal levels can only be achieved by giving salt in excess of water.[5, 9, 15] The administration of water to a patient with hyponatremia and oliguria will only lower the serum sodium further and aggravate the condition. To give isotonic saline solution to such a patient does not serve the purpose of restoring serum sodium to normal levels, since it contains very little sodium in excess of the concentration in the serum. An example will easily illustrate this. If, for instance, the serum sodium is 120 meq. per liter and it is desired to increase it to 140 meq. per liter, it would be necessary to give at least 20 meq. of sodium times the volume of the extracellular space. (The actual amount of sodium to give in order to increase the serum sodium level should be calculated on the basis of total body water rather than extracellular volume.) For convenience, we can consider that to be 15 L., which means that we want to give a total of 300 meq. of sodium. One liter of normal saline solution contains 155 meq. of sodium. If the patient is excreting no water, it will mean that each time we give 1 L. of normal saline solution we give only 15 meq. of sodium in excess. Since the patient needs 300 meq. of sodium, he would, in other words, require 20 L. of normal saline solution to restore the serum sodium to normal. Only if the patient can excrete water without sodium almost as fast as it is given is it possible to increase serum sodium with intravenously administered isotonic saline solution. If oliguria is present, only edema will result. To restore the serum sodium to normal, it is necessary that the organism gain sodium in excess of water.

The procedure to find out if the sodium retention which is seen following severe stress and shock is pathologic or physiologic could be to give such a patient, relatively soon following the trauma, a hypertonic sodium solution intravenously in an amount which is sufficient to restore the serum sodium to normal levels. If the patient then excretes sodium in the urine in a normal fashion on an adequate sodium intake, his condition was that of a physiologic salt retention, which is no longer existing. If he does not respond to the sodium load, we must consider that his salt retention is pathologic and is still existing, and consequently fluid and salt have to be administered with great precaution in order to avoid water intoxication.

Since a physiologic salt retention can lead to a pathologic one, if it persists for a certain period of time, it is only logical that if serum sodium is not restored to normal levels, a pathologic salt retention will very likely develop. The so-called postoperative salt retention, which has led a considerable number of surgeons to abolish completely the use of salt solutions in the immediate postoperative period, may simply be the result of a physiologic salt retention, which eventually turns into a pathologic one if no attempts are made to restore the serum sodium to normal levels soon after the operation.

Several investigators have reported that administration of isotonic sodium chloride or hypotonic sodium chloride postoperatively would lead to retention of sodium as well as water.[4, 7, 12, 14] This will, as previously mentioned, not correct the lowered serum sodium and, therefore, does not reveal the nature of the sodium retention.

The immediate infusion of hypertonic saline solution in acute cases of hyponatremia will usually improve the diuresis greatly, and no salt retention will be seen.[3, 5, 9] Several authors have reported excellent results in the treatment of postoperative oliguria by the use of hypertonic saline solution.[5, 9, 15]

All these reports seem to indicate that the salt retention which is seen following severe stress and shock is of the physiologic type, and that the pathologic sodium retention need not develop if the serum sodium is restored within a matter of twelve to twenty-four hours.

The adrenals are greatly stimulated under periods of stress, and since it is known that some of the adrenal cortical hormones are powerful stimulators of renal reabsorption of sodium, it might be assumed that the salt retention seen following severe stress and shock can be a result of increased adrenal activity. We have, however, as will be shown later, reason to believe that pathologic salt retention need not develop even when pronounced increase in adrenal activity is seen. It is well worth remembering, in this connection, that even desoxycorticosterone, which under normal conditions will cause salt retention, will, if administered to a patient with Cushing's disease, lead to an increase in sodium excretion.

It is a serious difficulty, however, that the normal serum sodium is usually unknown, especially in cases of acute trauma. If we find a serum sodium of 135 meq. per liter, we consider that within the normal range. Had we determined the serum sodium prior to the trauma, we may find that it has dropped from 145 meq. per liter. If the extracellular space is 15 L., it means that the patient had lost 150 meq. of sodium. Determination of serum sodium is, in other words, not of great value, unless we know what it was immediately prior to the trauma. This makes it difficult to estimate the exact amount of hypertonic sodium solution which should be given. Administration of sodium chloride in great excess can probably be dangerous, since it may lead to a condition in which sodium is pushed into the cells.

It would thus seem to be better to follow the sodium excretion in the urine, since by this method administration of sodium could be guided by the ability of the kidneys to excrete it. This, however, meets with certain difficulties. In the first place, it would involve an elaborate setup for immediate and continued sodium determinations in the urine and, second, it could be misleading, since sodium can be excreted in the urine despite the presence of sodium retention. If the filtration is greatly increased and if the load to the tubules is in excess of the maximum reabsorption capacity, urinalysis for sodium will not reveal the true nature of the condition, which may be that of a pathologic salt retention with consequent formation of edema despite some sodium excretion in the urine.[16]

The proper procedure would be to carry out a complete balance study in order to evaluate the exact amount of sodium retained.[17] This, however, is much too complicated and time-consuming to apply in the average case.

A simple method, which requires practically no laboratory setup and which is apparently more valuable than sodium determinations in the urine or in the serum, has recently been developed by us.[18, 19] Acidification of the urine, according to Pitts,[20, 21] takes place by means of a hydrogen ion-exchange mechanism whereby sodium and/or potassium[22] is exchanged for hydrogen ion. The hydrogen ion is available through the activity of the enzyme carbonic anhydrase, which will lead to formation of carbonic acid from carbon dioxide and water. Inhibition of carbonic anhydrase will cause an increase in urinary pH as well as a great increase in excretion of sodium and potassium.[22] This increase, however, can be greatly in excess of that which could be accounted for in terms of arrested hydrogen ion exchange. Consequently, it must be assumed that carbonic anhydrase is responsible in some additional way for a much greater reabsorption of sodium than has hitherto been assumed.[30]

If this is true, it would follow that maximum activity in the tubular systems involving carbonic anhydrase should result in maximum reabsorption of sodium and maximum production of hydrogen ion, the latter probably being responsible for a fixation of urinary pH on the acid side.

In a recent study,[18] it has been shown by us that patients with a sodium or potassium excretion below approximately 45 microequivalents per minute have a fixed urinary pH, the actual pH differing from individual to individual between 4.5 and 6.0. It seems from these experiments that the fixation of the urinary pH on the acid side represents maximum effort in base reabsorption. In a patient on a normal diet, the reaction of the urine will change in a fairly regular pattern, with an alkaline tide in the morning and alkaline tides a couple of hours following each meal (Fig. 1, *A*).[23-28] If the urinary pH is low and fixed, this will represent physiologic sodium retention if administration of sodium chloride in excess of possible loss results in an increase in urinary pH as well as an increase in urinary excretion of sodium. If administration of salt to a patient with a fixed acid urine in excess of a possible loss does not

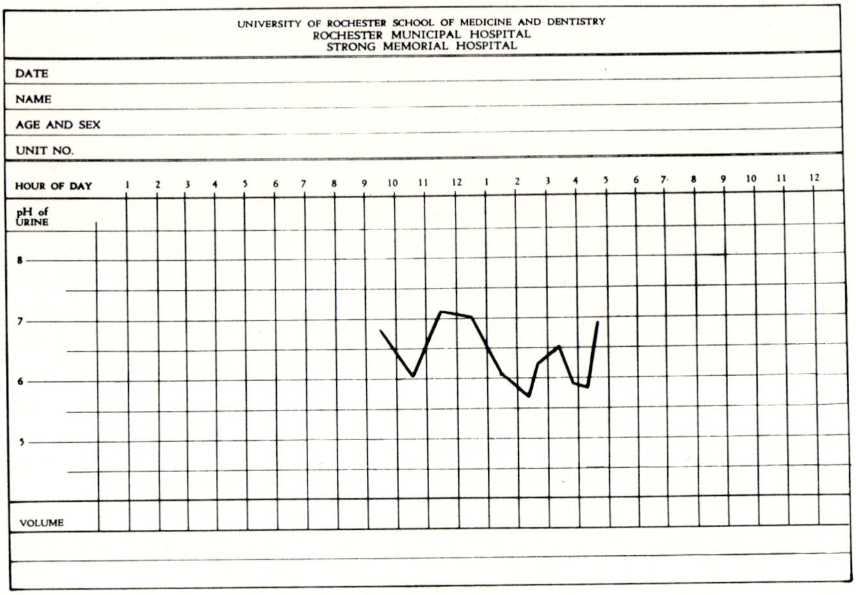

A.

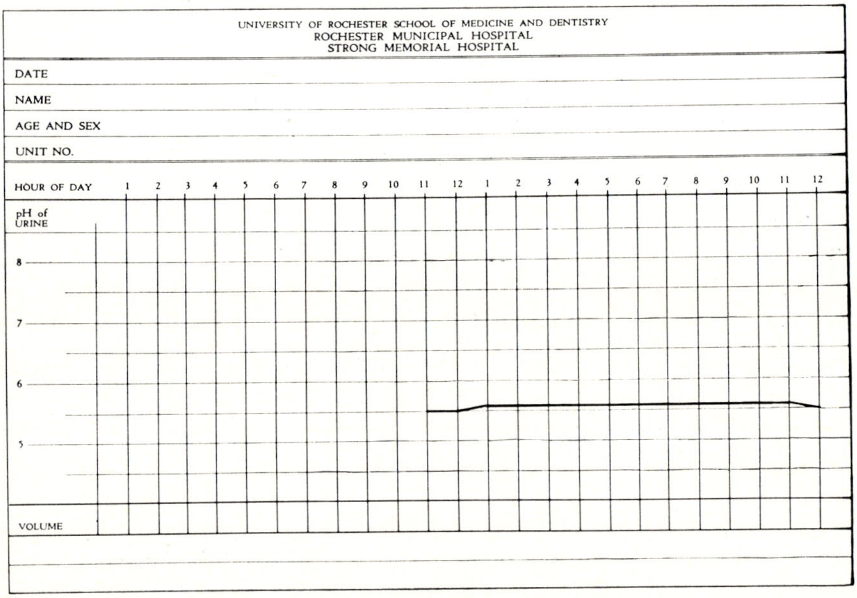

B.

Fig. 1.—Hourly urinary pH determinations plotted against time. In both cases, urine collection started in the morning. *A* is from a person with a normal sodium excretion in the urine. *B* is from a person who excreted practically no sodium in the urine.

result in any increased excretion of sodium and change in the urinary pH, this will represent pathologic salt retention.

Hourly determinations or continuous recordings of pH for a minimum period of six hours have now been performed on urine in approximately 100 cases. All urine samples have been analyzed for sodium, potassium, and ammonia, and most of them also for chloride and titratable acidity. In all the cases where a fixed urinary pH was present, and where titratable acidity was normal or low, the sodium and potassium excretion was low.

The method we now employ is as follows: at 10 A.M. the patient voids a specimen, and the pH of the urine is immediately determined using a pH meter. He then voids a urine sample for the next five consecutive hours, and urinary pH is determined immediately on each sample. The patient must be well hydrated to assure proper diuresis. If no fluctuation in the pH is seen, and the urine is acid, it indicates most often that little or no sodium is excreted in the urine (Fig. 1, *B*).

Occasionally a fixed acid urinary pH is seen despite a sodium excretion of reasonable magnitude. This happens, for instance, when ammonium chloride is administered to a normal person for several days. The reason for this is probably to be found in the increase in urinary titratable acidity whereby the buffer capacity of the urine is increased to such an extent that pH variations will be nullified as a result. However, in order to increase the urinary titratable acidity, a period of at least two to three days of a high acid load is required. Although this may well complicate the use of this method for evaluation of sodium excretion in patients with prolonged acidosis, it does not invalidate the use of the method in acute cases of shock. In preoperative evaluation of sodium balance, it can be said that if normal fluctuations are present, the patient is capable of excreting sodium in a normal manner. If urinary pH is fixed, pathologic salt retention is probably present, and at least it will warrant a more complete evaluation.

We have been using a specially constructed pH meter in which pH of the individual samples can be measured or, if desirable, the patient can be catheterized and the catheter connected directly to the machine so that the pH can continuously be read on the meter*[18, 19] (Fig. 2). A pH meter like the one described is a very stable instrument, and it is extremely simple to use.

This method can easily be applied to a preoperative evaluation of salt balance, which seems desirable, since a patient in salt retention probably is a greater surgical risk than one who is in a normal salt balance.[19]

It is probably impossible to avoid postoperative salt retention in a patient in whom such a condition existed prior to the operation. Postoperative treatment should therefore be completely different in patients who had normal salt balance and in patients who had pathologic salt retention prior to the operation. Only in the patient who was in normal salt balance preoperatively can we expect to find out whether the stress or the shock itself will cause physiologic or pathologic salt retention. In cases when an acute trauma has been inflicted, it

*Furnished through the courtesy of the Macbeth Instrument Company, Newburgh, N. Y.

naturally is impossible to know what the condition was prior to the trauma, but if the patient was healthy before, it is reasonable to assume that normal salt balance was present. This would indicate that most cases of burns and crush as well as other traumatic injuries should be treated as the postoperative cases in which normal salt balance was present prior to the operation.

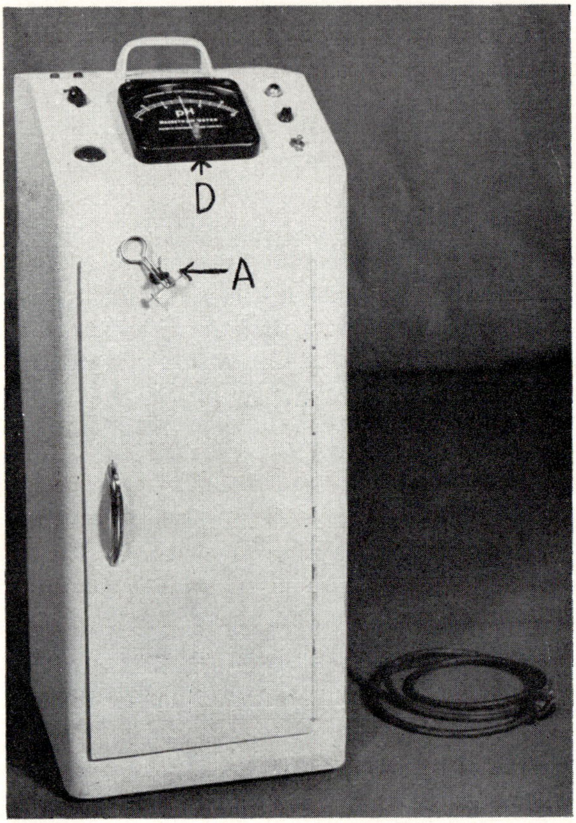

Fig. 2.—Macbeth pH meter constructed so that it can be used for continuous reading or recording of urinary pH in catheterized patients. For this use, the meter is connected with a rubber tubing (*A*) and the pH of the urine will continuously be registered by the electrodes in the flow chamber (*C*) (Fig. 2*B*). Determinations of pH on voided samples can be made simply by pouring the sample down into the beaker (*B*) and reading the meter (*D*). The machine operates on 110 volt A.C. current and can be standardized with commercially available buffer solutions (*E* and *F*).

We have recently treated three severely burned children, applying these principles.[16] The first case was of an 8-year-old boy with a 50 per cent burn, of which approximately 20 per cent was third degree. The second was of a 7-month-old child with a 22 per cent burn, almost all of it third degree. The third was of a 4-year-old girl who suffered a 50 per cent burn of which 30 per cent was third degree. All three were catheterized shortly following the trauma, and the urinary pH was continuously followed. The patients were oliguric at the time the catheterization was performed and remained so for the first ten to twelve hours. In this period, they were given plasma, normal saline solution, and dextrose to restore blood volume and decrease viscosity. During this whole period, the urinary pH remained relatively fixed. They were then given hypertonic sodium chloride in amounts which were calculated to increase the serum sodium level approximately 10 to 15 meq. per liter. As soon as the urinary pH started to rise, the hypertonic sodium chloride was discontinued. This procedure immediately increased the diuresis in all three cases, and the increase in urinary pH was found to correspond to a great increase in urinary

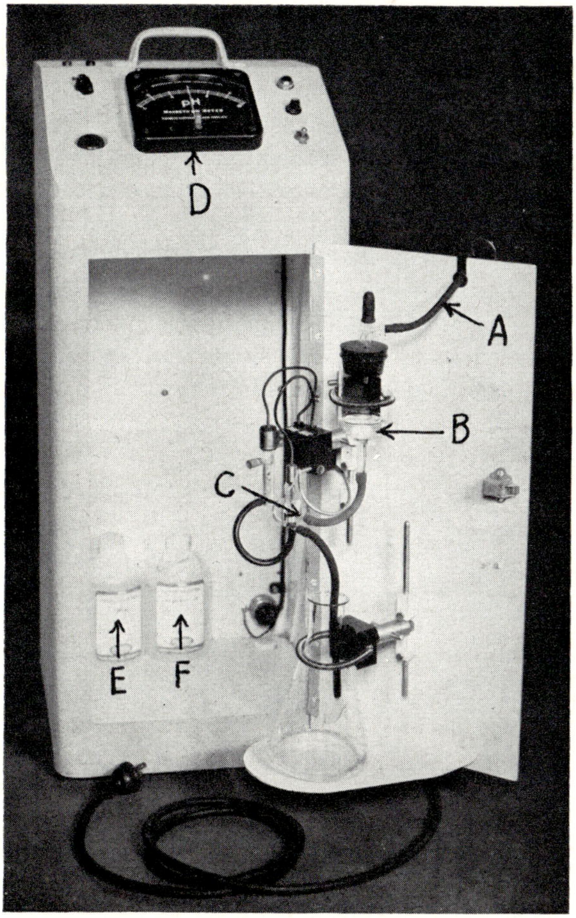

Fig. 2B. *(For legend, see opposite page.)*

excretion of sodium. Continued treatment was then carried out in the usual fashion with special emphasis placed on their sodium and potassium intake. Sodium was administered orally or intravenously in amounts which would maintain normal urinary pH fluctuations, and potassium was administered orally in almost equal dosages as sodium. It is probably extremely important to give sufficient amounts of potassium as soon as diuresis is re-established in order to facilitate the return of potassium into the damaged cells and to avoid excess uptake of sodium in the cells.[29] The children all responded very well to the treatment and exhibited no sign of water or pathologic salt retention. Except for edema in the burned areas, no clinical signs of edema, peripheral or in the lungs, were observed. We were told by the plastic surgeons that the burns appeared drier than they had anticipated. It might well be that this was a result of proper hydration.

In the 8-year-old boy, 17-ketosteroids were determined in the urine, and it was found that he excreted great amounts, indicating a high adrenal cortical function. Despite this, he exhibited no signs of pathologic salt retention.

In these three cases we must assume that the initial salt retention seen was physiologic since it could be reversed by administration of sodium, which apparently restored the serum sodium to normal levels. By the treatment employed, the administration of fluid was extremely simplified, since there was no sign of overhydration and the amounts of fluid given could be guided simply by the urinary output. It was found constantly that an increase in water load would result in an immediate increase in diuresis.

It is suggested that the method presented here be used as a simple tool for evaluation of sodium balance. Whether used preoperatively or as a guide for therapy in conditions following severe stress and shock, it seems possible to get a clear answer to the important question of whether a patient is in physiologic or pathologic salt retention.

If a pathologic salt retention is diagnosed, the patient should be treated accordingly, with restricted intake of water and sodium until urinary pH again starts fluctuating. In the case of a physiologic salt retention, fluctuations in urinary pH should be restored and maintained by proper administration of sodium and potassium to avoid development of a pathologic salt retention. In such a patient, there seems to be no danger of overhydration. The amount of sodium to be given can be determined by the fluctuations in urinary pH. If too little sodium is administered, urinary pH variations will disappear and the urine will remain acid.

CONCLUSIONS

A great deal of work still has to be done to provide us with a better understanding of electrolyte and water metabolism under normal as well as pathologic conditions. The described relationship between urinary sodium, potassium, and pH fluctuations, although fundamentally little understood, provides us nevertheless with an important tool in the treatment of acute electrolyte disturbances, as in shock and severe stress.

REFERENCES

1. Moritz, A. R.: Pulmonary Injury—Experimental, Symposium on Burns, National Academy of Sciences, Washington, D. C., 1951, National Research Council, p. 88.
2. Black, D. A. K., Platt, R., and Stanbury, S. W.: Regulation of Sodium Excretion in Normal and Salt-depleted Subjects, Clin. Sc. **9**: 205, 1950.
3. Winfield, J. M., Fox, C. L., Jr., and Mersheimer, W. L.: Etiologic Factors in Postoperative Salt Retention and Its Prevention, Ann. Surg. **134**: 626, 1951.
4. Ariel, I. M., Kremen, A. J., and Wangensteen, O. H.: An Expanded Interstitial (Thiocyanate) Space in Surgical Patients, SURGERY **27**: 827, 1950.

5. Zimmermann, B., and Wangensteen, O. H.: Observations on Water Intoxication in Surgical Patients, SURGERY **31**: 654, 1952.
6. Zimmermann, B.: Endocrine Mechanisms Concerned in Postoperative Electrolyte Changes, Proc. Surg. Forum., Clin. Congress Am. Coll. Surgeons, Philadelphia, 1950, W. B. Saunders Company, p. 447.
7. Ariel, I. M., and Kremen, A. J.: Compartmental Distribution of Sodium Chloride in Surgical Patients Pre and Postoperatively, Ann. Surg. **132**: 1009, 1950.
8. Wilson, W. C., MacGregor, A. R., and Stewart, C. P.: The Clinical Course and Pathology of Burns and Scalds Under Modern Methods of Treatment, Brit. J. Surg. **25**: 826, 1938.
9. Welt, L. G.: Edema and Hyponatremia, Arch. Int. Med. **89**: 931, 1952.
10. Cizek, L. J., and Huang, K. C.: Water Diuresis in the Salt-depleted Dog, Am. J. Physiol. **167**: 473, 1951.
11. Frieden, J., Rice, L., and Elisberg, E. I.: Renal Tubular Sodium Metabolism in Sodium Deficiency States, Am. J. Physiol. **168**: 93, 1952.
12. Moyer, C. A.: Acute Temporary Changes in Renal Function Associated With Major Surgical Procedures, SURGERY **27**: 198, 1950.
13. Wilkinson, B. M., and McCance, R. A.: The Secretion of Urine in Rabbits During Experimental Salt Deficiency, Quart. J. Exper. Physiol. **30**: 249, 1940-41.
14. Ariel, I. M., Abels, J. C., Pack, G. T., and Rhoads, C. P.: The Treatment of Hypochloremia Refractory to the Administration of Sodium Chloride, Especially in Patients With Gastrointestinal Cancer, J. A. M. A. **123**: 28, 1943.
15. Goodyer, A. V. N., and Glenn, W. L.: Excretion of Solutes Injected Into the Renal Artery of the Dog, Am. J. Physiol. **168**: 66, 1952.
16. Schlegel, J. U., Anderson, F. W., Madsen, P. O., and Betheil, J. J.: The Altered Response to Sodium Loading in Several Severely Burned Individuals After Initial Treatment With Hypertonic Sodium Containing Fluids. To be published.
17. Moore, F. D., and Ball, M. R.: The Metabolic Response to Surgery, Springfield, Ill., 1952, Charles C Thomas, Publisher.
18. Schlegel, J. U., Parry, W. L., Betheil, J. J., and Bloch, A. L.: A Study of the Relationship Between pH of the Urine and Sodium and Potassium Excretion, Proc. Soc. Exper. Biol. & Med. **84**: 223, 1953.
19. Schlegel, J. U.: Return of Sodium Loads in Normal Subjects Following Restricted Sodium Intake, SURGERY. To be published.
20. Pitts, R. F.: Modern Concepts of Acid Base Regulation, Arch. Int. Med. **89**: 864, 1952.
21. Pitts, R. F.: Effects of Adrenal Cortical Hormones on Renal Function, Adrenal Cortex, Trans. of the Third Conference, New York, 1951, Josiah Macy, Jr., Foundation, p. 11.
22. Berliner, R. W.: Tubular Secretion of Potassium and Acid, Renal Function, Trans. of the Third Conference, New York, 1951, Josiah Macy, Jr., Foundation, p. 174.
23. Jones, B.: Philos. Trans. **135**: 335, 1845.
24. Hubbard, R. S., and Steele, T. M.: Variations in the Morning Alkaline Tide of Normal Individuals, J. Biol. Chem. **84**: 199, 1929.
25. Ryberg, C. T. H.: The Physiological Variations in the Reaction of the Human Urine, Acta physiol. scandinav. **6**: 271, 1943.
26. Leathes, J. B.: Renal Efficiency Tests in Nephritis and the Reaction of the Urine, Brit. M. J. **2**: 165, 1919.
27. Nicolaysen, B.: Variations in Reaction and Salt Content of the Urine Independent of Food Intake, Norsk. mag. f. laegevidensk, **93**: 766, 1932.
28. Stanbury, S. W., and Thomson, A. E.: Diurnal Variations in Electrolyte Excretion, Clin. Sc. **10**: 267, 1951.
29. Bland, J. H.: The Clinical Use of Fluid and Electrolyte, Philadelphia, 1952, W. B. Saunders Company.
30. Pitts, R. F.: Renal Regulation of Acid Base Balance, A Symposium on Renal Function in Children, Buffalo, 1953.

SWELLING OF THE ARM AFTER RADICAL MASTECTOMY

A Clinical Study of Its Causes

William T. Fitts, Jr., M.D., John G. Keuhnelian, M.D., I. S. Ravdin, M.D., and Stanley Schor, Ph.D., Philadelphia, Pa.

(From the Department of Surgery, Hospital of the University of Pennsylvania, and the Harrison Department of Surgical Research, Schools of Medicine, University of Pennsylvania)

The incidence of swelling of the arm after radical mastectomy, as reported in recent articles, varies from 8 per cent to 95 per cent.[1, 2] It has been our experience that, if a careful examination is made, some degree of swelling will be noted following radical mastectomy in a high percentage of patients and that severe, crippling swelling associated with recurrent lymphangitis is not uncommon.

Swelling of the arm after mastectomy has been ascribed to various causes. Halsted[3] expressed the opinion that infection of the operative field, associated with necrosis of skin edges and adjacent cellulitis, leads to recurrent lymphangitis and progressive lymphatic obstruction. Veal,[4] on the other hand, stated that edema resulting from obstruction of the axillary and subclavian veins is by far the most common cause of such swelling. He thought that lymphatic obstruction was usually a secondary result of venous obstruction which, if prolonged, would lead to permanent blockage of lymphatic flow. It is difficult to reconcile Veal's conclusion with the reports of Neuhof,[5] Constantine,[6] and MacDonald,[2] all of whom noted no significant increase in the incidence of edema when ligation or excision of a portion of the axillary vein was performed as a part of a radical mastectomy. Obesity and postoperative roentgen therapy have also been cited as important causal factors in the development of edema.

In our experience, swelling may occur in the absence of any of these factors, and may be lacking when at least some of them have existed. In an attempt to measure the importance of certain factors that might produce swelling, we have made a detailed statistical study of all patients in whom radical mastectomy was performed by two of us (I. S. R. and W. T. F.) during a five-year period. Although the total number of patients (130) is small, we believe the following circumstances justify the analysis:

1. The operative procedure during this period did not vary in any major detail.
2. We personally examined all of the wounds at frequent intervals until healing was complete, and recorded the data concerning wound healing.
3. We have performed follow-up examinations of all 130 patients at intervals until July, 1952, or until the death of the patient, and have the exact time of development and the degree of swelling.

Supported by the A. Atwater Kent Fund.
Received for publication, Aug. 6, 1953.

4. A large number of the patients received penicillin prophylactically, a factor not considered by previous authors, to our knowledge, and one which might be expected to reduce the incidence of swelling if swelling were due largely to postoperative infection.

Analysis of Data.—In the five-year period between July, 1946, and July, 1951, we performed radical mastectomy on 130 patients with cancer of the breast. The operation consisted of removal of the breast, the pectoral muscles, and axillary contents caudad to the axillary vein, which was not ligated in any instance. Primary skin grafting was performed in fourteen instances because the skin flaps could not be closed without excess tension. All of the patients were dressed by us until the wound was healed, and have been examined at frequent intervals subsequently, usually at three- to six-month intervals, until death occurred or until July, 1952. The tissues removed at operation were examined in the Laboratory of Surgical Pathology of the University of Pennsylvania. The axillary nodes were removed in the laboratory and were examined microscopically for evidence of metastasis.

At examinations subsequent to operation, special attention was paid to swelling of the arm, and any degree of swelling was recorded. Some swelling developed in 49 per cent of the 130 patients. Table I classifies the patients with swelling into four groups according to the degree of swelling. Fourteen per cent of the patients developed swelling severe enough to be a significant complaint, but the remaining patients with swelling, 35 per cent, had no significant symptoms. If the swelling fluctuated, which was not infrequent, we classified it as its height.

TABLE I. SEVERITY OF SWELLING FOLLOWING RADICAL MASTECTOMY (130 PATIENTS)

GROUP	NUMBER	PER CENT
I. Minimal swelling; no symptoms; patient often unaware of swelling	28	21
II. Mild; patient aware of swelling but no disability	18	14
III. Moderate; some disability	9	7
IV. Severe; recurrent attacks of lymphangitis; severe disability	9	7
Total	64	49

For the purpose of this study, the 130 patients were divided into two groups: those who developed swelling (64 patients) and those who did not develop swelling (66 patients). Table II lists sixteen factors which might be related to swelling, and compares the incidence of these factors in the two groups.

For each of the seventeen possible causal factors, the difference between the swelling and the nonswelling groups was tested statistically. The differences were found to be significant at the 0.05 level for the following five factors: marginal necrosis, obesity, average number of axillary nodes removed, penicillin, and postoperative x-ray therapy. That is, if there were actually no difference between the patients with swelling and the patients without swelling as far as these five characteristics are concerned, the probability of getting a difference as large as the one observed for this size sample is 0.05 (that is, 5 times in 100) due to chance variations of sampling. At the 0.01 level, only the first four showed significant differences, and with further analysis* only the first three actually appeared to be important.

DISCUSSION

Our experience indicates that no one cause can be held entirely responsible for swelling of the arm after radical mastectomy. The three factors which appear to be most important from the preceding statistical analysis—marginal necrosis, average number of axillary lymph nodes removed, and obesity—are all factors which could predispose toward progressive lymphatic obstruction, considered by Halsted to be the cause of postoperative edema. From our data, lymphatics certainly appear to be closely related to swelling because in every category in which axillary lymph nodes are analyzed—number of nodes removed, degree of involvement with metastases—the greater the injury to lymphatics, the higher was the incidence of postoperative swelling. Similarly, wound healing appears closely related. In every instance, those factors indicating poor wound healing—marginal necrosis, infection, fluid collection, delayed healing time—were higher in the swelling group. It may seem that

*All significant differences observed are strictly valid, however, only if all factors are independent. If certain of the factors showing significant differences are dependent on other of these factors, then the one that actually caused swelling may not be apparent. For example, if obesity increases the probability of the development of marginal necrosis, then the significant difference attributed to obesity may in reality be due to marginal necrosis rather than to obesity per se. Similarly, some of the eleven factors showing no significant differences in Table II may have had actual differences of significance masked by dependence on other factors which are not significant. For example, let us assume that skin grafting actually increases the probability of swelling significantly. Let us also assume that skin grafting is more often performed in nonobese patients, and if nonobese patients have less chance of developing swelling, then the swelling caused by skin grafting might be masked by its dependence on nonobesity and would be shown only if obese and nonobese patients with skin grafting were tested separately.

For this reason, each of the sixteen possible causal factors was tested for dependency against every other possible causal factor. Those factors showing dependence significant at the 0.05 level were analyzed to determine whether or not this dependence actually affected the differences observed between the swelling and the nonswelling groups.

For the eleven factors yielding insignificant differences between the swelling and nonswelling groups, only one type of dependence has any real importance. In this type, the presence of one factor increases the probability of the absence of another, and a real difference may be hidden by combining these subgroups.

Only two factors yielding insignificant differences between swelling and nonswelling groups—side of lesion and fever—had the important type of dependence in which the presence of one factor increases the absence of the other. Fever proved to be less common when the lesion was on the left side, and thus homogeneous subgroups were tested. These tests showed that for patients having the lesion on the left side the difference between the per cent of swelling and nonswelling patients having fever and not having fever was insignificant. Thus, it appears that none of the eleven factors found insignificant at the 0.05 level was insignificant because of dependency on other factors.

For factors showing significant differences between swelling and nonswelling groups at the 0.01 level and exhibiting the other type of dependence—the presence of one factor increasing the probability of the presence of another—homogeneous subgroups were tested statistically. By this means it is possible to determine if any of the significant differences attributed to one factor are in reality caused by another factor associated with the first.

The significant difference observed for penicillin disappeared when tested by homogeneous subgroups of marginal necrosis and obesity. This implies that the significant difference observed for penicillin between the swelling and nonswelling groups was primarily due to its dependency with obesity and marginal necrosis.

The difference between the average number of nodes removed for homogeneous subgroups of marginal necrosis, no marginal necrosis, obesity, and no obesity showed significant difference between swelling and nonswelling groups; similarly, when obesity was tested within marginal necrosis groups and marginal necrosis within obesity groups, the probability that the difference observed was due to chance was only slightly higher than 0.05. It appears from this analysis, then, that the three primary factors in the occurrence of swelling after radical mastectomies are marginal necrosis, the numbers of axillary nodes removed, and obesity.

In an effort to strengthen these conclusions, an additional test was run between the patients who experienced moderate or severe swelling (Groups III and IV) and those without swelling. Once again, marginal necrosis, average number of lymph nodes removed, and obesity were the only factors significant at the 0.05 level.

infection itself should have had a more significant relationship. Yet full-blown infection was seen in only a few instances. Also, it may be that the chronic lymphangitis associated with marginal necrosis over a prolonged period of delayed wound healing is more effective in blocking off lymphatics than an acute cellulitis.

TABLE II. A COMPARISON OF FACTORS WHICH MIGHT CAUSE SWELLING OF THE ARM FOLLOWING RADICAL MASTECTOMY

POSSIBLE CAUSAL FACTORS	PATIENTS (64) WITH SWELLING	PATIENTS (66) WITHOUT SWELLING	DIFFERENCE SIGNIFICANT AT 0.05	0.01
1. Age	51.1 yr. (mean)	51.3 yr. (mean)	No	No
2. Obesity	43.8 %	19.7 %	Yes	Yes
3. Side of lesion (left)	53.0 %	50.0 %	No	No
4. Metastases to axillary nodes	51.5 %	38.0 %	No	No
5. Metastases to axillary fat	25.0 %	24.2 %	No	No
6. Average number of axillary nodes removed	19.1 (mean)	15.3 (mean)	Yes	Yes
7. More than ⅓ axillary nodes involved	31.3 %	16.7 %	No	No
8. More than ½ axillary nodes involved	18.7 %	13.6 %	No	No
9. Skin graft at primary operation	14.1 %	7.6 %	No	No
10. Penicillin given prophylactically	85.9 %	65.1 %	Yes	Yes
11. X-ray therapy given prophylactically	17.2 %	4.5 %	Yes	No
12. Fever after operation (at least 100° F. by mouth on any 3 days)	18.8 %	16.7 %	No	No
13. Fluid collection	59.4 %	45.5 %	No	No
14. Infection	14.1 %	6.1 %	No	No
15. Marginal necrosis	51.6 %	27.3 %	Yes	Yes
16. Time required for complete healing	41.3 days (mean)	32.2 days (mean)	No	No

A finding we had not anticipated was that related to the prophylactic administration of penicillin. If it had any effect at all, penicillin appeared to increase rather than to decrease the incidence of swelling. We were careful to include in the penicillin group only those patients who received it from the time of operation, and not only after wound complications were noted. Those patients not receiving penicillin prophylactically were, in most instances, those operated on early in the study, before penicillin was easily available. It is possible that in this period patients more likely to develop wound complications, for example, those with unusual tension on the flaps, were given penicillin. In any event, it seems clear that in our hands penicillin was not effective in decreasing postoperative swelling. Again, the chronic low-grade infection associated with marginal necrosis is the type least likely to respond to antibiotics.

It may appear that wound complications were unusually high in these patients. We were extremely strict in classifying complications. For example, several patients had notes on their hospital charts stating that the wound had healed primarily before their discharge from the hospital. Yet, these patients, when seen as outpatients for subsequent dressings, would be found to have small areas of marginal necrosis, and complete epithelization might require several weeks. No wound was considered healed until epithelization was absolutely complete and no dressing was required. As noted in Table II, full-blown infection, as manifested by redness, heat or suppuration, was uncommon.

Roentgen therapy was given prophylactically to only a few of our patients, and these were selected patients in that they were those who were more likely to have far-advanced cancer as manifested by extensive metastases to axillary lymph nodes. Accordingly, little can be concluded from our study concerning the effect of x-ray therapy on producing postoperative swelling. We can say that our high incidence of swelling was due largely to other factors.

SUMMARY

Almost one-half of a series of 130 patients developed swelling of the arm after radical mastectomy. No one factor was the determinant in the development of swelling, although several factors that might relate to lymphatic obstruction appeared important. The number of axillary lymph nodes removed, marginal necrosis, and obesity appeared to be the most important from a detailed statistical analysis. Other factors which might be related to lymphatic obstruction—percentage of lymph nodes involved with cancer, fever after operation, fluid collection, and definite infection—were only slightly higher in the swelling group. Penicillin given prophylactically to the majority of these patients did not appear to reduce the incidence of swelling.

REFERENCES

1. Guthrie, D., and Gagnon, G.: The Prevention and Treatment of Postoperative Lymphedema of the Arm, Ann. Surg. **123:** 925-936, 1946.
2. MacDonald, I.: Resection of the Axillary Vein in Radical Mastectomy: Its Relation to the Mechanism of Lymphedema, Cancer **1:** 618-624, 1948.
3. Halsted, W. S.: The Swelling of the Arm After Operations for Cancer of the Breast—Elephantiasis Chirurgica: Its Causes and Prevention, Bull. Johns Hopkins Hosp. **32:** 309-313, 1921.
4. Veal, J. R.: The Pathologic Basis for Swelling of the Arm Following Radical Amputation of the Breast, Surg., Gynec. & Obst. **67:** 752-760, 1938.
5. Neuhof, H.: Excision of Axillary Vein in the Radical Operation for Carcinoma of the Breast, Ann. Surg. **108:** 15-20, 1938.
6. Constantine, H.: Peut-on réséquer la veine axillaire dans le traitement du cancer du sein? Bull. et mém. Soc. nat. de chir. **58:** 1284-1286, 1932.

Case Reports

ESOPHAGEAL LEIOMYOMA

LOUIS G. BRIZZOLARA, M.D.,* AND CHARLES L. GERACI, M.D.,**
SAN FRANCISCO, CALIF.

(From the Surgical Service, United States Veterans Administration Hospital)

APPROXIMATELY twenty-eight patients with leiomyoma of the esophagus have received surgical treatment.[1-12] The procedures performed have been either local excision with or without entering the esophageal lumen or esophageal resection and esophagogastrostomy. Approximately nineteen cases have been reported in which patients were treated by local excision.[1-5] The purpose of this paper is to add to the literature another case of leiomyoma of the esophagus treated by local excision.

CASE REPORT

L. J. G., a 28-year-old white man, entered San Francisco Veterans Administration Hospital on Jan. 19, 1953, because of dysphagia. He had noted vague substernal pains and obstructionlike symptoms after eating solid foods three years previously, and at that time had received a general examination including a barium esophagogram, which revealed no abnormality. The symptoms had persisted, although he had never complained of vomiting, retching, hematemesis, or melena. His appetite was excellent and there had been no weight loss.

The patient had consulted his local physician one week prior to admission, at which time an esophagogram was reported to have revealed a long, smoothly lobulated filling defect in the middle and lower thirds of the thoracic esophagus. Esophagoscopy the same day had confirmed these findings, but had not revealed the presence of any intraluminal disease or mucosal involvement. The remainder of the past history was not remarkable.

Physical examination at the time of this admission revealed a healthy, young adult white man in no distress. There were no abnormal physical findings. Chest x-ray film was negative, and an esophagogram demonstrated a smoothly lobulated filling defect covering a 10 cm. segment of the midesophagus (Fig. 1). No mucous membrane involvement could be discerned.

Esophagoscopy was performed Jan. 27, 1953, revealing a smoothly multilobulated mass compressing the lumen from both right and left, beginning at the level of the aortic arch and extending inferiorly for approximately 10 cm. The esophageal mucosa was smooth and pale throughout its length, and there was no evidence of mucosal involvement in tumor. The esophagoscope could be passed through the compressed area without difficulty, the operator obtaining the impression that the mass was "spread apart" by the instrument. No biopsy was taken.

A tentative diagnosis of leiomyoma of the esophagus was made, and on Feb. 2, 1953, the esophagus was explored through a left-seventh-rib thoracotomy incision. A dumbbell-shaped mass was found in the wall of the esophagus at the level of and just beneath the

Received for publication, March 20, 1953.

*Chief of Surgical Service, United States Veterans Administration Hospital; Assistant Clinical Professor of Surgery, University of California Hospital.

**Senior Resident in Surgery, United States Veterans Administration Hospital.

aortic arch. After the esophagus was freed from its bed, the muscularis over the tumor mass was incised and a firm cartilaginous-appearing white mass was found lying within the muscle and the submucosa. This was dissected from the surrounding tissue bluntly with the aid of a Hawley dissector without difficulty. It was found to extend longitudinally for a short distance in the left wall, then cross the posterior wall and extend upward for about 9 cm. in the right wall of the esophagus. After complete removal there was no bleeding, and the muscularis was closed with interrupted 000 silk sutures. The thorax was closed in layers in the usual manner, with one posterior chest tube connected to underwater seal drainage.

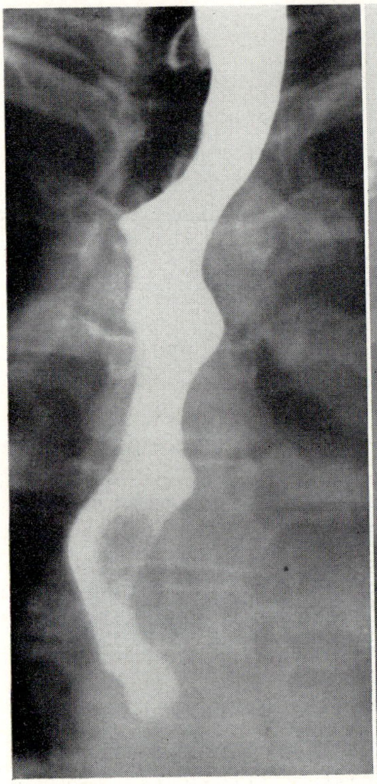

Fig. 1.

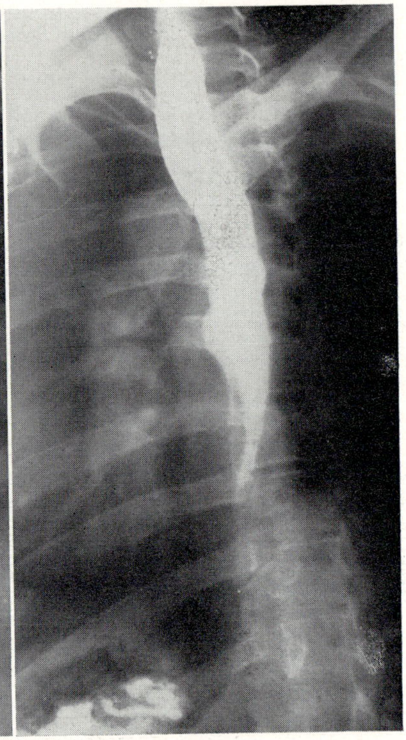

Fig. 2.

Fig. 1.—Preoperative esophagogram showing lobulated filling defect.
Fig. 2.—Postoperative esophagogram showing normal contour of lumen.

Postoperatively the patient convalesced rapidly and was ambulatory on the second day after surgery; the chest tube was removed on the fourth postoperative day, and all sutures were out by the tenth postoperative day. Liquids were started by mouth on the third day, with progression to a soft diet on the ninth day. Thereafter the patient progressed rapidly to a regular diet. A repeat esophagogram (Fig. 2) made fifteen days after surgery revealed no constriction or irregularity of the esophagus. The patient was discharged from the hospital sixteen days after surgery, completely asymptomatic, and he has since returned to his occupation.

The lesion measured 12 by 3 by 2.5 cm. and appeared as in Fig. 3. It was pale gray and was firm and cartilaginous, and apparently encapsulated. Microscopic sections showed numerous interlacing bundles of elongated, pale, staining cells with large regular nuclei. The appearance was typical of a leiomyoma, as shown in Fig. 4.

COMMENT

Leiomyoma of the esophagus is a benign lesion that causes dysphagia and partial esophageal obstruction. The histopathology and clinical picture have been well described.[2, 3, 14, 15] Once the lesion becomes symptomatic, some form of surgical intervention is indicated. The operation of choice is local excision of the lesion. This can be accomplished by enucleation from the muscularis

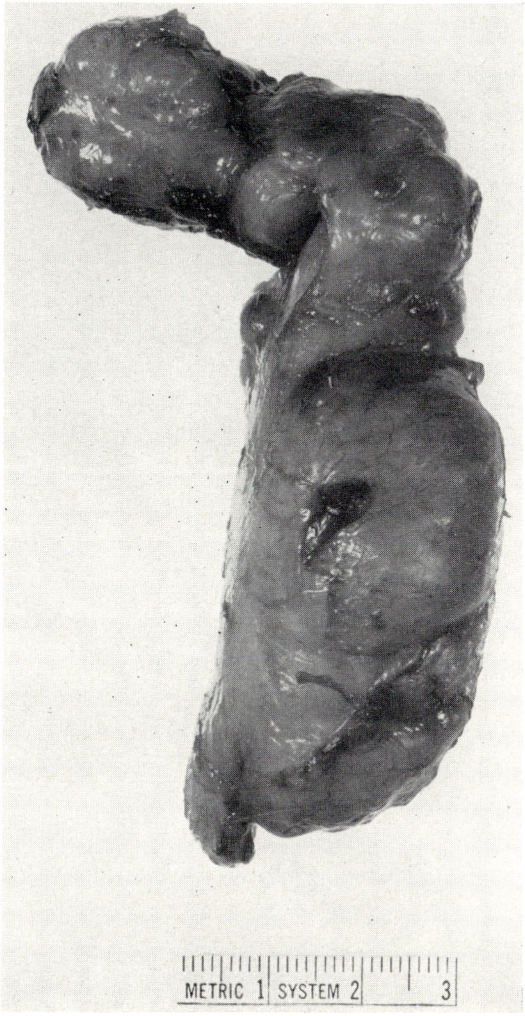

Fig. 3.—Gross appearance of tumor.

and submucosa of the esophageal wall without entering the mucosa, as was done in our case. Following removal in this manner the muscularis is reapproximated with interrupted nonabsorbable sutures. In some cases it may be necessary to excise a segment of the mucosa with the lesion, and then subsequent closure is accomplished in two layers with interrupted nonabsorbable sutures to both the mucosa and the muscularis. If local excision is not feasible, then some form of esophageal resection must be made, and in such cases continuity is re-established by esophagogastrostomy. This procedure is far less desirable in view of the high incidence of gastrointestinal disturbances and esophagitis which follows such a resection and anastomosis. Postoperative complications in patients having local excision without excision of mucosa are obviously lower than in patients in whom the esophageal lumen is entered or the esophagus resected.

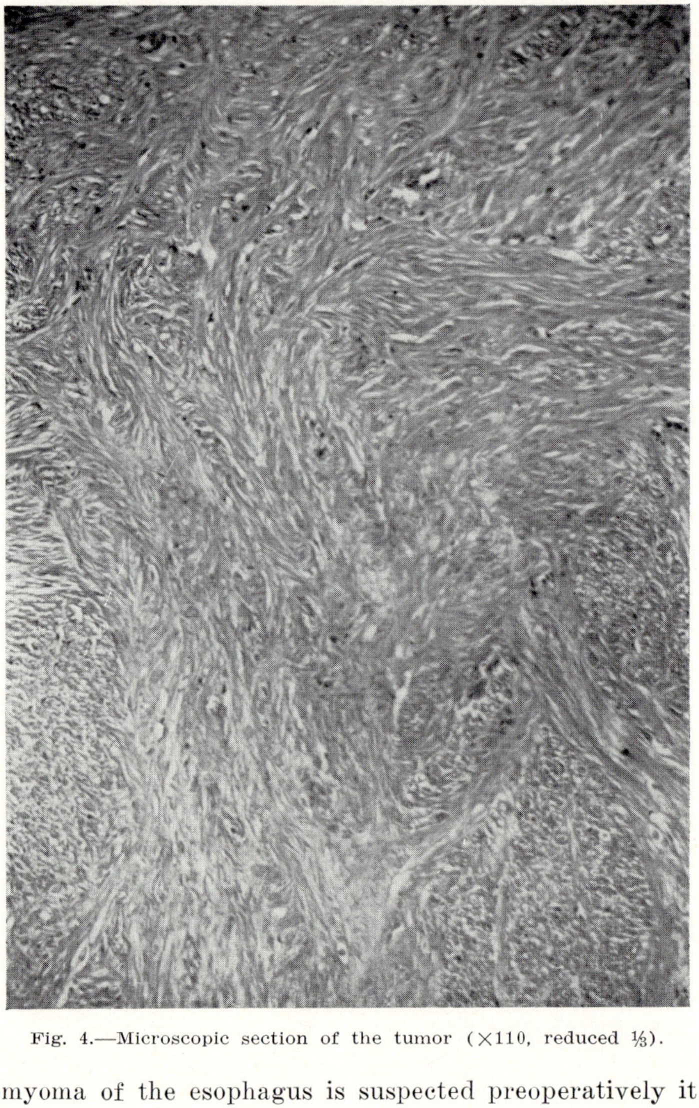

Fig. 4.—Microscopic section of the tumor (×110, reduced ⅓).

If leiomyoma of the esophagus is suspected preoperatively it is not advisable to attempt a biopsy via the esophagoscope, as the resulting scarring and adherence make dissection of the lesion from the mucosa difficult if not impossible, and the esophageal lumen is very likely to be entered. In this case it was found that a blunt dissector (Hawley or thyroid type) was a particularly suitable instrument to use to aid in freeing the lesion from its bed.

SUMMARY

A case report of the successful removal of a leiomyoma of the midthoracic esophagus is presented. This is the twenty-ninth reported case of such a removal and the twentieth reported case of excision by enucleation.

REFERENCES

1. Westerhorn, O.: Leiomyoma of the Esophagus, Acta chir. scandinav. **103**: 158, 1952.
2. Goldman, A., and Masters, H.: Leiomyoma of the Esophagus, Arch. Surg. **60**: 559, 1950.
3. Myers, R. T., and Bradshaw, H. H.: Benign Intramural Tumors and Cysts of the Esophagus, J. Thoracic Surg. **21**: 470, 1951.
4. Chi, P. S., and Adams, W. D.: Benign Tumors of the Esophagus, Arch. Surg. **60**: 92, 1950.
5. Daniel, R. A., and Williams, R. B.: Leiomyoma of the Esophagus, J. Thoracic Surg. **19**: 800, 1950.
6. Schnug, G. E.: Leiomyoma of the Cardioesophageal Junction, Arch. Surg. **65**: 342, 1952.
7. Garlick, W. L., and Stegmaier, J. G.: Benign Tumors of the Esophagus, SURGERY **29**: 109, 1951.
8. Dugan, D. J., and Meagher, C. S.: Esophageal Leiomyomas, Arch. Surg. **61**: 1066, 1950.
9. Kenworthy, R. A., and Welch, C. S.: Leiomyoma of the Esophagus and Cardia of the Stomach, SURGERY **23**: 745, 1948.
10. Schafer, P. W., and Kittle, C. F.: Esophageal Leiomyoma, J. A. M. A. **133**: 1202, 1947.
11. Calinenson, M., and Clagett, O. T.: Surgical Removal of Leiomyomas of the Esophagus, Am. J. Surg. **72**: 745, 1946.
12. Hurwitz, A.: Leiomyoma of the Esophagus, SURGERY **25**: 304, 1949.
13. Moersch, H. J., and Harrington, S. W.: Benign Tumors of the Esophagus, Ann. Otol., Rhin. & Laryng. **53**: 800, 1944.
14. Harrington, S. W.: Surgical Treatment of Benign and Secondarily Malignant Tumors of the Esophagus, Arch. Surg. **58**: 646, 1949.
15. Palmer, E. D.: The Esophagus and Its Diseases, New York, 1952, Paul B. Hoeber, Inc.

THE CASE FOR DE NOVO ORIGIN OF LATE RECURRENCE OF CANCER OF THE FEMALE BREAST

N. William Wawro, M.D., Hartford, Conn.

(From the Department of Surgery, Hartford Hospital)

INTRODUCTION

FORTY-SEVEN years ago, the problem of late recurrence of mammary cancer provoked Jordan[1] to ask, "Are we justified in ever pronouncing a patient cured after surgery for breast cancer?" Ransohoff[2] raised a similar question after reviewing the number of late recurrences in the long-term follow-up of this group of neoplasms.

The more immediate problem of early postoperative recurrence has claimed the attention of many surgeons.[3, 4] Large series[3, 5] of carefully documented records of breast neoplasms indicate that approximately 25 per cent of patients will develop recurrence on the ipsilateral chest wall involving either scar, axilla, parasternal zone, or supraclavicular nodes within 5 years. The rapidity of local recurrence appears to be related to several factors, singly or in combination—notably, size of original lesion, extent of skin and axillary node involvement, and thoroughness of the surgical procedure. Furthermore the presence of locally recurrent disease carries a grave prognosis, since 80 to 90 per cent of these patients ultimately die of metastatic disease. Handley's[6] concept of permeation of breast cancer cells into the lymphatic plexus of cutaneous superficial fascia with later extension toward the vertical skin lymphatics to form skin nodules has attracted the support of many physicians to explain both early and late recurrence.

The circumstances surrounding a late recurrence in a recent patient, 17 years after original mastectomy, suggest that, in addition to Handley's concept, it is possible that recurrent breast cancer may be explained by the development of a second primary carcinoma in residual breast tissue remaining in the original operative field.

CASE REPORT

H. W., a 58-year-old housewife, had a left radical mastectomy in 1932 for a small comedocarcinoma (Fig. 1) arising in area of cystic disease unassociated with metastases to regional axillary nodes. The subsequent course was uncomplicated. In 1949, seventeen years later, this patient noted a small left parasternal nodule 2 by 5 cm. over the third left rib, for which two courses of deep x-ray therapy were administered. The lesion failed to regress, and painful ulceration followed. When I saw the patient in December, 1950, she presented an oval, raised ulcerating lesion, 4 by 7 cm., fixed to underlying tissues, and unassociated with palpable regional or distant metastases. The right breast was free of any masses. Roentgen film of the chest was negative for pulmonary metastases.

A block resection of the ulcerating mass with underlying chest wall including the second, third, and fourth left ribs, internal mammary vessels, and lymphatics was carried out (Fig. 2).

Received for publication, April 6, 1953.

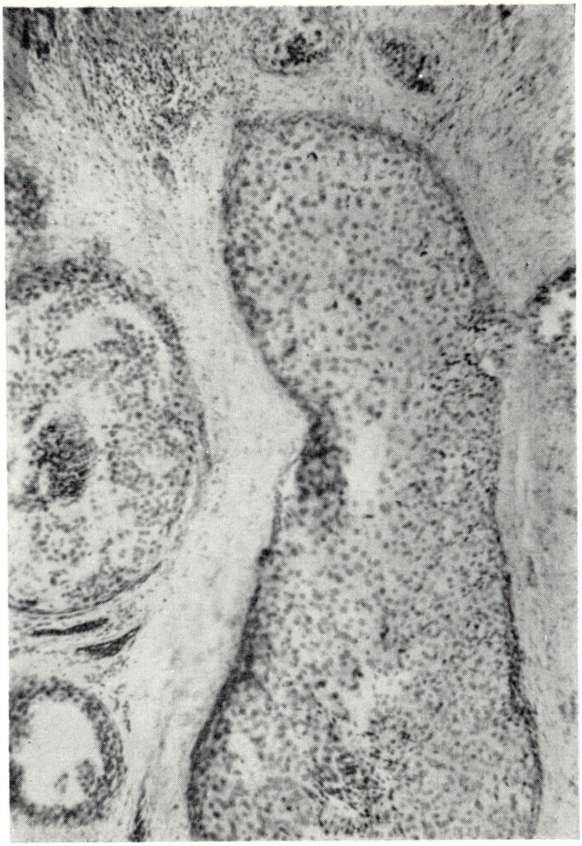

Fig. 1.—Photomicrograph of comedocarcinoma of left breast removed by mastectomy in 1932. (Magnification, ×200.)

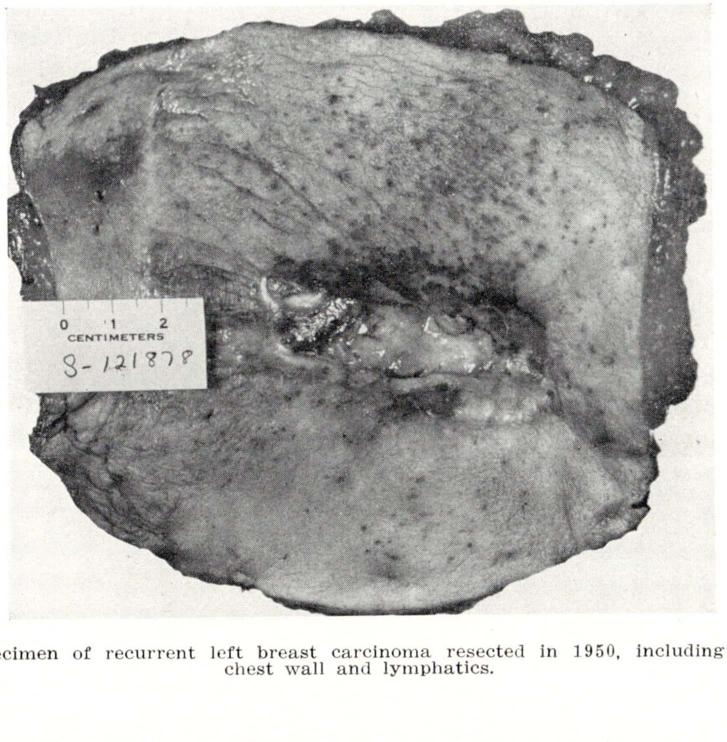

Fig. 2.—Specimen of recurrent left breast carcinoma resected in 1950, including underlying chest wall and lymphatics.

No involvement of underlying pericardium or parietal pleura was noted. Microscopic examination of submitted specimen revealed infiltrating carcinoma of breast (Fig. 3) without involvement of subjacent internal mammary lymph nodes. The large 10 by 15 cm. chest wall defect was repaired by sliding the opposite right breast medially as a flap.

In the process of resecting this lesion, it was noted that the skin flaps on the operative side were 2 to 4 cm. thick and contained white breast tissue to a thickness of 2 cm. Biopsy of this tissue adjacent to the neoplasm was reported as ''atrophic breast tissue'' (Fig. 4).

The operative procedure was well tolerated and patient was discharged without impairment of pulmonary function.

Fig. 4.

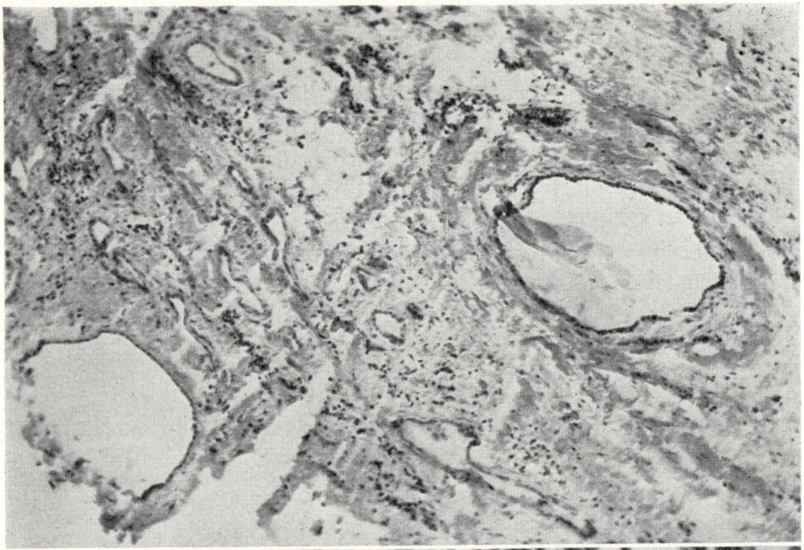

Fig. 3.

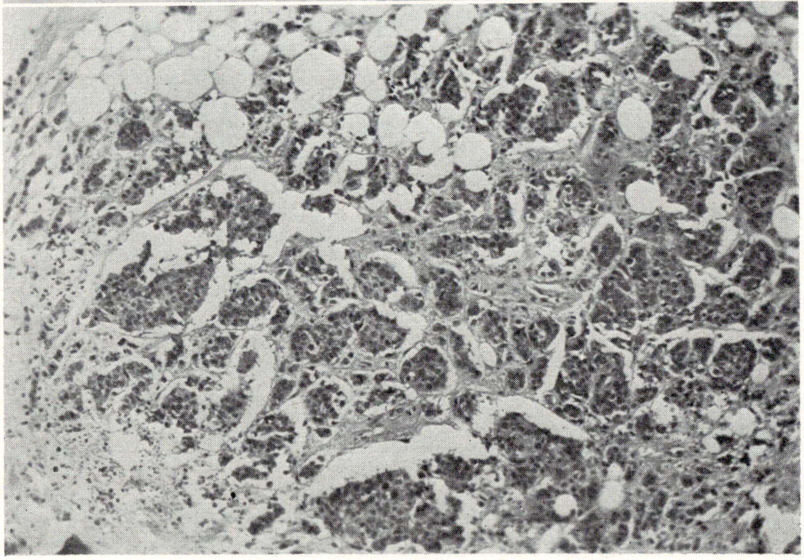

Fig. 3.—Photomicrograph of fibrocarcinoma of recurrent neoplasm removed in 1950 as demonstrated in Fig. 2. (Magnification, ×200.)

Fig. 4.—Photomicrograph of residual atrophic breast tissue found within skin flaps adjacent to recurrent neoplasm of 1950 (Fig. 2). (Magnification, ×200.)

DISCUSSION

If one will arbitrarily select 10 years as the dividing line between early and late recurrence, one then encounters several reports[7-10] in the literature dealing with late recurrence of mammary cancer. Daland has reported a recurrence 34 years after mastectomy, though no microscopic report of the original lesion was available.

It is not the author's desire to contest Handley's concept from experience derived in a single case. However, if normal breast tissue remains within skin flaps *following* mastectomy, that tissue constitutes a potential menace equal to that of the opposite breast. The very fact that cancer may arise in the opposite breast in approximately 10 per cent of women[11] who have survived 5 years or longer after radical mastectomy, lends credence to the danger of leaving non-neoplastic breast tissue in skin flaps after breast amputation.

Study of reports of late recurrence from the literature does not permit critical evaluation of the thoroughness of removal of breast tissue (and axillary nodes), but since many of these procedures were carried out several decades ago, when the radical mastectomy was undergoing clinical trial and evolution, and antedated the use of agents to combat shock, selective anesthesia, and high development of technical skill, it is logical to believe that some of these patients may have had varying amounts of uninvolved breast tissue left in the skin flaps.

It is suggested, therefore, that it is the surgeon's responsibility to leave no breast tissue in the operative field when radical mastectomy is carried out for mammary cancer. A very excellent description of such a meticulous technique is described by Haagensen.[12] Furthermore, adequate follow-up of the patient with mammary cancer is indicated since such a patient has no immunity to developing a second primary neoplasm in the opposite breast. In fact, a recent study indicates that the susceptibility for second breast cancer is higher than the normal incidence.[13]

CONCLUSION

1. A case report of a homolateral recurrence of breast cancer 17 years after radical mastectomy is presented.

2. Microscopic evidence of residual breast tissue in the original operative field is demonstrated.

3. It is suggested that a second primary breast carcinoma may arise in such an anatomic setting.

4. Complete removal of the breast tissue in the affected breast by radical mastectomy and adequate follow-up for the duration of the patient's life should improve the results in the treatment of this neoplasm.

REFERENCES

1. Jordan, A. B.: Deutsche Med. Wochenschrift, June 16, Pages 912-914, 1904.
2. Ransohoff, J.: Carcinoma of the Breast, Ann. of Surg. **46**: 72-80, 1907.
3. White, W. C.: Problem of Local Recurrence After Radical Mastectomy for Cancer, Surgery **19**: 149-153, 1946.
4. Oliver, D. R., and Sugarbaker, E. D.: Significance of Skin Recurrence Following Radical Mastectomy, Surg., Gynec. & Obst. **85**: 360-367, 1947.

5. Stout, A. P., and Haagensen, C.: Cancer of Breast, Results of Treatment, Ann. Surg. **116**: 801-815, 1942.
6. Handley, W. S.: Cancer of Breast and Its Treatment, ed. 2, London, 1922, John Murray.
7. Daland, E. M.: Some Unusual Aspects of Breast Cancer, New England J. Med. **233**: 515-519, 1945.
8. Woolsey, G.: Late Recurrence After Radical Operation for Carcinoma of Breast, Ann. Surg. **80**: 932-938, 1924.
9. Perry, T. J.: Adenocarcinoma. Case Recurring After 27 Years, Rhode Island M. J. **31**: 44-46, 1948.
10. Brown, A.: Late Recurrence in Skin Following Radical Amputation of Breast for Cancer, Tr. West. S. A. **53**: 293-307, 1946.
11. Haagensen, C.: Cancer of Breast, American Cancer Society Handbook, New York, 1950.
12. Haagensen, C.: Technique of Radical Mastectomy, SURGERY **19**: 100-131, 1946.
13. Mider, Burroughs, Schilling, J. A., Donovan, J. C., and Randall, E. S.: Multiple Cancer, A Study of Other Cancers Arising in Patients With Primary Malignant Neoplasms of the Stomach, Uterus, Breast, Large Intestine, or Hematopoietic System, Cancer **5**: 1104-1110, 1952.

TRANSORBITOCRANIAL FOREIGN BODY

Gordon M. Carver, Jr., M.D., Durham, N. C., and W. Patterson, M.D., Philadelphia, Pa.

FORTUNATELY, one does not frequently encounter a patient with a wooden stake protruding from the orbit. Recent foreign hostilities (Korean War) and the ever-increasing automobile and industrial accident rate significantly enhance the possibilities of having to treat such lesions and warrant the reporting of this unusual case with a review of the problems and principles of the treatment of orbitocranial wounds.

In transorbitocranial injury the surgeon is confronted with a compound, comminuted, infected cranial wound which may be complicated by involvement of the paranasal sinuses, the orbital contents, the carotid artery, and the cavernous sinus and the destruction of an undetermined amount of cerebral tissue with possible ventricular rupture. The frequent involvement of the paranasal sinuses in facio-orbitocranial wounds and the complications resulting from unrecognized and untreated communications between the subarachnoid space and the bacteria-laden sinuses characterize this type of head injury and prompt early surgical correction. Subsequent plastic restoration of orbitofacial contour is an important problem and may be one of the determining factors in the choice of the operative approach to be selected.

In general, radical débridement of cranial and cerebral wounds, closure of the dura, and suturing of the scalp without tension and without drainage are the cardinal principles of treating compound cranial wounds. Such wounds should be immediately converted into simple wounds, except when severe shock or a hopeless condition of the patient contraindicates operation.

Orbitocranial wounds involving the paranasal sinuses necessitate repair of the overlying dura (by fascia lata grafting when necessary), exenteration of the sinus mucous membrane, and drainage of the sinus into the nasal passage.[1-3] The operative approach in orbitocranial wounds must afford adequate exposure for complete débridement, investigation of intracranial pathology, exenteration and drainage of involved sinuses, and closure of the dura.

Calvert[4] discussed the pro and con of exposure by frontal bone flap with intradural repair of the torn dura, versus the direct orbital approach with exenteration of the sinuses and extradural repair. He favored turning a frontal bone flap in the majority of cases and repairing the dura from above, since the subsequent plastic repair is reduced to a minimum and repair of an unsuspected dural tear on the opposite side can be provided for.

The protagonists of the direct operative approach through the wound of entrance favor it because the procedure is less traumatic to an already

Received for publication, April 17, 1953.

severely injured patient, the line of approach is the same as that of the missile tract in the brain making it easier to follow and to remove damaged contaminated bone, the drainage of damaged air sinuses into the nose is facilitated, and the time required for the direct approach is much less.

In the patient to be reported on the large missile entering the orbito-frontal space required an osteoplastic flap above the frontal sinuses, similar to the frontal craniotomy exposure proposed by Dandy[5] for the removal of orbital tumors. This approach offered an excellent exposure to the frontal lobe area for removal of foreign bodies, bone chips, and necrotic cerebral tissue. The depth of penetration by the foreign body could be visualized, and the surgeon was in a position to control intracranial hemorrhage after removal of the wooden stake.

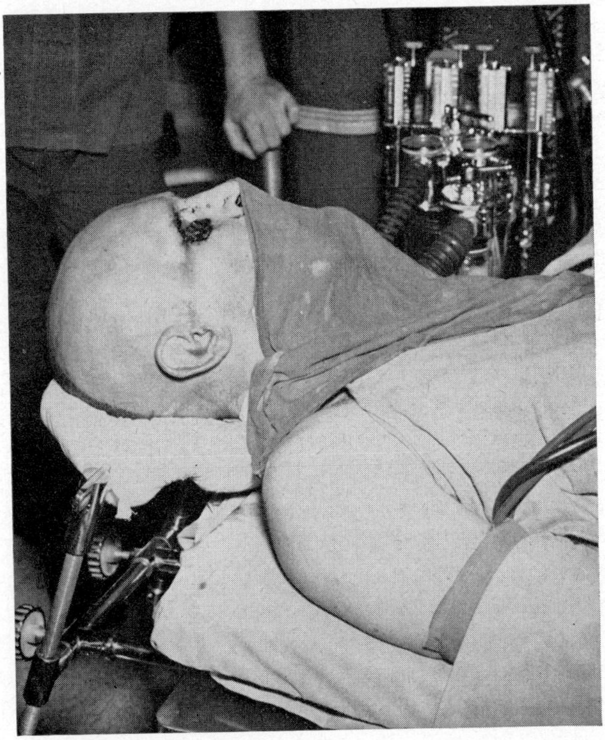

Fig. 1.—Photograph taken just prior to the operation showing the wooden stake protruding from the right orbit. The foreign body was wedged in the orbit breaking off flush with the infraorbital ridge.

The surgeon must select the operative approach best suited for the individual patient according to the presenting lesion, the available operating facilities, and his own surgical experience and training. If a complete definitive operation cannot be performed the patient should be given emergency supportive treatment and transferred to a general hospital, as it was demonstrated during World War II by Stewart and Botterell[6] that with administration of antibiotics a delay of one, two, or even three days was considered of less consequence than the dangers of earlier but incomplete operation.

CASE REPORT

A 19-year-old Marine was admitted to the Camp Lejeune Naval Hospital on Dec. 19, 1951, with a wooden stake protruding from the right orbit (Fig. 1). While driving a tank through a forest the stake was deflected upward, passing through the driver's port into the patient's right orbit. He was rushed to the hospital, arriving approximately twenty-five minutes after the accident.

Physical Examination.—The patient was slightly confused but was able to relate the details of the unfortunate accident. The pulse was becoming weak at 120 per minute, and with a blood pressure of 85/55 shock was imminent. Blood was drawn for cross-matching, and a unit of plasma was started with rapid peripheral circulatory adjustment.

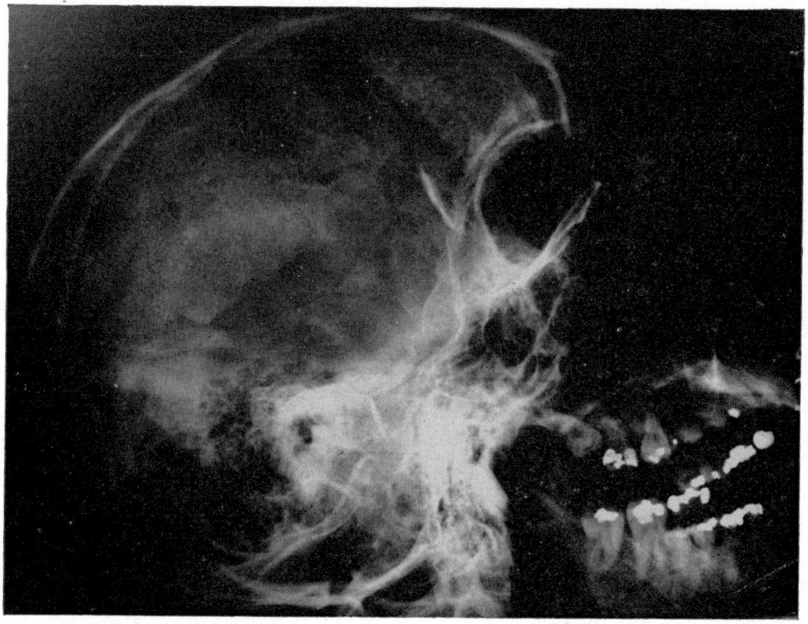

Fig. 2.—Lateral x-ray picture of the skull showing rupture of foreign body through the orbital roof with displacement of one large bone fragment posterior and inferior. Fracture of orbital roof extends into frontal sinus. A depressed fracture of the infraorbital ridge is also present on the right side.

Vision of the left eye was not impaired, and the patient was able to move all extremities without comparable weakness. There was no sensory disturbance, and reflexes were only slightly hyperactive on the left side. The remainder of the general physical examination was normal.

X-ray pictures of the skull revealed the foreign body to have ruptured through the bony orbital roof displacing the fragments into the inferior surface of the frontal lobe (Fig. 2). There was no x-ray evidence suggesting entry into the middle cranial fossa. The comminuted orbital roof fracture extended forward into the inferior surface of the right frontal sinus, and there was a depressed fracture of the right infraorbital ridge. No sphenoidal or ethmoidal fracture was noted.

Operation.—Under Pentothal Sodium anesthesia with intratracheal oxygen, a right frontal craniotomy was performed. The dura was opened just within the bony margin, and the frontal lobe retracted laterally; the foreign body was found to have entered the inferiomedial aspect of the frontal lobe preceded by the bone fragments of the orbital roof. The wooden stake was extracted through the orbit with considerable bleeding from the orbit but with very litle intracranial hemorrhage.

Bone fragments and wooden splinters were removed from the wound, some taken out through the craniotomy opening and some passed out through the orbit using the tips of the index fingers. The wound was copiously irrigated with warm saline solution until all necrotic brain tissue had been removed and no bone or wooden fragments could be visualized or palpated. Gentle palpation revealed no rupture into the anterior horn of the right ventricle.

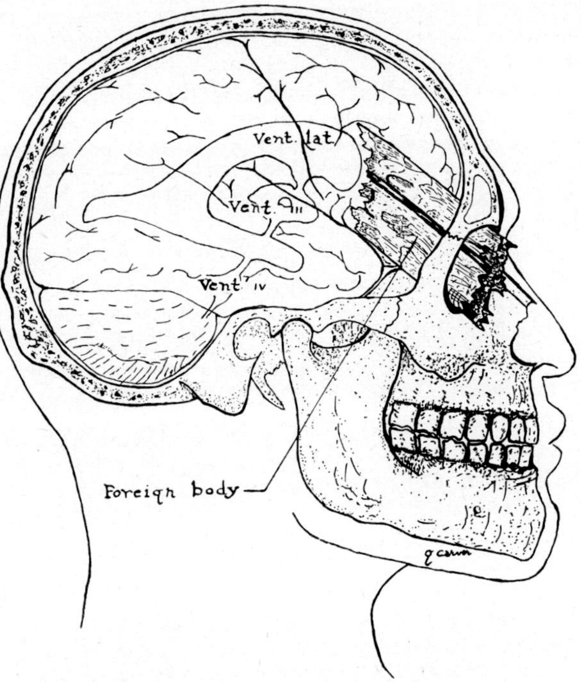

Fig. 3.—Diagrammatic sketch showing relative position and size of wooden stake to vital intracranial structures. The foreign body measured 9.4 cm. by 3.8 cm. not including the numerous wooden fragments that were removed from the frontal lobe.

It was now apparent that the direction of the wooden stake had been about thirty-five degrees upward from a horizontal plane, rupturing through the orbital roof into the inferiomedial aspect of the frontal lobe, severing the optic and olfactory nerves and miraculously missing the internal carotid artery, cavernous sinus, and optic chiasma. The tip of the foreign body was found to be beveled, and the long end of the bevel was directed superiorly into the frontal lobe while the short end was inferior and not long enough to damage these structures (Fig. 3).

There was no fracture into the ethmoid sinuses, but a fracture extending into the inferior portion of the frontal sinus from the orbital roof was noted. The mucous membrane of the frontal sinus was intact; therefore, its bone fragments were reapproximated, and the mucous membrane was left undisturbed.

The dura overlying the roof of the orbit was torn irregularly in an anterior-posterior direction, being intact over the ethmoid sinuses. A satisfactory closure of the dura was obtained, and the retro-orbital tissue was then sutured to the inferior surface of the dura to buttress the dural suture line.

The foreign body forced the orbital contents laterally, tearing through the inner canthal portion of the upper lid. The eye was enucleated, preserving the bulbar conjunctiva into which a glass prosthesis was placed, and the conjunctival sac was closed with a 00000 silk continuous suture.

A depressed segment of the fractured infraorbital ridge was grasped with a towel clip and elevated into position. The defect in the upper lid was repaired, and a median tarsorrhaphy performed.

The craniotomy wound was closed without drainage, and a pressure dressing was applied to the head and right orbit.

Postoperative Course.—The patient was mentally alert and oriented as soon as he recovered from the anesthesia. He ran a slightly elevated temperature up to 101° F. for three days after which it gradually returned to normal. There was no cerebrospinal rhinorrhea.

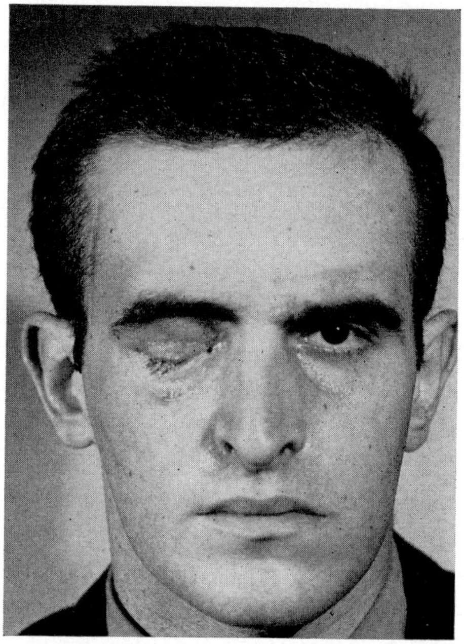

Fig. 4.—Patient's postoperative appearance at time of transfer to United States Naval Hospital, Bethesda, Md., for ocular prothesis.

The patient received 300,000 U. of procaine penicillin and 1 Gm. of streptomycin every twelve hours for ten days. He required only codeine for relief of an occasional headache. Phenobarbital, 60 mg., was given every four hours as an anticonvulsant and sedative. The operative wounds healed primarily without infection.

X-ray pictures revealed no evidence of intracranial infection or retained bone fragments.

There was no mental confusion or personality change postoperatively, and Wechsler-Bellevue and Grassi tests revealed no intellectual impairment. Neurological examinations showed loss of first, second, third, fourth, and sixth right cranial nerve function. On Jan. 2, 1952, a rubber conformer was inserted between the conjunctival surfaces of the globe and the eyelid to prevent symblepharon and obliteration of the supra- and infrapalpebral sulci.

A blepharoplasty was performed on Feb. 8, 1952, reconstructing the inner canthal portion of the right upper lid. The patient was subsequently transferred to the United States Naval Hospital, Bethesda, Md., for an ocular prosthesis (Fig. 4).

DISCUSSION

The direction and degree of cranial penetration by the wooden stake could not be exactly determined preoperatively, but from the history, physical findings, and x-ray pictures the intracranial damage was thought to be confined to the right frontal lobe. The frontal craniotomy offered excellent visability for removal of the foreign body, control of hemorrhage, débridement, and inspection of the carotid artery, paranasal sinuses, and dura overlying the orbit.

It was gratifying to find that the cavernous sinus and carotid artery had not been injured. In addition to the immediate devastating effect of rupture of these structures, unrecognized trauma often results in a lethal delayed intracranial hemorrhage.[7]

The possibility of ventricular perforation also had to be ruled out and, had the ventricle been entered, the problem of ventricular-system obstruction from necrotic brain tissue, foreign body, or hematoma would have been added to those already present. If the ventricle had been entered, the prognosis would perhaps not have been significantly changed, as Haynes[8] reported excellent results following transventricular wounds of the brain with early operation, meticulous removal of foreign bodies, necrotic brain tissue, and absolute hemostasis.

The roof of the orbit might have been reconstructed at the primary operation using a perforated tantalum plate or an iliac bone graft; however, in this particular case since there was gross contamination and severe tissue trauma it was thought too hazardous. If the orbital roof could have been repaired primarily it would have simplified subsequent ocular prosthetic insertion.

Of the many postoperative complications which follow cranial wounds of this nature, infection is the most frequent. Of 354 brain wounds treated by Cairns and Calvert[9] during World War II, 14 per cent showed major infections (abscess, meningitis, or both together) after débridement, primary closure, and chemotherapy. Approximately one-third of the patients with infection died.

The late effects of severe cerebral injury result from scar tissue formation and atrophy of the brain. Russell[10] studying 200 patients with cerebral wounds found that 32 (16 per cent) suffered from generalized convulsions after leaving the hospital. Over three-fourths of those who developed major epilepsy have fits at infrequent intervals and should have no great difficulty in obtaining suitable employment. Of those who develop fits, 70 per cent will probably have the first convulsion within eighteen months. Our patient is now sixteen months postoperative and has not as yet experienced an epileptic seizure.

With early definitive surgical treatment and the use of antibiotic drugs, the prognosis in orbitocranial wounds is good.

SUMMARY

1. An unusual case of a transorbitocranial wooden foreign body is presented, and the problems and principles of treatment of such lesions are reviewed.

2. Orbitocranial wounds should be operated upon as soon as circumstances will permit a complete primary surgical procedure.

3. Postoperative complications and sequelae are discussed.

REFERENCES

1. Schorstein, J.: Gunshot Wounds of the Fronto-orbital Region, Lancet **1:** 44, 1944.
2. McKenzie, D.: Head Injuries Involving Air Sinuses, Brit. M. J. **1:** 652, 1944.
3. Webster, J. E., and Gurdjian, E. S.: Penetrating Cranial Wounds—A Summary of Methods Used in Management—Collective Review—Internat. Abstr. Surg. **82:** 353, 1946.
4. Calvert, C. A.: Orbito-Facio-Cranial Gunshot Wounds, Brit. J. Surg. (War Surg. Supp. no. 1) p. 119, 1947.
5. Dandy, W. E.: Prechiasmal Intracranial Tumors of the Optic Nerves, Am. J. Ophth. **5:** 169, 1922.
6. Stewart, O. W., and Botterell, E. H.: Cranio-Facial-Orbital Wounds Involving Paranasal Sinuses—Primary Definitive Surgical Treatment, Brit. J. Surg. (War Surg. Supp. no. 1) p. 112, 1947.
7. Schorstein, J.: Intracranial Hematoma in Missile Wounds, Brit. J. Surg. (War Surg. Supp. no. 1) p. 96, 1947.
8. Haynes, W. G.: Transventricular Wounds of the Brain, J. Neurosurg. **2:** 463, 1945.
9. Cairns, H., Calvert, P. D., and Northcraft, G. B.: Complications of Head Wounds, With Especial Reference to Infection, Brit. J. Surg. (War Surg. Supp. no. 1) p. 198, 1947.
10. Russell, W. R.: Rehabilitation After Gunshot Wounds of the Brain, Brit. J. Surg. (War Surg. Supp. no. 1) p. 252, 1947.

CONGENITAL DUODENAL DIAPHRAGM

Report of Two Cases

Alexander H. Bill, Jr., M.D., and William M. Pope, M.D.,
Seattle, Wash.

(From the Department of Surgery, School of Medicine, University of Washington, and the Children's Orthopedic Hospital)

When one must deal with an obstruction of the duodenum in an infant, one thinks of the possible causes of such an obstruction as lying either outside or inside the bowel.

The conditions causing obstruction of the duodenum from outside the bowel include most frequently bands from an incompletely rotated cecum or else the presence of an annular pancreas. The most frequent causes of obstruction inside the duodenum are complete atresia and, more rarely, a duodenal diaphragm.

The lesions outside the duodenum can be readily recognized at surgery, and corrected without opening the duodenum. The lesions inside the duodenum, however, cannot be fully identified and differentiated without opening the bowel.

The following two patients proved to have duodenal diaphragms. They are reported on to illustrate the pitfalls which may be encountered and, in the second case, a surgical approach which we believe will be satisfactory in most instances.

A duodenal diaphragm is a septum partially or completely obstructing the bowel lumen. It is covered on both sides with intestinal epithelium, and is usually only a few millimeters thick. When a stoma is present, it may be small or large. Such a diaphragm may be redundant and may prolapse several inches into the adjacent intestine, as it did in one of our cases. A diaphragm may be found anywhere in the duodenum, from the pylorus to the jejunum, and at times multiple diaphragms are present. On occasion, the bile ducts go through the body of the diaphragm and open on either the upper or lower surface.

Case 1.—R. R. B., a 5-day-old boy, was admitted to the Children's Orthopedic Hospital on Nov. 22, 1950, because of persistent vomiting and upper abdominal distention since birth. X-ray pictures (Fig. 2) taken on the day of admission showed two large gas bubbles interpreted to be in the stomach and duodenum, respectively.

On the day of admision, a laparotomy was performed. At operation, a dilatation of the duodenum ending at the ligament of Treitz was found. What appeared to be an extrinsic band of peritoneum was divided, and gas was observed to proceed down through the previous area of obstruction.

Postoperatively the obstruction was unimproved. The infant was again explored on the tenth hospital day. At this operation, what were believed to be either residual or

Received for publication, April 20, 1953.

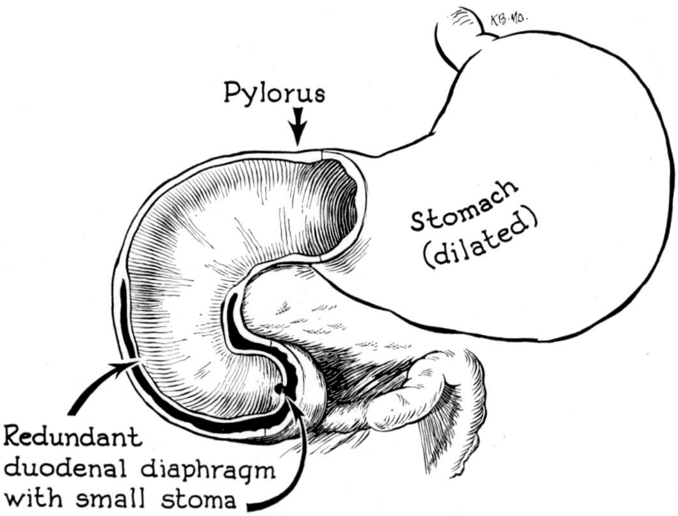

Fig. 1.—Diagram of pathology found in Case 1. The diagram shows a redundant duodenal diaphragm, the nature of which could not be ascertained from outside the bowel.

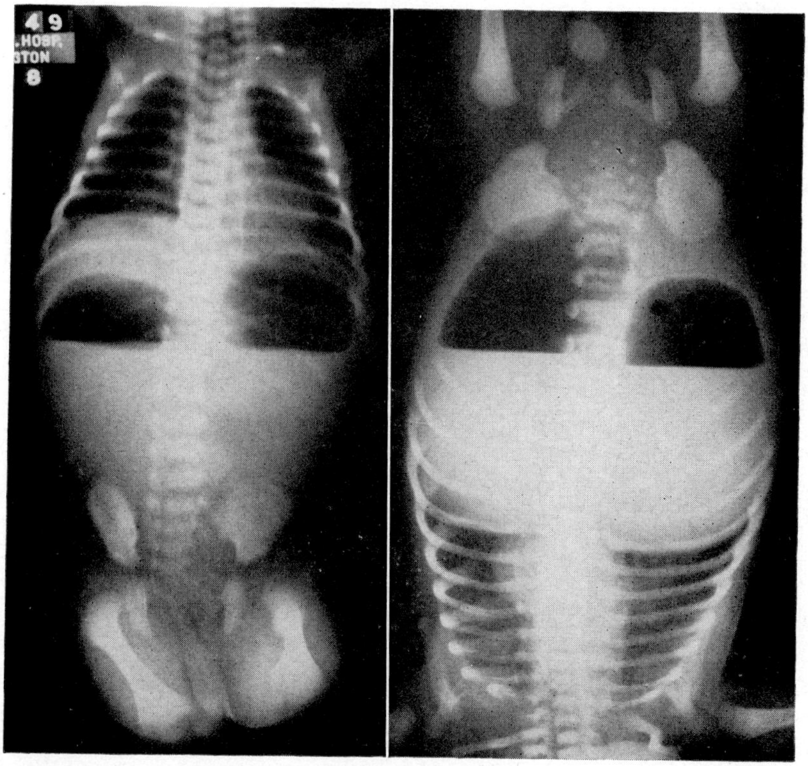

A. *B.*

Fig. 2.—*A*, Supine film of Case 1 shows obstructive dilatation which could be entirely stomach; however, *B*, an anteroposterior film with infant inverted demonstrates the pylorus and proves that there is also dilatation in the proximal duodenum.

postoperative adhesions were further divided, and again an apparently satisfactory lumen was left through which gas was seen to pass.

The infant continued to do poorly and was explored a third time on the twenty-fourth hospital day. At this time the obstruction seemed to be in approximately the same place, and a duodenotomy was performed in a longitudinal direction. The duodenum was explored proximally for the length of an instrument without any obstruction being felt, and the incision was then sutured transversely. On the following day the infant died.

At autopsy, a redundant duodenal diaphragm was found, shaped like an aviation "wind-sock." At its apex was a tiny aperture which permitted a small amount of gas to go through at the exploratory operations. At the third operation, the diaphragm had evidently been displaced upward by the exploring instrument until its apex was at or above the level of the pylorus.

The ampulla of Vater opened directly into the substance of the diaphragm with a stoma both above and below. Other findings at autopsy included an area of localized peritonitis at the site of the duodenotomy and generalized edema.

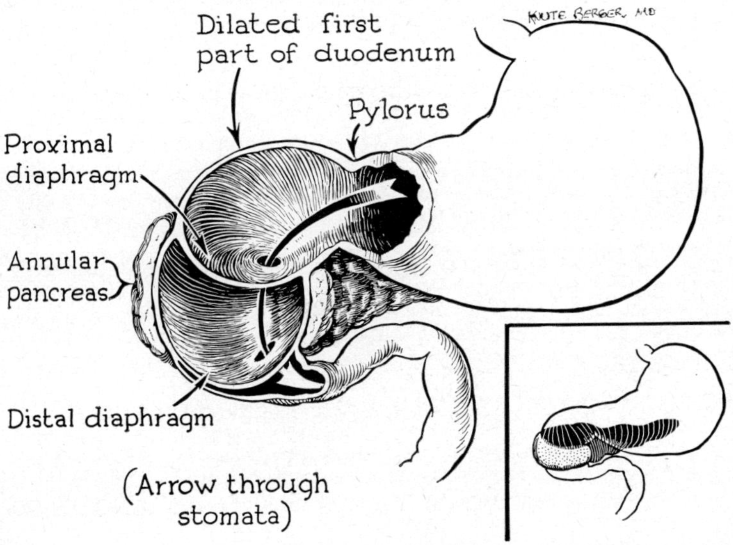

Fig. 3.—Diagrammatic representation of pathology found in Case 2, including the two incomplete duodenal diaphragms and the annular pancreas.

CASE 2.—C. L. R. was admitted to the Children's Orthopedic Hospital on Jan. 4, 1952. This 15-month-old girl was referred to the Hospital because of intermittent vomiting since birth. The vomitus consisted of feedings without bile. The infant was put on a formula five days after birth because of the vomiting, having been on mother's milk prior to this. She regained her birth weight of eight pounds in two months. She remained somewhat undernourished but developed fairly normally. The vomiting of part of her feedings continued almost daily, usually in the early evening. The infant was also constipated much of the time, requiring frequent enemas. During the two months prior to admission, she had had two abdominal explorations at another hospital. There had been no improvement in symptoms following either operation.

Examination revealed a female infant appearing normal except for slight undernourishment and a moderate distention of the upper abdomen. The physical examination was otherwise normal.

Roentgenologic examination of the upper gastrointestinal tract (Fig. 4) demonstrated the stomach to be markedly dilated with considerable gas and fluid. There was incompetency of the pyloric valve with rapid flow of barium between the dilated stomach and the proximal duodenum, which was extremely dilated secondary to the marked contriction in the mid-descending duodenum. Because of stasis and moderate dilation in the horizontal, or third portion, of the duodenum, a second point of obstruction near the ligament of Treitz was suggested.

The jejunum was small in caliber due to functional disuse. Barium enema revealed the colon to show no evidence of malrotation.

The child continued to vomit part of her feedings while under observation. She was operated upon on the fourth hospital day.

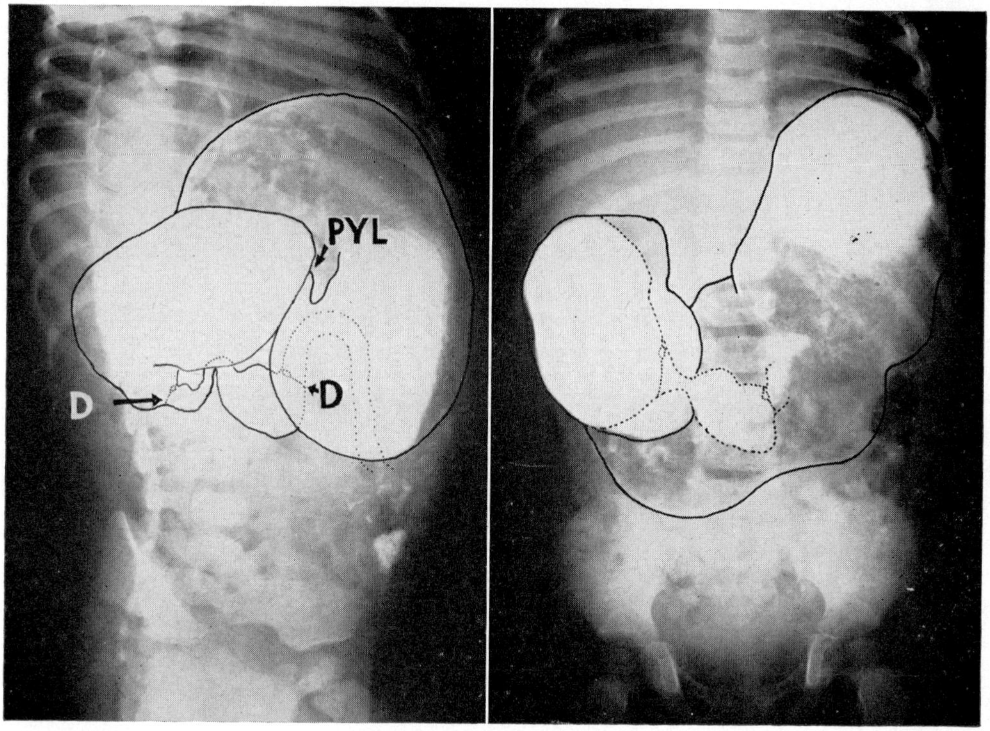

A. *B.*

Fig. 4.—*A*, Right anterior oblique film of Case 2 in the prone position reveals extreme enlargement of the duodenal cap and the tapering obstruction of the descending duodenum with stasis of barium in the horizontal third portion.

B, Anteroposterior supine film confirms the latter finding and also shows the moderate dilatation, with distention and obliteration of valvulae conniventes in transverse duodenum.

On opening of the abdomen, there was found to be marked dilation of the stomach and duodenum. Exploration of the small bowel below the ligament of Treitz showed relative collapse. Further exploration of the duodenum revealed a pancreatic ring which encircled the dilated descending portion of the duodenum without creating any constriction (as confirmed later when two fingers were easily inserted through the portion of the duodenal lumen which was surrounded by the pancreatic ring). The duodenum was opened in a longitudinal direction above the pancreas, and exploration inside revealed a diaphragm, extending slightly through the annular pancreatic channel, which had a small stoma on the lesser curvature side of the bowel. This stoma would admit only the end of a hemostat. The diaphragm was divided transversely with scissors. After division of this septum, a similar diaphragm was found about 2 cm. distally. This also was divided transversely in a lateral direction. After this, the operator's finger could be easily passed through the remainder of the duodenum and past the ligament of Treitz. The ampulla of Vater was never fully identified, but bile was present in the duodenum. The duodenum was closed with two layers of sutures, and an incidental appendectomy was performed. The child was given a transfusion of whole blood while on the table, and left the operating room in good condition.

Postoperatively she did well and was discharged on the eight postoperative day, taking a full diet. She was seen in the clinic five weeks later and had been eating well and had had no further vomiting.

Comment.—These two cases are presented to illustrate some of the pitfalls which may be found associated with cases of congenital duodenal obstruction. The first patient was operated upon three times by us, and a diagnosis was finally made at autopsy. The second patient was operated upon twice elsewhere and then once by us with final success.

We now feel that if an unexplained congenital duodenal obstruction is observed at operation, a duodenotomy should be performed above the site of obstruction. If a duodenal diaphragm is found, it may be divided. It should, of course, be divided in a radial direction with the line of incision going anteriorly or laterally in order to avoid the possibility of cutting across a bile duct in the body of the diaphragm. If, on the other hand, an atresia is demonstrated, a duodenojejunostomy may be performed using the exploratory incision in the duodenum for the proximal stoma of the anastomosis.

SUMMARY

Congenital duodenal diaphragms are defined. The difficulty in diagnosis, even at operation, is emphasized in two cases. A plan for surgical attack in cases of intrinsic congenital duodenal obstruction is suggested.

We wish to acknowledge the assistance of Dr. Byron Ward in interpreting the x-ray pictures and in selecting films for illustrations.

REFERENCES

1. Benson, C. D., and Coury, J. J.: Congenital Intrinsic Obtruction of the Stomach and Duodenum in the Newborn, Arch. Surg. **62:** 856 (June) 1951.
2. Forshall, I.: Duodenal Obstruction in the Newborn With a Description of Four Cases, Brit. J. Surg. **35:** 58 (July) 1947.
3. Krieg, E. G.: Duodenal Diaphragm, Ann. Surg. **106:** 33 (July) 1937.
4. Ladd, W. E., and Gross, R. E.: Abdominal Surgery of Infancy and Childhood, Philadelphia and London, 1941, W. B. Saunders Company.
5. Nelson, W. I.: Congenital Diaphragm of the Duodenum, Minnesota Med. **30:** 745 (July) 1947.
6. Saunders, J. B. deC. M., and Lindner, H. H.: Congenital Anomalies of the Duodenum, Ann. Surg. **112:** 321 (Sept.) 1940.

RUPTURE OF THE PREGNANT UTERUS DUE TO NONPENETRATING ABDOMINAL TRAUMA

Report of a Case

John N. McClure, Jr., M.D., Atlanta, Ga.

(From the Whitehead Department of Surgery, Emory University, and the Grady Memorial Hospital)

During the past several years, there have been numerous reports on the subject of abdominal wounds, both penetrating and nonpenetrating. Although rupture of the pregnant uterus as a result of nonpenetrating abdominal trauma remains a rarity, Lazard and Kliman[1] found forty-one cases in the literature up to 1936, added one of their own, and mentioned two others that occurred after their article was written. Several additional cases have been reported since their paper was published. The relative infrequency of this lesion, even in large city hospitals, is illustrated by the fact that Morrison and Douglass,[2] in a search of the combined records of the clinics of the University Hospital, Baltimore, from 1920 to 1943, and of the Baltimore City Hospital, from 1935 to 1943, were able to find only one case. Examination of the last ten years' records at the Grady Memorial Hospital failed to reveal a single case of ruptured pregnant uterus resulting from nonpenetrating abdominal trauma. Because of the rarity of such lesions, the following case is reported.

CASE REPORT

A 16-year-old, unmarried Negro girl was brought by ambulance to the emergency room of the Grady Memorial Hospital, July 29, 1951, soon after injury in an automobile accident. She had been riding in the back left side of the car with two other passengers on the same seat at the time the accident occurred, and she was rendered unconscious for a period thought to be approximately one to five minutes. Upon admission to the emergency room, however, the patient was alert and cooperative.

Past History.—Except for her statement that she had not menstruated during the preceding four months, the patient's past history was noncontributory.

Physical Examination.—The temperature was 98° F.; pulse, 104; respiration, 20; and blood pressure, 96/60. There was a clean laceration 4 cm. long through the scalp at the hairline of the forehead. The breasts were enlarged, firm, and slightly tender; their consistency was compatible with pregnancy. The abdomen was flat, with no abrasions or contusions of the skin. Slight tenderness and muscle spasm were present over the entire abdomen, but there was no rebound pain. The uterus was palpable approximately 6 cm. above the symphysis. Shifting dullness was absent; peristalsis was active with normal tone.

The external genitalia were normal. A small amount of chocolate-colored matter was found in the vagina. The cervix was small and soft, and the os was not dilated. On bimanual examination, the uterus was again palpated several centimeters above the symphysis. No blood or other abnormal conditions were found in the rectum. Digital examination of this area confirmed the findings of pregnancy obtained on vaginal examination.

Received for publication, April 21, 1953.

The right thigh was greatly enlarged and painful, with bone crepitus in the femur. Dorsalis pedis pulses were normal in both feet.

The other physical and neurological findings were within normal limits.

Roentgenograms of the skull were negative for fracture, but those of the right thigh revealed a transverse fracture in the mid-shaft of the femur.

Laboratory Examination.—A specimen of urine obtained by catheterization showed 2+ albumin. It was sugar-negative. Microscopic examination of an uncentrifuged sample disclosed seven to ten red blood cells per high-power field.

The admission diagnosis following these examinations was: (1) laceration of the scalp, (2) cerebral concussion, (3) transverse fracture of the mid-shaft of the right femur, (4) intrauterine pregnancy of approximately four months, with threatened abortion, and (5) possible ruptured intra-abdominal viscus. The patient was transferred to the surgical ward for further observation and treatment.

A Thomas splint with traction was applied to the right lower extremity. Five per cent dextrose in 1,000 c.c. of distilled water was given intravenously, and the blood pressure rose to 120/80, but the pulse remained around 104.

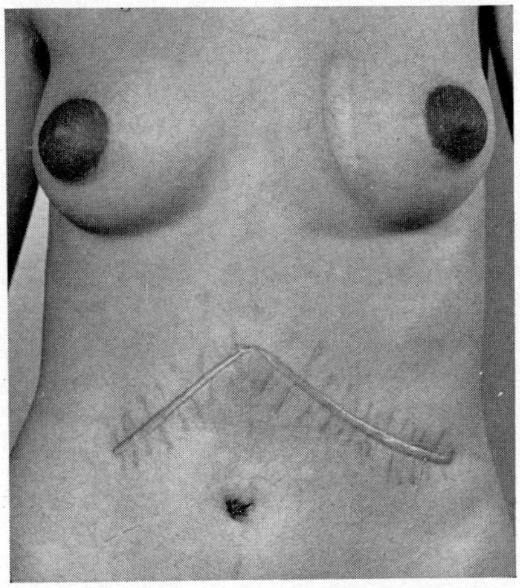

Fig. 1.—Photograph showing placement of the original incision in the left subcostal region. In order to obtain better exposure, this was extended downward across the right rectus muscle.

The next morning, the blood pressure was 114/70 and the pulse was 100. There was marked generalized tenderness and rebound pain in the abdomen, which was distended with free fluid. Peristalsis was present. The chocolate-colored vaginal discharge noted in the earlier examination had only slightly discolored one perineal pad during the night. Examination of the blood, fourteen hours after admission, showed the hemoglobin to be 8.3 Gm. per cent; the hematocrit, 28; and the white blood cell count, 9,800 with normal differentiation. The diagnosis of ruptured intra-abdominal viscus, probably spleen, liver, or uterus, was made, and the patient was prepared for laparotomy.

Operation.—Seventeen hours after admission to the hospital, a left subcostal incision was made under Pentothal Sodium with cyclopropane, ether, and oxygen anesthesia. When the peritoneal cavity was opened, there was a gush of blood, and approximately 600 c.c. of blood and clots was removed. The spleen and left lobe of the liver were carefully inspected, but no bleeding points were found. The operator's hand was then moved to the pelvis where the fetus and placenta were found lying free in the peritoneal cavity. To obtain better exposure, the original incision was angulated downward and extended across the right rectus muscle (Fig. 1). The uterus was elevated into the wound and isolated with warm, moist laparotomy pads. A 4 cm. laceration with irregular edges was present in the fundus of the uterus, adjacent to the right cornu (Fig. 2). The uterine cavity was filled with a clot, and blood oozed slowly from the wound. After removal of the clot, the rough edges of the wound were excised and two small arteries in the uterine wall were ligated with No. 00 chromic catgut. The wound was closed in two layers with continuous No. 0 chromic catgut. In the first layer, a simple suture was used to approximate the edges, and a continuous inverting mattress suture was employed in the second layer.

After all the blood was removed from the peritoneal cavity, the abdomen was closed without drainage in anatomic layers, using interrupted sutures of No. 00 surgical silk, except for the skin, where No. 000 silk was employed.

The operation was completed in one hour, twenty minutes. The patient received 1,000 c.c. of cross-matched blood during the procedure, and at no time did the blood pressure fall to shock level. She was returned to the ward in excellent condition.

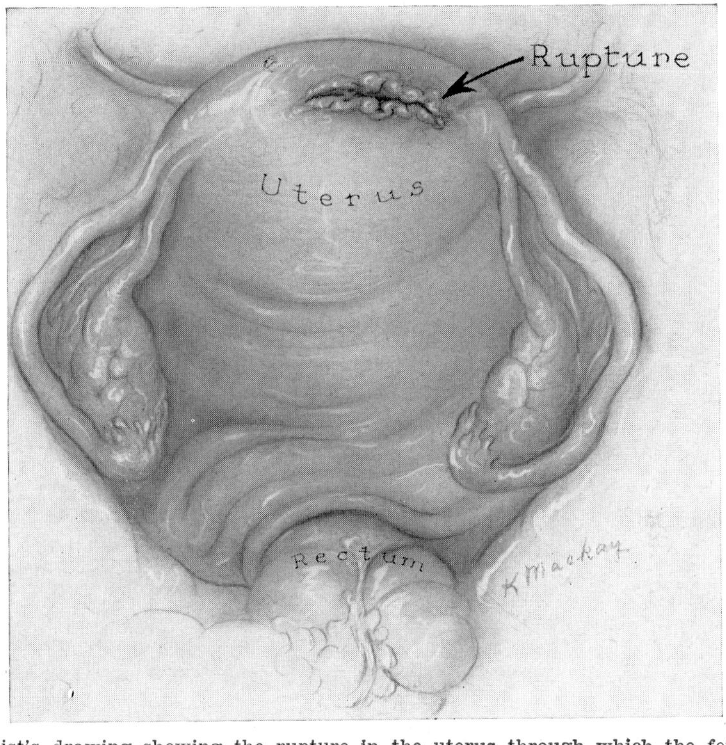

Fig. 2.—Artist's drawing showing the rupture in the uterus through which the fetus and the placenta were extruded.

Postoperative Course.—Nasogastric suction was continued for twenty-four hours, and the patient was then advanced on a diet.

The pathology report was a fetus consistent with menstrual age of eighteen weeks and immature placental tissue.

The right lower extremity was left in a Thomas splint until the eighth postoperative day, at which time the fractured femur was fixed with an intramedullary nail (Kuntscher) under spinal anesthesia. The postoperative course was again uneventful, and the patient began walking on crutches five days after the second operation and thirteen days after the first. She was discharged from the hospital on the twenty-third day.

The patient was followed in the surgery and orthopedic outpatient clinics for twelve months. No complications occurred, and menses returned normally eight weeks after repair of the uterus. There has been excellent bony healing of the femur.

DISCUSSION

According to DeLee and Greenhill,[3] "a healthy uterus will tear only under the most violent indirect injury." With the steadily increasing number of automobile accidents each year, it is surprising, as Woodhull[4] pointed out, that the condition is not reported more frequently. Doubtless many more cases occur than are described in the literature.

The diagnosis should certainly be suspected in any pregnant woman who has been in an automobile accident, or received other trauma to the abdomen, despite the lack of gross vaginal bleeding or the absence of severe prolonged shock. The case reported here is a notable example of this fact, and its management was made even more difficult by the presence of other injuries.

Repair of the uterus, rather than hysterectomy, was believed to be the operation of choice in this case, and the smooth postoperative course and uneventful recovery seem to justify this procedure.

Adequate exposure in this case was obtained by extending a left subcostal incision downward across the right rectus muscle.

REFERENCES

1. Lazard, E. M., and Kliman, F. E.: Traumatic Rupture of the Uterus in Advanced Pregnancy, California & West. Med. **45**: 482-485 (Dec.) 1936.
2. Morrison, J. H., and Douglass, L. H.: Rupture of the Uterus, Am. J. Obst. & Gynec. **50**: 330-335 (Sept.) 1945.
3. DeLee, J. B., and Greenhill, J. P.: Principles and Practice of Obstetrics, ed. 9, Philadelphia, 1947, W. B. Saunders Company.
4. Woodhull, R. B.: Traumatic Rupture of the Pregnant Uterus Resulting From an Automobile Accident, SURGERY 12: 615-620 (Oct.) 1942.

Editorial

The Mechanism of Action of Ergotamine in Hyperthyroidism

THE mechanism of action by which ergotamine prevents thyroid storms is based on an interrelationship of adrenalin and thyroxin. Brace and Reid,[2] in 1941, called attention to this relationship and to the great potentiating effect of adrenalin on thyroxin action. They mentioned Clark's[3] interesting pharmacologic experimental investigation, in which he found that adrenalin in a dilution of 1 in 10^8 (1 in one hundred million) gives characteristic and recognizable physiologic effects, and that similar effects can be produced by a dilution of 1 in 10^{16} (1 in ten thousand million million), if a like solution of thyroxin is used as well.

One sees here a tremendous potentiating effect of adrenalin on thyroxin. Reid poined out, however, that 1 c.c. of a solution in a dilution of 1 in 10^{16} (1 in ten thousand million million) will, in the case of adrenalin, contain 300,000 molecules, and in the case of thyroxin, 100,000 molecules. When these are distributed over the cells to be affected, only an extremely small percentage of the cell surface could receive even a monomolecular layer of the drug. This area of the cell where the drug is adsorbed is known as the pattern cell receptor, and this occupies one one-thousandth or less of the cell area.

The normal thyroxin-adrenalin relationship would be represented by one-half of the pattern cell receptor being occupied by adrenalin and one-half by thyroxin. In patients suffering from thyrotoxicosis, perhaps 75 per cent of the pattern cell area is occupied by thyroxin and 25 per cent by adrenalin, and the potentiating effect of the adrenalin on the thyroxin explains the patients' acute thyrotoxicosis. When ergotamine is given, it occupies the pattern cell receptor in place of the adrenalin, thereby diminishing the chances of a thyroid storm or acute thyrotoxicosis. The action of adrenalin is rather short-lived and probably does not exist beyond four to five minutes, while the effect of ergotamine probably lasts twenty to thirty minutes.

Thus, the mechanism of action of the ergotamine is its occupation of the pattern cell receptor with the thyroxin, blocking the adrenalin, which thereby loses its potentiating effect on the thyroxin. If ergotamine is given at the time of operation, it has immediate clinical effect in reducing the pulse rate of the patient anywhere from thirty to fifty beats within a five-minute period.

When the antithyroid effect of thiourea was demonstrated by the MacKenzies[4] and applied clinically with success by Astwood[1] and others, it was considered an agent that specifically inhibited the formation of the thyroid hormone. Reid,[5] in recent experimental observations on rats and mice, found that the effect of thiourea in these animals was due at least in part to the lowering of the oxygen consumption of all of the tissues with the exception of the myocardium. In other words, less thyroid hormone is formed with thiourea because the release of energy necessary for producing the hormone is restricted by interference with oxygen utilization.

This animal work, if it can be applied to human beings, would indicate that some patients, even though the metabolic rate has been reduced to normal, develop thyrotoxicosis postoperatively. Thus, they continue with a high pulse rate even though the metabolic rate has been appreciably reduced by thiourea. It is in these patients that ergotamine is particularly useful, as well as in those who do not respond satisfactorily to iodine therapy.

Ergotamine has been used during the past twelve years more than 150 times on patients with hyperthyroidism without any ill effects. Occasionally it is given for two to three days preoperatively in the dosage of 1 mg. three times daily. Just before anesthesia is begun, it can be used intravenously, giving ½ mg. and repeating this dose once, twice, or three times during the operative procedure if necessary. The clinical effects are most dramatic, and in many instances this has been a lifesaving measure in a critically ill patient.

—*J. William Hinton.*

REFERENCES

1. Astwood, E. B.: J. Pharmacol. & Exper. Therap. **78**: 79-89 (May) 1943; J. A. M. A. **122**: 78-81 (May 8) 1943.
2. Brace, D. E., and Reid, L. C.: Ann. Surg. **113**: 62-72 (Jan.) 1941.
3. Clark, A. J.: General Pharmacology, in Heffter, A.: Handbuch der experimentellen Pharmakologie, Berlin, 1937, Julius Springer, pp. 4, 22.
4. MacKenzie, C. J., and MacKenzie, J. B.: Endocrinology **32**: 185-209 (Feb.) 1943.
5. Reid, L. C.: Arch. f. experimentelle Path. u. Pharmakol. In press.

Recent Advances in Surgery

Conducted by Alfred Blalock, M.D.

TRAUMATIC RUPTURE OF THE NORMAL SPLEEN

Analysis of 28 Cases

Lawrence M. Knopp, M.D., and Henry N. Harkins, M.D., Seattle, Wash.

(From the Department of Surgery, University of Washington School of Medicine, and the Division of General Surgery, King County Hospital)

INTRODUCTION

TRAUMATIC injuries of the abdomen have always been among the most important surgical problems. In recent years, interest in these problems has assumed increasing importance because of, among other things, war and the rapid development of the automobile as a means of transportation. Both war wounds and the much more frequent wounds secondary to automobile accidents may produce serious subcutaneous abdominal injuries. Among these, injury to the spleen is said to be the most common. Wright and Prigot (1939) found that splenic injury accounted for 47.6 per cent of all subcutaneous injuries of the abdomen. These figures antedated World War II. In the same paper, splenic injury was reported to be present in one of each 666 accident cases admitted to Harlem Hospital to that date. Roettig and co-workers (1943) found that one of each 920 accident admissions to the Ohio State University Hospital had traumatic rupture of the spleen.

The first reported case of splenic rupture was that of Celsus in the fifteenth century A.D. (Blain, 1952). There were about 500 reported cases of ruptured spleen in the literature by 1923, and over 1,000 cases reported by 1950 (Blain, 1952). There can be no question that the increase in number of reported cases represents, in part, an increase in diagnostic techniques and acumen. There can also be no doubt that the increase in trauma of all types secondary to our modern way of life has contributed in large measure to the growth of reported cases of ruptured spleen in the literature. Zabinski and Harkins (1943) stated that trauma accounts for rupture of the normal spleen in almost every case, and in this matter they are in agreement with most authors on this subject.

In this paper, 28 cases of rupture of the normal spleen are analyzed with these ends in view: (1) to state the experience with such cases in the King County Hospital, Seattle, with particular reference to diagnostic criteria and diagnostic aids, and (2) to present a summary of methods of treatment used in this hospital. The cases reviewed occurred between the years 1938 and

Received for publication, July 14, 1953.

1951, inclusive, and all cases are in either Class 3 or Class 4, according to the classification of Harkins and Zabinski (1943), that is, traumatic rupture of the normal spleen or delayed rupture of the normal spleen (Table I).

TABLE I. CLASSIFICATION OF RUPTURE OF THE SPLEEN (HARKINS AND ZABINSKI, 1943)

CLASS	TYPE OF RUPTURE
1	Spontaneous rupture of the normal spleen
2	Spontaneous rupture of the diseased spleen
3	Traumatic rupture of the normal spleen
4	Delayed rupture of the normal spleen
5	Delayed rupture of the diseased spleen
6	Traumatic rupture of the diseased spleen

ANALYSIS OF CLINICAL MATERIAL

Age Incidence.—Among 28 cases of ruptured spleen reviewed, 20 (71.4 per cent) occurred in patients between the ages of 1 and 30 years. These 20 cases were distributed as follows: 5 in the first decade, 7 in the second, and 8 in the third. No ruptured spleens were detected in patients under 7 years of age. The remaining 8 patients were distributed as follows: 1 was under 30 years, 5 were between 31 and 50 years old, and there was 1 case each in the seventh and eighth decades. The oldest patient in our series was a woman, aged 79 years (Table II).

TABLE II. AGE INCIDENCE (YEARS)

AGE (YR.)	NUMBER OF PATIENTS
1-10	5
11-20	7
21-30	8
31-40	1
41-50	3
51-60	2
61-70	1
71-80	1

Sex Incidence.—The male-female ratio in this series was 1.8 to 1. Consideration of the sex incidence by age groups (Table III) shows that female patients predominated between the ages of 1 to 20 years, and 51 to 80 years, respectively, although male patients constituted 64.4 per cent of the total number. Between the ages of 21 and 50 years, there were 12 men and no women.

TABLE III. SEX INCIDENCE BY AGE GROUPS

AGE (YR.)	SEX	
	MALE	FEMALE
1-20	5	7
21-50	12	0
51-80	1	3
Totals	18	10

Trauma.—Twenty-six patients gave a history of trauma. One of the remaining two patients experienced the onset of symptoms while swimming, and the other could give no contributing history at all.

Automobile accidents accounted for 10 patients, of whom 7 were passengers and 3 were pedestrians. Falls contributed 8 cases to the total number. The shortest recorded fall was eight feet, while the longest was sustained by a patient who drove a truck off the fifth floor of a multilevel garage. Four patients received injuries which to them appeared to be trifling, tripping or stumbling against an unyielding object. One patient sustained a blow from a falling tree trunk. Bullet wounds of the upper abdomen were present in 3 patients (Table IV).

TABLE IV. TYPE OF TRAUMA PRODUCING SPLENIC RUPTURE

Automobile accidents	10
Falls	8
Blows	5
Bullet wounds	3

Symptomatology.—Two patients were comatose upon admission and were unable to relate a history. Three additional patients entered the King County Hospital at a time when the house staff was inadequate in number, and the charts of these patients are lacking in certain essential clinical details.

Of the 23 patients with well-documented histories, 16 (69.6 per cent) complained of generalized abdominal pain, while 7 (30.4 per cent) complained of left upper quadrant pain. Vomiting was noted one or more times in each of 7 patients (30.4 per cent). Kehr's sign (pain in the left shoulder) was noted in only 4 patients (17.4 per cent). Other symptoms recorded only once each in separate patients were pain in both shoulders, inspiratory pain, pain in the left upper abdominal quadrant, and dizziness.

Signs.—Generalized abdominal rigidity was present in 22 patients (78.6 per cent), and shock and generalized abdominal tenderness had the same frequency, each being present in 18 cases (64.4 per cent). Seventeen patients had visible evidence of trauma (60.7 per cent). Pallor was noted in 14 cases (50 per cent), and hypoactive or absent bowel sounds were found in each of 13 patients (46.4 per cent). Twelve patients (42.8 per cent) had left upper quadrant tenderness. Although dullness in one or both flanks was noted in 9 cases, and left upper quadrant swelling in 5 cases, there were five charts in which this information did not appear as either a positive or negative finding. Other low frequency signs were: left upper quadrant rigidity (5 cases) and abdominal distention (3 cases). Two patients were comatose secondary to head injury rather than to acute blood loss resulting from a ruptured spleen (Table V).

Associated Injuries.—Eighteen patients had other injuries in addition to rupture of the spleen. Fractured extremities were present in 6 cases, fractured ribs in 5 cases, craniocerebral injury in 5 cases, and lacerated kidney and traumatic paraplegia (1 each).

Onset of Abdominal Complaints.—McIndoe (1932) established forty-eight hours as the dividing line between acute and delayed ruptures of the spleen. The latent period is that time between injury and the onset of the signs and symptoms produced by splenic hemorrhage. In 18 of our 28 cases (64.4 per cent) there was no latent period. Two patients had a latent period of less than four hours, and two additional patients, of less than sixteen hours. Two patients represented true delayed ruptures of the spleen according to the criteria of McIndoe, having latent periods of forty-eight and seventy-six hours, respectively. No abdominal complaints were present in 4 patients. Thus, 92.8 per cent of patients of our total series had acute traumatic rupture of the spleen (Table VI).

TABLE V. PHYSICAL SIGNS

Generalized abdominal rigidity	22
Shock	18
Generalized abdominal tenderness	18
Visible evidence of trauma	17
Pallor	14
Absent or diminished bowel sounds	13
Left upper quadrant tenderness	12
Flank dullness	9
Left upper quadrant swelling	5
Left upper quadrant rigidity	5
Abdominal distention	3
Coma	2
Left upper quadrant dullness	1

TABLE VI. TIME OF ONSET OF ABDOMINAL COMPLAINTS*

Immediate	18
2-4 hours	2
4-8 hours	1
8-16 hours	1
$>$ 48 hours	2

*Four additional patients had no abdominal complaints.

Laboratory Aids.—The presence of anemia is of importance in the diagnosis of splenic rupture. In 18 of our 28 cases, anemia was found. There was moderate anemia in 10 of these 18 cases, and severe anemia in 8. Five patients had no anemia, and five additional patients had no admission red blood cell counts. Since some of our patients had hemoglobin determinations, others hematocrit determinations, and still others red blood cell count, but no patient all three, we established the following criteria as an estimate of the degree of anemia: severe anemia if the red blood cell count was less than 3,000,000, hemoglobin less than ten grams, or hematocrit less than 30 per cent; moderate anemia if the corresponding figures were, respectively, 4,000,000, twelve grams, or 40 per cent; and no anemia for figures above the latter.

White blood cell counts were taken in 19 cases. Three patients had less than 10,000, 11 had between 10,000 and 20,000, and 5 had a count greater than 20,000.

Urinalysis was not recorded for 10 patients. An additional 13 patients had hematuria, either gross or microscopic, while 10 patients had essentially normal urine.

The importance of abdominal roentgenograms in the diagnosis of splenic rupture has been stressed by Webb (1939), O'Neill and Rousseau (1945), and

Perisho and Steiner (1944). Webb reported the following changes in a typical case: (1) increased density in the left upper quadrant of the abdomen, (2) elevation of the left side of the diaphragm, (3) displacement of the stomach to the right side, (4) free fluid between intestinal loops. O'Neill and Rousseau added to these changes obliteration of the splenic shadow with serration of the greater curvature of the stomach. Only 4 of 25 patients in this series who received diagnostic roentgen studies of the abdomen had findings suggestive of splenic rupture according to these criteria. In each of these 4 cases, obliteration of the splenic shadow was noted, and in 2 the stomach was displaced to the right.

Evidence of free blood in the peritoneal cavity can often be determined by needle aspiration. This procedure was carried out in 8 of our cases, and revealed the presence of free blood in 6 cases.

Preoperative Diagnosis.—A correct diagnosis of splenic rupture was made in 19 cases. An additional 5 cases included rupture of the spleen in the differential diagnosis. The only incorrect diagnosis was pancreatic cyst, and for 3 patients the associated injury was diagnosed, but not the splenic rupture.

Results of Operation.—Twenty-three patients were operated upon, and 5 died shortly after admission to the hospital before the indications for surgery were clear. Splenectomy was performed in 21 patients, while 2 patients were treated by packing of the splenic fossa.

Eighteen patients recovered and 5 died, an operative mortality of 21.7 per cent. All five fatalities were among the patients treated by splenectomy. The average hospital stay was 20.5 days among the patients who recovered, and was somewhat less in those patients treated by splenectomy than in those treated by packing, averaging twenty days and twenty-four days, respectively (Table VII).

TABLE VII. RESULTS OF OPERATION

TYPE OF OPERATIVE TREATMENT	NUMBER OF CASES	RECOVERED	DIED	MORTALITY RATE (PER CENT)	AVERAGE HOSPITAL STAY (DAYS)
Splenectomy	21	16	5	23.8	20
Packing	2	2	0	0	24
Totals	23	18	5	21.7	20.5

Complications.—In our series, the following postoperative complications occurred: two wound infections, one subdiaphragmatic abscess, and one each of pleural effusion and pneumothorax. In both of the latter cases, the patient had fractured ribs.

DISCUSSION

The diagnosis of splenic rupture rests on the same basis as the diagnosis of any human ailment, namely, a good history and a good physical examination. In this syndrome, the laboratory is seen in its clearest light as an aid to and not a substitute for the clinical evaluation of the patient.

Certain features of the history should be emphasized when one is confronted with the differential diagnosis of splenic rupture. The age of the patient is of some interest. In the classic paper of McIndoe (1932), the age range was 8 to 63 years, but most of his patients were between the ages of 15 and 50 years. Zabinski and Harkins (1943) stated that the syndrome is most common in men during the third decade of life. The same age group predominated in the series of Roettig and associates (1943). Furthermore, it is generally agreed that men are affected more often than women, although the ratio varies. Thus, Zabinski and Harkins had a male to female ratio of 3.5 to 1, while Roettig and co-workers (1943) found a ratio of 10 to 1. In this series, the ratio was only 1.8 to 1. These data are perhaps made more clear when the male-female ratio is considered by age group. In this series, the ratio was reversed in the first two and the last three decades, while between the ages of 21 and 50 years there were no women. The preponderance of men in the middle age groups is explained by their traditional predominance in sports, heavy work, automobile driving, and activities in general. By the same token, youth and old age are much more democratic regarding these factors. Thus, women receive an equal or an increased number of splenic injuries during these periods of life.

The increasing pace of modern life, and particularly the higher horsepower automobile, is effecting a reversal in the types of trauma producing rupture of the spleen. Thus, both McIndoe (1932) and Zabinski and Harkins (1943) found that falls produced most cases, whereas Roettig and associates (1943) reported more than twice as many cases produced by automobile accidents as by falls. In spite of the number of cases in which severe trauma is sustained, the trauma may be so slight as to be considered negligible, as indeed it is in those patients who give no history of trauma at all.

Although rupture of the spleen may be present without clinical symptoms or signs (Perisho and Steiner, 1944), most patients do have symptomatology which will usually lead to a correct or a working diagnosis. McIndoe found two symptoms and signs in most cases: pain in the left upper abdominal quadrant and abdominal rigidity with left upper quadrant tenderness. These same findings, with the addition of shifting flank dullness and pain referred to the left shoulder (Kehr's sign), were cited by Blain (1952) as of outstanding importance. Roettig, Nusbaum, and Curtis (1943) stated that shock is a sign of high frequency, whereas Zabinski and Harkins found shock to be uncommon in their study of delayed rupture of the spleen. In our series, pain, either generalized abdominal or left upper quadrant, was present in most cases, and vomiting was often noted, although less common. Kehr's sign was decidedly uncommon. Most of the patients in our series had abdominal rigidity and tenderness, and were in shock. Pallor and hypoactive or absent bowel sounds were frequently noted, and well over one-half the patients had some visible evidence of trauma.

That the increased incidence of shock in our series was not mediated by delay in arrival at the hospital or in recognition of the acuteness of the emergency is made evident by the fact that the majority of the patients with acute ruptures who underwent surgery did so within five hours after trauma. The degree of shock and the number of abdominal findings appear to be in direct proportion to the degree of trauma sustained.

Zabinski and Harkins reported that delayed splenic rupture accounted for 14 per cent of all rupture of the spleen. One-half of these occurred by seven days, and an additional 25 per cent by the end of the second week. Delayed rupture was defined by McIndoe as occurring forty-eight hours or more after the initial injury. Bailey and Schreiber (1944) found an acute-delayed rupture ratio of 5.5 to 1, and Roettig and co-workers (1943) found a ratio of 10 to 1. In our series, the ratio was 13 to 1. Both of the patients in our series who had delayed splenic rupture considered their trauma negligible. The severity of trauma in automobile accidents may well lead to a decreased incidence of delayed rupture of the spleen, inasmuch as severe trauma is more likely to result in acute intra-abdominal injuries.

Leukocytosis and the anemia of hemorrhage have been discussed at length by Zabinski and Harkins (1943) and Blain (1952), among others. The importance of the complete blood count as an aid in the diagnosis of splenic rupture cannot be questioned.

Paracentesis has been recommended by Wright and Prigot (1939), who stress that it should be repeated if negative and the patient continues to show signs of internal bleeding. Only 8 of our patients had abdominal paracentesis, and free blood was obtained in 6 cases.

The most common associated injury reported by McIndoe (1932), Zabinski and Harkins (1943), Roettig and associates (1943), Waugh and Prior (1939), and Blain (1952) is fractured ribs. In our series, fractured extremities was a slightly more frequent coexistent injury, and craniocerebral injury had an equally high incidence.

The only treatment for a diagnosed case of splenic rupture is splenectomy, according to most authors. Hall (1951) stated that, of unoperated cases, 50 per cent die within one hour, and most within twenty-four hours. McIndoe had eight fatalities in 9 unoperated cases. Zabinski and Harkins cited a 77 to 100 per cent mortality in cases not treated surgically. Six of 7 patients in Roettig's series died without surgical treatment. The mortality rate with splenectomy is relatively low, as compared with the unoperated mortality rate. Bueerman (1943) stated that the operative mortality in reported series of cases was 33 per cent. McIndoe's operative mortality was 27 per cent, while Blain reported extremes of 15 to 25 per cent. Zabinski and Harkins had an operative mortality of 10 per cent, and Roettig and co-workers of 9 per cent. In our series the operative mortality was 21.7 per cent. Treatment by tamponade is mentioned only to state the opinion that it is not the treatment of choice, although both of the patients in our series who were so treated survived. It is uncertain insofar as control of bleeding is concerned, and in both our and Roettig's series, the morbidity is higher than in cases treated by splenectomy.

The higher mortality rate in this series is in direct proportion to the degree of trauma sustained. Although shock was an infrequent finding in the series of Zabinski and Harkins (1943) and Roettig and associates (1943), it was one of the more common findings in our series, and can well explain the higher operative mortality.

SUMMARY: "THE RUPTURED SPLEEN PATIENT"

The ruptured spleen patient is most commonly a man between the ages of 20 and 50 years. He has either been involved in an automobile accident or been injured in a fall, shortly before admission, although he may have sustained another type of blow to the left side of the abdomen. He complains of generalized abdominal pain, perhaps more severe in the left upper quadrant. He has vomited. He may have referred pain in the left shoulder. On physical examination, he is found to have generalized abdominal rigidity, and he is in shock. The abdomen is tender throughout, pallor is marked, and bowel sounds are hypoactive or absent. He dislikes palpation of the left upper quadrant. He has fractured ribs on the left side, and one or more extremities are fractured. Blood counts reveal anemia and leukocytosis, and there is likely to be blood in the urine. An abdominal paracentesis reveals free intraperitoneal blood. He is transfused and taken to surgery, where a ruptured spleen is removed. He responds well to surgery and will probably be discharged from the hospital in three weeks, having had an uneventful postoperative course.

REFERENCES

1. Bailey, H. A., and Schreiber, S. L.: Delayed Rupture of the Spleen, Am. J. Surg. **66**: 4-14 (Oct.) 1944.
2. Blain, A., III: The Diagnosis and Emergency Management of Ruptured Spleen, Alexander Blain Hosp. Bull. **11**: 19-29 (Feb.) 1952.
3. Bueerman, W. H.: The Latent Period and Delayed Hemorrhage Following Traumatic Rupture of the Spleen, U. S. Nav. M. Bull. **41**: 73-93 (Jan.) 1943.
4. Hall, D. P.: The Spleen, A Few Surgical Aspects, Ann. Surg. **17**: 376-390 (May) 1951.
5. Harkins, H. N., and Zabinski, E. J.: Traumatic Rupture of the Spleen, Am. J. Surg. **61**: 67-75 (July) 1943.
6. McIndoe, A. H.: Delayed Hemorrhage Following Traumatic Rupture of the Spleen, Brit. J. Surg. **20**: 249-268 (Oct.) 1932.
7. O'Neill, J. F.: and Rousseau, J. P.: Roentgenologic Examination of the Abdomen as an Aid in the Early Diagnosis of Splenic Injury, Ann. Surg. **121**: 111-119 (Jan.) 1945.
8. Perisho, G. M., and Steiner, M.: Traumatic Rupture of the Spleen, U. S. Nav. M. Bull. **43**: 216-222 (Aug.) 1944.
9. Roettig, L. C., Nusbaum, W. D., and Curtis, G. M.: Traumatic Rupture of the Spleen, Am. J. Surg. **59**: 292-319 (Feb.) 1943.
10. Waugh, R. L., and Prior, J. A.: Traumatic Rupture of the Spleen With Delayed Hemorrhage, SURGERY **14**: 125-133 (July) 1943.
11. Webb, R. C.: Traumatic Rupture of the Normal Spleen With Delayed Hemorrhage, Lancet **59**: 545-547 (Dec.) 1939.
12. Wright, L. T., and Prigot, A.: Traumatic Subcutaneous Rupture of the Normal Spleen, Arch. Surg. **39**: 551-576 (Oct.) 1939.
13. Zabinski, E. J., and Harkins, H. N.: Delayed Splenic Rupture: A Clinical Syndrome Following Trauma, Arch. Surg. **46**: 186-213 (Feb.) 1943.

Book Reviews

Das Klapp'sche Kriechverfahren. By Dr. B. Klapp. Pp. 70, with 115 illustrations. Georg Thieme Verlag, Agent for U. S. A.: Stuttgart, 1953, Grune & Stratton, Inc., New York, N. Y.

This small volume is written by the son of the originator of the Klapp crawling exercises. Presentation of the method is well done by means of numerous photographs. It describes in detail the corrective exercises for the development of the musculature of the back. It is of particular value to personnel of hospitals for crippled children and rehabilitation centers.

Surgery of Repair as Applied to Hand Injuries. By E. K. Rank and A. R. Wakefield. Baltimore, 1953, Williams & Wilkins Company. $8.00.

While most books on the surgery of the hand deal primarily with operative technique and methods of repair, there is a dearth of good material concerning the management of hand injuries, the timing of operations, and the planning of a program of reconstruction. This book fills this gap since it deals not with technique but with management. There is a thorough discussion of primary treatment, a section on intermediate treatment, and a final section on secondary treatment of hand injuries.

The authors write from a wide experience in civil and military surgery. Their experience is well documented with photographs and drawings. Emphasis is laid upon principles as illustrated by individual cases.

This is a very practical book for surgeons who encounter hand injuries. Its low price should make it available to surgical residents, for whom it has unusual value.

Gingivitis in Military Personnel With Special Reference to Ulceromembranous Gingivitis. By J. J. Pindborg. (Odontol. Tidskr., 1951, vol. 59, no. 6, pp. 405-499.)

The author reports on his examination of 9,659 male Danish recruits for the condition of their gingival tissues. He distinguishes between different forms of gingivitis, and conducts a statistical analysis of 4,503 case histories obtained in his examination. He relates the occurrence of gingivitis to seasonal influence, occupation, previous dental care, calculus, irregularity of teeth, consumption of tobacco, presence of third molars, and to the military service. There is an apparent significant correlation between gingivitis and presence of calculus and between the consumption of tobacco and the severity of ulceromembranous gingivitis. The incidence of ulceromembranous gingivitis is highest during the fall months.

These data may be of some interest to dental surgeons in the armed forces, public health officials, and research workers in the field of gingivitis epidemiology.

Orthopädische Konstruktionen. By Prof. Dr. Franz Schede. Pp. 98, with 141 illustrations. Stuttgart, 1953, Georg Thieme Verlag, Agent for U. S. A.: Grune & Stratton, Inc., New York, N. Y.

This book contains illustrations and discussions of equipment used in the treatment of orthopedic deformities. While some of the material will not appeal to American orthopedists, there are other parts which display great ingenuity and which could find wide acceptance in this country.

This book should be in the hands of surgeons directing the work of large orthopedic institutions. It has little to offer the surgeon engaged in the treatment of crippled children and the rehabilitation of adults.

The Surgery of Infancy and Childhood, Its Principles and Techniques. Edited by Robert E. Gross. Pp. 1,000. Philadelphia and London, 1953, W. B. Saunders Company.

Twelve years have elapsed since the predecessor of this splendid monograph appeared under the joint authorship of Dr. William E. Ladd and Dr. Robert E. Gross. New chapters of surgery have been opened up in the meantime, and suggestions of improvement in the results of surgery are very much in evidence in almost every chapter of the surgeon's interest.

The pediatric surgeon apparently deals with all areas of surgery except the brain and spinal cord, the eye, ear, and nose, and skeletal injuries and deformities. Apart from these areas of surgical interest, which by inference may be regarded as coming within the domain of the surgical specialist, the only field of surgery not covered in this monograph is plastic surgery. Yet, as is apparent from a perusal of this remarkable monograph, the pediatric surgeon deals with the formidable plastic problems of the alimentary and genitourinary tracts.

This book constitutes a significant contribution to the literature of the surgical management of congenital anomalies of the viscera. A study of this treatise makes it difficult to escape the impression that university clinics would do well to recognize pediatric surgery as a specialty. The results reported by Gross from the Children's Hospital in Boston in this important book could not be duplicated without the concentration of interest which Gross and his colleagues have lent *The Surgery of Infancy and Childhood.* That significant achievement warrants serious study and consideration by surgical groups everywhere. This magnificent monograph by Gross could be construed as a strong endorsement of the principle of pediatric surgery as a specialty.

ANNOUNCEMENT

American Goiter Association

The 1954 meeting of the American Goiter Association will be held at the Somerset Hotel, Boston, Mass., April 29 and 30 and May 1.

The program for the three-day meeting will consist of papers and discussions dealing with the physiology and diseases of the thyroid gland.

SURGERY

Vol. 35 April, 1954 No. 4

Original Communications

TRANSPARIETAL SPLENOPORTAL ROENTGENOGRAPHY AND RESEARCH ON PORTAL HYPERTENSION

Our Clinical Experience

A. M. Dogliotti, M.D.,* and S. Abeatici, M.D.,** Turin, Italy

PORTAL hypertension is the common denominator of several morbid processes, which differ from each other as to their site, etiology, and pathogenesis, although all are prone to cause some circulatory interference with the intrahepatic or extrahepatic portal vein or with any one of its roots. Therefore, the picture of portal hypertension does not form a well-defined nosologic unit, being only the symptomatic expression of a hemodynamic disorder consequent to the established venous obstruction. The pathoanatomic variety of all obstructive factors is reflected by a range of clinical features, all having the common background of portal stasis, but in varying degree, depending on the site, nature, and extension of the obstructive process and the capacity of a compensatory circulation. Thus one can see how serious cases, characterized by such dramatic features as digestive hemorrhage with splenomegaly and clear subcutaneous venous network, might fade away, through several steps, toward the latent or initial forms wherein a persistent meteorism or a moderate splenic tumor are the only revealing signs. Only with the aid of the diagnostic means we now have can we locate, with sufficient accuracy, the site of the portal lesion and appraise the degree of the circulatory alteration, even in those cases which are clinically silent, atypical, or monosymptomatic. It is generally agreed that a classification of the causes of the portal block should be worked out upon the basis of topographic principles; this seems to be justified to some extent by the variety of pathogenic, clinical, and therapeutic features. Thus, we have two major groups of obstructive factors: extrahepatic and intrahepatic. A more precise differentiation is given by pathoanatomic considerations, which allow us to divide the causes of the portal block according to the classification in Table I.

A morphologic study of all these obstructive factors and a sound evaluation of the consequent circulatory disorders can be safely carried out through a preoperative phleboroentgenographic examination of the portal system; this we

Received for publication, Aug. 20, 1953.
*Professor of Surgery and Director of the Surgical Clinic of the University of Turin.
**Assistant Professor of Surgery, University of Turin.

usually do following the method of "transparietal splenoportography," which was conceived and worked out in our School (Abeatici and Campi), and which is now commonly performed.

TABLE I

1. *Extrahepatic obstructive factors*		
(a) Congenital lesions	Stenosis	
	Angiomatosis of the smaller omentum	
	Cruveilhier-Baumgarten syndrome	
(b) Thrombosis		
(c) Compressions (by)	Inflammatory processes	Acute
		Chronic
	Benignant tumors	
	Malignant tumors	Primary
		Secondary
2. *Intrahepatic obstructive factors*		
(a) Congenital lesions		
(b) Infiltrations		
(c) Parenchymatous hepatitis	Acute	
	Subacute	
	Chronic	
(d) Biliary lesions (cholestatic fibrosis)		
(e) Circulatory lesions (hepatic stasis)		
(f) Focal lesions	Inflammatory	
	Parasitic	
(g) Neoplasms	Primary	
	Secondary	

Technique for Transparietal Splenoportography.—This technique is based on visualization of the portal system by means of a percutaneous injection of a radiopaque preparation into the splenic parenchyma. Experimental research, trials on corpses, and clinical experiences enabled us to establish some technical details which make this type of examination easier and quicker.

The splenic area being delimitated by percussion, we locate the ninth or tenth intercostal space; here, on the middle axillary line generally, we give a local novocaine anesthesia including the skin and underlying tissues. Then we perform the splenic puncture employing a needle 12 cm. (five inches) in length and 1.5 mm. (one-sixteenth of an inch) external gauge. The needle, having entered the peritoneal cavity, must be directed upward medially and backward; after a few centimeters we feel a soft elastic resistance, beyond which we continue further for from 4 to 5 cm. (about two inches). At this point, the mandrin being withdrawn from the needle, the dripping of the blood assures us of the right position. The radiopaque preparation, a 70 per cent solution of Joduron, may then be injected with a common 50 c.c. syringe; the quantity injected varies from 15 c.c. to 40 c.c. The injection must be performed very quickly and should never last more than three to four seconds; it is easily performed without any resistance. The introduction of the liquid is practically painless, so that we have abandoned general anesthesia, which we used in earlier cases (Fig. 1).

Also in order to get a functional evaluation of the portal system, we must have serial roentgenograms made according to the following chronological classification: One, two, three, five, eight, and eleven seconds after the beginning of the injection. The hemodynamic conditions of the splenoportal circulus can thus be determined with sufficient accuracy, since we have a graphic survey of changes of the opacifying time in different segments of the venous branching, and we are able to determine actual diffusion curves.

Fig. 1.

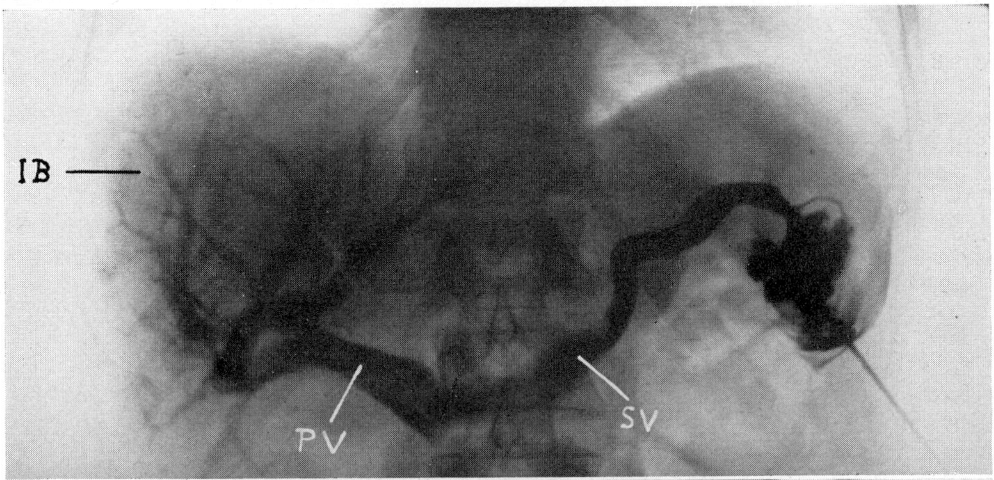

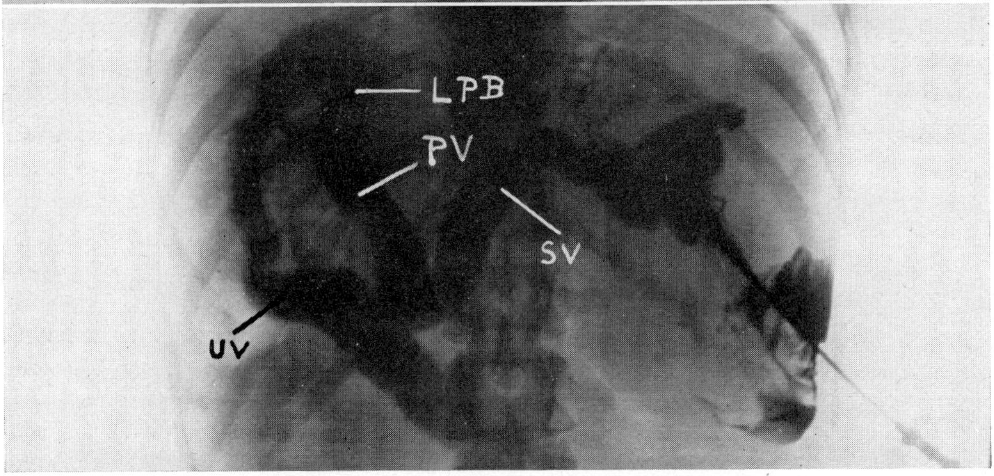

Fig. 2.

Fig. 1.—Normal splenoportal roentgenography. *SV*, Splenic vein; *PV*, portal vein; *IB*, intrahepatic branches.

Fig. 2.—Cruveilhier-Baumgarten syndrome. *SV*, Splenic vein; *PV*, portal vein; *LPB*, left portal branch; *UV*, umbilical vein.

Considerations of Some Cases of Portal Hypertension.—Both clinical and phleboroentgenographic examinations made in twenty-one cases of portal stasis (1952 to 1953) have given us new evidences of the multitude of obstructive factors and of the variety of nosologic features which seem to be bound to the nature of the morbid process, to the site of the portal block, and to the capacity of collateral circulation. The etiological features, which we happened to recognize in our patients, are thus far from constant, and not at all alike in all cases. Ascitic liquid, for instance, was present in twelve cases, and it is not easy to determine its origin. The supposition, put forward by Caroli, Paraf, and Schwarzmann, that the presence of ascitic liquid might be a consequence of insufficient natural portacaval connections seems to be rather fascinating, and sustained by findings on corpses; even our portographic researches seem to add more value to it; however, we think it needs a deeper study and further confirmation. We must bear in mind the parts played in the pathogenesis of the abdominal effusion by both hepatargy and protein unbalance.

Fig. 3.

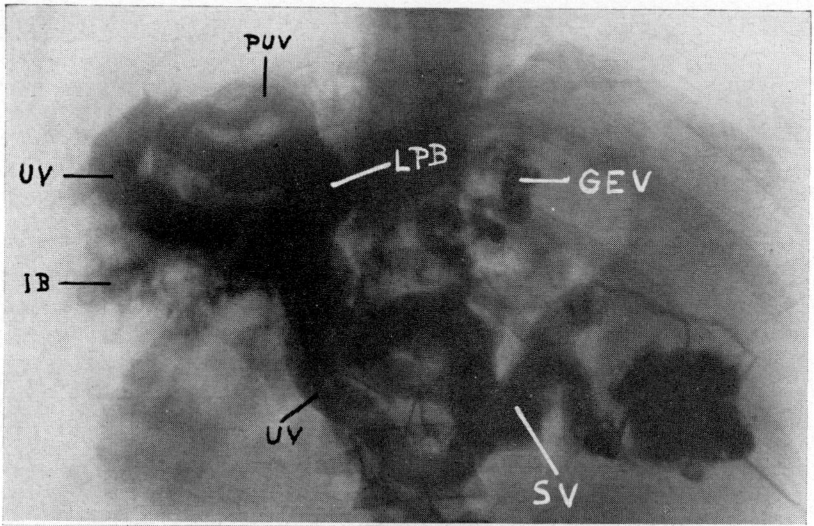

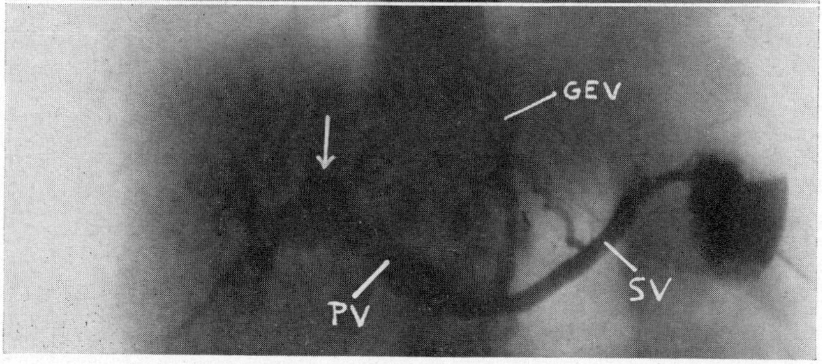

Fig. 4.

Fig. 3.—Cruveilhier-Baumgarten syndrome. *SV*, Splenic vein; *GEV*, gastroesophageal veins; *LPB*, left portal branch; *UV*, umbilical vein; *PUV*, paraumbilical vein; *IB*, intrahepatic branches.

Fig. 4.—Thrombosis of the left portal branch. *SV*, Splenic vein; *GEV*, gastroesophageal veins; PV, portal vein.

Gastroenteric hemorrhage, which is by far the most dramatic feature of portal hypertension, was seen in five cases of extrahepatic obstruction and in one case of intrahepatic obstruction. The pathogenesis of this type of hemorrhage, either in the form of hematemesis or in the form of melena, is normally ascribed to the breaking off of gastroesophageal phlebectasia. Notwithstanding the importance of portal stasis, the vascular fragility should never be underestimated nor should the concomitant alterations regarding prothrombinemia and the hematic proteins.

Fig. 5.

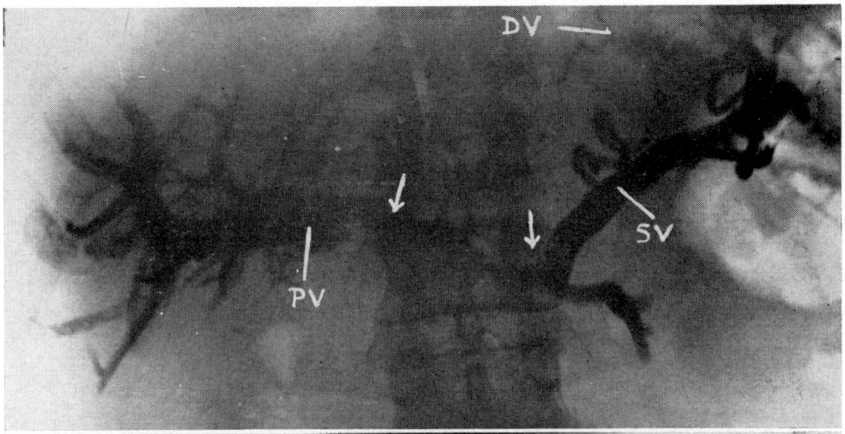

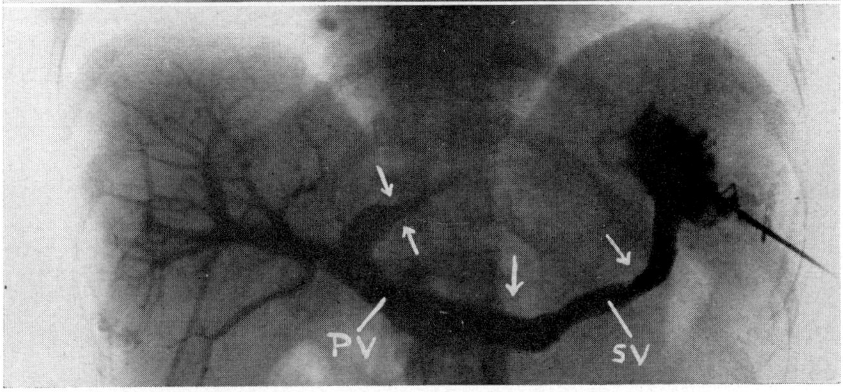

Fig. 6.

Fig. 5.—Pancreatic carcinoma. Compression of splenic vein. *DV*, Diaphragmatic veins; *SV*, splenic vein; *PV*, portal vein.

Fig. 6.—Pancreatic pseudocyst. Displacement of the splenic vein, compression of the left portal branch. *SV*, Splenic vein; *PV*, portal vein.

Another interesting feature of portal hypertension lies in the lienal behavior. We noticed that the size of this organ is likely to change widely from one case to the other, so that we had forms with a clear splenomegaly while in many other instances the size of the spleen was virtually normal or only slightly above average. This varying behavior of the spleen may be related to the greater or lesser availability of the compensatory collateral circulation, the latter depending on the site of the portal obstruction.

The multitude of factors involved in portal hypertension and the many individual variations of venous stasis are both directing the choice for surgical treatment toward eclecticism. The ideal therapeutic action should be represented by the complete removal of the venous obstruction. However, this can be done quite rarely, only in a few forms with extrahepatic compression or with suprahepatic stasis. More frequently, the surgical therapy must be directed only toward mitigating the existing hypertension either in the whole portal area or in a part of it. Such a palliative aim can be reached through a series of surgical interventions, ranging from simple splenectomy to the various types of portacaval venous anastomoses.

Fig. 7.

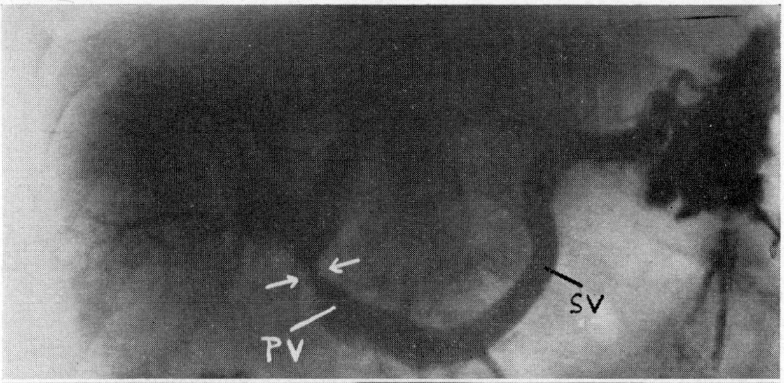

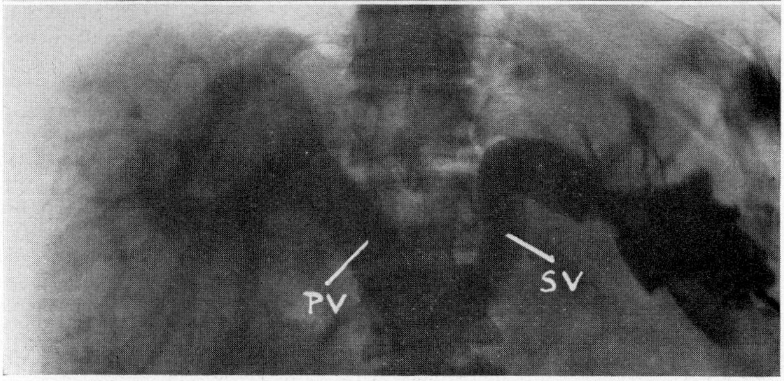

Fig. 8.

Fig. 7.—Lymphadenal metastasis of the hepatic hilus from ovarian carcinoma. Ring compression of the portal vein. *SV*, Splenic vein; *PV*, portal vein.

Fig. 8.—Hepatic fibrosis in multilobular liver. Reduction of the intrahepatic branching, missing opacification of the left lobe, displacement of the very short left portal branch. *SV*, Splenic vein; *PV*, portal vein.

Splenectomy, considered a minor therapeutic intervention in the treatment of portal stasis, is clearly advisable in cases where an obstruction can be found before the confluence of the lienal vein with the coronary vein (vena coronaria ventriculi); these are cases where hypertension is confined to a short portion of the lienal vein, so that it is clearly unnecessary to perform a shunt afterward.

A noticeable reduction of blood supply within the portal area can also be obtained by means of splenic artery ligature, thus producing a fall of one-third of the whole stream. Besides, the stagnant blood from the portal area is likely to flow back through the lienal veins which are left undamaged and to reach some collateral way through the already existing anastomosis. Ligature of the splenic artery is particularly recommended for depauperated patients who are bodily unable to suffer surgical interventions of greater importance; moreover, it is recommended in patients with congestive splenopathy and high pressure in the portal area where, for some reason or another, it is not possible to perform normal splenectomy and portacaval shunting.

Fig. 9.

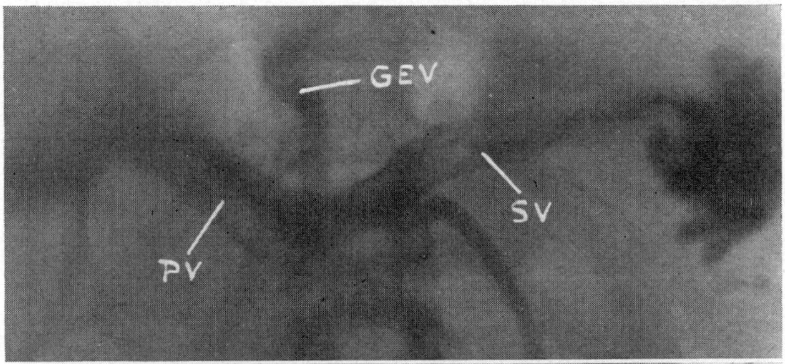

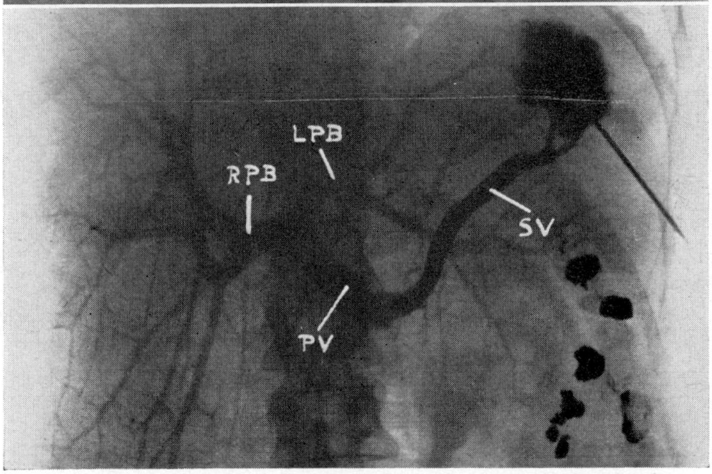

Fig. 10.

Fig. 9.—Hepatic fibrosis in multilobular liver. Splenoportal roentgenography three months later. *SV,* Splenic vein; *GEV,* gastroesophageal veins; *PV,* portal vein.

Fig. 10.—Hepatic steatosis: hepatomegalia, thinned intrahepatic branches. *SV,* Splenic vein; *PV,* portal vein; *RPB,* right portal branch; *LPB,* left portal branch.

Among the several surgical interventions devised to relieve portal stasis by creating new ways for the blood to discharge, portacaval anastomosis (and its variant, splenorenal anastomosis) offers the best therapeutic possibilities. Portacaval anastomosis produces an effective and long-lasting palliative action, especially in those cases where all important disturbances are related to the portal hypertension. This venous shunting is then likely to establish a wide drain to the flowing down of the stagnant blood, and the implied amendment to the circulation removes the serious danger of gastroesophageal hemorrhage which has, in these cases, a purely mechanical origin.

Indeed, our most satisfactory result was obtained by splenorenal shunt in a case of Cruveilhier-Baumgarten syndrome with repeated massive hemorrhages from esophageal varices and developed periumbilical venous network (Fig. 3). The patient had significant relief, and the lowering of the portal hypertension was evidenced by the stopping of the gastroesophageal hemorrhages and by the disappearance of the abdominal veins.

Fig. 11.

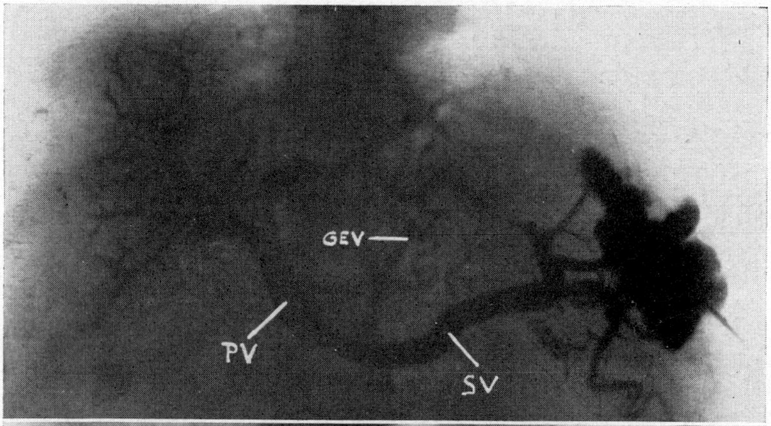

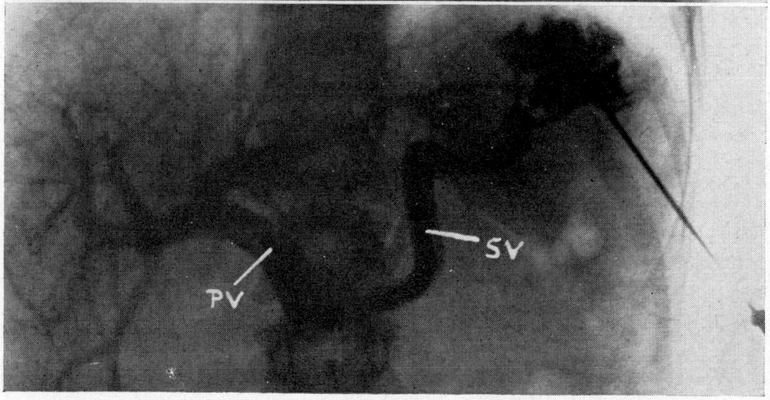

Fig. 12.

Fig. 11.—Atrophic cirrhosis: strong reduction and thinning of the intrahepatic branches. *SV*, Splenic vein; *GEV*, gastroesophageal veins; *PV*, portal vein.

Fig. 12.—Cholestatic fibrosis: hepatomegalia, reduction and thinning of the secondary intrahepatic branches. *SV*, Splenic vein; *PV*, portal vein.

Portacaval anastomosis is not to be recommended, on the contrary, in cases of intrahepatic obstruction and in cases of cirrhosis of the liver, where portal hypertension is a second-rate feature, the most important disturbances being related to the liver involvement, and the circulatory alterations being far more complex. Other interventions have been suggested for the treatment of cirrhosis; among them is ligature of the hepatic artery, founded on the assumption, merely theoretical, of an overturn of relationships between arterial circulation and portal circulation within the course of the pathologic process. Ligature of the hepatic artery would produce a reduction of the arterial pressure within the intrahepatic arterial branching, thus making easier the portal reflux. Besides, the ligature, being made at the origin of the hepatic artery, would promote a drop of the portal pressure, especially when associated with the similar ligature of the lienal artery. However, the method of action of the hepatic artery ligature has not yet been ascertained, nor have the theoretical foundations of this intervention been confirmed.

More practical seems to be the arterialization of the portal vein, as suggested by Paterni and as performed by Pettinari and associates, by means of anastomosis between the splenic artery and vein or between the splenic artery and portal vein. The arterial blood flowing in through the whole portal area produces an increase of the venous circulation, thus improving the oxygenation of the hepatic parenchyma; experimental data and early clinical results seem to support this possible way of improving the circulatory conditions of a diseased liver.

CONCLUSIONS

As a conclusion, we believe we can safely state that the surgical treatment of portal hypertension, being subordinate to the characteristics of the primary lesion and to the importance of circulatory stasis, always requires a thorough preoperative study of the circulatory conditions and a careful examination of the morphologic features of the venous branching in this area. A vague diagnosis of hypertension is not sufficient as a rule, the diverse nature of the morbid process and the different sites of the consequent obstruction giving way to several surgical problems. To the solution of these problems, transparietal portal roentgenography adds, in our opinion, an important and definite contribution. It enables the surgeon to determine, prior to intervention, the characteristics of the primary lesion, the importance of the hemodynamic disorder, and the possibilities for a compensatory circulation to the portal one. Therefore, we hope that this procedure may gain a wider clinical application.

REFERENCES

1. Abeatici, S., and Campi, L.: Sur les possibilités de l'angiographie hépatique. La visualisation du système portal, Acta radiol. **36**: 383, 1951.
2. Abeatici, S., Campi, L., and Ferrero, R.: Valore clinico ed indicazioni della splenoportografia transparietale, Minerva med. **43**: 1370, 1952.
3. Blakemore, A. H.: Indications for Portacaval Anastomosis, Surg., Gynec. & Obst. **84**: 645, 1947.
4. Blakemore, A. H.: Portacaval Anastomosis, Surg., Gynec. & Obst. **87**: 277, 1948.
5. Blakemore, A. H., and Lord, J. W.: The Technic of Using Vitallium Tubes in Establishing Porta-Caval Shunts for Portal Hypertension, Ann. Surg. **122**: 476, 1945.
6. Boulvin, R., Chevalier, M., Gallus, P., and Nagel, M.: La portographie par voie splénique transpariétale, Acta chir. belg. **50**: 534, 1951.
7. Brombart, M., Boulvin, R., and Chevalier, M.: Radiologie et hypertensions portales, Acta gastro-enterol. belg. **15**: 383, 1952.
8. Campi, L., and Abeatici, S.: La portographie par la voie splénique, J. sciences méd. de Lille **69**: 676, 1951.

9. Caroli, J., Paraf, A., and Schwarzmann, V.: Rôle de l'hypertension portale dans la pathogénie des ascites cirrhotiques; sa démonstration par la radiomanométrie portale, Semaine hôp. Paris **27**: 1761, 1951.
10. Dogliotti, A. M.: Ipertensione portale grave trattata mediante anastomosi spleno-renale: documentazione splenoportografica, Comunic. Soc. Piem. di Gastroent., Torino, XII: 15, 1952.
11. Leger, L., Albot, G., and Arvay, N.: La phlébographie portale dans l'exploration des affections hépato-spléniques, Presse méd. **59**: 1230, 1951.
12. Linton, R. L., Hardy, I. B., and Volwiler, W.: Porta-caval Shunts in Treatment of Portal Hypertension, Surg., Gynec. & Obst. **87**: 129, 1948.
13. Paterni, L.: Il disordine circolatorio nella cirrosi epatica e possibilita di nuovi metodi di terapia chirurgica, Policlinico (Sez. prat.) **56**: 253, 1949.
14. Pettinari, V.: Moderni indirizzi e realizzazioni nella terapia chirurgica della cirrosi epatica, Boll. e mem. Soc. Piem. Chir. **22**: 616, 1952.
15. Rousselot, L. M.: Combined Splenectomy and Portacaval Shunts in Portal Hypertension, J. A. M. A. **140**: 282, 1949.
16. Santy, P., and Marion, P.: Portographies per-opératoires pour syndrome de Banti, Presse méd. **59**: 221, 1951.
17. Scoville, A., and Leroux, G.: Réflexions sur la portographie par voie splénique transpariétale, Acta chir. belg. **51**: 193, 1952.
18. Sousa Pereira, A.: La méthode phlébographique dans l'étude des troubles de la circulation du système porte, Lyon chir. **46**: 291, 1951.

LYMPH NODE METASTASES: EXPERIENCE WITH AORTIC LIGATION OF INFERIOR MESENTERY ARTERY IN CANCER OF THE RECTUM

JACK W. MCELWAIN, M.S., M.D.,* HARRY E. BACON, M.D., AND HOWARD D. TRIMPI, M.D., PHILADELPHIA, PA.

(From the Department of Proctology of Temple University Medical School)

INTRODUCTION

SINCE Reybard[68] performed the first resection and anastomosis for cancer of the large bowel in 1832, surgeons have been striving to extend the scope of operations to combat this regrettable condition. With the ever-increasing knowledge of anesthesia, blood replacement, and sepsis control, more radical surgery is becoming possible. In order to utilize most effectively these recent advances in regard to the treatment of large bowel malignancy, certain anatomic and pathologic limitations must be understood.

Because extended surgical procedures for cancer of the colon, rectum, and anus are instituted in an effort to remove the dispersion routes of malignant cells as well as to extirpate the local growth, it is important for the colonic surgeon to know fully the methods and pathways of tumor dissemination. One of the most important routes of cancer spread is via the lymphatic system. Indeed, Moynihan[57] in 1908 stated that "the surgery of malignant disease is not the surgery of organs, it is the anatomy of the lymphatic system." There has been some monumental work on the lymphatic system in recent years, especially in regard to cancer of the distal colon and rectum. Most of these studies, however, have only embraced that section of the lymphatic pattern distal to the left colic branch of the inferior mesenteric artery.

Extended surgical procedures on the colon, rectum, and anus frequently involve ligation of large supplying vessels. There is little disagreement as to the safety of this course of action when large branches of the superior mesenteric artery are ligated, but some controversy still exists regarding the advisability of ligating the inferior mesenteric artery above its left colic branch when an attempt is being made to preserve the blood supply to the distal large bowel. Recent work by Ault[3] has stimulated renewed interest in this subject.

The purpose of this paper is to report the results found in the clearing of intramesenteric lymph nodes from 90 cases of cancer of the colon, rectum, and anus in which a ligation of the inferior mesenteric artery was performed at its aortic origin. No attempt has been made to study the extramesenteric lymph nodes, although a discussion of their importance will be made.

Received for publication, Aug. 3, 1953.

*Thesis submitted in partial fulfillment of requirements for the degree of M.S. in Proctology.

ARTERIAL BLOOD SUPPLY

The blood supply to the colon and rectum has been well demonstrated by many authors.[2, 22, 35, 38, 76] The left half of the transverse colon, the descending and sigmoid colons, and the upper rectum are supplied by the inferior mesenteric artery. It arises from the anterior surface of the aorta 3 to 4 cm. above the junction of the common iliac arteries. This is usually about 4 cm. below the duodenum, but in rare instances the origin may be directly behind that organ. As it crosses the left common iliac artery and continues into the pelvis, it is renamed the superior hemorrhoidal artery.

The first branch of the inferior mesenteric artery is the left colic, which originates 2 to 4 cm. from the aorta and courses beneath the peritoneum. Arising from the inferior mesenteric artery below the left colic are the sigmoidal branches. These vary from two to four in number and run beneath the peritoneum to supply the lower ascending and sigmoid colons. The superior hemorrhoidal artery divides into two branches at the third piece of the sacrum. These in turn redivide to supply the rectum.

Of particular interest to the surgeon performing a ligation of the inferior mesenteric artery at its aortic origin is the anastomotic potential of the marginal artery. This artery originates in the cecal arcades and courses along the entire large bowel to end in the sigmoidal arcades. It is located 1 to 8 cm. from the bowel wall, being somewhat nearer to it from the transverse colon to the rectum. Frequently it forms secondary arcades, but rarely tertiary. The only site where this artery may be inconstant is along the ascending colon where, in 5 per cent of cases, numerous separate branches terminate in the bowel.

Its function as a collateral blood channel between the two sides of the colon was questioned by Litten in 1875, who found that cutting the superior mesenteric artery in dogs led to gangrene due to poor anastomosis with the inferior mesenteric. In 1893, Morestin (as quoted by Archibald) ligated the inferior mesenteric artery without causing gangrene. This work was substantiated by Archibald,[2] who discovered that material could be injected into the superior mesenteric artery of cadavers and then be found in the superior hemorrhoidal vessels despite the ligation of all the branches of the inferior mesenteric artery some distance from the bowel. In 1907, Sudek,[77] being annoyed at the frequent failure of distal blood supply following perineal resections of the rectum, studied the various colonic anastomotic channels by injections and roentgenography and then defined his well-known "critical point." Sudek claimed that ligation of the superior hemorrhoidal artery distal to the last sigmoidal branch would not permit dye injected into the inferior mesenteric artery to flow into the upper rectal blood vessels. His original studies were not made in reference to the Miles procedure or to end-to-end resections. He concluded that perineal resections of the rectum should be supplemented by transabdominal ligation of the superior hemorrhoidal artery proximal to the last sigmoidal branch, which would have the added benefit of permitting more adequate mobilization of the bowel. This work was confirmed by Hartmann[44] in 1909. However, he placed the level of the ligation at the sacral promontory. In 1910, Rubesch,[70] while studying gangrene of the rectum after operations, stressed the importance of this artery near the bowel. In 1913, Drummond[22] ligated all the main arteries to the colon and reported that material injected into the ileocolic artery entered the sigmoidal vessels without interruption. It was he who most accurately described the location and course of the marginal artery which now rightfully bears his name.

Other authors have added a word of caution, however, about the indiscriminate ligation of large colic vessels. Manasse[48] felt that the marginal artery, although present in the sigmoid area, was weak, and communicated poorly with the last sigmoidal branch. Pope and Buie[63] have shown a varying pattern in the pelvic colon vessels, and pointed out the frequent paucity of anastomosis with the marginal artery. Desmarest[20] and Jamieson and Dobson[45] do not advocate the generalization that the marginal artery is infallible. Steward and Rankin[76] point out that care must be taken not to draw too many conclusions from cadaver studies alone, as the smooth muscle of fixed vessel walls often contracts. Others who rely moderately on the anastomotic function of the marginal artery are Pope and Judd,[64] Sunderland,[79] Bacon and Smith,[9] and Muir.[58]

LYMPHATIC DRAINAGE

The lymphatic drainage system of the large intestine originates in the mucosa, where tiny, blind-end lymph capillaries begin in the superficial epithelium. These pathways anastomose to form a subepithelial plexus, which in turn joins the more coarse tubules of the submucosa. Some of the primary lymphatics contain smooth muscle fibers which contract and milk the lymph toward the collecting channels. From the submucosa, the lymphatics course in a radial direction through the muscle coats to ramify in a subserous plexus. A few channels run for a short distance longitudinally between the circular and longitudinal muscle coats, but for the most part the initial direction of flow is in a radial direction. This is an important concept in approaching the problem of intramural spread of tumor cells. The flow of lymph is aided also by the presence of intermittent constrictions in the lymph channels which correspond to the valves of the venous system. Located in the subserous plexus of lymphatics are small lymph follicle aggregations called epicolic nodes by Jamieson and Dobson.[45] The lymph stream filters through these nodes and collects into larger channels which course into the para-colic nodes located about 1 cm. from the bowel wall. As the lymphatics embryologically bud from veins, it is not difficult to understand why the course of the lymphatic system parallels that of the vascular for the most part. From the paracolic glands, efferent lymph follows along ever-enlarging pathways to the intermediate nodes. These are fewer in number, and located at the branches of the large arteries such as the colic and superior hemorrhoidal vessels. Principal nodes are a fourth line of filtration found at the origin of the main large bowel arteries, such as the superior and inferior mesenteries. As a rule, the foregoing is the usual route taken by lymph. However, as reported by Rouvière[69] and more recently by State,[75] there may be skip patterns of drainage. Rouvière demonstrated that pathways from the hepatic flexure and especially the sigmoid colon may drain directly to the intermediate or principal nodes. Jamieson and Dobson[45] stated, however, that the paracolic nodes in the distal two-thirds of the transverse colon and the splenic flexure are never by-passed. When lymphatic blockage occurs because of tumor metastases, the lymphatic spread is from paracolic to paracolic nodes.

Colon.—The ileocecal region is rich in lymphatics. Many paracolic and intermediate nodes are also in existence, with large principal nodes occurring at the origin of the ileocecal artery. The ascending colon is less rich, but intermediate nodes can be demonstrated along the ascending and descending branches of the right colic artery. A principal node is present at the superior mesenteric angle. The transverse colon and the flexures are drained through several paracolic and intermediate nodes with large principal aggregations at the middle colic origin. The descending colon is poorly endowed with nodes except for a few paracolics and one or two intermediates. The sigmoid colon, however, subtends many lymph nodes. Epicolic lymph follicles are found in abundance in the appendices epiploicae. Large principal nodes exist at the origin of the inferior mesenteric and left colic vessels. Grinnell[42] has discovered as many as ten nodes in this angle, which has been called by some the "axilla of the abdomen."

Rectum.—The lymphatic anatomy of the rectum and anus does not follow completely the vascular pattern, and although many research workers have written extensively on the subject, some confusion still exists. There are three pedicles of spread as clarified by Sauer and Bacon[71]: superior, lateral, and inferior.

Superior pedicle: This pedicle contains more lymphatics than the other two and is the main drainage system of the rectum. The entire rectum and the anal canal are drained by this pedicle, which follows the distribution of the inferior mesenteric artery in the mesocolon. It is a constant system, for dye injected anywhere in the rectal or anal canal mucosa can be demonstrated in inferior mesenteric lymph nodes. Channels from the anus and rectum pass through the pararectal nodes of Gerota, which are from four to ten in number, and located above the levator muscles on the posterolateral rectal wall, to the intermediate nodes about the superior hemorrhoidal bifurcation. One large node situated directly in the angle of the bifurcation receives nearly all the lymphatic channels and, consequently, has been named the "principal node of the rectum." Effects from there travel along the superior hemorrhoidal artery to reach the principal nodes at the origin of the inferior mesenteric artery. These nodes are from five to ten in number, and lie in the superior angle to the left of the aorta. A few tracts follow the inferior mesenteric vein to the pancreaticoduodenal nodes higher in the abdomen. Rouvière[69] stated that a few lymphatic pathways from the low rectum may by-pass the pararectal nodes to enter the intermediate nodes, but that only a rare pathway will be found to extend directly from the rectum to the inferior mesenteric nodes. This was also noted by Villemin.[81]

Lateral pedicle: This pedicle, often called the middle, consists of four drainage patterns: the middle hemorrhoidal, the lateral sacral, the anterior, and the middle sacral.

The most important of these is the middle hemorrhoidal, which consists of paired groups of channels draining the distal 4 cm. of the rectum. These lymphatics rarely extend into the anal canal. They gather in one or two lymph nodes situated in the lateral rectal ligaments. These nodes may be located directly on the bowel wall or 1 to 2 cm. laterally. Efferents course laterally and cephalad in these ligaments beneath the superior wing of the endopelvic fascia to nodes along the internal iliac artery. An inconstant obturator lymph node may receive some channels. A few pathways may extend directly from the rectum to the iliac nodes. Proximal drainage then enters the nodes on either side of the aorta.

The second group of lateral pathways of spread is along the lateral sacral vessels. Lymphatics from the coccygeal area, anastomosing with those of the middle sacral, drain the distal 4 cm. of rectum and anal canal. They follow the anterior branches of the paired lateral sacral vessels along the hollow of the sacrum beneath the inferior wing of the endopelvic fascia to the internal iliac nodes and thence to the aorta. On occasion, large nodes may be found just distal and lateral to the promontory of the sacrum, receiving many of these channels.

A third group of channels classified as lateral spread is the anterior. Reinhold[67] in his thesis on pelvic lymphatics has described paired tracts draining the distal few centimeters of rectum which arch anteriorly in the layers of rectogenital septum ascending behind the rectourethralis muscle of Roux in the male and the rectovaginal septum in the female. The tracts course laterally over the upper portion of the rectogenital septum toward the internal iliac vessels, anastomosing in some instances with the middle hemorrhoidal lymphatics. The lower vaginal and prostatic lymphatics also may be joined by small numbers of anterior coursing lymphatics, according to Nesselrod.[59]

The fourth group of lymphatic channels composing the lateral mode of drainage is the middle sacral. These channels from the posterior 4 cm. of the rectum and anterior coccygeal area follow the course of the middle sacral artery to the aorta. One or two intercepting nodes are situated just below the sacral promontory.

There is no lateral lymphatic drainage demonstrable higher than 4 cm. above the anorectal line. This level corresponds to the usual location of the middle valve of Houston, 7 cm. from the anal verge. Early workers have called it the "plica transversalis of Kohlrausch," as related by De Oliveira.[19] The absence of lateral spread is abrupt at that level, as demonstrated by a failure of dye to appear in the lateral zones of spread when injection has been made just above. This level of the rectum, therefore, becomes surgically important in the treatment of rectal malignancies.

Inferior pedicle: The columns of Morgagni, the anal canal, and the perianal integument are drained along bilateral lymph channels which follow the course of the inferior hemorrhoidal artery. Pathways extend through the ischiorectal fossa to the internal iliac and aortic lymph nodes in some instances. A more frequent course of drainage, however, does not follow the vascular supply, but extends beneath the subcutaneous tissue of the buttocks and groin to empty into the superficial and thence the deep inguinal lymph nodes. Most tracts enter the superior and internal group of nodes. These pathways anastomose in the anal canal with the superior hemorrhoidal and to a lesser degree the middle hemorrhoidal lymphatics.

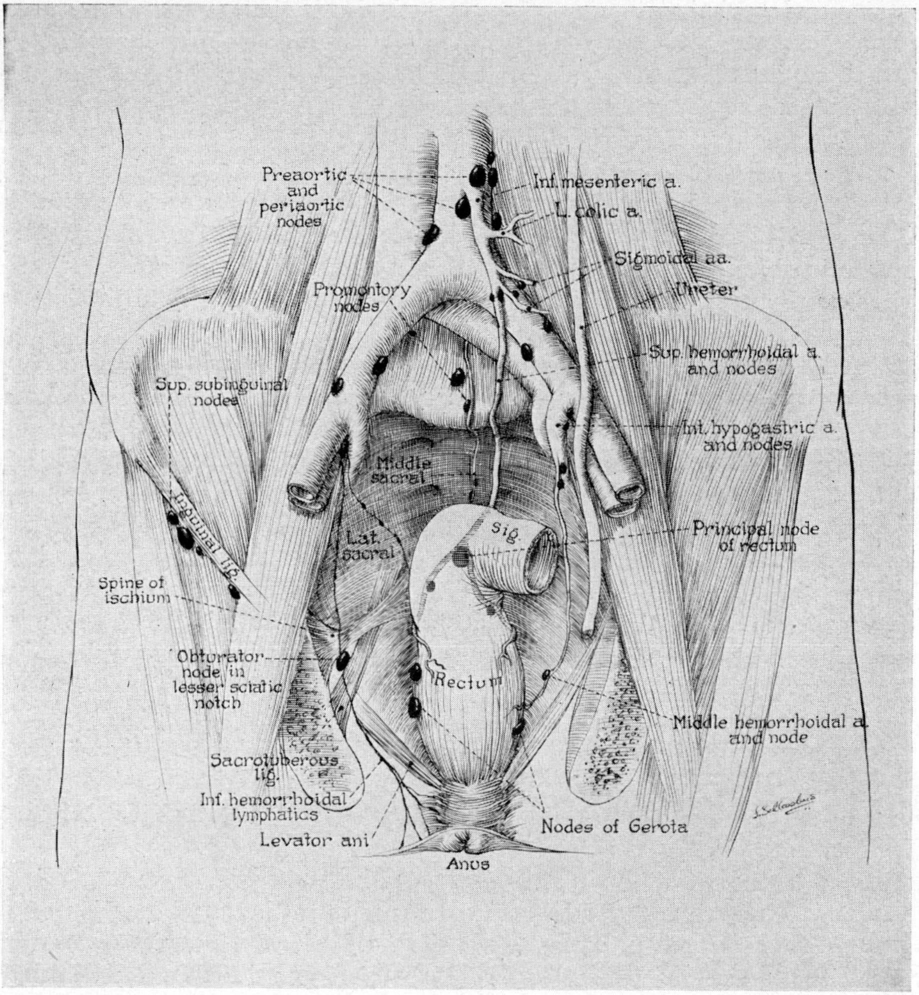

Fig. 1.—Some of the tracts of the lymphatics of the rectum and anus.

Fig. 1 depicts some of the tracts mentioned.

RESEARCH

One hundred fifty patients with carcinoma of the colon, rectum, and anus were subjected to an aortic ligation of the inferior mesenteric artery. Ninety

Fig. 2.

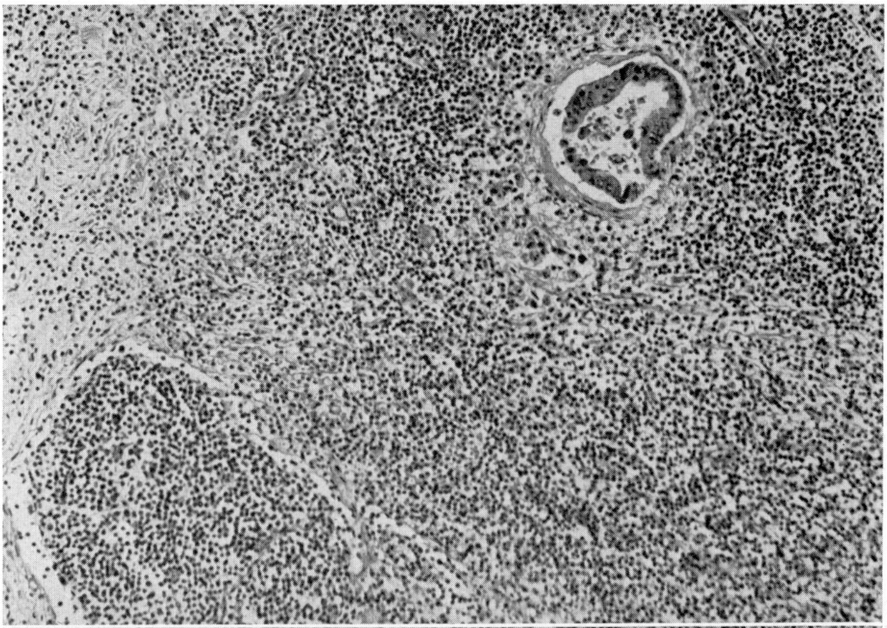

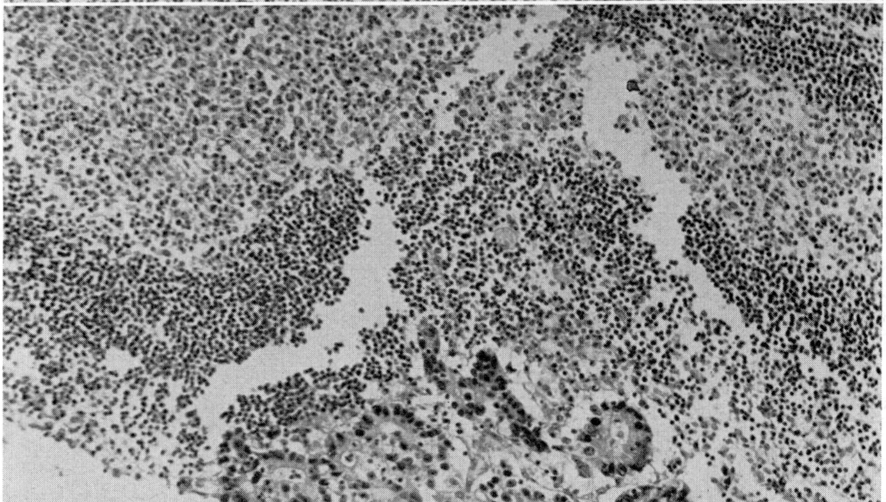

Fig. 3.

Figs. 2 and 3.— Photomicrographs illustrating the appearance of metastases in two nodes.

of the specimens were cleared of lymph nodes by a modified Spalteholz technique[74] with special attention directed toward intermediate and principal node metastases from the variously located lesions. All nodes were sectioned pseudoserially, and questionable areas of metastases were submitted to staff members in the Department of Pathology of the Temple University School of Medicine for consultation. The lymph nodes were removed from the specimens by sharp dissection under transillumination. No attempt was made to study nodes from the lateral routes of spread. Also, no nodes under 2 mm. in diameter were sectioned. Peltier in a recent study[61] on similar material found no metastases in nodes of this size or less, and Grinnell in a personal communication stated that it occurred only in rare instances. Microtome sections were made at 150 micron intervals, and the slides stained with hematoxylin and eosin. No less than three sections of any given mode were made. In some instances, as many as fifteen cuts were made. The average number of fields per node was five to seven.

RESULTS

In all 90 cases, the blood supply to the distal bowel proved adequate despite the ligation of the inferior mesenteric artery at its origin. The only complication encountered was a hematoma in the retroperitoneal space in one instance. Forty-three of the patients were men and forty-seven women. This is in sharp contrast to the usual 3 to 2 ratio of men over women. The average age of the men was 60 years, of the women, 58 years. Of the 90 patients, 54 (60 per cent) evidenced lymph node metastases. Thirty-one of these, or 57.4 per cent, were women, and 23 were men. Eighty-six specimens were of adenocarcinomas, 3 were of squamous cell carcinomas, and 1 was of sarcoma. The last was a malignant mesenchymoma of the distal rectum with 1 regional node metastasis.

Operative procedures instituted included 33 abdominoperineal resections of the rectum with preservation of the sphincters, 31 abdominoperineal excisions of the rectum of the extended Miles type, 25 anterior resections of the bowel with end-to-end anastomosis, and 1 total colectomy. The colectomy was performed on a patient with chronic ulcerative colitis, and an unexpected adenocarcinoma of the sigmoid was discovered. An interesting sidelight was the finding of adenomata in 20 per cent of all the operative specimens. In 3 cases, or 3.3 per cent, a double primary cancer existed. In each case the second tumor was located in the sigmoid colon and was subtended by the same lymphatic drainage pattern as the primary.

The number of lymph nodes dissected from each specimen varied considerably from 4 to 68, with the average being 31 per case. When positive nodes were present, the average number was 33. With negative nodes it was 27. The most nodes positive in a given specimen was 26, the mean being 5.7 per specimen.

Figs. 2 and 3 illustrate the appearance of metastases in two nodes.

Twenty-eight of the specimens with positive nodes contained three or less involved nodes for an incidence of 5.3 per cent. The remaining 26 specimens evidenced metastases in more than three nodes.

The pathologic classification of cancer of the colon and rectum into the A, B, and C groups of Dukes was utilized in this study throughout. Group A encompasses those tumors which are confined to the mucosa and submucosa. Group B includes those tumors which have penetrated into the muscle layer of the bowel wall, but not entirely through it. Group C describes that group of tumors which has invaded to or through the serosal coat. This last group has been subdivided into C_1, which allows lymph node metastases to exist in regional nodes only, and C_2, which includes positive lymph nodes up to the line of mesenteric division. In the 28 specimens which showed three or less positive nodes, 89 per cent were classed as C_1.

Eleven, or 12.2 per cent, of the 90 specimens were removed in the presence of liver metastases. Easily palpable, mesenteric nodes were felt in all these cases but two. Interestingly enough, one specimen with an involved liver had negative lymph nodes upon clearing.

Table I compares the location of the tumors with the type of pathology.

TABLE I

LOCATION	NO.	PER CENT	SQUAMOUS	ADENO-CARCINOMA	SARCOMA
Anus	3	3.3	3		
Low rectum	31	34.4		30	1
Upper rectum	38	42.4		38	
Sigmoid	18	20.1		18	
Total	90	100.0	3	86	1

TABLE II. POSITIVE NODES

LOCATION	A	B	C_1	C_2	TOTAL NUMBER	TOTAL PER CENT
Low rectum	0	4	6	4	14	46.6
Upper rectum	0	4	13	8	25	65.8
Sigmoid	0	1	9	4	14	70.7
Total	0	9	28	16	53	

TABLE III

LOCATION	NUMBER (GRADE C)	C_1	C_2
Low rectum	14	10	4
Upper rectum	25	17	8
Sigmoid	14	10	4
Total	53	37	16

The cases of adenocarcinoma were classified as follows (three squamous cell tumors and one sarcoma were excluded):

	A	*B*	*C*	*Total*
Anus				
Low rectum	2	8	16	26
Upper rectum	3	7	28	38
Sigmoid	1	2	19	22
Total	6	17	63	86

The 54 specimens which contained positive lymph nodes are compared with the grade of tumor in Table II (sarcoma and squamous cell tumors excluded).

Here it may be noted that the 6 tumors of the A group were localized in the bowel and did not metastasize to any lymph nodes. A study of the metastatic pattern of the 9 positive B group tumors revealed only regional node

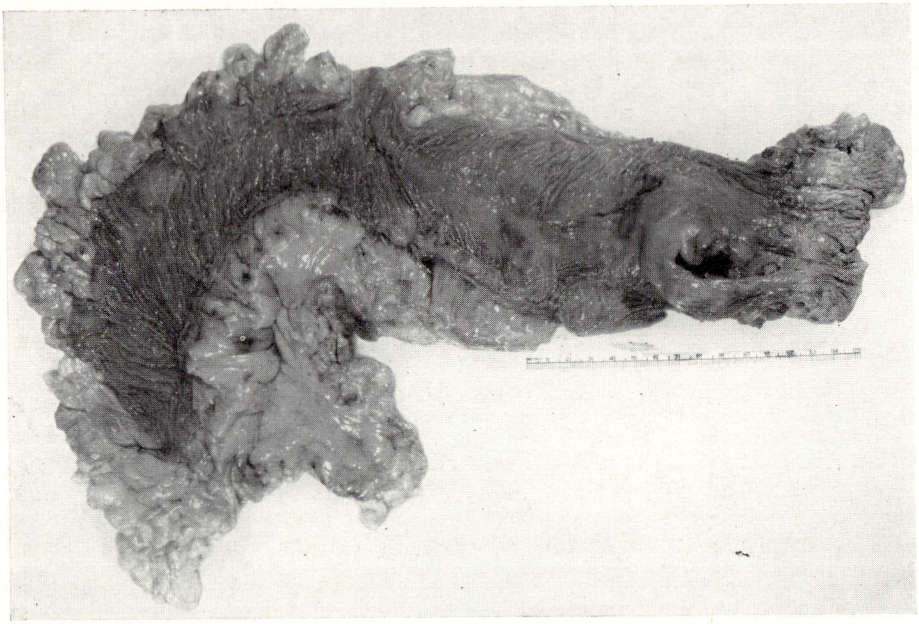

Fig. 4.—Postoperative specimen in case of E. A., 53-year-old man with malignant mesenchymal tumor involving the rectal wall at 6 cm.

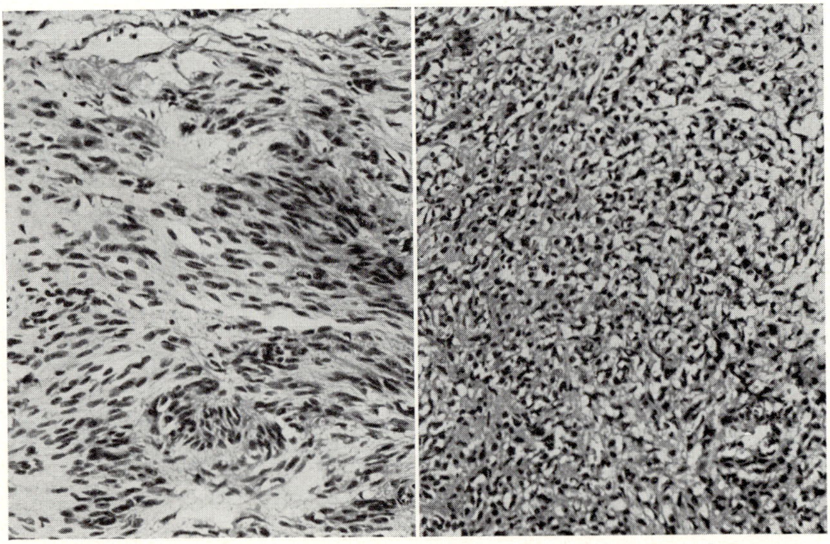

A. *B.*

Fig. 5.—Microscopic appearance of tumor in same case as Fig. 4.

involvement. Thus, in all the cases studied only the C group gave rise to metastases proximal to the intermediate nodes, as may be noted in Table III (sarcoma excluded).

Here it can be noted that 63.6 per cent of all positive nodes from Grade C tumors were regional. Only 16 specimens, or 17.8 per cent of the total 90, evidenced metastatic disease in the principal nodes of the origin of the inferior mesenteric artery. Six of these were from men and 10 from women. The average number of lymph nodes cleared from each of these 16 specimens was 33. The number of positive nodes per specimen was 9.8, or nearly twice as many as in the other positive node cases. All evidenced an orderly pattern of spread through the paracolic and intermediate nodes. One of the high positive nodes from a sigmoid lesion revealed a positive regional, but no intermediate node, and another showed only one positive node directly at the inferior mesenteric root (see Figs. 4 and 5).

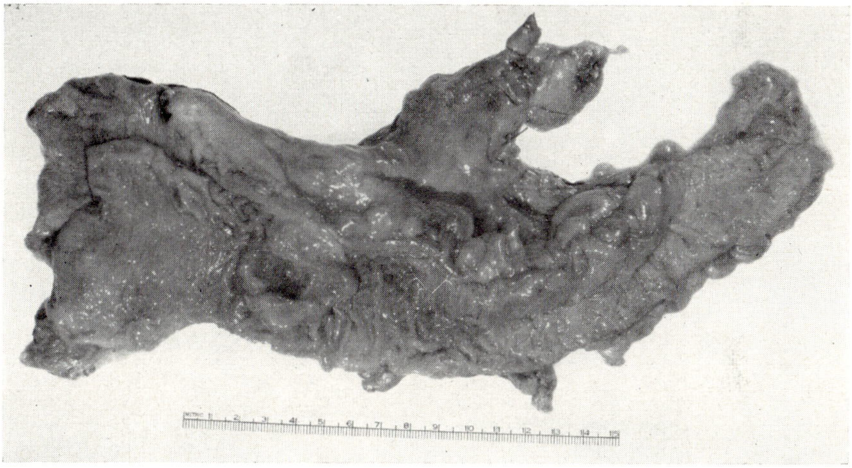

Fig. 6.—Postoperative specimen in case of D. E., 65-year-old man with C_2 lesion at 11 cm.

Figs. 4 and 5 illustrate the case of E. A., a 53-year-old man, with a malignant mesenchymal tumor involving the rectal wall at 6 cm.

Table IV reveals the location of the tumor in regard to high positive nodes and after exclusion of the cases with liver metastases.

Therefore, it may be realized that of 90 operative cases, 12 evidenced involved nodes near the origin of the inferior mesenteric artery without liver metastases.

The nodes from 4 of these 12 positive cases feasibly could have been extirpated by ligating the inferior mesenteric artery just distal to the left colic branch. The remaining 8, however, could be adequately removed only by means of a high ligation. Thus, positive nodes would have been left behind in 9 per cent of all the operative cases if a high ligation had not been carried out.

In these 8 cases, 4 evidenced grossly enlarged nodes at surgery, while 4 did not. The average age of these patients was 52 years. Five were women. All 8 primaries were located in the rectum, 5 low and 3 high.

Figs. 6 through 16 illustrate the pattern of spread in the remaining patients with a high number of positive nodes.

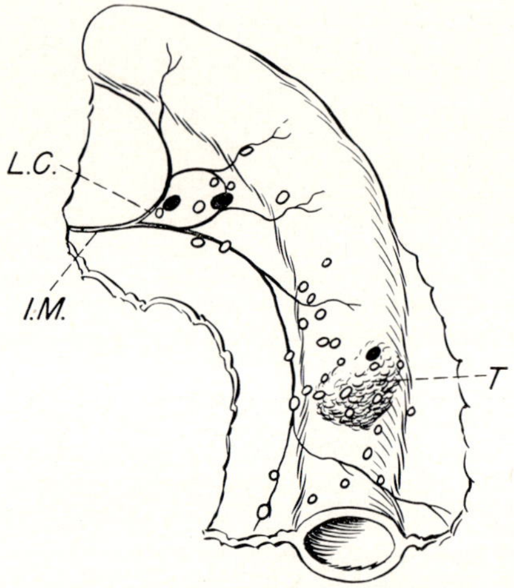

Fig. 7.—Pattern of lymph node spread in same case as Fig. 6.

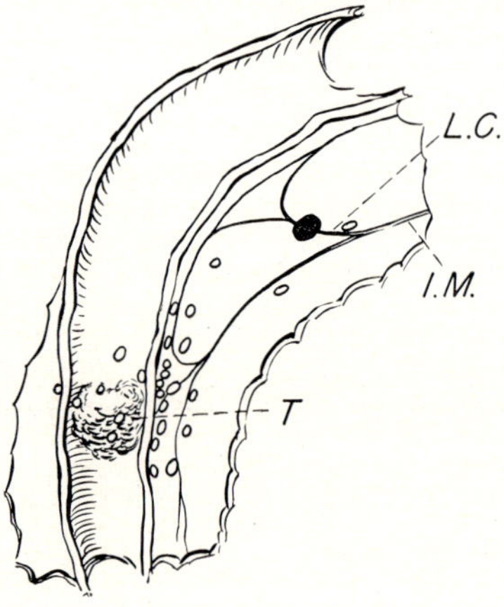

Fig. 8.

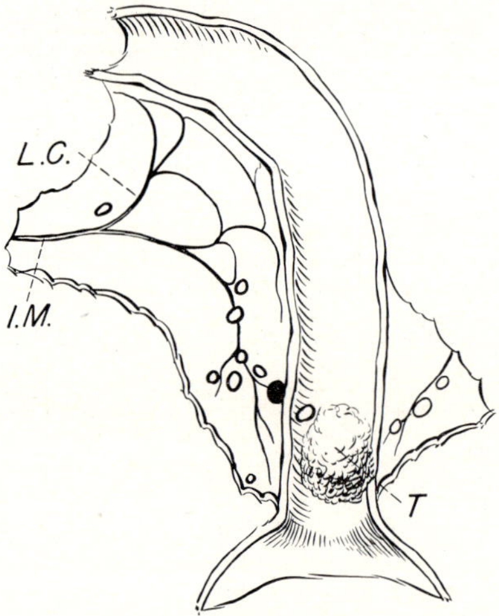

Fig. 9.

Fig. 8.—Pattern of lymph node spread in case of C. McE., 47-year-old man with C_1 lesion at 15 cm.

Fig. 9.—Pattern of lymph node spread in same case as Fig. 8.

The case of D. E., a 65-year-old man with a C_2 lesion at 11 cm., is illustrated in Figs. 6 and 7.

The case of D. McE., a 47-year-old man with a C_1 lesion at 15 cm., is illustrated in Figs. 8 through 10.

Mrs. P. F., a 52-year-old white woman with a type C_2 lesion at 8 cm., underwent abdominoperineal proctosigmoidectomy with preservation of the sphincters (seven nodes positive). (Fig. 11.)

G. A., a 52-year-old white man with a type C_2 lesion at 10 cm., underwent abdominoperineal proctosigmoidectomy with preservation of the sphincters (ten nodes positive). (Fig. 12.)

J. B., a 54-year-old white man with type C_2 lesion at 10 cm., underwent abdominoperineal proctosigmoidectomy with preservation of the sphincters (twenty-six nodes positive). (Fig. 13.)

Mrs. R. S., a 50-year-old white woman with type C_2 lesion at 4 cm., underwent an abdominoperineal excision of the rectum, extended Miles type, plus a panhysterectomy and removal of posterior vaginal wall (seventeen nodes positive). (Fig. 14.)

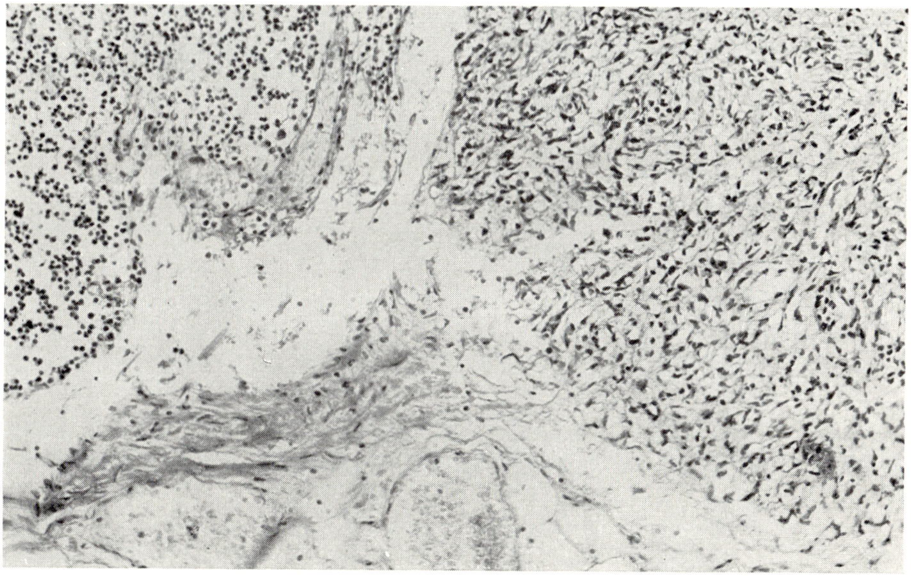

Fig. 10.—Microscopic appearance of the metastasis in same case as Fig 8.

Mrs. M. M., a 63-year-old white woman with a type C_2 lesion at 16 cm., underwent an anterior resection of the sigmoid and rectosigmoid with end-to-end anastomosis (five nodes positive). (Fig. 15.)

Mrs. E. S., a 70-year-old white woman with a type C_2 lesion at 16 cm., underwent an anterior resection of the sigmoid and recotsigmoid with end-to-end anastomosis (five nodes positive). (Fig. 16.)

Table V points out the results of other authors in the over-all clearing of nodes.

Grinnell[42] recently cleared 37 specimens of colonic and rectal cancer removed by high ligations and found 7 instances of positive nodes at the origin of the inferior mesenteric artery. This represents an incidence of 17 per cent in the present study. Grinnell believed that a high ligation was imperative in all his cases in order to remove these nodes. These findings conform to the

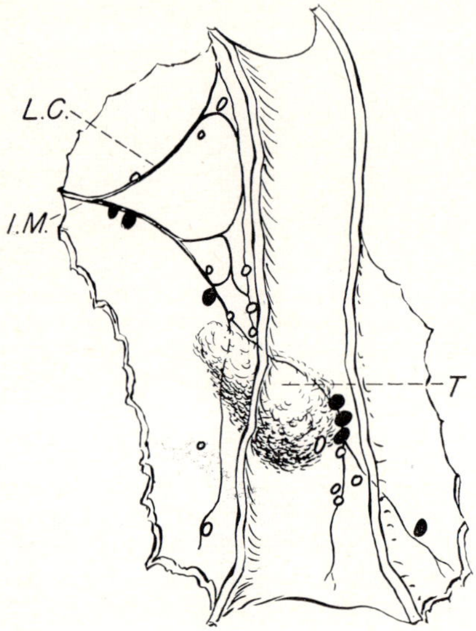

Fig. 11

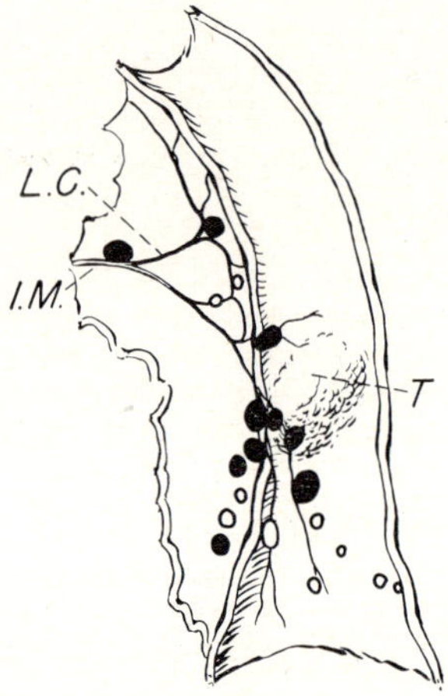

Fig. 12.

Fig. 11.—Pattern of lymph node spread in case of Mrs. P. F., 52-year-old woman with C_2 lesion at 8 cm.

Fig. 12.—Pattern of lymph node spread in case of G. A., 52-year-old man with C_2 lesion at 10 cm.

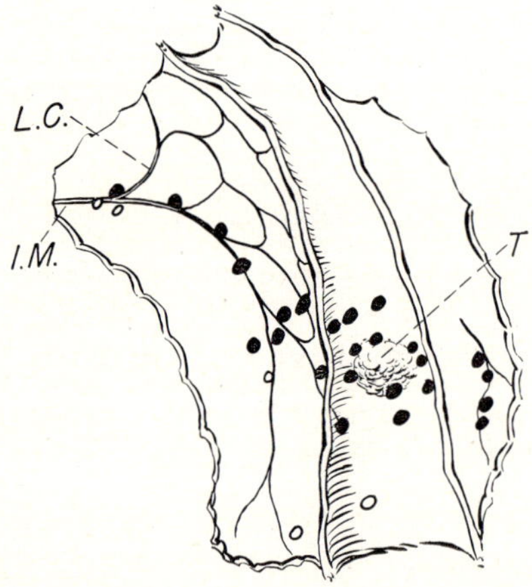

Fig. 13.

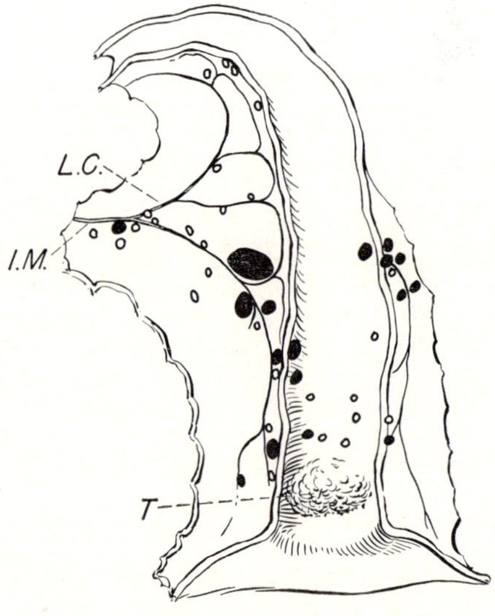

Fig. 14.

Fig. 13.—Pattern of lymph node spread in case of J. B., 54-year-old man with C_2 lesion at 10 cm.

Fig. 14.—Pattern of lymph node spread in case of Mrs. R. S., 50-year-old woman with C_2 lesion at 4 cm.

opinons of Ault,[3] State,[75] and others who recommend the high ligation almost as a routine.

It is interesting to note in this present series that the spread of tumor cells in a superior direction through the lymphatic system from the lower and upper rectum appears to be orderly. No skip areas were demonstrated even to the intermediate nodes. Lesions in the sigmoid colon, however, differ somewhat. Two cases have been demonstrated, one showing a skip of the intermediate nodes and the other of both the intermediate and the regional.

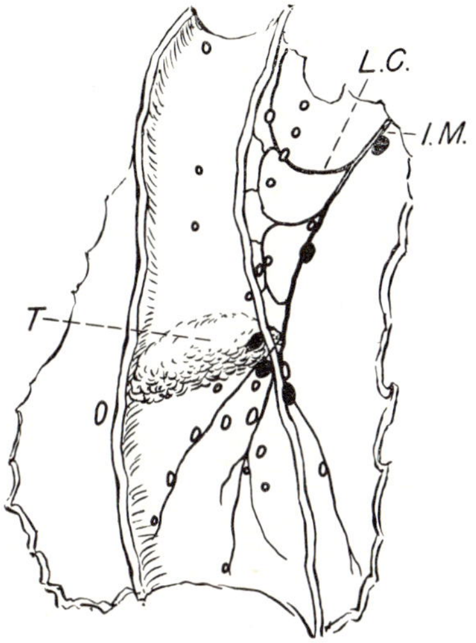

Fig. 15.

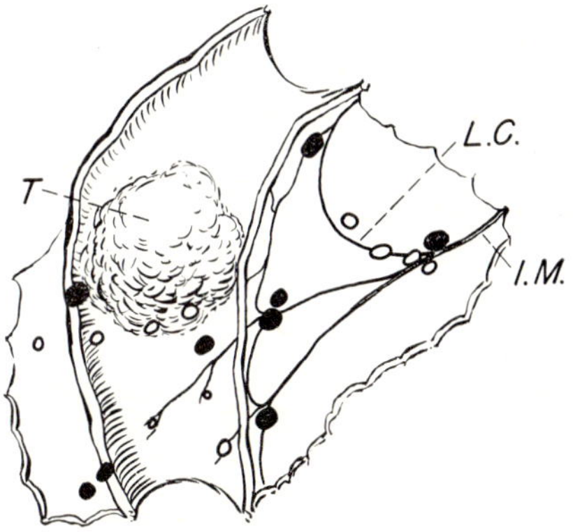

Fig. 16.

Fig. 15.—Pattern of lymph node spread in case of Mrs. M. M., 63-year-old woman with C_2 lesion at 16 cm.

Fig. 16.—Pattern of lymph node spread in case of Mrs. E. S., 70-year-old woman with C_2 lesion at 16 cm.

Table IV

LOCATION	POSITIVE HIGH NODES	LIVER CASES EXCLUDED
Anus	0	0
Low rectum	3	3
Upper rectum	8	6
Sigmoid	5	3
Total	16	12

Table V

AUTHOR	NUMBER OF SPECIMENS	NUMBER OF NODES	PER CENT POSITIVE
McVay[50]	100	6	47
Wood and Wilkie[87]	100	11	51
Westhues[85]	74	25	59
Gabriel, Dukes, and Bussey[28]	100	28	62
Gilchrist and David[32]	200	52	62.5
Coller, Kay, and MacIntyre[13]	53	67	64
Grinnell[41]	322	38	47
Peltier[61]	25	52	52

Also of interest is the difficult correlation between enlarged lymph nodes at surgery and the possibility of metastases. Gilchrist[33] and Dukes[25] have stated that a 50 per cent error is to be expected. In this series, one-half of the high positive lymph nodes were accompanied by grossly palpable nodes.

SUMMARY

The routes and methods of cancer dissemination in lesions of the colon, rectum, and anus have been discussed, and a review of the vascular and lymphatic supply to the area has been made with special reference to the advisability and practicality of ligating the inferior mesenteric artery at its aortic origin.

Ninety cases of distal bowel resections for cancer with a high ligation of this artery have been presented, and the findings in the cleared specimens reviewed. Sixty per cent of these cases revealed positive lymph nodes, 17.8 per cent of which were located at the origin of the inferior mesenteric artery. Three cases of squamous cell carcinoma of the anus failed to exhibit nodal metastases, but the malignant mesenchymoma of the low rectum did involve a regional node. All the rectal lesions initiated an orderly pattern of lymphatic spread, but the sigmoidal lesions in at least 2 cases revealed a skip pattern. No correlation was attempted between the presence of high positive nodes and lateral lymphatic spread. In at least 8 cases, a ligation of the inferior mesenteric artery below the left colic branch would not have removed positive nodes in the upper portion of the mesentery. Thus, 9 per cent of the operative procedures would have been failures without a high ligation.

CONCLUSIONS

1. Ligation of the inferior mesenteric artery at its aortic origin in the treatment of cancer of the distal colon, rectum, and anus appears to be a safe procedure.
2. The presence of positive inferior mesenteric lymph nodes in cancers of the distal colon, rectum, and anus is frequent.
3. A ligation of the inferior mesenteric artery at its origin should be included in the extirpation of all cancers of the distal colon and rectum.

REFERENCES

1. Abel, A. L.: Discussion on Advanced Carcinoma of the Rectum, Proc. Roy. Soc. Med., Lond. **43**: 1087, 1950.
2. Archibald, E.: Operative Treatment of Cancer of the Rectum, J. A. M. A. **50**: 573, 1908.
3. Ault, G. W., Castro, A. F., and Smith, R. S.: Carcinoma of Upper Rectum and Rectosigmoid; Clinical Report on High Inferior Mesenteric Ligation, Postgrad. Med. **8**: 176, 1950.
4. Bacon, H. E.: Evolution of Sphincter Muscle Preservation and Re-establishment of Continuity in the Operative Treatment of Rectal and Sigmoidal Cancers, Surg., Gynec. & Obst. **82**: 434, 1946.
5. Bacon, H. E., McElwain, J. W., and Trimpi, H. D.: Surgical Management of Large Bowel Lesions, Bull. New York Acad. Med. **29**: 34, 1953.
6. Bacon, H. E., and Rowe, R. J.: The Radicability of Methods to Eliminate Colostomy: A Critical Review, J. Internat. Coll. Surgeons **11**: 243, 1948.

7. Bacon, H. E., and Sauer, I.: Selection of Surgical Procedure in Treatment of Cancer of the Rectum, J. Internat. Coll. Surgeons **13**: 24, 1950.
8. Bacon, H. E., and Sauer, I.: Surgical Treatment of Cancer of the Lower Bowel, Cancer **3**: 773, 1950.
9. Bacon, H. E., and Smith, C. H.: The Arterial Supply of the Distal Colon, Ann. Surg. **127**: 28, 1948.
10. Black, W. A., and Waugh, J. M.: Intramural Extention of Carcinoma of Descending Colon, Sigmoid, and Rectosigmoid; Pathological Study, Surg., Gynec. & Obst. **87**: 457, 1948.
11. Brown, C. E., and Warren, S.: Visceral Metastases From Rectal Carcinoma, Surg., Gynec. & Obst. **66**: 611, 1938.
12. Cole, W. H.: Recurrence in Carcinoma of the Colon and Proximal Rectum Following Resection for Carcinoma, Arch. Surg. **65**: 264, 1952.
13. Coller, F. A., Kay, E. B., and MacIntyre, R. S.: Regional Lymphatic Metastases of Carcinoma of the Rectum, SURGERY **8**: 294, 1940.
14. Connell, J. F., and Rottino, A.: Retrograde Spread of Carcinoma in the Rectum and Rectosigmoid, Arch. Surg. **59**: 897, 1949.
15. Cuneo, B., and Marcille, M.: Lymphatiques illiaques, Bull. Soc. anat. de Par. **12**: 281, 1901.
16. Deddish, M. R.: Discussion on Advanced Carcinoma of Rectum, Proc. Roy. Soc. Med. **43**: 1075, 1950.
17. Deddish, M. R.: Abdomino-pelvic Lymph Node Dissection in Cancer of the Rectum and Distal Colon, Cancer **4**: 1364, 1952.
18. Delamere, G., Poirier, P., and Cuneo, B.: The Lymphatics, Chicago, 1904, W. T. Keener & Co.
19. De Oliveira, E.: Observações sobre os linfáticos ano-retais, Thesis, 1947.
20. Desmarest, E.: Technique de la resection de l'angle gauche du colon pour cancer, J. de chir. **14**: 575, 1917-18.
21. Dixon, C. F.: Anterior Resection for Malignant Lesions of the Upper Part of the Rectum and Lower Part of the Sigmoid, Ann. Surg. **128**: 425, 1948.
22. Drummond, H.: Some Points Relating to the Surgical Anatomy of the Arterial Supply of the Large Intestine, Proc. Roy. Soc. Med., Lond. **7**: 185, 1913.
23. Drummond, H.: The Arterial Supply of the Rectum and Pelvic Colon, Brit. J. Surg. **1**: 677, 1914.
24. Dukes, C. E.: The Hereditary Factor in Polyposis Intestini or Multiple Adenomata, Cancer Rev. **5**: 241, 1930.
25. Dukes, C. E.: Spread of Cancer of the Rectum, Brit. J. Surg. **68**: 64, 1930.
26. Dukes, C. E.: The Surgical Pathology of Rectal Cancer, Proc. Roy. Soc. Med., Lond. **37**: 131, 1944.
27. Dunphy, J. E., and Broderick, E. G.: A Critique of Anterior Resection in the Treatment of Carcinoma of the Rectum and Pelvic Colon, SURGERY **30**: 106, 1951.
28. Gabriel, W. B., Dukes, C., and Bussey, H. J. R.: Lymphatic Spread in Cancer of the Rectum, Brit. J. Surg. **23**: 395, 1935.
29. Gerota, D.: Die lymphgefasse des rectum und des anus, Arch. f. anat. u. Physiol. **14**: 240, 1895.
30. Gilchrist, R. K.: Indications Regarding Operations for Carcinoma of Distal Colon and Rectum, SURGERY **27**: 787, 1950.
31. Gilchrist, R. K., and David, V. C.: Lymphatic Spread of Carcinoma of the Rectum, Ann. Surg. **109**: 621, 1938.
32. Gilchrist, R. K., and David, V. C.: Prognosis in Carcinoma of the Bowel, Surg., Gynec. & Obst. **86**: 359, 1948.
33. Gilchrist, R. K., and David, V. C.: Cancer of the Large Bowel, Ann. Surg. **126**: 421, 1948.
34. Glover, R. P., and Waugh, J. M.: The Retrograde Lymphatic Spread of Carcinoma of the Rectosigmoid Region, Surg., Gynec. & Obst. **82**: 434, 1946.
35. Goligher, J. C.: The Blood Supply of the Sigmoid Colon and Rectum, Brit. J. Surg. **37**: 157, 1949.
36. Goligher, J. C., Dukes, C. E., and Bussey, H. J. R.: Local Recurrences After Sphincter Saving Excision of Carcinoma of the Rectum and Rectosigmoid, Brit. J. Surg. **39**: 199, 1951.
37. Gordon-Watson, C.: Origin and Spread of Cancer of the Rectum in Relation to Surgical Treatment, Lancet **1**: 239, 1938.
38. Gray's Anatomy, ed. 25, edited by C. M. Goss, Philadelphia, 1948, Lea & Febiger.
39. Grinnell, R. S.: The Grading and Prognosis of Carcinoma of the Colon and Rectum, Ann. Surg. **109**: 500, 1939.
40. Grinnell, R. S.: The Lymphatic and Venous Spread of Carcinoma of the Rectum, Ann. Surg. **116**: 200, 1942.

41. Grinnell, R. S.: Lymphatic Metastases of Carcinoma of Colon and Rectum, Ann. Surg. **131**: 494, 1950.
42. Grinnell, R. S., and Hiatt, R. B.: Ligation of the Inferior Mesenteric Artery at the Aorta in Resections for Carcinoma of the Sigmoid and Rectum, Surg., Gynec. & Obst. **94**: 526, 1952.
43. Guernsey, D. E., Waugh, J. M., and Dockerty, M. B.: Carcinoma of the Rectum; Prognosis Based on the Distance of Lesions From, or Involvement of, the Levator Ani Muscle, and Involvement of the Anal Sphincters, Surg., Gynec. & Obst. **92**: 529, 1951.
44. Hartmann, H.: Some Considerations Upon High Amputations of the Rectum, Ann. Surg. **50**: 1091, 1909.
45. Jamieson, J. K., and Dobson, J. F.: The Lymphatic System of the Caecum and Appendix, Lancet **1**: 1137, 1907.
46. Jamieson, J. K., and Dobson, J. F.: The Lymphatics of Colon, Proc. Roy. Soc. Med., Lond. **2**: 149, 1909.
47. Maguire, F. A.: The Anatomy of the Female Pelvis, ed. 4, Sydney and London, 1949, Angus & Robertson, Ltd.
48. Manasse, P.: Die arterielle gefassversorgung des s. romanum in ihrer bedentung für die operative verlagerung desselben, Arch. f. klin. Chir. **83**: 999, 1907.
49. McKittrick, L. S.: Principles, Old and New, of Resection of the Colon for Carcinoma, Surg., Gynec. & Obst. **87**: 15, 1948.
50. McVay, J. R.: Involvement of Lymph Nodes in Carcinoma of Rectum, Ann. Surg. **76**: 755, 1922.
51. Miles, W. E.: A Method of Performing Abdominoperineal Excision for Carcinoma of the Rectum and of the Terminal Portion of the Pelvic Colon, Lancet **2**: 1812, 1908.
52. Miles, W. E.: Cancer of the Rectum, London, 1926, Harrison & Sons, Ltd.
53. Miles, W. E.: Rectal Surgery, London, 1939, Cassell & Co., Ltd.
54. Mondor, H.: Contribution a l'étude du cancer du rectum, Thèse de doct., 1914.
55. Monsarrat, K. W., and Williams, K. J.: Intramural Extension in Rectal Cancer, Brit. J. Surg. **1**: 173, 1913.
56. Morgan, C. N., and Lloyd-Davies, O. V.: Discussion on Conservative Resection in Cancer of the Rectum, Prog. Roy. Soc. Med., Lond. **43**: 701, 1950.
57. Moynihan, B. G. A.: The Surgical Treatment of Carcinoma of the Sigmoid Flexure and the Rectum, Surg., Gynec. & Obst. **6**: 463, 1908.
58. Muir, E. G.: Rectal Cancer and Preservation of Function, Brit. M. J. **2**: 286, 1948.
59. Nesselrod, J. P.: Anatomy of Pelvic Lymphatics, Ann. Surg. **104**: 905, 1936.
60. Paitre, F., Giraud, D., and Dupret, S.: Pratique anatomo-chirurgicale illustrée, Paris, 1935, Gaston Doin & Cie.
61. Peltier, L. F.: The Search for Lymph Node Metastases in Cancer of the Rectum, SURGERY **30**: 443, 1951.
62. Poirier, P., Cueno, B., and Delamere, G.: The Lymphatics, Chicago, 1904, W. T. Keener & Co.
63. Pope, C. E., and Buie, L. A.: A Description of the Arterial Blood Supply of the Pelvic Colon, Tr. Am. Proct. Soc. (1929) **30**: 78, 1930.
64. Pope, C. E., and Judd, E. S.: The Arterial Supply of the Sigmoid, Rectosigmoid and Rectum, S. Clin. North America **9**: 957, 1929.
65. Quenu, E.: Extirpation abdomino-perineale de cancer du rectum, Bull. et mém. Soc. de chir. de Par. **27**: 185, 1901.
66. Quenu, E.: Vaisseaux lymphatiques de l'anus, Bull. Soc. anat. de Par. 309, 1893.
67. Reinhold, P.: Contribution a l'étude des récidives post-opératoires du cancer rectal, Thèse de doct., 1924.
68. Reybard, J. F.: Memoire sur une tumer cancereuse affectant l'illiaque du colon, Bull. Acad. de méd., Par. **9**: 1031, 1844.
69. Rouvière, H.: Anatomie des lymphatiques de l'homme, Paris, 1932, Masson & Cie.
70. Rubesch, R.: Ueber die vermeidung der Darmgangran bie Rectum operationen, Beitr. z. klin. Chir. **67**: 480, 1910.
71. Sauer, I., and Bacon, H. E.: Influence of Lateral Spread of Cancer of the Rectum on Radicability of Operation and Prognosis, Am. J. Surg. **81**: 111, 1951.
72. Sauer, I., and Bacon, H. E.: A New Approach for Excision of the Lower Portion of the Rectum and Anal Canal, Surg., Gynec. & Obst. **95**: 229, 1952.
73. Seefield, P. H., and Bargen, J. A.: The Spread of Carcinoma of the Rectum: Invasion of Lymphatics, Veins, and Nerves, Ann. Surg. **118**: 76, 1943.
74. Spalteholz, W.: Ueber das Durchsichtigmachen von menschlichen und tierischen Praparaten, Leipzig, 1911, S. Hirzel.
75. State, D.: Combined Abdominoperineal Excision of the Rectum; a Plan for Standardization of the Proximal Extent of Dissection, SURGERY **30**: 349, 1951.
76. Steward, J. A., and Rankin, F. W.: Blood Supply of the Large Intestine: Its Surgical Considerations, Arch. Surg. **26**: 843, 1933.

77. Sudek, P.: Ueber die Gefaessnersorgung das Mastarmes in Hinsicht auf die operative Gangraen, München. med. Wchnschr. **2**: 1314, 1907.
78. Sugarbaker, E. D., and Wiley, H. M.: Significance of Fixation in Operative Carcinoma of Large Bowel, SURGERY **27**: 343, 1950.
79. Sunderland, S.: Blood Supply of the Distal Colon, Australian & New Zealand J. Surg. **11**: 253, 1942.
80. Uhlenhut, E., Day, E. C., Smith, R. D., and Middleton, E. B.: The Visceral Endopelvic Fascia and the Hypogastric Sheath, Surg., Gynec. & Obst. **86**: 9, 1948.
81. Villemin, F., Huard, P., and Montagné, M.: Recherches anatomiques sur les lymphatiques du rectum et de l'anus, Rev. de chir. **63**: 39, 1925.
82. Wangensteen, O. H.: Primary Resection (Closed Anastomosis) of Rectal Ampulla for Malignancy With Preservation of Sphincteric Function, Surg., Gynec. & Obst. **81**: 1, 1945.
83. Wangensteen, O. H.: Cancer of the Colon and Rectum, Wisconsin M. J. **48**: 591, 1949.
84. Waugh, H. M., and Kirklin, J. W.: The Importance of the Level of the Lesion in the Prognosis and Treatment of Carcinoma of the Rectum and Low Sigmoid Colon, Ann. Surg. **129**: 22, 1949.
85. Westhues, H.: Die pathologisch-anatomischen Grundlagen der Chirurgie des Rektumkarzinoms, Leipzig, 1934, Georg Thieme.
86. Willis, R. A.: The Spread of Tumors in the Human Body, London, 1952, Butterworth & Co. (publishers), Ltd., St. Louis, Mo., The C. V. Mosby Company.
87. Wood, W. Q., and Wilkie, D. P. D.: Carcinoma of the Rectum: an Anatomicopathological Study, Edinburgh M. J. **40**: 321, 1933.

AN EXPERIMENTAL STUDY OF THE BUFFERING CAPACITY OF THE CONTENTS OF THE UPPER SMALL BOWEL*

Lawrence B. Kiriluk, M.D.,** and K. Alvin Merendino, M.D.,
Seattle, Wash.

(From the Department of Surgery, University of Washington School of Medicine)

The merits of using a short afferent loop in the Billroth II plan of gastric resection have been emphasized.[1-3] It has been shown in this laboratory that the mucosal sensitivity of the small bowel, per se, is not an important factor influencing the increased incidence of stomal ulcers accompanying long afferent loops.[4] It appeared reasonable to explore the thesis that as the length of the afferent loop was increased, the buffering capacity of the small bowel contents was decreased, in other words, that the neutralizing capacity of the alkaline juices decreased progressively as the distance was increased from the pylorus. Cross[5] has shown that in profusing alkaline solutions of known formula, the volume which is returned and the buffering capacity of the solution which is returned are both decreased as the length of the perfused loop is increased.

More exact information regarding the buffering capacity of the contents within the upper small bowel found in the normal animal seemed desirable. A simple, direct approach to the problem was used.

METHODS AND MATERIALS

A series of 32 adult mongrel dogs was used. All animals were being sacrificed incident to other experiments which in no way involved the gastrointestinal tract. The animals were fasted eighteen hours and anesthetized, using 15 mg. of Nembutal intravenously per pound of body weight. A midline laparotomy incision was made. The duodenum and jejunum were isolated and cross-clamped every 10 cm. for 80 cm. The first clamp was placed 3 cm. distal to the pylorus. An intact blood supply was maintained. A clamp also was placed across the hepatoduodenal ligament to prevent continued emptying of bile into the first segment.

Forty cubic centimeters of distilled water was used to lavage each 10 cm. segment. The lavage was performed through the bowel wall using a 15 gauge needle and a 50 c.c. syringe. The lavage solution was injected into and aspirated from each segment five times, over a period of less than one minute. In one-half of the cases, the lavage was begun in the most proximal segment and continued distally. In the remainder, the procedure was reversed. The clamping

Received for publication, Aug. 19, 1953.

*Supported by University of Washington Initiative 171 Funds for research in biology and medicine.

**Trainee, American Cancer Institute.

and lavage were carried out as rapidly as possible. The animals were sacrificed at the close of the experiment.

The pH of each specimen then was determined by means of the Beckman Model G pH Electrometer, using glass electrodes. Portions of each specimen were then titrated.

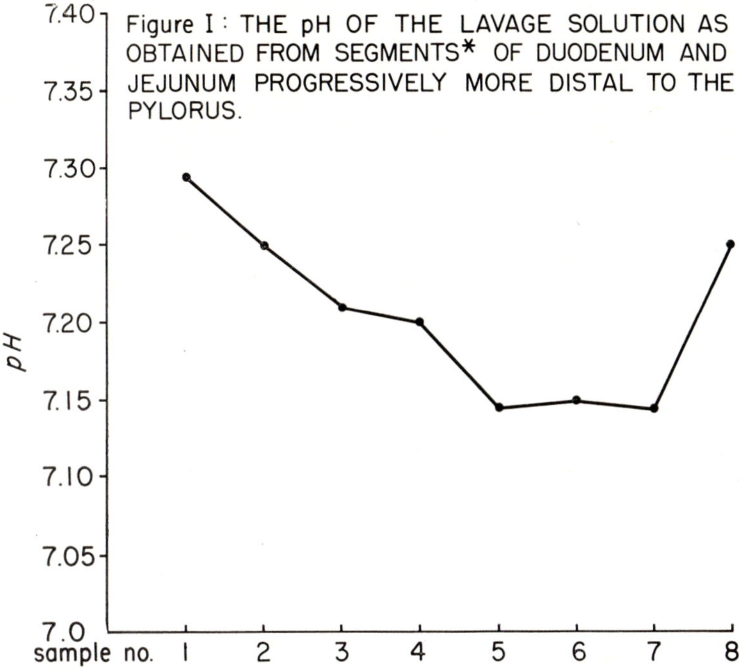

Figure I: THE pH OF THE LAVAGE SOLUTION AS OBTAINED FROM SEGMENTS* OF DUODENUM AND JEJUNUM PROGRESSIVELY MORE DISTAL TO THE PYLORUS.

*Each sample represents a 10 cm. segment of intestine analyzed. Sample no. 1 represents the segment 3 to 13 cm. distal to the pylorus. Sample 8 represents 10 cm. segment at 73 to 83 cm.

Samples from 8 dogs were titrated with 0.01 normal HCl to a pH of 2.9, using Töpfer's reagent (dimethyl-amino-azobenzene) as the indicator. Samples from 24 dogs were titrated with 0.01 normal NaOH to a pH of 8.4, using phenolphthalein as the indicator. The amount of HCl required to counteract the buffering effect of the lavage solution was obtained by subtracting from the total used the amount of HCl which would be required to carry a NaOH solution through the same pH change. The amount of NaOH required to counteract the buffer capacity of the lavage solution was obtained by subtracting from the total used the amount which would be required to carry a HCl solution through the same pH change.

RESULTS

The determinations of the buffering capacity and the pH within each segment are illustrated in Figs. 1 through 3. The figure plotted is the average obtained from the series of animals used.

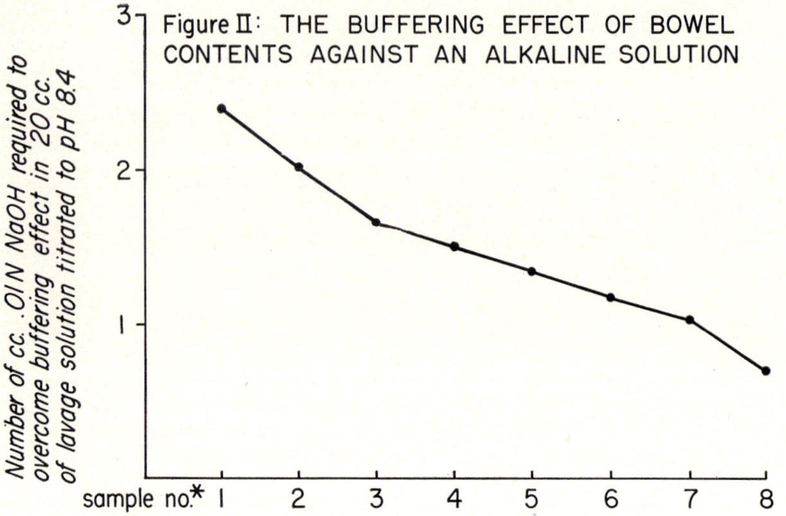

*Each sample represents a 10 cm. segment of intestine analyzed. Sample no. 1 represents the segment 3 to 13 cm. distal to the pylorus. Sample 8 represents 10 cm. segment at 73 to 83 cm.

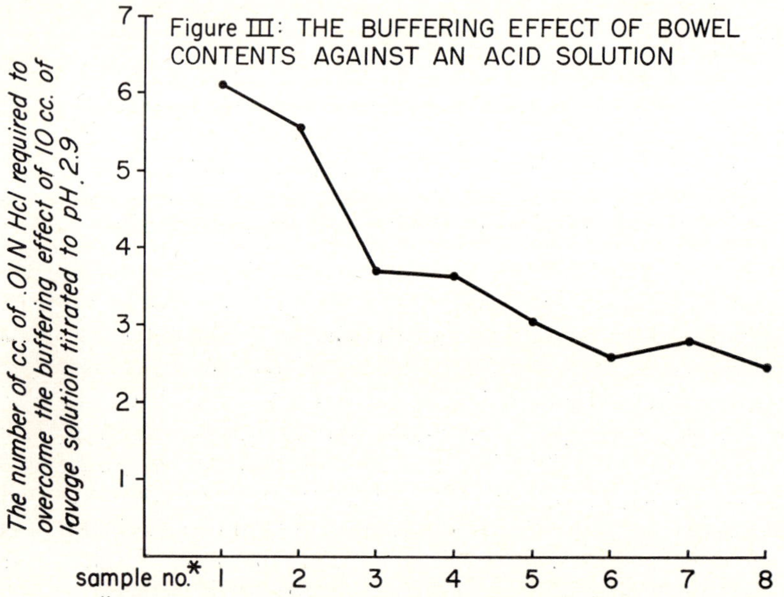

*Each sample represents a 10 cm. segment of intestine analyzed. Sample no. 1 represents the segment 3 to 13 cm. distal to the pylorus. Sample 8 represents 10 cm. segment at 73 to 83 cm.

The average pH of the lavage solutions obtained at 10 cm. intervals varied from 7.14 to 7.29 in the first 83 cm. of the bowel. There appeared to be a progressive decrease in the alkalinity of the contents as the distance from the pylorus was increased (Fig. 1). The first 10 cm. segment had the highest pH. This would appear reasonable, since the ampulla of Vater and the pancreatic ducts empty into this segment. In the dog, the major pancreatic duct empties singly into the duodenum, while the minor duct enters with the bile duct. Even though the animals were fasted eighteen hours prior to the test, and the hepatoduodenal ligament was clamped, it must be assumed that some pancreatic juice entered the bowel after the clamps had been applied. A sudden rise in the pH in the eighth sample, in the 10 cm. segment at 73 to 83 cm. distal to the pylorus, was noted. The reason for this occurrence is not known. The rise in the pH was not supported by similar changes in the buffering capacity (Figs. 2 and 3). However, the pH alone is not an indicator of buffering capacity of any solution.

The results shown in Figs. 2 and 3 indicate that the buffering capacity of the contents of the duodenum and jejunum decreased progressively as the distance from the pylorus increased. This decrease appears almost linear. The buffering capacity of the contents in the first duodenal segment was approximately two and one-half times that in the segment 73 to 83 cm. distally. This relationship was essentially the same against acid and alkaline solutions. In turn, the capacity against an acid solution, as plotted in this experiment, was approximately five times that against an alkaline solution. However, the titration of the lavage solutions with HCl was carried through a wider pH range. The exact relationship of the buffering capacity of the lavage solutions against acid and base was not determined.

DISCUSSION

Buffers, by definition, are substances which, when present in a solution, maintain the latter at a relatively constant pH when an acid or an alkali is added to it. In short, a buffer has the power to "soak up" or "tampon" acid or base. Because of the multiplicity of substances found in the juices in the region of the ampulla of Vater, the buffering system is undoubtedly very complex in nature. From this, it may be assumed that the complete "buffer system" has multiple isoelectric points, and therefore prevents any precipitous change in pH. In the normal animal, the buffer system is present in the first portion of the duodenum, and as the acid juices enter they are neutralized before any major change in the pH of the local environment can occur. Consequently, the pH remains at or near the neutral range.

The progressive loss of buffering capacity as the intestinal contents traverse the bowel lumen is probably dependent upon several factors. It is not unlikely that the nature of the contents is altered by a two-way exchange of ions, variable in type and amount between the blood and intestinal contents.[6] Furthermore, no attempt was made in these studies to determine the ionic content of the lavage solutions obtained at various levels. The addition of mucosal secretions such as succus entericus into the lumen would influence both the pH and buffering capacity of the bowel contents.

Cantarow and Trumper[7] stated that, under normal conditions, approximately 90 per cent of the bile salts entering the intestine is reabsorbed into the portal circulation by the lymphatics. If it is assumed that the remainder of the constituents of the juices are capable of being absorbed in a similar fashion, then the results obtained from these experiments and those of Cross tend to indicate that the majority of the absorption occurs in the proximal portion of the small bowel. Cross stated that there is a sharp drop in buffering capacity of perfusion solutions from the intestinal loops longer than 20 cm. The work herein reported indicates an almost linear decrease in buffering capacity as the distance from the pylorus is increased.

This pattern of the loss in buffering capacity of the bowel contents is important when the Billroth II plan of gastric resection is contemplated. In this circumstance, care must be taken to insure as short an afferent loop as possible. The effective buffering capacity of the loop contents delivered at the gastroenterostomy is less and less as the length of the afferent loop is increased. This same mechanism would be existent when a gastroenterostomy is performed without gastrectomy. In view of other results from this laboratory, which cast real doubt upon the thesis of differential intestinal sensitivity to acid-pepsin mixtures, and in view of the results of others, which seem to minimize the secretin factor in this regard, it appears to us that the buffering capacity of the intestinal contents delivered at the gastroenteric stoma is the most important protective mechanism against the development of stomal ulcer when the Billroth II plan of gastrectomy is carried out.

The rationale of a short afferent loop in the Billroth II plan of gastrectomy appears to be closely related to the fact that the closer the gastroenteric stoma is to the pylorus, the greater is the buffering capacity of the luminal contents, and therefore in this situation there exists the greatest protection against the development of stomal ulcers.

SUMMARY AND CONCLUSIONS

1. A series of pH and buffering capacity determinations was made of bowel contents found at various levels of the small intestine up to 83 cm. from the pylorus.

2. There is a progressive decrease in the pH and in the buffering capacity of the bowel contents as the distance from the pylorus is increased.

3. By increasing the length of the afferent loop in the Billroth II plan of gastrectomy, less buffering capacity is available for the neutralization of acid secretion at the gastroenteric stoma.

REFERENCES

1. Merendino, K. A., Varco, R. L., Litow, S. S., Kolouch, F., Baronofsky, I., and Wangensteen, O. H.: Stomal Ulcer Attending Complete Intragastric Regurgitation Influenced by Length of Afferent Duodenojejunal Loop, Proc. Soc. Exper. Biol. & Med. **58**: 222, 1945.
2. Wangensteen, O. H.: The Criteria of a Satisfactory Operation for Ulcer and Causes of Failure After Gastric Resection for Ulcer, Minnesota Med. **24**: 66, 1945.

3. Merendino, K. A., Lannin, B. G., Kolouch, F., Baronofsky, I., Bratrud, T. E., and Wangensteen, O. H.: Length of Afferent Duodenojejunal Loop in Gastric Resection, a Factor in Stomal Ulcer, Proc. Soc. Exper. Biol. & Med. **58**: 226, 1945.
4. Kiriluk, L. B., and Merendino, K. A.: Unpublished data.
5. Cross, F. S.: The Loss of Buffering Capacity of Alkaline Solutions After Passage Through Long and Short Duodenojejunal Loops, Proc. Surg. Forum, Clin. Congress Am. Coll. Surgeons, Philadelphia, 1951, W. B. Saunders Company, p. 89.
6. Visscher, M. B., Fetcher, E. S., Jr., Carr, C. W., Gregor, H. P., Bushey, M. S., and Barker, D. E.: Isotopic Tracer Studies on the Movement of Water and Ions Between Intestinal Lumen and Blood, Am. J. Physiol. **142**: 550, 1944.
7. Cantarow, A., and Trumper, M.: Textbook of Clinical Biochemistry, ed. 4, Philadelphia, 1949, W. B. Saunders Company.

AN ELUCIDATION OF THE INTESTINAL SENSITIVITY FACTOR AND THE DISTANCE FACTORS IN THE INCIDENCE OF STOMAL ULCER IN THE BILLROTH II TYPE GASTRECTOMY*

LAWRENCE B. KIRILUK, M.D.,** AND K. ALVIN MERENDINO, M.D., SEATTLE, WASH.

(From the Department of Surgery, University of Washington School of Medicine)

THE importance of a short afferent duodenojejunal loop in the Billroth II plan of gastric resection has been emphasized.[7-10] Several possible theories have been propounded for the increased incidence of stomal ulcers when a long afferent loop is utilized. The factors conceived to be important in the genesis of stomal ulcer are as follows: (1) the secretin factor, (2) the factor of altering the effective neutralizing capability of alkaline juices the further they progress down the intestine from their portal of entry into the lumen, and (3) the sensitivity factor, implying an increased susceptibility of the mucosa of successively lower segments of the small intestine to injury by the acid gastric secretions.

Matthews and Dragstedt[4] studied the factor of intestinal sensitivity by anastomosing an isolated gastric pouch obtained from the greater curvature to various levels of the intestinal tract. They concluded that the chemical action of pepsin hydrochloric acid can by itself produce typical chronic progressive ulcer in the stomach, duodenum, jejunum, ileum, or colon, and further that the resistance of these organs to the digestive action of pure gastric juice decreases progressively from the stomach to the colon. McMaster,[6] following a series of experiments in which the intact stomach was anastomosed to various segments of small and large intestine, concluded that "the intestinal mucosa was increasingly more sensitive to gastric content from the duodenum to the colon." He found no duodenal ulceration following gastroduodenostomy. Following gastrojejunostomy, jejunal ulceration occurred in 45 per cent of the animals. Iliac ulceration developed in 80 per cent of animals after gastroileostomy. Each of ten dogs developed a marked hemorrhagic colitis subsequent to a gastrocolostomy. The longest survival of the latter group was twenty days. Kolouch[3] concluded, from a series of complicated experiments wherein he employed a long afferent loop so arranged as to insure complete intragastric drainage of the afferent loop contents, that it was difficult to separate out with finality the role of the various factors contributing to the development of stomal ulcers, and that the secretin factor could not be divorced completely from the "distance" factor.

A previous report by one of us (K. A. M.)[7] indicated that following a 75 per cent gastrectomy of the Billroth II type, an afferent loop less than 27 cm.

Received for publication, Aug. 19, 1953.

*Supported by University of Washington Initiative 171 Funds for Research in Biology and Medicine.

**Trainee, National Cancer Institute.

long was unattended by complications, while the utilization of an afferent loop 27 cm. or longer frequently resulted in stomal ulcers in dogs subjected to histamine stimulation. Furthermore, as the length of the afferent loop increased so did the incidence of stomal ulcer. This observation has been substantiated by others.[3, 5]

While the three factors alluded to initially undoubtedly play roles of varying importance in such an experimental preparation, it seems unlikely that the secretin factor is significant quantitatively. On the other hand, the buffering capacity of the material presented at the stoma (in part influenced by secretin) and the inherent sensitivity factor appear to be of greater importance.

The present project was proposed to utilize the experimental preparation of a 75 per cent gastrectomy and alteration of the length of the loop in various manners which would allow the interposition of various segments of the small intestine to be used for the gastroenterostomy stoma.

In this fashion, it is possible to compare and separate the factors of the length of the afferent loop and the intestinal sensitivity as each influences the incidence of stomal ulcer following the Billroth II type of gastrectomy.

MATERIALS AND METHODS

Forty-five adult mongrel dogs weighing an average of approximately thirty pounds were operated upon. Anesthesia was effected by the intravenous administration of 15 mg. of Nembutal per pound of body weight. All surgical procedures were carried out aseptically.

Each animal was subjected to a Billroth II type subtotal gastric resection, 75 per cent by weight. A Hofmeister closure was made on the lesser curvature side, and the duodenum was inverted. All intestinal anastomoses were performed by the closed method, utilizing a single row of interrupted No. 60 black cotton sutures. The gastroenterostomies were made by the open technique, using two rows of interrupted No. 60 black cotton sutures. The stoma measured 5 cm. in length in each case. The jejunal segments to be tested for sensitivity were selected at a distance of 27 cm. (the critical length) or more from the inverted duodenal stump.

The group of 45 dogs was divided into three series of 15 each. Each series was subdivided into five groups of 3 dogs each. The constant factor in all animals was a 75 per cent subtotal gastrectomy following the Billroth II plan. The three major series to be listed differ in that the length of the afferent loop and the source of intestinal mucosa utilized in the gastroenterostomy are varied.

Series I (Fifteen dogs, Fig. 1, *A*).—The duodenum was transected 15 cm. distal to the inverted duodenal stump. A 10 cm. segment of jejunum, in each series of 3 animals, then was isolated from progressively lower segments of the intestine. The blood supply was preserved carefully to each segment. In the first group of 3 animals, the 10 cm. segment represented the area 27 to 37 cm. from the inverted duodenal stump. In each succeeding group of 3 animals, the jejunal segments were obtained at progressively lower levels by 10 cm. increments. In the fifth group of 3 animals, the jejunal segment represented the area 67 to 77 cm. from the inverted duodenal stump. Each isolated jejunal segment was interposed between the ends of the transected duodenum, and anastomosed in an isoperistaltic fashion. The gastroenterostomy then was made into the proximal end of the transplanted jejunal segment. Thus, the afferent loop was kept constant at 15 cm., and consisted entirely of duodenum. The variable factor from group to group was the site of origin of the transplanted jejunal segment.

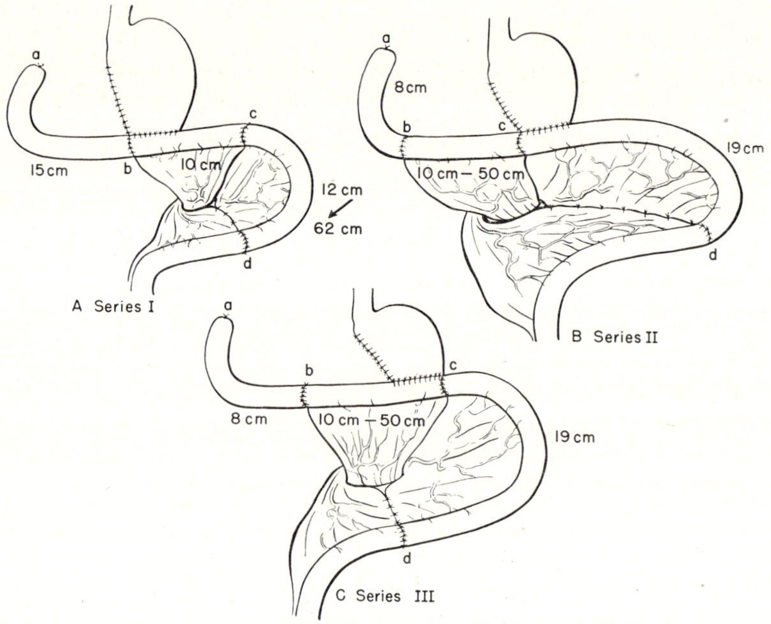

Fig. 1.—Schematic representation of the three plans of jejunal transplantation to test for differences in mucosal sensitivity to gastric juices. *a* to *b* is a segment of proximal duodenum. *b* to *c* is the transplanted jejunal segment anastomosed between the two ends of the transected duodenum. Segment *b* to *c* was obtained from site *d*. *c* to *d* is the distal portion of duodenum and/or the jejunum in normal continuity (see text).

Series II (Fifteen dogs, Fig. 1, *B*).—The duodenum was transected at a distance of 8 cm. from the duodenal inversion. In this series, the transplanted jejunal segment varied in length from 10 to 50 cm. In the first group of 3 animals, a 10 cm. segment of jejunum was isolated at 27 to 37 cm. distal to the duodenal inversion. In the second group, a 20 cm. segment was isolated at 27 to 47 cm. from the inversion. Progressively increasing lengths were isolated so that in the fifth group of animals, a 50 cm. length was isolated at 27 to 77 cm. from the inverted duodenal stump. Each jejunal segment was interposed between the two ends of the transected duodenum in an isoperistaltic fashion. The gastroenterostomy was made into the proximal end of the distal segment of the duodenum. Thus, the afferent loop varied in length from 18 to 58 cm. Each afferent loop contained 8 cm. of duodenum and a variable length of jejunum. In each case, the enteric portion of the gastroenterostomy consisted of duodenum originally located at 8 to 13 cm. from the inverted duodenal stump; therefore, anatomically this represented a gastroduodenostomy.

Series III (Fifteen dogs, Fig. 1, *C*).—The plan in this series was the same as that used in Series II, except that the gastroenterostomy was made into the distal end of the transplanted jejunal segment. The afferent loop consisted of 8 cm. of duodenum and a variable length of jejunum. The loop varied from 13 to 53 cm. in length. Postoperatively, the animals were injected daily for four days with 150,000 units of procaine penicillin. Intravenous 5 per cent glucose was administered for two days, following which the animals were allowed milk, progressing to a routine kennel diet within seven days.

A postoperative recovery and rest period of at least forty-five days was allowed. The animals then were subjected to daily intramuscular injections of 30 mg. of histamine phosphate base in beeswax for a maximum period of forty-five days. The histamine-in-beeswax was prepared and injected in the usual fashion.[1] Injections were made at approximately the same time each evening. The animals were routinely fed between 2:00 P.M. and 3:00 P.M. each day. The food pans were allowed for approximately one hour after feeding time and then were removed. Water was allowed at all times.

All animals dying during, or being sacrificed at, the end of the forty-five day injection period were autopsied carefully. The ulcers were measured, and the residual stomachs were weighed. The weight of the remaining stomach pouch and the weight of the resected specimen were used to determine the percentage of gastric resection.

RESULTS

The results are briefly summarized in Tables I, II, and III.

Series I.—Each of the 15 animals received a total of forty-five injections of histamine phosphate in beeswax. There were no deaths. The animals were sacrificed twenty-four hours after the last injection. At autopsy, only minimal findings were noted. Superficial erosions of the esophageal mucosa were noted in 2 animals, and of the gastric mucosa in 1 animal. Petechial hemorrhages were found in the gastric mucosa of 1 animal. No stomal pathology was noted. These findings are considered important in that some of the gastroenterostomies were made with the jejunal segments obtained at a distance of 77 cm. from the pylorus.

Series II.—The results in this series varied. Histamine stimulation caused no effect in the animals with short afferent loops. However, as the length of the afferent loop increased, the mortality and severity of pathology increased. In the series of 15 dogs, there were seven stomal ulcers. This is of particular import when it is realized that the gastroenterostomy was anatomically a gastroduodenostomy of duodenum which in normal continuity was 8 to 13 cm. from the pylorus. It is of interest to note that 2 animals (C-20 and C-43) died due to esophageal complications. One of these animals had a large stomal ulcer; the other had no stomal ulceration. No stomal obstruction was noted in any case.

Table I. Series I. (Fig. 1, *A*.) Seventy-five Per Cent Gastric Resection With the Gastroenterostomy Made to the Transposed Jejunal Segment; Each Dog Was Injected Daily With 30 mg. of Histamine-in-Beeswax

DOG NUMBER	WEIGHT (POUNDS)	SITE OF TRANSPOSED SEGMENT* (CM.)	LENGTH OF AFFERENT LOOP (CM.)	LENGTH OF SURVIVAL (DAYS†)	RESULTS
B-40	38	27-37	15	45	No findings
B-41	29	27-37	15	45	No findings
B-49	40	27-37	15	45	No findings
B-54	30	37-47	15	45	No findings
B-56	34	37-47	15	45	A few scattered petechial hemorrhages in the gastric mucosa
B-60	56	37-47	15	45	Several small superficial gastric erosions
B-61	38	47-57	15	45	Small superficial esophageal erosion
B-69	36	47-57	15	45	No findings
B-78	32	47-57	15	45	No findings
B-79	30	57-67	15	45	No findings
B-80	36	57-67	15	45	Two small esophageal superficial erosions
C-16	48	57-67	15	45	No findings
B-76	34	67-77	15	45	No findings
B-88	32	67-77	15	45	No findings
B-99	44	67-77	15	45	No findings

*Indicates the measured distance distal to the inverted duodenal stump. Each segment measured 10 cm. in length.

†Survival in days after beginning of daily histamine-in-beeswax administration.

Table II. Series II. (Fig. 1, *B*.) Seventy-five Per Cent Gastric Resection With the Gastroenterostomy Made to the Proximal End of the Distal Duodenal Segment; Each Dog Was Injected Daily With 30 mg. of Histamine-in-Beeswax

DOG NUMBER	WEIGHT (POUNDS)	SITE OF TRANSPOSED SEGMENT* (CM.)	LENGTH OF AFFERENT LOOP (CM.)	LENGTH OF SURVIVAL (DAYS†)	RESULTS
B-100	42	27-37	18	45	No findings
B-98	42	27-37	18	45	No findings
C-17	37	27-37	18	45	No findings
C-4	30	27-47	28	45	No findings
C-14	30	27-47	28	45	0.5 cm. shallow stomal ulcer; no bleeding
C-39	32	27-47	28	45	Small superficial esophageal erosion
C-20	24	27-57	38	9	Perforated esophageal ulcer; deep indurated stomal ulcer
C-22	42	27-57	38	45	No findings
C-43	32	27-57	38	27	Large bleeding esophageal ulcer; no stomal ulcer
C-21	28	27-67	48	14	Perforated stomal ulcer
C-23	27	27-67	48	35	Large, bleeding and penetrating stomal ulcer
C-61	40	27-67	48	0‡	—
C-25	44	27-77	58	11	No pathology noted at autopsy
C-28	34	27-77	58	11	Perforated stomal ulcer
C-57	34	27-77	58	45	Large, chronic stomal ulcer

*Indicates the measured distance distal to the inverted duodenal stump. The segments varied from 10 to 50 cm. in length.

†Survival in days after beginning of daily histamine-in-beeswax administration.

‡Animal died on thirty-ninth postoperative day. Four large stomal ulcers (76 per cent gastric resection by weight).

TABLE III. SERIES III. (FIG. 1, *C*.) SEVENTY-FIVE PER CENT GASTRIC RESECTION WITH THE GASTROENTEROSTOMY MADE TO THE DISTAL END OF THE TRANSPOSED JEJUNAL SEGMENT; EACH DOG WAS INJECTED DAILY WITH 30 MG. OF HISTAMINE-IN-BEESWAX

DOG NUMBER	WEIGHT (POUNDS)	SITE OF TRANSPOSED SEGMENT* (CM.)	LENGTH OF AFFERENT LOOP (CM.)	LENGTH OF SURVIVAL (DAYS†)	RESULTS
C-100	44	27-37	13	45	No findings
K-14	34	27-37	13	45	No findings
K-16	28	27-37	13	45	No findings
K-12	32	27-47	23	7	Bleeding stomal ulcer; two small superficial esophageal erosions
K-3	38	27-47	23	45	No findings
K-19	40	27-47	23	45	Chronic stomal ulcer
K-8	32	27-47	33	27	Perforated stomal ulcer
K-9	32	27-47	33	45	No findings
K-11	30	27-47	33	10	Perforated stomal ulcer
K-5	44	27-67	43	45	Small stomal erosion
K-7	36	27-67	43	40	Chronic, bleeding stomal ulcer
K-15	50	27-67	43	45	Chronic stomal ulcer
K-2	32	27-77	53	9	Perforated stomal ulcer
K-3	34	27-77	53	30	Large chronic stomal ulcer
K-4	32	27-77	53	6	Bleeding stomal ulcer

*Indicates the measured distance distal to the inverted duodenal stump. The transposed segments varied from 10 to 50 cm. in length.

†Survival in days after beginning of daily histamine-in-beeswax administration.

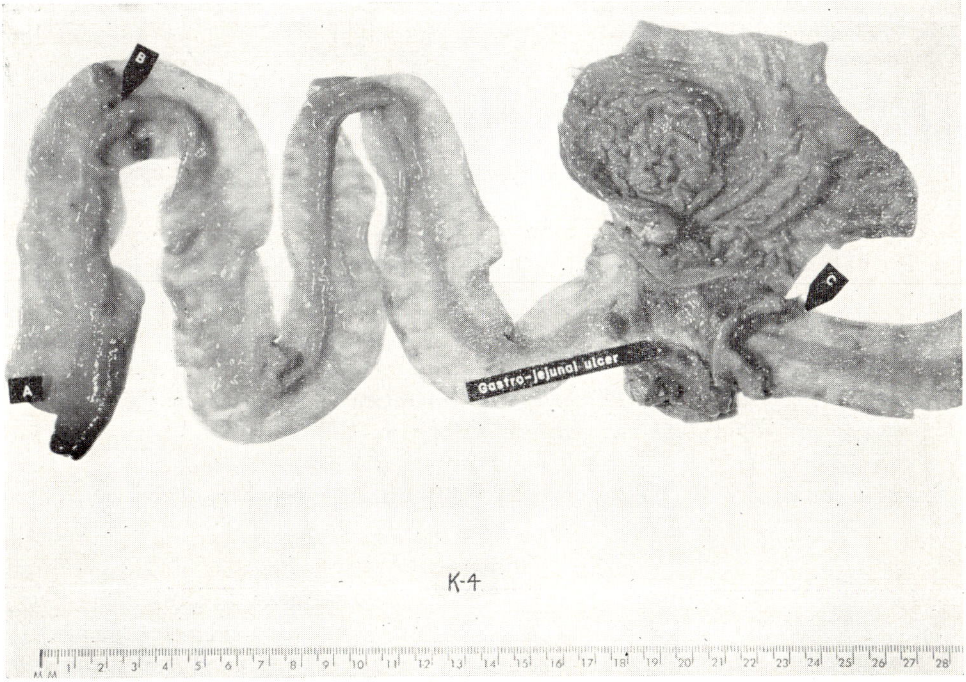

Fig. 2 (K-4, Series III).—Photograph showing a large stomal ulcer. *A*, Inverted duodenum; *A* to *B* represents 8 cm. of duodenum; *B* to *C* represents a 50 cm. segment of transplanted jejunum. Note that the ulceration does not extend to the anastomotic line. In no case did the ulcer involve the gastroenteric anastomosis. The reason for this is not known. It would appear, however, that avascularity was not a factor of ulcer formation since the enteric wall in juxtaposition to the anastomotic line has the poorest blood supply.

Series III.—This series of 15 animals underwent a similar procedure as Series II, except that the gastroenterostomy was made to a jejunal segment. The animals with short afferent loops tolerated the period of histamine stimulation well. The mortality and the incidence of stomal ulcers increased directly as the length of the afferent loop was increased. There were nine stomal ulcers in this group (Fig. 2).

DISCUSSION

The total lack of stomal pathology in Series I, wherein following a subtotal (75 per cent) gastrectomy the gastroenterostomy was fashioned with interposed jejunum obtained 27 to 77 cm. from the inverted duodenal stump, is of considerable importance. This experimental preparation parallels a previously reported series[8] wherein a gastrectomy of similar magnitude was performed with the gastrojejunostomy effected to identical jejunal segments, which however were in continuity, rather than interposed. The latter series resulted in a 100 per cent incidence of stomal ulcer, with a 43 per cent incidence of perforation with generalized peritonitis. The only difference between the series was the length of the afferent loop. In the present series it was constant at 15 cm. from the inverted duodenal stump, while in the early series the length of the afferent loop was dependent upon the site of the gastrojejunostomy. The striking contrast obtained by a comparison of these two series of experiments highlights the importance of a short afferent loop following the Billroth II plan of gastrectomy.

When the length of the afferent loop was increased as in Series II and III, the incidence of stomal ulcer increased pari passu in both series regardless of whether the gastroenterostomy was made to duodenum or jejunum as far as 77 cm. from the inverted duodenum. The incidence of stomal ulcer was practically the same in both groups of animals. It is of interest to note that in Series II, the gastroenterostomies were made to duodenum which originated only 8 to 13 cm. from the pylorus. The length of the proximal loop was the single variable factor.

One thing is certain, namely, that the secretions from the residual (25 per cent) gastric pouch delivered to the stoma have erosive potentialities. Furthermore, a protective mechanism or mechanisms are present which prevent stomal pathology when a short afferent loop is utilized.

These protective mechanisms have been alluded to previously. No definite conclusions may be drawn from these experiments regarding the secretin factor. However, if the entire duodenal mucosa is necessary for maximum secretin production, then the experimental preparations of McMaster, Dragstedt, and Matthews were ideal in this regard. In their preparations, the duodenum was intact. Consequently, the acid peptic juices, by implication, liberated an essentially optimal amount of secretin and therefore secondarily exerted a maximal protective action at the stoma. In view of the fact that stomal ulcers developed in their experiments with regularity, it must be assumed that the secretin factor is unimportant to this problem.

The results herein reported indicate that the factor of inherent intestinal mucosal sensitivity is likewise unimportant. While it cannot be assumed that segments of the small intestine lower than 77 cm. from the pylorus are relatively insensitive to gastric juice, certain facts should be presented which may not be apparent. The length of the dog's jejunum and ileum is approximately 290 cm. In man, the length of the small intestine from the ligament of Treitz to the ileocecal valve represents jejunum and ileum. Arbitrarily, the upper two-fifths is designated jejunum and the lower three-fifths is ileum. If these same relationships are applied to the dog, the jejunum extends 116 cm. from the ligament of Treitz. Therefore, the 10 cm. interposed loops obtained from 67 to 77 cm. levels represented small intestine exposed to acid juice from approximately the mid-jejunum. As evidenced by the results in all series, there is little, if any, evidence of increased mucosal sensitivity to acid peptic juice down to this level in the small intestine. Furthermore, recent experiments regarding the comparative sensitivity of the mucosa of the various segments of the gastrointestinal tract to acid peptic action in drip experiments indicate that there is actually little, if any, differential sensitivity in the entire small intestine.[2] Therefore, the factor of intestinal mucosal sensitivity seems to be of little or no importance with regard to the length of the afferent loop and the incidence of stomal ulcers.

By exclusion, then, one must concentrate primarily on the buffering capacity of the material delivered at the stoma as the major factor protecting against the development of stomal ulcers. In view of the increased incidence of stomal ulcer as the length of the afferent loop is increased, it must be assumed that the buffering capacity of bile, pancreatic, and bowel secretions is decreased the greater the length of bowel it must traverse.

Studies from this laboratory soon to be published[2] demonstrate that the buffering capacity of the bowel contents does actually decrease as the distance from the pylorus increases.

CONCLUSIONS

1. The importance of a short afferent loop in the prevention of stomal ulcers following the Billroth II plan of gastric resection has been reaffirmed.

2. Inherent mucosal sensitivity of the upper small intestine is relatively unimportant as a factor influencing the incidence of stomal ulcers under these conditions.

3. Contrary to previous opinion, the mucosa of the mid-jejunum does not appear to be more sensitive to gastric secretions than more proximal segments.

REFERENCES

1. Code, C. F., and Varco, R. L.: Chronic Histamine Action, Proc. Soc. Exper. Biol. & Med. 44: 475, 1940.
2. Kiriluk, L. B., and Merendino, K. Alvin: An Experimental Study of the Buffering Capacity of the Contents of the Upper Small Bowel, SURGERY 35: 532, 1954; The Comparative Sensitivity of the Mucosa of the Various Segments of the Alimentary Tract in the Dog to Acid-Peptic Action, SURGERY 35: 547, 1954.
3. Kolouch, F., Jr., Moreno Castellanos, M., Dubus, A. T., Baronofsky, I., and Wangensteen, O. H.: Mechanism of Stomal Ulcer as Related to Length of Afferent Duodenojejunal Loop, Proc. Soc. Exper. Biol. & Med. 58: 275-280, 1945.

4. Matthews, W. B., and Dragstedt, L. R.: The Etiology of Gastric and Duodenal Ulcer, Surg., Gynec. & Obst. **55**: 265-286, 1932.
5. Mayo, H. W., Jr.: Relationship of the Length of the Afferent Loop to the Incidence of Histamine-Induced Jejunal Ulcer in Gastrectomized Dogs, Proc. Surg. Forum, Clin. Congress Am. Coll. Surgeons, Philadelphia, 1950, W. B. Saunders Company, pp. 89-94.
6. McMaster, P. E.: Effects of Diverting the Gastric Contents to the Lower Intestinal Levels, Arch. Surg. **28**: 825-836, 1934.
7. Merendino, K. Alvin, Varco, R. L., Litow, S. Kolouch, F., Baronofsky, I., and Wangensteen, O. H.: I. Stomal Ulcer Attending Complete Intragastric Regurgitation Influenced by Length of Afferent Duodenojejunal Loop, Proc. Soc. Exper. Biol. & Med. **58**: 222-225, 1945.
8. Merendino, K. Alvin, Lannin, B. G., Kolouch, F., Baronofsky, I., Litow, S. S., and Wangensteen, O. H.: II. Length of Afferent Duodenojejunal Loop in Gastric Resection, a Factor in Stomal Ulcer, Proc. Soc. Exper. Biol. & Med. **58**: 226-230, 1945.
9. Wangensteen, O. H.: The Importance of a Short Afferent Duodenojejunal Loop in Gastric Resection for Ulcer, Bull. Minnesota M. Found. **4**: 82 (May) 1944.
10. Wangensteen, O. H.: The Criteria of a Satisfactory Operation for Ulcer and Causes of Failure After Gastric Resection for Ulcer, Minnesota Med. **24**: 66-70, 1945.

THE COMPARATIVE SENSITIVITY OF THE MUCOSA OF THE VARIOUS SEGMENTS OF THE ALIMENTARY TRACT IN THE DOG TO ACID-PEPTIC ACTION*

Lawrence B. Kiriluk, M.D.,** and K. Alvin Merendino, M.D., Seattle, Wash.

(From the Department of Surgery, University of Washington School of Medicine)

The problem of gastrointestinal ulceration has been a subject of much discussion and investigation for many years. A matter of great concern to the surgeon is related to the recurrent or stomal ulcer attending operations specifically designed to cure the patient with ulcer diathesis. Such stomal ulcers occur in segments of the intestinal tract which rarely develop ulcerations "spontaneously." By subtotal gastrectomy in the Billroth II plan, a segment of intestine which in the normal situation is not subjected to the trauma of the acid-peptic mixture is placed in direct opposition to acid-producing mucosa. Furthermore, it has been shown that when the gastrectomy is made to progressively lower segments of the intestinal tract the incidence of stomal ulcer increases.[1, 2] This work suggests that there exists a differential susceptibility of the mucosa of the intestinal tract to injury, either chemical or physical. Consequently, segments of the gastrointestinal tract have been subjected to various physical and chemical agents in an effort to determine the degree of differential mucosal susceptibility or resistance to trauma at the various levels.[3-6] Kolouch[7] exposed the antral and duodenal mucosa, and made comparative studies on these two segments by exposing them to a drip of an acid-peptic mixture. He noted a marked difference in the reaction of the mucosa at these two sites. In this laboratory, attention has been drawn to the extreme degree of sensitivity of the esophageal mucosa to regurgitated gastric juices,[8] and to the lack of differential sensitivity of small intestine down to the mid-jejunum.[9]

Basically, the resistance to ulcer formation and the perpetuation of an ulcer once formed within a segment of the gastrointestinal tract will depend on the ability of the mucosa at that site to resist injury or, if injured, its ability to recover and heal. To our knowledge, no studies have been made evaluating the mucosal resistance of the esophagus, stomach, duodenum, jejunum, and ileum exposed to chemical trauma, and the ability of each of these segments to recover and heal. The problem to be resolved, then, is the differential susceptibility and the response to trauma of the mucosa at the various levels within the esophagus, stomach, and small intestine when exposed to an acid-peptic mixture.

MATERIAL AND METHODS

Twelve adult mongrel dogs were used. The animals were fasted for eighteen hours prior to surgery. They were anesthetized, using 15 mg. of Nembutal intra-

Received for publication, Aug. 19, 1953.

*Supported by University of Washington Initiative 171 Funds for Research in Biology and Medicine.

**Trainee, National Cancer Institute.

venously per pound of body weight. Respiration was maintained by a mechanical respirator supplying oxygen.

A thoracoabdominal approach was used. The left thorax was entered through the tenth intercostal space, and the incision was extended distally across the costal cartilages and the abdominal wall. The left lung was retracted upward with wet laparotomy sponges. The diaphragm was divided from the hiatus in the direction of the thoracotomy incision. The lower esophagus was exposed at the cardiac juncture, and a 6 to 7 cm. longitudinal incision proximal to the esophagogastric sphincter was made on the left lateral aspect. The mucosa was exposed by elevation and the proper placement of a wet laparotomy sponge. A gastrotomy was performed to expose a segment of the gastric mucosa. A segment of the duodenum 10 cm. distal to the pylorus, the jejunum 10 cm. distal to the ligament of Treitz, and the ileum 10 cm. proximal to the ileocecal valve were exposed by making a longitudinal incision of similar length through the antimesenteric wall. This allowed the mucosa of the mesenteric wall of the bowel to be exposed.

In each case, a wet laparotomy sponge was placed so that the area exposed to drip was elevated and no "puddling" of acid-peptic mixture occurred at the exact site of the drip. The blood supply to each segment was carefully maintained. A black cotton suture was placed superficially in the serosa opposite the site of the drip. The suture served as a landmark to find the exact site of the drip at the time of autopsy.

An acid-peptic mixture of 0.1 normal HCl and 1 per cent pepsin was selected as the irritative "drip" solution since it has a pH of 1.2, approximately that of the gastric juice in the normal dog. One per cent pepsin was arbitrarily used. An increase in the percentage of pepsin up to 3 per cent does not appear to increase the irritative properties of the mixture. The acid-peptic mixture was dripped at the rate of 1 c.c. per minute to each of the five exposed segments. The mixture was dripped from burettes at a height of two inches. The excess of the drip mixture was absorbed by sponges, overflowed into the drapes, or aspirated from pools as it collected. The duration of the drip varied from fifteen minutes to fifteen hours.

An attempt was made to establish the optimal duration of drip. This would, of necessity, consist of a time interval which would produce mucosal damage of sufficient degree to evaluate both grossly and microscopically and yet not be so severe that a total lack of regeneration or healing would occur in the immediate postoperative period. Judging from the changes which occurred in the initial cases, it was felt that a drip period of sixty minutes would produce the desired specimens for study.

Three of the animals were sacrificed immediately following the experiment; the remaining animals were allowed to recover. The bowel incisions were repaired, and the peritoneal and pleural cavities were lavaged with warm saline solution. The chest and abdominal walls were closed in the usual manner. Procaine penicillin, 300,000 units, was given immediately postoperatively. Intravenous glucose solution was administered daily. The animal which was allowed to survive for fifteen days postoperatively was eating a routine kennel diet by the fifth postoperative day. The animals were sacrificed at varied post-operative intervals.

Gross examination was made at the time of autopsy, and multiple sections were taken for microscopic study.

RESULTS

The results are briefly summarized in Table I. The application of the acid-peptic mixture by drip produced a similar tissue response at the corresponding levels within the alimentary tract in all animals.

Esophagus.—A thin layer of mucus covered the esophageal mucosa at the time of exposure. The layer persisted throughout the entire period of drip, even up to fifteen hours. Following the start of the drip, petechial hemorrhages appeared within the mucosa at approximately fifteen minutes. Blanching then occurred, followed by a translucent appearance of the superficial layers. The subepithelial vessels were observed grossly at approximately twenty minutes. The vessels darkened and appeared coagulated at approximately thirty minutes. Subsequently, the site of the drip darkened, but no new changes occurred during that period of exposure.

Animals were sacrificed at one, two, three, and fifteen days. All esophagi exhibited frank erosions or ulcers. In general, the site of injury appeared hyperemic, rough, and raw. Two animals (S-5 and S-10) had lesions covered by a plaque of necrotic tissue. A raw surface was found on dislocation of the plaque. Microscopic evidence of injury was noted in every instance. Definite changes were noted in the esophagi of the animals sacrificed immediately following the drip period. After fifteen minutes of drip, the stratified epithelium was absent over most of the drip site. Occasional islands remained. The lamina propria lost some cellular detail and became more homogeneous in appearance than is normal. The remainder of the esophageal structures appeared normal. After thirty minutes of drip, the epithelium was completely absent. The lamina propria was homogeneous in appearance and the blood vessels within it were distorted and coagulated. The lamina muscularis mucosae appeared normal, but the submucosa became distorted and areas of homogeneity with loss of cellular characteristics appeared. The most superficial portions of the esophageal glands lost cellular detail and regularity. Following fifteen hours of drip, evidence of severe injury was found. The entire esophageal wall was edematous, detailed cellular characteristics were absent, and all of the blood vessels were coagulated. The mucous glands appeared to be the most resistant to injury. Although the general contour of the glands was retained, the cellular detail was lost.

Evidence of esophageal injury persisted in the animals which were allowed to survive for variable periods postoperatively (Fig. 2). The edema and homogeneity noted immediately postdrip subsided, and the cellular detail became more apparent. Cellular infiltration was present twenty-four hours postoperatively and became more prominent at seventy-two hours. Small irregular areas of pale-staining squamous epithelium were noted at seventy-two hours. This was considered to be evidence of re-epithelization occurring from the margins.

TABLE I. A DIRECT COMPARISON OF THE SENSITIVITY OF THE MUCOSA OF THE ESOPHAGUS, DUODENUM, JEJUNUM, AND ILEUM TO ACID-PEPTIC ACTION

DOG NO.	DURATION OF DRIP IN MINUTES	POSTDRIP SURVIVAL IN HOURS (SACRIFICED)	POSITIVE FINDINGS OF INJURY AT AUTOPSY*					POSITIVE FINDINGS OF INJURY ON MICROSCOPY*				
			ESOPHAGUS	STOMACH	DUODENUM	JEJUNUM	ILEUM	ESOPHAGUS	STOMACH	DUODENUM	JEJUNUM	ILEUM
S-1	6,300 (15 hr.)	0	+	0	+	+	+	+	0	+	+	+
S-3	15	0	+	0	+	+	+	+	0	+	+	+
S-2	30	0	+	0	+	+	+	+	0	+	+	+
S-4	30	360 (15 days)	+	0	0	0	0	+	0	0	0	0
S-5	60	24	+	0	0	0	0	+	0	0	0	0
S-7	60	24	+	0	0	0	0	+	0	0	0	0
S-12	60	24	+	0	0	0	0	+	0	0	0	0
S-6	60	48	+	0	0	0	0	+	0	0	0	0
S-11	60	48	+	0	0	0	0	+	0	0	0	0
S-8	60	72	+	0	+	0	0	+	0	0	0	0
S-9	60	72	+	0	0	0	0	+	0	0	0	0
S-10	60	72	+	0	0	0	0	+	0	0	0	+

*Indicates gross and microscopic changes in structure as a result of injury. The changes are described in the text under Results.

The suture line was not bridged by epithelium at seventy-two hours. Microscopic study of the esophagus of the animal (S-4) sacrificed fifteen days after a thirty-minute drip revealed cellular infiltration through all layers. Infiltration was most marked in the submucosa. The epithelium showed regeneration, but had not covered the entire surface of the drip site. Complete epithelization had occurred across the suture line.

Stomach.—The area of stomach mucosa exposed to the drip mixture became covered by a persistent layer of mucus, and revealed no gross changes at the time of the exposure or at the time of autopsy. No changes were noted on microscopic study.

Intestine.—The mucosa blanched almost immediately following the start of the drip. No significant time difference was noted in the onset of blanching of the mucosa of the duodenum, jejunum, or ileum. Petechial hemorrhages appeared in the ileal mucosa in approximately two to three minutes, in the duodenal mucosa in approximately three to four minutes, and in the jejunal mucosa in approximately four to five minutes after the start of the drip mixture. The petechial hemorrhages remained for two to three minutes and then darkened as if blood coagulation had occurred. No further hemorrhaging appeared. The entire area of the drip became covered by mucus or mucinlike exudate shortly after the start of the drip. The area became progressively more necrotic in appearance. After approximately one hour, a small depression appeared at the site of the drip but never extended into the submucosal layers, even after fifteen hours. At the time of the autopsy of the animals which were allowed postoperative survival, only one lesion was noted on gross examination. A 4 mm. depressed, red area was noted in the duodenal mucosa of S-8. This lesion was not found in the sections taken for microscopic study.

Microscopic evidence of injury was noted in the small bowel segments in each animal sacrificed immediately following the experiment and in S-10, in which an ileal ulceration was found seventy-two hours postoperatively. In general, the findings of injury were very similar and indistinguishable in the duodenum, jejunum, and ileum.

Following fifteen minutes of drip, the villi became distorted, and the most superficial parts were absent. Necrotic debris covered the surface. The remaining, superficial epithelial cells as well as the cells of the propria lost cellular characteristics and became more homogeneous. Evidence of extravasated blood was seen, but no coagulated vessels were noted.

Following thirty minutes of drip (Fig. 1, *A, B, C,* and *D*), the damage to the superficial mucosal layers increased. The erosion of the superficial epithelium and the lamina propria of the villi was marked. The capillary network and the central arteries and veins became damaged and appeared coagulated, taking a dark stain. The cellular detail was maintained in all remaining layers; however, the thickness of the bowel wall was increased, and in general a more homogeneous appearance was noted.

Following fifteen hours of drip, severe damage to all layers was evident. The villi were absent. The crypts of Lieberkühn became distorted and appeared empty and small as if dehydrated. The muscularis mucosae and the submucous layers blended into one homogeneous distorted layer having no cellular detail. The muscular layers were distorted, homogeneous, and lacked cellular detail. The entire wall was thickened by edema. The blood vessels were identified, but the contents were homogeneous and represented destroyed and coagulated bloods.

A.

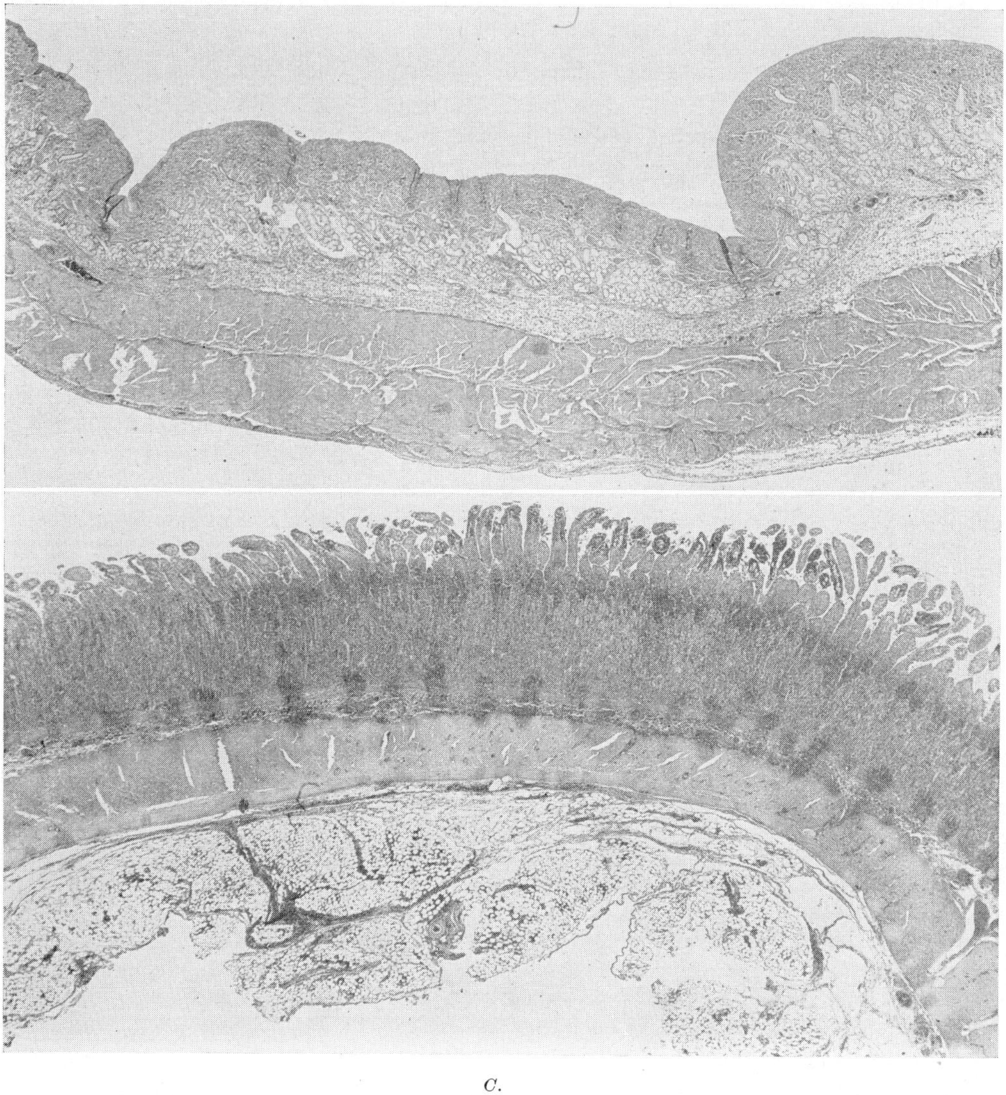

C.

Fig. 1.—Dog S-2. Photomicrographs of specimens exposed to thirty minutes of acid-peptic drip. *A*, Esophagus. Note the absence of the epithelium, the homogeneity of the lamina propria, and the coagulation of the surface vessels. *B*, *C*, and *D*, Duodenum, jejunum, and ileum. Note the distortion of the villi with loss of cellular characteristics of the superficial epithelium and lamina propria. Also, the superficial portion of the central blood vessels is damaged and takes a dark stain.

In the animals allowed to survive, microscopic evidence of mucosal injury was found in one instance only, S-10. This animal had been subjected to a sixty-minute drip and was allowed seventy-two hours for recovery. At autopsy, an ulceration of the ileal mucosa was overlooked. Upon microscopy, however, complete denudation of the mucosa and an acute cellular infiltration of the mucosa were noted.

B.

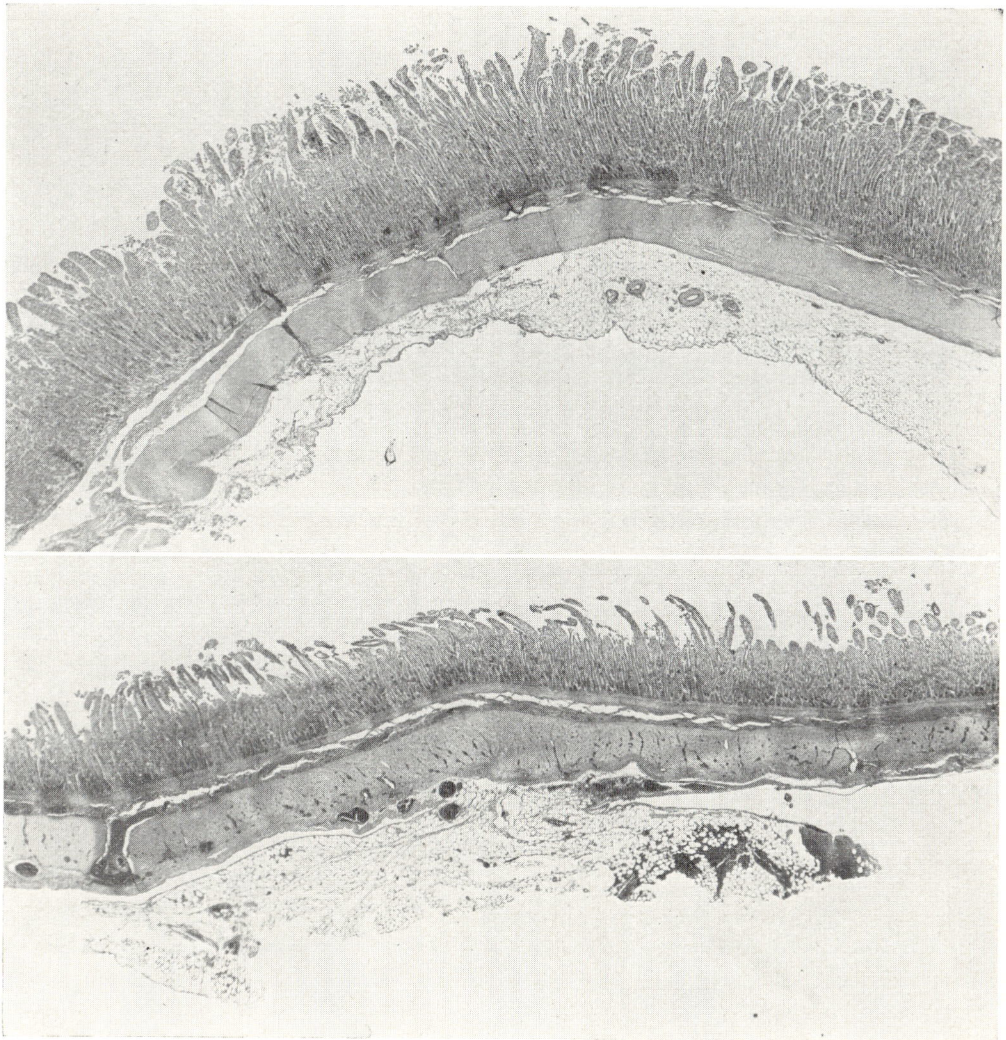

D.

Fig. 1, *B* and *D*. (*For legend see opposite page.*)

DISCUSSION

The mucosal susceptibility to injury, either chemical or physical, at the various levels within the alimentary tract has been recognized. However, the extreme degree of sensitivity of the esophageal mucosa to acid-peptic injury has not been fully appreciated. The sensitivity of the esophageal mucosa to the regurgitated gastric digestive mixture has been noted in this laboratory. Wangensteen,[10] an early proponent of the acid-peptic theory of the etiology of esophagitis, stated that the squamous epithelium of the esophagus is more vulnerable to injury by the acid-peptic digestive juice than is the glandular epithelium of the stomach. This statement may be expanded to include the small bowel.

A.

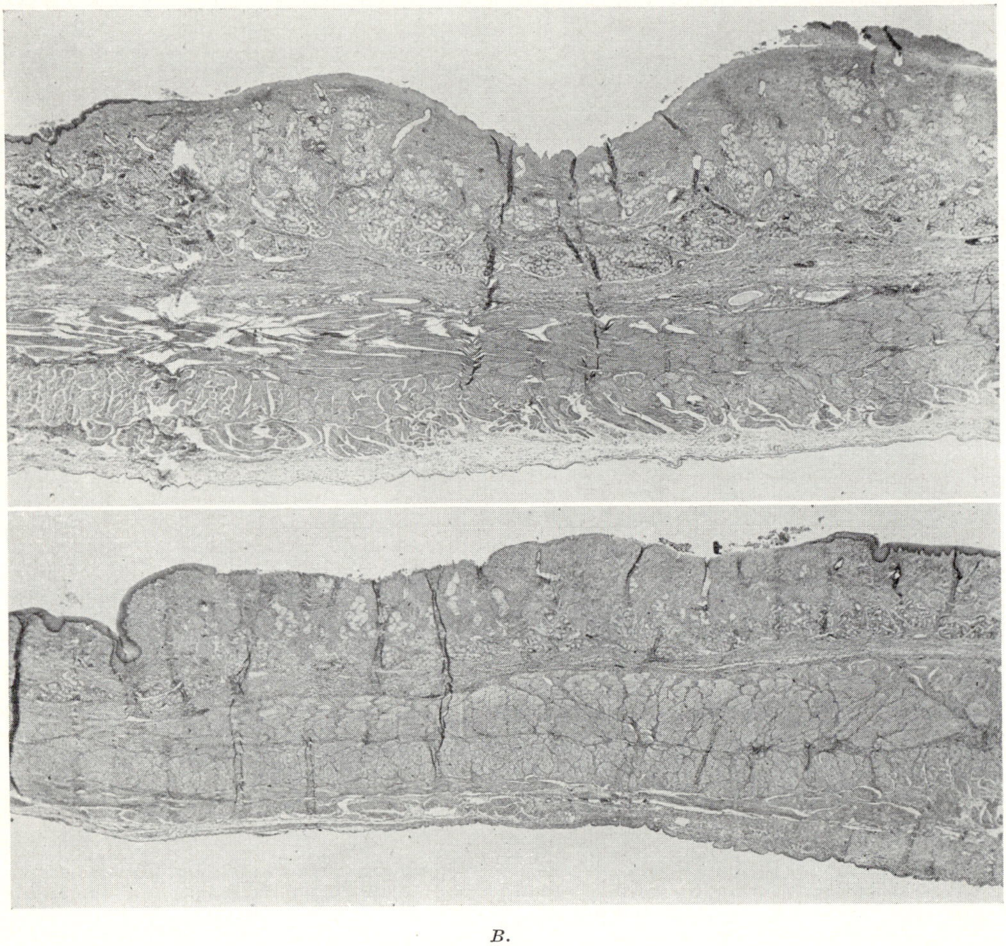

B.

Fig. 2.—*A*, Dog S-11, sacrificed forty-eight hours following a sixty-minute drip. Photomicrograph of the esophagus shows the epithelium to be absent. There is lack of loss of cellular detail in the lamina propria, lamina muscularis mucosae, and portions of the submucosa. Cellular infiltration is prominent, and a superficial necrotic plaque is noted. *B*, Dog S-10, sacrificed seventy-two hours following a sixty-minute drip. Photomicrograph of the esophagus shows similar changes as noted in *A*. Note the island of pale epithelium in the center. This is considered evidence of regeneration.

The ability of a mucosal surface to maintain "normality" depends on its ability to withstand insult or repeated irritative insults, and its ability to regenerate or heal. From the experimental work herein described, a comparative evaluation can be made of the mucosa of the esophagus, the stomach, and the small bowel, as each reacts to the irritative properties of an acid-peptic mixture and as each responds in recovery. The mucosa of the stomach appeared very stable and showed no appreciable signs of injury either grossly or microscopically. Others have found the mucosa of the stomach to be very resistant to various forms of trauma. The mucosa of the small bowel was the first to show gross signs of injury. This appeared as "blanching," hemorrhage, and necrosis. However, the process was limited. The layer of mucus and cellular debris over the crypts may be the protective mechanism. The regenerative power of the small bowel epithelium is enormous.

The rapidity of regeneration of the mucosa of the small bowel is demonstrated in this experiment by the lack of gross or microscopic evidence of mucosal damage on examination twenty-four hours following a sixty-minute acid-peptic drip. The one exception was noted in Dog S-10.

It appears that the structural composition of the surface lining of the various sections of the alimentary tract is important. The glandular epithelium of the stomach was very resistant to injury. The mucosa of the small bowel consisting of villi and crypts was injured, but "healed" rapidly. No differential sensitivity of the duodenum, jejunum, and ileum to the acid-pepsin drip was observed either immediately or delayed. All responded in like fashion to the initial trauma and healed rapidly when the drip was discontinued. Apparently, the stratified squamous epithelium of the esophagus is very susceptible to injury by acid-peptic digestive mixture. Once injured, the regeneration is slow. This was demonstrated in this experiment by Dog S-4, in which mucosal regeneration was incomplete fifteen days following a thirty-minute drip.

SUMMARY

1. A method of studying the isolated effects of acid-peptic trauma to various segments of the alimentary tract has been presented.

2. This study revealed: (a) that the mucosa of the stomach is very resistant to trauma by an acid-peptic mixture; (b) that the mucosa of the duodenum, jejunum, and ileum is sensitive to acid-peptic injury, but that the injured area "heals" rapidly; and (c) that the esophageal mucosa is the most susceptible to injury and that the recovery rate is slow.

3. Under the conditions of this experiment, no significant differential sensitivity to the acid-peptic mixture was observed in the duodenum, jejunum, or ileum. All underwent similar changes in their initial response to the injury and in healing.

REFERENCES

1. Matthews, W. B., and Dragstedt, L. R.: The Etiology of Gastric and Duodenal Ulcer, Surg., Gynec. & Obst. 55: 265-286, 1932.
2. McMaster, P. E.: Effects of Diverting the Gastric Contents to the Lower Intestinal Levels, Arch. Surg. 28: 825-836, 1934.
3. Miller, J. R., Herrick, J. F., Mann, F. C., Grindley, J. H., and Priestly, J. T.: Resistance of Explanted Gastric Mucosa to Various Chemical and Physical Agents, SURGERY 28: 1, 1950.
4. Ferguson, D. J., Sanchez-Palomera, E., Sako, Y., Clatworthy, H. W., Toon, R. W., and Wangensteen, O. H.: Studies on Experimental Esophagitis, SURGERY 28: 1022, 1950.
5. Florey, H., and Webb, R. A.: Mucus Secretion in Acute Experimental Inflammation of the Colon, and Other Mucous Membranes of the Cat; Histological Changes, Brit. J. Exper. Path. 12: 286, 1931.

6. Driver, R., Chappel, R., and Carmichael, E.: Effect of Concentration of Pepsin and the Differential Susceptibility of Jejunal Segments to Experimental Jejunal Ulcers in Dogs, Am. J. Digest. Dis. **12**: 166, 1945.
7. Kolouch, F., Jr.: A Direct Visual Technique for Studying Chemical and Other Injury to Exposed Mucosal Surfaces, SURGERY **17**: 641, 1945.
8. Kiriluk, L. B., and Merendino, K. A.: An Experimental Evaluation in the Dog of Esophago-Gastrectomy for the High Lying Gastric Ulcer, Ann. Surg. **134**: 918-923, 1951.
9. Kiriluk, L. B., and Merendino, K. A.: Unpublished data.
10. Wangensteen, O. H., and Leven, N. L.: Gastric Resection for Esophagitis and Stricture of Acid-Peptic Origin, Surg., Gynec. & Obst. **88**: 560, 1949.

THE EFFECT OF PARTIAL EXCLUSION OF BILE AND PANCREATIC JUICE ON THE ACIDITY OF THE GASTRIC CONTENTS IN THE POSTGASTRECTOMY PATIENT

Douglas A. Farmer, M.D., and Reginald H. Smithwick, M.D., Boston, Mass.

(From the Departments of Surgery, Massachusetts Memorial Hospitals and Boston University School of Medicine)

In four recent cases of duodenal ulcer patients subjected to partial gastrectomy plus vagotomy, we have utilized duodenostomy tubes as an added safeguard to hazardous duodenal stump closure. This preparation has afforded an unusual opportunity to study the neutralizing effect of regurgitant pancreatic, biliary, and duodenal secretions on the acidity of the gastric contents in the postgastrectomy patient. Opinions regarding the importance of enterogastric regurgitation in the modification of gastric acidity have varied widely. Most studies of this factor have been performed upon experimental animals, and in the majority, attention has been directed toward the development or prevention of jejunal ulcers in animals subjected to a variety of procedures which have aided or prevented regurgitation. Few such studies have been made in human beings, and only rarely have careful acidity studies been performed. We have been unable to find reference to another study similar to that reported here.

In 1923, the introduction of a method by which peptic ulcers could be produced in animals by the diversion of the duodenal contents to the lower small bowel[1] aroused considerable interest in the degree of protection against peptic ulcer afforded by the alkaline secretions contained in the duodenum. McCann[2] in 1929 reported the development of jejunal ulcers in 80 per cent of twenty-six dogs in which the method of anastomosis provided total regurgitation into the fundus of the stomach. He felt that jejunal ulcers could be as easily produced by introducing duodenal contents directly into the stomach as by draining them into the lower ileum. Methods reported by Graves[3] and Ivy,[4] however, in which duodenal contents were shunted into the antrum rather than the fundus failed to substantiate McCann's findings. Maier[5] modified McCann's procedure by anastomosing the proximal cut end of jejunum to the fundus of the stomach with a side-to-side anastomosis. In anastomosing the pyloric end of the stomach to the distal cut end of jejunum, both apposing ends were cut at an angle in order to obtain a large stoma and to interfere to some extent with the sphincteric action of the pyloric muscle. In McCann's preparation, the proximal cut end of jejunum was attached end to side to the gastric fundus, and the pyloric end of the stomach and the distal cut end of jejunum were joined with a simple end-to-end anastomosis. In Maier's hands, only one jejunal ulcer developed in several preparations, and he suggested

---

This investigation was supported in part by a research grant (G-3394 C) from the National Institute of Health, Public Health Service.

Received for publication, Aug. 14, 1953.

that the discrepancy between his results and those of McCann might be explained by the fact that his maneuver provided for rapid emptying of the stomach due to the much larger gastrojejunostomy stoma, while in McCann's experiment the stoma was small, and delayed gastric emptying had been noted. Wilhelmj[6] further modified the duodenogastric drainage by creating a side-to-side anastomosis between the anterior gastric wall and almost all of the duodenum in such a way that the duodenum virtually formed a part of the anterior wall of the stomach. With this method, the development of jejunal ulcers was prevented. Owings and Smith[7] very logically carried the problem a step further, and having produced jejunal ulcers in animals using the Mann-Williamson preparation, they demonstrated that a certain percentage of these ulcers could be healed by shunting the duodenal contents back into the stomach. Lannin,[8] on the other hand, performed antral resection and established total regurgitation in four dogs, and found that jejunal ulcers developed in all.

Statements regarding the effect of enterogastric regurgitation on gastric acidity in the experimental animals are likewise contradictory. Neither McCann[2] nor Kesavalu and Mann[9] found significant change in the pre- and postoperative acidity curves after promoting intragastric duodenal drainage. Maier,[5] however, found considerable reduction in acidity in his animals after operation, while Wilhelmj,[10] who likewise found a reduction, concluded that the efficacy of duodenal secretions in lowering acidity is due more to dilution than to neutralization; "on the average 75 per cent of the reduction in acidity was due to dilution and 25 per cent to neutralization." Recently, Kanar and associates[11] have shown that in dogs prepared with Heidenhain pouches, gastroenterostomy resulted in a significant rise in volume and free-acid content of pouch secretion. Zubiran and co-workers[12] established Heidenhain pouches and then performed vagotomy. With this preparation, they demonstrated a rise in acid secretion by the pouch after gastroenterostomy in which the jejunum was anastomosed to the antrum. In animals in which they established a denervated Heidenhain pouch and, in addition, excised the antrum and anastomosed the duodenum to the distal end of the stomach, no change in acid secretion by the pouch occurred if the jejunum was then anastomosed to the body of the stomach.

Only a limited amount of evidence exists concerning the effect of duodenal secretions on the acidity of the gastric contents in man. Such evidence as is available is indirect in nature. Schmilinsky[13] is generally credited with the first attempt at total intragastric regurgitation in human beings. In a personal communication to Maier,[5] he described results in three patients with jejunal ulcer following posterior gastroenterostomy upon whom he reoperated and instituted total regurgitation. One died postoperatively, another died within one year of a new perforated jejunal ulcer, and the third developed a severe and distressing gastritis. An additional five patients with duodenal ulcer who were thus handled all developed severe postoperative gastrointestinal symptoms. Wangensteen[14] reported on three patients upon whom he performed antral excision with total intragastric regurgitation, with development of jejunal ulcers in two of the three. Cholecystgastrostomy has been performed in an attempt to control gastric acidity by Babcock[15] and Braithwaite.[16] The latter described a recurrence of symptoms in 40 per cent of his cases within two years after operation.

Although total regurgitation has failed in human beings, this does not necessarily imply that the partial intragastric regurgitation which occurs after gastrojejunal anastomosis is an insignificant factor in the modification of gastric acidity. The possible importance of this factor is often minimized or overlooked in discussions of the effect of various maneuvers designed to reduce gastric acidity. Points more frequently stressed are complete antral excision, removal of a large segment of the acid-bearing portion of the stomach, removal of most of the lesser curvature, establishment of a short jejunal loop, and the possible beneficial effects of vagotomy. Although the bathing of the stoma by alkaline juices in high local concentration is recognized to have a protective neutralizing effect on acid gastric contents ejected through the stoma, the actual reduction of intragastric acidity by regurgitation may be of real importance in certain cases. We have recently[17, 18] pointed out our interest in the physiologic effect of various operative maneuvers on the acidity of the gastric contents, and have stated that if, as a result of operation, the pH can be maintained above 3.5 we believe the likelihood of recurrent ulceration is negligible. The evidence to be presented in this report suggests that in an occasional case the neutralizing effect of duodenal contents may be the deciding factor as to whether or not the operation performed fulfills our own criteria of acceptability.

METHOD OF STUDY

Our routine for the study of pre- and postoperative gastric acidity in ulcer patients has been previously presented.[17, 18] To recapitulate briefly, gastric contents are continuously aspirated and collected for one hour under "basal" or fasting conditions and for one hour after stimulation of the stomach by peptone beef broth. Sufficient intravenous insulin to effect a good clinical reaction is given, and four thirty-minute aliquots are collected over the course of the next two hours. With each aliquot, pH is detected using a Beckman pH meter, and free acid is determined by electrometric titration to a pH of 3.5. Above this pH level, no free acid is present. Volume is recorded and acidity is calculated in terms of total milliequivalent output per hour.

In two of the four patients referred to in this report, satisfactory preoperative studies were obtained, but in the others, massive hemorrhage necessitated emergency surgery and precluded routine evaluation. In each case, scarring, inflammation, and edema made dissection distal to the pylorus difficult, and resulted in an unsatisfactory duodenal stump closure. To protect against possible leakage, a Foley catheter was inserted into the duodenum through a stab wound distal to the suture line in such a way that the tip of the catheter lay near the ampulla of Vater. The Foley bag was inflated, and a purse-string suture applied to secure the catheter. In each case we removed an estimated one-half of the stomach and resected the vagus nerves below the diaphragm, a combination which in our hands has given more uniformly successful results than any other procedure.[18] Convalescence was uneventful in each case. Postoperative studies were made both with the duodenostomy tube in place on suction and later, after its removal. Thus we obtained data concerning the acidity of the gastric contents during a period of at least partial exclusion of bile and pancreatic juice for comparison with values obtained when regurgitation, such as was afforded by the Hofmeister type of anastomosis, was taking place.

RESULTS AND DISCUSSION

Table I lists the pre- and postoperative acidity figures. Postoperative I values were obtained with the duodenostomy tube on suction and Postoperative II values, after its removal. Acidity is recorded in terms of pH and total milliequivalents of free acid per hour. The latter is calculated by the formula $\frac{\text{units of free acid} \times \text{volume}}{1,000}$. The volume of duodenal contents aspirated during the first postoperative studies is also tabulated.

TABLE I. THE EFFECT OF PARTIAL EXCLUSION OF BILE AND PANCREATIC JUICE ON ACIDITY OF THE GASTRIC CONTENTS

		ACIDITY GASTRIC CONTENTS						
		PREOPERATIVE		POSTOPERATIVE I (WITH DUODENAL SUCTION)			POSTOPERATIVE II (WITHOUT DUODENAL SUCTION)	
CASE NUMBER	TEST	pH	MEQ. PER HOUR	pH	MEQ. PER HOUR	VOLUME OF DUODENAL CONTENTS ASPIRATED (C.C.)	pH	MEQ. PER HOUR
1 (E. R.)	Basal	1.3	5.3	1.9	0.24	21	7.3	0
	Broth	1.1	9.4	2.8	0.9	13	6.6	0
	Insulin	1.0	17.9	1.9	0.3	11	6.9	0
2 (M. L.)	Basal	1.4	4.4	4.0	0	12	6.5	0
	Broth	1.0	19.9	5.8	0	3	6.6	0
	Insulin	1.1	19.3	4.1	0	20	6.4	0
3 (C. S.)	Basal	–	–	3.7	0	2	5.2	0
	Broth	–	–	3.7	0	2	6.3	0
	Insulin	–	–	3.7	0	40	6.2	0
4 (H. C.)	Basal	–	–	6.0	0	7	5.2	0
	Broth	–	–	6.3	0	2	6.6	0
	Insulin	–	–	6.2	0	38	6.5	0

The values in Case 1 (E. R.) are most striking. With partial exclusion of the duodenal contents in the postoperative period it will be noted that the pH of the gastric contents is in a strongly acid range. Viewing these figures alone, one would say that the operation had failed to reduce gastric acidity to a point where recurrent ulceration could be considered highly improbable. The later studies, on the other hand, with regurgitation taking place reveal the gastric contents to be very nearly neutral. In this pH range, recurrent ulceration will almost certainly not occur. The reduction in acidity due to the presence of duodenal buffer substances is emphasized if hydrogen ion concentration is considered in terms of milligrams per cent. For example the shift in postoperative pH under basal conditions from 1.9 to 7.3 represents a reduction in concentration from 1.3 to 0.000005 mg. per cent. We feel that it is unlikely that this marked difference in acidity, in otherwise identical studies performed five days apart in the postoperative period, is due to artefact. In our experience, the postoperative results check closely in the same patient tested at different times.

Fig. 1.

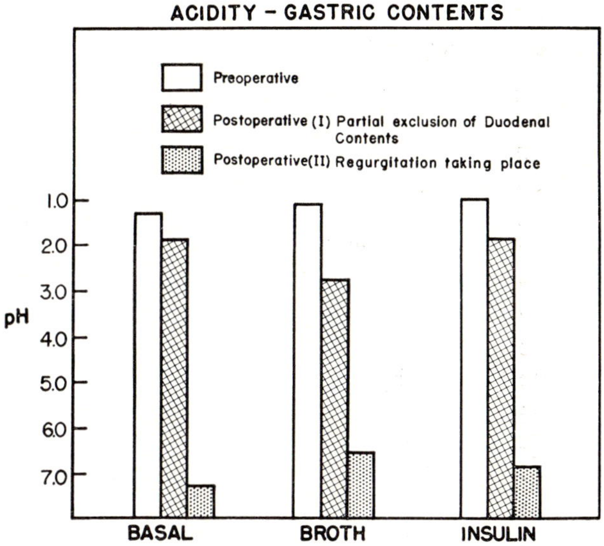

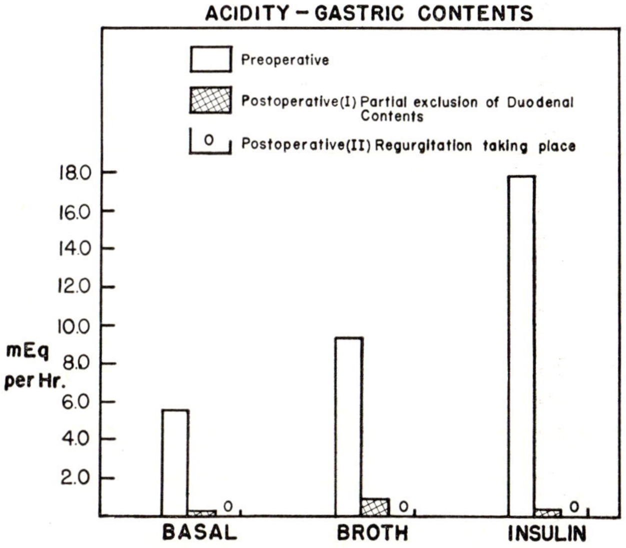

Fig. 2.

Fig. 1 (Case 1, E. R.).—The effect of bile and pancreatic juice on pH of the gastric contents following hemigastrectomy combined with vagotomy.

Fig. 2 (Case 1, E. R.).—The effect of bile and pancreatic juice on acidity of the gastric contents in terms of total milliequivalents of free acid per hour following hemigastrectomy combined with vagotomy.

The results in Case 1 are depicted graphically in Figs. 1 and 2. The marked quantitative reduction in acidity noted if the preoperative and Postoperative I values are considered in terms of total milliequivalents is due not only to some reduction in hydrogen ion concentration, but also to a marked reduction in volume of gastric contents. In Cases 2 and 3 (M. L. and C. S.), the results are less striking. The pH values in the first postoperative tests ranged between 3.7 and 5.8. In the second postoperative tests they were somewhat higher under all conditions of study. In Case 4 (H. C.), despite removal of a portion of the duodenal contents the postoperative pH levels were high.

The method of diversion of duodenal contents used in this study was such that a variable portion of the pancreatic and biliary secretions could proceed, unhindered, to the gastroenterostomy stoma. This probably accounts for the variation in the postoperative findings from case to case. Significant traces of bile were found in the gastric aspirations of Case 2, and to an even greater extent in Case 4. Failure of sufficient exclusion may well explain the high initial postoperative pH levels found in the latter case. In Cases 1 and 3, little evidence of bile was detected in the gastric contents. Although pancreatic juice unaccompanied by bile has been shown to reflux back through a normal intact pylorus,[19] it seems most unlikely that selective regurgitation would occur through a gastroenterostomy stoma, and therefore in Cases 1 and 3 diversion of the duodenal contents was apparently more effective.

We have previously indicated our satisfaction with the uniform reduction in gastric acidity effected by hemigastrectomy and vagotomy, a maneuver which, if properly performed, should largely eliminate both the chemical and neurogenic phases of gastric secretion. Among the patients discussed in this report, however, we would classify the physiologic results in Case 1 as poor and in Cases 2 and 3 as fair if we considered only the initial postoperative studies carried out with regurgitation prevented. On the other hand, all of the results based on the later postoperative studies with regurgitation permitted would be classified as entirely satisfactory. Small quantities of duodenal contents, seemingly insignificant in some instances, appear to have made a considerable difference. The volume which was diverted varied not only in different patients, but also from time to time in the same patient. The hourly volumes and the marked variation are not dissimilar to those recorded for biliary and pancreatic output under experimental conditions.[20] It appears that if the operative procedure performed greatly reduces the total amount of acid in the gastric contents by reducing both free acidiy and volume, as occurred in Case 1 (Fig. 2), but permits a small residue whose pH is low, this residue can be easily neutralized by a small quantity of bile and pancreatic juice. If, however, during the postoperative period there is a considerable volume of moderately acid gastric contents, then the small amount of buffer material regurgitated into the stomach might be completely overwhelmed with little or no change in gastric acidity. This would explain the results of Holman and Sandusky,[21] who found gastric acidity not appreciably altered in

92 per cent of seventy-five patients subjected to posterior gastroenterostomy, a procedure which provides regurgitation but either leaves unaltered or, according to some evidence, augments the mechanisms by which the stomach produces acid. It might further explain the failure of Schmilinsky's total enterogastric regurgitation and Wangensteen's enterogastric regurgitation plus antrectomy. It is to be borne in mind that duodenal ulcer patients, in general, produce large quantities of highly acid gastric contents both on fasting and under stimulation, but we have no evidence that in these same patients the production of bile or pancreatic juice is increased in a proportionate fashion. In a simple posterior gastroenterostomy, there is a single stoma between the stomach and jejunum which is the site of high local concentration of bile and pancreatic juice. In such a preparation, although gastric acidity may be insignificantly modified by regurgitation, sufficient neutralization takes place at the stoma to prevent gastrojejunal ulcers in the majority of instances. In total regurgitation procedures, the two stomas are separated from one another, and all of the duodenal contents are emptied into the stomach and diluted. As the quantity is probably insufficient to modify effectively the large volume of highly acid gastric contents characteristic of most ulcer patients, the full brunt of this acidity is then brought to bear upon the efferent stoma.

In Case 3, the initial postoperative pH values indicate achlorhydria but fall in a range in which peptic activity is not negligible. The relatively low hydrogen ion concentration is reduced to almost nothing when regurgitation is allowed. Peptic activity appears to become negligible when pH values are 4.5 or more.[22, 23] On the other hand, even though peptic activity may be significant in the range 3.5 to 4.5, we have yet to see a jejunal ulcer in a patient whose pH values were 3.5 or more under all of the conditions of study employed. To our knowledge, the old adage "no free acid, no peptic ulcer" is still valid.

SUMMARY

1. Suction applied to a duodenostomy tube inserted at the time of gastrectomy will remove at least a portion of the duodenal contents which normally bathe the stoma and regurgitate to a variable degree into the gastric lumen. We have studied postoperative gastric acidity in four such preparations with the duodenostomy tube on suction, and later after its removal.

2. In one case, diversion of bile and pancreatic juice appeared to have a profound effect on hydrogen ion concentration. In two others, the effect was slight but definite. In the fourth case, perhaps because of inadequate aspiration of duodenal contents, no appreciable change was noted.

3. Recurrent ulceration is highly unlikely if achlorhydria results from an operation performed for the relief of duodenal ulcer. The factor of regurgitation, frequently overlooked or minimized in discussions of the effect of various operative maneuvers on acidity of the gastric contents, may, in some instances, be decisive in the achievement of achlorhydria.

REFERENCES

1. Mann, F. C., and Williamson, C. S.: The Experimental Production of Peptic Ulcer, Ann. Surg. **77**: 409-422, 1923.
2. McCann, J. C.: Experimental Peptic Ulcer, Arch. Surg. **19**: 600-659, 1929.
3. Graves, A. M.: Combined and Separate Effects of Bile, Pancreatic Secretion and Trauma in Experimental Peptic Ulcer, Arch. Surg. **30**: 833-853, 1935.
4. Ivy, A. C., and Fauley, G. B.: Factors Concerned in Determining Chronicity of Ulcers in the Stomach and Upper Intestine; 1. Susceptibility of Jejunum to Ulcer Formation; 2. Effect of Diet on Healing of Acute Gastric Ulcer, Am. J. Surg. **11**: 531-543, 1931.
5. Maier, H. C., and Grossman, A.: Relation of Duodenal Regurgitation to the Development of Jejunal Ulcers, SURGERY **2**: 265-274, 1937.
6. Wilhelmj, C. M., O'Brien, F. T., McCarthy, H. H., and Hill, F. C.: The Role of Duodenal Secretions in the Prevention of Experimental Jejunal Ulcer, Am. J. Physiol. **117**: 79-85, 1936.
7. Owings, J. C., and Smith, I. H.: Experimental Production and Cure of Jejunal Ulcers, Proc. Soc. Exper. Biol. & Med. **29**: 832-833, 1931-32.
8. Lannin, B. G.: Experimental Evaluation of a Satisfactory Operation for Ulcer, SURGERY **17**: 712-741, 1945.
9. Kesavalu, A., and Mann, F. C.: The Influence of Duodenal Contents on Intragastric Acidity, SURGERY **14**: 578-587, 1943.
10. Wilhelmj, C. M., Henrich, L. C., and Hill, F. C.: The Influence of Duodenal Secretions on Acid Gastric Contents, Am. J. Physiol. **111**: 293-304, 1935.
11. Kanar, E. A., Schmitz, E. J., Sauvage, L. R., Storer, E. H., and Harkins, H. N.: The Secretory Response of the Stomach to Gastroenterostomy as Measured by a Heidenhain Pouch, Proc. Surg. Forum, Clin. Congress Am. Coll. Surgeons, 1952, Philadelphia, 1953, W. B. Saunders Company.
12. Zubiran, J. M., Kark, A. E., Montalbetti, A. J., Morel, C. J. L., and Dragstedt, L. R.: Quantitative Studies on the Effect of Gastrojejunostomy on Gastric Secretion, Proc. Surg. Forum, Clin. Congress Am. Coll. Surgeons, 1952, Philadelphia, 1953, W. B. Saunders Company.
13. Schmilinsky, H.: Dei einleitung der gesamten Duodenalsafte in den Magen (inner Apotheke), Centralbl. f. Chir. **45**: 416, 1918.
14. Wangensteen, O. H., and Lannin, B.: Criteria of an Acceptable Operation for Ulcer, Arch. Surg. **44**: 489-500, 1942.
15. Babcock, W. W.: Control of Hyperchlorhydria and Its Consequences by Cholecystogastrostomy, Med. Rec. **98**: 476, 1920.
16. Braithwaite, L. R.: The Role of Bile in Duodenal Regurgitation, Brit. J. Surg. **31**: 3-13, 1943.
17. Farmer, D. A., and Smithwick, R. H.: The Effect of Various Surgical Procedures Upon the Acidity of the Gastric Contents of Ulcer Patients, Ann. Surg. **134**: 319-331, 1951.
18. Farmer, D. A., and Smithwick, R. H.: Hemigastrectomy Combined With Resection of the Vagus Nerves, New England J. Med. **247**: 1017-1022, 1952.
19. Medes, G., and Wright, C. B.: Studies on Duodenal Regurgitation, J. Clin. Investigation **6**: 403-425, 1928.
20. Babkin, B. P.: Secretory Mechanism of the Digestive Glands, New York, 1950, Paul B. Hoeber, Inc.
21. Holman, C., and Sandusky, W. R.: Gastric Acidity After Gastroenterostomy, Am. J. M. Sc. **195**: 220-230, 1938.
22. Hollander, F.: What Is pH? Gastroenterology **4**: 497-508, 1945.
23. Northrop, J. H., Kunitz, M., and Herriott, R. M.: Crystalline Enzymes, New York, 1948, Columbia University Press.

THE RELATION OF BACTERIA IN THE BILE TO BILIARY DYNAMICS, CHOLANGITIS, AND POSTCHOLECYSTECTOMY SYNDROME

S. Albert Sarkisian, D.M.D., M.D., Brockton, Mass., and John M. McGowan, M.D., M.S. (Surg.), Quincy, Mass.

(From the Department of Surgery, Tufts Medical College, Boston, Mass., the Boston and Quincy City Hospitals)

IN PREVIOUS communications,[1, 2] one of us (J. M. McG.) has shown that many gall bladder patients demonstrate a sensitivity of the bile ducts to perfusion of normal saline solution under pressure. We have routinely measured perfusion pain pressure and resting intrabiliary pressure after gall bladder operations in patients with T tubes in the common bile ducts for over fifteen years. We have learned to expect a perfusion pain pressure of 550 mm. of water or more, and a resting pressure of 30 mm. of water or less. In most cases, the perfusion pain pressure is below the level of 550 mm. of water, and the resting pressure is above 30 mm. of water above the ensiform two weeks postoperatively. The biliary dynamics tend to reach normal levels after a period of T-tube drainage. The duration of drainage necessary to restore the "biliary dynamics" to normal is variable. We have come to learn that it is very essential that normal dynamics exist before the T tube is removed in order to avoid recurrence of biliary symptoms after operation.

With T-tube drainage, the biliary dynamics usually return to normal after variable periods, in some cases in six weeks, in others up to one year.

In two cases of cholangitis occurring postoperatively, we were impressed with the rapid return to normal of the biliary dynamics after injection of streptomycin through the T tube into the biliary tree.

These observations led us to believe that a low perfusion pain pressure indicated residual infection in the bile duct, that is, cholangitis. The pain produced by perfusion of the bile duct is of the same nature as pain which patients with biliary disease experience before surgery. For that reason we believe that a low perfusion pain pressure in the common bile duct indicates infection, that is, cholangitis.

Reasons for this belief are as follows: (1) pain on pressure is a cardinal sign of infection, and (2) invariably, tolerance to perfusion improves with common bile duct drainage, a fact in agreement with the surgical axiom that infection improves with drainage.

The purpose of this study, therefore, was to determine (1) the relationship between biliary dynamics and bacteria in bile, (2) the nature of bacteria in the common duct, and (3) the effect of antibiotic agents on (a) biliary dynamics and (b) bacteria in bile.

Received for publication, Aug. 10, 1953.

Although there has been a great deal of research carried out on the bacteriology of gall bladder bile and to a lesser degree on duodenal drainage bile, there has been very little work of this nature reported on common duct bile.

REVIEW OF LITERATURE

Twiss[3] studied the bacteriology of the biliary tree. One hundred twenty patients with chronic biliary tract disease were studied. In each case a preoperative duodenal drainage was carried out with sterile precautions. A sterile duodenal tube covered with a gelatin capsule, so as to prevent contamination by organisms from the nasopharynx and laryngeal areas, was used. The basis of the study assumes that the normal fasting duodenum is sterile.

In 120 cases, Twiss found twenty-eight positive cultures from duodenal bile, and all of these were verified at operation. The organisms were found to be identical in the two types of cases. The types of bacteria found, in the order of frequency, were *Bacillus coli,* colon-Streptococcus group, *Bacillus typhosus,* nonhemolytic Streptococcus, Staphylococcus and Streptococcus, and an unidentified Enterococcus group.

Mirizzi[4] obtained bile for culture at operation by introducing an olive-tipped catheter through the stump of the cystic duct; in addition, he obtained bile from the gall bladder and duodenum, and cultured a piece of tissue from the gall bladder wall. He concluded that bile from the common duct is sterile in a large number of patients with disease of the extrahepatic biliary tract, and also that stone in the common bile duct is the most frequent cause of infection of the bile.

Zollinger and Cutler[5] emphasized the importance of *Bacillus coli* infection of the biliary tree. Of 146 patients operated upon for acute cholecystitis, four deaths were recorded, and the cause of death in three of these patients was infection. One had a definite septicemia due to *Bacillus coli,* and the other two had peritonitis due to the same organism.

METHOD OF STUDY

A series of cases of patients in whom T tubes had been placed in the common bile duct at the time of cholecystectomy was studied at the Boston City Hospital. The patients were seen at intervals of two to three days during the postoperative period, at which time the following studies were made: (1) cultures of the T-tube bile were taken, (2) intrabiliary pressure studies were recorded, and (3) the effect of antibiotics on the bacteria in bile was studied.

1. *Bacteriology.*—The bile was taken from the T tube by a sterile technique. The following method was found to be quite effective in excluding contamination after numerous bacterial checks: the exposed end of the T tube is washed with green soap, then alcohol (70 per cent), and finally painted with a 7 per cent tincture of iodine, with care being taken to paint the first 0.5 cm. of the inner portion of the T tube. After this has dried, another application of 7 per cent iodine is used. Then a 10 c.c. sterile syringe is attached to the prepared end of the T tube, and the bile allowed to enter the syringe at its own secreting pressure. About 3 to 5 c.c. of the bile is collected for culture.

2. *Biliary Dynamics.*—The biliary pressure studies were carried out by the method suggested previously by one of us (McGowan[6-8]). Briefly, the apparatus is assembled around an ordinary Y-shaped glass tube. The stem of the Y is attached by means of a rubber tube to a bottle of intravenous saline solution. To each limb of the Y tube is attached a rubber tube, one of which is to be connected to the T tube of the patient and the other to an upright manometer. The tubing is filled with normal saline solution from the reservoir bottle before it is connected to the patient, and all the air bubbles in the rubber tubing are removed. The zero level of the manometer is placed at the level with the xiphoid process of the sternum, with the patient lying flat on the back. Two separate pressure readings are made: (1) the resting intrabiliary pressure and (2) the perfusion pain pressure level.

The resting intrabiliary pressure is an index of the patency of the lower end of the bile duct. It is taken as follows: After the manometer is connected to the T tube as described, some saline solution is allowed to perfuse into the duct by allowing saline solution to flow from the reservoir bottle sufficient to raise the pressure to 100 to 200 mm. of water. The pressure is allowed to fall several times until an average level has been obtained. The resting intrabiliary pressure under normal conditions has been found to be less than 30 mm. of water above the xiphoid level. Elevated pressure may be due to various conditions, such as, inflammation of the head of the pancreas, spasm of the duodenal wall, a missed stone in the common duct, or edema of the duodenal mucosa at the ampulla of Vater.

If obstruction is due to spasm, it will be relieved by four deep inhalations of amyl nitrite. If this medication reduces the pressure to normal, the obstruction is due entirely to spasm. If it fails to do so, it is due to some other process. If there is a partial reduction of the resting intrabiliary pressure, then the obstruction is due partially to spasm and partially to a more permanent factor.

The perfusion pain pressure level is defined as the lowest hydrostatic pressure that the common duct can tolerate before the patient experiences discomfort. Some patients experience pain when the biliary tree is exposed to relatively low perfusion pressures at times not over 70 mm. of water, whereas in other cases pressures of 500 mm. and even 700 mm. can be tolerated without discomfort. This difference in pain pressure is explained as follows: If the bile ducts are dilated, high tension is developed by relatively low pressures; if the ducts are inflamed, the slightest intraductal pressure will produce pain. The bile passages should be able to withstand a pressure of 500 mm. without discomfort. If the T tube is removed while the perfusion pain level is below 300 mm. of water, subsequent distress can be expected. Previous experience has indicated that if the bile ducts are decompressed long enough by T-tube drainage, the tolerance to water pressure invariably improves up to 500 mm. of water or better. It is believed that the T tube can then be removed without the probability of postcholecystectomy syndrome. Experience with over 200 cases of T-tube drainage tends to bear this out.

Biliary pressure studies as described were carried out initially fourteen days after operation. We believe that studies should not be carried out before this time because of the danger of intra-abdominal leakage. The fistulous tract around the T tube at the end of fourteen days is well sealed off.

Biliary pressure studies were then carried out at least once and sometimes twice weekly depending on the individual patient. For the most part, patients were discharged from the hospital as soon as possible and then seen weekly at the Surgical Follow-Up Clinic.

Three criteria were used as an indication for T-tube removal: (1) *clinically,* the patient had no postoperative distress after the T tube had been clamped consistently for three weeks; (2) *bacteriologically,* bile cultures for pathogenic organisms were negative; (3) *physiologically,* the resting intrabiliary pressure was below 30 mm. of water and the pain perfusion level above 500 mm. of water.

3. *Antibiotics.—*

The administration of antibiotics intraductally was carried out in those patients who had a continual positive bile culture and a disturbance of biliary dynamics after fourteen days. Penicillin was instilled as 100,000 U. of aqueous type in 15 c.c. of sterile saline solution at least three times daily for two days, and then cultures were taken after twenty-four hours. The T tube was clamped off for two hours following each instillation. Streptomycin was also used in a few cases in doses of 1 Gm. four times a day, and instilled as described previously. Bacitracin was used also, but only as a preliminary study. Our aim in this paper is not to evaluate the relative merits of various antibiotics but instead to correlate the bacteriology with the biliary dynamics.

RESULTS

Twenty-seven cases of patients with T-tube drainage in all were used for this study. Twenty-one of these cases were studied in detail as far as the bacteriology of bile was concerned. Table I shows the quantity and types of bacteria found.

TABLE I. AN ANALYSIS OF THE BACTERIOLOGY OF BILE OBTAINED BY T-TUBE DRAINAGE

	NUMBER OF CASES	PER CENT OF TOTAL CASES
Cases with bacteria	18	85
Cases showing no growth	3	15
Total cases studied	21	
Cases with pure culture	2	10
Cases with mixed cultures	16	90
Total cases	18	
Types of organisms (in order of frequency)		
Escherichia coli	13	
Bacillus proteus	8	
Aerobacter aerogenes	6	
Bacillus pyocyaneus	5	
Bacillus welchii	3	

It is interesting to note that we had no growth of streptococci or staphylococci, which may be explained by the inhibitory effect of bile on these organisms.

Bile cultures were taken at various intervals ranging from the first day postoperative to as long as the sixtieth day. The cultures became negative at various time intervals. The average time was calculated to be thirty-five days after operation; this, of course, includes all cases regardless of whether the patient received any antibiotics or not. With the use of streptomycin in doses of 1 Gm. intraductally, four times a day for two days or eight doses, making a total of 8 Gm., the average time for negative bile cultures was about twenty-six days postoperative. Although this does not appear to be a great difference, each case must be considered individually because of the number of variable factors, such as, the age, duration, and severity of the disease, postoperative complications, whether or not there were stones, and finally the type and potency of the bacteria cultured from the bile.

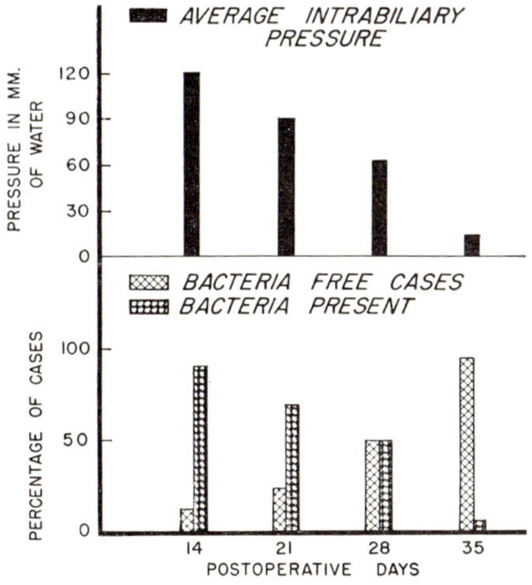

Fig. 1.

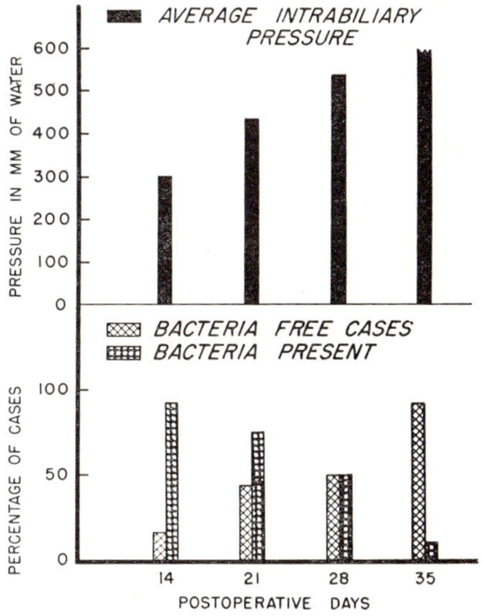

Fig. 2.

Fig. 1.—Graph representing the correlation between the average resting intrabiliary pressures and the bacteria of the bile in T-tube patients not receiving antibiotics intraductally. The intrabiliary pressures are resting ones and are averaged on the fourteenth, twenty-first, twenty-eighth, and thirty-fifth postoperative days. Note that on the twenty-eighth day one-half the patients have bacteria in the bile, and the resting intrabiliary pressure is above normal (30 mm.).

Fig. 2.—Graph representing the average pain perfusion levels as compared with the bacteriology of the bile in patients not receiving antibiotics intraductally. The pain perfusion levels are again average readings on the fourteenth, twenty-first, twenty-eighth, and thirty-fifth postoperative days. Compare with Fig. 4.

In comparing the relationship between the bile cultures, the resting intrabiliary pressure, and the pain perfusion level, there was a consistent and definite finding that when the bile cultures became negative, irrespective of how soon or whether or not antibiotics were used, the resting intrabiliary pressures and pain perfusion pressure were always within normal limits. The exceptions to the findings occurred in three cases in which the underlying pathology was chronic pancreatitis and carcinoma of gall bladder, respectively. In these three cases, there was a definite permanent obstruction to the lower end of the common duct. In all of these cases, the bile cultures became negative

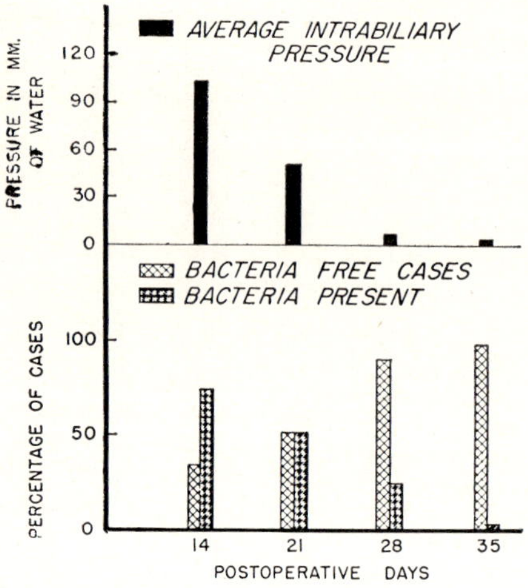

Fig. 3.

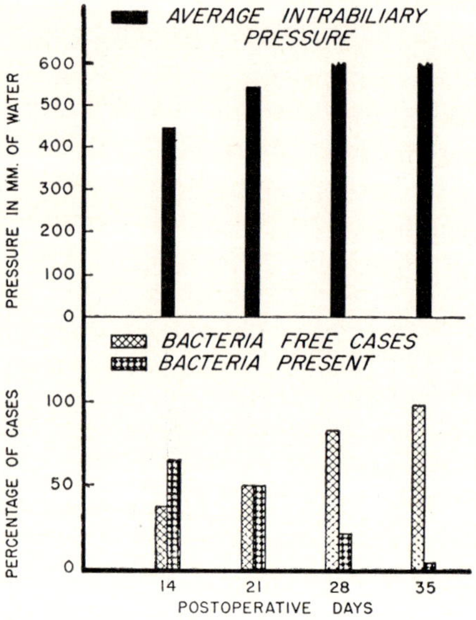

Fig. 4.

Fig. 3.—Graph representing the resting intrabiliary pressure correlated with the bacteria in bile in an average of patients who have received antibiotics intraductally. The averages are shown for the fourteenth, twenty-first, twenty-eighth, and thirty-fifth postoperative days. Compared with Fig. 1, the patients receiving streptomycin tended to be bacteria-free earlier, and the resting intrabiliary pressure tended to return to normal sooner.

Fig. 4.—Graph representing average pain perfusion levels correlated with the bacteria in bile in an average of patients who have received antibiotics intraductally. The averages are shown for the fourteenth, twenty-first, twenty-eighth, and thirty-fifth postoperative days. Compared with Fig. 2, one notes that there is increased tolerance to pressure in the duct by increased perfusion pain level and at the same time the patients tend to become bacteria-free sooner.

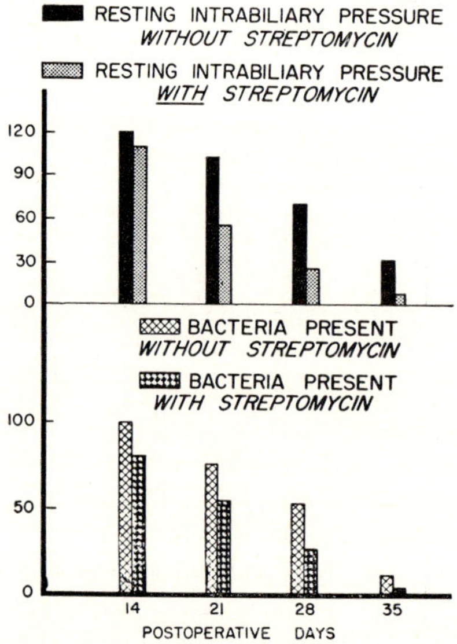

Fig. 5.—Graph representing a correlation of the resting intrabiliary pressures with and without streptomycin intraductally as compared with the bacteria in bile. The averages are from the fourteenth, twenty-first, twenty-eighth, and thirty-fifth postoperative days. The resting intrabiliary pressure tends to return to normal sooner in the patients receiving streptomycin through the T tube. Relaxation of spasm parallels disappearance of bacteria.

while the resting intrabiliary pressure remained elevated, while in sharp contrast the pain perfusion level was normal. In one of these cases, adenocarcinoma of the gall bladder had spread to the lymphatics about the common duct and caused an obstruction to the lower end of the duct.

Our findings are also represented by Figs. 1 through 4. We have attempted to show graphically the relationship between resting intrabiliary pressures, the pain perfusion levels, and the bacteria in bile on the fourteenth, twenty-first, twenty-eighth, and thirty-fifth postoperative days.

Figs. 1 and 2 represent the patients receiving no streptomycin and Figs. 3 and 4 represent those patients receiving streptomycin. It will be noted that as the bile cultures became negative in general, the resting intrabiliary pressure became normal, and likewise the pain perfusion level became normal. It will also be noted that in those cases in which patients received streptomycin intraductally the cultures tended to become negative earlier. A comparative study of both groups of cases is shown in Fig. 5.

Routine bile study forms were used for each case, which served as a very effective method of following the course of the patient postoperatively.

DISCUSSION

We have noted now for many years that patients with common duct drainage tend to improve, in so far as the biliary dynamics are concerned, on T-tube drainage alone. That is, the perfusion pain level, which may be low, as low as 70 mm. of water, postoperatively, will improve as drainage is continued, and on the other hand the ability of the patient to stand pressure within the bile duct improves. Concurrently with this, spasm of the lower end of the common bile duct tends to disappear.

The reasonable conclusions from these observations are: (1) Prolonged biliary drainage tends to permit cholangitis to improve, therefore increasing tolerance to intrabiliary pressure rises. (2) With improvement in cholangitis, a reflex spasm of the duodenal musculature tends to disappear.

The inferences which can be gathered from these observations are that the postcholecystectomy syndrome or biliary dyskinesia, so long known to be associated with spasm of the sphincter of Oddi, actually is secondary to infection in the upper radicles of the biliary tract, and the sphincter spasm is secondary as a result of reflex. If these conclusions are correct, then it would be expected that a shorter period of T-tube drainage would be necessary to restore biliary dynamics if antibiotics were used at the same time. In this paper, we are mainly concerned with correlating the bacteria in bile with biliary dynamics. The results have strengthened our opinion concerning the relationship of cholangitis to biliary dynamics. Also, the limited degree to which we have studied the effect of antibiotics administered parenterally and into the T tube tends to show that the duration of T-tube drainage is decreased with the use of antibiotics, that is, the patient's biliary dynamics return to normal sooner when they are used than when they are not.

The bacteriology of bile and its significance serve as a continual source of debate among workers in this field, as do the bacterial flora and its origin. For the most part, the organisms cultured are usually of enteric origin. This is easily explained when it is considered that any trauma or disturbance in the physiology of the common duct, cystic duct, and hepatic duct could encourage a retrograde spread of organism from the duodenum along the biliary tree.

The culture of *Clostridium welchii* from the bile has been obtained in many cases by other workers, as discussed previously. We have cultured this organism in a few cases, but only as a mixed culture and not as a pure culture. It is hard to evaluate the significance of *Clostridium welchii,* but clinically in those cases in which we obtained this organism, the patients were those presenting a history of symptoms extending over a long period of time, often associated with jaundice, chills, and fever in repeated attacks over a period of years.

There seemed to be a definite relationship between *Bacillus coli* and gallstones. In all of the cases of cholelithiasis, a positive culture of *Bacillus coli* was obtained from the bile. This observation is not a new one by any means; it has been previously noted that any obstructive element associated with the biliary tree, whether it be in the common duct or the cystic duct, seems to encourage the growth of *Bacillus coli.*

The intrabiliary pressure studies showed a definite correlation to the degree of infection in the biliary radicles. In those cases in which the bacteria in bile was abundant, the resting intrabiliary pressure was elevated above normal, and when the bacterial flora began to return to normal, the resting intrabiliary pressure returned to normal. Likewise, the pain perfusion level was also related directly to the degree of infection as manifested by the bacteria in bile. Patients who tolerated perfusion pressures up to 700 mm. of water without experiencing discomfort were found to have no bacteria in the bile.

A reduction in perfusion pain pressure below 550 mm. of water indicates the presence of infection in the bile ducts, that is, cholangitis. Supportive evidence includes these factors:

1. There is a correlation between low perfusion pain levels and bacteria; as bacteria disappears from the bile, the tolerance to pressure increases.

2. The perfusion pain pressure improves with T-tube drainage invariably. The measurement of perfusion pain pressure is the application of a basic principle in the study of the process of inflammation, no different from that employed by the clinician when he measures degree of inflammation in a felon by applying pressure with the examining finger.

The true role of antibiotics in our cases is hard to evaluate. Those patients receiving streptomycin intraductally had an earlier diminution of bacteria in bile than the controls. By the same token, the biliary dynamics were restored to normal much sooner. As to the relative value of different types of antibiotics, we are in no position to discuss this factor at this time. Study along this line is being continued by Dr. Walter Carrigan and one of us (J. M. McG.) at the Boston City Hospital.

As a practical clinical application concerning removal of the T tube, this work confirms what we have already shown, namely, that the T tube should be left in until (1) biliary dynamics have been restored to normal, that is, resting pressure is 30 mm. or less, and perfusion pain level is 550 mm. or more, and (2) cholangiograms show absence of stone or extrinsic pressure. Bile culture, while valuable in correlating data for research purposes, may not be necessary clinically, since results parallel biliary dynamics which are more easily measured.

SUMMARY

1. A review of the literature on the bacteriology of bile is presented.

2. A method of study of bacteriology of bile in T-tube patients is presented, with special emphasis on our method of collecting bile for cultures.

3. The biliary dynamics studies are described with recording of resting intrabiliary pressures and pain perfusion pressures in twenty-seven cases on T-tube drainage.

4. Twenty-one cases are reported in detail from the bacteriologic point of view. The most common bacteria found in bile were (in order of frequency) *Escherichia coli, Bacillus proteus, Aerobacter aerogenes, Bacillus pyocyaneus,* and *Bacillus welchii.*

5. Two of the common antibiotics, penicillin and streptomycin, were given intraductally to some of the patients. Their order of efficiency is as follows: streptomycin (most effective) and then penicillin. However, only a limited number of cases studied are here reported. Further studies are in progress, and at a later time more cases are to be reported.

REFERENCES

1. McGowan, J. M.: Dynamics of Biliary Drainage, SURGERY **18:** 470-478, 1945.
2. McGowan, J. M.: Complications and Sequelae of Gallbladder Disease, Rev. Gastroenterol. **17:** 649, 1950.
3. Twiss, J. R.: A New Type of Duodenal Tube Tip, Am. J. M. Sc. **135:** 107-110, 1933.
4. Mirizzi, P. L.: A Study of the Bacteriology of the Common Bile Duct in Comparison With the Other Extrahepatic Segments of the Biliary Tract, Surg., Gynec. & Obst. **76:** 242 (March), 1934.
5. Zollinger, R., and Cutler, E. C.: The Treatment of Acute Cholecystitis, J. A. M. A. **121:** 481-485, 1943.
6. McGowan, J. M., and Henderson, F. F.: Prevention and Management of Pain Following Cholecystectomy, New England J. Med. **222:** 948-953, 1940.
7. McGowan, J. M., Butch, W. L., and Walters, W.: Pressure in the Common Bile Duct of Man: The Relation to Pain Following Cholecystectomy, J. A. M. A. **106:** 2227-2230, 1936.
8. McGowan, J. M., Keeley, J. K., and Henderson, F.: Pathological Physiology of Biliary Drainage: The Description of the Use of a New Type of T-tube and the Criteria for Its Removal, Surg., Gynec. & Obst. **84:** 174-180, 1947.

APPROACH TO MIDTHORACIC ESOPHAGEAL CARCINOMA FOR ITS RADICAL SURGICAL TREATMENT

KOMEI NAKAYAMA, M.D.,* CHIBA, JAPAN

TO LOOK back on the history of esophageal surgery in Japan, the first reports on the radical removal of esophageal carcinoma were made in April, 1933, by our distinguished predecessor, the late Professor Seo, and by Professor Osawa at the Thirty-third Annual Assembly of the Japanese Surgical Association.

Since these reports were made, there had been no noticeable progress in this field of surgery in Japan until we succeeded in the radical removal of cancer of the lower thoracic esophagus by the abdominal approach in the use of so-called "*incomplete anastomosis*" with adaptation of esophageal tissue and gastric tissue by few sutures.

Since our first successful operation in February, 1946, the number of radical removals of thoracic esophageal cancers in the past seven years has amounted to 399 cases, including 101 cases of upper or midthoracic esophageal carcinoma (Table I). During these eight years, remarkable changes were made in the operative technique by the employment of positive pressure anesthesia and antibiotics which were introduced from the United States. Recently, we have succeeded in operating upon carcinoma of the thoracic esophagus almost as easily as performing gastrectomies in the past, in so far as the operative technique and operative mortality are concerned.

The operative methods applying to these carcinomas in our clinic differ according to the localities, and we have succeeded with each operative method, and we trust this report may prove worthy of consideration and reference.

Total or subtotal thoracic esophagectomy in the radical surgical treatment of upper and midthoracic esophageal cancer requires re-formation of the gastric tube as a secondary operative procedure in order to re-establish the continuity of the digestive tract.

Esophagogastric Anastomosis.—We have devoted especial attention in our cases of total or subtotal esophagectomy to the re-formed gastric tube in an attempt to clarify the question of where the gastric vessels should be ligated to avoid interference with or interruption of an adequate blood supply. We would like to report the results of this study.

Garlock and his associates have previously reported that necrosis of the stomach can be prevented if the right gastroepiploic artery alone is not ligated (Fig. 1). However, there was no report by these investigators describing details concerning any of the other gastric arteries in relation to the circulation of the stomach. We have noted that ligation of the right gastric artery excessively influences subsequent necrosis at the apex of the gastric wall (gastric cardia).

Received for publication, Sept. 18, 1953.

*Professor of surgery, School of Medicine, Chiba University.

Until recently, in our clinic, ''antethoracic esophagogastric anastomosis'' was employed as the routine operative procedure for re-establishing the gastrointestinal canal following total or subtotal esophagectomy. The subcutaneous gastric tube could thus be observed with comparative ease for the circulatory effects in question.

TABLE I. OPERATIVE CASES OF RADICAL ESOPHAGECTOMIES (FEBRUARY, 1946, TO JULY, 1953), NAKAYAMA SURGICAL CLINIC

OPERATIVE METHOD	TOTAL CASES	CANCER	ULCER	CORROSIVE STRICTURE	BENIGN STENOSIS
Cervical esophagectomy	13	13			
Total or subtotal esophagectomy	109	101	1	7	
Esophagocardiectomy intrathoracic esophagogastric or esophagojejunal anastomosis	80	73	2	1	4
Intra-abdominal esophagogastric anastomosis	48	41	4		3
Total gastrectomy with esophagectomy	140	130	10		
So-called incomplete anastomosis	48	41			7
Totals	438	399	17	8	14

Postoperatively, we have seen extensive necrosis of the gastric tube in three cases; this is illustrated in Fig. 2. One patient had a cicatricial healing of the gastric ulcer on the lesser curvature (Fig. 3) which had eroded through the blood vessels in this region. The other two cases were those of aged persons with a lesser curvature of short length but a long thorax. This necessitated individual ligation of the arteries along the lesser curvature to mobilize the stomach sufficiently to form a long gastric tube (Fig. 1). Such ligations were employed in other cases also. In most of them, a tiny necrosis or infection developed at the site of the anastomosis, which resulted in a small fistula extending to the skin. The patients who did not develop either the necrosis or infection subsequent to this type of ligation were relatively young people with better over-all circulation. On the other hand, where the method of individual ligation was not employed, none of the operative patients retained sufficient blood circulation of the mobilized gastric tube. This resulted in either necrosis or infection. Therefore, it is concluded that surgeons must apply the ligatures with great caution since improper ligation results in subsequent necrosis or infection of the mobilized gastric tube by virtue of inadequate gastric blood supply.

It is natural for surgeons to preserve as many gastric vessels as possible in order to prevent necrosis secondary to mobilization of the stomach. However, adequate mobilization for anastomosis of the gastric tube to the esophageal remnant requires extensive ligation of gastric vessels. With improper ligations, the hazard of unexpected operative death from necrosis or infection is great; this hazard may happen in the procedure which leaves only the right gastroepiploic artery unligated. The hazard is more marked when the length of the lesser curvature is short, thus requiring more extensive mobilization of this portion for the formation of the gastric tube, or when it is necessary to ligate the arteries along the lesser curvature in order to extirpate lymphatic metastasis in the celiac axis.

To determine more accurately the effects of various types of ligation procedures on the circulation of the gastric arteries, we have injected opaque

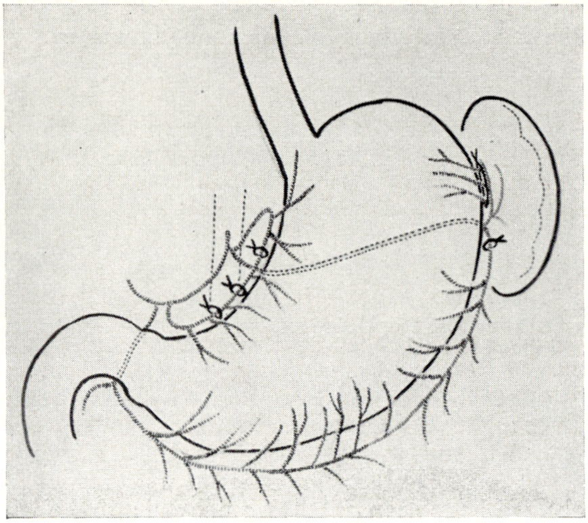

Fig. 1.—The right gastroepiploic artery is left, and the other gastric arteries are ligated. Each individual arterial arch along the lesser curvature is ligated.

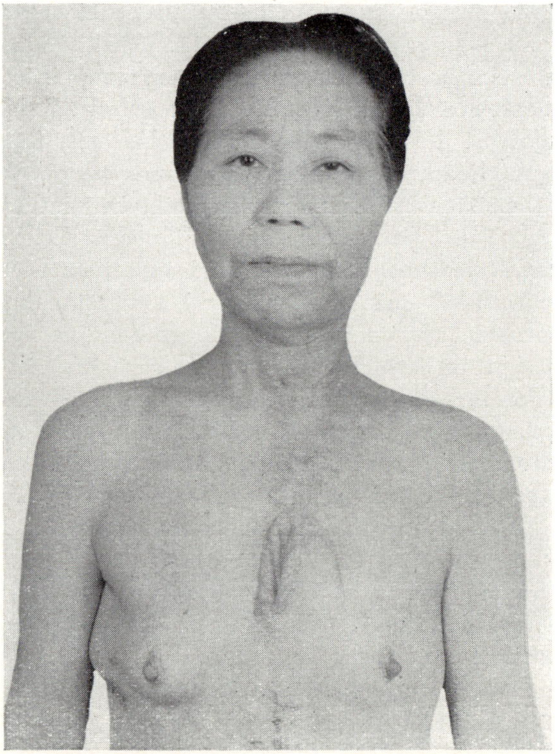

Fig. 2.—Photograph showing the cicatricial healing of extensive necrosis of antethoracically mobilized stomach, and resultant fistula.

chemicals into one patent artery after the ligation of all other arteries in the stomachs of post-mortem specimens. This has been carried out in order to map the areas of stomach wall supplied by each of the various arteries involved.

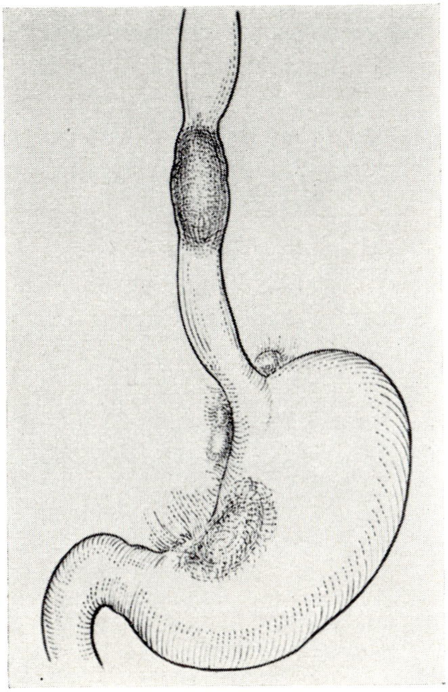

Fig. 3.—Midthoracic esophageal carcinoma with cicatricial healing of a gastric ulcer on the lesser curvature.

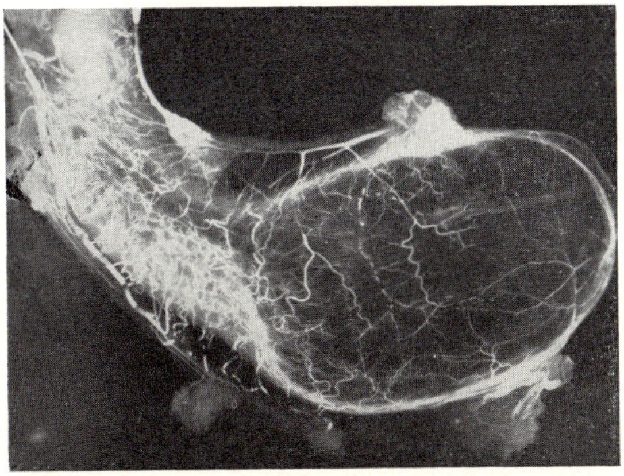

Fig. 4.—Roentgenogram of mobilized post-mortem gastric tube injected with contrast material into the right gastroepiploic artery following the ligation shown as in Fig. 5. Indicates that a sufficient amount of the material reaches the apical portion of the stomach.

As shown in Fig. 4, the mobilized gastric tube has a sufficient supply of the contrast material up to the apical zone following injection of the right gastroepiploic artery. In this instance, the arteries of the greater curvature and gastric cardia were all ligated, but the arteries of the lesser curvature were left patent (Fig. 5). It is seen that it is not necessary to inject the right gastric artery in order to fill all the gastric arterial circulation, provided none of the branches of the right gastric artery are ligated.

In the second instance, we injected the right gastroepiploic artery with the opaque substance following ligations of the arteries along the lesser curvature (Fig. 6). Here again, we obtained sufficient supply of the substance up to the apical zone of the gastric wall. This demonstrates that the opaque substance injected into the right gastroepiploic artery flows into the apical portion of the mobilized gastric wall through the arteries along the lesser curvature (Fig. 7).

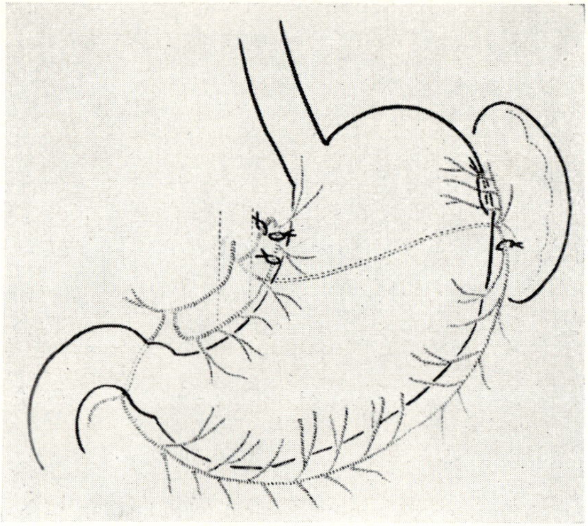

Fig. 5.—The right gastric and gastroepiploic artery are left.

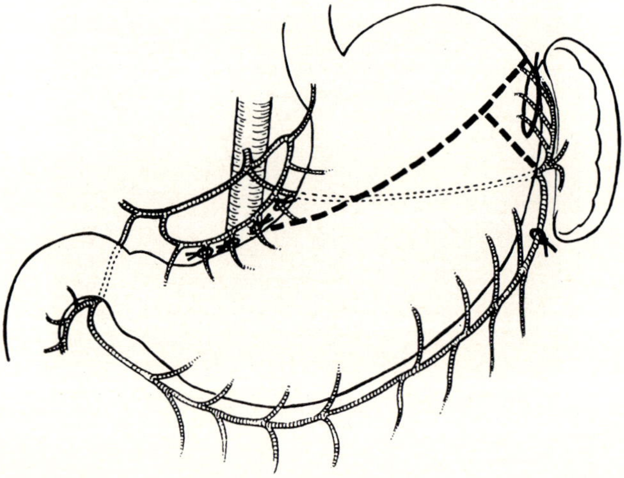

Fig. 6.—The arteries along the lesser curvature are ligated.

The third method of investigation was to ligate each individual arterial arch along the lesser curvature at the time of the mobilization of the stomach (as in Fig. 1). Injection of the contrast material into the right gastroepiploic artery following such ligation shows only a very slight amount of the substance reaching the apical portion of the mobilized gastric wall (Fig. 8) as opposed to a sufficient supply as noted in the previous two instances. The results of this third investigative approach explain the high potential for extensive necrosis of the mobilized gastric wall when the procedure was carried out on aged persons with sclerotic arteries and poor circulation in general. Even necrosis may not occur; the circulation is so poor that the area can be easily infected, with resultant fistula formation.

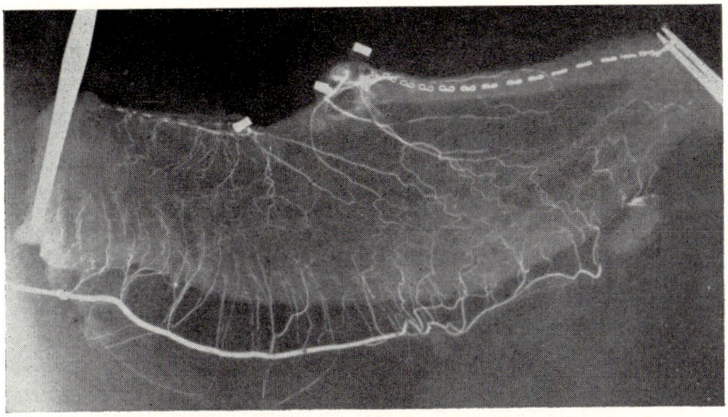

Fig. 7.—Roentgenogram of mobilized post-mortem gastric tube injected with contrast material into the right gastroepiploic artery following ligations of the arteries along the lesser curvature. The injected material flows into the apical portion through the arteries along the lesser curvature.

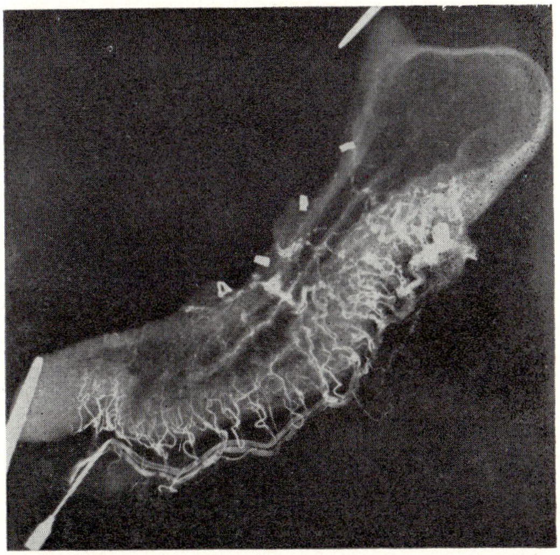

Fig. 8.—Roentgenogram of mobilized post-mortem gastric tube injected with contrast material into the right gastroepiploic artery following the ligation of the individual arches of the right gastric artery and other gastric arteries except the right gastroepiploic artery. Only a very slight amount of the material injected reached the apical portion of the stomach.

A considerable number of these fistulas was seen in previous cases. Therefore, we performed our total or subtotal esophagectomies using the antethoracic esophagogastric anastomosis or pulling the gastric tube up to the cervical esophagus extrathoracically, thus making the anastomosis in the neck. This avoided intrathoracic anastomosis with the attendant danger of death from leakage through such fistulas into the thorax.

Another very interesting result was obtained in the investigation by injecting the opaque substance into the right gastric artery. The injection was performed after first ligating the right gastroepiploic artery at its axis, leaving the arterial arches along the lesser curvature untouched. The contrast material was seen to flow from the arteries along the lesser curvature to the arterial arches along the greater curvature, finally filling the vascular network in the apical zone of the mobilized gastric wall. Of course, the quantity of contrast material which flowed into the apical zone was visibly smaller than that in the former investigation.

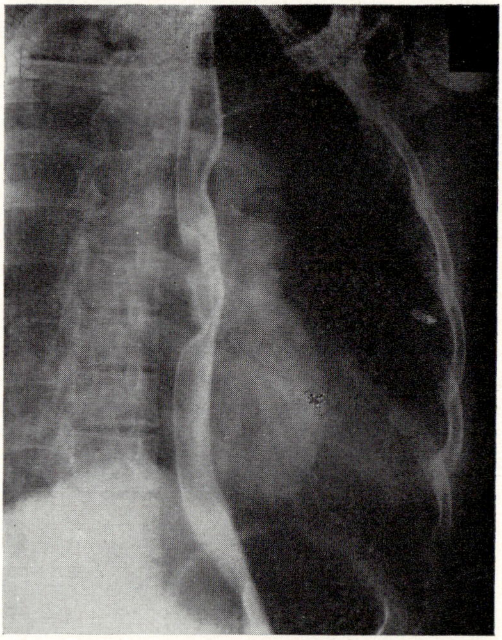

Fig. 9.—Preoperative roentgenogram of midthoracic esophageal carcinoma.

The conclusion which became apparent from the results of these studies of the gastric circulation is as follows: In order to maintain sufficient blood circulation in the apical zone of the mobilized gastric tube in total or subtotal thoracic esophagetcomy, it is essential for the surgeon to leave the arterial arches along the greater and lesser curvatures completely untouched, and to leave unligated either the right gastric artery along the lesser curvature or the right gastroepiploic arteries along the greater curvature.

The following case is presented in illustration.

CASE 1 (Figs. 9 through 12).—A subtotal esophagectomy with antethoracic placement of the stomach for esophageal carcinoma. In the operative procedure, the patient's right gastroepiploic artery was ligated at its axis, but arches of the arteries along the lesser and greater curvatures were left untouched at the time of gastric mobilization. The patient recovered following the complete removal of the mid-esophageal carcinoma without the formation of any fistulas from the re-formed gastric tube.

The patient was a 41-year-old male physician who presented with a chief complaint of dysphagia. Clinical diagnosis was midthoracic esophageal cancer.

History of present disease: Three months prior to admission to the hospital, the patient noted retrosternal discomfort on swallowing. The condition progressed rapidly and caused the patient to visit the Medical College for examination on Jan. 12, 1951. By this time he could not swallow solid food. Fluoroscopic studies with accompanying radiographs showed signs of an esophageal cancer. He was sent to our clinic with this diagnosis and was admitted to the hospital on Jan. 25, 1951.

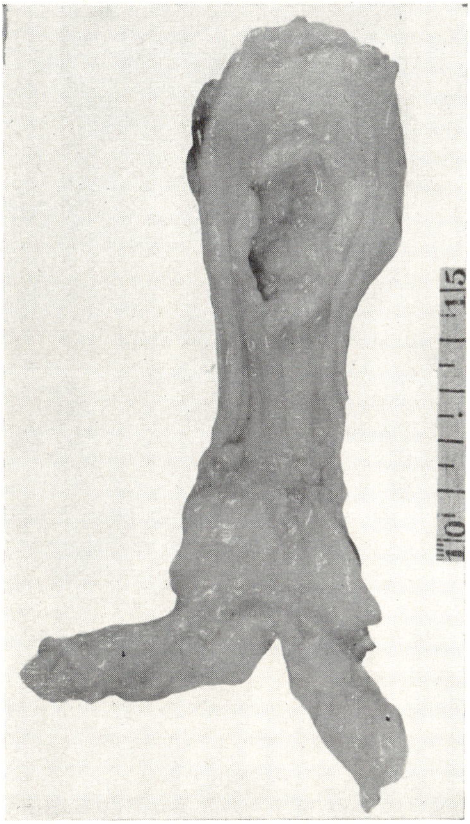

Fig. 10.—Removed specimen.

Examination on admission revealed a thin patient of medium height with hemoglobin, 85 per cent; red blood count, 4,200,000; white blood count, 6,700; urine, no specific findings; stool, positive for occult blood.

Surgery was performed on Feb. 1, 1951. The operative method was total thoracic esophagectomy with antethoracic esophagogastric anastomosis.

The patient was positioned face down for thoracotomy performed from the left thorax with resection of the fifth and sixth ribs. The carcinoma lay under the azygos vein, with infiltration toward the gastric cardia. An abdominal approach was therefore made by midline incision. Lymphatic metastases were found both at the axis of the celiac artery and at the hiatus of the diaphragm. Another metastasis was found at the axis of the right gastroepiploic artery. In the process of extirpation of these lymph nodes, the gastroepiploic artery was ligated. Therefore, ligation of the right gastric artery was avoided. The anastomosis was made between the gastric tube and the esophageal remnant in the cervical region, with the tube raised antethoracically through a skin tunnel to the neck superficial to the sternum.

The postoperative course was uneventful and satisfactory. The patient was discharged from the hospital one month following admission without the formation of a fistula having taken place from the anastomosed part. The postoperative roentgenogram is shown in Fig. 11.

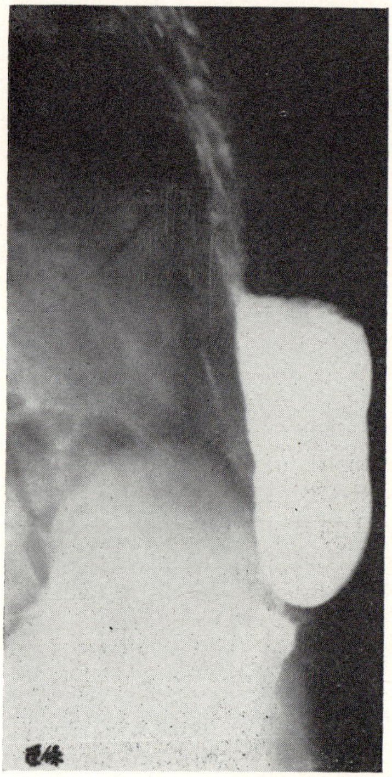

Fig. 11.—Postoperative roentgenogram which shows the re-establishment of alimentary tract with antethoracic esophagogastrostomy.

The operative handling of the gastric blood vessels was illustrated whenever total or subtotal esophagectomy required re-establishment of the continuity of the digestive tract by esophagogastric anastomosis which utilized the whole stomach for the gastric tube after complete mobilization. Recently, we have been applying the method of handling the gastric blood vessels suggested by the studies with the opaque material. This has been done so as to minimize the injury to the arterial arches along both the lesser and greater curvatures. Careful operative treatment of the gastric artery protects the anastomosis both from secondary infection and from fistula formation, thus helping to promote success in the primary cure accomplished by antethoracic esophagogastric anastomosis.

Let us now turn our attention to the problem of which operative approach is most advantageous for the complete removal of carcinoma in the mid- and upper-thoracic esophagus.

In the United States and Europe, MacManus, Kent, and Mathewson have been insisting upon the operative convenience of the right thoracic approach. However, this approach has a great disadvantage as compared to the left

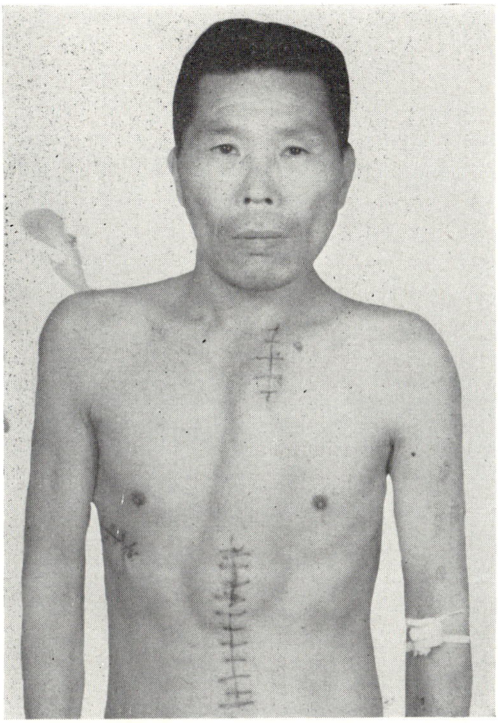

Fig. 12.—Photograph of patient after operation.

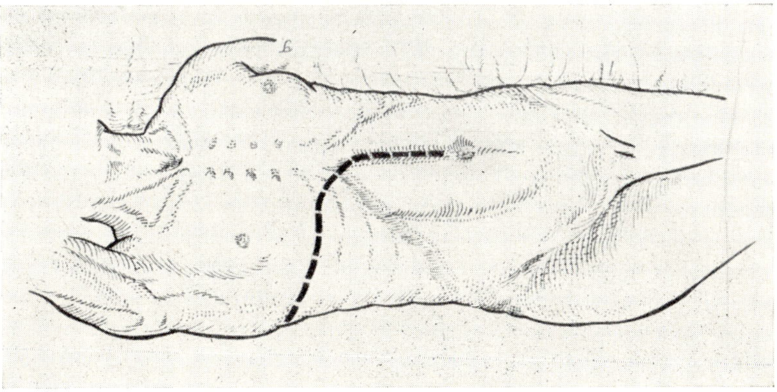

Fig. 13.—The dotted line shows continuous right thoracoabdominal incision.

thoracoabdominal approach, since the former requires two separate skin incisions, one from the abdomen and the other from the thorax. With this double incision, the difficulty is frequently encountered that, following the mobilization of the stomach through the abdominal incision, the thoracic incision reveals an inoperable lesion lying in the thoracic cavity. The simultaneous approach from the right (thoracoabdominal approach) is similar to the procedure we have been using from the left to complete removal of carcinoma of the lower esophagus

Fig. 14.

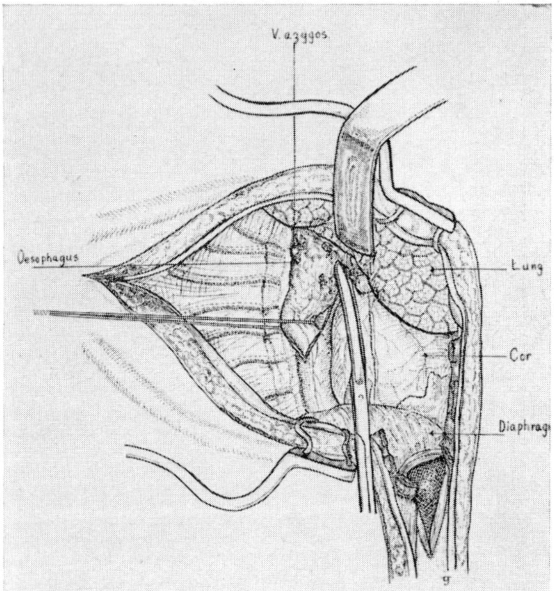

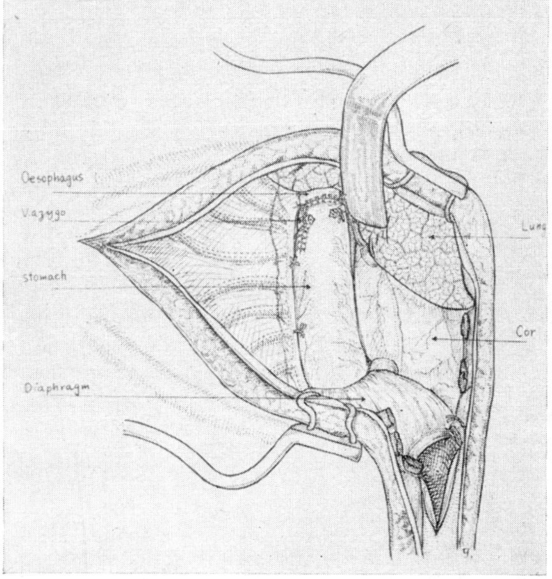

Fig. 15.

Fig. 14.—Diagram of completed anastomosis (right thoracoabdominal approach).

Fig. 15.—After ligation of the azygos vein, whole esophagus can be mobilized easily from the right thorax.

in a one-stage operation. This simultaneous approach from the right has been impossible and has resulted in objections by R. H. Sweet and others who prefer the left thoracoabdominal approach, even for the treatment of the upper and midthoracic esophageal lesions.

Since we have demonstrated, through our investigations just described, that the complete mobilization of the stomach can be carried out with ease and security, we have been struggling to establish a new approach from the right thorax for the radical surgical treatment of carcinoma of the upper- and midthoracic esophagus. We have finally succeeded in establishing a transdiaphragmatic approach from the right for the removal of carcinoma of the upper- and midthoracic esophagus. This approach eliminates both the costectomy and one unnecessary incision. It also simplifies the whole operative technique, while the approach from the left requires a blind operative technique for the removal of a lesion in this portion. The surgical procedures have been so simplified by this approach that the amount of bleeding during the operation has been reduced and the time for the entire operation has been amazingly shortened to approximately one hour.

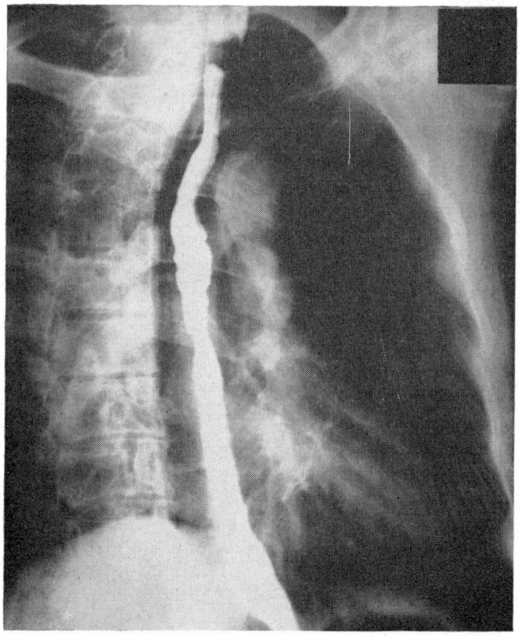

Fig. 16.—Preoperative roentgenogram which shows midthoracic esophageal carcinoma.

Following is a brief explanation of the operative procedure: An incision is made from thorax to abdomen, as illustrated in Fig. 13, thus opening the thoracic and abdominal cavities through one continuous incision. Severance of the sixth and seventh or the seventh and eighth costal arches lays open the site of the lesion and allows us to identify the state of the malignant lesion in the thoracic cavity or the degree of the lymphatic metastasis at the axis of the celiac artery in the abdominal cavity. This twofold evaluation can be performed at one and the same time. In addition, an evaluation of the gastric blood vessel arrangement may be made, and the mode of ligation can be decided upon. If it is seen that there is a likelihood that the operation may produce some interference with the blood circulation of the mobilized stomach, antethoracic esophagogastric anastomosis must be the procedure of choice to follow

Fig. 17.

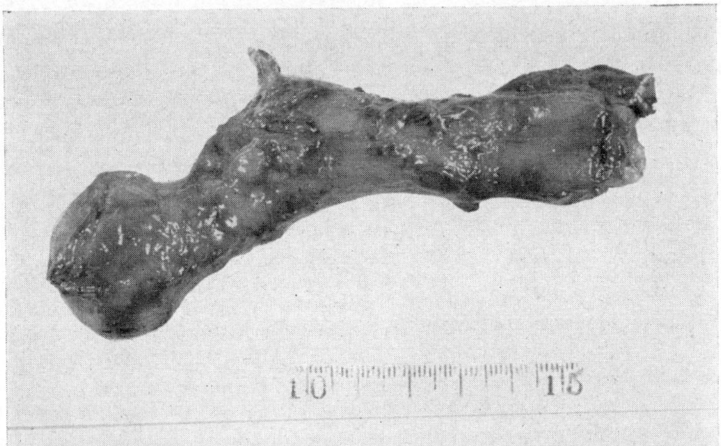

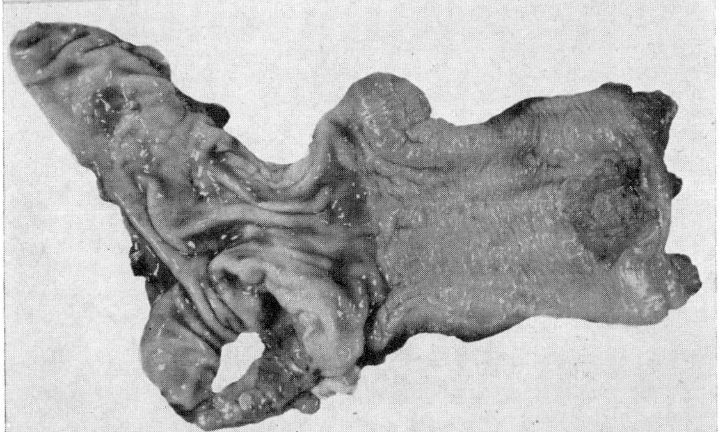

Fig. 18.

Fig. 17.—Outside of removed specimen.
Fig. 18.—Inside of removed specimen.

extirpation of the lesion. However, if the arrangement of the gastric vessels is such that it lends itself well to a ligation which leaves an adequate blood supply, then intrathoracic esophagogastric anastomosis is preferable.

The first step of the procedure within the abdominal cavity is the mobilization of the esophagus from its surrounding tissue, following the ligation and division of the azygos vein (Fig. 14). The esophagus is then amputated above the level of infiltration, and the amputated esophagus is pulled to the abdominal cavity through the hiatus of the diaphragm. This is done without making an incision in the diaphragm.

Radical extirpation of the lesion after careful evaluation of the infiltrations is followed by mobilization of the stomach and fashioning of a gastric tube. The gastric tube is brought to the upper remnant of the esophagus through the hiatus of the diaphragm and positioned for anastomosis within the thoracic cavity (Fig. 15). Anastomosis of the posterior wall is carried out with one layer of suture (Albert). Three anchoring sutures are placed, which secure the posterior wall of the gastric tube to the mediastinal pleura or to the aortic adventitia. Interrupted silk is used. The anterior wall is usually anastomosed in two layers, Albert and Lembert suturing being used. The gastric serosa is united with the mediastinal serosa.

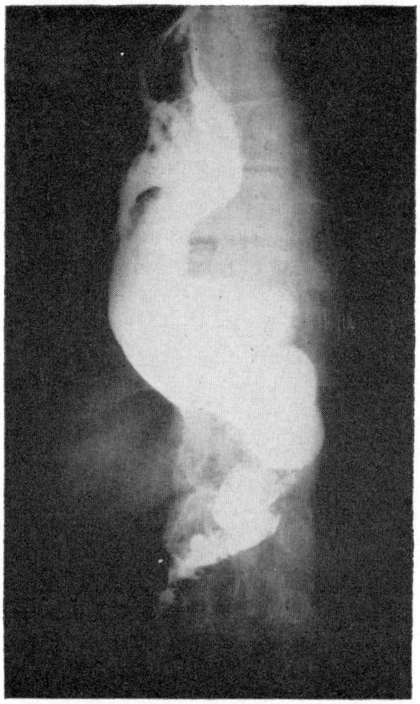

Fig. 19.—Postoperative roentgenogram demonstrating anastomosis being observed at the level of aortic arch.

(This technique for esophagogastric anastomosis is usually utilized in lower thoracic esophagectomy also.)

The thoracic and abdominal walls are closed by two layers of suture, following the insertion of a T tube into the thoracic cavity. A stomach tube is also inserted to be utilized both for suction of excess gas and fluids in the stomach and also for feeding purposes after the third postoperative day.

Recently, 22 cases (until July, 1953) of radical esophagectomies for middle and upper thoracic esophageal cancers have been performed, using this new approach. There has been no operative death in our clinic as yet.

CASE 2 (Figs. 16 through 20).—The patient was a 59-year-old man who presented himself with the chief complaint of dysphagia. Clinical diagnosis was midthoracic esophageal cancer.

Clinical history: The patient gave a history of dysphagia with onset three months prior to admission and with sudden increase in severity twenty days prior to admission. The patient experienced the feeling of stagnation of food and retrosternal burning. By the time of admission, the patient could not digest solid food.

On admission Aug. 30, 1952, examination revealed a man of medium height, but thin. Hemoglobin count was 75 per cent; red blood count, 4,000,000; white blood count, 7,800; stool examination, positive for occult blood. Operation was performed Sept. 5, 1952. The operative method was subtotal esophagectomy by the right transdiaphragmatic approach with intrathoracic esophagogastric anastomosis.

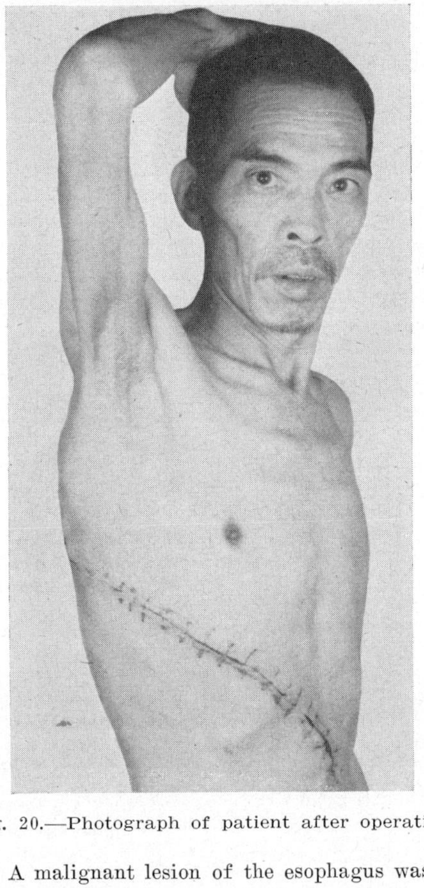

Fig. 20.—Photograph of patient after operation.

Operative findings: A malignant lesion of the esophagus was discovered at the level of the azygos vein. Infiltration of the lesion into both the anterior and the posterior wall of the esophagus was noted. Adherence of the lesion to the surrounding tissue was present, and lymphatic metastases were also found at the axis of the celiac artery. Following the extirpation of these lymph nodes, the esophagus was removed, together with a portion of the gastric cardia. The anastomosis was performed in the right thoracic cavity.

The postoperative course of this patient was smooth and uneventful. Fig. 19 shows a postoperative roentgenogram of the patient, the anastomosis being observed at the level of the aortic arch.

SUMMARY

There have been many varying techniques used for the approach and for the anastomosis when subtotal esophagectomy has been necessary in the radical surgical treatment of malignancy of the esophagus. However, the operative method which we have introduced in this report appears to us to be the best. This opinion is based on the fact that we have utilized a variety of methods in many esophageal operations in the past seven years, not a single one of them having proved satisfactory until this new approach was devised.

This operative method necessitates only one incision, the thoracoabdominal extending from the right thorax, although incisions of the costal angles may be utilized to get complete exposure of the esophagogastric canal. However, neither costectomy nor incision of the diaphragm is required. In addition, the operative technique has shortened the operative time because of the simplified procedure, and reduced the amount of bleeding throughout the entire operative procedure.

However, this operation is applicable only for those patients whose gastric blood supply is not dangerously interfered with by the mobilization. If cicatricial healing of the gastric ulcer on the lesser curvature is noticeable, or if it is seen that ligation of the arterial arches on the lesser curvature is essential to increase the scope of the operation, then esophagogastric anastomosis is to be preferred. Since we have obtained such satisfying and enlightening results in our examination of the gastric blood circulation and can thus determine which arteries may be safely ligated without jeopardizing the blood supply of the gastric wall, we feel that intrathoracic esophagogastric anastomosis can be performed without any fear.

In conclusion, subtotal esophagectomy can be performed with ease and assurance. Both this operation and resection of the esophagus and cardiac portion of the stomach for lesions of the lower esophagus can be performed from the left thoracoabdominal approach as easily as our predecessors were able to perform them over ten years ago.

It is my hope that this report will be of some benefit to surgeons who, now or presently, will have occasion to perform these operations.

REFERENCES

1. Gasper, M. R.: Am. J. Surg. **84:** 306 (Sept.) 1952.
2. Kent, E. M.: J. Thoracic Surg. **19:** 559, 1950.
3. MacManus, J. E.: SURGERY **24:** 9, 1948.
4. Sweet, R. H.: Surg., Gynec. & Obst. **94:** 46 (Jan.) 1952.

HUMAN MEASUREMENTS INVOLVED IN TRACHEOBRONCHIAL RESECTION AND RECONSTRUCTION PROCEDURES

Report of a Case of Bronchial Adenoma*

K. Alvin Merendino, M.D., and Lawrence B. Kiriluk, M.D.,** Seattle, Wash.

(From the Department of Surgery, University of Washington School of Medicine)

IN THIS laboratory, problems related to tracheobronchial resection and reconstruction have been investigated.[1-4] Important phases of the experimental aspects of this problem have been concluded.

The clinical application of tracheobronchial resection and reconstruction would appear to be important in traumatic injuries of the bronchi and in tuberculosis. Such procedures for bronchogenic carcinoma would appear to have merit only in unusual circumstances. Most instances would fall into the group of palliative rather than curative operations for obvious reasons. Although tracheobronchial reconstructive procedures are applicable to the clinical entities listed previously, the work in this laboratory has been directed toward the problem of benign bronchial tumors.

TRACHEOBRONCHIAL MEASUREMENTS IN THE HUMAN BEING

In order to bridge the hiatus between the experimental facts and the clinical application of tracheobronchial reconstructive operations, certain additional anatomic knowledge is necessary. One bit of missing information relates to the spatial relationship of the tracheobronchial tree and the luminal diameters of bronchi which conceivably might be anastomosed to each other. In order for a theoretical plan of action to be meaningful, information relating to the following items is of importance: (1) the distance between the carina and the major bronchial take-offs; (2) the luminal diameters of various areas of the lower trachea and bronchi.

Consequently, 136 fresh human cadavers were studied at autopsy. The distances between the various take-offs of the bronchi and segments were measured. There were fifty-seven female cadavers with an age range of 13 to 86, the average age being 68 years, and seventy-nine male cadavers with an age range of 18 to 90, with an average age of 66 years. The measurements are schematically presented in Fig. 1.

In another group of fifty-five fresh human cadavers, measurements were made of the luminal diameters in various areas. There were thirty-three female cadavers with an age range of 13 to 86, the average age being 67 years and twenty-two male cadavers in an age range from 46 to 83, with an average age of 68 years. These measurements are presented in Fig. 2.

Received for publication, July 23, 1953.

*Supported by a grant from the National Institutes of Health, Project RG-2015 (R).

**Trainee, National Cancer Institute.

In evaluating the luminal diameters, particularly of the lower bronchus, it should be pointed out that the measurements may seem greater than might be expected. This is due to the fact that in the area under question flattening of the bronchi occurs. The data were obtained by sagittal section of the bronchi with removal of the top half and measurement of the bottom portion in situ. Therefore, the measurement is accurate but the greatest diameter has been obtained of an ovoid sphere. If the lower bronchus were distended, undoubtedly the cross-sectional area would be smaller than a segment of the main bronchus with a comparable diameter as recorded.

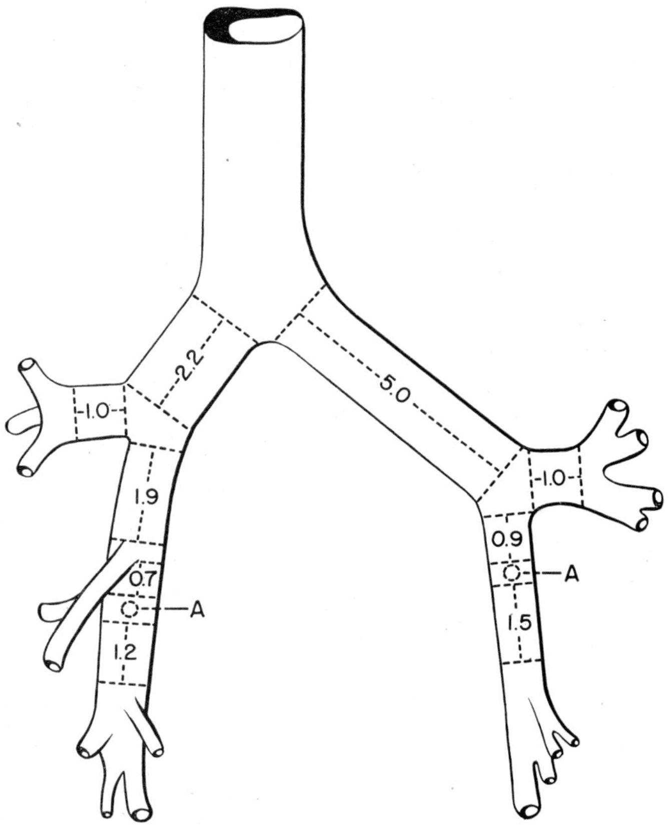

Fig. 1.—Average measurements in 136 fresh cadavers of the spatial relationship of the carina and bronchial tree. *A* indicates the orifice of the dorsal or superior segment of the lower lobes.

From human measurements, together with the experimental data in animals, it is possible to evolve various plans of excision and reconstruction dependent not only on the location of the tumor, but also on other important circumstances existent in each patient. It is apparent that if a peripheral adenoma were encountered, a lobectomy or segmental excision would be advisable.

In addition to tumor location and luminal and spatial relationships, further attention must be paid to the volume requirements of the preserved pulmonic tissue. In "tailoring" the distal bronchus, care must be taken so that the spared lung lies comfortably in position with sufficient room to allow for its complete expansion.

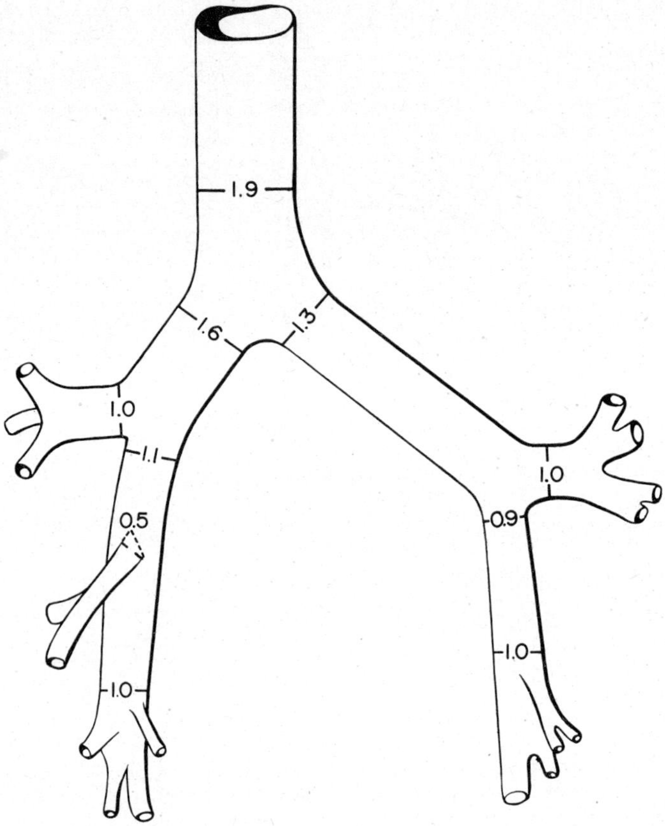

Fig. 2.—Average luminal diameters of the various areas which might be utilized for anastomotic procedures. These figures represent the averages in fifty-five fresh cadavers with the exception of the diameter of the lower lobe bronchus before it divides into the basal segments. This latter diameter represents the average measurement in twenty cadavers.

CLINICAL APPLICATION

Planned bronchial excision with reconstruction of the bronchial tree has been accomplished in patients with tuberculous stenosis by Gebauer.[5] He has shown the feasibility of the resection of a stenotic area on both right and left sides combined with a resection of either upper lobe and the anastomosis of the main bronchus on either side with the distal bronchus. Tuttle[6] in 1947 performed an unplanned reconstructive procedure similar to that to be reported in a patient with bronchiectasis who had been subjected to a left lower lobectomy some years before.

CASE REPORT

The patient, a 64-year-old white man, was admitted to the hospital for the first time on Nov. 27 1951, with a chief complaint of shortness of breath.

Approximately five weeks prior to admission he had developed an upper respiratory infection with blood-streaked sputum and pleuritic pain at the left posterior base. There was a twenty-pound weight loss.

Physical Examination.—The patient was thin and gaunt with a markedly emphysematous chest. Diaphragms were depressed bilaterally. There were decreased breath sounds, vocal sounds, and tactile fremitus at the left lateral base with some sticky inspiratory râles and an expiratory wheeze locally.

Except for a moderate leukocytosis, the laboratory findings were unremarkable.

X-ray examination of the chest on Nov. 28, 1951, revealed moderate pulmonary emphysema. In addition, a triangular area of moderate opacity in the posterior inferior portion of the left lower lobe was noted with some apparent infiltrative changes seen in this same area. It was felt that this was possibly due to atelectasis secondary to a bronchial lesion.

At bronchoscopic examination, Dec. 14, 1951, a granular appearing lesion was noted in the intermediate bronchus of the left lung approximately 1½ cm. distal to the left upper lobe take-off. This lesion appeared to be raised and to extend to or into the bifurcations of the left lower lobe. Microscopic diagnosis was possible carcinoma of the lung.

The patient was sent to the Cardiology Laboratory, where the following findings were noted:

Vital capacity	3.25 L. in 4.9 seconds
Vital rate	0.67 L. per minute
Resting ventilation	17.0 L. per minute
Respiratory rate	20
Maximum breathing capacity	54.2 L. per minute (about one-third normal)
Respiratory reserve	69 per cent
Physical fitness index	11.3 (normal range, 13 to 16)

The consultant concluded that exploration could be attempted, but by all means the most limited excision possible should be performed.

Operation.—A left exploratory thoracotomy was performed on Jan. 14, 1952. The operative procedure planned prior to surgery was carried out without event. A left lower lobectomy was performed with a portion of the left main bronchus and approximately 1 cm. of the left upper bronchus resected, en masse. The distal upper lobe bronchus was anastomosed by means of interrupted 0000 silk to the proximal left main bronchus, end to end. All blood supply to the upper lobe was preserved (Fig. 3).

The lung expanded well with positive pressure, and the left upper lobe realigned itself in the chest filling the pleural cavity considerably more satisfactorily than if a routine left lower lobectomy had been performed with the normal bronchial arrangement.

Postoperative Course.—The patient was able to cough up mucus fairly well. The highest temperature was 101.8° rectally, which occurred on the second postoperative day. At this time, the radial pulse was 120; respiration was 35. By the fourth postoperative day, the temperature and pulse were normal, although the respiratory rate was 25. On Jan. 19, 1952, the fifth postoperative day, the patient was dyspneic. A relatively large amount of mucus was aspirated, and the nasal oxygen catheter, which was plugged, was reopened, following which the patient was more comfortable. Some subcutaneous emphysema was noted over the left chest extending up to the neck. On Jan. 20, 1952, the subcutaneous emphysema was noted to have extended down the right arm, trunk, and medial aspect of both thighs. Physical examination revealed a collapsed left lung. A portable x-ray film of the chest confirmed this. There was a slight tracheal shift to the right. However, the patient was comfortable if the trachea was kept clean. The following day, Jan 21, 1952, the patient was much less dyspneic and the subcutaneous emphysema was noted to have receded. An x-ray film taken on Jan. 22, 1952, revealed the left upper lobe to be re-expanded. The anterior catheter was removed and the stitches were taken out. The patient was ambulated.

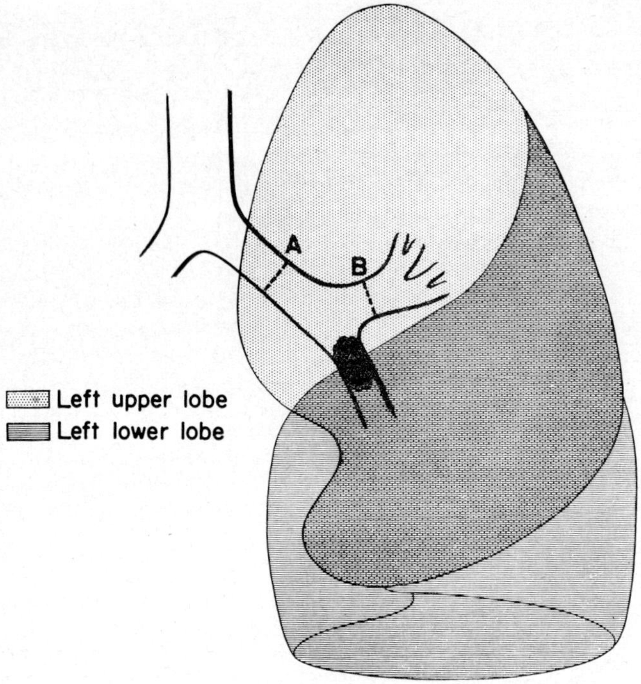

A.

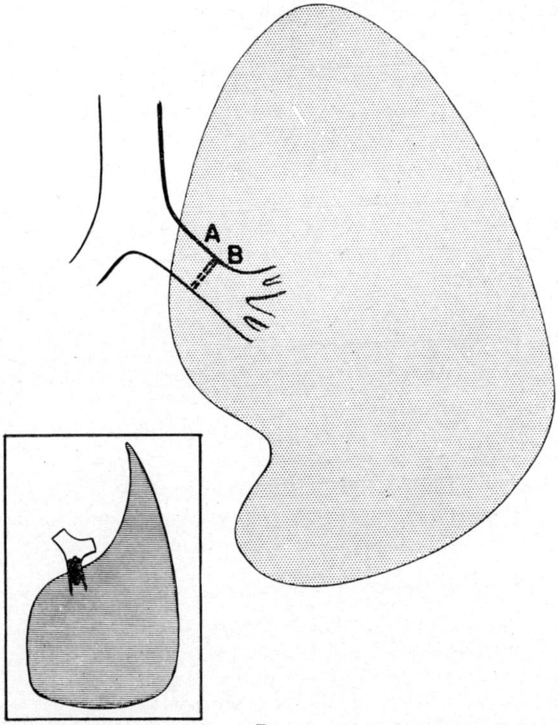

B.

Fig. 3.—*A*, This schematic drawing indicates the location of the bronchial adenoma. The lines *A* and *B* indicate the lines of transection. *B*, The reconstructive procedure is depicted. The inset sketch represents the component parts of the excised specimen.

A.

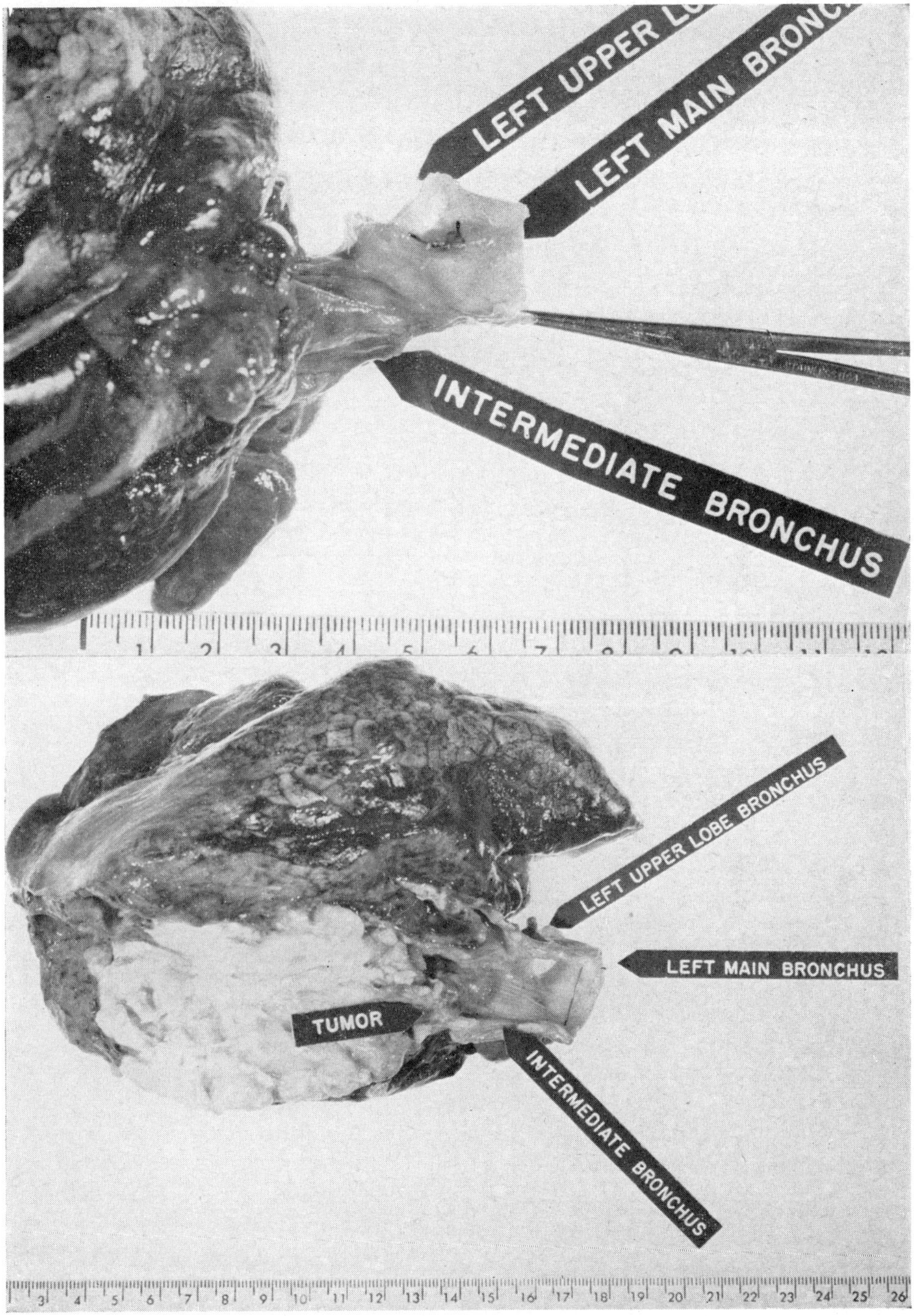

B.

Fig. 4.—Excised specimen. *A*, Close-up view of the proximal bronchial excision of the lower bronchus with the lower lobe, left upper, and distal left main bronchus. *B*, Opened view of lower lobe and tumor.

By the en masse excision of the structures indicated, an additional 4 cm. of the bronchus proximal to the tumor was excised than could have been removed with a lower lobectomy alone.

The microscopic report of the resected specimen was bronchial adenoma (doubtfully malignant) (Fig. 4).

He was discharged on the twenty-second postoperative day.

Progress Report.—Early following discharge, there was slight difficulty in raising sputum in the recumbent position. This, however, created no problem. An x-ray film taken on Feb. 26, 1952, revealed the left upper lobe to occupy comfortably the left half of the chest, and appeared normally aerated.

The patient was readmitted to the hospital on March 10, 1952, for bronchoscopy. A No. 7, 45 cm. bronchoscope was passed without difficulty. The right main-stem bronchus was normal. The carina was sharp and cords normal. The suture line in the left main bronchus was clear and without stenosis. The bronchus distal to the suture line continued in a straight line with the main-stem bronchus. For all practical purposes, one gained the impression that the scope was being passed into a normal left lower lobe. There was no evidence of recurrence. The distal bronchus was patent and appeared to function normally.

On June 25, 1952, bronchospirometry studies were carried out.*

Bronchospirometry

Barometric pressure, 755 Temperature, 22° C. Correction factor (S.T.P. 760 and 0°), 0.9193

Gas Exchange	*Normal Values*	*Right Result*	*Per Cent*	*Left Result*	*Per Cent*	*Totals*
O_2 consumption (c.c./min.)	Dependent on BMR	199.0	62	121.0	38	320
Ventilation (L./min.)	5.0 L./min.	4.8	53	4.2	47	9
Ventilation equivalent	2.4-2.6	2.4		3.5		2.8
C.c. O_2/L. ventilation	42-45 c.c./min.	42.0		28.0		36
*Lung Volume**						
Vital capacity		1480	61	956	39	2703 2436

*In the normal person, 55 per cent of lung volume is on the right and 45 per cent on the left.

Summary.—There was 62 per cent oxygen consumption, right with 53 per cent ventilation on that side. On the left side, there was 38 per cent oxygen consumption with 47 per cent ventilation. Vital capacity studies with and without catheter checked within 267 c.c. It was felt that there was no block on either side.

The patient is alive and well without complaints at the present time, almost two years after surgery. The dyspnea is no longer a problem. He continues to be a somewhat garrulous individual, and he now states that he is able to talk continuously without stopping for breath, as was the case preoperatively.

Comment.—By resecting the lower lobe with portions of the left upper lobe and left main bronchus, approximately 4 cm. of additional bronchial tissue was removed proximally than could have been obtained by a lower lobectomy alone. In retrospect, an immediate tracheotomy following surgery would have lessened the problems associated with retained bronchial secretions.

SUMMARY

1. The average human measurements at autopsy of the tracheobronchial tree pertinent to the problem of resection and reconstruction have been presented.

2. A case of bronchial adenoma with the patient undergoing a bronchial resection with reconstruction has been presented. The respiratory function of

*Courtesy of Dr. Frank Cline, Jr., Firland Sanatorium.

the distal lung has been shown to be normal. To our knowledge, no other report has been made of a bronchial adenoma treated in this fashion.

3. We believe that bronchial resection and reconstruction is the operation of choice in selected cases of bronchial adenoma.

Acknowledgment.—We wish to acknowledge the assistance of Dr. Lloyd M. Nyhus, Dr. John W. Finley, Dr. Ralph J. Schlosser, and Dr. Donald G. Fletcher in obtaining at autopsy the measurements of the bronchial relationships.

REFERENCES

1. Kiriluk, L. B., and Merendino, K. A.: An Experimental Evaluation of Bronchial Anastomosis and Healing With Special Consideration of the Plane of Transection, Surg., Gynec. & Obst. **96**: 175-182, 1953.
2. Kiriluk, L. B., and Merendino, K.: An Experimental Evaluation in the Dog of Bronchial Transplantation, Bronchial, Tracheal and Tracheobronchial Resection With Reconstruction, Ann. Surg. **137**: 490-503, 1953.
3. Kiriluk, L. B., and Merendino, K. A.: An Experimental Evaluation of Pulmonary Function and Lung Substance Distal to Transection or Resection of Tracheobronchial Segments, Surg., Gynec. & Obst. **96**: 617-624, 1953.
4. Kiriluk, L. B., and Merendino, K. A.: Experimental Bronchial Transection, Resection, and Transplantation in the Growing Dog, Proc. Surg. Forum, Clin. Congress Am. Coll. Surgeons, Chicago, 1953. To be published.
5. Gebauer, P. W.: Pulmonary Surgical Salvage by Bronchial Resection, Surg., Gynec. & Obst. **94**: 347-357, 1952.
6. Tuttle, W. M.: Personal communication, 1953.

THE SYNDROME OF PERIPHERAL ARTERIAL INSUFFICIENCY WITH PARTIAL OCCLUSION OF THE ILIAC ARTERY

A Study of Nine Cases

Rutherford S. Gilfillan, M.D.,* Jesse L. Steinfeld, M.D.,** and Frank H. Leeds, M.D.,*** San Francisco, Calif.

In 1940 Leriche[8] described a syndrome produced by obstruction of the terminal aorta and characterized by absent pulses in both lower limbs, sexual impotency, and an atypical intermittent claudication. Clinical and arteriographic studies since that time have shown that similar manifestations develop with partial obstruction of the common or external iliac arteries.

The syndrome due to partial occlusion of the iliac artery is one of intermittent claudication with a characteristic radiation of pain. With exercise, the pain begins in the calf and then may radiate to the thigh, hip, and buttock. The pain occurs in the presence of easily palpable peripheral pulses. A systolic bruit may be heard over the terminal aorta or iliac arteries.[13] Comparison of the femoral and the carotid pulses reveals that the femoral pulse is weaker and more easily obliterated by pressure. With exercise of the involved extremity there is disappearance of the pedal pulses and blanching of the foot and ankle. The blood pressure of the thigh is lower than that of the arm.

Sexual impotence, a characteristic finding in the Leriche syndrome,[9, 10] is uncommon in partial obstruction of the common iliac artery. Global atrophy of the lower limbs, also characteristic of the Leriche syndrome,[9, 10] is not found in partial iliac obstruction, although localized muscular atrophy may be present.

We have had occasion to study nine patients who met the clinical criteria of partial occlusion of the iliac artery. Six of these patients were studied before and after lumbar sympathectomy. The investigations included arteriography, reflex vasodilatation, plethysmography, oscillometry, ballistocardiography, and muscle clearance of radioiodine. The aims of the investigation were twofold: (1) to find, within the limits of readily available clinical and laboratory procedures, physiologic alterations which might serve to identify the syndrome and to differentiate it from the Leriche syndrome, and (2) to obtain information which might add to the understanding of certain aspects of vascular physiology.

Received for publication, July 31, 1953.

*Vascular Research Laboratory, Marin General Hospital, and Department of Surgery, University of California School of Medicine.

**Laboratory of Experimental Oncology, National Cancer Institute, National Institutes of Health, Public Health Service, Department of Health, Education and Welfare, and the Cancer Research Institute and Department of Medicine, University of California School of Medicine.

***Department of Surgery, University of California School of Medicine.

MATERIALS AND METHODS

To determine the anatomic site of the initial pain and its subsequent radiation, we had the patients walk at a rate of 120 steps per minute until pain occurred. Before and after exercise, the extremities were compared with respect to elevation pallor and dependent rubor.

Plethysmographic tracings and pulse recordings with gelatin tambour were made with the Burch Winsor Plethysmograph.[1] Records were obtained both with the patient at rest and following exercise to the point of pain. Arteriograms were obtained in all cases by direct injection of 35 or 70 per cent Diodrast into the aorta.[4]

Oscillometry was carried out before and after exercise with the Tycos Recording Oscillometer or with the Collens Oscillometer. The disappearance of pulses following exercise (jumping on one leg at the rate of two jumps per second), the appearance of pain in the calf, and the reappearance of pulses were carefully timed.

Muscle clearance was measured using the method first described by Kety[6] and later modified by Wisham and Yalow.[14] Approximately 10 microcuries of I^{131} buffered to pH 7.5 and in a constant volume of 0.25 ml. was injected through a 25 gauge 2½ inch needle into the gastrocnemius and quadriceps muscles of the involved leg. A lead shielded and collimated scintillation counter using a thallium activated sodium iodide crystal was placed over the injected area, and the counts per minute were continuously recorded by an Esterline Angus Recorder, which was driven by the relay of a Tracerlab Autoscaler. Approximately 5,000 counts were recorded for each plotted point, readings having been taken every two minutes for forty-five to sixty minutes.

The rate of disappearance of I^{131} was determined for approximately ten minutes, and then the subject exercised by hopping on one leg for 100 hops in from sixty to ninety seconds in the control group, or until severe pain appeared in the case of the patients (fewer than 100 hops). The subject was then placed in exactly the same position, and the remaining activity was recorded for approximately thirty minutes. A plot of the log of external counts per minute against time, corrected for the nonmoving clearance component, Figs. 7 and 8, yielded a line with negative slope, k. This may also be expressed as percentage of ion cleared per minute, K.

Ballistocardiograms were obtained in six cases.

Reflex vasodilatation tests were made after the method of Gibbon and Landis,[5] using an electric blanket as the stimulus to reflex heating rather than water at 43° to 45° C.

Unilateral or bilateral sympathetic blocks were performed in six cases.

RESULTS

Severe pain during minimal or moderate exercise in all cases began invariably in the calf and radiated to the ipsilateral thigh, hip, and buttock

TABLE I. CLINICAL SUMMARY

CASE	AGE (YR.)	LESION	CLAUDICATION	POTENCY	BRUIT	ELEVATION PALLOR		PULSE RETURN FOLLOWING EXERCISE (DORSALIS PEDIS)	BLOOD PRESSURE		ATROPHY OF CALF OR THIGH	BLANCHING DURING EXERCISE (FOOT)
						AT REST	FOLLOWING		ARM	LEG		
1. A. L.	54	Partial right common iliac occlusion	Calf to thigh to hip	+	+	0	+	5′ 0″	140/110	80/60	+	+
2. N. D.	47	Partial right common iliac occlusion	Calf only	+	+	0	+	2′ 15″	160/90	140/80	-	+
		Partial left common iliac occlusion	Calf only		+	0	+	2′ 0″	160/90	148/80	-	+
3. J. K.	47	Partial right common iliac occlusion	Calf to thigh to hip	+	+	0	+	2′ 0″	160/90	150/110	+	+
4. R. N.	57	Partial right common iliac occlusion	Calf to thigh to hip	0	+	0	+	3′ 20″	150/80	140/90	-	+
5. A. Y.	48	Partial left external iliac occlusion	Calf to thigh to hip	+	+	+	+	4′ 30″	140/90	70/0	+	+
6. J. H.	43	Partial right external iliac occlusion	Calf to thigh to back	+	0	0	+	4′ 30″	140/80	—	-	+
		Partial left external iliac occlusion	Calf to thigh to back			0	+	5′ 0″	—	—	-	+
7. W. W.	60	Partial right common iliac occlusion	Calf only	+	+	0	+	5′ 10″	160/90	140/70	-	+
8. L. H.	56	Partial left common iliac and external iliac occlusion	Calf only	+	+	0	+	6′ 10″	120/80	100/60	-	+
9. F. C.	34	Partial left iliac occlusion	Calf only	+	+	0	+	4′ 20″	140/90	100/60	+	+

(Table I). In no instance was the site of the original pain other than the calf. There was no elevation pallor at rest, but following exercise elevation pallor was found, and persisted for from one to three minutes. Blanching of the involved foot during exercise also occurred in all cases. The pedal pulses disappeared during exercise and did not reappear for two to six minutes following the cessation of exercise.

A.

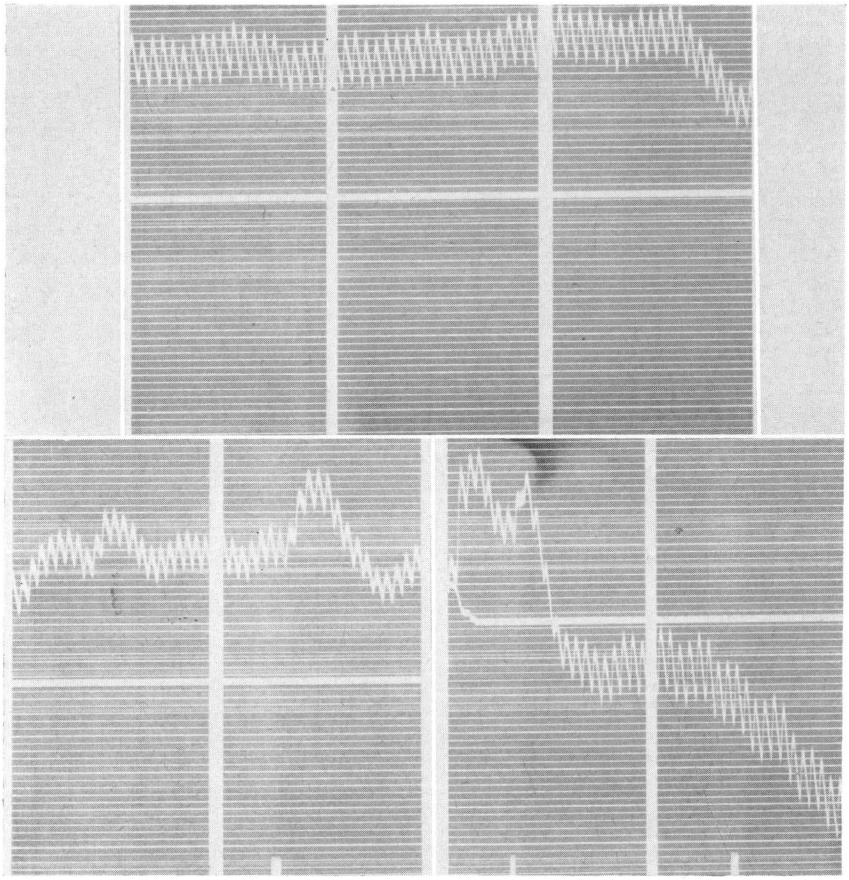

B. *C.*

Fig. 1 (Case 2, N. D.).—Plethysmographic tracing, right second toe (postsympathectomy). *A,* At rest. *B,* Two minutes following exercise to claudication (eighty jumps on right leg at two jumps per second). *C,* Six minutes later, return to normal.

The plethysmograph (Fig. 1) and pulse tracings (Fig. 2) both demonstrated the decrease in pulse amplitude attendant upon exercise, and clearly indicated the time of return following exercise.

In all patients, a narrowing of the arterial lumen could be demonstrated by contrast roentgenography. Representative arteriograms are shown in Figs. 3 and 4.

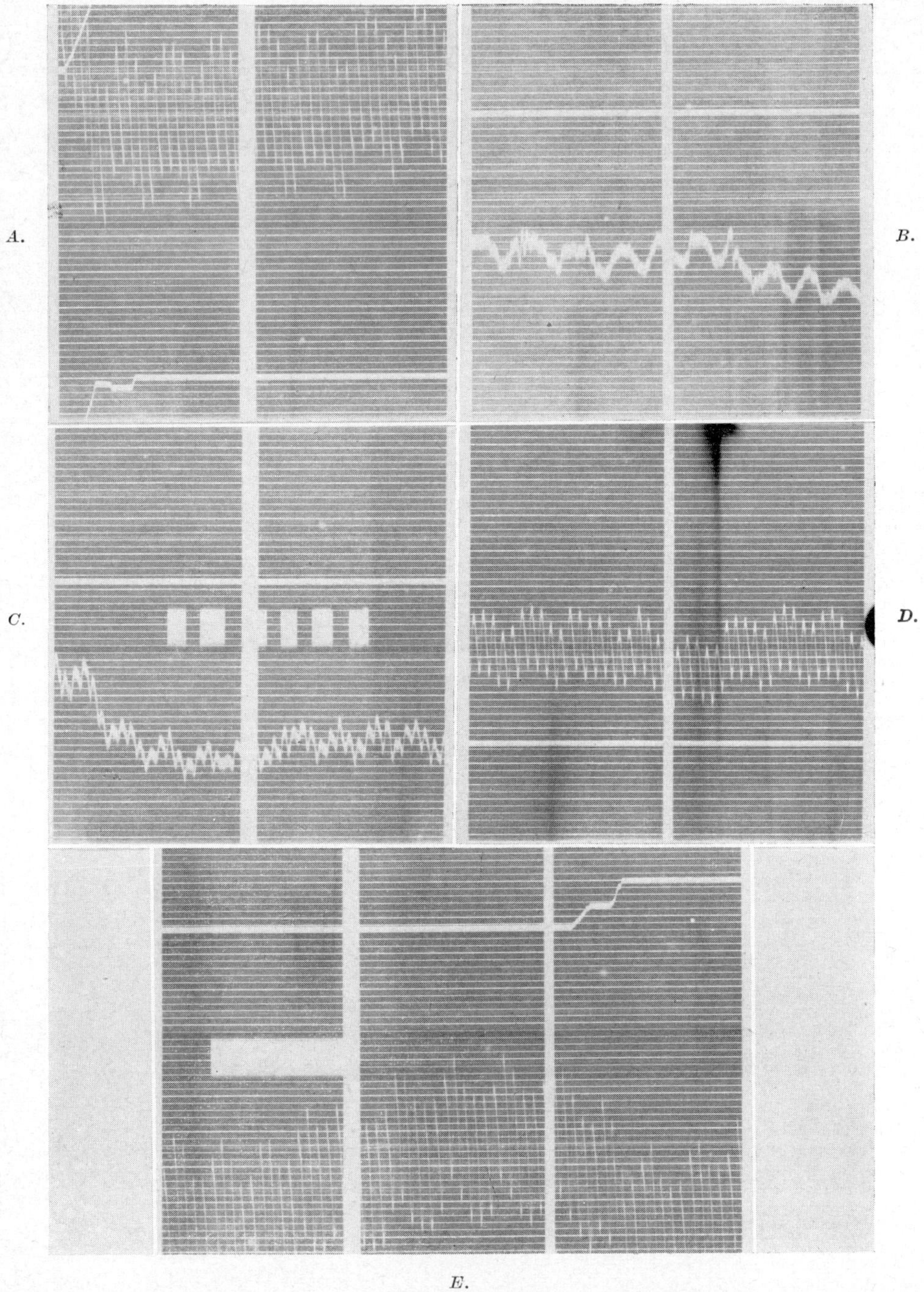

Fig. 2 (Case 2, N. D.).—Pulse tracing made with gelatin tambour over right dorsalis pedis artery (postsympathectomy). *A,* At rest. *B,* Thirty seconds following exercise to claudication (eighty-six jumps on right leg at two jumps per second). *C,* Five minutes following exercise. *D,* Ten minutes following exercise. *E,* Fifteen minutes after exercise. Interval marker indicates ten-second startle reaction (loud bell rung beside patient's head) with no response.

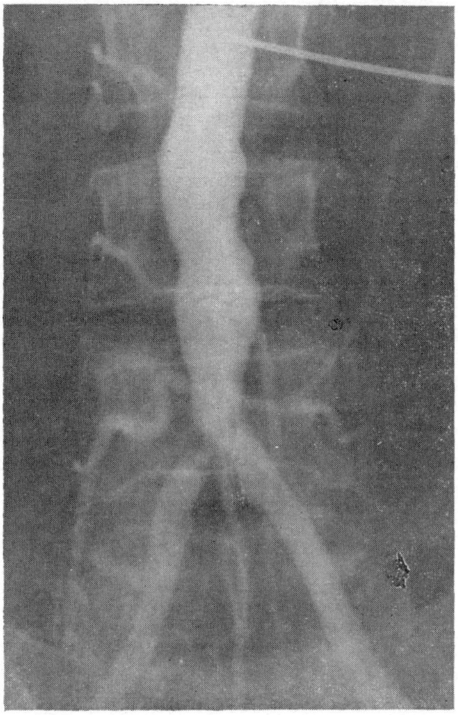

Fig. 3 (Case 3, J. K.).—Right common iliac artery, partial occlusion.

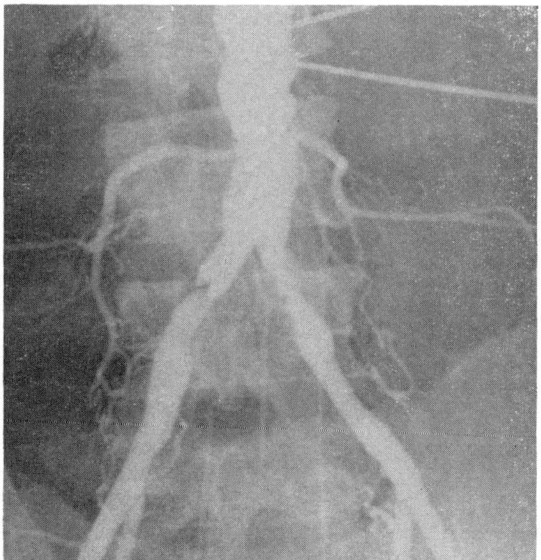

Fig. 4 (Case 2, N. D.).—Bilateral partial iliac occlusions.

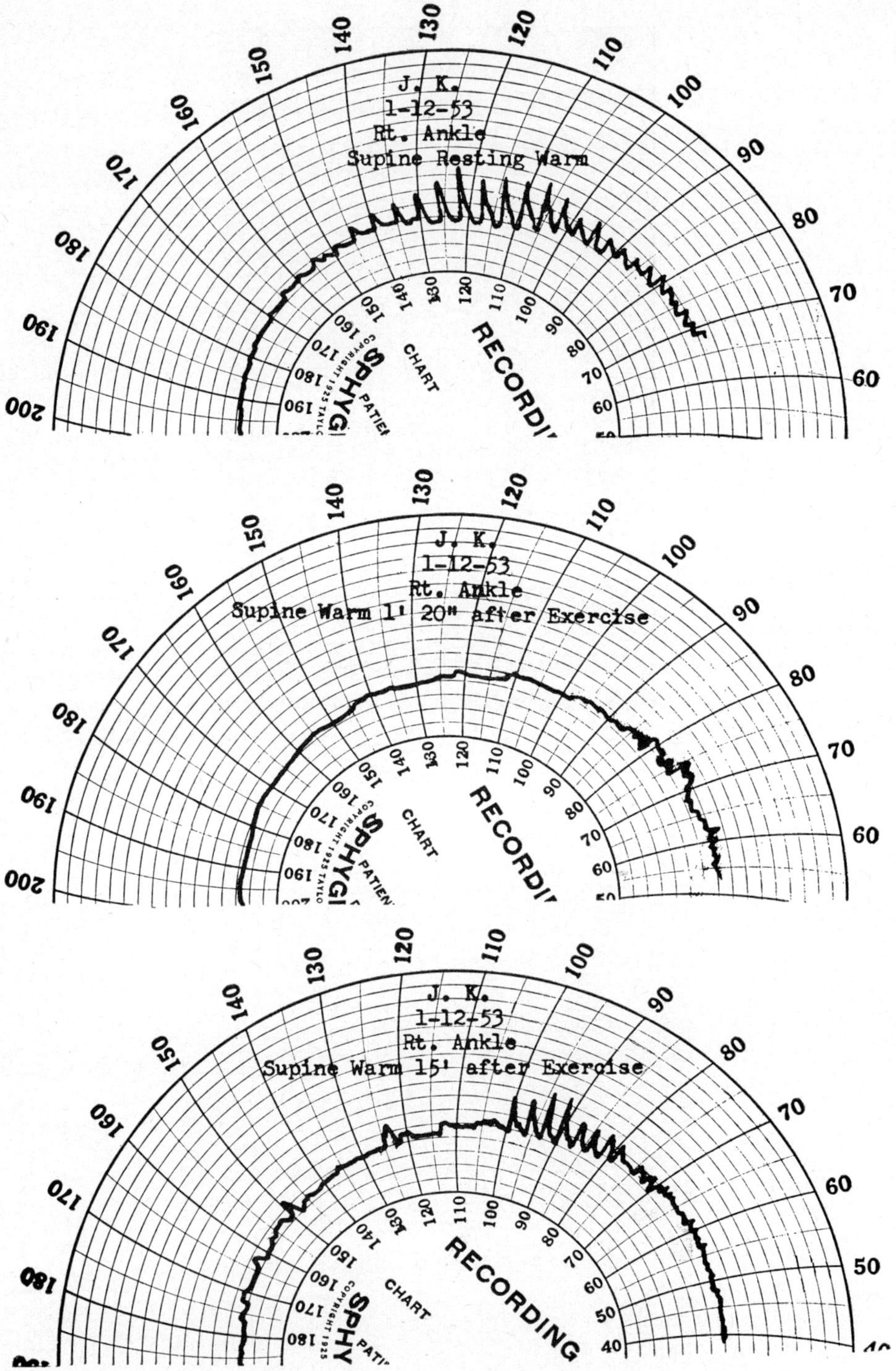

Fig. 5 (Case 3, J. K.).—Oscillometric tracing, right ankle, showing decrease in pulsations following exercise with incomplete return after fifteen minutes.

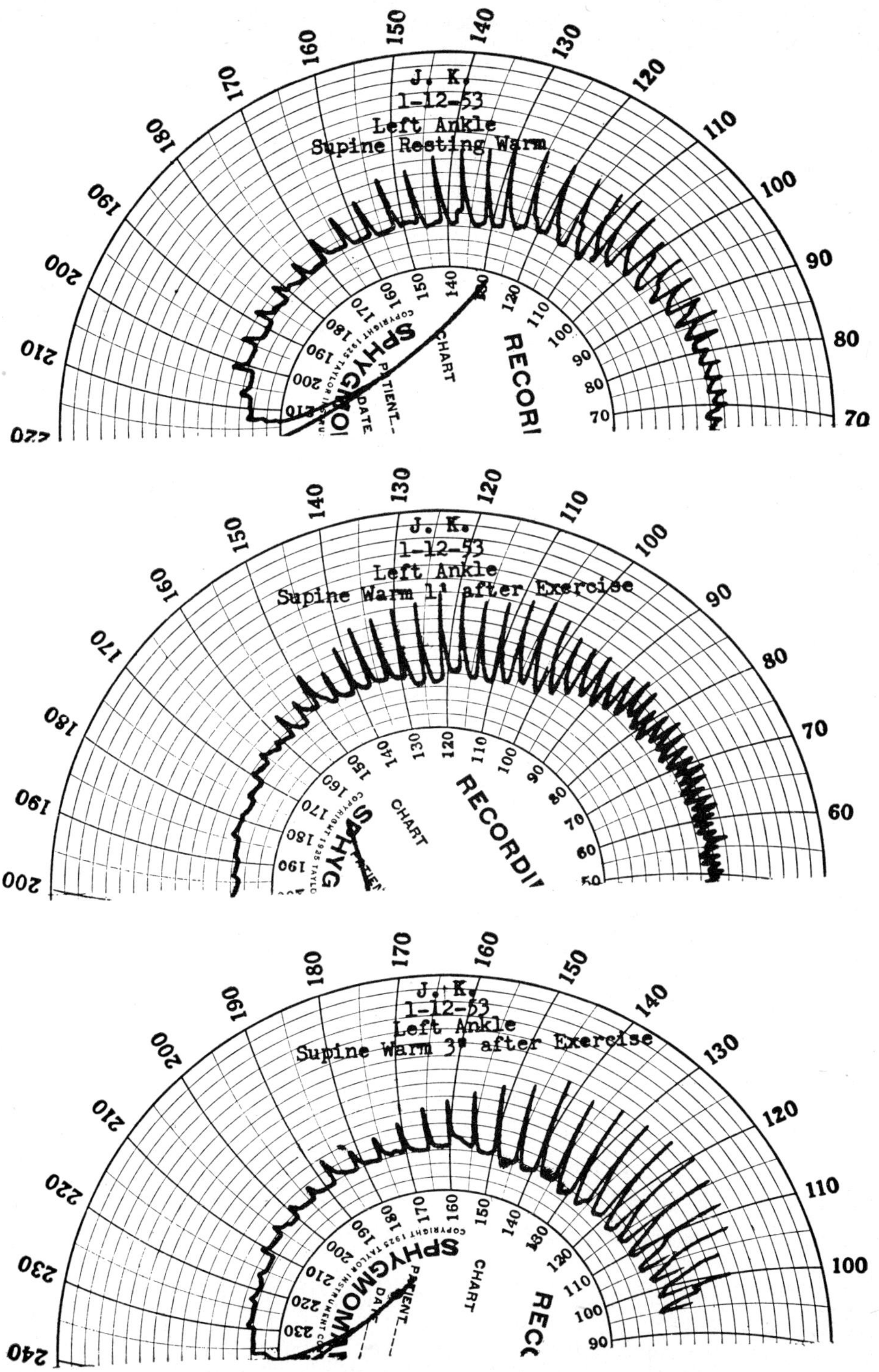

Fig. 6 (Case 3, J. K.).—Oscillometric tracing, left ankle, showing normal response.

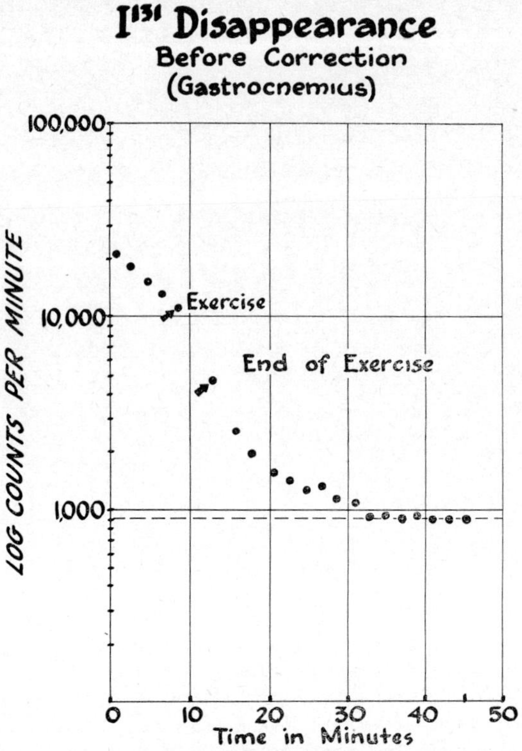

Fig. 7.—Graph showing variation of logarithm of counts per minute of I^{131} with time.

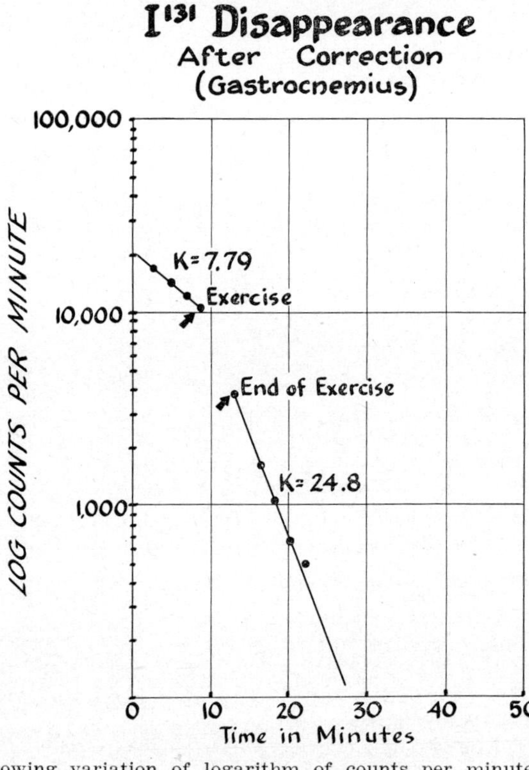

Fig. 8.—Graph showing variation of logarithm of counts per minute of I^{131} with time, corrected for nonmoving component.

Oscillograms of the calf showed a decrease in the oscillations following exercise, with the decrease persisting for over one minute in all nine cases (Fig. 5). The normal response following exercise, an increase of oscillations or a short decrease followed by an increase, is shown in Fig. 6.

Table II shows that there is no obvious difference in the percentage of I^{131} cleared per minute between resting control patients and those with intermittent claudication. Furthermore the rate of disappearance of the ion following exercise compared with the resting disappearance rate was approximately the same in the control and experimental groups.

TABLE II. PERCENTAGE OF I^{131} REMOVED PER MINUTE: $K = 100 \frac{\Delta N/N}{\Delta t}$

		K BEFORE EXERCISE	K FOLLOWING EXERCISE	$R = \frac{\text{AFTER EXERCISE}}{\text{BEFORE EXERCISE}}$
		Controls		
1-J.	Quadriceps;	3.46	5.55	1.60
	gastrocnemius	3.92	13.80	3.54
2-G.	Quadriceps;	4.75	8.78	1.93
	gastrocnemius	7.79	24.80	3.19
3-C.	Quadriceps;	9.00	24.70	2.75
	gastrocnemius	11.20	28.80	2.58
		Patients With Partial Iliac Artery Occlusion		
4-D.	Quadriceps;	2.31	7.3	3.16
	gastrocnemius	6.12	13.3	2.18
5-K.	Quadriceps;	14.40	14.4	1.00
	gastrocnemius	4.84	15.0	3.10
6-S.	Quadriceps;	4.72	11.5	2.44
	gastrocnemius	3.74	14.7	3.94

Ballistocardiograms on six patients were abnormal in each instance, but exhibited no characteristic pattern.

The vasodilatation tests were normal in all cases studied.

Following sympathetic block and lumbar sympathectomy in six patients there was no change in the clinical findings, response to exercise, oscillometry, plethysmography, or pulse tracings.

DISCUSSION

Each of the nine patients with partial occlusion of the common iliac artery had a characteristic intermittent claudication on exercise in the presence of easily palpable femoral and pedal pulses. This is in contrast to the situation found in the Leriche syndrome, where the pedal pulses are not palpable and the femoral pulse is not palpable or very feeble. In this group of patients, the blood pressure in the thigh was lower than in the arm, whereas in the Leriche syndrome, blood pressure is not obtainable in the thigh. Inability to maintain an erection is a characteristic finding in the Leriche syndrome (progressing to actual sexual impotence in long-standing cases),[9] but this finding of decreased sexual power was found in only two of the nine patients in this group. Localized muscular atrophy in the lower limbs with partial iliac artery occlusion may occur in contrast to global atrophy of both lower extremities found in the Leriche syndrome. Elevation pallor was found in partial iliac obstruction only after exercise to the point of pain, whereas elevation pallor is present at rest in the patients with the Leriche syndrome.[9] In both syndromes a bruit may be heard over the terminal aorta or common iliac arteries.

Patients with the Leriche syndrome have an atypical intermittent claudication described as a feeling of extreme weakness or weariness in both lower limbs immediately on walking or while standing.[8, 9] If these patients are encouraged to walk to the point of appearance of actual pain, a "true" intermittent claudication will occur. The pain will, however, begin in the buttock and then radiate to the hip, thigh, and calf. This radiation of pain on exercise in the Leriche syndrome (and in total obstruction of the common external iliac artery) differs from that of partial iliac artery obstruction, where the pain begins in the calf and radiates successively to the thigh, hip, and buttock.

Two laboratory procedures are of importance in the differential diagnosis. The oscillogram shows no pulsations in the calf in the Leriche syndrome, but shows decreased or normal pulsation at rest in partial iliac obstruction. Following exercise, however, there is a decrease in the pulse in these patients rather than the increase found in the normal persons. This inverse relation of the oscillometric tracings was also found by Ejrup[2, 3] in his study of 660 cases of peripheral arterial obliterative disease. The arteriogram or aortogram actually demonstrates the lesion and represents the measure by which the definitive diagnosis is reached.

The ballistocardiogram, plethysmograph, reflex vasodilatation, and I^{131} clearances did not aid in the differential diagnosis.

Radioiodine clearances in these patients were made in an attempt to correlate the occurrence of pain with a decrease in clearance (representing blood flow). The fact that no decrease in clearance was found either before or after exercise may be correlated with the patients' experiencing no pain at those times, and with the pain of intermittent claudication ceasing almost immediately on termination of exercise. It would be of interest to measure muscle clearance during the actual period of exercise when the patient is experiencing pain.

The disappearance of the dorsalis pedis pulse during exercise where one was previously palpable points to either (1) a lack of sufficient blood to distend the peripheral artery or (2) vasoconstriction distally. Pearl[11] in 1937 described disappearance of the pulses in the extremities following exercise, which he attributed to a vasomotor phenomenon. Some of Pearl's patients, however, were later found to have an organic obstruction.[12]

Because thrombosis of the terminal aorta may begin as common iliac artery thrombosis, recognition of this syndrome followed by appropriate therapy may prevent or delay aortic thrombosis.[10] Accordingly, despite the failure of sympathetic block to alter the patient's symptomatology favorably, lumbar sympathectomies were performed in six of the nine cases.[9, 10] There was no discernible effect on the symptoms, although the adequacy of sympathectomy was proved by the lack of a startle reaction during plethysmography and by the maintenance of digital temperatures five to ten degrees above a room temperature of 18° to 20° C. Specifically, sympathectomy did not affect the occurrence of pain during exercise, reappearance of pulses following exercise, oscillometry, or the plethysmographic or pulse tracings.

Kinmouth and associates[7] have shown in the rabbit and cat that there is little if any sympathetic control of the major arteries down to and including the femoral artery, and that change in caliber of these vessels followed blood pressure change only. It is our feeling that the syndrome presented here is attributable to changes occurring on an obstructive basis, and is not due to vasomotor effects mediated via the lumbar sympathetic nervous system.

CASE REPORT

J. K., a 37-year-old engineer, was admitted to the neurological service of the University of California Hospital on Feb. 15, 1952, with a chief complaint of severe right leg pain. Eight months prior to admission, the patient first noted onset of calf pain, which appeared after walking three or four blocks. When the patient continued to walk, this pain increased in severity, radiating to the thigh, hip, and buttock. This progressed until at the time of admission the pain appeared after the patient walked approximately one block. The patient stated that he had smoked approximately fifteen cigarettes a day for many years.

Physical examination revealed a well-developed, obese white man; blood pressure was 160/80, right arm. Pertinent physical findings included the following: (1) There were palpable pulsations of equal intensity in brachial, radial, and ulnar arteries bilaterally. (2) The femoral, dorsalis pedis, and posterior tibial pulses were all palpable bilaterally, but were markedly diminished on the right. (3) When compared with the right carotid artery, the right femoral pulse was more easily obliterated by pressure. (4) The feet were moist and cool, but there was no dependent rubor or elevation pallor. (5) There was a 2 to 3 cm. atrophy (circumference measurement) of the right thigh and calf when compared with the left. (6) Ophthalmologic examination showed the discs to be flat, of normal color, with the edges clear and well defined; retinal vessels were of normal caliber and distribution; no exudates or hemorrhages were seen. Laboratory tests revealed a negative serologic test for syphilis. Hemoglobin was 15.7 Gm. per 100 c.c. Serum cholesterol was 234 mg. per cent.

The following procedures were performed: (1) Exercise: When the patient hopped on the affected leg (right) at the rate of two hops per second, the right foot blanched immediately, pain appearing in the right calf at the end of thirty seconds. As the patient continued to hop, pain appeared in the right thigh at forty seconds and in the right buttock at forty-five seconds. At this point the patient was unable to exercise further. (2) Pulse recordings: Palpation of the pedal pulses was attempted at forty-five seconds, but no pulse could be found. The pedal pulses could not be palpated in the right foot until three and one-half minutes after cessation of exercise, while color returned to the foot approximately twenty seconds after completion of the exercise. Finally, with the patient at rest, oscillometric tracings revealed diminished pulse amplitude in the right calf and thigh as compared to the left. A reflex vasodilatation test revealed a normal response with a slight delay in the upper extremity and a normal rise of temperature to full levels of vasodilatation in the toes of both feet. Plethysmographic tracings revealed a decrease in amplitude of the pulse waves following exercise. This decrease persisted for one and one-half minutes. Also, pulse tracings of the dorsalis pedis artery following exercise revealed a decrease in amplitude which did not return to normal for over seven minutes.

On Feb. 21, 1952, a direct puncture aortogram was carried out under general anesthesia. Six serial films were taken at approximately eight-second intervals. These revealed a constriction of the right common iliac at its take-off from the aorta. There was dilatation of the aorta for 3 to 4 cm. above its bifurcation. Arteriosclerotic changes on the lower abdominal aorta and left common iliac artery were also present.

Following conservative therapy, the patient was discharged from the hospital on Feb. 24, 1952.

On March 6, 1952, the patient was admitted to Franklin Hospital, and on March 7, 1952, a right lumbar sympathectomy was performed (first, second, and third lumbar ganglia). The postoperative course was uneventful, and the patient was discharged from the hospital on March 14, 1952. At that time, a reflex vasodilatation test showed maintenance of the temperature of the toes at 28° to 32° C. despite exposure to an environmental temperature of 19° C. Clinical examination following discharge from the hospital revealed little or no change in the clinical or laboratory findings described previously, with the exception that the right pedal pulses were more easily palpable at rest. On Dec. 23, 1952, the hopping test was repeated, and again revealed pain in the calf at thirty seconds and in the thigh at forty seconds. Palpation immediately following exercise revealed the pulses to be absent for over two minutes. Color did not return to the foot following exercise for approximately fifteen seconds. Measurement of the right thigh and calf still showed 2 to 3 cm. of atrophy.

Despite the appearance of pain during hopping at approximately the same time as before sympathectomy, the patient felt he could walk a greater distance without pain than before the operation. There were, however, no quantitative laboratory data to support the patient's statement.

SUMMARY

1. A syndrome due to partial obstruction of the common or external iliac artery was studied in nine patients.

2. The clinical and laboratory criteria for differentiating partial iliac artery obstruction from the Leriche syndrome are discussed.

3. Sympathectomy had no effect in six cases, indicating that the basis for the phenomena observed is obstructive rather than vasomotor in origin.

REFERENCES

1. Burch, G. E.: A New Sensitive Portable Plethysmograph, Am. Heart J. **33**: 48-75, 1947.
2. Ejrup, B.: Tonoscillography After Exercise as an Early Diagnostic Method in Organic Peripheral Arterial Disease, Acta med. scandinav. (supp. 239) **138**: 347-366, 1950.
3. Ejrup, B.: Tonoscillography After Exercise, Acta med. scandinav. (supp. 211) **130**: 1-272, 1948.
4. Freeman, N. E., Gilfillan, R. S., Fullenlove, T. M., and Leeds, F. H.: Surgery of the Large Arteries, Monographs on Surgery, Baltimore, 1952, Williams & Wilkins Company, pp. 385-415.
5. Gibbon, J. H., Jr., and Landis, E. M.: Vasodilatation in the Lower Extremities in Response to Immersing the Forearms in Warm Water, J. Clin. Investigation **11**: 1019-1036, 1932.
6. Kety, S.: Measurement of Regional Circulation by the Local Clearance of Radioactive Sodium, Am. Heart J. **38**: 321-327, 1949.
7. Kinmouth, J. B., Simeone, F. A., and Perlow, V.: Factors Affecting Diameter of Large Arteries With Particular Reference to Traumatic Spasm, SURGERY **26**: 452-471, 1949.

8. Leriche, R.: De la résection du carrefour aortico-iliaque avec double sympathectomie lombaire pour thrombose artéritique de l'aorte; le syndrome de l'oblitération termino-aortique par artérite, Presse méd. **48**: 601-604, 1940.
9. Leriche, R., and Morel, A.: The Syndrome of Thrombotic Obliteration of the Aortic Bifurcation, Ann. Surg. **127**: 193-206, 1948.
10. Beaconsfield, P., and Kunlin, J.: Insidious Thrombosis of the Aortic Bifurcation, Arch. Surg. **66**: 356-364, 1953.
11. Pearl, F.: Angiospastic Claudication, Am. J. M. Sc. **194**: 505-513, 1937.
12. Pearl, F.: Personal communication.
13. Popkin, R. J.: Systolic Murmurs Heard Over the Lower Abdominal Aorta: Its Significance, in Peripheral Vascular Diseases, Angiology **1**: 244-246, 1950.
14. Wisham, L. H., and Yalow, R. S.: Some Factors Affecting the Clearance of Na^{24} From Human Muscle, Am. Heart J. **43**: 67-76, 1952.

BENIGN CYSTADENOMA OF PANCREAS

Report of Four Treated Cases, One by Whipple Type of Resection

Harold A. Zintel, M.D., Horatio T. Enterline, M.D., and Jonathan E. Rhoads, M.D., Philadelphia, Pa.

(From the Harrison Department of Surgical Research, Schools of Medicine, University of Pennsylvania, and the Department of Surgery of the Hospital of the University of Pennsylvania)

BENIGN cystadenoma of the pancreas is a rare lesion. Mozan[1] reviewed the literature in 1951 and concluded that only forty-nine definite cases, including one of his own, were reported in the literature. Since Mozan's report, Sawyer,[2] Tagariello,[3] and Haukohl[4] have recorded a total of four additional cases, making the total of reported definite cases fifty-three. Because of the apparent relative rareness of this lesion it was thought worth while to record four additional cases treated surgically and followed from two and one-half to ten and one-half years. One of these patients had a Whipple type resection of the head of the pancreas.

The report of Mozan[1] establishes the frequency of symptoms in patients with benign cystadenoma of the pancreas. In the case reports reviewed in his report, a palpable mass was present in 82 per cent of the patients, dyspepsia in 73 per cent, and pain in 57 per cent. When very large tumors were present, premature gastric satiation, gaseous distension, belching, nausea, and vomiting were the most frequent symptoms. Fourteen per cent of the patients had associated diabetes mellitus. Only the case reported by Mozan had jaundice and ascites. There were seven times as many female patients as male patients. Only thirty-one of the patients reviewed by him had been operated upon, and the apparent operative mortality was 26 per cent, with the fate of three patients unknown. Only twenty-two of the patients had complete surgical extirpation of the lesions.

Case 1.—The patient, F. W., was a 59-year-old white woman, who for four months had had intermittent cramplike pains of the lower abdomen. The pain occurred one hour after eating and lasted for two to three minutes. During this same period of four months she had noted indigestion, anorexia, belching, passage of excessive amounts of flatus, dizziness, and occasional nausea not related to the abdominal pains. For one month, swelling of the abdomen with retraction of the umbilicus had been noted. She had lost fifteen pounds in the four months of illness.

Other than progressive deafness, palpitation, and nervousness, the systemic review of her history was negative. Physical examination demonstrated a tender, firm, upper abdominal midline mass extending from the palpable liver edge to just below the umbilicus.

An x-ray study of the stomach and small intestine showed the existence of an epigastric soft tissue mass which displaced the antral portion of the stomach and the first portion of the duodenum downward (Fig. 1). The gall bladder was visualized by the

Received for publication, Sept. 14, 1953.

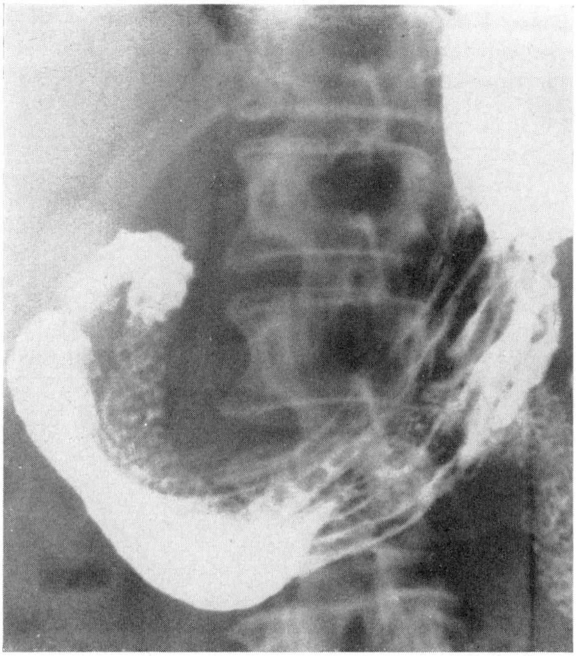

Fig. 1.—Downward displacement of stomach shown by x-ray film in Case 1, F. W.

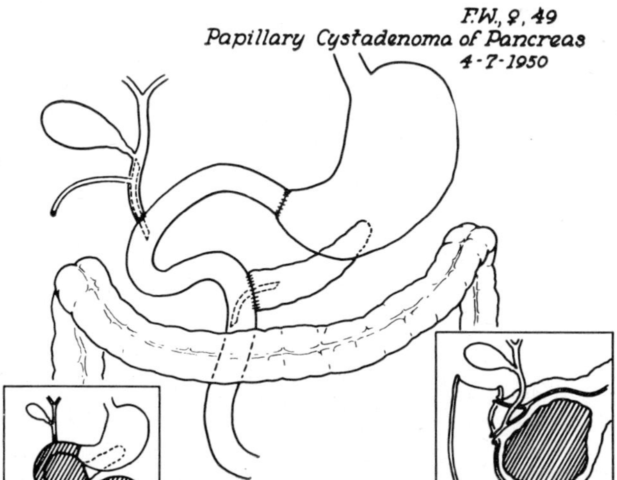

Fig. 2.—Diagrammatic representation of the reconstruction of stomach, jejunum, and remaining pancreas and common bile duct, Case 1, F. W. *1,* Insert showing the extent of the tissue removal. *2,* Insert showing the location of the lesion in the head of the pancreas.

Graham-Cole test, and was thought to be normal. There was no evidence of intrinsic abnormality of the stomach or duodenum. An electrocardiogram showed relatively early changes of the type which develop in the hypertensive state, the so-called left ventricular strain. A complete blood count and urinalysis were normal. The fasting blood sugar was 100 mg. per cent. The serum bilirubin level was 0.15 mg. in one minute and 0.53 mg. total. The prothrombin time was 74 per cent of normal.

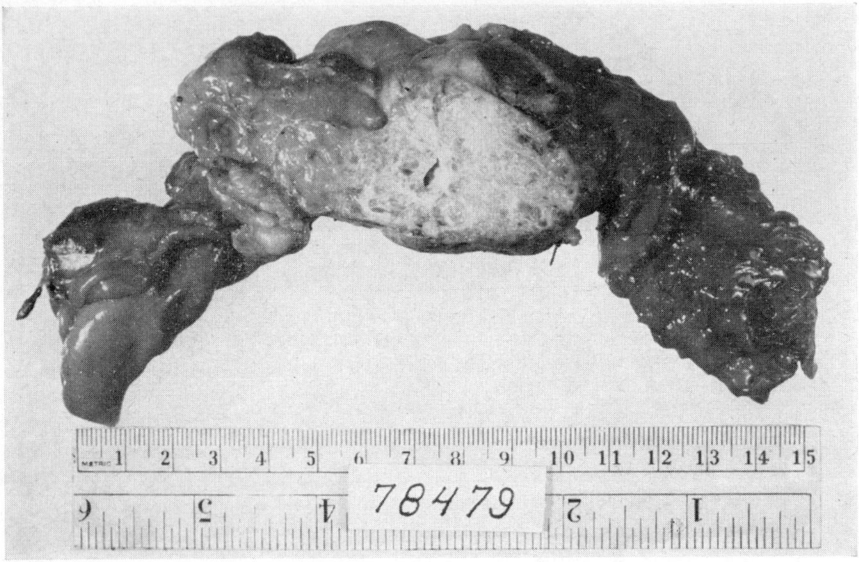

Fig. 3.—Gross appearance of the sectioned lesion in relation to the duodenum in Case 1, F. W.

With a preoperative diagnosis of palpable carcinoma of the head of the pancreas, operation was performed (by H. A. Z.) on April 4, 1950. At operation the head of the pancreas was distorted, especially in the anterior-posterior plane, so that the head of the pancreas was a rounded mass approximately 8 cm. in diameter. Numerous large blood vessels coursed over the surface of the head of the pancreas. The common duct was not dilated. Several enlarged lymph nodes in the gastrocolic omentum were removed for biopsy. Frozen histologic sections of these lymph nodes were reported to show normal lymph node structure. A small portion of the stomach, the entire duodenum, the head of the pancreas, including all of the tumor, and the distal portion of the common duct were removed (Fig. 2). The proximal end of the jejunum was brought through the transverse mesocolon and anastomosed to the distal end of the stomach. Approximately eight inches below this anastomosis, a choledochojejunostomy was effected, and six inches below this the main pancreatic duct was anastomosed to jejunal mucous membrane. Through a separate opening in the common bile duct, a T tube was placed so that one limb of the tube protruded through the stoma into the jejunum. The entire operative procedure required four and one-half hours to complete. The cut surface of the gross original specimen is shown in Fig. 3. The postoperative course was uneventful. The patient's temperature was as high as 100.4° F. on only one occasion. She was discharged from the hospital on the twenty-first postoperative day.

Pathologic Report.—The specimen consisted of the head of the pancreas, which was largely replaced by a well-circumscribed, rounded, multiply loculated, cystic mass 5 cm. in diameter. Twenty-three centimeters of duodenum extended around one side of the pancreas. The duodenum and a portion of the common bile duct were loosely attached to the mass. The surrounding pancreatic tissue, of whoch there was only a small amount remaining, appeared normal. A small portion of undilated, main pancreatic duct was seen. In section, the tumor was seen to be composed of a honeycombed mass of thin-walled cysts containing clear, watery fluid. Their size varied from 1 to 10 mm. in diameter.

The histologic sections (Fig. 4) showed the cysts to be lined by low cuboidal, uniform epithelial cells. In many areas, the lining wall became piled up, forming multiple papillary festoons. The pancreas surrounding the lesion appeared intact, with perhaps some increase in fibrous connective tissue around the larger ducts. A few islands of Langerhans were seen. The pancreatic lesion appeared to be more like a benign neoplasm than a congenital or a malignant disease. Diagnosis was papillary cystadenoma of pancreas.

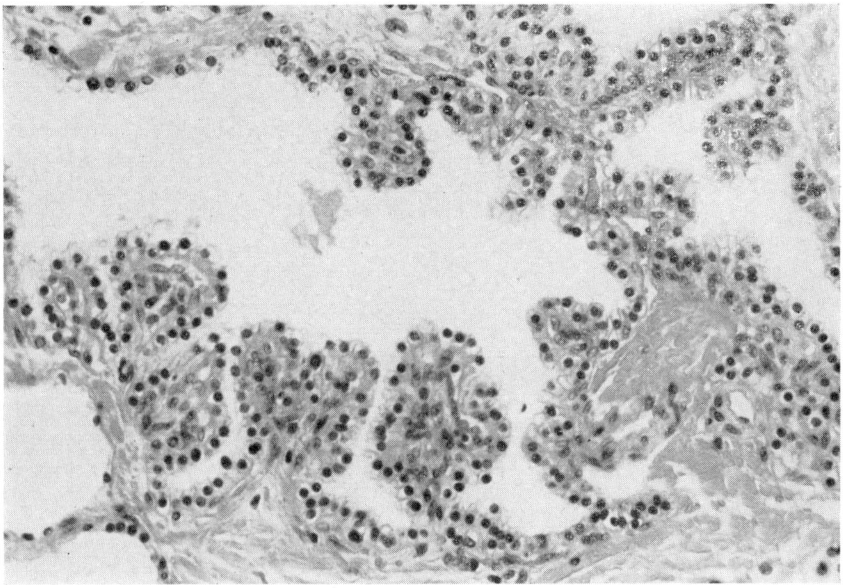

Fig. 4.—Photomicrograph, lesion of Case 1, F. W. (×200, reduced ⅓.)

During the first ten months following operation, on seven or eight occasions the patient had shaking chills, drenching sweats, nausea, and vomiting lasting four to six hours. Thereafter, she had jaundice and pruritis lasting approximately one week. It was apparent that she had intermittent hepatocholangitis. During this time she also frequently had indigestion, which she feels was partly the result of ''nerves.'' During the last twenty-four months (of the thirty-four month period of postoperative observation), she had no recurrence of the jaundice, pruritis, or the other symptoms of which she had previously complained. She had gained eighteen pounds in weight. Her only complaints when last observed were excessive belching and the passage of excessive amounts of flatus.

Case 2.—The patient, S. Z., was a 40-year-old white woman, who was first admitted to the hospital Dec. 4, 1942. She gave a history of a more or less constant burning pain along the left costal margin and precordium. This pain was not related to food or exercise. The pain had been present for varying periods for the previous four years. More recently, pain tended to radiate to the right thigh and upper third of leg. One month before admission, a mass was discovered in the left upper quadrant by her family physician, who referred her to the hospital. The findings of note on this admission consisted of a firm, nontender, readily palpable mass in the left upper quadrant. The mass was freely movable and descended with respiration. Laboratory studies were essentially negative, except for a moderate anemia. X-ray examinations revealed an extrinsic mass displacing the stomach to the right and anteriorly, and displacing the kidney downward. The patient was transferred to the surgical ward and operated upon (by J. E. R. and H. A. Z.) on Jan. 12, 1943. The gastrocolic omentum was divided to gain access to a large retroperitoneal cyst which was seen to arise from the tail of the pancreas. During efforts to remove the most posterior portion of the cyst, however, the cyst ruptured, and attempts to free this lowermost portion were unsuccessful. The cyst contents were therefore aspirated, and the free portions of the cyst were excised. A cigarette drain and a rubber tube drain were sewn into the remaining adherent portion of the cyst wall and exteriorized through a left stab wound. The cyst measured 11 cm. in diameter and its external surface was smooth. The internal surface was slimy, with numerous small areas of hemorrhage. There were several low ridges in the lining of the cavity and numerous bulbous papillary projections, which were soft, thin-walled, and cystic. Secondary cysts contained clear, mucoid material. Microscopic examination showed the cyst wall to be composed of a dense, fibrous, partly hyalinized connective tissue. The cyst wall was lined with an interrupted layer of tall columnar epithelium thrown into numerous folds (Fig. 5). Similar cells lined the papillary masses and secondary cysts. Occasionally these cells showed nucleoli compressed into a crescent in the base of the cell. In some, the cell surfaces were ruptured with the cytoplasmic contents bursting into the lumen of the cyst. Similarly lined acini were also present beneath the surface epithelium. The pathologic diagnosis made at this time was cystadenoma of the pancreas.

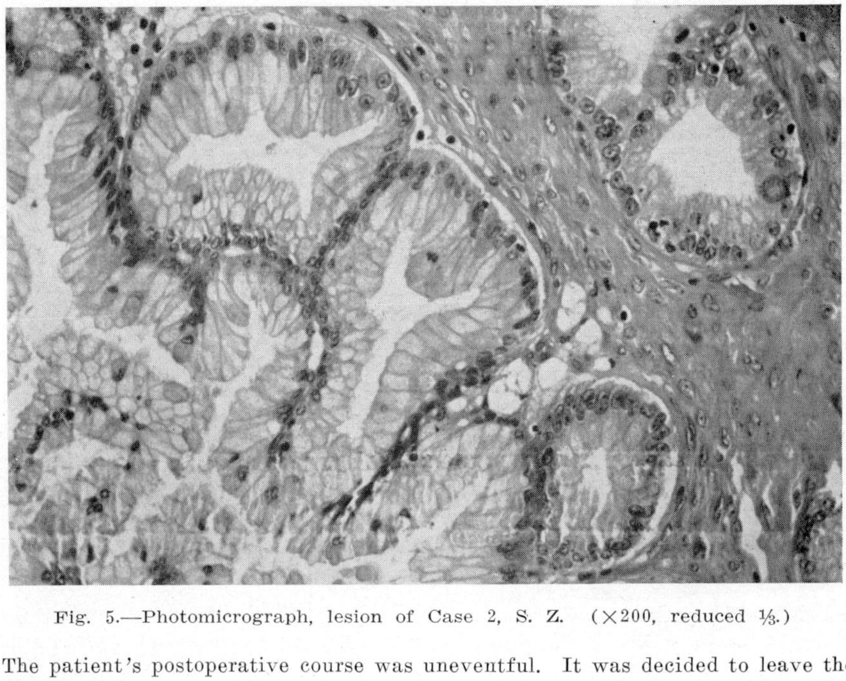

Fig. 5.—Photomicrograph, lesion of Case 2, S. Z. (×200, reduced ⅓.)

The patient's postoperative course was uneventful. It was decided to leave the rubber drain in place for an indefinite period. The patient was discharged on the nineteenth postoperative day. She was readmitted in the eleventh postoperative month for study and possible removal of the drain. X-ray studies at this time showed no connection of the fistulous tract to any viscus, and were otherwise negative except for slight displacement of a portion of jejunum to the right. The possibility of a recurrent pancreatic cyst was considered to explain this finding, but thought not likely. The drain was removed and the patient discharged, following which procedure the sinus closed. The patient was readmitted to the hospital five years later. She had noticed tarry stools several weeks previously. Examination at this time again revealed a smooth firm mass, which was movable and palpable on deep inspiration, present in the left upper quadrant. Gastroscopy revealed deformity of the posterior wall of the stomach interpreted as probably due to extrinsic pressure. Laboratory studies revealed a strongly positive benzidine test for blood in the stool. Other laboratory studies were essentially negative. A second operation was performed Aug. 14, 1948 (by J. E. R.). At this time, a firm but cystic mass was present on the posterior wall of the greater curvature of the stomach. It was smooth and freely movable. Due to close adherence of the cyst wall to the surrounding structures, it was not possible to remove the cyst completely, and therefore the cyst was again marsupialized. The postoperative course was uneventful. Since the second operation the patient has been well and continues to gain weight. Ten and one-half years after the original operation she continues to have small amounts of discharge through the rubber drainage tube, which has been kept in place.

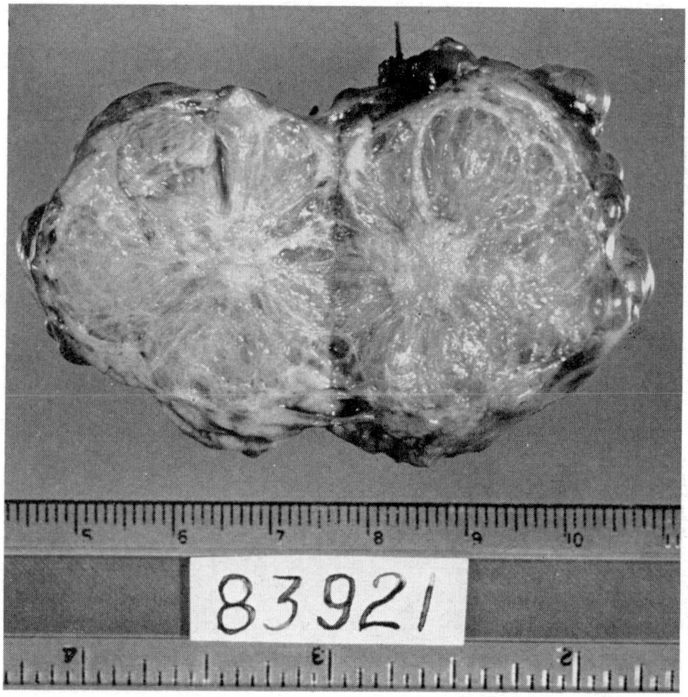

Fig. 6.—Gross appearance of sectioned lesion, Case 3, E. C.

CASE 3.—The patient, E. C., was a 42-year-old white woman who was admitted on Dec. 4, 1950, to the Hospital of the University of Pennsylvania on the Gynecologic Service of Dr. Franklin Payne. The patient's chief complaint was of metrorrhagia and dysmenorrhea. Her family physician had palpated a right adnexal mass.

The family history and past medical history were not contributory. Systemic review was negative with the exception of a mild upper respiratory infection one month previously. Physical examination revealed a somewhat tender, orange-sized mass just to the right of the umbilicus. This did not descend with respiration.

After a dilation and curettage of the uterus and cervical biopsy, the abdomen was opened through a subumbilical, midline incision. On exploration of the abdomen, an encapsulated, spherical mass 3.5 cm. by 3 cm. was found arising from the head of the pancreas. The external surface of the mass was studied with clear cysts about 6 mm. in diameter. A frozen section was performed by Dr. Robert C. Horn. He made the diagnosis of a papillary cystadenoma of the pancreas. One of us (J. E. R.) excised the mass in toto with a surrounding cuff of normal pancreatic tissue. The gross cut specimen is shown in Fig 6. There was no evidence of spread of the tumor. A Penrose drain was placed in the bed of the pancreas and the wound closed. The drain was removed on the seventh postoperative day. The postoperative course was uneventful except for persistent clear discharge from the sinus tract remaining after removal of the drain. Grossly the tumor was well encapsulated. On section it was seen to be composed of myriads of small cysts separated by thin septa. Centrally there was a firm granular core of pale tissue 1 cm. in diameter resembling the center of an orange. Microscopic examination of the tumor confirmed the diagnosis of cystadenoma of the pancreas (Fig. 7). The lesion was composed of cystic spaces of irregular shape, which were lined by a layer of epithelial cells. These were for the most part cuboidal, but in numerous areas columnar and much vacuolated. Between the cysts were coarse septa of connective tissue. At the periphery, the lesion seemed to merge with pancreatic parenchyma. The surrounding pancreatic ducts were distended. The patient was discharged from the hospital on the eighteenth postoperative day. The drainage gradually diminished. When seen three months postoperatively, the patient was asymptomatic. The wound was completely healed. She has been symptom-free for the two and one-half years since operation.

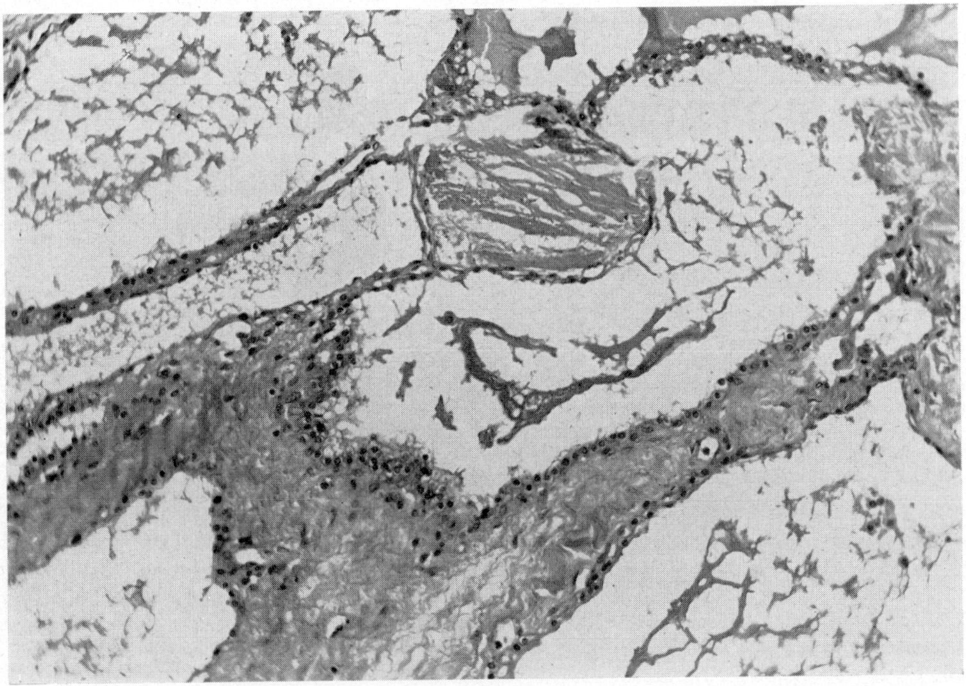

Fig. 7.—Photomicrograph, lesion of Case 3, E. C. (×200, reduced ¼.)

CASE 4.—D. D., a 47-year-old Negro woman, had chief complaints of pain and swelling beneath the left breast of six months' duration. She described the pain as being episodic and sharp in the right upper quadrant of the abdomen and with radiation toward the left axillary area. She had had "excessive" gas, flatulence, and vague abdominal discomfort for nearly one year. On physical examination a large hard mass was palpable in the left upper quadrant. It extended 7 cm. below the costal margin and from the midline to the anterior axillary line. She had a hemoglobin level of 66 per cent and a lymphocytosis of 49 per cent. A gastrointestinal x-ray film showed the stomach to be displaced anteriorly and to the right by a soft tissue mass. The urogram showed the left kidney to be distorted, presumably by a kidney tumor. At laparotomy, March 10, 1949, a cystadenoma measuring 14 by 10 by 4 cm. was excised from the body of the pancreas. The tumor was a multiloculated cyst containing a watery mucinous fluid. On histologic examination a great deal of fibrosis and necrosis was evident. Ducts lined by cuboidal epithelium and groups of islet cells were seen. A few glandlike structures lined by columnar epithelium were present. Epithelium and cuboidal and columnar types lined the cystic spaces, which contained much debris. The epithelial nuclei were regular. There was no evidence of invasion of the stroma. The histologic diagnosis was cystadenoma of pancreas and hematoma of pancreas. The patient was entirely free of symptoms after operation and at the time of her last follow-up visit three years after operation.

DISCUSSION

Although it has been suggested that those lesions which show papillary projections on histologic section be regarded as malignant, the more common practice has been to consider such lesions benign, in the absence of direct evidence of malignancy.[2] The fact that three of the patients here reported had the papillary type of cystadenoma and have been followed for from two and one-half to ten and one-half years without evidence of metastasis would tend to justify the opinion that a diagnosis of malignancy is not justified on the basis of the finding of papillary projections. None of the patients reported here had evidences of jaundice or diabetes. It would appear that the most satisfactory type of treatment of benign cystadenoma of the pancreas is complete surgical extirpation whenever this can be safely accomplished. It is recognized that the patient reported in Case 1 might develop ulceration of the jejunum because the gastric juices are unneutralized in the first portion of the jejunum. Ordinarily we would prefer to have the common bile duct and pancreatic anastomoses proximal to the gastroenterostomy.

SUMMARY

Fifty-three cases of definite benign cystadenoma of the pancreas have previously been reported in the literature. The most common symptoms associated with this lesion, as described by Mozan, are given. The case reports of four female patients with benign cystadenoma of the pancreas treated by surgery are recorded. These patients are alive and well two and one-half to ten and one-half years after the operation. Photographs of the gross and histologic findings are included. Evidence is presented to support the view that histologic papillary projections alone do not indicate malignancy in cystadenoma of the pancreas.

ADDENDUM

Since this article was submitted for publication, the patient reported in Case 1 had several additional episodes of hepatocholangitis. At operation on Jan. 30, 1953, a stricture at the site of the previous choledochojejunostomy was found and repaired. A cholecystojejunostomy was also performed. Exploration of the abdomen revealed no evidence of recurrence of the cystadenoma. During the same hospital admission, a left radical mastectomy was performed for carcinoma of the breast. The patient was well when seen on Feb. 2, 1954.

REFERENCES

1. Mozan, A. A.: Cystadenoma of Pancreas, Am. J. Surg. **81**: 204, 1951.
2. Sawyer, K. C., Spencer, J. R., and Lubchenco, A. E.: Proliferative Cysts of the Pancreas, Ann. Surg. **135**: 549, 1952.
3. Tagariello, P.: L'Adenoma cistico del pancreas, Arch. ital. mal. app. diger. **17**: 325, 1951.
4. Haukohl, R. S., and Melamed, A.: Cystadenoma of Pancreas; Report of 2 Cases Showing Calcification Am. J. Roentgenol. **63**: 234, 1950.

Case Reports

RECURRING MYXOMATOUS CUTANEOUS CYST

Norman H. Isaacson, M.D.,* and Dennis McCarty, M.D.,** Washington, D.C.

(From the Department of Surgery, George Washington University Medical School)

Myxomatous cutaneous cysts or so-called "synovial lesions of the skin" were originally described by Jones and Markins[2] in 1880. Succeeding cases, although usually presented to dermatologic societies, have received scant attention in the medical literature. Only some thirty cases have been reported. The scarcity of adequate description of this condition, together with the fact that these peculiar cysts are usually extirpated by surgeons who have the embarrassment of seeing them recur repeatedly, has prompted the following report.

CASE REPORT

A. P., a 44-year-old white woman, first noted a growth on the dorsoulnar side of the right middle finger, at the level of the distal interphalangeal joint in July, 1951. (See Fig. 1.) No history of trauma preceded the tumor, which gradually attained the size of a "pea." Thinking it to be a blister, she "pricked" it open several times, each time discharging a small amount of syrupy clear fluid, and each time developing a prompt recurrence in one to two weeks' time. In November, 1951, the lesion was surgically drained and again recurred in four weeks' time. Complete excision of the lesion in January, 1952, was followed by a recurrence six weeks later. The lesion, at first asymptomatic, became somewhat tender to touch after excision, although it never showed any signs of inflammation. Pressure failed to collapse the lesion, although the wearing of a tight bandage around it seemed to prevent its continued growth, according to the patient. X-ray films of the finger showed no connection to the underlying bone or joint.

The patient was submitted to radiation therapy, receiving a total dose of 1,000 r in three treatments on June 21, 1952, July 22, 1952, and Aug. 21, 1952, respectively. Within four weeks following the last treatment, the cyst began to shrink and the skin overlying it became shriveled. By December, 1952, the cyst had completely disappeared and has not recurred to date. (See Fig. 2.)

The case presented is typical of those reported in the literature.[2-8] The patients are usually women (75 per cent) in their forties (average age, 48 years) with a history varying from a few months to a few years.

The cyst occurs on the dorsal surface of the fingers (one of Gross' cases occurred on a toe), usually in close proximity to and a little to the side of the distal interphalangeal joint. They vary from 5 to 12 mm. in greatest diameter, although usually are about the size of a pea. They are smoothly rounded, thin-walled structures and often can be transilluminated. The color is that of normal skin, although if the wall is thin it may have a bluish cast or a vesicular appearance. The surrounding skin is normal in appearance, unless altered by

Received for publication, April 23, 1953.

*Clinical instructor in surgery, George Washington University Medical School.
**Present address: Front Royal, Va.

superimposed secondary infection. Pressure does not reduce the size of the mass, for the cyst cavity does not communicate with a joint, bursa, or tendon sheath. Tenderness is usually mild or absent. The patients frequently state that they have pricked the cyst open on several occasions, believing it to be a vesicle. The fluid released is clear and colorless and has a syrupy consistency. In every instance, the individual was surprised to find that such drainage gave only temporary relief and was followed by recurrence in two to four weeks' time.

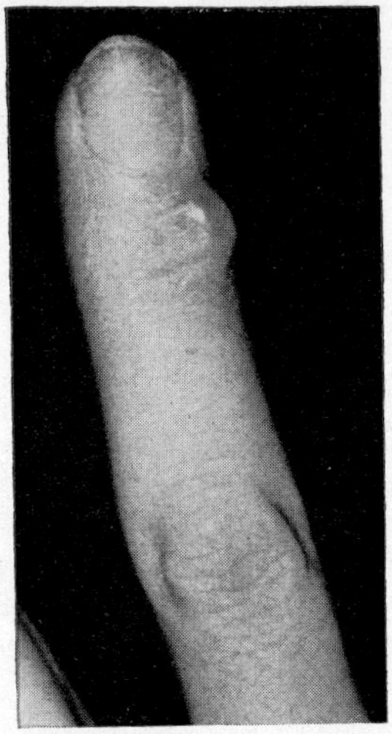

Fig. 1.—Myxomatous cutaneous cyst showing characteristic location and appearance.

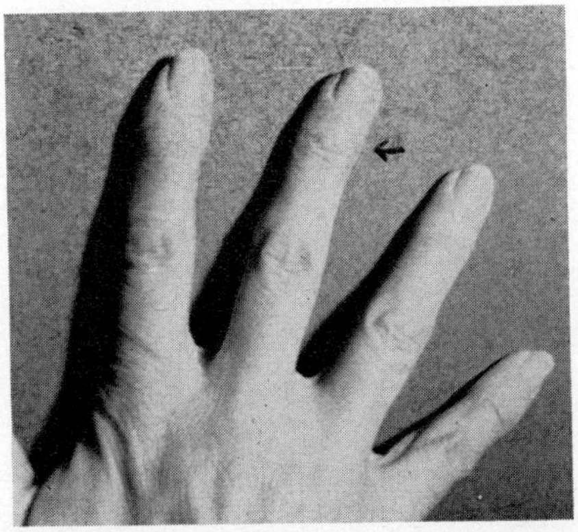

Fig. 2,—Same patient four months after x-ray therapy (1,000 r).

Pathologically the condition represents a localized degeneration in the corium. The connective tissue in this area undergoes a myxomatous change, the collagen gradually disappears, and a basic staining mucoid material collects between the remaining fibroblasts. As the process continues, liquefaction occurs in the central portion of this myxomatous tissue, resulting in a cavity filled with semifluid material. The cavity has no epithelial or endothelial lining, does not communicate with any subjacent structure, and shows no evidence of inflammatory change, nor is there appreciable pathology in surrounding blood vessels.

The etiology of this degenerative process has remained obscure. The various theories, which suggest that it is due to localized repeated trauma, vascular insufficiency, or degenerated connective tissue tumors, a variant of Heberden's nodes, or an outpocketing of a synovial membrane, remain unproved.

Electrocoagulation, fulguration, incision and drainage, curettage, chemical cauterization, freezing with carbon-dioxide snow, surgical excision, and amputation have all been tried alone or in combination in the treatment of myxomatous cutaneous cysts. Excluding amputation as an utterly needless procedure, recurrence was practically universal in two to three weeks following these forms of treatment. In several of the reported cases, recurrence occured as many as eight times.

By contrast, permanent disappearance of the cyst resulted when an adequate amount of radiation therapy was used. A cosmetically perfect result is obtained by this means, with no perceptible residuum or scarring. Jacox and Freedman[8] recommended a dose of 1,400 to 1,600 r (physical factors: 100 kv. constant potential, 4 Ma., 30 cm. focal skin distance, no added filtration, intensity, 120 r per minute, portal size as determined by the lesion), and in their series they saw no undesirable side effects and permanent regression of the cyst in four to six weeks.

SUMMARY AND CONCLUSIONS

A case is presented of an uncommon cutaneous condition, characterized by the formation of a small recurring myxomatous cyst of the skin of a finger or toe. The lesion is produced by a mucoid degeneration of the connective tissue of the corium, the cause of which is unknown. It is resistant to all surgical forms of therapy and recurs promptly when incised, excised, cauterized, or fulgurated. It responds best to radiation therapy, which usually effects a permanent cure.

REFERENCES

1. Hyde, J. N., and Montgomery, R. H.: Diseases of the Skin, ed. 1, Philadelphia and New York, 1897, Lea Brothers and Co., p. 444.
2. Lingenfelter, G. P.: A Case for Diagnosis, J. Cutan. Dis. incl. Syph. **31**. 647, 1913.
3. Ormsby, O. S.: Synovial Lesions of the Skin, J. Cutan. Dis. incl. Syph. **31**: 943, 1913.
4. Sutton, R. L.: Radium in the Treatment of Synovial Lesions of the Skin, J. A. M. A. **66**: 565, 1916.
5. Montgomery, D. W., and Culver, G. D.: The Pathologic Anatomy of Synovial Lesions of the Skin, Arch. Dermat & Syph. **5**: 329, 1932.
6. Savatard, L.: Peri-articular Fibroma of the Skin ("Synovial" Lesion of the Skin), Arch. Dermat. & Syph. **9**: 441, 1924.
7. Gross, R. E.: Recurring Myxomatous, Cutaneous Cysts of the Fingers and Toes, Surg., Gynec. & Obst. **65**: 289, 1937.
8. Jacox, H. W., and Freedman, L. J.: Roentgen Treatment of Myxomatous Cutaneous Cysts, Radiology **36**: 695, 1941.

TOTAL TRANSPLANT OF THYROID GLAND USING VASCULAR ANASTOMOSES

Report of Successful Result in Chronic Tetany

Julian A. Sterling, M.D., and Ralph Goldsmith, M.D., Philadelphia, Pa.

(From the Surgical Service of the Albert Einstein Medical Center [Northern Division])

PARATHYROID gland transplant was accomplished experimentally[1] in 1929 (Cattell). In 1934, Stone[2] and his colleagues used an isotransplantation technique of thyroid and parathyroid tissue in ten cases. Two of these were successful. These authors introduced the tissue culture method[3] of preparing the graft for transplant. However, others are not convinced that this technique[4] helps the viability of the graft. The "free" transplant has been most successful. A transplant to the left axilla was successful in the symptomatic relief of a patient for at least six months.[5] Another technique was used in dogs[6] whereby the parathyroid gland was fragmented and injected into the jugular vein, these emboli being deposited in the pulmonary tissue. This parathyroid tissue remained in the lung parenchyma.

The present consensus[7, 8] is that a small transplant obtained by flawless technique and transplanted to an avascular area not subject to excessive trauma is most likely to remain viable and active.

The human parathyroid gland up to the age of 10 years contains the "chief" cell, which is the active secreting cell. It is most desirable, then, to obtain parathyroid tissue from a child for transplant to a patient who has tetany. Since, in such young and tiny tissue, the parathyroid glands could be easily injured, it was thought preferable to obtain such tissue as a portion of the intact thyroid gland. It was thought further that the blood vessels between gland and host could be anastomosed.

Because of the good result achieved by this method of transplant, its use is reported in a case of chronic tetany.

CASE REPORT

E. M., a 28-year-old white woman, was admitted to the Northern Division of the Albert Einstein Medical Center on Nov. 21, 1952, for the purpose of transplanting freshly procured thyroid gland tissue. She was blood type AB, Rh positive. Past history dated for over ten years to a thyroidectomy. Following this, it was noted that she was suffering from bilateral recurrent laryngeal nerve palsy, severe hypothyroidism, and severe hypoparathyroidism. Tetany had been progressively continuous. By November, 1952, it was necessary for this patient to take daily from 30 to 80 c.c. of calcium gluconate intravenously in order to overcome tetany. An attempt to transplant parathyroid tissue using the tissue culture technique in 1949 was unsuccessful.

On Nov. 21, 1952, she had a serum calcium of 8.8 mg. per cent. There were positive Chvostek and Trousseau signs, and the patient was very miserable psychologically. Table I, which lists the blood chemistries, indicates that when not taking calcium this patient had

Received for publication, April 27, 1953.

a serum calcium level of 5.2 mg. per cent. While on calcium therapy, the calcium rose to 8.8 mg. per cent. Ionizable calcium was always measured at normal levels.

TABLE I. BLOOD CHEMISTRY STUDIES

DATE	TOTAL CALCIUM (MG. PER CENT)	PHOSPHORUS (MG. PER CENT)	TOTAL PROTEINS (GM. PER CENT)	CHOLESTEROL (MG. PER CENT)	REMARKS
December, 1947	5.2		5.7		Tetany
August, 1948	5.7	6.4	6.9		Tetany
February, 1950	7.8	4.5			Tetany
November, 1952	8.8		6.0	130	Tetany
Nov. 21, 1952					Operation
Nov. 24, 1952	15.6	3.4			Tetany
Nov. 28, 1952	10.1		5.0		Tetany
Dec. 8, 1952	9.2	4.2	6.6		No tetany
Dec. 11, 1952	9.7	3.6	7.2		No tetany
Feb. 18, 1953	9.4	4.0	6.4	278	No tetany

The pediatric department of the Albert Einstein Medical Center had been alerted to the possibility of transplant in this case. On the morning of Nov. 21, 1952, a 3-week-old boy died following sudden decompression of a myelomeningocele. Within one hour after death, the body was brought to the operating room. Under aseptic precautions, the entire thyroid gland including its vascular pedicles was removed (Fig. 1). The vascular pedicles consisted of the middle thyroid vein and its attachment to the external jugular vein on each side, plus the superior thyroid artery attached to the external carotid and its continuation as the common carotid artery bilaterally. The carotid arteries (approximate diameter was 5 mm.) and the jugular veins (approximate diameter was 4 mm.) bilaterally were secured against bleeding from their branches. Polyethylene tubing was inserted. The gland was bathed in and perfused with Darrow's solution containing 1 mg. of heparin per cubic centimeter. The gland was less than 2 cm. in diameter. Its weight was estimated at 1.5 Gm.

Within two hours, the patient for whom the gland was intended was brought to the operating room. A skin incision was made one-half inch above and parallel to the left Poupart's ligament and extending up approximately three inches from the pubis. The subcutaneous tissue was dissected to expose two large veins and an artery. The patient's veins were approximately 4 mm. in diameter and the artery approximately 3 mm. in diameter. It is probable that these vessels were the superficial external pudendal vein and the superficial external epigastric artery and vein. The superficial external epigastric vein was cut, thus presenting medial and lateral ends.

The left carotid artery of the transplant was joined by end-to-side anastomosis to the superficial pudendal vein, using interrupted through-and-through sutures of fine silk. The left jugular vein was joined by end-to-end anastomosis to the lateral segment of the superficial epigastric vein, using interrupted sutures of fine silk (Fig. 2). Immediately after completion of this portion of the anastomosis, the color of the transplanted gland changed from pale yellow to reddish purple. The right jugular vein was joined by end-to-end anastomosis to the medial segment of the superficial epigastric vein. The right carotid artery was anastomosed by end-to-end anastomosis to the available artery. Each anastomosis was inspected and leakage controlled by tiny pieces of Gelfoam. The artery-to-artery anastomosis was not completely satisfactory because of disparity in size and the partial obstruction to flow presented by the inversion of the wall of the larger vessel. However, blood did flow through it. The skin was closed with interrupted sutures of fine Dermalon.

The donor had died at 8:15 A.M.; operation for removal of transplant began at 9:15 A.M.; the procedure of vascular anastomosis and reimplantation was completed at 2:30 P.M.

Following the transplant, the patient's requirement for intravenous calcium remained almost unchanged for eight days. It was still necessary to use intravenous calcium gluconate

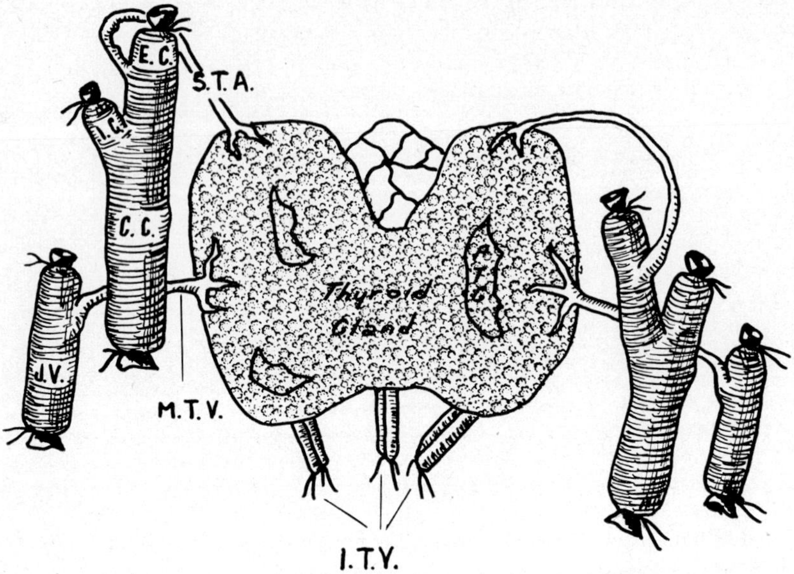

Fig. 1.—Drawing of thyroid gland and vascular pedicles removed from infant. *J.V.*, Jugular vein; *M.T.V.*, middle thyroid vein; *I.T.V.*, inferior thyroid veins and thyroid ima; *S.T.A.*, superior thyroid artery; *E.C.*, external carotid artery; *I.C.*, internal carotid artery; *C.C.*, common carotid artery.

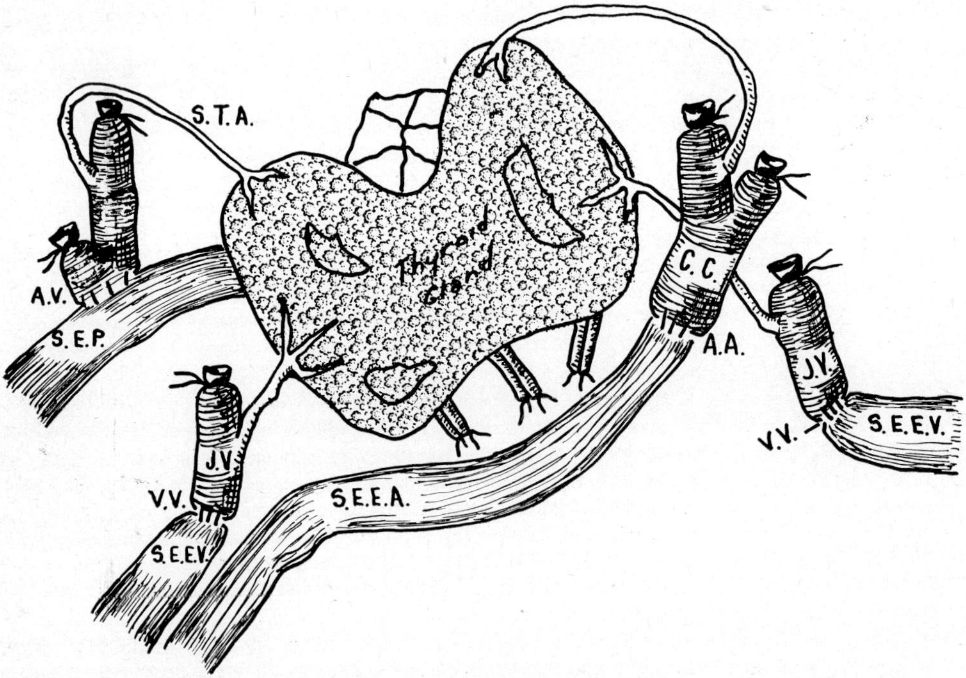

Fig. 2.—Drawing of anastomoses: vascular pedicles of gland and patient's vessels. *A.V.*, End-to-side anastomosis, comomn carotid artery to superficial external pudendal vein; *S.E.P.*, superficial external pudendal vein; *S.T.A.*, superior thyroid artery; *V.V.*, end-to-end anastomosis, internal jugular vein to superficial external epigastric vein; *J.V.*, jugular vein; *S.E.E.V.*, superficial external epigastric vein; *A.A.*, end-to-end anastomosis, common carotid artery to superficial external epigastric artery; *S.E.E.A.*, superficial external epigastric artery; *C.C.*, common carotid artery.

in doses of 20 to 40 c.c. once or twice daily. This was not readily understood. Finally, it was found that the patient's total blood protein had dropped from a level of 6.0 Gm. per cent four days prior to hospital admission to a level of 5.0 Gm. per cent. As soon as the blood protein level was brought to within normal limits by intravenous plasma and forced protein feedings, no further medication was needed. The patient had been taking small amounts of calcium and 2 c.c. of viosterol by mouth daily during the interval immediately postoperatively when she was still requiring calcium gluconate for relief of tetany. All medication was stopped on Dec. 11, 1952, except oral calcium, which was stopped on Jan. 6, 1953.*

Isotope (I^{131}) uptake was determined on the eighth postoperative day. It was found that the transplanted gland behaved as normal thyroid tissue (9 per cent uptake).

Since operation, the patient had normal menstrual periods, has had multiple teeth extractions, and has sustained other stresses with no ill effect. She has returned to normal activities. Previous signs of calcium deficiency have disappeared. The incision in the left groin healed; the site of the graft had been slightly indurated for one week, but there was no evidence that the tissue had become cystic, abscessed, or necrotic.

Re-evaluation was made Feb. 18, 1953. This was three months after operation, nearly eleven weeks after the last intravenous injection of calcium gluconate, and over one month after any medication whatsoever had been given. A.T. 10 and thyroid extract had been discontinued at operation in November, 1952.

There are complaints of coldness in the extremities, and the patient, when under emotional stress, notes occasional fleeting cramps in the calves and fingers. These subside spontaneously. She is able to complete her day's waitress duties. The only major complaints are backache and frequency, with occasional dysuria. It is felt that slight residual deformity from fracture of the thoracic spine (1948) and a chronic pyelonephritis are the causative factors. On occasion, the patient feels dyspneic and notes periodic ankle edema.

At present, temperature, pulse, respiration, and blood pressure are normal. Weight is 135 pounds (no change in three months). There is no edema, dyspnea, pallor, cyanosis, or tremor. Chvostek and Trousseau signs are not elicited. Skin and hair are of normal texture. The outlines of the transplanted gland are still palpable and the pulsations in the area are still present.

Complete blood count is normal. Blood calcium (9.4 mg.), phosphorus (4.0 mg.), and protein (6.2 Gm. per cent) are within normal limits (Table I). Pyuria is present. Sulkowitch test shows a faint trace of urinary calcium. Determination of radioactive iodine uptake now (6.2 per cent) reveals the presence of functioning thyroid tissue at the site of the transplant. Rate of basal metabolism on March 5, 1953, was reported at -9 per cent. The serum cholesterol is 280 mg. per cent.

DISCUSSION

Fortunately, in this case the patient's blood type is AB (Rh positive), thus permitting the transplant of tissue from a donor of any blood type. The transplantation in accordance with the method reported in this case is very tedious and exacting. Technically, it was possible to place only four or five sutures in end-on fashion to anastomose the vessels. These anastomoses were functioning when they were completed. It cannot be stated unequivocally that these are still patent. That the glandular tissue has functioned satisfactorily for three months can be inferred from the patient's clinical status and freedom from symptoms of hypothyroidism and hypoparathyroidism.

As indicated by Peer and Walker[10] in accordance with Roux's law, highly specialized tissue such as a secreting gland can continue to survive provided there is functional stimulation. Their study also demonstrated that cells can

*At the advice of Dr. Abraham Cantarow.[9]

stay alive for four days at body temperature if the grafts are merely humid. In addition, they demonstrated that the vascular system in free grafts tends to survive transplantation. They alluded to the skin, but it is felt that any effort made to assure the circulation of blood to new tissue will assist in the maintenance of viability for a longer time. As Cantarow[9] and others have indicated, only a few cells are needed in order to maintain the parathyroid function in the body.

It is understood that the follow-up interval since transplant is a short one. Nonetheless, there is sufficient evidence to indicate that the procedure was successful in that symptoms of hypothyroidism and hypoparathyroidism were relieved. The patient may be on the verge of myxedema at this time, since the cholesterol is high normal at 278 mg. per cent. It was never expected that the thyroid tissue would continue to function, so that the evidence, three months later, by tracer study that the transplanted tissue retained iodine was, indeed, surprising. Further observations on this patient will be forthcoming.*

SUMMARY

The case is reported of a 28-year-old woman who had suffered severe tetany of ten years' duration due to surgical trauma. This tetany was relieved by transplant of thyroid and parathyroid glands using vascular anastomoses. The gland was procured from an infant of 25 days.

In such critical glandular deficiencies as in the reported case, the utilization of very young thyroid and parathyroid tissue is efficient. It is suggested that the carotid and jugular vessels be anastomosed with the host's vessels to provide the gland with some nutrition until local circulation is adequate.

We express appreciation for their cooperation to the pediatrician (Dr. G. Elson) and to the parents of the child from whom the gland was obtained.

REFERENCES

1. Cattell, R. B.: Parathyroid Transplantation, Am. J. Surg. **7**: 4-8, 1929.
2. Stone, H. B., Owings, J. C., and Gay, G. O.: Transplantation of Living Grafts of Thyroid and Parathyroid, Lancet **1**: 625-626, 1934.
3. Stone, H. B., Owings, J. C., and Gay, G. O.: Living Grafts of Thyroid and Parathyroid, Surg., Gynec. & Obst. **60**: 390-393, 1935.
4. Pinkus, H. K., Maddock, W. G., and Color, F. A.: Clinical and Experimental Observations on Parathyroid Transplants, Tr. Am. A. Study Goiter pp. 65-70, 1937.
5. Houghton, B. C., Klassen, K. P., and Curtis, G. B.: Studies in Human Thyroid Gland Transplantation, Ohio State M. J. **35**: 505-508, 1939.
6. Reid, M. R., and Rausohoff, J.: Intravascular Thyroid Grafts, Am. J. M. Sc. **206**: 731-735, 1943.
7. Peycolin, R., Latarjet, M., and Guillet, E.: On the Treatment of Postoperative Tetany by a Parathyroid Graft, Lyon chir. **42**: 467-470, 1947.
8. Bland, W. H., Chesson, A. L., and Crow, J. B.: Parathyroid Gland Transplantation, North Carolina M. J. **11**: 501-504, 1950.
9. Cantarow, A.: Personal communication.
10. Peer, L. A., and Walker, J. C.: The Behavior of Human Tissue Grafts, Plast. & Reconstruct. Surg. **7**: 6-23, 73-84, 1951.

*The patient, fifteen months following transplantation, is well.

MUCOCELE OF INVERTED APPENDICEAL STUMP FOLLOWING APPENDECTOMY

Report of a Case

George C. Rasch, M.D., and Dempsey C. Strange, M.D., Indianapolis, Ind.

(From the Department of Surgery, Indianapolis Veterans Administration Hospital, and the Indiana University Medical Center)

ALTHOUGH mucoceles of the vermiform appendix have been described since early in the nineteenth century, we have been unable to find recorded in the literature a case of mucocele occurring in the wall of the cecum at the site of a ligated and inverted appendiceal stump. The following is a report of such a case.

CASE REPORT

The patient was a white man, aged 58 years, who was admitted to the Indianapolis Veterans Hospital in October, 1952, complaining of right lower abdominal pain present for almost four years following an appendectomy performed elsewhere. The pain was described as being a continuous dull ache, not related in any way to eating. The patient had had nausea and vomiting prior to the appendectomy, but not since that time. There had been no hematemesis, melena, or change in bowel habits, and he had lost no weight. Physical examination was negative except for deep tenderness in the right lower quadrant of the abdomen. No masses were palpable. Blood count was normal and urinalysis negative. A gastrointestinal series revealed no abnormality, and cholecystograms showed good visualization of the gall bladder. Films of the barium enema revealed a smooth deformity of the inferior medial border of the cecum with a suggestion of a pressure defect on the terminal ileum (Fig. 1).

Records obtained from the previous hospital admission indicated that the appendectomy had been performed as an interval procedure, with an operative diagnosis of an old perforated appendix. The operative note stated that the base of the appendix was ligated with chromic catgut and inverted into the cecum with several interrupted silk sutures. Films following a barium enema two months after the appendectomy had been interpreted as normal. The patient's abdominal pain began shortly after this barium enema.

Because of the persistence of pain and the constant finding of a cecal deformity following barium enema, an exploratory laparotomy was thought to be indicated. It was performed on Oct. 21 after preparation of the large bowel with neomycin. When the abdomen was opened through a transverse incision, a firm smooth mass was palpated in the cecum. There was no gross evidence of tumor extending through the cecal wall or involving structures adjacent to the bowel. Therefore, the cecum was opened and the mass found to be submucosal with no evidence of growth through the mucosa. The mucous membrane was incised, and grayish jellylike material was found within the tumor. Several silk sutures were noted on the external surface of the cecum, presumably at the site of inversion of the appendiceal stump. Resection of the cecum was necessary in order to remove the entire mass. The terminal ileum was transected and an end-to-side ileocolostomy performed. The patient was discharged after two weeks without symptoms and with normal bowel function. Films of a barium enema, prior to discharge, revealed only the deformity created by removal of the cecum.

Pathologic examination of the resected specimen showed the cecal wall to be markedly thickened with increase in the amount of connective and muscular tissue. Large amounts of

Reviewed by the Veterans Administration and published with the approval of the Medical Director. The statements and conclusions published by the authors are a result of their own studies and do not necessarily reflect the opinion of the Veterans Administration.

Received for publication, May 11, 1953.

mucous material, occurring in lakes of considerable size, were seen. Fibrosis and occasional groups of normal mucous-secreting cells were found. The nuclei of the mucous-secreting cells did not appear neoplastic. A mild lymphocytic inflammatory reaction was present. Chemical examination of the mucoid material indicated that it contained true mucin with a complex carbohydrate component. The diagnosis was mucocele of the cecum, postappendectomy.

DISCUSSION

There is some difference of opinion in the literature concerning the first description of a mucocele of the appendix. Some authors[2, 6, 7, 9] credited Virchow with the first report in 1863, while others[2, 10] stated that Rokitansky first described the condition in 1842. All agreed, however, that Fere in 1877 first applied the term mucocele to describe a dilation of the appendix containing mucous material.

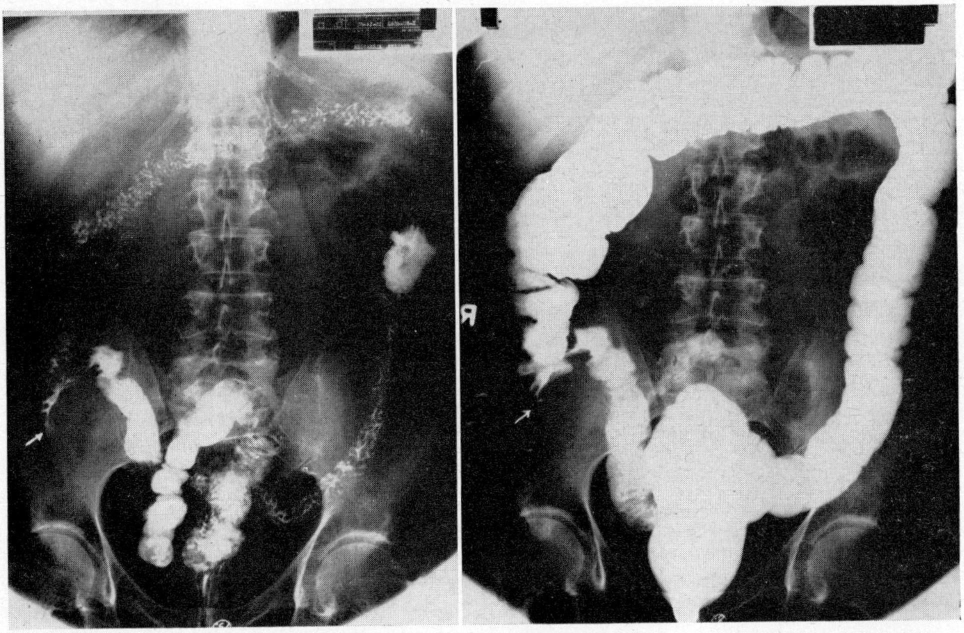

A. B.

Fig. 1.—Films of the barium enema showing smooth, constant deformity of the cecum.

Three conditions have been mentioned as necessary to produce a mucocele of the appendix. These include stenosis of the lumen of the appendix, continuous secretion of mucin, and an absence of virulent infection. Grodinsky and Rubnitz[7] found that mucoceles could be produced experimentally in rabbits by washing out the lumen of the appendix and completely ligating the organ. There is also some mention made of the importance of an intact blood supply to the appendix, at least in the production of experimental mucocele.[1]

Grossly, mucoceles vary greatly in size. They may be only several centimeters in length or may be as large as the 30 cm. specimen reported by Kelly.[12] Usually the dilated cyst contains a yellowish to gray colored jellylike material.

This contains pseudomucin and has also been known to contain true mucin.[2] Mucicarmine and safranine stains may demonstrate the presence of pseudomucin.[2] Certain chemical tests may demonstrate true mucin, as was possible in our case. Microscopic examination of a mucocele may show hyperplastic mucosa, although atrophy usually occurs as the cystic dilation increases. The involved wall may be replaced with fibrous tissue containing spaces filled with mucous material.[7]

The usual symptoms of an appendiceal mucocele are vague and not at all diagnostic.[3, 4, 6, 7, 9] Abdominal pain, usually in the right lower abdomen, and present for some time, is often noted. Occasionally, a mass may be palpated in the abdomen.[6, 9] Barium enema examinations may reveal a pressure defect in the cecum. Gastrointestinal symptoms, such as nausea, vomiting, change of bowel habits, and so forth, are usually absent.

The prognosis for mucocele of the appendix uncomplicated by pseudomyxoma peritonaei is excellent if the lesion is completely removed.[1, 3, 7] Bowel resection, as in this case, sometimes is necessary to assure complete removal.

Although the mucocele in our case occurred in the cecal wall at the site of an inverted appendiceal stump, rather than in the appendix itself, the symptomatology and pathologic findings were similar to those of mucocele of the appendix. The vague right lower abdominal pain and the pressure defect on barium enema were present, and constituted, in fact, the reasons for exploratory laparotomy. Other significant symptoms were absent. The history of previous appendectomy in our case made a correct preoperative diagnosis even more unlikely than in the usual case of mucocele. The pathologic picture of the removed specimen was similar to that described for mucocele of the appendix. The three factors previously mentioned as being necessary for the development of a mucocele also seem to have been present in this case. Yeager[13] has pointed out that the usual inversion of an appendiceal stump after ligation is not an inversion at all, but actually is simply the burying of the stump in a small blind pouch created by the inverting suture. A closed space is thus formed. If mucous-secreting cells should remain in the buried stump of the appendix, a mucocele might conceivably develop. Why such a condition occurs so rarely is unknown, although there are several possible explanations. The absence of blood supply to the crushed and tightly ligated stump may cause its intraluminal sloughing. Furthermore, if an absorbable material is used for ligation, its resorption may obviate the persistence of a blind pouch.

The possibility that our patient had originally a mucocele which was incompletely removed was considered unlikely, since the patient's hospital record indicated clearly that the appendix was small, the only abnormalities being adhesions and evidence of previous perforation.

SUMMARY

A case is reported of a mucocele present in an inverted and ligated appendiceal stump four years after appendectomy. The symptomatology and pathology of mucocele of the appendix is discussed briefly in relation to the reported case.

REFERENCES

1. Cianos, J. N., Garrison, A. S., and Stewart, G. A.: Mucocele of the Appendix, Bull. School Med. Univ. of Maryland **35**: 72, 1950.
2. Norment, W. B.: Tumors of the Appendix, Surg., Gynec. & Obst. **55**: 590, 1932.
3. Van Buskirk, W. C.: Mucocele of the Appendix, J. Missouri M. A. **47**: 613, 1950.
4. Phemister, D. B.: Pseudomucinous Cyst of the Appendix, J. A. M. A. **64**: 1834, 1915.
5. Ward-McQuaid, J. N.: A Case of Compound Intussusception of a Mucocele of the Appendix, Brit. J. Surg. **37**: 109, 1949.
6. Latimer, E. O.: Mucocele of the Appendix, Am. J. Surg. **47**: 125, 1940.
7. Grodinsky, M., and Rubnitz, A. S.: Mucocele of the Appendix and Pseudomyxoma Peritonei, Surg., Gynec. & Obst. **73**: 345, 1941.
8. Dodge, G. E.: Cystic Dilation of the Vermiform Appendix, Ann. Surg. **63**: 334, 1916.
9. Mayo, C., and Fauster, J. U.: Mucocele of the Appendix, Minnesota Med. **15**: 254, 1932.
10. Weaver, C. H.: Mucocele of Appendix With Pseudomucinous Degeneration, Am. J. Surg. **36**: 523, 1937.
11. Miller, D.: Mucocele and Myxoglobulosis of the Appendix, S. Clin. North America **27**: 337, 1947.
12. Kelly, J. A.: Cystic Dilatation of the Vermiform Appendix, Ann. Surg **49**: 524, 1909.
13. Yeager, G.: The Appendiceal Stump, Ann. Surg. **126**: 814, 1947.

ASCARIASIS OF THE COMMON BILE DUCT

Report of a Case Causing Symptoms After Cholecystectomy

Samuel Shore, M.D., Harvey N. Lippman, M.D., and Robert A. Weber, M.D.,
Los Angeles, Calif.

(From the Department of Surgery, University of California Medical Center at Los Angeles, and the Division of Surgery, Los Angeles County Harbor General Hospital, Torrance, Calif.)

ASCARIS lumbricoides, the common roundworm, is believed to be the most common parasite found in man.[4, 5, 8] Reports of instances of ascaris infestations of surgical significance are found infrequently in the literature. Complications associated with this disease include intestinal obstruction due to a bolus of entangled ascarides,[2, 7] acute pancreatitis due to obstruction of the duct of Wirsung,[4] bowel perforation, obstructive appendicitis,[7] cholelithiasis caused by a nidus of ascarides,[1] obstruction of the common bile duct,[4] ascending cholangiohepatitis, and multiple liver abscesses.[2, 3]

We wish to present a case of choledochal ascariasis which was characterized by symptoms of biliary tract disease. The symptoms occurred three years after cholecystectomy, and the cause of the complaint was not discovered until after surgical exploration and T-tube drainage of the common duct. The unusual nature of this case lies in the fact that the worm, undiscovered at operation, presented itself at the cutaneous opening of the T tube on the twelfth postoperative day. As far as we can determine, this is the first case demonstrating this peculiar sequence of events to be reported in the literature.

CASE REPORT

A 40-year-old, 220-pound white woman was first admitted to the Los Angeles County Harbor General Hospital in July, 1950, complaining of right upper abdominal pain of fourteen hours' duration. She presented a twenty-five year history of symptoms suggestive of gall bladder disease for which a cholecystectomy had been performed at another institution in 1947. Following this operation, the patient was purportedly asymptomatic until January, 1950. From this date and during the succeeding six months prior to admission, she suffered at least nine attacks characterized by pain in the right upper abdomen radiating to the right infrascapular area and accompanied by nausea and vomiting. These episodes lasted from twenty-four to forty-eight hours and were increasing in degree of severity and duration. Jaundice, biliuria, and acholic stools were not observed with these attacks. The past history and systemic review were not contributory except as indicated in the present illness. The patient was born and raised in Nebraska, and for the fourteen years prior to the first admission had resided in California. On admission, the patient's temperature was 101° F. The positive physical findings were limited to the abdomen. The patient was markedly obese. Healed right subcostal and right lower rectus incisions were noted. The right upper abdominal quadrant was tender on deep palpation, but no masses, guarding, or rigidity was present. The white blood cell count was 11,700 with 64 per cent neutrophils and 13 per cent nonsegmented forms. No eosinophils were seen on this examination. The serum amylase and urinary diastase were reported to be within normal limits. The urinalysis was not contributory. A flat film of the abdomen revealed no abnormality. The patient's symptoms

Received for publication, June 22, 1953.

subsided under conservative management, and she was discharged after thirteen days to be followed in the outpatient department.

The patient was admitted to the hospital for the second time on Aug. 24, 1950, with essentially the same complaints and findings, and was discharged thirteen days later after a similar course of treatment. The provisional diagnosis at this time was possible calculus of the common bile duct or mild relapsing pancreatitis. An upper gastrointestinal roentgenographic study performed in the outpatient department was noncontributory. A double-dose oral cholecystogram revealed no gall bladder shadow. One month later, the patient was admitted for the third time under similar circumstances and after four days was discharged on a low caloric diet in preparation for a proposed common duct exploration if the symptoms recurred.

We had no occasion to see her again until June, 1951, when she sought admission for right upper abdominal pain of three days' duration. The physical findings were essentially the same as noted on previous admissions. When the symptoms had subsided, she was subjected to abdominal exploration. No abnormalities other than a surgically absent gall bladder and numerous upper abdominal adhesions were noted. The common bile duct was normal in size and consistency, and on supraduodenal exploration a No. 8 Bakes dilator passed with ease through the papilla of Vater without revealing any obstruction. A No. 18 T tube was inserted into the common duct, and a cholangiogram was performed at the operating table. The films confirmed the clinical impression and disclosed a normal extra- and intrahepatic biliary tree.

The patient's subsequent course was uneventful until the twelfth postoperative day, at which time the apparent cause of the prolonged complaint, a roundworm (Ascaris lumbricoides), presented itself at the open cutaneous end of the T tube and was extracted by an attending physician. It measured 17.5 cm. in length. After a course of hexylresorcinol, the patient was discharged from the hospital with the T tube in place.

She was admitted for the fifth time on July 11, 1951, because of difficulty in maintaining adequate drainage from the T tube. Ascaris ova were identified in the biliary drainage, but were not found in the stools. A second course of hexylresorcinol was administered. One month after operation, a follow-up cholangiogram was found to be negative. The T tube was inadvertently removed by the patient on the sixty-second postoperative day. The fistula closed spontaneously, and the patient has remained asymptomatic to date. The stools have remained free of ascaris ova.

SUMMARY

A case of Ascaris lumbricoides infestation of the common bile duct which caused symptoms of biliary tract disease three years after cholecystectomy is reported. The diagnosis was consistently missed, even after surgical exploration of the common bile duct and operative cholangiography, until the worm presented itself at the open cutaneous end of the T tube on the twelfth postoperative day.

REFERENCES

1. Aviles, J.: Role of Ascariasis in Gall Bladder Disease, Surg., Gynec. & Obst. **27**: 459, 1918.
2. Bochus, H. D.: Gastroenterology, ed. 3, Philadelphia, 1947, W. B. Saunders Company, p. 272.
3. Crowell, B. C.: Dangers of Ascariasis, Am. J. M. Sc. **159**: 380, 1920.
4. Gallagher, W. J.: Ascaris Lumbricoides Causing Common Duct Obstruction, J. Missouri M. A. **27**: 170, 1930.
5. Morton, C. B.: Ascariasis of the Gall Bladder, Arch. Surg. **17**: 324, 1928.
6. Pribram, E. E.: Diseases of the Biliary Passages Caused by Ascarides, Deutsche med. Wchnschr. **45**: 655, 1919.
7. Wangensteen, O. H.: Intestinal Obstruction, Springfield, Ill., 1948, Charles C Thomas, Publisher, pp. 316-322.
8. Yang, S. C. H., and Laute, P. J.: Biliary Ascariasis, Report of 19 Cases, Ann. Surg. **123**: 299-303, (Feb.) 1946.

ADENOCARCINOMA OF THE ESOPHAGUS

Report of a Case of Glandular Metaplasia of the Esophageal Mucosa

John V. Thomas, M.D., and Lyle J. Hay, M.D., Minneapolis, Minn.

(From the Department of Surgery of the Veterans Administration Hospital)

We wish to report a case of adenocarcinoma occurring in the lower end of the esophagus, distinctly separated from the stomach by uninvolved esophagus, and originating from glandular epithelium which lined the esophagus from the esophagogastric junction to at least the level of the aortic arch.

True adenocarcinoma of the esophagus is rare, and the number of reported cases is in sharp contrast to the oft-quoted incidence of this lesion. Most observers conclude that adenocarcinoma in the esophagus represents an extension from a gastric carcinoma.[3, 4, 8] Ackerman and Regato[1] agreed with this concept and doubted that adenocarcinoma of the esophagus constitutes an entity. Hewlett,[7] writing in 1900, reported that he had collected from available literature six cases of adenocarcinoma of the esophagus, four located in the upper two-thirds, and two located just above but separate from the stomach.[7] Feldman[6] in 1939 reported an esophageal polyp at the level of the sternal notch which proved to be an adenocarcinoma. In the same year, Carrie[5] reported an adenocarcinoma of the upper half of the esophagus which he believed had originated from a patch or island of ectopic gastric epithelium. He believed that this was the second authentic esophageal adenocarcinoma to be found in the literature, and called attention to Feldman's report.

CASE REPORT

F. C., a 66-year-old white, single, male farmer, was first admitted to the Minneapolis Veterans Hospital on Feb. 24, 1953. He had enjoyed good health until four months before admission, when he experienced dysphagia to solid foods. The dysphagia progressed until he was able to swallow only liquids. One month before admission he sought relief from his physician. Roentgenologic and esophagoscopic examinations revealed an ulcer of the esophagus. The symptoms continued, and he was admitted to this hospital. A sixteen-pound weight loss had been noted. There was no family history of cancer. Physical examination was negative except for evidence of recent weight loss. Laboratory examinations were within normal limits. There was no anemia. Roentgenologic examination of the esophagus revealed a sharp filling defect in the lower third of the esophagus with normal esophagus between the lesion and the stomach (Fig. 1). The esophagoscopist noted no mucosal abnormalities above the level of the lesion. During this latter procedure, inadvertent perforation of the distal end of the esophagus occurred. The patient experienced immediate severe epigastric and substernal pain, and the procedure was terminated. The patient was taken to the operating room immediately. Transthoracic exploration of the distal esophagus revealed evidence of perforation and a mass 2 cm. in diameter involving the esophagus but not fixed to any adjoining structures. The lesion was discrete, and between its lower border and the esophagogastric junction there was 5 cm. of apparently normal esophagus. The stomach was normal. The esophagus was resected from 8 cm. proximal to the lesion to just below the cardiac orifice.

Received for publication, June 26, 1953.

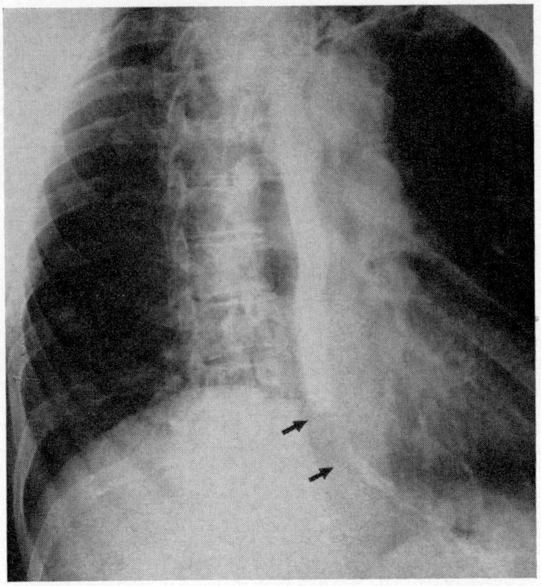

Fig. 1*A*.—Right anterior oblique roentgenogram after barium swallow illustrating sharp filling defect in lower esophagus with a normal esophageal mucosal pattern between the lesion and the gastric cardia.

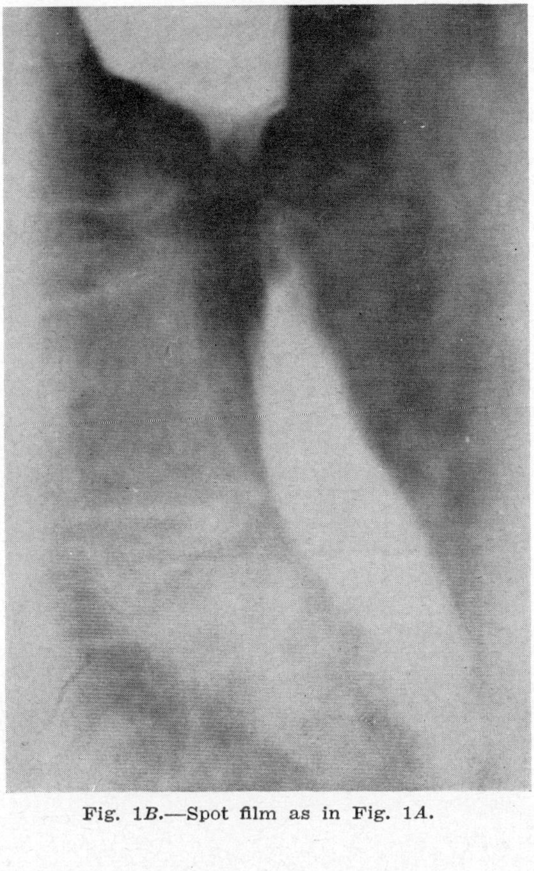

Fig. 1*B*.—Spot film as in Fig. 1*A*.

An anastomosis was made between the fundus of the stomach and the proximal esophagus just below the aortic arch. The patient's immediate postoperative course was uneventful.

Pathologist's Description of the Resected Specimen.—The resected specimen included the distal portion of the esophagus and a small portion of the cardiac end of the stomach, and measured 10 cm. in length. In the mid-portion of the resected esophagus, a hard mass 3 cm. in diameter was found. Approximately 3 cm. of uninvolved esophagus was measured both proximal and distal to the tumor. Except in the area of the tumor, the mucosa appeared normal to gross inspection.

A.

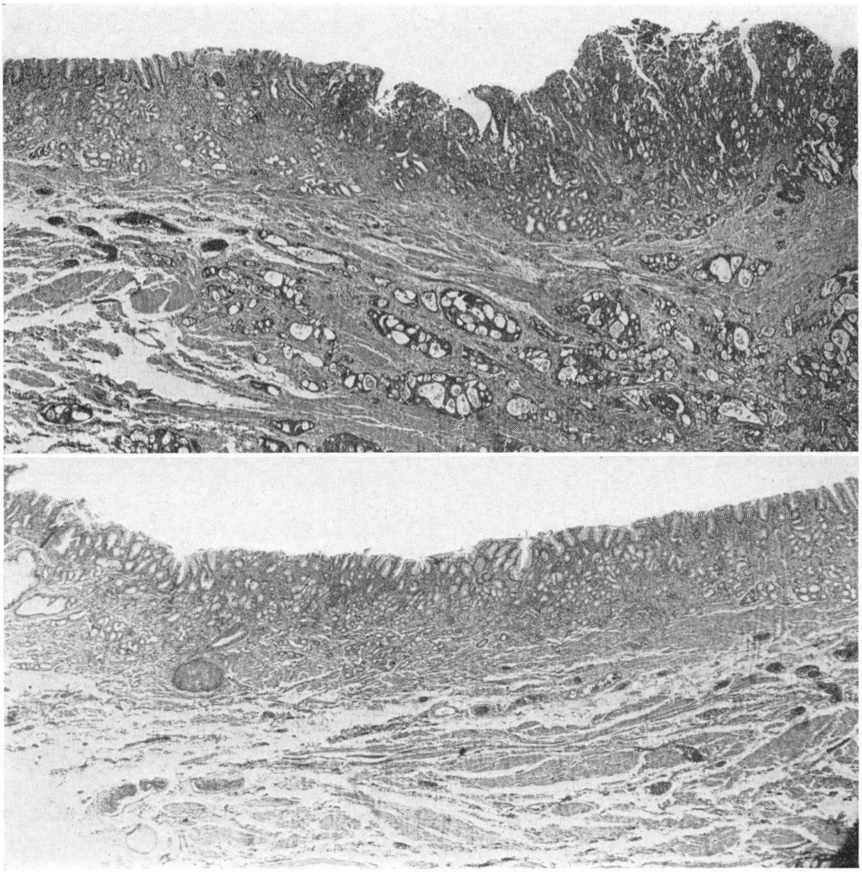

B.

Fig. 2.—*A*, Section through the distal edge of the tumor illustrating the well-differentiated adenocarcinoma infiltrating the muscular layers of the esophagus. On the left side is seen the benign glandular epithelium lining the esophagus distal to the lesion. (Photomicrograph, × 24; reduced ⅓.)

B, Section through the proximal end of the resected esophagus (just below the aortic arch). The esophagus is lined by columnar epithelium compatible with the gastric cardia. No squamous epithelium was found. (Photomicrograph × 24; reduced ⅓.)

Microscopic sections through the tumor revealed a well-differentiated adenocarcinoma which was invading the muscularis mucosae. Clumps of tumor were also seen in lymphatic channels (Fig. 2, *A*). The esophageal mucosa distal to the lesion was benign glandular epithelium with many goblet cells (Fig. 2, *A*). The proximal line of esophageal resection revealed columnar epithelium which was compatible with the mucosa of the gastric cardia

(Fig. 2, *B*). Additional sections were made to confirm the fact that the normal squamous epithelium had been replaced by this columnar type throughout the length of the resected esophageal segment. No parietal cells were found. An area of perforation was identified just proximal to the tumor.

COMMENTS

This case is of interest for at least two reasons. First, we believe it to be an authentic adenocarcinoma originating in the esophagus, which is not to be confused with the common lesions of this type originating in the gastric cardia and involving the esophagus by direct extension. Second, the presence of normal-appearing glandular epithelium rather than squamous epithelium throughout the specimen, both proximal and distal to the malignant lesion, has interesting embryologic and pathologic implications.

In the human embryo, the trachea separates from the esophagotracheal primordium at about the 4 mm. stage.[9] At this time, both trachea and esophagus are lined by ciliated columnar epithelium, but at about the eleventh week of development, squamous transformation of the esophagus begins, and usually all of the columnar cells have disappeared by the time of birth,[11] although occasionally a full-term infant will exhibit ciliated cells in the esophageal mucosa.[2] In addition to this normal embryologic transition of the esophageal mucosa, we must consider the normal histology of the adult esophagus, which reveals two types of glands. The esophageal glands proper begin to develop during the fourth intrauterine month, and in the adult are found unevenly distributed throughout the length of the esophagus. The glands consist of mucous cells and are located in the submucous layer. The esophageal cardiac glands[11] or Kardiadrüsen,[7] so named because they resemble the glands in the gastric cardia, lie superficial to the muscularis mucosa and are thus differentiated from the normal esophageal glands. These islands of gastric mucosa were first described by Schmidt in 1805.[12] When present, they are found most commonly in the upper portion of the esophagus between the level of the cricoid cartilage and the fifth tracheal ring, but are also frequently seen in a narrow zone just above the esophagogastric junction. Lubarsch[10] considered these areas to be identical to gastric mucous membrane and commented that he had not seen or read of a tumor of or related to these islands of gastric mucosa. Taylor[13] considered these aberrant patches of gastric mucosa in the esophagus to be a type of congenital heterotopia, and he emphasized the fact that all of the different epithelial cells lining the gut arise from the same layer of endoderm, and thus these areas represented a slight error in development. He described six patients who showed patches of gastric epithelium in the esophagus ranging from one-eighth to three-fourths inch in diameter, easily visible at autopsy. His patients varied in age from 7 to 74 years, and he concluded that heterotopic tissue once formed persists indefinitely.

Rector and Connerly[12] reasoned that these islets of gastric mucosa might represent nests of cells destined to form gastric glands. They made microscopic sections of the esophagus in 1,000 consecutive autopsies of infants and children ranging in age from prematurity to 14 years. In sixty-three cases, they observed gastric mucosa without parietal cells, and fifty-six of these areas were located in the upper two-third of the esophagus. Twenty-six patients showed patches of gastric mucosa with parietal cells, and none of these occurred in the distal one-third of the organ. Thus 7.8 per cent of their patients exhibited gastric mucosa in the esophagus, and they believed that a higher figure would have been the result if serial sections had been made. They suggested the role that might be played by these areas in the genesis of carcinoma, papilloma, and peptic ulcer.

CONCLUSION

Review of the literature revealed no case report of such extensive replacement of the normal esophageal mucosa by glandular epithelium as shown in the case reported. The relationship of the adenocarcinoma encountered here to the ectopic epithelium seems too obvious to be coincidental.

REFERENCES

1. Ackerman, L. V., and Regato, J. A.: Cancer—Diagnosis, Treatment and Prognosis, St. Louis, 1947, The C. V. Mosby Company.
2. Arey, L. B.: Developmental Anatomy, ed. 5, Philadelphia, 1947, W. B. Saunders Company.
3. Bell, E. T.: Textbook of Pathology, ed. 5, Philadelphia, 1944, Lea & Febiger.
4. Bockus, H. L.: Gastroenterology, vol. 1, Philadelphia, 1946, W. B. Saunders Company.
5. Carrie, A.: Adenocarcinoma of the Upper End of the Esophagus Arising From Ectopic Gastric Epithelium, Brit. J. Surg. **37**: 474, 1939-40.
6. Feldman, M.: Adenocarcinomatous Pedunculated Polyp of the Esophagus, Am. J. Digest. Dis. **6**: 453, 1939.
7. Hewlett, A. B.: The Superficial Glands of the Esophagus, J. Exper. Med. **5**: 319, 1900-01.
8. Jackson, C.: Carcinoma and Sarcoma of the Esophagus. A Plea for Early Diagnosis, Am. J. M. Sc. **169**: 625, 1925.
9. Jordan, H. E., and Kindred, J. E.: Textbook of Embryology, ed. 5, New York and London, 1948, D. Appleton-Century Company, Inc.
10. Henke, F., and Lubarsch, O.: Handbuch der speziellen pathologischen Anatomie und Histologie, vol. 4, Berlin, 1926, Julius Springer.
11. Maximov, A. A., and Bloom, W.: Textbook of Histology, Philadelphia, 1952, W. B. Saunders Company.
12. Rector, L. E., and Connerly, M. L.: Aberrant Mucosa in the Esophagus in Infants and Children, Arch. Path. **31**: 285, 1941.
13. Taylor, A. L.: The Epithelial Heterotopias of the Alimentary Tract, J. Path. & Bact. **30**: 415, 1927.

STRESS SYNDROME AND PERFORATED PEPTIC ULCER

Report of Two Cases

Alex W. Ulin, M.D., and John B. Cancelmo, M.D., Philadelphia, Pa.

(From the Department of Surgery, Hahnemann Medical College and Hospital)

INTRODUCTION

In his classic and prophetic article in 1932, Cushing[1] had marked the hypothalamic area of the brain as significant in the etiology of peptic ulcer. Over a decade later, Dragstedt[2] focused attention on the vagus nerve and the importance of the neural mechanism on gastric secretion. More recently, Seymour Gray and his associates[3] demonstrated the importance of stress and a humoral mechanism through the pituitary-adrenal axis. In 1951, they summarized case reports as well as the results of their own clinical investigation which proved the effect of corticotrophin (ACTH) as well as cortisone on gastric secretion. They were able to show that (1) this medication, in normal subjects, in doses of 100 to 160 mg. daily for a period of three to four weeks, increased the gastric acid secretion to the active duodenal ulcer level, and (2) in patients with peptic ulcer, the administration of 100 mg. of corticotrophin daily produced definite evidence of impending perforation.

It seems to us that the report of Gray heralds a new chapter in the experimental and clinical investigation of peptic ulcer. It may be that the total answer of the pathophysiology of peptic ulcer will come only when we have fully studied and correlated the knowledge of the humoral and neurogenic mechanisms in question. Porter and his associates[4] have made good progress in this direction in their recent work on monkeys. Their results show a true dual influence of the hypothalamus: the first originating in the anterior hypothalamus and being conducted through the vagus and blocked only by vagotomy, and the second originating in the posterior hypothalamus and being conducted humorally through the pituitary-adrenal axis and being blocked only by adrenalectomy. Consequently, we think it important to report two cases in which the stress syndrome caused perforation of a duodenal ulcer: (1) a 42-year-old man who had been on cortisone therapy for three months, and (2) a 6-year-old boy with fractures of the femur and humerus. Neither of these patients gave any previous history of ulcer or indigestion.

Case 1.—A 45-year-old white, male dye tester was admitted on Aug. 18, 1951, with a chief complaint of abdominal pain of nine hours' duration, sudden in onset, generalized, with nausea but no vomiting. For three months prior to admission he had been taking cortisone, 150 mg. daily, for arthritis of the hands and wrists. Blood pressure was 196/106, pulse 112, respirations 24, and temperature 99.4°. He appeared acutely ill, and positive findings were limited to the abdomen, which was distended, tympanitic, and rigid in the

Received for publication, July 27, 1953.

epigastrium. Liver dullness was present and peristalsis absent. A Levin tube was passed to the stomach for continuous suction. A survey film of the abdomen did not show any free air within the peritoneal cavity. Emergency laboratory studies showed a red blood count of 4,500,000 with 13.2 Gm. of hemoglobin, a white blood count of 11,350 with 76 per cent neutrophils, 23 per cent lymphocytes, and 2 per cent monocytes. A urinalysis was negative. Two hours after admission, celiotomy was performed and a perforated duodenal ulcer closed. The perforation was neatly punched out with little adnexal reaction. In spite of copious gastric content in the peritoneal cavity, the reaction was remarkable in that there was no purulent or fibrinous exudate. Progress during the first eight postoperative hours was poor. A pleural friction rub was heard in the right anterior chest in the fourth intercostal space; he was lethargic, toxic, and hypopyrexic. Circulating eosinophils were 462 per cubic millimeter. In addition to the daily intravenous intake, 20 mg. of ACTH was added to 1 L. of 5 per cent glucose in water, and infused over an eight-hour period.

First Postoperative Day.—Temperature was 99.6° (rectal). He was well oriented, and peristalsis was faintly audible. The circulating eosinophils were 380 per cubic millimeter, plasma chlorides 81 meq. per liter, carbon-dioxide combining power 50 volumes per cent, and blood urea nitrogen 11.4 mg. per cent. Twenty milligrams of ACTH was infused over an eight-hour period in addition to the fluids given for maintenance and correction of the lowered chloride value. During this period the patient became increasingly more alert and comfortable.

Second Postoperative Day.—Temperature was 99.2° (rectal). The patient was resting comfortably with very little pain. The circulating eosinophils were zero. The carbon-dioxide combining power was 48.5 volumes per cent, chlorides 88 meq. per liter, sodium 146 meq. per liter, and potassium 3.4 meq. per liter. An electrocardiogram showed no confirmatory evidence of the potassium deficiency. He was given 500 c.c. of whole blood, 1,000 c.c. of Ringer's lactate, and 500 c.c. of 1.14 per cent potassium chloride for this period.

Third Postoperative Day.—Temperature was 99.6° (rectal). Peristalsis was active; the patient was passing flatus. The Levin tube was removed, and the patient was started on liquid feedings. Laboratory studies were as follows: chlorides 100 meq. per liter and potassium 4.4 meq. per liter.

From this point, the patient's postoperative course progressed satisfactorily, being marred only by a febrile reaction which was due to atelectasis of a portion of the right lower lobe. The patient responded well to expectorants and Terramycin by mouth, and he was discharged on the twenty-first postoperative day on a strict ulcer regimen.

CASE 2.—A 6-year-old white boy was admitted Dec. 22, 1951, because of persistent vomiting of thirty-six hours' duration and epigastric pain. He had been discharged three days previously in a body cast including the left arm and left leg for fractures of the left humerus and femur suffered on Dec. 2, 1951, in an automobile accident. Temperature was 101° (rectal), and he exhibited abdominal rigidity with marked tenderness in the right upper and lower quadrants. Faint peristalsis was audible. A white blood count was 7,700 with 75 per cent neutrophils and 25 per cent lymphocytes, and a red blood count was 4,780,000 with 12.4 Gm. of hemoglobin. Two hours after admission, celiotomy was performed, and a perforated ulcer in the first portion of the duodenum was closed. Postoperatively he was treated with parenteral fluids, blood transfusions, and Wangensteen suction, and he made a good recovery. Hospital convalescence was complicated by pharyngitis and pylorospasm. Further orthopedic procedures delayed discharge until the twenty-fourth day following the abdominal surgery.

COMMENT

We feel that these two cases of perforated duodenal ulcer are probably related to the stress syndrome. In the first case, the prolonged administration of cortisone was a positive factor in this man's ulcer perforation. The fact that the response to ACTH was so dramatic and efficacious would seem to indicate that the adrenal gland had been made idle by the cortisone medication. Concerning the second patient, we believe that the perforation was due to stress associated with the accident.

SUMMARY

1. The stress syndrome and its relation to peptic ulcer have been discussed.

2. Two cases of perforated peptic ulcer, implicating a humoral etiology, have been presented.

REFERENCES

1. Cushing, H.: Peptic Ulcers and the Interbrain, Surg., Gynec. & Obst. **55**: 1, 1932.
2. Dragstedt, L. R., and Schafer, P. W.: Removal of the Vagus Innervation of the Stomach in Gastro-Duodenal Ulcer, SURGERY **17**: 742-749 (May) 1945.
3. Gray, S. J., Benson, J. A., Reifenstein, R. W., and Spiro, H. M.: Chronic Stress and Peptic Ulcer. I. Effect of Corticotropin (ACTH) and Cortisone on Gastric Secretion, J. A. M. A. **147**: 1529, 1951.
4. Porter, R. W., Movins, H. J., and French, J. D.: Hypothalamic Influences on Hydrochloric Acid Secretion of the Stomach, SURGERY **33**: 875-880 (June) 1953.

Editorial

Surgical Anesthesia

THE advances in surgical anesthesia in the last twenty-five years have been phenomenal. The number of anesthetics available, together with the number of supplementary ancillary drugs, gives the anesthetist a wide choice of anesthetics and enables him to carry the patient with a minimum of the anesthetic agent. This is highly desirable and has resulted in a remarkable decrease in our postoperative pulmonary complications.

In spite of this, there are still certain things left to be desired in the management of the surgical anesthetic. Frequently, in an effort to carry the patient "light," the anesthetist allows straining and struggling, which markedly handicaps the work of the surgeon. While it is extremely desirable to give the patient as little of the anesthetic agent as necessary, it is also desirable to have him "deep" enough to enable the surgeon to accomplish the mission which he has set out to accomplish.

A great many anesthetists feel that the patient should be almost awake at the end of the operation. This is fine, provided he does not go into an excitement stage and start struggling on the way back to his room. Patients should have a narcotic as soon as they start moving around during the period of awakening from the anesthesia. It is in this period that they are likely to do their suture line damage. They are still enough under the influence of the anesthetic to be oblivious to pain, and any struggling or jerky movements may break suture lines. If they have the narcotic early, they will sleep the anesthetic off instead of struggling it off. If at the end of the operation they are so light that it is felt they are not likely to stand the trip through long corridors back to their room without struggling, the narcotic should be given before they leave the operating room. If it is not given before they leave the operating room, floor nurses should be instructed to give the narcotic as soon as the patient starts moving or struggling.

It is generally agreed that too much narcosis following operation invites pulmonary complications. After the first dose, narcotics can as a rule be given sparingly. It is the first dose that is important in order to prevent unconscious struggling while the patient is under the influence of the anesthetic agent. By such struggling, abdominal suture lines are often broken and the postoperative hernia starts right then and there. Furthermore, it is probable that a great many inguinal hernias recur before the patient is out of the anesthetic, when injudicious struggling is allowed, thus breaking suture lines. Mattress sutures of heavy black silk in the abdominal fascia have been seen to break with a loud report before the wound was closed, when the patient was allowed to become light and struggle. One wonders how many times this occurs after the wound has been closed, when the surgeon cannot see what is going on.

At the close of abdominal operations with the patient very light, anesthetists often introduce a catheter to suck out the trachea. This frequently causes spasmodic struggling with its consequent bad effect on the abdominal suture line. At the conclusion of abdominal and hernia operations, the degree of anesthesia of the patient should be discussed by the surgeon and the anesthetist. It should be determined between them whether the best interest of the patient will be served by giving a little more of the anesthetic agent or of some ancillary drug in order to carry the patient back to his room, or whether a narcotic should be administered before he leaves the operating room.

It is obvious that the paramount objective of both the anesthetist and the surgeon is the welfare of the patient. This involves the patient's being kept light enough to maintain physiologic balance but deep enough to prevent interfering with the work of the surgeon.

—*Amos R. Koontz*

Recent Advances in Surgery

Conducted by Alfred Blalock, M.D.

BLOOD OXYGENATORS: THEORY AND STUDIES IN DESIGN

Nicholas S. Gimbel, M.D.,* and Joseph Engelberg, B.M.E., M.S.,**
Philadelphia, Pa.

(From the Harrison Department of Surgical Research, Schools of Medicine, University of Pennsylvania)

GENERAL CONSIDERATIONS OF BLOOD OXYGENATORS

The current interest in oxygenators stems from the need to divert the circulation from the heart so that intracardiac surgery may be accomplished under direct vision without hurry. This paper discusses the theoretical basis of artificial oxygenators, and presents the results obtained from tests of three particular oxygenators.

Modern Oxygenators.—Most mechanical oxygenators in current use operate by exposing thin films of blood to an atmosphere of oxygen. The *spinning disk oxygenator* of Crafoord described by Björk[1] consists of a series of rotating disks mounted on a common horizontal shaft. As the disks turn, they dip into a pool of blood, forming a film at the periphery of the disk. The film is changed with each revolution. The *spinning screen oxygenator* of Dennis and associates[2] consists of a series of rotating wire mesh disks also mounted on a common horizontal shaft. Blood is distributed onto each disk near its center, and is filmed over the whole surface of the disk by gravity and centrifugal action. In the *stationary screen oxygenator* of Miller and co-workers,[3] blood flows by gravity down a set of stationary, vertically oriented wire mesh screens. The *Stedman packing oxygenator* of Bailey[4] consists of a stack of horizontal perforated and embossed wire mesh plates. The blood flows downward through the stack while oxygen is passed upward. In the *Archimedes' spiral oxygenator* of Joengbloed,[5] the blood is filmed on the inside surface of a tube which is wound into a helix. The blood film is propelled forward through the tube when the helix is rotated about its axis.

These oxygenators disperse blood in oxygen. Other oxygenators, however, disperse oxygen in the blood. In the *small bubble oxygenator* of Clark and associates,[6] minute oxygen bubbles are introduced into the blood. The blood and residual bubbles are then passed through a chamber filled with Antifoam†-coated polyethylene shreds. Here the small bubbles coalesce, and a separation

Supported in part by funds made available for applications of engineering to medicine by Mr. John Ware.

Received for publication July 27, 1953.

*Present address: Wayne University, College of Medicine, Detroit, Mich.

**Present address: Benjamin Franklin Institute, Philadelphia, Pa.

†Compound XC-110, Dow-Corning Corporation, Midland, Mich.

of the blood from the residual gas is effected. Lary[7] uses even smaller bubbles, but manages to dispense with defoaming facilities by avoiding an oxygen surplus. This apparatus is the purest of "oxygenators," since no carbon dioxide can be eliminated. Thomas'[8] *large bubble oxygenator* uses bubbles large enough to separate from the blood by buoyancy. In the *foam oxygenators* of Waud[9] and Gimbel and Engelberg,[10] the blood is oxygenated as it cascades down a densely packed column of foam.

Physical and Chemical Aspects of Gas Exchange.—Oxygen is carried by the blood both as a solute and as oxyhemoglobin within the erythrocytes. The quantity of oxygen which is dissolved in the plasma is normally about one-fiftieth of that bound by the hemoglobin, and will at normal barometric pressures be neglected in considering the oxygen-carrying capacity of blood.

The combination of hemoglobin and oxygen may be represented by the equation

$$Hb + O_2 \rightleftharpoons HbO_2 + \text{Heat}.$$

From this equation it is apparent that a high oxygen tension and a low temperature favor the formation of HbO_2. This equilibrium is also influenced by the pH (Bohr effect). As the pH drops, the reaction moves toward the left. At an oxygen tension of 100 mm. Hg and normal pH, hemoglobin is approximately 97 per cent saturated.

The erythrocyte equilibrates with great rapidity with the oxygen tension of the adjacent plasma.[11] In the subsequent discussion it will therefore be assumed that the oxygen tension in the erythrocyte and in the plasma is the same.

The fundamental problem involved in the operation of blood oxygenators is the transfer of oxygen across a gas-blood interface. If blood and oxygen were exposed to one another without any turbulence within the liquid or gas, movement of the gas would depend solely on the kinetics of the individual gas molecules. This process is generally referred to as molecular diffusion. When the gas and liquid phases are subject to turbulence, the process is called eddy diffusion. Eddy diffusion, more rapid because distribution occurs through mixing, is the transfer mechanism of mechanical oxygenation. The situation is that of a gas phase and a liquid phase in contact at an interface, each of which has associated with it a certain degree of turbulence. The partial pressure of the oxygen in the gas phase is P_G and that in the liquid phase is P_L. If N_{O_2} equals the number of oxygen molecules which enter the plasma per unit time, then

$$N_{O_2} = K_{O_2}A\ (P_G - P_L)$$

where A is the area at the interface.

The factor K increases with turbulence and temperature.

Several observations may be made about the preceding equation:

1. *Turbulence:* In order to explain the variation of K with turbulence, two films—one consisting of stagnant gas, the other of stagnant liquid—are postulated at the interface.[12] The gas traverses these films by the relatively slow process of molecular diffusion, which is the rate-limiting factor

in the oxygenation process. The greater the turbulence in each phase, the thinner these films become, with a consequent increase in the diffusion rate across the interface. Certain phases offer more resistance to eddy diffusion than others. It is of particular importance to provide turbulence to the high resistance phase. In blood oxygenators, the resistance of the blood phase is large compared to that of the gas phase, a phenomenon which is said to be due to the low solubility of oxygen in plasma.[12] Producing turbulence in the blood results in a substantial increase in the speed of oxygenation, while turbulence in the gas phase has practically no effect.* In the *vertical cylinder oxygenator,* a several-fold increase in oxygenation is noted when wire mesh screens are used instead of smooth metal plates.[13] This may be attributed to the turbulence produced by the blood flowing down the uneven wire mesh surfaces.

2. *Temperature:* With increasing temperature, the factor K in the diffusion equation becomes larger, and this increases the rate of diffusion. On the other hand, at higher temperatures, oxyhemoglobin is more dissociated. This results in a greater value of P_L for any given saturation, with a consequent decrease in the rate of diffusion. In all perfusion systems, P_G is maintained at a value quite far above the value of P_L which is required for complete saturation. Under these conditions, the increase in K considerably outweighs the decrease in $P_G - P_L$, and the net result is an increase in the rate of oxygenation with increasing temperature.[1] However, since the oxygen requirements of the perfused subject also vary with his temperature, it is questionable whether the subject's oxygen debt is reduced by oxygenating the blood at, say, 37° C. instead of 30° C.

3. *Oxygen tensions:* The equation shows that the rate of diffusion is proportional to the difference in oxygen tensions between the gas and liquid phases. The value of P_G is directly proportional to the absolute pressure of the ventilating gas. Thus, operating the oxygenator above atmospheric pressure increases the rate of diffusion. If the blood becomes saturated with oxygen under these conditions, some of the dissolved gas may be expected to come out of solution when the blood is returned toward atmospheric pressure. Whether a limited amount of minute oxygen bubbles would be injurious is uncertain. On the other hand, operating the oxygenator below atmospheric pressure allows simplification of the extracorporeal circuit. Because in this case the oxygenator may draw its own blood, the pumps that carry the blood from the veins and from the coronary sinus of the opened heart may be dispensed with. The decrease in rate of oxygen diffusion is compensated by the reduced blood holdup resulting from the elimination of two pumps.

Carbon Dioxide Elimination.—It is desirable, although it does not appear to be essential in short-term perfusions, to maintain a constant pH in the blood by eliminating CO_2 at an appropriate rate. The equation which describes CO_2

*Since the pulmonary capillaries are approximately the same diameter as the erythrocytes, it is not unreasonable to suppose that the layer of stagnant plasma adjacent to the capillary wall is swept away as the erythrocyte squeezes through. From the previous considerations, this should make a material contribution to the gas exchange.

elimination is

$$N_{CO_2} = K_{CO_2}A\ (P'_L - P'_G)$$

where P′ represents the partial pressure of CO_2, and K_{CO_2} is the proportionality constant. From data for the diffusion of O_2 and CO_2 through water, K_{CO_2} is estimated to be approximately twenty-five times K_{O_2}. This explains why elimination of CO_2 may be readily achieved in spite of the fact that the diffusion gradient can never exceed the plasma CO_2 tension (normally 40 mm. Hg). In film oxygenators, CO_2 elimination usually surpasses formation unless P'_G is maintained between 1 per cent and 3 per cent in the ventilating gas. In the bubble and foam oxygenators, however, the gas flow may be limited by the capacity of the defoaming system, so that adequate CO_2 elimination may not be achieved. However, the debt in CO_2 elimination tends to be self-limiting because as the CO_2 tension mounts, the available gas can transport a larger quantity.

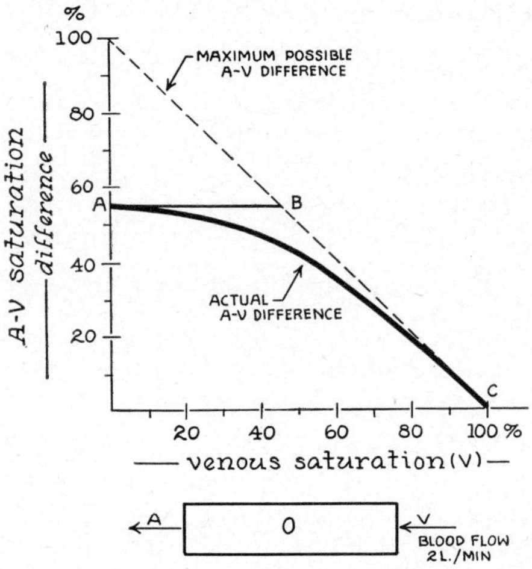

Fig. 1.—Saturation gain of a typical oxygenator as a function of the saturation of the venous blood.

Work Function.—Consider a typical oxygenator *O* (Fig. 1), through which blood is flowing at a constant rate. The performance of this oxygenator at varying venous saturations is shown by the heavy line, the *A-V difference* in per cent of saturation being plotted against the *venous saturation (V)* in per cent. The dotted line, representing 100 – V, indicates the maximum increase in saturation possible for any V. If the oxygenator were equally effective at all saturations, it might be anticipated that the path of performance for bloods of varying venous saturations would follow the line *ABC*. Thus, equal increments of oxygen would be added up to the point *B*, after which the arterial blood would always be saturated. The actual path of the oxygenator, however, described by the heavy line, is seen to lie below the anticipated performance. What is the explanation for this defection?

There are two reasons for dropping off oxygenation at higher saturations:

1. Since at higher saturations the average value of P_L in the diffusion equation is greater, there will be a decrease in the rate of diffusion. However, changes in P_L have little effect on the rate of oxygenation when P_G is of the order of 700 mm. Hg. With pure oxygen at atmospheric pressure, the loss in diffusion gradient as blood passes from 0 to 80 per cent saturation is 5 per cent. Hence, this does not explain the relatively large decline in oxygenation which is actually encountered.

2. The important factor arises because, unlike pulmonary capillaries, the films of present-day oxygenators are several erythrocytes thick. Only the plasma and erythrocytes actually at the gas-blood interface are immediately exposed to the oxygen; the deeper blood is relatively anoxic. Blood is at the interface for a certain time, T, characteristic of the particular apparatus, before turbulence remixes it with the subsurface blood. When T is longer than is required to saturate the film, exposure time will be wasted.

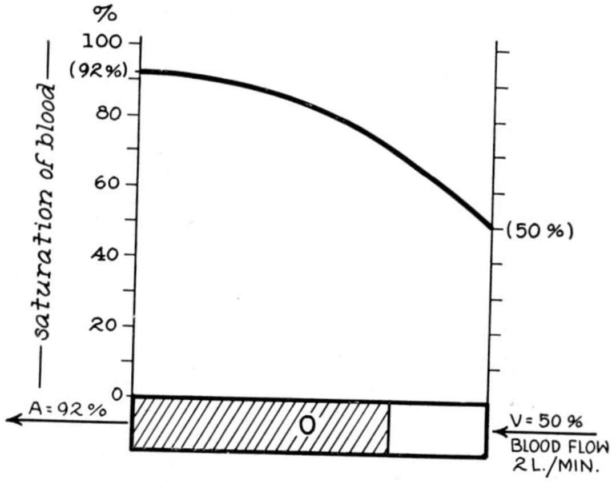

Fig. 2.—Saturation of blood as a function of distance through the oxygenator. In the region of the oxygenator indicated by shading, each film is exposed for a longer time than is necessary for it to absorb all the oxygen it can carry.

In Fig. 2 we show an oxygenator which at a flow of 2 L. per minute takes blood from a venous saturation of 50 per cent to an arterial saturation of 92 per cent. As the blood moves along the oxygenator, the saturation of the blood increases from 50 to 92 per cent. Hence, under steady-state conditions it should be possible to associate with every point along the oxygenator a particular saturation between 50 and 92 per cent. In Fig. 2 the saturation has been plotted as a function of the distance along the oxygenator. Consider the point in the oxygenator at which the saturation is 60 per cent. The film exposed at this point cannot increase more than 40 per cent in saturation. If the time T is such that the saturation of the film can increase only 30 per cent, then up to the point along the oxygenator where the average saturation becomes 70 per cent, each film will introduce an equal quantity of oxygen corresponding to a saturation difference of 30 per cent. Above 70 per cent, each film is exposed longer than is necessary for it to pick up the maximum amount of oxygen it can carry, and hence the oxygenation process becomes less efficient. Thus, the rate of oxygenation decreases at higher saturations because the film exposure time is progressively wasted as the capacity of the film to take oxygen falls. Karlson and associates[14] encountered the same phenomenon when they observed that, when oxygenating blood by filming it on the inside of a vertical revolving cylinder, the saturation at any given blood flow did not increase in proportion to the height of the cylinder. In one experiment, blood flowing at 200 ml. per minute into a certain cylinder rose in saturation from 68 to 86 per cent, an increment of 18 per cent. When the cylinder was doubled in length, the additional increment in saturation was only 7 per cent.

It becomes desirable to find a criterion by means of which it is possible to determine the relative difficulty or "work" involved for a given oxygenator in going from one level of saturation to another. Specifically, we are interested in a function W, which we may call the "work function," which will associate with every level of saturation a number in such a way that the relative difficulty for oxygenating blood from a saturation S_V to a saturation S_A, is proportional to the difference $W_A - W_V$ of the work functions for the two saturations.

Table I lists the work function for the spinning disk oxygenator. This was obtained as will be described in the section on this apparatus. As an example of the use of the work function let us consider the relative difficulty of oxygenating from 40 per cent to 70 per cent as compared to 65 per cent to 95 per cent. As shown in Table I, the difference in work function between 40 per cent to 70 per cent is 70.6 – 40.9, or 29.7, work function units (wfu). Similarly for the interval 65 to 95 per cent, the work done is 115.9 – 65.4 = 50.5 wfu. The relative difficulty of oxygenation in the two regions is $\frac{50.5}{29.7} = 1.7$.

TABLE I. WORK FUNCTION FOR SPINNING DISK AND STEDMAN PACKING OXYGENATOR (BEEF BLOOD AT 37° C., 95 PER CENT O_2, 5 PER CENT CO_2 AT 760 MM. HG)

SATURATION PER CENT	WORK FUNCTION (wfu)	SATURATION PER CENT	WORK FUNCTION (wfu)
15	22.4	76	77.3
20	25.6	78	79.8
25	29.0	80	82.3
30	32.8	81	84.0
35	36.7	82	85.2
40	40.9	83	86.8
42	42.6	84	88.0
44	44.3	85	90.0
46	46.1	86	91.7
48	48.0	87	93.4
50	50.0	88	95.5
52	52.1	89	97.4
54	54.3	90	100.0
56	56.3	91	102.1
58	58.2	92	105.7
60	60.3	93	108.6
62	62.3	94	111.7
64	64.3	95	115.9
66	66.4	97	124.5
68	68.3	99	135.9
70	70.6		
72	72.7		
74	74.8		

Suppose now that an experiment shows that the spinning disk oxygenator at a certain blood flow rate oxygenated the blood from 40 per cent to 70 per cent. The question might arise: What would have been the arterial saturation had the venous saturation been 65 per cent? We have seen that the work done in the 40 per cent to 70 per cent interval is 29.7 wfu. Hence, we are dealing with an oxygenator which is capable of an output of 29.7 wfu. The work function of 65 per cent is 65.4 wfu. To this we add the work done, 65.4 + 29.7 = 95.1 wfu, and thus obtain the work function of the arterial blood for this case. Table I shows the saturation corresponding to 95.1 wfu to be 88 per cent. This then would be the arterial saturation with an input of 65 per cent venous blood.

The familiar form for expressing the oxygenation accomplished by an apparatus is the volume of oxygen introduced per minute. The appropriate formula is:

$$\text{Flow (in 100 ml./min.)} \times \frac{(\text{final saturation in \%-initial saturation in \%})}{100}$$
$$\times \text{ oxygen capacity of the blood (in ml. } O_2\text{/100 ml. of blood)} = O_2 \text{ introduced (in ml./min.).}$$

It is apparent from this formula that there is an inverse relationship between the saturation increase and the oxygen capacity (hemoglobin concentration) of the blood; other conditions remaining the same, the more anemic the blood, the greater will be the saturation change. Since oxygenation is easier at lower saturations, as has been already discussed, oxygen introduced cannot provide a unique description of the oxygenating capacity at different saturation ranges. Work function units are, in effect, saturation units corrected to give a unique description of the oxygenator in question which is independent of the saturation range. Therefore, if the final and initial work functions are substituted for the final and initial saturations in the preceding formula, the resulting equation becomes independent of the saturation range:

Flow (in 100 ml./min.) × (final work function − initial work function) × oxygen-capacity of the blood (in ml. O_2/100 ml. blood) = work function introduced (in work function units).

Application of this formula makes possible the comparison of experiments performed with bloods of different hemoglobin concentrations or in different saturation ranges.

Example: An oxygenator will raise the saturation of blood of 20 volumes per 100 ml. oxygen capacity flowing at 3.0 L. per minute from 40 per cent to 70 per cent saturation. What final saturation might be anticipated for blood of 16 volumes per 100 ml. oxygen capacity flowing at the same rate and starting at a saturation of 60 per cent?

Steps: 1. Calculation is made of increase in work function units. The work function of the initial saturation is subtracted from that of the final saturation.

2. Work function units introduced are obtained by multiplying flow × increase in work function units × capacity.

3. Solve for unknown new wfu increase; add to wfu of new initial saturation; then convert sum to corresponding saturation.

a. 70 per cent saturation – work function 70.6 wfu
40 per cent saturation – work function 40.9 wfu
29.7 increase

in work function units.

b. 30 × 29.7 × 20 = 11,880.

c. 30 × X × 16 = 11,880.

d. X = 37.1 work function units.

Work function of 60 per cent = 60.3 wfu.

60.3 + 37.1 = 97.4 wfu.

Saturation analogue of 97.4 wfu is 89 per cent saturation. It is important to note that such calculations are based on assumptions that are only approximately true. It is assumed that the work function of the oxygenator is exactly known, and that the work function and the efficiency do not change within the range of hemoglobin concentrations encountered. Since these assumptions are not entirely correct, the calculations based on them can only be approximations. The question arises as to the applicability and usefulness of the work function described. Does it apply to different oxygen tensions and to different oxygenators? Since the function is obtained empirically, only experiments can define its applicability. Thus, it appears that the function used previously also describes the performance of the Stedman packing oxygenator. However, a different function is obtained with the foam oxygenator. Large variations in the gas oxygen tension also change the function. Experiments have shown the variations in performance at various blood flows to be too large to permit the comparison of experiments in which flow changes.

Practical Considerations of Mechanical Oxygenators.—The ideal oxygenator accomplishes its work while holding a relatively small amount of blood. It should be simple, safe, and reliable.

Holdup: The blood holdup of an oxygenator may be defined as the entire blood volume which is within the oxygenator during its operation. This includes blood volume which is in the oxygenator distributor, in the collecting pool, and in the defoaming chamber if present. In most oxygenators the holdup varies with the blood flow rate. In the case of the film oxygenators, this results from a thickening of the film, in the foam oxygenator, from a wider separation of the bubbles. It is inevitable that as the oxygenator gains blood, the subject loses it, and vice versa.

Miller and co-workers[3] have been able to overcome fluctuations in blood volume due to holdup by use of a recirculating pump which maintains a constant flow of blood through the oxygenator.

Comparative efficiency: Karlson and associates[14] introduced the concept of comparative efficiency as a criterion for the comparison of different oxygenators. The efficiency was defined as the ratio of the milliliters of oxygen introduced into 100 ml. of blood per milliliter of blood film holdup. To make this definition unique, several additional specifications should be made. First, since the efficiency of most oxygenators varies with the blood flow rate, this should be stated. Second, the holdup used in the definition should be the total holdup in the oxygenator, including the systems which distribute the venous blood and collect the arterial blood. Third, since the amount of oxygen introduced is influenced by the degree of venous saturation (the work function consideration), the venous saturation should be specified. In view of these considerations Karlson's definition might be modified to read: *The comparative efficiency of a blood oxygenator is the ratio: the largest flow of blood of 15 Gm. per cent hemoglobin which can be raised from 60 to 90 per cent saturation*/the total holdup at that flow rate.*

The comparative efficiencies of the oxygenators described in this paper are presented for purposes of comparison in the summary. These efficiencies are an index of the amount of oxygen which an oxygenator is capable of introducing into blood for a given amount of holdup. Since any oxygenator can be made to produce an arbitrary saturation change for an arbitrary blood flow, provided it is made large enough, it is clear that efficiency is simply an index of the relative holdup. To lay stress on a small holdup may appear unreasonable when one considers the use of these oxygenators for operations where cost and availability of donor blood do not play an important part. There are, however, a number of other considerations which give the question of holdup its importance. First, the more donor blood that has to be used, the graver the danger of transfusion reactions and serum hepatitis. Second, the greater the holdup, the greater the problem of homeostasis; a small fluctuation in holdup becomes a significant variation in the subject's blood volume. Third, in experimental surgery the obtaining of large quantities of donor blood becomes a time-consuming annoyance.

Film characteristics: In the stationary screen oxygenator and the Stedman packing oxygenator, the blood tends to course down in channels without wetting the surface evenly and making full use of the filming surface. Such oxygenators show an improved performance if the filming surfaces are completely flooded with saline solution prior to the admission of blood, and if the surfaces are kept wet with blood throughout the perfusion by means of a recirculating pump.

In the spinning disk oxygenator, on the other hand, good filming is obtained without special measures.

Blood trauma: Hemolysis, as an index of trauma to the blood, is not a problem with the oxygenators under discussion. All oxygenators decrease the platelet count of the circulating blood to some extent, but little comparative information is available.

Humidification and heating of the gas: Many heart-lung machines provide for the heating and the humidification of the oxygen prior to its entrance into the oxygenator. To decide whether it is desirable to incorporate accessories for this purpose, the following facts should be taken into consideration:

The saturation of 1 L. per minute of dry gas results in a loss of about 3 Gm. of water per hour from the blood. The heat of vaporization of 3 Gm.

*This saturation range, arbitrarily chosen, combines the virtues of clinical interest and experimental sensitivity.

of water represents a loss of 1.6 kilogram calories. If this gas must also be warmed from room temperature to 37° C., an additional 0.3 kilogram calorie per hour will be lost from the blood.

Warming and humidifying 1 L. of dry cool gas per minute therefore represents a loss of 1.9 kilogram calories per hour, or approximately 6 per cent of the heat production of a 20 kilogram subject.

EXPERIMENTAL STUDIES IN OXYGENATOR DESIGN

Experimental Techniques (General).—To achieve precision in the technique of evaluating oxygenators, in vitro tests with beef blood were carried out. This made it feasible to hold a steady state and to control the flow and saturation of blood entering the apparatus, and was of great value in obtaining data under controlled conditions.

Fifteen to thirty liters of beef blood were collected in one-fifth their volume of citrate-dextrose solution at an abattoir. The hemoglobin concentration of the citrated blood was between 9 and 12 Gm. per cent. In order to make the results immediately applicable to normal blood, the data presented were corrected by means of the work function to a hemoglobin concentration of 15 Gm. per cent. Penicillin was added to the blood. Experiments and analyses were completed within eight hours of the bleeding. The experiments were carried out in a constant temperature hood at 37° C.

To provide unsaturated blood for testing, the Stedman packing column, to be described subsequently, was employed. The blood was recirculated through the column, which was ventilated by either 5 per cent CO_2-95 per cent N_2, or by 100 per cent CO_2 followed by 100 per cent N_2. The 5 per cent CO_2–95 per cent N_2 mixture was preferred since the CO_2 tension was thereby maintained at 36 mm. Hg tension and variations in Bohr effect were avoided. Pure carbon dioxide followed by pure nitrogen to return the pH to the normal range proved the more rapid method, however. No precise method was available for producing any desired unsaturation for study; approximations could be achieved on the basis of experience.

Sufficient unsaturated blood was prepared so that conditions within the oxygenator would be in a steady state for at least three minutes before samples were taken. The oxygenator was ventilated with 95 per cent O_2–5 per cent CO_2 at a flow of 7 L. per minute, unless otherwise noted. Constant, reproducible blood flows were obtained by driving the blood by direct air pressure, adjusted by a solenoid, mercury pressure switch combination, to maintain a uniform pressure drop across a resistance in the blood circuit leading to the oxygenator. Samples of the blood before and after passage through the oxygenator were analyzed in duplicate. When carbon dioxide and oxygen determinations were desired, the technique of Van Slyke was employed. In general, however, analyses were for oxygen only; these were performed spectrophotometrically by the technique of Gordy and Drabkin,[15] modified to hemolyze the blood as suggested by Hickman and Frayser.[16] Hemolysis was obtained under anaerobic conditions by using a three-way stopcock for adding the saponin solution and mercury. The hemolyzed samples were examined in cuvettes having a 1 mm. light path in a Beckman DU spectrophotometer.

An attempt was made in each experiment to adjust the conditions of blood flow and oxygenator so that an increase in saturation of at least 20 per cent would be achieved. This minimized the influence of experimental or analytic inaccuracies. In view of work function considerations, testing is less sensitive when blood leaves the apparatus at saturations over 90 per cent, and this range was generally avoided.

Experimental Techniques Used for the Spinning Disk Oxygenator.—
Ranges studied:

Holdup:	500 to 900 ml.
Disk speed:	50 to 125 r.p.m.
Oxygen tension:	700 and 1,000 mm. Hg.

Because of the nature of this oxygenator, a simple and informative testing procedure is available that cannot be readily applied to other oxygenators. It is true of all circulatory systems that, provided the fluid moves along with even progression and without channeling or dallying in stagnant pools, the following formula applies:

$$\frac{\text{Volume of a chamber in the circuit}}{\text{Transit time of fluid through the chamber}} = \text{flow of fluid through circuit.}$$

Thus, any particular minute flow will designate what the transit time through a chamber of given volume must be; a blood flow of 2,000 ml. per minute through an oxygenator of 500 ml. content will require a transit time through the oxygenator of fifteen seconds. Hence, the oxygenation of 500 ml. of stationary blood achieved in fifteen seconds should be equivalent to that obtained with an active circulation of 2,000 ml. per minute.

A collecting catheter of low dead space is placed at the bottom of the oxygenator in a central location. The desired volume of blood is placed in the oxygenator and reduced to a low saturation by passing 5 per cent O_2 – 95 per cent N_2 above the rotating disks. The disks are stopped, the atmosphere is flushed with 5 per cent CO_2 – 95 per cent O_2, and the disks are rotated once more. Five milliliter blood samples are collected at the rate of 1 ml. per second, with five seconds intervening between samples, so that there are six samples per minute and each mirrors the average saturation of a five-second interval. The experiments are made with varying amounts of blood in the apparatus and varying rates of disk rotation. When the saturations are plotted against time, the change in saturation for any exposure time may be read, and the change in saturation at the flow rate corresponding to the exposure time estimated.

Experimental Techniques Used for the Stedman Packing Oxygenator.—
Ranges studied:

Column height:	0.25 to 2.75 feet.
Blood flow:	200 to 5,200 ml. per minute.
Oxygen tension:	700 and 1,000 mm. Hg.

Holdup in the Stedman packing oxygenator was determined by passing blood at varying flow rates through two feet of packing that had been removed from its casing. When a steady state was achieved, the isolated packing was weighed; the holdup was obtained by subtracting the weight of the dry packing.

Experimental Techniques Used for the Foam Oxygenator.—

Ranges studied:

Column height:	1 to 3 feet.
Blood flow:	600 to 3,000 ml. per minute in 1½ inch diameter column.
Oxygen tension:	140 and 700 mm. Hg.
Gas flow:	100 to 3,500 ml. per minute in 1½ inch diameter column.
Column diameter:	1.5, 2, 3 inches.
Bubble orifices:	Sizes 17, 20, 21, 23, 25 hypodermic needles.

The work function for the foam oxygenator was determined as follows: The blood was passed at a rate of 1,000 ml. per minute into a 12 inch high, 1½ inch diameter column using 25 gauge hypodermic needles for gas dispersion. The gas used was a mixture of 95 per cent O_2-5 per cent CO_2. Batches of blood having venous saturations varying between 24 and 64 per cent were passed through the oxygenator. Holdup in the foam oxygenator was determined at varying gas and blood flows in a 1½ inch diameter, three-foot-high column by simultaneously closing the inlet and outlet of the oxygenator and then measuring the volume of the defoamed blood.

THE SPINNING DISK OXYGENATOR

Description of Apparatus.—The oxygenator tested was closely modeled on that employed by its originator, Crafoord.[1] The oxygenator (Fig. 3) consists of a horizontal cylinder with blood entering at one end and leaving at the other. Within the cylinder are a series of fifty disks of 19.7 cm. diameter, mounted 0.4 cm. apart on a horizontal shaft. The disks dip into the blood that is in transit through the cylinder so that an annular film of blood forms at the periphery of the disk. Oxygen is passed through the space above the blood. There are two principal variables in the use of the apparatus: 1. The height or amount of blood in the oxygenator determines the width of the annular film on the disk and also the segment of the disk which will be exposed to the oxygen above the surface of the blood. 2. The rate at which the disks rotate determines the frequency with which the films are renewed in the blood trough.

Practical Operation.—The more blood that is present in the oxygenator and the more rapidly the disks rotate, the greater is the tendency toward formation of foam and the formation of films that bridge from one disk edge to the next. The apparatus cannot be rotated at a peripheral speed of 130 cm. per second (125 r.p.m.) for more than short periods of time without prohibitive foaming, and 110 cm. per second (105 r.p.m.) was found to be the highest speed for practical operation, although even here a few bubbles formed. Smearing Dow-Corning Antifoam on the inside of the cylinder and along the disks did not prove helpful.

An increase in blood content of the oxygenator from 800 to 900 ml. causes a rise of 4 mm. in the level of blood in the cylinder. The task of keeping constant the blood volume of the oxygenator, and therefore of the subject, becomes difficult, since most control devices employ changes in blood height as their reference.

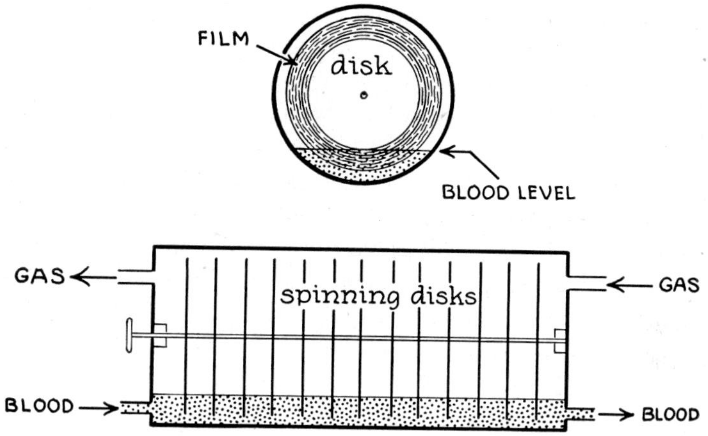

Fig. 3.—Spinning disk oxygenator: schema.

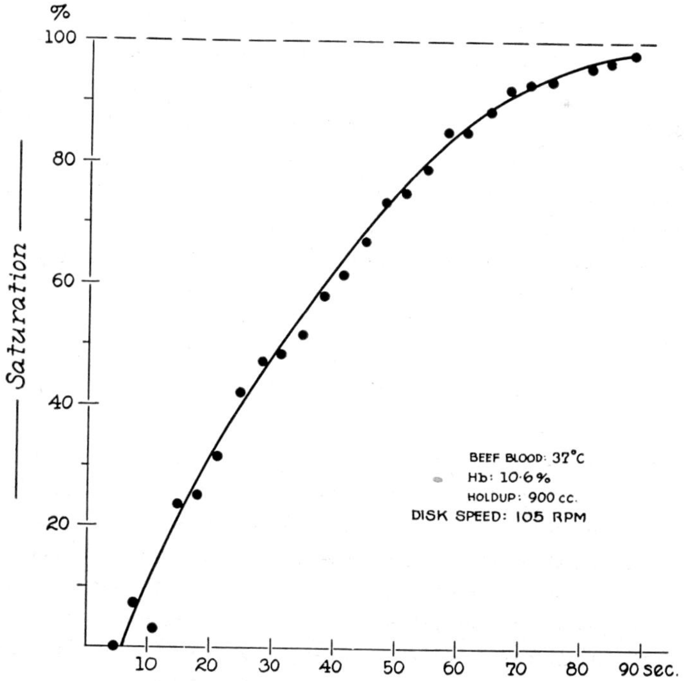

Fig. 4.—Spinning disk oxygenator: saturation as a function of film exposure time.

Results.—The characteristics of the spinning disk oxygenator have been described in detail in a comprehensive monograph by Björk.[1]

Work function: Fig. 4 plots saturation versus time for 900 c.c. of beef blood at 37° C. in the spinning disk oxygenator operating at 105 r.p.m.

Take two saturations, S_1 and S_2, on this curve and let the corresponding times be T_1 and T_2. Since the time interval, $T_1 - T_2$, is indicative of the relative difficulty in oxygenating from S_1 to S_2, we define the difference in work function $W_1 - W_2$ between the two levels of saturation as

$$W_1 - W_2 = C\ (T_1 - T_2)$$

where C is an arbitrary constant. However, to provide a basis of comparison for various work function curves of different oxygenators, the work function level of 50 per cent saturation has been arbitrarily set at 50 work function units (wfu), the 90 per cent saturation level at 100 wfu. This determines the value of C. The work function for the spinning disk oxygenator is given in Table I.

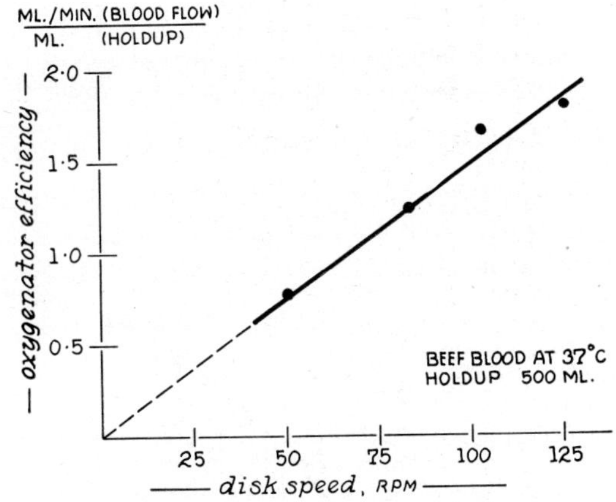

Fig. 5.—Spinning disk oxygenator: efficiency as a function of disk speed.

Overpressure operation: Two experiments were performed in which the oxygen tension was 1,000 mm. Hg instead of 700 mm. Hg (Table II). These experiments may be compared with those in which 900 ml. of beef blood at 37° C. was exposed at a disk rotation rate of 105 r.p.m., since the conditions were identical except for the oxygen pressure. The time required for hemoglobin saturation to rise from 50 to 90 per cent is almost exactly inversely

TABLE II. SPINNING DISK OXYGENATOR; OXYGENATION AS A FUNCTION OF OXYGEN TENSION (BEEF BLOOD, 900 ML., 105 R.P.M., 37° C.)

	EQUIVALENT FLOW (50-90%) (ML./MIN.)	GRADIENT O_2 (MM. HG)
	2,850	940
	2,000	630
Ratio:	1.42	1.50

proportional to the oxygen gradient. Consequently, the corresponding blood flow is directly proportional to the gradient. This correlation of oxygenation power with oxygen tension of the gas is predicted by the diffusion equation and demonstrated experimentally by Björk[1] for oxygen tensions below 700 mm. Hg.

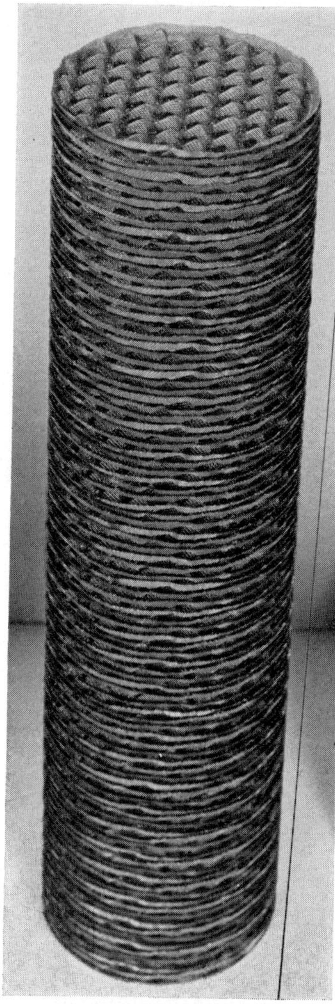

Fig. 6.—Stedman packing oxygenator.

Efficiency: The comparative efficiency of our spinning disk oxygenator with a holdup of 900 ml. and at 105 r.p.m. was $\frac{1.7 \text{ ml./min. (blood flow)}}{\text{ml.} \quad \text{(holdup)}}$. The comparative efficiency of Björk's oxygenator is estimated at $\frac{1.0 \text{ ml./min.}}{\text{ml.}}$. The difference between these two oxygenators may be attributed to the fact that our disks were 19.7 cm. in diameter, while Björk's disks were 13 cm. in diameter.

Thus our minute area per disk was 2.6 square meters per minute, while Björk's minute area per disk was about 1.5 square meters per minute.

The linear variation of efficiency with disk speed (Fig. 5) concurs with the findings of Björk.[1] Thus the efficiency of this oxygenator is limited by the highest disk speed at which it can be operated without foaming.

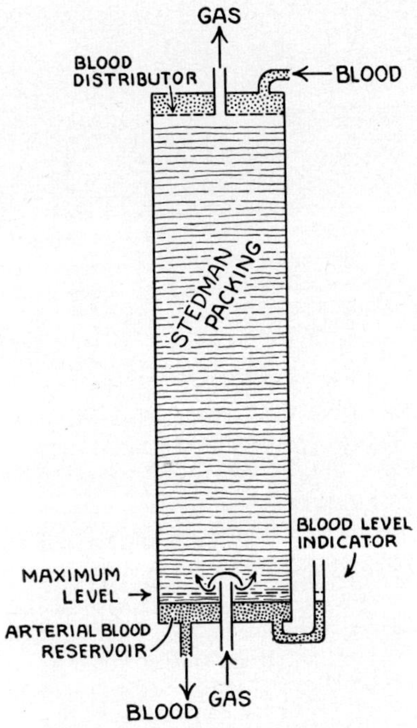

Fig. 7.—Stedman packing oxygenator: schema.

THE STEDMAN PACKING OXYGENATOR

Description of Apparatus.—The Stedman packing oxygenator was introduced by Bailey.[4] Stedman packing is a tower packing used by the chemical industry in processes requiring intimate contact between liquids and gases. It consists of stacks of 60 by 40 mesh stainless steel wire cloth disks of six-inch diameter. Each wire disk is embossed and perforated so that it presents a pattern of pyramids, valleys, and holes (Fig. 6). There are 100 disks per foot of column height, providing an effective area of thirty-four square feet. Blood is distributed at the top of the column, and flows downward in a continuous stream from disk to disk. The oxygen is delivered at the bottom of the column, just above the blood pool that runs off the column. A tight fit between the disks and the casing assures that the oxygen passes upward through the disks. A diagram of this oxygenator is shown in Fig. 7.

Practical Operation.—The oxygenator does not foam since there are no moving parts and the oxygen moves past the blood rather than through it. If the sheets are not wet, the filming of the blood is imperfect because of channeling. Since the sheets are spot-welded together, it is possible to inspect only the exterior surfaces, and it is necessary to rely on strong alkaline solutions for cleanliness.

TABLE III. WORK ACCOMPLISHED AS A FUNCTION OF COLUMN HEIGHT FOR THE STEDMAN PACKING

RUN NO.	BLOOD FLOW (ML./MIN.)	DIFFERENCE IN WORK FUNCTION (wfu)	RATIO OF DIFFERENCE IN WORK FUNCTION	COLUMN HEIGHT (FT.)	RATIO OF COLUMN HEIGHT
G3	4,000	52.1	1.84	2.75	1.84
H6	4,000	28.4		1.50	
H2	2,700	32.5	1.52	1.50	1.50
D5	2,700	21.4		1.00	
H1	1,330	51.3	1.42	1.50	1.50
B5	1,400	36.2		1.00	

Results.—

Work function: The work function for this oxygenator is given in Table I. The identity of the work functions of the spinning disk and Stedman packing oxygenators was established by the close correlation prevailing between the experimental results obtained for the Stedman packing oxygenator and those predicted by the work function of the spinning disk oxygenator.

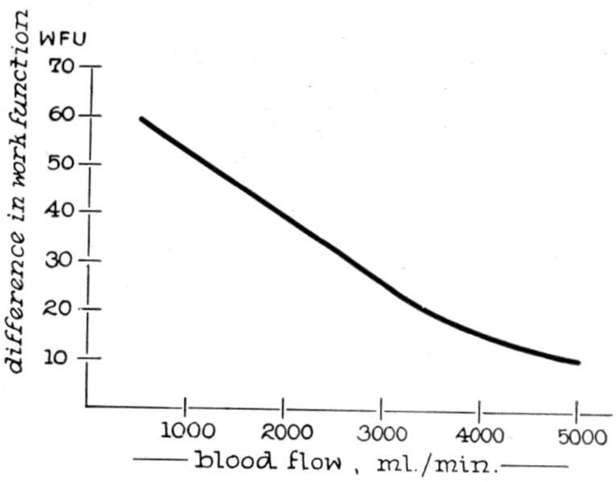

Fig. 8.—Stedman packing oxygenator: work done as a function of blood flow.

For example, since each disk in the column may be considered an individual oxygenator, the difference in work function produced by a column may be expected to be proportional to the column height. In Table III, pairs of experiments performed at the same flow but at different column heights are listed. The ratio of the column heights and the ratio of the change in work function are substantially equal.

Oxygenating characteristics: The change in work function which this oxygenator accomplishes per foot of column height is shown as a function of blood flow in Fig. 8. This curve can be used to estimate the change in saturation of blood at various flow rates. To illustrate its use, suppose one wishes to estimate the approximate length of column required to oxygenate a 2 L. per minute flow of blood from a saturation of 70 per cent to 95 per cent. Table I shows the required change of work function to be 115.9 – 70.6 = 45.3 wfu. From Fig. 8 it is seen that the work done by one foot of six-inch diameter packing at a flow of 2 L. per minute is 40 wfu. The length of column needed then is 45.3/40.0 = 1.1 feet.

Holdup: The holdup of blood in the packing at varying flow rates is shown in Fig. 9. This curve is linear within the range of anticipated flows. When

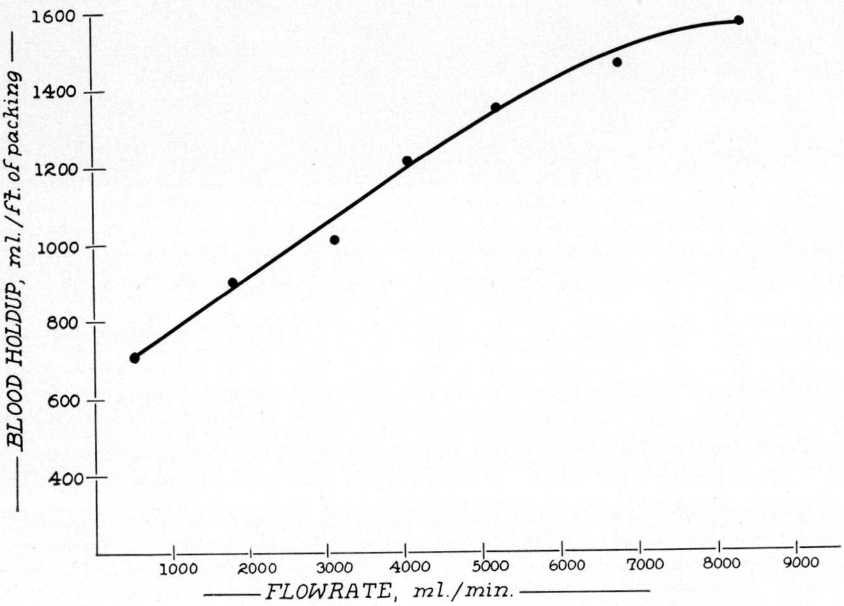

Fig. 9.—Stedman packing oxygenator: holdup as a function of blood flow.

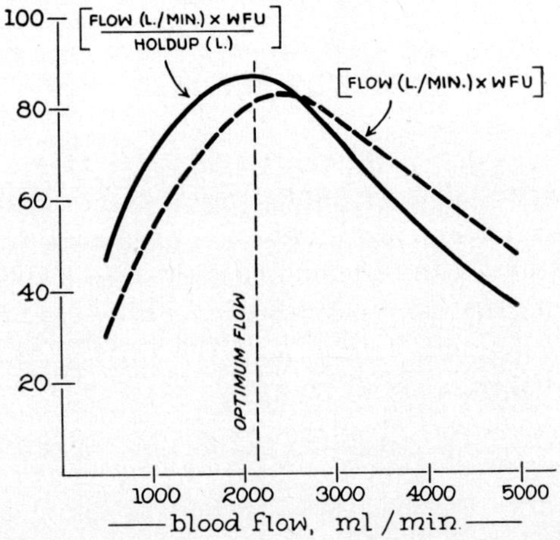

Fig. 10.—Stedman packing oxygenator: efficiency as related to blood flow.

the curve is extrapolated to zero flow, it becomes apparent that there is a holdup of about 600 ml. of blood per foot of packing that persists even at negligible flow.

Optimum blood flow: By multiplying the change in work function at a given flow, Fig. 8, by the flow itself and plotting the product against flow, we obtain the dotted curve of Fig. 10. This curve gives the number of work function units which are introduced for any given flow. The solid curve of Fig. 10 represents the work function units introduced, divided by the holdup. The flow at which the maximum of this curve appears represents the point of highest efficiency. This occurs at approximately 2,100 ml. per minute. Since this flow is distributed over a six-inch diameter circle, an area of twenty-eight square inches, the blood flow for peak efficiency should be 110 ml. per minute per square inch. (This is a useful design figure since Stedman packing is available in various diameters.)

Overpressure oxygenation: In Table IV, the results for two experiments performed at the same flow and column height but at different oxygen tensions are recorded. An appreciable gain in oxygenation is noted with the higher oxygen tension. This gain is compared to the ratio of the oxygen diffusion gradients (P_{O_2} in gas – average P_{O_2} in plasma).

TABLE IV. OVERPRESSURE OXYGENATION WITH STEDMAN PACKING

RUN NO.	BLOOD FLOW (ML./MIN.)	SATURATIONS (PER CENT) INITIAL	SATURATIONS (PER CENT) FINAL	DIFFERENCE IN WORK FUNCTION (wfu)	RATIO OF DIFFERENCE IN wfu	AVERAGE OXYGEN GRADIENT (MM. HG)	RATIO OF GRADIENT
D9	2,700	47	72	25.7	1.7	630	1.5
M2	2,700	35	78	43.1		940	

Efficiency: The comparative efficiency is $\frac{1.8 \text{ ml./min. (blood flow)}}{\text{ml. (holdup)}}$ when the oxygenator is operated at its most efficient flow.

THE FOAM OXYGENATOR

Description of Apparatus.—The foam oxygenator,[10] shown schematically in Fig. 11, consists of a two-inch diameter commercial Pyrex pipe* which has at its top a six-inch diameter bowl. At the bottom of the pipe there is an oxygen manifold consisting of 125 2½ inch long 25 gauge hypodermic needles. Blood is slowly admitted at the bottom of the column, and is permitted to rise above the tips of the needles. The oxygen passing through the needles bubbles through the blood, forming foam as it emerges from the blood. The foam continues to rise until the whole column above the blood is filled. When the foam contacts the Antifoam-coated vertical baffles in the bowl, it breaks, the gas from each bubble passing upward through the baffles and out of the oxygenator, and the blood surrounding each bubble trickling down through the column until it reaches the pool of blood at the bottom. Venous blood is now admitted through the showerhead distributor and cascades down through the

*Available from Sentinel Glass Company, Hatboro, Pa.

foam being oxygenated in the process. The arterialized blood is withdrawn from the bottom of the oxygenator. Three distinct gas-liquid phases are apparent when the oxygenator is in operation: 1. At the bottom there is a pool of blood through which bubbles are rising freely as they are emitted from the oxygen manifold. In order to prevent oxygen embolism, the bubbles must have a rate of ascent greater than the rate of descent of the blood being withdrawn from the oxygenator. The larger the bubble, the more rapidly it climbs. At low oxygen flows, the bubble size is determined largely by the size

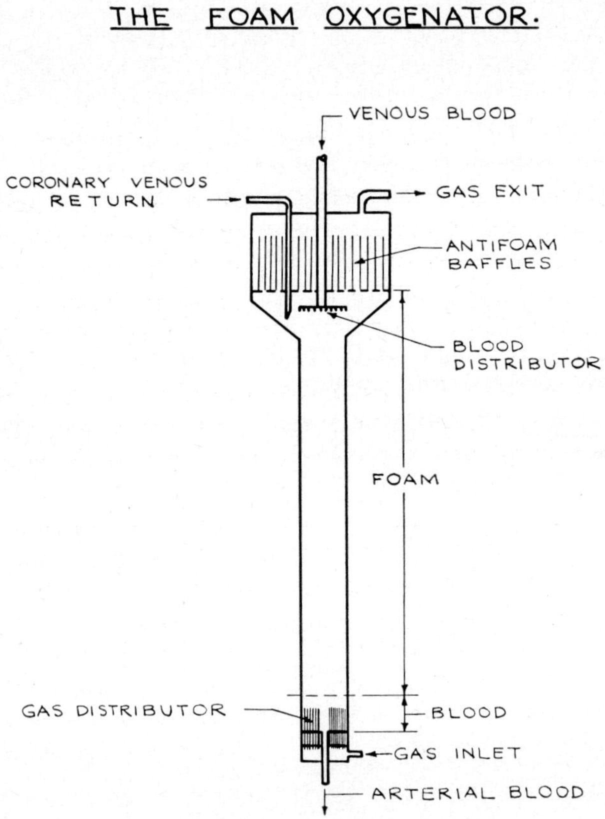

Fig. 11.—Foam oxygenator: schema.

of the orifice; the diameter of the bubble is proportional to the cube root of the diameter of the needle.[17] (Bubbles released from coarse sintered glass disks are not consistently large enough to avoid gas embolism under normal operating conditions.) 2. Above the blood pool there is a foam column where the bubbles are separated by rather heavy blood films. 3. The bubbles above the blood distributor are bound by thin blood films since only the blood released by the defoaming baffle passes down through them.

The maximum gas flow which can be passed through the oxygenator is determined by the capacity of the defoaming system. A defoaming baffle consisting of one-quarter inch diameter plastic tubes cut into three-inch lengths coated with Antifoam and packed vertically into the defoaming bowl is capable of defoaming a gas flow of 6.5 ml. per minute per square centimeter of defoamer cross section with dog blood. Another type of stationary baffle is formed by a three-inch-wide stainless steel sheet wound into a helix with one-eighth inch spacing between the turns. In the large bubble oxygenator of Thomas, defoaming is accomplished by pulsatile, high-velocity jets of air which mechanically break up the foam. This system has the advantage over the stationary defoamers described in that no antifoam compound need be used.

Practical Operation.—When this oxygenator is used in a perfusion circuit, the arterial pump is continuously adjusted to maintain the blood-foam interface about two inches from the bottom of the column. At the site at which the interface is to be observed, the glass should not be siliconed, or else static bubbles will adhere and obscure the view.

To obviate channeling, the oxygenator should be aligned vertically.

If the oxygenator is not used at atmospheric pressure, a large flow resistance placed between the oxygen tank and the oxygen manifold will reduce fluctuations in the gas flow due to fluctuations in the pressure within the oxygenator. We have used a filtration candle* submerged in water for this purpose. To gauge the gas flow it is desirable to use a flowmeter.†

Results.—In contrast to film oxygenators, the operation of the foam oxygenator is greatly affected by the magnitude of the gas flow. This additional variable makes the specification of the conditions for its operation more complex.

Gas flow: The gas flow which combines optimum oxygenation with a low holdup is of the order of 70 ml. per minute per square centimeter of cross-sectional area. At higher flows there is a steep increase in holdup, while at lower flows the oxygenator eliminates less carbon dioxide.

To eliminate the CO_2 production of a twenty kilogram dog, a gas flow of about 140 c.c. per minute per square centimeter is needed. At lower flows the tendency toward respiratory acidosis is self-limiting, however, since the higher the CO_2 tension of the blood, the more CO_2 any given volume of oxygen will be able to carry away.

Blood flow: The blood flow through the column should not exceed 140 ml. per minute per square centimeter if an orderly foam column is to be maintained. At higher flows the blood-foam interface becomes difficult to distinguish.

Work function: The work function for the foam oxygenator is shown in Fig. 13. It differs from the work function of the Stedman packing and spinning disk oxygenators in that it falls off less rapidly at higher saturations.

Oxygenating characteristics: With the blood flow and gas flow as given previously, this oxygenator will introduce a work function difference of 1.8 wfu per inch of column height for blood of 15 Gm. per cent hemoglobin.

*No. 03 filter candle, Selas Company, Philadelphia, Pa.
†Rotameter type instrument, Fisher and Porter Co., Hatboro, Pa.

Design procedure: Suppose one wants a foam oxygenator which will oxygenate a maximum blood flow of 4,000 ml. per minute from 60 per cent to 90 per cent. The work function difference from 60 per cent to 90 per cent is found from Fig. 13 to be 100 – 60 = 40 wfu. The height of the oxygenator therefore should be $\frac{40}{1.8} = 22$ inches. The cross-sectional area of the oxygenator is found to be $\frac{4{,}000}{140} = 28.5$ cm.[2] This is equivalent to a 2.4 inch diameter tube. The gas flow is $70 \times 28.5 = 2{,}000$ c.c. per minute.

Holdup: The holdup for beef blood having a concentration of 12 Gm. per cent hemoglobin at 37° C. is given as a function of blood flow in Fig. 12. The holdup is expressed as the fraction of the total oxygenator volume which is occupied by the blood. The holdup for undiluted blood may be expected to be somewhat higher than that shown in Fig. 12 because of the increased viscosity.

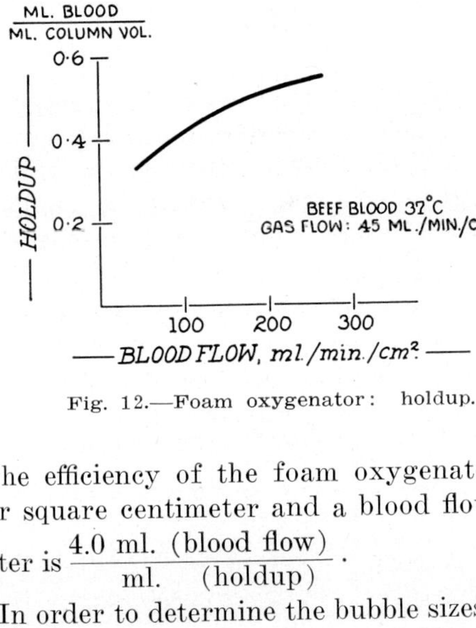

Fig. 12.—Foam oxygenator: holdup.

Efficiency: The efficiency of the foam oxygenator for a gas flow of 70 ml. per minute per square centimeter and a blood flow of 140 ml. per minute per square centimeter is $\frac{4.0 \text{ ml. (blood flow)}}{\text{ml. (holdup)}}$.

Bubble size: In order to determine the bubble sizes for maximum efficiency, experiments were carried out with oxygen manifolds consisting of Nos. 17, 21, 22, 23, and 25 hypodermic needles.

The number of needles in each manifold was chosen so that the total cross-sectional area of the needles was the same in each manifold. Since bigger needles produce bigger bubbles and since the ratio of surface area to volume decreases with increasing bubble size, one would expect a lower efficiency with the bigger needles. The holdup, however, is less for larger bubbles. The combined effect of these two opposing tendencies was found to be a drop in efficiency for the larger bubbles. Thus, the efficiency for the Nos. 21, 22, and 23 needles was 20 per cent lower than that for the No. 25 needles. The possibility remains that the greater ease of defoaming large bubbles may indicate the use of the larger needle sizes despite their drop in efficiency. The use of needles smaller than No. 25 (.010 inch internal diameter) would be more efficient but raises additional problems. The needles are difficult to handle and to clean, defoaming becomes more difficult, and embolism is a possibility.

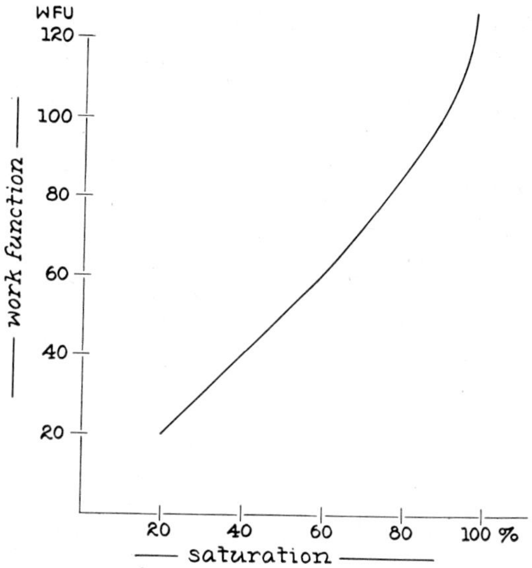

Fig. 13.—Foam oxygenator: work function curve.

SUMMARY AND CONCLUSIONS

1. The major physical problem for artificial oxygenators is the rapid introduction of oxygen into the plasma. A high oxygen diffusion gradient and a high degree of turbulence in the blood are the principal means of expediting oxygen transfer.

2. Oxygenators expose individual blood films for periods of time without regard to the degree of hemoglobin unsaturation. Thus, this time is used less efficiently at high saturations since the surface blood is saturated before the termination of the exposure time. Thus, more oxygenator working space and time are required to increase the hemoglobin saturation from 80 to 100 per cent than from 60 to 80 per cent. As a means of quantitating the relative difficulty in oxygenating over various saturation ranges the work function is introduced.

3. To increase the precision of the concept of oxygenator efficiency, it appears desirable to compare oxygenators working within the same saturation range, and that of 60 to 90 per cent is arbitrarily chosen. We therefore define comparative efficiency as follows: The largest flow of blood of 15 Gm. per cent hemoglobin which the oxygenator can raise from 60 to 90 per cent saturation divided by the total blood holdup at this flow rate.

4. Some experimental techniques of evaluating oxygenators through in vitro studies are outlined. The power to control and stabilize blood flow and

oxygen saturation is of great value in obtaining results for comparison of apparatus.

5. The efficiency of the spinning disk oxygenator varies directly with minute exposure area. Larger disk area and greater speed of rotation increase oxygenation linearly. With disks of 19.7 cm. diameter, foaming renders operation at over 105 r.p.m. impractical.

6. The Stedman packing oxygenator operates with a peak efficiency at a blood flow of about 2,100 ml. per six-inch diameter circle.

7. The efficiency of both spinning disk and Stedman packing oxygenators is increased by 50 per cent when the oxygen diffusion gradient is increased by 50 per cent.

8. The foam oxygenator operates most efficiently with an oxygen flow of 70 ml. per minute and a blood flow of 140 ml. per minute per square centimeter. Larger bubbles decrease oxygenating efficiency by almost 20 per cent, but are more readily defoamed.

9. The comparative efficiencies of the three oxygenators studied are as follows: spinning disk, 1.7, Stedman packing, 1.8, foam, 4.0.

Acknowledgments.—The spinning disk oxygenator used in this study was generously made for us by the General Precision Laboratories, Pleasantville, N. Y., through the offices of Mr. Ivan Greenwood. The Stedman packing oxygenator was loaned to us by Dr. L. B. Bragg of the Packed Column Corporation, New York, and by Dr. John Gibbon. The Sentinel Glass Company, Hatboro, Pa., gave material assistance in the formation of the foam oxygenator. Polyethylene used for the defoaming baffle in the foam oxygenator was donated by Mr. Peter Seckel of the Anchor Plastic Company, New York. Polyvinyl tubing was generously supplied by the Sunlite Manufacturing Company, Milwaukee, Wis. Needle tubing was obtained through the kindness of Mr. Oscar Schwidetzky, Becton, Dickinson and Company, Rutherford, N. J. The blood pump used in many in vitro experiments is made by the Vanton Corporation, New York, and was generously supplied by Mr. J. J. Ashton and Mr. Gerald Lewis of that organization.

We are greatly indebted to many workers in the field of mechanical pump-oxygenators who advised us, showed us the detailed operation of their laboratories, and saved us from many futilities. We are especially obliged to Dr. John Gibbon and Dr. Bernard Miller, of the Jefferson Medical College, to Dr. Clarence Dennis and Dr. Dwight Spreng, of the New York State Medical College, to Dr. Leland Clark, Jr., and Dr. Frank Gollan of Antioch College, and to Dr. W. J. Kolff and Dr. Frederick Olmsted, of the Cleveland Clinic Research Institute. We are deeply indebted to Dr. David L. Drabkin and Dr. Edward Gordy for having introduced to us their method for the spectrophotometric determination of oxyhemoglobin. We wish to thank Dr. Harry M. Vars and Dr. James M. Walker of the Harrison Department of Surgcal Research for much advice and assistance.

We thank Miss Betsy Hoffer and Miss Florence Conway for the secretarial assistance which we received from them, and finally we wish to express our indebtedness to our technician Mrs. Frances Philips for her selfless and devoted contributions to our project.

REFERENCES

1. Björk, V. O.: Brain Perfusions in Dogs With Artificially Oxygenated Blood, Acta chir. scandinav. (supp. 137) **96**: 1-122, 1948.
2. Dennis, C., Spreng, D. S., Nelson, G. E., Karlson, K. F., Nelson, R. M., Thomas, J. V., Eder, W. P., and Varco, R. L.: Development of a Pump-Oxygenator to Replace the Heart and Lungs; An Apparatus Applicable to Human Patients and Application to One Case, Ann. Surg. **134**: 709-721, 1951.
3. Miller, B. J., Gibbon, J. H., Jr., and Gibbon, M. H.: Recent Advances in the Development of a Mechanical Heart and Lung Apparatus, Ann. Surg. **134**: 694-708, 1951.
4. Heart-Lung Device Ready for Test of Reviving Those Clinically Dead, The New York Times, Dec. 4, 1950.
5. Jongbloed, J.: Mechanical Heart Lung System, Surg., Gynec. & Obst. **89**: 684-691, 1949.
6. Clark, L. C., Gupta, V. B., and Gollan, F.: Dispersion Oxygenation for Effective Survival of Dogs Breathing Pure Nitrogen for Prolonged Periods, Proc. Soc. Exper. Biol. & Med. **74**: 268-271, 1950.
7. Lary, G. G.: Experimental Maintenance of Life by Intravenous Oxygen: Preliminary Report, Proc. Surg. Forum, Clin. Congress Am. Coll. Surgeons, 1951, Philadelphia, 1952, W. B. Saunders Company, pp. 30.
8 Thomas, J. A.: Les possibilités actuelles du coeur-poumon artificiel destiné à la perfusion totale du corps humain, 14th Congress, International Surgical Society, 1951, Brussels, 1952, Imprimerie Médicale et Scientifique, pp. 1004.

9. Waud, R. A.: A Mechanical Heart and Lung, Canad. J. M. Sc. **30**: 130-135, 1952.
10. Gimbel, N., and Engelberg, J.: An Oxygenator for Use in a Heart-Lung Apparatus, Proc. Surg. Forum, Clin. Congress Am. Coll. Surgeons, 1952, Philadelphia, 1953, W. B. Saunders Company, pp. 154.
11. Roughton, F. J. W., Legge, J. W., and Nicolson, P.: The Kinetics of Hemoglobin in Solution and in the Red Blood Corpuscle, New York, 1949, Hemoglobin, Interscience Publishers, Inc., pp. 67.
12. McCormack, H.: The Applications of Chemical Engineering, New York, 1940, D. Van Nostrand Company, Inc.
13. Stokes, T. L., and Flick, J. B.: An Improved Vertical Cylinder Oxygenator, Proc. Soc. Exper. Biol. & Med. **73**: 528, 1950.
14. Karlson, K. E., Dennis, C., Westover, D. E., and Sanderson, D.: Pump Oxygenator to Supplant the Heart-Lungs for Brief Periods. I. Evaluation of Oxygenator Techniques; An Efficient Oxygenator, SURGERY **29**: 678-696, 1951.
15. Gordy, E., and Drabkin, D. L.: A Simplified Spectrophotometric Technique Applicable to Standard Equipment for the Determination of O_2 Saturation of Blood, Am. J. M. Sc. **221**: 231-232, 1951.
16. Hickman, J. B., and Frayser, R.: Spectrophotometric Determination of Blood Oxygen, J. Biol. Chem. **180**: 457, 1949.
17. Maier, C. G.: The Ferric-Sulphuric Acid Process, U. S. Bureau of Mines Bulletin 260, 1927.

Book Reviews

Surgery for Nurses. By James Moroney, M.B., Ch.B., F.R.C.S. (Eng.), L.R.C.P. (Lond.), with a Foreword by Miss Dorothy M. Smith, O.B.E., Chairman of General Nursing Council for England and Wales, Matron, Guy's Hospital, London. Ed. 2. Edinburgh and London, 1952, E. & S. Livingstone. $6.00.

A surgical textbook of nursing, in order to achieve wide utility, must provide in a single treatise a broad discussion of all of the surgical specialties and the nursing requirements related to them. Despite the inherent disadvantages which this prerequisite creates, the author here has done admirably well.

As an introduction, the nurse is reminded of her increased responsibilities and the contributions, especially to surgical diagnosis, which are accomplished by her careful observation of the patient. There follows a detailed discussion of the fundamentals of preoperative and postoperative care, of the principles of surgical bacteriology and immunology, a description of the basis of inflammation, and a chapter on observations related to hemorrhage. These discussions on the principles of surgery are well done and are complemented by an adequate review of antibiotic therapy and an excellent description of surgical dressing techniques.

The clinical discussions of the General and Thoracic Surgery entities are quite adequate, as are those of the other surgical specialties, which include Urology, Neurosurgery, Fractures and Orthopedics, Otolaryngology, Ophthalmology, and Gynecology. There is besides this a brief ''Introduction to Obstetrics.'' The correlation of the basic nursing functions and problems with these didactic clinical descriptions is an outstanding feature of the book.

There are certain differences from American textbooks which this book of English origin preserves. For example, there is a chapter devoted to the surgical forms of tuberculosis and a brief, but excellent, summary of the chemotherapy of tuberculosis. Such a presentation is probably uncommon in similar American textbooks.

On the other hand, some methods of surgical therapy are recommended or emphasized which are not largely acceptable in this country; they include a wider use of radiotherapy for malignant tumors of the head and neck, and an apparent enthusiasm for colonic restoration of the stomach following gastrectomy. There is a notable failure to emphasize the significance of nodular goiter as a precursor of carcinoma of the thyroid. These differences are not crucial and do not significantly influence the utility which the book is designed to have.

This is a well-recommended textbook for nurses.

Physiological Foundations of Neurology and Psychiatry. By Ernst Gellhorn, M.D., Ph.D., Pp. 556. Minneapolis, 1953, University of Minnesota Press.

In this volume Dr. Gellhorn has summarized over 100 of his own previously published investigations, as well as a large amount of other related work. The aim of the book, as stated in the preface, is more modest than the title implies. ''By no means all, but only some, physiological foundations of neuropsychiatry are treated, those with which the writer is familiar through his own experimental work . . . it is hoped that significant topics have been selected, of interest to physiologists, endocrinologists, internists, neurologists and neurosurgeons, psychiatrists and students of human behavior.''

After a review of current knowledge about neuronal activity, the motor cortex, and the physiology of movements, there is an outline of the physiologic basis of consciousness, in which the author takes the position that "understanding the mind from the point of view of neurophysiology is not an entirely hopeless task." Then there is a discussion of autonomic functions, with an interesting chapter on the eye as an indicator of autonomic activity.

The section on "Integrations" includes chapters on the principles of neuroendocrine action, on the physiologic basis of emotion, and on homeostasis.

In the concluding section, entitled "Applications," one of the important topics discussed is the relation of mental processes to the central autonomic balance, and the use of autonomic tests in the analysis of psychoses. The effectiveness of shock therapy is shown to be related to increased and prolonged reactivity of the sympathetic hypothalamic centers.

The discussions of the topics chosen are lucid and thorough, and reveal the extensive experience and authority of the author.

Grenzen des Normalen und Anfänge des Pathologische im Röntgenbilde des Skelettes. By Dr. A. Köhler. Ed. 9. Pp. 672, with 1,282 illustrations. Stuttgart, 1953, Georg Thieme Verlag, Agent for U.S.A.: Grune & Stratton, Inc., New York, N. Y.

The boundaries between the normal, the anomalous, and the pathologic remain poorly defined. This is especially true of the anatomy of the skeleton as displayed on roentgenographs. Köhler published this monograph as a guide for use in interpreting x-ray photographs which were not entirely normal or obviously pathologic. The ninth edition is as valuable today as was the first edition in 1910. The normal variations and anomalies of the skeleton are catalogued in a systematized manner well designed for easy reference. In addition to reproductions of typical examples, there are comprehensive charts and drawings which summarize this information. A large number of examples of various disease processes of bone in their earliest stages are inserted throughout to aid in differential diagnosis. The bibliography has been brought up to date and includes a large number of references from the recent European medical literature. This is a necessary reference book for roentgenologists, orthopedists, and fracture surgeons. It is not necessary to have a fluent reading knowledge of German to utilize the information presented. The publishers have used good paper, and the illustrations are clear and well chosen.

ANNOUNCEMENTS

Third International Congress on Diseases of the Chest

The Third International Congress on Diseases of the Chest, sponsored by the American College of Chest Physicians every second year, will be held in Barcelona (Spain) Oct. 4-8, 1954.

Communications will be held on diseases of the chest and thoracic surgery, including anesthesiology, experimentation, tuberculosis, cancer, thoracic wall, lung, pleura, mediastinum, esophagus, pericardium, heart, great vessels, and diaphragm.

During the celebration of the Congress, an exposition of surgical, clinical, radiologic, and photographic materials, as well as pharmaceutic products, books, and arts related to medicine, will be held at the Hospital de la Santa Cruz y de San Pablo of Barcelona, meeting place of the Congress.

All physicians and surgeons who wish to attend the Congress should write for application and any other information to Dr. A. Caralps, General Secretary of the Congress, Córcega, 393, 4.º, 1.ª, Barcelona (Spain).

Sixth Congress of the Pan-Pacific Surgical Association

The Sixth Congress of the Pan-Pacific Surgical Association will be held in Honolulu, Hawaii, Oct. 7-18, 1954. Doctors are cordially invited to attend and are urged to make arrangements as soon as possible if they wish to be assured of adequate facilities.

An outstanding scientific program with over 100 leading surgeons, including sessions in all divisions of surgery and related fields, promises to be of interest to all members of the profession.

The Association office has been appointed as travel agent for those attending the Congress and it is important that all hotel and travel reservations be made through the Honolulu headquarters of the Pan-Pacific Surgical Association.

For further information, write to F. J. Pinkerton, M.D., Director General, Pan-Pacific Surgical Association, Suite Seven, Young Building, Honolulu, Hawaii.

SURGERY

Vol. 35 May, 1954 No. 5

Original Communications

SURGICAL CORRECTION OF AORTIC INSUFFICIENCY

Charles A. Hufnagel, M.D.,* W. Proctor Harvey, M.D.,**
Pierre J. Rabil, M.D.,*** and Thomas F. McDermott, M.D.****
Washington, D. C.

(From the Georgetown University Medical Center)

THE treatment of aortic insufficiency has always offered a serious problem in medical management once the signs of failure have appeared. Like many of the other acquired valvular diseases, the onset of failure is to a large measure the end result of the mechanical defect, which after a prolonged period of time imposes an insurmountable strain upon the myocardium. This, in effect, is a reflection of the excessive work-load imposed by free insufficiency. A reduction or complete correction of the valvular defect would, therefore, offer great hope for these otherwise incapacitated patients. Ideally, such correction of the valvular defect, if instituted early, might prevent the development of myocardial damage, or, if achieved later, might permit the changes which have occurred to be reversed.

The surgical treatment of aortic insufficiency has been extensively investigated in experimental animals. In our laboratory and in others, attempts have been made to reconstruct the aortic valve.[1-3] While many of these experiments have shown early promise, the late results have not appeared sufficiently good for application in the clinic. Other attempts have been made to replace the aortic valve with transplanted tissue. In most cases this transplanted tissue has been a homologous transplant of either the aortic or pulmonary valve as a unit. Again, the late results have been less satisfactory than had been hoped. Still other methods have been devised to reconstruct a valve with segments of pericardium, veins, arteries, or a combination of these structures. While some of these methods may be useful ultimately, we have felt that they have been distinctly less satisfactory than another line of endeavor which we have been pursuing since 1946.

This research was supported by a grant-in-aid from the National Heart Institute of the National Institutes of Health of the United States Public Health Service (H-914).
Received for publication, Sept. 14, 1953.
*Professor of surgical research.
**Assistant professor of medicine.
***Fellow in cardiovascular surgery.
****Professor of anesthesiology.

In 1944, an investigation of the feasibility of replacement of major portions of the arterial tree with plastic materials was begun. During the course of this study, in the past, a number of significant facts were established. It was found that properly designed tubes of methyl methacrylate could be used permanently to replace portions of the aorta. It was established that the surface properties of methyl methacrylate inhibited coagulation of blood, and this gave further evidence that the concept of Hirschboeck[4] was correct. It was postulated that nonwettability of the surface was related to inhibition of clotting, and that plastic materials other than methyl methacrylate having a similar property showed similar results, but the best results were obtained only when the surface was highly polished.[5] Later this concept of nonwettability was investigated further by Walter and Murphy,[6] who termed this property hemorepellency.

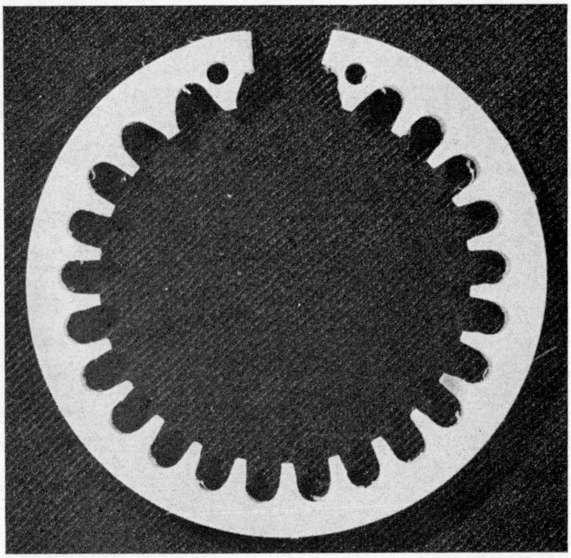

Fig. 1.—The details of the multiple-point fixation ring are shown. The openings for the ring-holder are adjacent to the split. The split allows the ring to be placed around the aorta before it is divided.

A further outgrowth of this early investigation was the development of the concept of multiple-point fixation.[5, 7, 8] In order to fix permanently a rigid prosthesis in the aorta, it was necessary to devise a method other than simple ligature. Many types of ligatures were tried in this investigation. Essentially, all of these which utilize continuous circumferential pressure for fixation produce necrosis of the aortic wall distal to the ligature. This uniformly produced fatal hemorrhage or aneurysm with delayed hemorrhage. In order to obviate this difficulty, continuous circumferential pressure was abandoned, and a device was designed which exerted pressure at discrete points on the circumference of the aorta while leaving intervening areas in which no pressure was exerted. We termed this multiple-point fixation. At the present time it is obtained using a nylon ring with multiple teeth projecting from its inner surface. The teeth are of sufficient length to elevate the body of the fixation ring below the outer aortic surface. The teeth are sufficiently close together to coapt the aortic wall to the prosthesis without leakage between the projecting points. The ring is split at one point so that it can be opened and placed around the intact aorta. Other details of the construction of the ring are shown in Figs. 1 and 2. The small holes adjacent to the split serve a dual purpose. They are used to admit the points of a holding instrument which firmly close the ring around the prosthesis and permit immediate fixation of the aorta to the prosthesis when the instrument is closed (Fig. 3). After fixation is made permanent by tying the ligature which surrounds the body of the ring, the holding instrument can be withdrawn, and a stainless steel wire (Surgaloy) is passed through these

A.

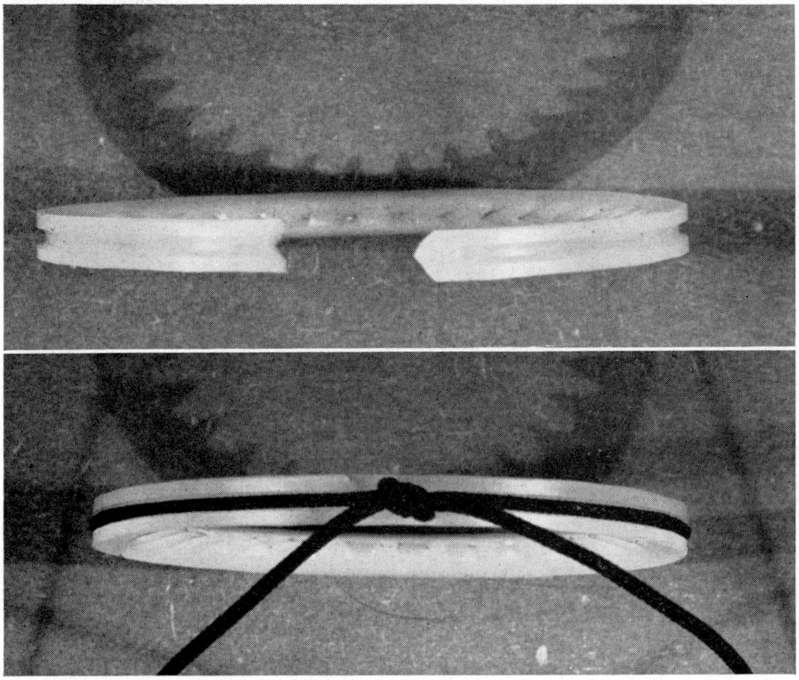

B.

Fig. 2.—The beveled construction of the split ring is shown in *A*. The closed ring with the tied ligature is shown in *B*.

holes and tied for further security. This method prevents the necrosis of the distal portion of the aorta, and is now used routinely to maintain the position of the prosthesis in the aorta. This type of fixation has been used experimentally several hundred times with no fatality caused by erosion or slippage of the fixation device. To date, it is the only method to be entirely satisfactory for the fixation of a rigid prosthesis in major vessels. It has been employed throughout this study and has been to a large extent responsible for the success of the permanent intubation method employed.

The plastic valve naturally evolved following the success of the permanent intubation of the aorta. The valve is essentially a modification of the tube. Many types of plastic valves have been employed experimentally. The majority of these have been some modification of a ball-type valve, although a number of flexible- and rigid-type valves have also been used. To date, the most useful

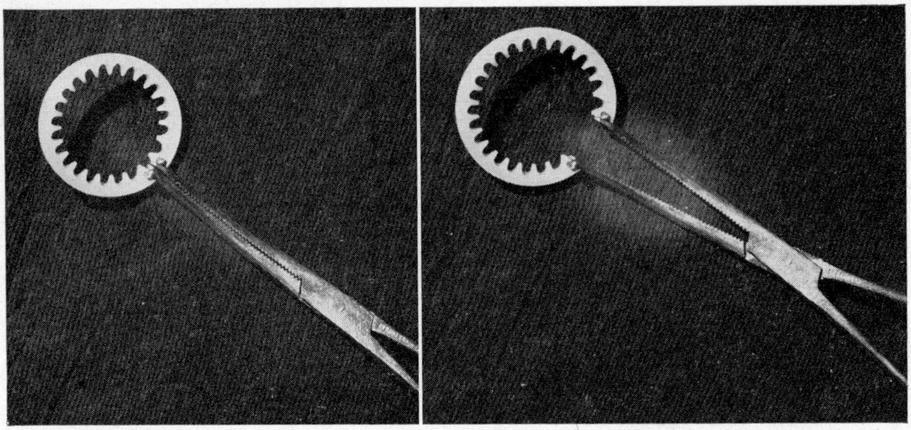

A. *B.*

Fig. 3.—The ring-holding instrument is shown in the closed position in *A* and in the open position in *B*.

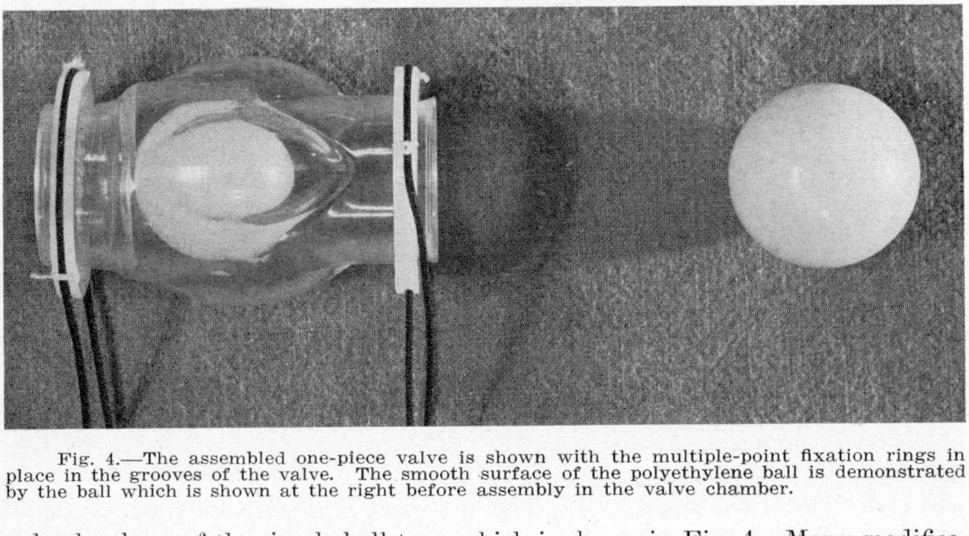

Fig. 4.—The assembled one-piece valve is shown with the multiple-point fixation rings in place in the grooves of the valve. The smooth surface of the polyethylene ball is demonstrated by the ball which is shown at the right before assembly in the valve chamber.

valve has been of the simple ball type which is shown in Fig. 4. Many modifications of this basic design were used before the development of this current design. The valve is composed of an inlet, a chamber which contains the ball, and an outlet. The entire valve is molded in a single piece so that the inner surface can be made extremely smooth and without seams. The ball itself which rests in the chamber has been made of methyl methacrylate and later of polyethylene. The design of the chamber is such that the ball is guided from the seat to the valve stops in an essentially straight line. When the ball is constructed of methyl methacrylate, it is made hollow so that its specific gravity is slightly less than one. This ball is also made without an outside seam. Polyethylene balls are made solid since the specific gravity of polyethylene is quite satisfactory. However, in order to decrease further the weight of the ball, polyethylene balls can also be made hollow without external seams. The relation of the total cross-sectional area of the chamber is adjusted to prevent serious impedance to flow through the valve. Thus, under given pressure the flow through the valve is essentially equal to that which would flow through a simple tube of a diameter equal to the inlet of the valve. The valve will function in any position. The pressure differential necessary to open or close the valve completely is 5 mm. Hg. At each end of the valve there is a groove on the outer surface. This is immediately adjacent to the inlet and outlet ends. The grooves are sufficiently deep to hold the aorta and the fixation rings without slippage. The fixation rings and the grooves are matched so that there is a constant relation between the inner diameter of the ring and the groove. This allows for the passage of the aortic wall between the inner end of the teeth and the groove. The fixation ring is made of solid semiflexible nylon. The outer surface of the body of the fixation ring is grooved. The purpose of this groove is to maintain the position of the heavy braided silk ligature on the fixation ring. From the inner surface of the ring, the multiple teeth project. The body of the ring is split between two of the teeth. This split was made in the form of a V so that when the ring is closed the ends dovetail. Immediately adjacent to the split of the ring, two small holes are drilled through the body of the ring. These holes permit the insertion of an instrument to open and close the ring. The use of this instrument has the further advantage of producing immediate fixation of the prosthesis in the aorta when the instrument is closed. It also allows the fixation suture to be tied without tension.

A valve-holding instrument is also used in placing the valve. This instrument fits the contours of the valve and holds it firmly while it is being inserted.

This method, the prostheses, and the instruments employed have been developed through extensive experiments in the laboratory. During the course of these investigations such plastic valves have been placed into the thoracic aorta of 300 dogs for varying lengths of time. Some dogs are still living five years after the insertion of the valve. Others have been sacrificed at various intervals. When the valves have been made properly, we have had no instance of clotting. Imperfections of the inner surface of the valve, however, are very harmful. Failure to remove foreign substances such as wax, grease, or other materials used in the manufacture may result in clotting in the small-size valves. However, after obtaining uniformly good results by the elimination of these variables, a series of patients with severe aortic insufficiency was selected for a clinical trial with this method. For clinical use the valve* is made in four

---

*The valves and fixation rings are manufactured by the Brunswick Manufacturing Company, Boston, Mass. We wish to acknowledge the extremely helpful cooperation of Mr. Carl Hewson, whose continuing efforts have made possible the production of this valve.

We wish to acknowledge the assistance of Dr. Herbert Broida of the Bureau of Standards and Mr. Phillip Pfaff of the Bureau of Standards for their many efforts and suggestions in the investigation and study of the valve, and in particular Mr. Pfaff's help in the design of the ring-holding device.

sizes, ranging from three-quarters inch to one and one-eighth inch in inside diameter. Each size is one-eighth inch larger than the one smaller. It has been our experience that such variation in size is essential to meet the requirements of the different diameters in the human aorta. We have employed each of these sizes in patients.

PROCEDURE

The descending aorta just beyond the left subclavian artery has been chosen for the site of the valve for several reasons. In this site it is not necessary to occlude total blood flow, and this greatly reduces risk of operation in critically ill patients. In this site the aortic occlusion is well tolerated for rather prolonged periods so that the margin of safety is great; also, approximately 75 per cent of the total regurgitant flow is controlled in this site and the dangers of air embolization are minimized. We feel that this site offers the ideal relationship between maximum benefit and minimum risk.

The left chest is opened through the bed of the fifth rib, and the aorta is freed from its bed from the base of the left subclavian artery over a distance of 6 to 8 cm. The intercostal vessels are ligated and divided. The nylon rings together with their attached ligatures are passed around the intact aorta. The closing instrument is then inserted into each of the nylon rings. The valve is carefully inspected and washed with saline solution. These valves have been sterilized by soaking for eighteen hours in 1:500 Zephiran, and triply rinsed in sterile saline solution prior to being placed on the operating table. The valve holder is then applied to the valve so that it is prepared for insertion. The aorta is then occluded with Potts aortic clamps, and the aorta divided. A segment of aorta is removed. The distal end of the aorta is then grasped at equidistant points in Judd-Allis clamps and held open widely. The valve is inserted into the opened aortic end, and the ring closed into the groove with the holding clamp. The ligature is then tied. Great care is taken to see that the ring fits well and that the edges of the ring are well approximated when the ring is closed. The ring-holding clamp is removed. The Judd-Allis clamps are applied to the proximal aorta. The proximal end of the valve is inserted, and the ring similarly closed and tied. The ring clamp and valve holder are then removed. The valve is filled with saline solution containing 1 mg. of heparin per 10 c.c. As much air as possible is removed from the valve. The distal aortic clamp is then removed, and following this the proximal clamp is removed. These clamps are taken off slowly, and blood flow to the aorta is now resumed. A twisted Surgaloy No. 000 suture is placed through the holes in the ring and tied. This gives further security to the valve and to the ring, insuring against any slippage, giving additional support in case the ligature should break. The same process is repeated at the distal end. Immediately following the removal of the aortic clamps, the valve can be heard to open and close. A pleural flap is then turned down from the lateral chest wall and sutured over the valve after a small square of Gelfoam is placed between the valve and vertebral bodies. After the pleural flap has been sutured in place, the valve is covered completely. The chest is then closed in the usual fashion.

Since September, 1952, twenty-three patients have had this type operation for aortic insufficiency, using the currently acceptable valve and multiple-point fixation.[9] Most of these patients have been in the terminal stages of their disease. Actually, all have shown signs of cardiac failure, ranging from mild to severe. All have had diastolic gallop rhythms and Austin Flint murmurs associated with their severe aortic insufficiency. In almost all of these patients the cardiac enlargement has been extreme. In several instances, technical difficulties were encountered because the heart filled almost the entire left chest. Three patients have had clinical and x-ray evidence of mitral stenosis and have had exploration of the mitral valve at the same procedure. We have attempted to select patients whose predominant lesion was that of aortic insufficiency, with the exception of the three cases listed previously. All of the patients selected have had extremely wide pulse pressures, none having a diastolic pressure higher than 40 mm. Hg. Many of the patients have had angina pectoris. Further evidence of the severe disease in most of these patients is shown by conduction defects which were present in almost all. Liver disease secondary to cardiac disease has been common. One patient has had complete coarctation of the aorta associated with severe aortic insufficiency, and both lesions were corrected at the same procedure.

These patients have been classified using a grading similar to that used clinically for mitral stenosis, with the necessary allowances for the differences between aortic and mitral disease. All except four of these patients have been Class IV, the remainder Class III. It is interesting that in a patient* with a coarctation of the aorta, it was not possible to place the valve into the stump of the aorta since the area of coarctation extended to the take-off of the left subclavian artery. This made fixation of the valve in this location extremely difficult, if not completely impossible. Therefore, a portion, two inches long, of the distal aorta was dissected free and removed as a free aortic segment. This was then transplanted into the proximal aortic stump by direct suture technique. The valve was placed between this graft and the distal aorta. In essence, this constituted an autogenous aortic graft. This represents what we believe to be the first instance in which such an autogenous aortic graft has been placed in the human being. This patient has done extremely well postoperatively.

Anesthesia is a serious problem in such patients who are already suffering from conduction difficulties and who are, in the normal course of their disease, prone to sudden death. Two patients not included in this series were offered operation and died during induction of anesthesia before operation had begun. A technique has been developed† for induction and maintenance of these patients on an extremely light anesthesia, which has been most encouraging and which represents a major achievement in the control of these patients.

Among the first ten patients, there were four deaths. In the second series, Table I shows the distribution and the cause of death in the various categories. In the first group of ten patients, there was one death on the operating table

*Kindly referred to us by Dr. H. Shumacker.

†By Dr. Thomas McDermott, professor of anesthesiology, Georgetown University Medical Center.

of a terminal patient who had been bedridden for the past year. He had multiple decubiti and other evidences of severe debility. Death occurred during operation, but prior to the insertion of the aortic valve. This patient represents one in whom the operative procedure was not feasible because of the late stage of disease. Operation was offered to this patient as a last resort. One patient succumbed to subacute bacterial endocarditis some six weeks following operation. This apparently had been present preoperatively and had been in part responsible for his rapid decline prior to operation, although repeated blood cultures had been negative. The diagnosis was made at post-mortem examination. The patient had been treated with multiple antibiotics in large doses, all without results. One patient in this first group also died of an intractable pneumonitis, which was a causative agent in the onset of ventricular fibrillation in a patient with a severely impaired conduction system. This patient died several days after operation. One other patient succumbed ten days after operation, apparently of an acute cardiac arrhythmia. Autopsy showed no anatomic causes. Except for the death on the operating table, these deaths represent essentially complications of underlying disease.

TABLE I

	TOTAL	OPERATIVE MORTALITY	POSTOPERATIVE MORTALITY	LIVING AND IMPROVED
Series I (10 cases)				
Class III	1	0	0	1
Class IV	9	1 cardiac standstill	3: arrhythmias, 2; subacute endocarditis, 1	5
Series II (13 cases)				
Class III	3	0	0	3
Class IV	10	0	2: myocardial failure, 1; acute rheumatic fever, 1	8
Totals	23	1	5	17

In the second series of patients, one patient died of congestive failure several days postoperatively. This was another patient who was treated rather late in the course of disease with great difficulty in the control of failure. The second patient died of what appeared to be an acute exacerbation of rheumatic fever following operation associated with other complications not directly related to operation. We have thought that the most common cause of death in the postoperative period has been ventricular arrhythmia, and this has always been associated with serious degrees of conduction difficulties known preoperatively. We feel that patients with such conduction defects offer a very serious risk in contrast to those in whom there has been no serious change in rhythm.

There has been no case to date in which there has been evidence of failure of the valve to function or of clotting. The pulse contours in the lower extremities have become normal while those in the upper extremities have remained Corrigan in type. Electrocardiograms have shown no evidence of myocardial ischemia after or during operation, except as it existed prior to operation. Murmurs which have been present preoperatively have diminished after operation. There has been an increased exercise tolerance in all patients and a great decrease or absence of the necessity of mercurials. In all surviving patients there has been a dramatic improvement, which has been associated with a reduction in cardiac size as measured by x-ray film, as shown in a representative case in Fig. 5. This change in cardiac size can be noted in the first six weeks after operation. The rate at which this continues is not fully established because of the relatively short duration of the follow-up. It is believed that this decrease in cardiac size is due to decrease in dilatation of the left ventricle. In some patients there have been certain systolic murmurs at the apex which have been clinically interpreted as mitral insufficiency. No evidence of organic mitral insufficiency, however, could be found on exploration or on palpation of the auricle at operation. This type of murmur has diminished in relation to cardiac size.

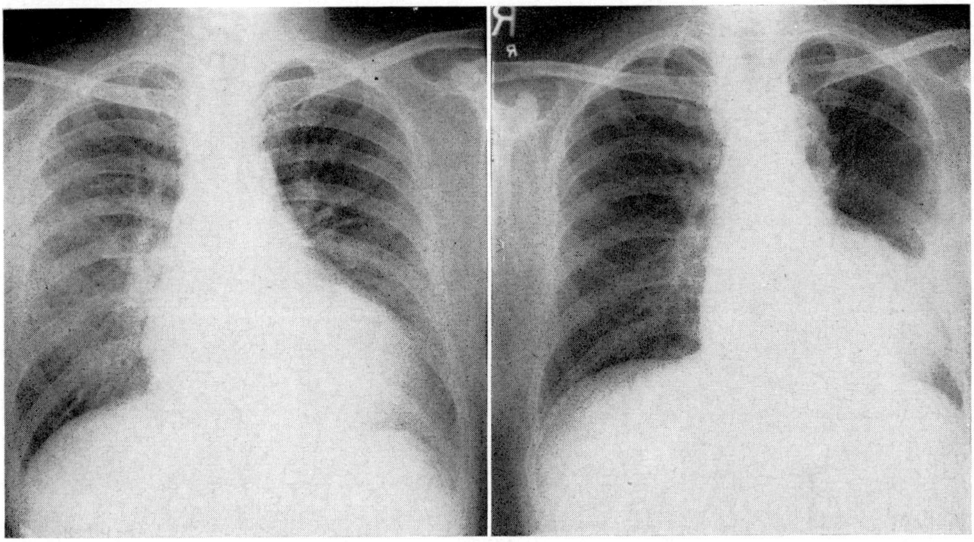

A. *B.*

Fig. 5.—*A* shows preoperative x-ray film of heart. Patient had an Austin Flint murmur and a diastolic gallop. *B* shows same patient one month after operation.

DISCUSSION

It is interesting to note that in the patients who comprise this series, the vast majority of cases of relatively pure aortic insufficiency are of rheumatic origin. Syphilitic disease has constituted only about 20 per cent of this group. The age of the patients has varied from 17 to 57 years. This is in sharp contrast to the common concept that rheumatic valvular involvement is predominantly that of aortic stenosis with little or no aortic insufficiency. One patient with syphilitic aortitis had an extremely thick aortic wall, which presented serious technical problems. However, it was possible to insert the valve and utilize the multiple-point fixation technique. Similarly, in the older age group of patients in whom there has been arterial atherosclerotic disease concomitant with the rheumatic process the use of multiple-point fixation has been most satisfactory.

The valve has been inserted into the descending aortic arch for several reasons. At this level there is a relatively long period of safety in which the aorta can be occluded without serious difficulty in the normal patient. We consider twenty minutes to be the maximal safe period. The actual insertion of the aortic valve usually requires between three and six minutes. The total period of occlusion in actual practice is within this range of time. In this location, approximately 75 per cent of the reflux is controlled. Attempts to place it in a more physiologic position were met with extreme difficulty. Technical difficulties which occlude the blood supply to the brain during insertion of the valve are very real. Air embolization by failure to eliminate all of the air from the valve is another serious problem. From techniques for deviation of the circulation, it would certainly be possible to place this valve in the ascending arch. On the basis of evidence from certain animal experiments which are not reported in detail here, we are questioning the validity of placing the valve in this location even if it were simple technically. However, we feel very strongly that these patients are in an extremely precarious physiologic state. Major manipulations near the heart and the great vessels are extremely hazardous. Attempts to explore the aortic valve during operation are always associated with serious arrhythmias. We feel that placing the valve in the aortic arch makes for minimal risk to the patient while maintaining almost all of the benefits by correcting the great majority of regurgitation.

In patients with combined aortic stenosis and insufficiency, it is very reasonable to suppose that by first placing the aortic valve in the aorta one might then proceed with an aortic valvulotomy. We have not encountered a patient in whom this appeared to be indicated; however, in the correction of aortic stenosis the dangers of producing insufficiency might be greatly minimized by the use of the valve.

After the valve has been inserted in the patient, the sound of the opening and closing of the prosthesis is readily audible, using the stethoscope. During the first few days postoperatively, the sound may be audible to the unaided ear. Patients are informed of this prior to operation. It has given rise to no difficulties in any patient to date. After the passage of several weeks to months, the sound gradually diminishes. This apparently is associated with covering of the valve with fibrous tissue. Proximity of the valve to the left main-stem bronchus always makes the valve audible if one listens to the patient who has the mouth open in a very quiet room. It is rather striking to note that most patients volunteer the information that while, prior to operation, they had the sensation of great throbbing throughout their entire body with each heart beat, and that at night the bed would usually pulsate with each cardiac contraction, this no longer occurs following operation.

CONCLUSION

Seventeen patients are now living and well following the insertion of an aortic valvular prosthesis. These patients have now been followed for periods of up to eleven months. These patients are greatly improved by the subjective and objective criteria. Currently, other types of prostheses are under study and further investigations as to the optimum site for the insertion of a valvular prosthesis are still under way. However, this group of patients represents the first attempt at the surgical correction of aortic insufficiency in patients. The results are extremely encouraging at this time.

REFERENCES

1. Hufnagel, C. A.: Resection and Grafting of the Thoracic Aorta With Minimal Interruption of the Circulation, Proc. Surg. Forum, Clin. Congress Am. Coll. Surgeons, 1948, Philadelphia, 1949, W. B. Saunders Company.
2. Hufnagel, C. A., and Eastcott, H. H. G.: Homologous Arterial Grafts, Bull. Georgetown Univ. Med. Center **4**: 119, 1952.
3. Bailey, C. P., Lacy, M. M., and Harris, J. S. A.: Surgical Treatment of Acquired Heart Disease, S. Clin. North America **31**: 1821, 1951.
4. Hirschboeck, J. S.: Delayed Blood Coagulation Time in Methyl Methacrylate Vessels, Proc. Soc. Exper. Biol. & Med. **47**: 311, 1941.
5. Hufnagel, C. A.: Permanent Intubation of the Thoracic Aorta, Arch. Surg. **54**: 382-389, 1947; Proc. Surg. Forum, Clin. Congress Am. Coll. Surgeons, 1946, Philadelphia, 1947, W. B. Saunders Company.
6. Walter, C. W., Murphy, W. P., Jr., Jessiman, A. G., and Ahara, R. M.: The Retardation of Clotting of Whole Blood on Contact With Stainless Steel, Proc. Surg. Forum, Clin. Congress Am. Coll. Surgeons, Philadelphia, 1951, W. B. Saunders Company, p. 289.
7. Hufnagel, C. A.: Plastic Valvular Prostheses, Proc. Surg. Forum, Clin. Congress Am. Coll. Surgeons, 1949, Philadelphia, 1950, W. B. Saunders Company.
8. Hufnagel, C. A., and Gillespie, J. F.: The Treatment of Aneurysms of the Aorta, Bull. Georgetown Univ. Med. Center **4**: 124, 1952.
9. Hufnagel, C. A., and Harvey, W. P.: The Surgical Correction of Aortic Regurgitation: Preliminary Report, Bull. Georgetown Univ. Med. Center **6**: 3, 1953.

TEMPORARY AORTIC OCCLUSION IN ABDOMINAL SURGERY

B. H. Burch, M.D., D. W. Traphagen, M.D., M. J. Folkman, D. A. Rosenbaum, and E. C. Mueller, M.D., Columbus, Ohio

(From the Department of Surgery, Ohio State University Medical School)

DURING the past year we have been interested in the use of aortic occlusion as a means of facilitating surgical procedures within the abdomen, and have suggested its trial in uncontrollable hemorrhage. Since all the viscera within the abdomen ultimately receive their blood supply from the aorta, it would appear that even the most furious of arterial hemorrhages within the abdomen could be controlled by aortic occlusion just above the celiac level. It is also apparent that regardless of the risk of aortic occlusion it cannot be greater than that of uncontrolled hemorrhage. In a previous report, aortic and portal vein occlusion as a method of obtaining hemostasis during partial hepatectomy was presented.[1] We have since used occlusion just above the bifurcation for one hour to facilitate the procedure of pelvic evisceration with minimal bleeding and without any complications.

Except for otherwise fatal conditions (aneurysms, emboli, and so forth), occlusion of the abdominal aorta has received little attention. Furthermore, we have been unable to find detailed studies which would indicate how long and at what levels the abdominal aorta may be occluded safely. We wished to determine the answer to this question (Series 1), record the effects on the cardiorespiratory system (Series 2), study the effect on blood electrolytes (Series 3), and attempt to improve survival by physical and chemical means (Series 4). In the latter three phases of the problem we have restricted our study to the celiac level for lethal periods of occlusion. Routine autopsy and microscopic sections were taken of each animal upon sacrifice or death. In this study, 114 dogs were employed.

PROCEDURE

Series 1.—The maximum safe time the aorta could be occluded above the celiac axis, superior mesenteric artery, renal arteries, and above and below the inferior mesenteric artery was determined by occluding the aorta with a Potts coarctation clamp for varying lengths of time. The time intervals employed are shown in Table I. Sterile operative procedures were carried out in each of 70 dogs. No special methods were employed to prolong their survival.

Series 2.—(a) Carotid and jugular pressures, pulse, and respiratory rates were determined in 5 dogs during a forty-minute period of aortic occlusion above the celiac axis and for one hour after release of the clamp (Table II).

Received for publication, Aug. 24, 1953.

Readings were taken every ten minutes, and the arterial pressures were recorded with a 0 to 760 mm. Hg pressure Statham gauge. Venous pressures were measured with a 0 to 300 mm. Hg pressure Statham gauge. These gauges were connected to a BL-320 Brush amplifier, and the output of the amplifiers was recorded simultaneously on a Brush Model BL-202 double-channel oscillograph. The pressure heads were connected to the animal by heavy-walled transparent plastic tubing, the latter being filled with heparinized isotonic saline solution. Arterial pressures were recorded from the left carotid artery, and venous pressures from the right jugular vein.

TABLE I. EFFECT ON SURVIVAL OF AORTIC OCCLUSION AT DIFFERENT LEVELS (70 DOGS)

MINUTES OCCLUDED	ABOVE CELIAC		ABOVE SUPERIOR MESENTERIC		ABOVE RENALS		ABOVE INFERIOR MESENTERIC		BELOW INFERIOR MESENTERIC	
	N	S	N	S	N	S	N	S	N	S
5	2	2								
10	2	2								
15	2	2								
20	2	2*								
30	2	1								
40	4	0								
60	4	0	2	2*	4	4*				
75			2	1	4	3				
90	4	0	2	0	4	1				
120			2	0	4	2				
150					4	2				
180					4	1	2	2*		
240							2	1		
300							2	1		
Ligation							5	0	5	3

N = number of dogs receiving aortic occlusion.
S = number of dogs surviving aortic occlusion.
*Maximum safe time.

TABLE II. MEAN VALUES DURING AND FOLLOWING FORTY MINUTES OF AORTIC OCCLUSION ABOVE THE CELIAC AXIS (5 DOGS)

	NORMAL	CLAMP ON	10 MIN.	20 MIN.	30 MIN.	40 MIN.	CLAMP OFF	10 MIN.	20 MIN.	30 MIN.	40 MIN.	50 MIN.	60 MIN.
Carotid pressure	155/123	181/152	207/157	211/166	206/161	196/157	96/59	120/94	116/89	113/88	115/84	114/83	110/79
Pulse per minute	137	111	104	127	136	137	141	128	130	135	137	139	139
Respiration per minute	22	22	21	26	25	24	29	26	25	25	22	24	24
Venous pressure (jugular in mm. H_2O)	23.2	26.0	31.1	22.1	19.5	26.0	11.7	9.1	9.1	1.30	15.6	22.2	24.8

(b) In another group, 3 dogs were employed in which the celiac, renal, and femoral pressures were measured simultaneously with carotid blood pressure while the aorta was occluded at different levels. These levels were just above the celiac axis, superior mesenteric artery, renal arteries, and above and below the inferior mesenteric artery (Table III).

Series 3.—Blood chemistries were taken in 5 dogs following sixty to ninety minutes' occlusion above the celiac axis when the animals were in profound shock just prior to death.

TABLE III. THE EFFECT OF VARIOUS LEVELS OF AORTIC OCCLUSION ON CAROTID BLOOD PRESSURE WHEN MEASURED SIMULTANEOUSLY WITH CELIAC, RENAL, OR FEMORAL PRESSURE; EACH SECTION REPRESENTS AN AVERAGE OF THREE DOGS

	NORMAL	BELOW INFERIOR MESENTERIC	ABOVE INFERIOR MESENTERIC	ABOVE RENALS	ABOVE SUPERIOR MESENTERIC	ABOVE CELIAC	CLAMP OFF	1 MIN. LATER
Carotid	123/86	134/95	130/88	145/95	175/119	188/137	66/47	136/92
Celiac	106/77	123/87	118/78	130/83	132/104	1	115/69	116/86
Carotid	141/107	146/112	132/99	145/114	159/130	189/155	78/49	139/99
Renal	130/94	142/101	131/92	18/0	9	9	122/90	119/85
Carotid	153/107	147/100	142/96	156/113	168/128	184/121	85/52	138/99
Femoral	156/101	21	22	13	23	16	136/85	134/99

Series 4.—(a) To determine whether or not cooling of the liver would aid in prolonging survival, the liver was cooled by means of rubber-covered copper tubing placed around the organ. A refrigerant solution of alcohol and acetone was cooled by passing it over dry ice and through the copper tubing by means of a pump. The liver temperature of the 9 dogs employed was kept between 10° and 20° C. by changing the speed of the pump. The aorta was clamped above the celiac axis for varying lengths of time, as recorded in Table IV.

TABLE IV. EFFECT OF AORTIC OCCLUSION ABOVE CELIAC AXIS ON SURVIVAL WHEN THE LIVER IS COOLED AND DRUGS ARE ADMINISTERED (31 DOGS)

MINUTES OF OCCLUSION	COOLED LIVER		DIBENZYLINE (MG./KG.) 1 MG.		3 MG.		4 MG.		5 MG.		6 MG.		AUREOMYCIN		ALLOXAN		VITAMIN E	
	N	S	N	S	N	S	N	S	N	S	N	S	N	S	N	S	N	S
40			1	0	2	2*	2	2*	1	0	1	0	1	0	1	1*	1	0
50			1	0	2	0	2	0	1	0	1	0	1	0	1	0	1	0
60	3	3*											1	0			1	0
75	2	1																
90	2	0																
120	2	0																

N = number of dogs receiving aortic occlusion.
S = number of dogs surviving aortic occlusion.
*Maximum safe time.

(b) Dibenzyline* in varying doses (1, 3, 4, 5, and 6 mg. per kilogram) was given intravenously to 14 dogs thirty minutes before occlusion of the aorta above the celiac axis. Aureomycin was given intravenously (30 mg. per kilogram) in another group of 3 dogs. Alloxan in doses of 15 mg. per

*Courtesy of the Smith, Kline & French Laboratories.

kilogram was given to 2 dogs thirty minutes before aortic occlusion above the celiac axis. Vitamin E was also tried on 3 dogs (1 Gm. intravenously). The length of occlusions is given in Table IV.

DATA AND DISCUSSION

Series 1.—It may be seen from Table I that the maximum safe time of occlusion just above the celiac axis is twenty minutes; the superior mesenteric artery, sixty minutes; above the renal arteries, sixty minutes; above the inferior mesenteric artery, three hours. It is apparent from the difference in the safe time of the celiac and renal series that it is safer to occlude below the celiac axis than above it, and that the organ probably responsible for this difference is the liver. It would appear that the kidneys are not the limiting factor at the celiac level, as the safe time at the renal arteries is one hour. In addition, survivals were observed when the aorta had been occluded just above the renal arteries for as long as three hours, indicating that there is considerable variability in the amount of kidney damage produced by occlusion. Hind limb paralysis was noted sporadically when the aorta was occluded longer than one hour above the renal arteries. When this occurred the animals always expired within a few days. It is interesting to note the survival time following occlusion. The dogs which expired following occlusion above the celiac axis did so within twelve hours. In the renal series, the dogs which expired did so on the third to fifth day. Bloody diarrhea, vomiting, and anuria appeared in the latter group, and were of grave prognostic significance.

Since the safe time above the inferior mesenteric artery was so long (three hours), it was decided to divide the aorta above the inferior mesenteric in 5 dogs. This was followed by 100 per cent mortality, with findings at autopsy of a gangrenous rectosigmoid and urinary bladder in each case. However, when 5 dogs had a ligation and division of the aorta just below the inferior mesenteric artery, the mortality was reduced to 40 per cent. A necrotic urinary bladder was found in the dogs which expired.

The microscopic findings in the animals which died following occlusion of the aorta above the celiac axis may be briefly summarized as focal necrosis of the liver with little evidence of renal damage. In the animals which died following occlusion just above the renal arteries, no liver damage was noted; however, renal damage strongly suggestive of lower nephron nephrosis was observed.

Series 2.—The average values of blood pressure, pulse, respiration, and venous pressure may be seen in Table II during and following forty minutes of occlusion of the abdominal aorta, just above the celiac axis.

The effects of thoracic aortic occlusion on blood pressure, pulse, respiration, and venous pressure were noted as long ago as 1886.[2] However, the cardiovascular response as affected by the duration of the occlusion has not been found, nor have the effects of systematic clamping at various levels within the abdomen. Our findings are similar to those obtained when the thoracic aorta is occluded, namely, a rise in carotid blood pressure followed by a fall upon release of the clamp.[2-5] Most important is the failure of blood pressure to reach the normal pressures at one hour. We have repeatedly observed marked hypotension prior to death. Pulse rate decreased markedly on application of the clamp above the celiac axis, and increased shortly after the removal of the clamp. This is probably due to the effects of the carotid and aortic sinus reflexes. Respiration and venous pressure were variable. It may be seen from inspection of Table II that venous pressure increases temporarily on application of the clamp and falls suddenly on removal.

The average values for the blood pressures measured in the celiac, renal, and femoral arteries simultaneously with carotid arterial pressures can be seen in Table III. The effect of clamping the aorta at higher and higher levels was a progressive increase in the carotid blood pressure. The same effect was noted in the renal and celiac arteries, except when the aorta was occluded above them, which resulted in a marked fall in blood pressure (Table III).

Series 3.—Blood chemical determinations in 5 dogs receiving aortic occlusion above the celiac axis for sixty to ninety minutes were made before occlusion and shortly before the animals expired. Comparing the postocclusion chemistries with the dogs' predetermined normals indicates no change in the cephalin flocculation time, thymol turbidity, total protein and albumin-globulin ratio, and prothrombin time. A moderate rise in the blood urea nitrogen and fall in CO_2 volumes per cent accompanied by a slight rise of potassium were noted in 2 dogs. It was our impression that these blood chemical changes were not of sufficient magnitude to account for the deaths resulting from occlusion above the celiac axis.

Series 4.—(a) At the present time, cooling the liver appears to be the most promising method of increasing the safe time of aortic occlusion above the celiac axis. It should be noted, however, that occlusion above the celiac axis cannot, even with cooling, be prolonged beyond one hour (Table IV). Sacrifice, at one month, of each of the survivors showed no gross changes, and microscopic sections showed minimal changes of the liver and kidneys.

(b) The effects of drugs in prolonging the maximum safe time of occlusion above the celiac axis may be seen in Table IV. Dibenzyline is seen to give protection in 3 to 4 mg. per kilogram doses, increasing the safe time to forty minutes of occlusion above the celiac axis. Alloxan appears promising, but Aureomycin and vitamin E were not effective in providing protection against the effects of aortic occlusion in the dose employed (Table IV).

It should be stated that the exact mechanism of death following aortic occlusion above the celiac axis is unknown. It seems clear, however, that the liver and kidneys play a predominant role in the outcome following aortic occlusion and that hypotension results from prolonged aortic occlusion above the celiac axis. We suspect that the mechanisms outlined by Shorr and associates[6] are involved when the aorta is occluded above the celiac axis and that VDM is one of the factors leading to fatalities when the time of occlusion is too long.

CONCLUSIONS

1. The maximum safe time of aortic occlusion just above the celiac axis is twenty minutes, above the superior mesenteric artery sixty minutes, above

the renal arteries sixty minutes, and above the inferior mesenteric artery three hours (60 dogs).

2. The mortality rate of ligation and division of the aorta just above and just below the inferior mesenteric artery is 100 per cent and 40 per cent, respectively (10 dogs).

3. Following lethal occlusions of the aorta above the celiac axis, carotid blood pressure does not return to normal, and continues to decline until death (5 dogs).

4. There is a progressive rise of celiac, renal, and carotid arterial pressures when occlusion of the aorta approaches these vessels from below, and a prompt fall in pressure occurs when the occlusion site is above them (3 dogs).

5. Cooling of the liver (10° to 20° C.) allowed sixty minutes of occlusion above the celiac axis without fatalities (9 dogs).

6. Dibenzyline and alloxan appear to exert protection from the effects of occlusion above the celiac axis; Aureomycin and vitamin E did not offer lasting benefit in the doses employed (22 dogs).

7. The liver and kidneys appear to play a dominant role in determining the outcome following aortic occlusion. Microscopic evidence of focal liver necrosis and renal tubular damage occurs in lethal occlusions above the celiac axis (all dogs).

8. Blood chemistries just before death in fatal aortic occlusions above the celiac axis were not of sufficient magnitude to account for the deaths (5 dogs).

Acknowledgment.—We wish to express our appreciation to Dr. Mel A. Davis for his careful review of the microscopic sections and helpful suggestions.

REFERENCES

1. Burch, B. H., Traphagen, D. W., and Folkman, M. J.: The Use of Aortic Occlusion in Abdominal Surgery With a Report of Two Human Cases, SURGERY **34**: 672, 1953.
2. de Jager, S. J.: Experiments and Considerations on Haemodynamics, J. Physiol. **7**: 130, 1886.
3. Barcroft, H. J.: Cardiac Output and Blood Distribution, J. Physiol. **71**: 280, 1931.
4. Watkins, E.: Circulatory Changes Produced by Clamping of Thoracic Aorta, SURGERY **22**: 530, 1947.
5. Clatworthy, H. W., and Varco, R. L.: A Small Bore Polythene Shunt to Prevent Mechanical Shock After Prolonged Cross-Clamping Thoracic Aorta, Proc. Soc. Exper. Biol. & Med. **74**: 434, 1950.
6. Shorr, E., Zweifach, B. W., and Furchgott, R. F.: On the Occurrence, Sites and Modes of Origin and Destruction, of Principles Affecting the Compensatory Vascular Mechanisms in Experimental Shock, Science **102**: 489, 1945.

COMPARISON OF LATE SEQUELAE OF COMMON AND SUPERFICIAL FEMORAL VEIN LIGATIONS

JOHN R. ROBINSON,* M.D., AND CARL A. MOYER, M.D., ST. LOUIS, MO.

(From the Department of Surgery, Washington University School of Medicine)

THE purpose of this clinical investigation was the examination of the physical consequences of ligation and division of the superficial and the common femoral veins of human beings. The clinical indications for the interruption of these veins are shown graphically in Fig. 1.

This study consists of observations of two groups of patients treated at the Wayne County General Hospital between 1944 and 1947. Between the first days of September, 1944, and January, 1946, thirty-one ligations of the common femoral veins of twenty-eight persons were performed (Series I).

From March 1, 1946, to Nov. 1, 1947, forty-three ligations of the superficial femoral veins of thirty-six persons were completed (Series II). All but three† individuals of both series were examined repeatedly until Nov. 1, 1952, or until they died. Consequently, the follow-up period of Series I is roughly eight years long and for Series II it is six and one-half years.

The selection of the site of ligation was not varied between Sept. 1, 1944, and April 1, 1945; the common femoral vein was always interrupted. Between April 1, 1945, and Jan. 1, 1946, the ligation and transection of the common femoral vein were performed only when clotted blood was found in it; when no clot was found in it, the superficial femoral vein was interrupted. After Jan. 1, 1946, only ligations of the superficial femoral systems were carried out, even though the clot extended into the common vein. When clotting extended proximal to the point of junction of the deep with the superficial vein, proximal aspiration was performed through an opening into the superficial vein. Afterward it was ligated above and below the incision and divided. Whenever free backflow was not attained after aspiration, the superficial vein was ligated and divided and anticoagulants were given.‡

The actual lengths of the observation periods are shown in Table I.

No operative deaths occurred in either series, although the operation was performed upon twelve persons while they were critically ill.

The age distribution of both series were statistically the same. The combined age distribution is shown in Fig. 2. Seemingly, thrombosis in the Wayne County General Hospital was somewhat associated with aging.

The ligations and divisions of the veins were performed through vertical incisions in order to minimize the transection of major lymphatic vessels and to provide adequate exposure. The femoral artery was meticulously avoided.

Received for publication, Sept. 19, 1953.

*Kankakee, Ill.

†The status of these three individuals as of Nov. 1, 1952, was determined by correspondence because change of residence made it impractical to see them.

‡In a number of instances when free backflow was not obtained, the hole in the vein was closed with sutures, and sole reliance was placed in anticoagulants; these cases are not included in this study.

TABLE I

YEAR	SERIES I: COMMON FEMORAL VEIN,* NUMBER OF PATIENTS	SERIES II: SUPERFICIAL FEMORAL VEIN, NUMBER OF PATIENTS
Original group	28	36
1 yr.	22	36
2 yr.	16	36
3 yr.	15	34
4 yr.	12	33
5 yr.	10	32
6 yr.	10	18
7 yr.	8	
8 yr.	7	

The progressive decline in numbers of individuals in Series I during the eight-year period is due to death; that in Series II is due to the same cause up to the sixth year. The difference in the number of patients between the five- and six-year periods of Series II is due to the fact that fourteen of the thirty-two had been operated upon between March 1 and Nov. 1, 1947, and therefore had not yet lived six years after the operation by Nov. 1, 1952.

*Number of patients of the series living at end of year.

It was never freed from its bed because of the impression that such a maneuver was a possible cause of the vasospasm observed in a number of instances prior to the beginning of this effort.

The sequelae of particular interest of the ligation of the superficial and common femoral veins were: (1) persistent brawny edema, (2) dermatitis and cellulitis, (3) varicose veins, and (4) ulceration.

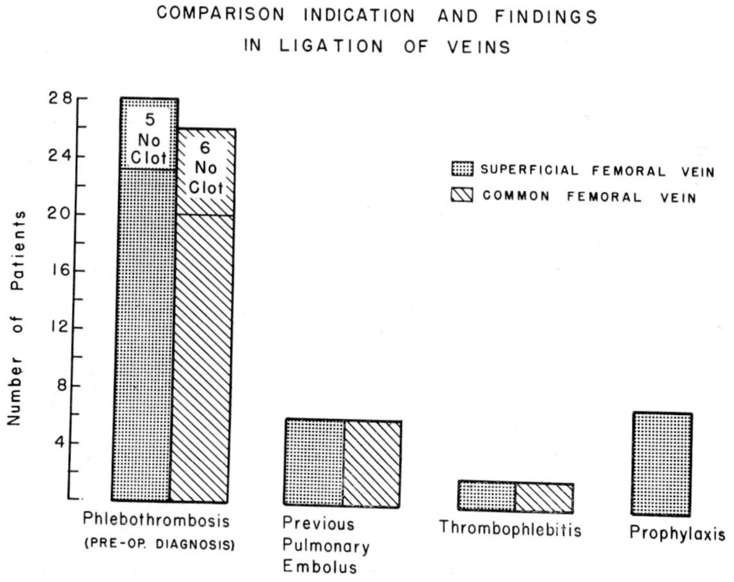

Fig. 1.

Table II contains the incidence of these sequelae at one, four, and eight, and one and five years for ligations of the common and superficial femoral veins, respectively. The percentile occurrences of edema, dermatitis, cellulitis, varicose veins, and ulceration after ligation of the superficial and common femoral veins are shown in Figs. 3 through 6.

TABLE II. INCIDENCE OF SEQUELAE OF LIGATION AND DIVISION OF COMMON FEMORAL VEIN AND SUPERFICIAL FEMORAL VEIN

SITE OF INTERRUPTION	COMMON FEMORAL VEIN			SUPERFICIAL FEMORAL VEIN	
YEARS AFTER OPERATION	1	4	8	1	5
Brawny edema	19 of 22	10 of 12	6 of 7	2 of 36	2 of 32
Varicose veins	12 of 22	12 of 12	7 of 7	2 of 36	6 of 32
Ulceration	10 of 22	10 of 12	5 of 7	1 of 36	1 of 32
Dermatitis and cellulitis	6 of 22	5 of 12	7 of 7	2 of 36	2 of 32

DISCUSSION

The ligation and division of the common femoral veins of man are followed by an inordinately high incidence of undesirable physical phenomena relative to the incidence of the same obtaining after ligation and division of the superficial femoral veins. The probability that chance alone could account for the observed differences is so small (see Table III) that the difference between the incidences of complications in the two series is significant. These late complications of ligations of the common femoral vein are of sufficient magnitude to collectively prevent the self-support of most of the individuals suffering them (see Fig. 7).

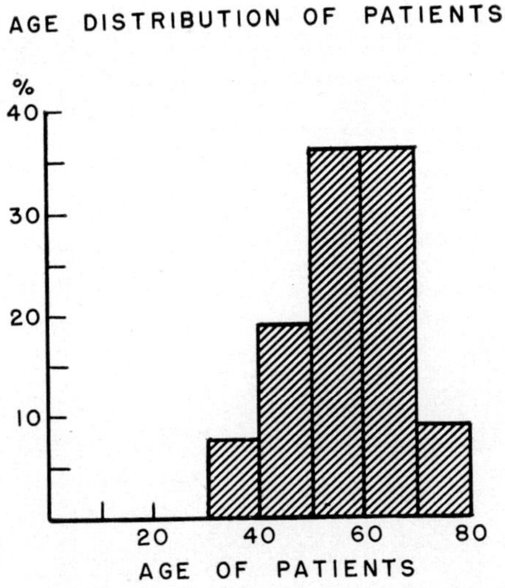

Fig. 2.

TABLE III. STATISTICAL COMPARISON

COMPLICATIONS	CHI SQUARE VALUES	PROBABILITY
Edema	26.000	< 0.001
Varicose veins	42.6297	< 0.001
Dermatitis	7.885	< 0.01
Ulcers	29.93946	< 0.001
Rehabilitation	18.0053	< 0.001

The reasons for the inordinately high incidence of late complications of ligation and division of the common femoral vein relative to that following the same procedures upon the superficial femoral system are not apparent.

Fig. 3.

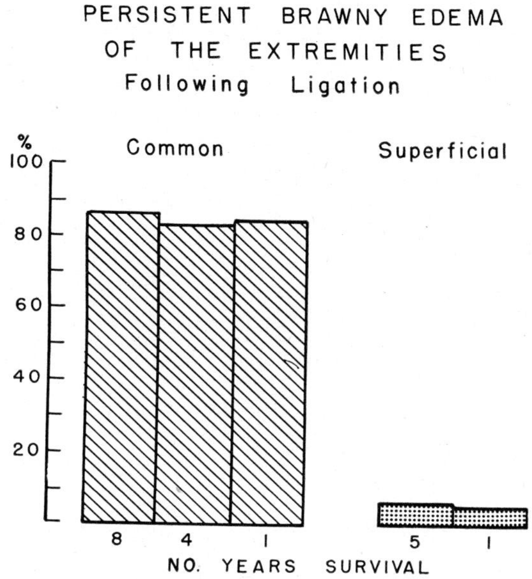

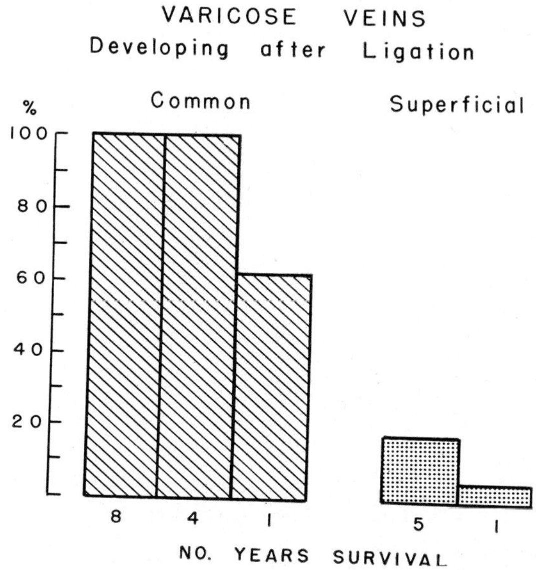

Fig. 4.

Conjecturally, the frequency and magnitude of the sequelae that follow the interruption of the deep veins of an extremity have been ascribed to the extent of the venous disease existing at the time of the ligation. A study of Table IV leads to doubt concerning this concept, for, although the cases are few, they indicate that the site of the ligation of the deep venous system is more significant than the extent of the thrombosis prior to the ligation.

Fig. 5.

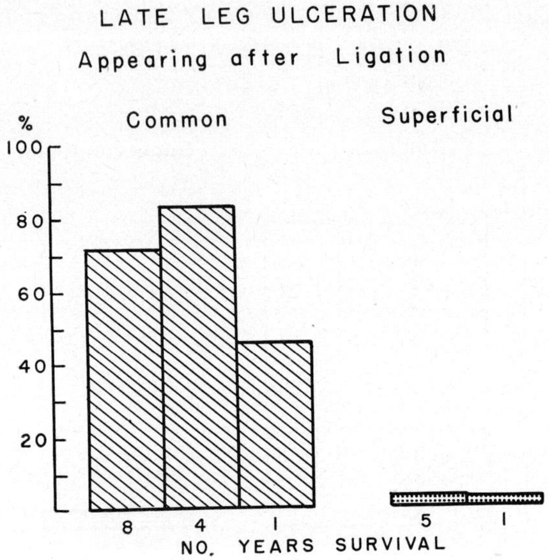

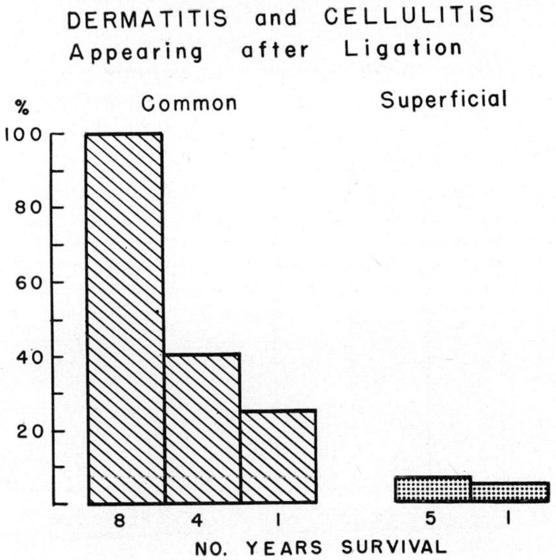

Fig. 6.

Although four patients of the six who had the common femoral veins interrupted when no clot was present in them died before one year had passed, all of them had developed varicose veins and brawny edema before they died. The two others suffered from all of the complications by the end of the first postoperative year. On the other hand, one year after ligation and division of the superficial femoral vein in the absence of clot in the vein at the groin, none of twelve individuals had varicose veins, dermatitis, brawny edema, or ulcers, and only two of eight had varicose veins alone at the end of five years.

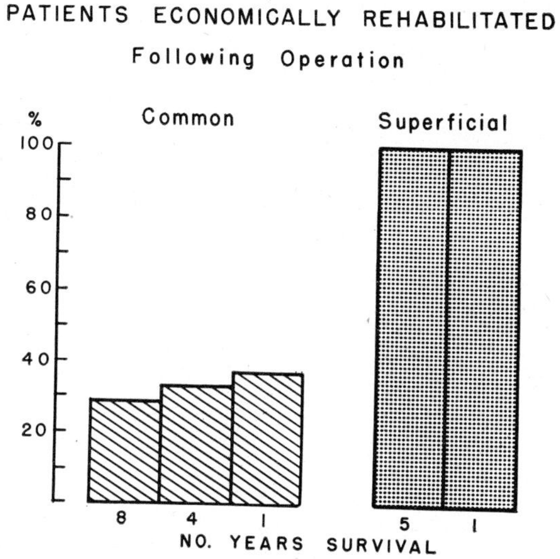

Fig. 7.

The temporal relationships between the various postligational sequelae are interesting in that they may be indicative of the etiological relationship of one to the other. Brawny edema appears first in practically all instances; nineteen of twenty-two persons showed it within one year after the ligation of the common femoral vein. Varicose veins tend to appear next, and dermatitis and ulceration follow. Postligational varicosities are not the sole factors in

TABLE IV. RESULTS OF BOTH TYPES OF LIGATIONS WHEN NO CLOT WAS PRESENT AT OPERATION

	COMMON FEMORAL VEIN — ERROR IN DIAGNOSIS — NO. OF CASES AND YR.			SUPERFICIAL FEMORAL VEIN — ERROR IN DIAGNOSIS — NO. OF CASES AND YR.				SUPERFICIAL FEMORAL VEIN — PROPHYLACTIC — NO. OF CASES AND YR.			
SEQUELAE	ORIGINALLY 6	ONE YR. 2	FOUR YR. 1	ORIGINALLY 5	TWO YR. 5	THREE YR. 4	FIVE YR. 4	ORIGINALLY 7	ONE YR. 7	THREE YR. 5	FIVE YR. 4
Edema		2	1		0	0	0		0	0	0
Varicose veins		2	1		0	0	1-2		0	0	1-2
Cellulitis, dermatitis		2	1		0	0	0		0	0	0
Ulcers		2	1		0	0	0			0	0
Economically rehabilitated		0	0		5	4	4		7	5	4

the etiology of brawny edema, ulceration, and dermatitis. All of the seven persons who lived eight years after the ligation and division of the common femoral vein had the acquired varices ligated and excised repeatedly, and yet five developed ulcers and six developed brawny edema. The chronic edema, ulceration, and dermatitis were checked to some extent, but not prevented or cured by removal and ligation of the varicose veins as they came. Therefore, the relationship of varicose veins to the other postligational sequelae is still speculative.

The causes of the hard edema which usually precedes ulceration are unknown. The hypertrophy of the epidermis, the subepidermal fibrosis and hyaline degeneration in it, the dilatation of the superficial lymphatic channels, and the hypertrophy of the superficial investing fascia of muscle which characterize the histologic picture of long-standing brawny edema are accompaniments of chronic lymphatic obstruction. However, no objective evidence for the existence of lymphatic stasis prior to the onset of brawny edema was obtained in these cases, so that no definitive statement can be made regarding the possible etiological role that might be played by postligational disturbances in lymphatic flow. Studies are now in progress in regard to this.

For a time, vasospasm was considered the primary etiological factor in the inception of the postligation syndrome. However, lumbar sympathectomy had no objective, long-term ameliorating, or curative effect on it. Between the second and fifth postoperative years, the lower lumbar ganglionic sympathetic chain was excised from six of the seven persons who were alive and who suffered from ulceration eight years after common femoral interruption. No prolonged improvement was noted in any case: universally the hard edema and ulcers recurred or persisted. Conceivably, in a few cases inadequate sympathectomy could have accounted for the failure to effect any prolonged beneficial influence on the postligational sequelae, but it is improbable that it could account for the universal failure. Therefore, it appears that vasospasm may be fairly safely discounted as the predominant cause of the edema, ulceration, and dermatitis following interruption of the common femoral vein. No transposition of the conclusions drawn from these observations to postphlebitic and varicose ulcerations should be made. The additional conditions imposed by ligation and division of the common vein may mitigate the possible effects of sympathectomy.

In so far as the selection of the site for the interruption of the deep venous system when indications for it exist, ligation of the common femoral system is to be avoided. A small personal experience* with individuals upon whom ligations of the inferior vena cava have been performed below the renal veins for extensive acute thrombotic disease with repeated pulmonary embolization provides us with the tentative conviction that ligation of the cava below the renal veins is less conducive to the induction of incapacitating complications than are ligation and division of the common femoral system.

*Three patients, all of whom have remained free of brawny edema and ulceration for four to eight years. All of them have extensive varices of both lower extremities.

Ligation and division of the superficial femoral vein can be performed with relative impunity.

CONCLUSIONS

1. Within one to eight years after ligation and division of the common femoral vein, incapacitating sequelae appear in more than three-fourths of the persons operated upon; however, ligation and division of the superficial femoral vein are attended by the same sequelae, with a frequency of less than one in ten.

2. Interruption of the common femoral vein is to be avoided.

3. Lumbar sympathectomy has no long-term curative influence on postligational ulceration, dermatitis, varicosities, or brawny edema.

4. The etiologies of the postligational sequelae are unknown. Apparently, the site of ligation is the primary determinant of ulceration, dermatitis, and brawny edema attending ligation and division of the deep veins of the lower extremity.

Acknowledgments.—We wish to thank Dr. M. Musselman and Dr. R. Gillespie of the Wayne County General Hospital, Eloise, Mich., for their cooperation in helping us to obtain part of the material used in this study.

AN EFFECTIVE CLINICAL METHOD FOR DETERMINING COAGULATION TIME OF BLOOD

Its Significance in the Presence of Intravascular Clotting

Patrick C. Shea, Jr., M.D., Roy L. Robertson, M.D., and D. C. Elkin, M.D., Atlanta, Ga.

(From the Whitehead Department of Surgery, Emory University, and the Grady Memorial Hospital)

The coagulation time of blood is frequently utilized in the study of hemorrhagic diseases and in the evaluation of heparin therapy. Its reliability as a clinical test has often been questioned because of the variability of the results obtained. This dissatisfaction is manifested by the large volume of papers offering new techniques or modifications of others. Lee and White,[1] as early as 1913, citing Cohen, wrote, ". . . in a very complete paper on the 'Coagulation Time,' . . . (he) has discussed thirty-one methods and their modifications." To add to the confusion, no uniformity is found even among the descriptions of particular modifications of specific methods.

This report presents a method which is believed to be more effective clinically than previously reported ones. More elaborate ones are available, some utilizing electromechanical recording devices.[2] This method can be performed with simple apparatus in the laboratory, doctor's office, or at the bedside. It is practical and economical, and requires only such equipment as is already available in every clinic or hospital. It has been used by a variety of staff personnel under diverse conditions, including daily and room temperature variations, and has been found to give consistent, accurate results on like samples of blood.

A survey of the literature was first made, and several methods of coagulation time determinations were selected for trial. After a number of these proved inadequate in one respect or another, the method reported here was devised from several by incorporating portions which seemed desirable. This procedure, therefore, is not entirely original.

EQUIPMENT AND METHOD

The necessary equipment consists of five serially numbered, standard Wassermann tubes (12 by 75 mm.), a 10 c.c. Luer syringe, a small serologic tube rack, a 19 gauge needle, alcohol or acetone sponges, tourniquet, and stop watch.

All coagulation times were performed at room temperature with seasonal variations indoors ranging from 72° to 90° F. The syringe and needle were dry and sterile; the tubes were chemically clean, oven-dried, and allowed to at-

The study reported herein was supported in part by a contract from the Veterans Administration on recommendation of the National Research Council's Committee on Veterans Medical Problems.

The heparin used in this study was supplied by The Upjohn Company, Kalamazoo, Mich.

Received for publication, Sept. 8, 1953.

Fig. 1.

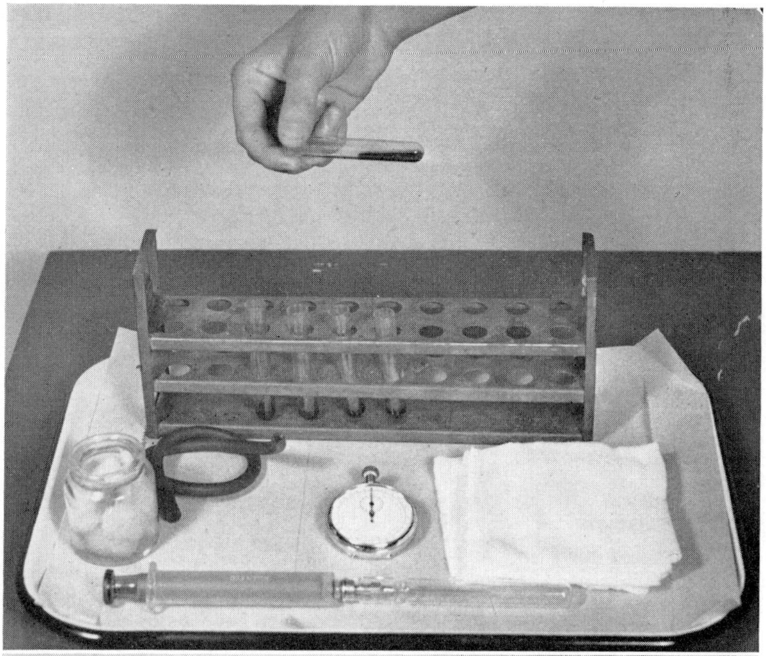

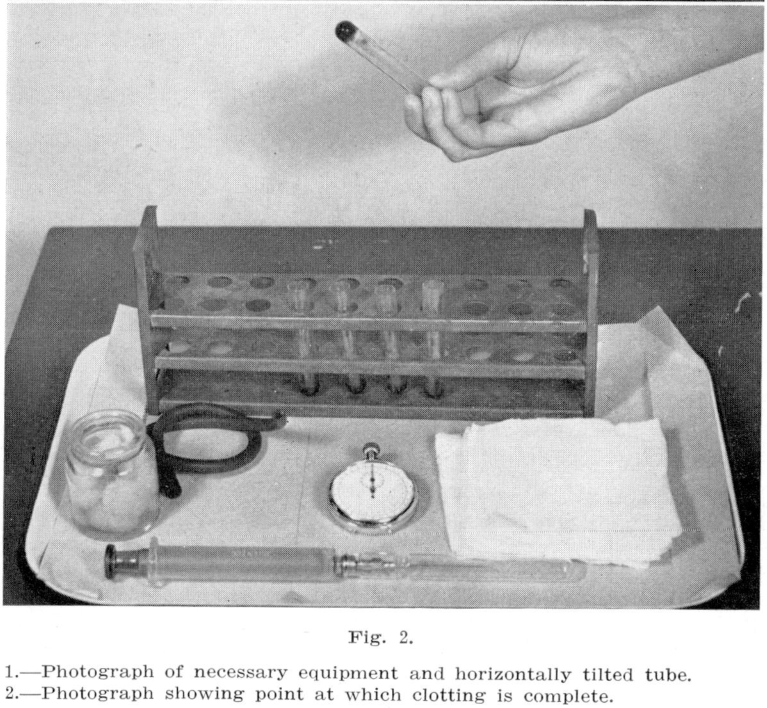

Fig. 2.

Fig. 1.—Photograph of necessary equipment and horizontally tilted tube.
Fig. 2.—Photograph showing point at which clotting is complete.

tain room temperature before being used. If the glass surfaces of any of the tubes or syringes which were to come in contact with the blood were etched, scratched, or broken, they were discarded.

The needle, with syringe attached, was inserted into a suitable arm vein after the usual preparation for venipuncture. Simultaneously with the appearance of blood in the syringe tip, the tourniquet was released and the stop watch was started. Aspiration was begun only after blood appeared in the syringe. Three to four cubic centimeters of blood was then rapidly, but gently, aspirated and the needle was withdrawn. Only those samples obtained by clean venipuncture were considered acceptable for the determination. If the syringe or needle was contaminated by tissue juice which contains thromboplastin, the blood sample was discarded, new equipment was obtained, and the procedure was repeated. Quick and associates[3] have stated that "even in taking blood by venipuncture enough tissue thromboplastin may occasionally gain entrance to reduce significantly the coagulation time, as Jacques and his co-workers have recently demonstrated."

The needle was removed from the syringe and 0.5 c.c. of blood was decanted carefully into each of the five glass tubes held upright in the test-tube rack. The tubes were filled in the reverse order of their intended examination (5, 4, 3, 2, 1).

Three minutes from the instant that blood first appeared in the syringe, Tube 1 was tilted from vertical to horizontal and replaced in the rack (Fig. 1). This process was repeated every thirty seconds until complete clotting occurred. The end point was defined as that time at which blood no longer ran along the surface of the horizontally tilted tube (Fig. 2). If the serum and cells separated into layers, the end point was defined as the time at which clotting became complete in all the layers. As soon as the end point was reached in the first tube, Tube 2, heretofore undisturbed, was tilted similarly every thirty seconds until its end point was reached. Serially, in like manner, the end points of the other three tubes were obtained. The end point of the fifth tube was recorded as the coagulation time of the blood.

CLINICAL STUDY

To determine the efficacy of the method, the study was submitted to clinical trial and statistical analysis of the data. Because the majority of thromboembolic diseases occur among hospitalized patients, both the diseased and control groups were selected from hospital patients. Several variables were thus eliminated. Control patients were on a similar diet, and the majority were in bed at least one-half of their waking hours. Excluded from the control group were patients recovering from operations, and those who had hepatic or renal disease, proved or suspected hemorrhagic diathesis, thrombosis or embolism (suspected or known), and those who were receiving or had recently received anticoagulants.

In many instances, duplicate examinations were made by different technicians on the same blood sample and on samples drawn at different periods. Daily variations and temperature effects were recorded. Among control patients with coagulation times of twenty to twenty-two minutes, the daily variation was less than one minute in repeated examinations. The variation between similar samples run in a water bath at 37° C. and those run at room temperature was one-half minute or less. In similar samples run by different technicians, it was never greater than one to one and one-half minutes.

These variations were considered of minor importance, since the error with commonly used methods is frequently as high as 10 per cent. Such slight deviations proved even less significant among the diseased patients, in whom the desired therapeutic range would be approximately three times normal, or pretreatment, coagulation time. If, with adequate dosage of heparin, the coagulation time of a patient whose pretreatment time was twenty minutes should be increased to approximately sixty minutes, a variation as great as three minutes would give an error of only 5 per cent.

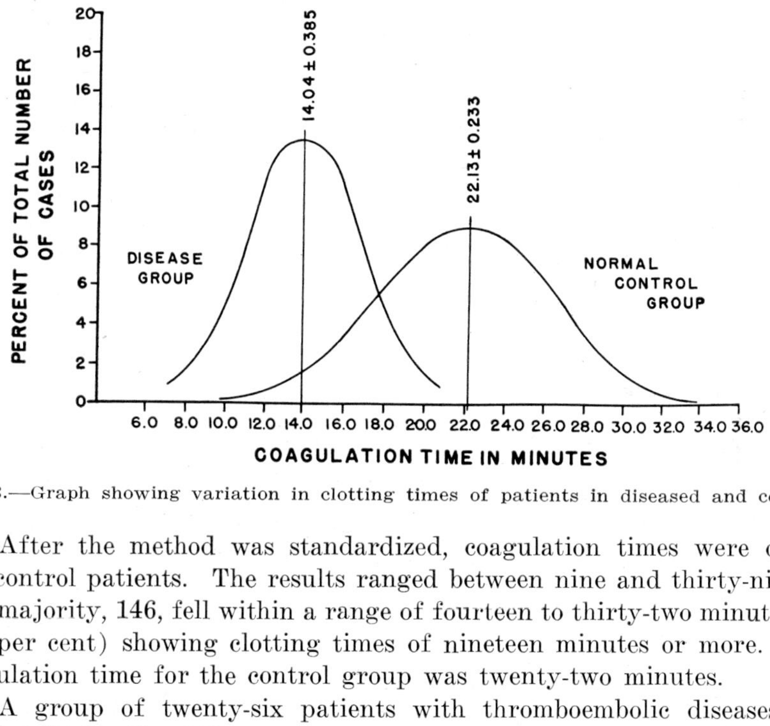

Fig. 3.—Graph showing variation in clotting times of patients in diseased and control groups.

After the method was standardized, coagulation times were obtained on 150 control patients. The results ranged between nine and thirty-nine minutes. The majority, 146, fell within a range of fourteen to thirty-two minutes, with 129 (86 per cent) showing clotting times of nineteen minutes or more. The mean coagulation time for the control group was twenty-two minutes.

A group of twenty-six patients with thromboembolic diseases was then studied (Table I). Whereas the mean coagulation time for the control patients was twenty-two minutes, it was only fourteen minutes for this group with intravascular clotting (Fig. 3).

Statistically, this variation between health and disease was significant.* An increased rate of clotting time as determined by this method would, therefore, draw attention to the possibility of intravascular clotting, or confirm it if sus-

*Statistical analysis of the data showed the sigma of the mean to be 0.363 for the control group and 0.587 for the diseased group; the sigma of the difference was 0.690. The critical ratio was found to be 11.6. When Fisher's t was calculated, the probability was found to be less than 0.001.

These findings indicate that the data subjected to analysis were of statistical significance.

pected. It would likewise influence both the heparin tolerance curve and the calculated dose of heparin. If the clotting time of a patient is to be maintained with heparin at or above three times his normal or pretreatment level, the desired rate becomes a relative figure rather than one arbitrarily set for all patients.

In a concurrent study, the height and duration of the rise in clotting time following administration of heparin were found by this method to be roughly proportional to the quantity injected, its physical state and medium, and the patient's tolerance for heparin.[4]

TABLE I. CLOTTING TIMES OF PATIENTS WITH THROMBOEMBOLIC DISEASES

CASE NUMBER	DISEASE	COAGULATION TIME (MINUTES)
1	Thrombosis, right femoral artery	11
2	Thrombosis, left popliteal artery	16.5
3	Embolus, left popliteal artery	16
4	Embolus, left popliteal artery	13
5	Embolus, right femoral artery	16
6	Embolus, bifurcation of aorta	14
7	Thrombosis, left popliteal artery	11
8	Thrombosis, right subclavian artery	6.5
9	Thrombosis, left femoral artery	17.5
10	Superior mesenteric artery thrombosis	17
11	Superior mesenteric artery thrombosis	14.5
12	Venous mesenteric thrombosis	13.5
13	Pulmonary infarct	11.5
14	Pulmonary infarcts	14
15	Pulmonary infarct	10
16	Pulmonary infarcts	10
17	Pulmonary infarct	14
18	Bilateral thrombophlebitis, femoral	19.5
19	Superficial and deep femoral thrombophlebitis, left	16
20	Superficial and deep femoral thrombophlebitis, right	13.5
21	Thrombophlebitis, axillary vein (postoperative)	15.5
22	Phlebothrombosis, lower extremity	17.5
23	Thrombophlebitis, lower extremity	13.5
24	Lateral sinus thrombosis	14.5
25	Priapism	17
26	Gangrene, right foot, arterial thrombosis	9
Mean		14

DISCUSSION

Quick,[3] in referring to coagulation time methods, has stated that "trustworthy results can be obtained only by performing the test under constant and rigidly controlled conditions and by excluding all outside agents that influence the coagulation reaction." He has also mentioned the need for a simple, uniform procedure. In discussing the Lee-White test, he said: "This procedure . . . yields as much and as accurate information as any test of coagulation so far devised, but unfortunately 'the test has not been rigidly standardized and at present there is no strict uniformity in the details of the procedure.' "

Ideally, coagulation time should be determined by withdrawing blood without trauma, allowing it to remain in a clean tube unmolested by air currents or motion until that precise instant when the coagulation end point is about to be reached, then suddenly inverting the tube and confirming the presence of a well-formed clot. This may only be approximated in actual practice. By increasing the number of tubes to five and allowing the last one to remain for a longer time undisturbed by agitation or tilting, it is more nearly approached than when fewer tubes are used and the factor of agitation has a greater effect on shortening the coagulation time. The brief interval frequently observed between the clotting times of the fourth and fifth tubes indicates that the last tube was often ready to clot spontaneously when its turn for agitation came (Fig. 3).

The temperature gradient appears to have little influence on the results of this test, which has more tubes and increased accuracy. When the variation in clotting time between similar samples which are run in a water bath at 37° C. and at room temperature, within the seasonal range of extremes mentioned, was found to be one-half minute or less, the water bath was eliminated. With certain other methods,[1, 4] it has also been found that room temperature does not significantly affect the clotting time.

Consistent results on similar samples of blood were obtained by this method by different personnel under different conditions. Such slight variations as occurred represented smaller percentile errors than those usually found with other methods. If a method is accurate to only one minute, when a one-tube procedure is used wherein the tube is gently tilted every thirty seconds to produce a normal clotting range of five to eight minutes, an error of one minute equals 12.5 to 20 per cent. Using three tubes, with a range between nine and fourteen minutes, a one-minute error equals 7 to 11 per cent. With the described five-tube method, however, having a range between eighteen and twenty-six minutes, an error of one minute decreases the percentile difference to between four and five. Certainly, if a shortened coagulation time is to be considered a possible indication of intravascular clotting, a method with 5 per cent error or less is preferable to one with 10 to 20 per cent.

Many clinicians have preferred Dicumarol (3,3′-methylenebis [4-hydroxycoumarin]) to heparin in anticoagulant therapy because the method of determining prothrombin times has been well standardized, whereas methods of coagulation time determinations have varied widely when performed by different personnel in different hospitals. Furthermore, because adverse results can also occur during heparin therapy, it is important to have a method which is consistent and from which as many variables as possible have been removed. Altered coagulation times as determined by the method described here provide an accurate laboratory control in the use of heparin.

SUMMARY

A method for determining the coagulation time of blood is presented. The essentials are atraumatic transfer of blood from vein to receptacle, the use of clean, dry, unscarred glass tubes of uniform size, and minimal agitation or exposure of the final tube.

The method is simple, effective, and as useful clinically as it is in the experimental laboratory. Because it requires only readily available apparatus and eliminates the need for constant temperature, it can be used at the bedside, in the home, office, or hospital with comparable results. It gives reproducible results in the hands of both well-trained and relatively inexperienced personnel, and has been found to give checks of within one minute when performed by different technicians from day to day.

It has produced uniform, accurate results of statistical significance in a group of 150 hospital patients without evidence of intravascular clotting and in a second group of twenty-six patients with thrombosis or embolism, in whom a significant lowering of coagulation time was observed.

It is emphasized that valid and comparable results can be obtained only if a uniform method is used with strict adherence to the selected technique.

We wish to express our appreciation to Mary Elizabeth Shannon, B.S., for her technical assistance in this study.

REFERENCES

1. Lee, R. I., and White, P. D.: A Clinical Study of the Coagulation Time of Blood, Am. J. M. Sc. **145**: 495-503, 1913.
2. Barker, N. W., and Barker, D. N.: A Coagulochronometer: A Device for Automatically Recording the Coagulation Time of Whole Blood, Proc. Staff Meet., Mayo Clin. **23**: 230-233 (May) 1948.
3. Quick, A. J., Honorato, C., and Stefanini, M.: Value and Limitations of Coagulation Time in Study of Hemorrhagic Diseases of Blood, Blood **3**: 1120-1129 (Oct.) 1948.
4. McCleery, R. S., Yarborough, J. A., and Weidner, M. G.: The Silicone-Tube Coagulation Time as an Aid in the Diagnosis of Phlebothrombosis, Surgery **31**: 28-42 (Jan.) 1952.
5. Robertson, R. L., and Shea, P. C.: The Effect of Intravenous Heparin Upon the Prothrombin Time. To be published.

NUTRITION FOLLOWING SUBTOTAL GASTRECTOMY OF FOUR TYPES (BILLROTH I AND II, SEGMENTAL, AND TUBULAR RESECTIONS)

LLOYD D. MACLEAN, M.D., JOHN F. PERRY, M.D., WILLIAM D. KELLY, M.D., DONN G. MOSSER, M.D.,* ANGELINE MANNICK, B.S.,** AND OWEN H. WANGENSTEEN, M.D., MINNEAPOLIS, MINN.

(From the Departments of Surgery, Radiology, and Nutrition, University of Minnesota Medical School)

ABNORMAL weight loss after subtotal gastrectomy is a frequent occurrence. Ivy, Grossman, and Bachrach[1] collected 864 cases from the literature, in 42 per cent of which the patients had lost weight following subtotal gastrectomy. In a recent report from this hospital, the average weight after operation of 893 patients who had undergone subtotal gastrectomy was 15.3 pounds below the usual preoperative weight.[2] Many of these patients are asymptomatic except for an inability to gain weight.

This investigation has been conducted to determine the etiological factors of importance causing weight loss after gastric resection so that therapeutic measures may be more intelligently applied. The relative importance of the following factors have been assessed: abnormal fat and nitrogen loss in the stool, decreased oral intake, pancreatic function as assessed by the secretin test following subtotal gastrectomy, and the possible significance of gastrojejunal anastomosis versus gastroduodenal anastomosis with and without preservation of vagus nerve continuity.

Many opinions in the literature concerning postgastrectomy nutrition are clinical impressions. The only reliable methods of investigation presently available to obtain objective information on this subject are metabolic (intake-output balance) studies and accurate records of weight change after operation.

METHODS

This investigation was conducted on thirty-five patients who had undergone the following operations three months to five years previously: Billroth I and Billroth II subtotal gastrectomy, segmental gastric resection,[3] and tubular gastric resection[4, 22, 23] Fig. 1). The patients chosen for investigation were not specially selected as being nutritional problems, nor as having particularly good results. The decision of who should be admitted to the hospital for study rested entirely with the patients.

All patients were admitted to the hospital for a period of eight to ten days, during which time the following studies were performed:

Supported by funds made available to the investigators through institutional grants from the American Cancer Society and the Damon Runyon Fund.

Received for publication, Sept. 26, 1953.

*Department of Radiology.

**Department of Dietetics.

1. Routine history and physical examination with special inquiry into eating habits and gastrointestinal symptoms.

2. Determination of hemoglobin, erythrocytes, leukocytes, and differential, mean cell diameter, reticulocytes, blood urea nitrogen, and total serum protein.

3. Roentgenologic examination with barium of the esophagus and upper gastrointestinal tract, as well as estimation of the transit time to the cecum in most cases.

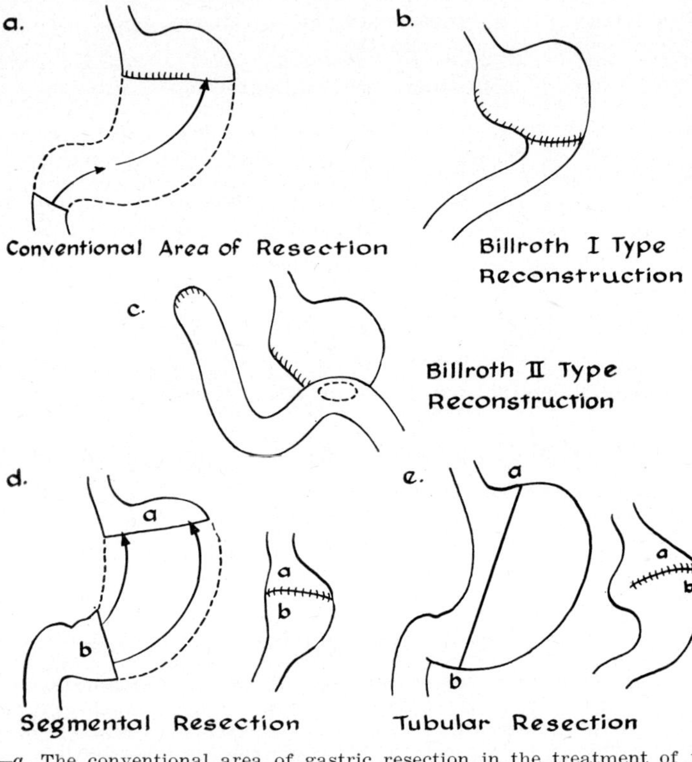

Fig. 1.—*a*, The conventional area of gastric resection in the treatment of peptic ulcer is the distal three-quarters of the stomach.

b, Billroth I reconstruction is an end-to-end anastomosis between the duodenum and cut end of the stomach with a Hofmeister closure of the lesser curvature.

c, Billroth II reconstruction with gastrojejunostomy and short afferent loop.

d, Segmental gastric resection is a three-quarter resection principally of the acid-producing area. Anastomosis is performed between the antrum and a very small fundic pouch. A Heineke-Mikulocz pyloroplasty is mandatory to permit satisfactory gastric emptying.

e, Tubular gastric resection is an excision of two-thirds of the stomach. The area of excision is the entire length of the greater curvature. Reconstruction is by means of transverse gastroplasty without interruption of the vagus nerves. The antrum remains. A pylorotomy is optional, and is performed only for obstruction and in the presence of massive hemorrhage for a duodenal ulcer. Duodenal ulcer is the chief indication for tubular resection.

4. Measurement of fecal fat and nitrogen excretion. Three- to four-day stool collections were used, with carmine dye orally to mark the interval. A weighed diet containing 145 Gm. of carbohydrate, 80 Gm. of fat, and 80 Gm. of protein with a total of 1,620 calories was offered, and the amount eaten was calculated. Intake was charted as for a person with diabetes, so that the actual quantity ingested was known. Fecal fat was determined by the method of Fowweather,[8]

and fecal nitrogen by the method of Kjeldahl.[9] Fat excretion in the stool was reported as percentage of ingested fat. Fecal nitrogen was reported in grams per day in the stool.

5. Study of pancreatic function by aspiration of the intestinal content below the gastric pouch before and after administration of secretin intravenously. Two tubes were placed in the gastrointestinal tract under fluoroscopy. One tube with a mercury balloon at the tip was placed as close as possible to the ampulla of Vater. A nine-hole gastric tube was positioned in the gastric pouch. Both tubes were placed on suction. The intestinal aspirate was collected under ice and frozen, and the following determinations were made: volume, pH, amylase, lipase, trypsin, and bicarbonate. Two thirty-minute fasting samples were collected, following which secretin, 1 unit per kilogram, was administered intravenously, and three twenty-minute samples were collected. The division of samples after secretin stimulation serves no useful purpose; therefore, all results are combined for the one-hour collection period. The pH was determined with a glass electrode. Amylase was determined by the method of Somogyi,[10] trypsin by the method of Dorothy Anderson,[11] and lipase by a modification of the method of Cherry and Crandall.[12]

RESULTS

Metabolic Studies Following Billroth II Procedure.—Nine patients who had undergone Billroth II resection were studied by intake-output balance methods. The weight loss, fat and nitrogen excretions in the stool, and estimated percentage of normal food intake since operation are tabulated in Table I. The normal fat excretion on a diet containing 80 Gm. of fat is 5 per cent of intake.[5] Over 10 per cent fecal excretion of fat intake is distinctly abnormal; 7.5 to 10 per cent is a borderline abnormality. On this basis, three of the nine patients were excreting abnormally large quantities of fat in the stool, one was borderline, and five were within normal limits. One patient, J. M., was excreting 37 per cent of ingested fat in the stool—the greatest loss encountered in this study. Weight loss was not entirely due to fat loss since two patients with normal fat excretion lost twenty-five and eighteen pounds, respectively. These patients were eating only 60 to 75 per cent of the amount ingested prior to surgery.

After the Billroth II procedure, three patients were excreting an excessive amount of nitrogen in the stool. The upper limit of normal excretion is 2 Gm. of nitrogen per day when the diet does not contain an excess of indigestible nitrogenous or nonnitrogenous roughage.[6] Diarrhea was prominent in only two of the patients; one of these patients was excreting an abnormal amount of both fat and nitrogen.

Metabolic Studies Following Billroth I Procedure.—Following Billroth I procedure, five patients underwent investigation as outlined (Table II). Four of the five lost an excessive amount of weight. Only one of the five patients excreted an abnormal amount of fat (10 per cent of intake). Nitrogen excretion was normal in all cases. Weight loss in all instances was closely related to decreased oral intake.

Table I. Fecal Fat and Nitrogen Loss in Relation to Weight Change After Billroth II Gastric Resection

Patient	Age (yr.)	Weight loss (pounds)	Interval between operation and study (mo.)	Fat loss* as per cent of intake	Nitrogen† loss in stool (grams per day)	Per cent of normal food intake	Small bowel transit time	Gastric emptying time (min.)	Diagnosis
1. H. E.	66	10	16	4.4	0.53	75+	2 hr.+	10	Duodenal ulcer
2. R. C.	59	15	10	9.0	1.27	75+	2 hr.+	10	Duodenal ulcer
3. T. W.	40	18	24	3.4	0.50	60	6 hr.	Immediate	Carcinoma of stomach
4. A. A.	68	5	36	6.8	1.30	100	5 hr.	15	Carcinoma of stomach
5. O. G.	56	7	42	17.7	2.45	100	2 hr.	—	Carcinoma of stomach
6. J. M.	67	30	26	37	6.67	75	20 min.	5	Gastric ulcer
7. W. W.	66	0	82	3	0.31	100	2 hr.+	60	Duodenal ulcer
8. A. R.	51	25	14	4	0.67	75	30 min.	15	Gastric ulcer
9. J. F.	56	25	24	10	2.30	50-75	—	30	Gastric ulcer

*Normal fat loss in stool when patient is ingesting 80 Gm. of fat in diet is 5 to 7.5 Gm. (7.5 to 10 Gm. is borderline, over 10 Gm. is abnormal).

†Normal fecal nitrogen excretion is under 2 Gm.

Table II. Fecal Fat and Nitrogen Loss in Relation to Weight Change After Billroth I Gastric Resection

Patient	Age (yr.)	Diagnosis	Weight changes (pounds)	Interval between operation and study (mo.)	Fat loss in per cent of intake	Nitrogen loss (grams per day)	Per cent of normal food intake	Small bowel transit time	Gastric emptying time (min.)
1. D. E.	24	Duodenal ulcer	–18	7	4.5	0.66	50	30 min.	10
2. A. A.	77	Gastric ulcer	–15	18	6	1.68	75	7 hr.	20
3. I. M.	70	Jejunal ulcer	–20	18	7	0.5	50	3.5 hr.	10
4. C. H.	67	Gastric ulcer	–20	8	5	1.06	75	2 hr.+	20
5. A. K.	65	Duodenal ulcer	–25	6	10	1.2	50	6 hr.	30

TABLE III. FECAL FAT AND NITROGEN LOSS IN RELATION TO WEIGHT CHANGE AFTER SEGMENTAL GASTRIC RESECTION

PATIENT	AGE (YR.)	DIAGNOSIS	WEIGHT CHANGE (POUNDS)	INTERVAL BETWEEN OPERATION AND STUDY (MO.)	FAT LOSS IN PER CENT OF INTAKE	NITROGEN LOSS (GM./DAY)	PER CENT OF NORMAL FOOD INTAKE	SMALL BOWEL TRANSIT TIME	GASTRIC EMPTYING TIME (MIN.)
1. F. B.	61	Duodenal ulcer	–28	12	6	—	75	3 hr.	120
2. E. A.	52	Duodenal ulcer	–42	9	7.3	1.21	50	2 hr.	10
3. O. L.	52	Duodenal ulcer	–80	17	12	2.2	50	40 min.	40
4. H. M.	36	Duodenal ulcer	–30	12	11.6	1.4	60	2 hr.+	5
5. A. L.	65	Duodenal ulcer	–30	14	10.5	0.68	75	—	30
6. C. S.	69	Duodenal ulcer	–15	13	9.2	0.95	75	3 hr.	20
7. F. O.	53	Duodenal ulcer	–20	17	5.8	1.2	75	4 hr.	40
8. E. M.	50	Duodenal ulcer	+16	8	5.6	1.58	100	1.5 hr.	90
9. A. R.	50	Duodenal ulcer	–20	24	3.5	1.2	50	2 hr.	30
10. E. G.	63	Duodenal ulcer	–10	17	7	1.2	60	6 hr.	40
11. J. W.	60	Duodenal ulcer	–20	16	9	1.1	100	—	30
12. W. O.	51	Duodenal ulcer	–35	13	2.1	—	50	2 hr.+	45
13. L. L.	64	Duodenal ulcer	–15	16	5	0.75	75	4.5 hr.	90
14. J. P.	49	Duodenal ulcer	–30	26	12	0.98	60	4 hr.	10
15. F. R.	58	Duodenal ulcer	–50	23	5	0.90	60	9 hr.+	60
16. F. E.	46	Duodenal ulcer	–18	18	11	1.4	60	4 hr.	30

TABLE IV. FECAL FAT AND NITROGEN LOSS IN RELATION TO WEIGHT CHANGE AFTER TUBULAR GASTRIC RESECTION

PATIENT	AGE (YR.)	WEIGHT LOSS (POUNDS)	INTERVAL BETWEEN OPERATION AND STUDY (MO.)	FAT LOSS IN PER CENT OF INTAKE	NITROGEN LOSS IN STOOL (GRAMS PER DAY)	PER CENT OF NORMAL FOOD INTAKE	SMALL BOWEL TRANSIT TIME	GASTRIC EMPTYING TIME (MIN.)	DIAGNOSIS
1. W. H.	44	20	4	4	1.36	75	—	—	Duodenal ulcer
2. L. L.	40	20	5	6	2.6	75	2 hr.+	30	Duodenal ulcer
3. G. Cl.	39	25	6	4.5	0.4	50-60	—	—	Duodenal ulcer
4. G. C.	44	30	6	5	0.5	50-60	30 min.	30	Duodenal ulcer
5. Y. R.	46	10	5	4.3	1.3	90	—	40	Duodenal ulcer

Metabolic Studies Following Segmental Resection.—Following segmental gastric resection,[3] sixteen patients underwent intake-output balance tests (Table III). Five were excreting distinctly abnormal quantities of fat in the stool, three were borderline, and eight patients were excreting normal quantities of fat in the stool.

Only one patient excreted a slightly elevated quantity of nitrogen in the stool.

Metabolic Studies Following Tubular Resection.—Five patients, four of whom had lost an excessive amount of weight following tubular gastric resection,[4, 22, 23] were investigated (Table IV). No abnormal or borderline abnormality of fat excretion exists. One patient excreted a slightly elevated quantity of nitrogen in the stool. Diarrhea is not present, but decreased oral intake is prevalent in this group of five patients.

Results of Metabolic Studies.—On the basis that 5 to 7.5 per cent of fat intake excreted in the stool is normal, 7.5 to 10 per cent is borderline, and over 10 per cent is distinctly abnormal, thirty-five patients who had undergone subtotal gastrectomy were studied. Eight of the thirty-five patients were excreting abnormal quantities of fecal fat (up to 37 per cent of oral intake in one patient). Five of the thirty-five patients were excreting borderline quantities of fecal fat, and the remaining twenty-two patients were within normal limits.

A distinctly abnormal loss of nitrogen in the stool (6.67 Gm. per day) was found in only one patient.

On the basis of the patients' opinion of the quantity of food ingested compared to the amount ingested preoperatively, when well, one can state that weight loss following gastrectomy is often due to decreased caloric intake. All patients were repeatedly questioned on oral intake and closely observed while in the hospital in order to obtain a reliable approximation of oral intake. While this method is subject to error in individual cases, we feel it supplies excellent information on groups such as this. Of 172 cases of tubular and segmental gastric resection, all patients who weighed the same as before operation (within five pounds of their usual weight) volunteered they were eating 100 per cent of what they did before operation. Many patients who had lost an excessive amount of weight (over twenty pounds) either could not ingest the 1,620 calorie diet while in the hospital or felt uncomfortably full after doing so. The dumping syndrome or early postprandial distress was precipitated by single large meals, which was a limiting factor in some cases, preventing a larger total caloric intake. These patients had learned that they could avoid the distress of palpitation, perspiration, nausea, drowsiness, and weakness by eating smaller quantities of food. Smaller meals at frequent intervals only partially compensates for the decreased caloric intake in these patients. Diets with the caloric content composed of variable amounts of fat and carbohydrate are being investigated at the present time.

Pancreatic Function Following Subtotal Gastrectomy.—In addition to intake-output balance study of fat and nitrogen excretion, secretin tests were performed on twenty-eight of the previously mentioned patients and on five normal persons, as outlined under Methods. It is not unreasonable to assume that pancreatic secretion would be reduced after subtotal gastrectomy. The effective stimuli to pancreatic secretion are (1) vagus nerve stimulation, (2) secretin mechanism—lowering of the pH of the duodenum to 4 leads to the production of secretin, which in turn stimulates external pancreatic and biliary secretion.

Following subtotal gastrectomy the acid-producing capacity of the stomach is markedly lowered and the vagus nerve supply to the pancreas is probably interrupted. Two patent sources of pancreatic stimulation are thereby lost or diminished in effect.

Since patients with steatorrhea on a pancreatic basis with excessive fat loss in the stool do show a marked depression of response to secretin, this test was used to evaluate pancreatic function following subtotal gastrectomy.

Results of Pancreatic Function Tests.—A group of five young normal persons was given the secretin test as outlined. The results are illustrated in Table V. The tests performed on patients who had undergone subtotal gastrectomy are illustrated in Tables VI, VII, VIII, and IX.

TABLE V. SECRETIN TEST ON NORMAL HUMAN BEINGS

PATIENT	VOLUME (C.C.)	pH	HCO_3 (C.C.)	AMYLASE (SOMOGYI UNITS)	TRYPSIN (GELATIN TUBES LIQUEFIED)	LIPASE (C.C. OF 0.05 N NaOH*)
1. F. S.	222	7-9	155	45,600	2-9	0.55
2. P. L.	110	8	63	16,550	6-9	—
3. M. E.	31.5	7-8	81	17,450	3-9	0.50
4. K. S.	73	7-8	28	15,200	4-9	0.38
5. B. J.	93	7+	30	46,400	4-6	0.90

Dilutions of duodenal juice used:

Tube		*Duodenal Juice*
1	0.125	1-100
2	0.25	1-100
3	0.5	1-100
4	1.0	1-100
5	0.2	1-10
6	0.4	1-10
7	0.8	1-10
8	1.6	1-10
9	0.32	undiluted
10		

*The lowest dilution in which the gelatin has liquefied in one or both tubes (duplicates) is considered as the reading.

All pancreatic function tests performed on the Billroth I group of patients are completely within normal limits in all respects. One patient, J. M., showed no pancreatic response to secretin stimulation following the Billroth II procedure. This patient has severe diarrhea with excessive fat excretion in the stool (37 per cent of intake), which has been partially relieved by pancreatin in large doses. A corrective diet for sprue and Banthine were ineffective in the treatment of this patient. This was the only patient examined in whom reduced pancreatic function probably is of importance in increased fat loss in the stool following subtotal gastrectomy. Following Billroth II gastrectomy, two other patients, H. E. and T. W., had below average volume responses to secretin; however, fat excretion is well within normal limits and nitrogen loss in the stool in the patients is completely normal.

TABLE VI. RESULTS OF SECRETIN TEST FOLLOWING BILLROTH II SUBTOTAL GASTRIC RESECTION

PATIENT	VOLUME (C.C.)	pH	HCO_3	AMYLASE (SOMOGYI UNITS)	TRYPSIN (GELATIN TUBES LIQUEFIED)	LIPASE (C.C. OF 0.05 N NaOH)	FAT EXCRETION (PER CENT OF INTAKE)	WEIGHT CHANGE (POUNDS)	PANCREATIC FUNCTION
1. H. E.	3.5	7	0	133,750	qns	qns	4.4	–10	Abnormal
2. B. C.	100	7+	109.1	111,600	5.6	1.9	9	–15	Normal
3. T. W.	14	7.3	0	31,100	4-9	0.72	3.4	–18	Abnormal
4. J. M.	0.5	8	—	—	—	—	37	–30	Abnormal
5. J. F.	43	7+	35	173,700	—	—	10	–25	Normal
6. A. S.	208	7+	6.2	56,250	7-9	0.2	4	–25	Normal

TABLE VII. RESULTS OF SECRETIN TEST FOLLOWING BILLROTH I SUBTOTAL GASTRIC RESECTION

PATIENT	VOLUME (C.C.)	pH	HCO_3	AMYLASE (SOMOGYI UNITS)	TRYPSIN (GELATIN TUBES LIQUEFIED)	LIPASE (C.C. OF 0.05 N NaOH)	FAT EXCRETION (PER CENT OF INTAKE)	WEIGHT CHANGE (POUNDS)	PANCREATIC FUNCTION
1. D. E.	235	7-8	58	140,000	5-7	0.6	4.5	–26	Normal
2. A. A.	84	7+	24	111,600	5-7	1.0	6	–15	Normal
3. I. M.	172	6.5	68	100,500	5-6	0.5	7	–10	Normal
4. C. H.	57	8+	134	130,500	5-7	1.3	5	–25	Normal
5. A. K.	33	7.5	85	63,200	4-5	0.09	10	–25	Normal

TABLE VIII. RESULTS OF SECRETIN TEST FOLLOWING SEGMENTAL GASTRIC RESECTION

PATIENT	VOLUME (C.C.)	pH	HCO_3	AMYLASE (SOMOGYI UNITS)	TRYPSIN (GELATIN TUBES LIQUEFIED)	LIPASE (C.C. OF 0.05 N NaOH)	FAT EXCRETION (PER CENT OF INTAKE)	WEIGHT CHANGE (POUNDS)	PANCREATIC FUNCTION
1. J. P.	8.2	7-8	0	3,840	7		12	–40	Abnormal
2. F. E.	72.5	7-7.5	22	70,450	4-7	3.3	11	–24	Normal
3. A. R.	76	8.5-9.3	154.1	98,400	—	9.9	3.5	–20	Normal
4. E. G.	24.5	8.1-8.5	69.0	78,050	—	2.0	7	–10	Normal
5. J. W.	220	7.6-7.9	55	73,500	4-6	0.5	9	–20	Normal
6. C. A.	63	8.9-9.1	96.3	22,740	7-8	0.04	—	–15	Normal
7. E. A.	60	7.4-7.6	13.6	3,650	4-9	13.4	7.3	–22	Normal
8. E. M.	44	7.0	59	4,100	3-9	0.45	5.6	+16	Normal
9. O. L.	21.9	8-8.4	92	45,000	6	3.9	12	–80	Abnormal
10. H. M.	199	8.8-8.6	52	51,400	6-7	9.5	11.6	–30	Normal
11. A. L.	110	7.3-8.7	54.2	54,040	6-7	0.4	10.5	–50	Normal
12. C. S.	72	7.8-7.9	149	47,400	7-8	0.2	9.2	–20	Normal
13. F. D.	11.2	8.2	97	42,350	—	2.0	5.8	–20	Abnormal

TABLE IX. RESULTS OF SECRETIN TEST FOLLOWING TUBULAR GASTRIC RESECTION

PATIENT	VOLUME (C.C.)	pH	HCO_3	AMYLASE (SOMOGYI UNITS)	TRYPSIN (GELATIN TUBES LIQUEFIED)	LIPASE (C.C. OF 0.05 N NaOH)	FAT EXCRETION (PER CENT OF INTAKE)	WEIGHT CHANGE (POUNDS)	PANCREATIC FUNCTION
1. W. H.	47.7	7-8	50.1	318,700	6	2.3	4	–20	Normal
2. L. L.	0.9	+8		441,600			6	–30	Abnormal
3. G. C.	56.1	7.6-9.6	0	157,200	8	0.5	5	–30	Normal
4. Y. R.	124	+7	66	328,000	4	0.1	4.3	–10	Normal

Of sixteen patients who were examined following segmental resection, two (J. P. and O. L.) had excessive fat loss and showed a subnormal pancreatic response to secretin (Table VIII). Neither patient was excreting excessive quantities of nitrogen in the stool.

Following tubular gastric resection, one patient, L. L., had a subnormal response to secretin; however, this patient's excretion of fat in the stool was within the normal range.

Summary.—The pancreatic function of twenty-eight patients following subtotal gastrectomy of four types was examined by means of the secretin test. Eleven of these patients were excreting distinctly abnormal or borderline quantities of fecal fat. In only three of the eleven patients could excessive fat loss possibly be attributed to pancreatic insufficiency on the basis of the secretin test. In only one of these patients was there an excessive excretion of nitrogen in the stool, characteristic of pancreatic insufficiency.

DISCUSSION

The possible causal factors of weight loss following gastrectomy have been stated by many authors[6, 16-18] to be one or more of the following: increased fat loss in the stool due to diminished pancreatic flow or imperfect mixing of foods and ferments; increased intestinal motility; loss of gastric digestion; and loss of gastric reservoir.

For the purposes of this investigation, normal weight is the usual weight of the patient for five years prior to operation, so that abnormal changes due to diet or obstruction immediately preceding the operation are eliminated. On this basis, thirty-two of the thirty-five patients lost weight. The average loss was twenty-one pounds.

Gastroduodenal continuity does not prevent excessive fat loss in the stool, since this occurred following segmental gastric resection.

Increased fat loss is not constantly accompanied by diarrhea or increased small bowel motility on roentgen examination. One patient who excreted 37 per cent of fat intake had a twenty-minute small bowel transit time, while a patient, following the same operation, who had a thirty-minute small bowel transit time was excreting only 4 per cent of fat intake (Table I). A thin barium meal was used in all cases. A mixture of barium and food possibly would give a more accurate picture of small bowel motility after partial gastric resection. Many patients, after partial gastrectomy, experience abdominal cramps after eating, which last for ten to thirty minutes and are aggravated by further eating. This probably represents hypermotility of the upper small bowel and may be important in separating the ingested food from pancreatic enzymes.

The gastric emptying time following Billroth II resection is rapid, usually being under thirty minutes (Table I). This circumstance is corroborated by Dr. Rigler and Dr. Nice of the Radiology Department of the University of Minnesota, who have examined a much larger series than is here reported.[21] Gastric emptying time after tubular and segmental gastric resection is usually thirty minutes or longer (Tables III and IV). No correlation exists, however, between rapid gastric emptying and weight loss or increased fecal fat excretion.

Increased fecal fat excretion occurs frequently following segmental resection and Billroth II subtotal gastric resection. With one exception, however, the fat losses were not great and cannot account entirely for major weight losses in patients. Excessive fat loss has not occurred after tubular gastric resection where vagus nerve continuity is preserved. The possibility exists that vagus nerve continuity is of importance in preventing excessive fecal fat excretion.

That these effects of vagotomy are not due to pancreatic insufficiency is suggested by the predominantly normal secretin tests and a normal stool nitrogen in all but one patient in this study. Furthermore, Routley and co-workers,[14] working with dogs, found that vagotomy had no effect on pancreatic functions when secretion was stimulated by food, acid, and alcohol in the upper gastrointestinal tract.

Fox and Grimson[13] studied nine patients who had lost weight following vagotomy. Three of the patients had undergone vagotomy alone, six vagotomy and gastroenterostomy. Eight of the nine patients were excreting an excessive amount of fat. One patient was excreting 33 per cent of intake (normal is 5 per cent).

Vagotomy may adversely affect intestinal enzyme secretion. Savich and Soshestvensky[15] have demonstrated an increased secretion of succus entericus in the cat on vagal stimulation both in volume and enzyme concentration. A large dose of atropine diminished or even completely arrested the intestinal secretion of these enzymes. This problem deserves further investigation.

Of the factors assessed to account for weight loss in the thirty-five patients who had undergone partial gastrectomy, decreased oral intake or loss of gastric reservoir is of greatest importance. Many patients whose fecal fat and nitrogen excretion were within normal limits had lost over ten pounds of weight. These patients were eating considerably less in twenty-four hours, however, than prior to surgery. A disagreeable feeling of fullness or precipitation of the dumping syndrome or rapid satiety prevented many of these individuals from ingesting greater quantities even with six meals a day.

Increased fecal fat excretion is an additional cause of weight loss in some patients. Excessive fat excretion may be caused by improper mixing of food and pancreatic enzymes due to rapid upper small bowel motility or due to the effects of intestinal vagotomy in some cases. Pancreatic insufficiency as a cause of weight loss after partial gastrectomy is not tenable for the following reasons: (1) normal secretin tests were obtained in the vast majority of cases tested; (2) pancreatin is of little or no value in the treatment of abnormal fat loss in the stool after gastrectomy;[16] (3) normal stool nitrogen excretion was uniformly found; (4) weight loss occurs regularly in the absence of either excessive fat or nitrogen loss in the stool.

The weight loss in this group of patients is high when postoperative weight is compared to the usual preoperative weight. The weight loss below ideal weights,[19, 20] as calculated for height and body build and considered in terms of longevity, is considerably less in most cases. A comparison of usual weight, present weight, and ideal weight for all cases is illustrated in Table X. In many instances, the postoperative weight loss has brought patients from an overweight state to within ideal weight range.

TABLE X. WEIGHT CHANGE IN ALL PATIENTS

NAME	TYPE OF OPERATION	USUAL PREOPERATIVE WEIGHT	PRESENT POSTOPERATIVE WEIGHT	IDEAL WEIGHT[19, 20]
1. J. W.	Segmental	170	150	145-156
2. E. G.	Segmental	135	125	136-147
3. E. A.	Segmental	180	138	153-164
4. E. M.	Segmental	130	146	153-164
5. L. L.	Segmental	145	130	137-147
6. O. L.	Segmental	250	170	157-168
7. F. E.	Segmental	138	120	133-143
8. F. O.	Segmental	175	155	157-168
9. F. R.	Segmental	200	150	157-168
10. C. S.	Segmental	165	150	153-164
11. F. B.	Segmental	178	150	153-164
12. H. M.	Segmental	185	155	153-164
13. R. C.	Billroth II	160	145	134-144
14. D. E.	Billroth I	118	100	107-115
15. O. G.	Billroth II	175	168	161-173
16. A. And.	Billroth I	130	115	145-156
17. C. H.	Billroth I	135	115	137-147
18. A. A.	Billroth II	145	140	134-144
19. T. W.	Billroth II	148	130	141-151
20. J. M.	Billroth II	140	110	145-156
21. A. K.	Billroth I	110	85	110-118
22. I. M.	Billroth I	175	155	145-156
23. J. F.	Billroth II	150	125	141-151
24. H. E.	Billroth II	155	145	117-125
25. W. O.	Segmental	190	155	157-168
26. A. S.	Billroth II	130	105	127-135
27. J. P.	Segmental	180	150	176-189
28. W. W.	Billroth II	220	220	166-178
29. A. L.	Segmental	160	130	124-132
30. W. H.	Tubular	160	140	156-164
31. Y. R.	Tubular	160	150	156-164
32. L. Lig.	Tubular	160	140	141-151
33. G. Cl.	Tubular	170	145	130-140
34. G. C.	Tubular	165	135	137-149
35. A. R.	Billroth II	150	125	124-132

TABLE XI. SUMMARY OF WEIGHT, FECAL FAT, FECAL NITROGEN LOSS, AND AVERAGE ORAL INTAKE

TYPE OF OPERATION	AVERAGE WEIGHT LOSS (POUNDS)	AVERAGE* PER CENT OF WEIGHT LOSS	AVERAGE FECAL FAT LOSS (GRAMS)	AVERAGE FECAL NITROGEN LOSS (GRAMS)	AVERAGE ORAL INTAKE PER CENT OF PRE-OPERATIVE INTAKE
Billroth I	19.6	16.2	6.50	1.05	65
Billroth II	15	10.3	9.50	1.79	80
Segmental	28.7	15	7.66	1.04	67
Tubular	21	12.8	4.76	1.23	66

*Per cent of weight loss is calculated as follows: $\frac{\text{Weight loss}}{\text{Usual preoperative weight}} \times 100$ and allows comparison of weight loss in patients of all weights.

A summary of average weight loss, average percentage of weight loss, average fat loss in the stool, average nitrogen loss, and average estimated oral intake is given in Table XI. The smaller average weight loss after the Billroth II operation is probably due to the fact that these patients had been operated upon many years prior to the study and had had opportunity to adjust to the altered gastrointestinal continuity. These patients could eat more, 80 per cent of the previous amount, than patients operated upon recently—segmental and tubular gastric resection patients.[4, 22, 23]

The hemogram made on all patients was normal in each instance, with one exception—a hypochromic, iron-deficiency anemia which occurred in a female patient following a Billroth II type gastric resection. A hemoglobin under 12 Gm. was considered abnormal.

From these studies, it would appear that a more effective therapeutic accomplishment is to be achieved by directing the attention and the interest of the patient to the goal of an increased caloric intake following subtotal gastrectomy, rather than toward efforts directed at increasing fat absorption from the gastrointestinal tract.

SUMMARY AND CONCLUSIONS

1. Thirty-five patients with subtotal gastrectomy were studied from three months to five years following operation to determine the etiological factors of importance causing weight loss.

2. Fat and nitrogen excretion in the stool was determined while the patients were hospitalized on a weighed intake of fat 80 Gm., protein 80 Gm., and carbohydrate 145 Gm. Three of nine patients excreted an abnormally large amount of fecal fat after Billroth II gastrectomy. One of five patients excreted a borderline quantity of fat after the Billroth I procedure. Segmental resection resulted in an abnormally large fat loss in the stool in five of sixteen patients. Fat excretion was normal in the five patients who underwent tubular resection.[4, 22, 23]

3. Excessive stool nitrogen loss is an infrequent occurrence following subtotal gastrectomy.

4. Thirty-two of the thirty-five patients who were studied lost weight. The average loss was twenty-one pounds. Large weight losses are possible with normal fat and nitrogen excretion in the stool and are closely related to decreased food intake despite many meals per day. Weight loss is considerably less when compared to ideal weights for each individual concerned.

5. Large weight loss is not closely related to rapid small bowel transit time or diarrhea.

6. Gastroduodenal continuity does not prevent excessive fat loss in the stool, since this occurred following segmental gastric resection.

7. Pancreatic function, as assessed by the secretin test, following subtotal gastric resection is completely normal in most patients. The possibility exists that rapid small bowel transit separates the food and enzymes in the presence of normal pancreatic function.

8. Of the factors assessed to account for weight loss in thirty-five patients after subtotal gastrectomy, decreased oral intake or loss of gastric reservoir capacity is of greatest importance. Increased fecal fat excretion is an additional cause of weight loss in some patients.

9. Investigation for the future would be most advantageously directed toward increasing caloric intake in patients following subtotal gastrectomy.

REFERENCES

1. Ivy, A. C., Grossman, M. I., and Bachrach, W. N.: Peptic Ulcer, Philadelphia, 1950, The Blakiston Company.
2. Rauch, R. F.: An Evaluation of Gastric Resection for Benign Lesions of the Esophagus, Stomach and Duodenum, Master's Thesis, University of Minnesota, 1952.

3. Wangensteen, O. H.: Segmental Gastric Resection for Peptic Ulcer, J. A. M. A. **149**: 18-23, 1952.
4. MacLean, L. D.: Tubular Gastric Resection: A Preliminary Evaluation, Bull. University of Minnesota Hospitals and Minnesota Medical Foundation **24**: 255-273, 1953.
5. Wollaeger, E. E., Comfort, M. W., Weir, J. F., and Osterberg, A. E.: The Total Solids, Fat and Nitrogen in the Feces: I A Study of Normal Persons and Patients With Duodenal Ulcer on a Test Diet Containing Large Amounts of Fat, Gastroenterology **6**: 83-92, 1946.
6. Everson, T. C.: Nutrition Following Gastrectomy, With Particular Reference to Fat and Protein Assimilation, Internat. Abstr. Surg. **95**: 209-230, 1952.
7. Diamond, J. S., Siegel, S. A., and Myerson, S.: The Secretin Test as an Aid in the Differential Diagnosis of the Steatorrhea With a Report of Fourteen Cases, Rev. Gastroenterol. **7**: 429-442, 1940.
8. Fowweather, F. S., cited by Peters, J. P., and Van Slyke, D. D.: Methods, vol. 2, Baltimore, 1932, Williams & Wilkins Company.
9. Kjeldahl, J., cited by Peters, J. P., and Van Slyke, D. D.: Methods, vol. 2, Baltimore, 1932, Williams & Wilkins Company.
10. Somogyi, M.: Micromethods for the Estimation of Diastase, J. Biol. Chem. **125**: 399-414, 1938.
11. Anderson, D. H., and Early, M. U.: Method of Assaying Trypsin Suitable for Routine Use in Diagnosis of Congenital Pancreatic Deficiency, Am. J. Dis. Child. **63**: 891-896, 1942.
12. Cherry, I. S., and Crandall, L. A., Jr.: Specificity of Pancreatic Lipase: Its Appearance in Blood After Pancreatic Injury, Am. J. Physiol. **100**: 266-273, 1932.
13. Fox, N. J., and Grimson, K. S.: Defective Fat Absorption Following Vagotomy, J. Lab. & Clin. Med. **35**: 362-365, 1950.
14. Routley, E. F., Mann, F., Bollman, J. L., and Grindlay, J. H.: Effects of Vagotomy on Pancreatic Secretion in Dogs, Surg., Gynec. & Obst. **95**: 529-536, 1952.
15. Savich and Soshestvensky, quoted by Babkin, B. P.: Secretory Mechanism of the Digestive Glands, P. B. Hoeleer, New York, 1950, Paul B. Hoeber, Inc.
16. Rekers, P. E., Pack, G. T., and Rhoads, C. P.: Metabolic Studies in Patients With Cancer of the Gastrointestinal Tract, SURGERY **14**: 197-215, 1943.
17. MacDonald, R., Ingelfinger, F. J., and Belding, H. W.: Late Effects of Total Gastrectomy in Man, New England J. Med. **237**: 887-896, 1947.
18. Wollaeger, E. E., Comfort, M. W., Weir, J. F., and Osterburg, A. E.: The Total Solids, Fat and Nitrogen in the Feces: II. A Study of Persons Who Had Partial Gastrectomy With Anastomosis of the Entire Gut End of the Stomach and the Jejunum (Palya Anastomosis), Gastroenterology **6**: 93-104, 1946.
19. Ideal Weights for Men. Statistical Bulletin, Metropolitan Life Insurance Co. **24**: 6, 1943.
20. Ideal Weights for Women. Statistical Bulletin, Metropolitan Life Insurance Co. **23**: 6, 1942.
21. Rigler, L. G., and Nice, C.: Personal communication.
22. Wangensteen, O. H.: Evolution and Evaluation of an Acceptable Operation for Peptic Ulcer (Including Description of the Technique of Tubular Gastric Resection With Transverse Gastroplasty and Extrapleural Sternotomy for Operations in the Attic of the Abdomen), Rev. Gastroenterol. **20**: 611-626 (Sept.) 1953.
23. Wangensteen, O. H.: The Peptic Ulcer Problem, Minnesota Med. **36**: 924-934 (Sept.) 1953.

THE EFFECT OF PERORAL BARIUM IN PARTIAL OBSTRUCTION OF THE SMALL BOWEL

An Experimental Study

Henry Donato, M.D., Henry W. Mayo, Jr., M.D., and L. H. Barr, M.D.,
Charleston, S. C.

(From the Departments of Surgery and Radiology, Medical College of South Carolina, and the Roper Hospital)

IT HAS been recognized for many years that the oral administration of barium in the presence of a potentially obstructing lesion of the colon is a dangerous practice which may result in complete obstruction. Such occurrences have been reported by Stalker,[5] Orgel,[4] and others, who have emphasized the value of performing a barium enema before the upper gastrointestinal series if there is any indication that the patient may have a lesion of the large bowel. Golob[3] has noted that barium remaining in the normal colon will become a stony, hard impacted mass, if not evacuated in a reasonable length of time, because of the function of the colon in absorption of water, and he has reported cases of complete obstruction developing on this basis. From a rational point of view, it would seem unlikely that the same process would occur in the partially obstructed small bowel since the small bowel is concerned primarily with secretion, digestion, and absorption of nutriments, rather than with fluid absorption. According to Best and Taylor,[1] "As a result of the sensitivity of the mucosa to mechanical stimuli, undigested food residues or other unabsorbable solid material will in their passage through the (small) bowel cause excitation of the glands and so increase the fluidity of the intestinal contents." Nevertheless, quite recently Cantor and his associates[2] condemned the use of the upper gastrointestinal series in the presence of suspected partial obstruction of the small intestine, because of the fear that the obstruction might be made complete, unless a long intestinal tube was first passed to the point of obstruction so that the dilute barium could be recovered promptly by suction, after the site of obstruction was demonstrated radiologically.

The present study was undertaken as a result of experiences with several clinical cases of chronic progressive small bowel obstruction, which in most instances were later proved to be on the basis of small bowel neoplasm. The radiologists concerned advocated the administration of oral barium as a diagnostic measure, and felt that there was no likelihood of the barium producing complete obstruction. However, certain of the clinicians concerned felt that the possibility of the development of complete obstruction was a real one.

METHODS

Unselected mongrel dogs of various sizes were used, and all operative procedures were carried out under aseptic conditions with veterinary Nembu-

Received for publication, Aug. 21, 1953.

tal anesthesia. The animals were kept in a fasting state for twelve hours before each operation, and given only liquids for twenty-four hours after recovery from anesthesia, after which the regular kennel diet was resumed. As the initial procedure in each animal, a double thickness of reactive cellophane about 2 cm. in width was placed circumferentially around the terminal ileum 5 to 20 cm. proximal to the ileocecal valve. The cellophane strip, which was placed snugly against the bowel wall without constricting the bowel, was fixed in place by two nonabsorbable sutures at the ends, which were then buried in mesentery so that a smooth surface presented to the peritoneal cavity. It had been planned to follow the development of obstruction with scout films of the abdomen, but the latter were found to be rather difficult to interpret in the earliest studies, and this method was therefore abandoned in favor of re-exploration, merely to determine the presence and degree of obstruction. The second exploration was carried out in most instances seven to fourteen days after implantation of cellophane, except for two animals observed six and seven weeks, respectively. A short time (one to eleven days) after re-exploration, barium sulfate, in the usual dilution, was given through a Levin tube passed into the stomach. The volume of the barium suspension administered varied between 100 and 150 c.c., depending on the size of the animal. Films of the abdomen were taken twelve or twenty-four hours after barium administration, and when there was marked stasis of barium in the small bowel, the progress of the meal was followed longer, in two cases for five days, with repeated films. Shortly after the last x-ray film was taken, the animal was sacrificed and autopsied, or subjected to laparotomy, at which time the involved portion of the intestine was resected between clamps. In some instances, this was done immediately after the last film was made, so that a direct comparison could be made between the roentgenologic findings and the autopsy material. In other animals, an interval of two to five days elapsed between the last film and inspection of the bowel. The degree of obstruction, the fluidity and character of the intestinal contents, and the size of the lumen of the bowel at the site of obstruction were noted in each instance.

RESULTS

Reactive cellophane was wrapped around the terminal small bowel of 38 dogs. Partial small bowel obstruction developed at the site of the cellophane in 30 animals, but because of the death of 14 animals for various reasons, only 16 animals were carried through the complete series of studies.

The gross picture seen at operation and at autopsy after snug encirclement of the small bowel by cellophane was a remarkably uniform one of chronic partial small bowel obstruction. Characteristically, the cellophane was covered, even one week after its application, by serosa, and surrounded by slightly edematous tissue, showing microscopically a marked inflammatory reaction, as well as fibrosis. In most animals, the lumen of the bowel at the site of obstruction was 3 to 6 mm. in diameter (Fig. 1). No mucosal ulceration was seen in any case. The bowel proximal to the obstructing lesion was dilated to two to three times normal size with thick hypertrophic walls, but distal to the site of obstruction, the bowel was collapsed slightly (Fig. 2). The proximal dilatation usually involved 30 to 40 cm. of small bowel, although in a few cases much more of the bowel was involved. Although regular observations in the kennels were not made, in so far as could be determined, the dogs continued to take food and to have bowel movements, and vomiting was a rare occurrence. This preparation was an effective means of producing a high grade of partial small bowel obstruction fairly consistently.

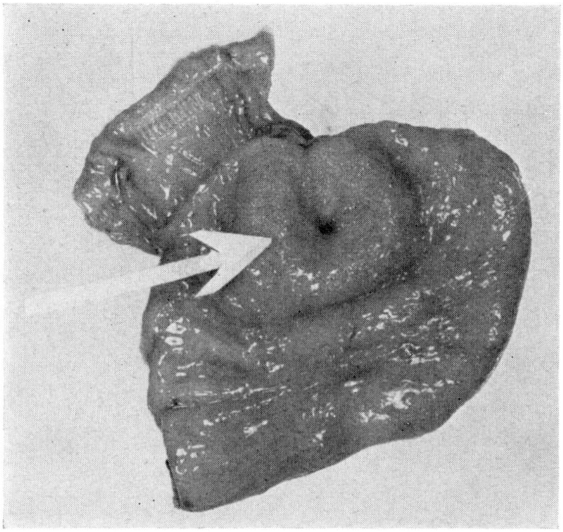

Fig. 1.—Open bowel showing diameter of the lumen at the site of obstruction.

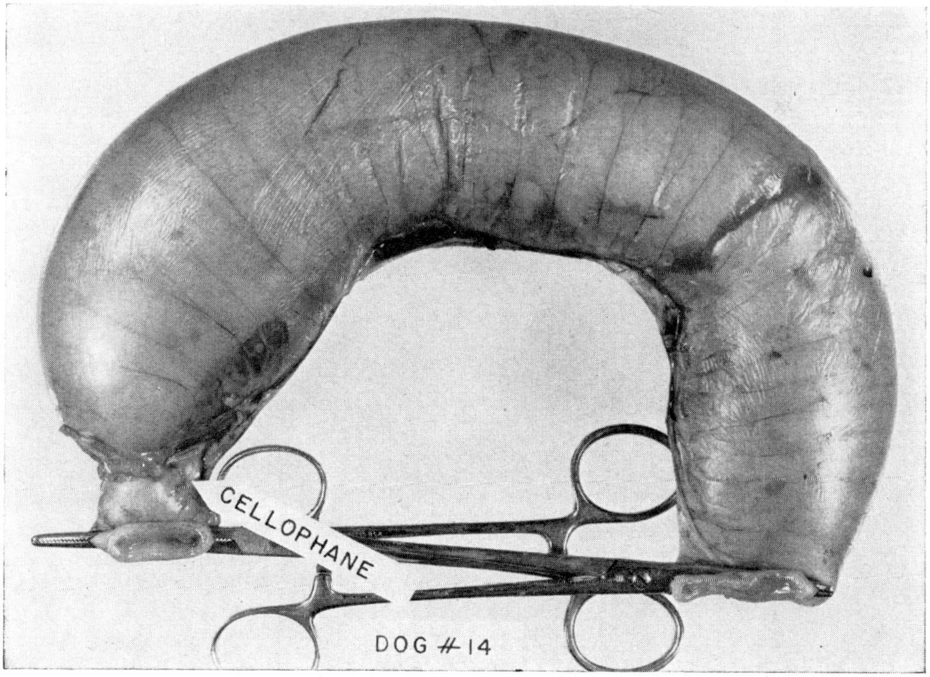

Fig. 2.—Resected bowel showing dilatation and hypertrophy proximal to obstruction with distal collapse.

In 13 of the 16 animals studied completely, a high degree of obstruction was produced, with marked proximal dilatation and hypertrophy, and lumina less than 6 mm. in diameter. The other 3 animals had definite obstruction which was classified as minimal, with lumina at the obstructive site ranging between 1 and 3 cm. In 2 of the latter animals there was a small amount of barium still noted in the terminal ileum on the twenty-four hour film, while in the third, the barium was still in the colon at twenty-four hours. Several nonobstructed dogs were given barium for comparison, and in each of these, no barium remained in the small bowel at twenty-four hours, and in only 1 animal was barium demonstrated in the colon at that time. The majority of the x-ray films taken of the other 13 dogs twelve and twenty-four hours after administration showed stasis of barium in the dilated terminal ileum, but with two exceptions, as the animals were followed over a period of time, the barium was gradually evacuated. Two dogs were followed for five days, during which time almost all of the barium remained in the terminal ileum, but at autopsy the intestinal contents containing barium were in a liquid state and there was no evidence that obstruction had been completed. Increasing distention or vomiting was not noted after barium administration. In 11 animals, the contents of the proximal dilated bowel at autopsy were in a fluid state, but were classified as semisolid in 5. It is particularly significant that complete obstruction did not develop in any instance.

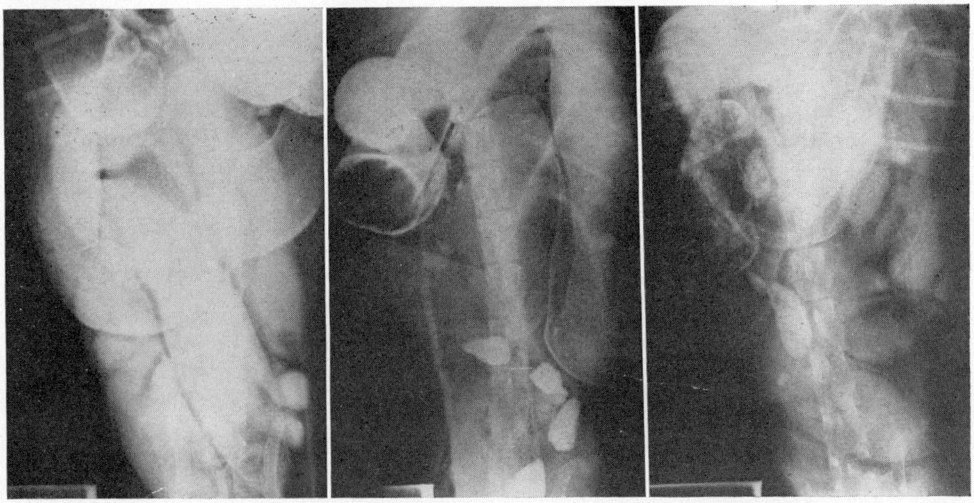

A. *B.* *C.*

Fig. 3.—Series of films showing progressive dilution of barium. *A*, Twenty-four hours; *B*, forty-eight hours; *C*, eighty-four hours.

In those animals in which there was marked stasis of barium in the bowel proximal to the obstruction (Fig. 3), as the animals were followed, even if little barium passed the site of obstruction, the barium became less dense, presumably due to an increase in fluidity of the intestinal contents and "scattering" of the barium.

DISCUSSION

These experiments demonstrate clearly that barium does not form a puttylike impacted mass when stasis occurs proximal to obstruction in the small bowel, nor does it render a partial obstruction complete. It is possible that the fluidity of the intestinal contents is later increased due to the mechanical stimulation of the presence of the barium. Unquestionably, the stasis proximal to obstruction is temporarily increased by the presence of the barium, but this should have little deleterious effect. The administration of barium by mouth to patients with chronic partial small bowel obstruction (after obstruction of the colon has been ruled out) should be safe and, by the manipulations of the radiologist and his fluoroscopic observations, might result in a fairly high percentage of correct radiologic diagnoses. However, the administration of barium in cases of complete obstruction, or in cases of acute obstruction due to adhesions, as described by Cantor and others,[2] or due to incarcerated hernia or volvulus, seems unnecessary, since the diagnosis should be made on the basis of clinical findings and scout films. It is also unwise, because unless the barium is evacuated before operation, it will interfere with the resumption of intestinal motility during the postoperative period.

SUMMARY

A satisfactory method for producing partial high-grade intestinal obstruction in the experimental animal has been presented. Animals prepared in such a way were studied by x-ray films at varying intervals after the administration of barium through a Levin tube. The animals then were autopsied, and the character of the bowel contents and size of the lumen at the site of obstruction were correlated with the x-ray findings. It was noted that complete obstruction due to impaction of barium did not occur and, in most cases, the barium remaining in the small bowel was in a fluid state.

CONCLUSIONS

Under the conditions of these experiments, barium failed to produce complete obstruction after entering the small bowel proximal to a previously produced partial obstruction.

REFERENCES

1. Best, C. H., and Taylor, N. B.: The Physiological Basis of Medical Practice, ed. 5, Baltimore, 1950, Williams & Wilkins Company, p. 536.
2. Cantor, M. O., McCollum, B. E., and Hodges, J.: Intestinal Intubation for Barium Produced Small Bowel Obstruction, Am. J. Digest. Dis. **19**: 148-150, 1952.
3. Golob, M.: The Advisability of Immediate Colonic Irrigation Following a Barium Enema, Radiology **22**: 486-489, 1934.
4. Orgel, D. H.: A Barium Meal Simulating Intestinal Obstruction, M. J. & Rec. **129**: 396-398, 1934.
5. Stalker, L. K.: Barium as a Factor in Intestinal Obstruction, Am. J. Surg. **72**: 756-757, 1946.

THE SIGNIFICANCE OF LOCAL VASCULAR CHANGES IN BLEEDING PEPTIC ULCER

CALVIN R. MACKAY, M.D.,* NEW ORLEANS, LA.

DESPITE the many advances and additions to the armamentarium in the conservative treatment of peptic ulcer, including various antacids and dietary regimens, as well as the newer anticholinergic drugs and the psychosomatic approach to the problem, chronic peptic ulcer remains a major disease, recurrences are frequent, and complications, including hemorrhage, are not uncommon.

It has been noted by Wangensteen[1] that evidence of peptic ulcer can be found in one of every twenty autopsies that are carefully performed; moreover, 10 per cent of all ulcer patients enter the hospital because of hemorrhage. Herbut[2] estimated that 19 per cent of all peptic ulcer patients have one or more hemorrhages, and Eusterman[3] has indicated that of all cases of gross hemorrhage from the upper gastrointestinal tract, peptic ulcer is responsible at least 85 per cent of the time.

While the reasons usually alluded to in explaining the failure to produce a permanent cure with medical therapy are inadequate dietary or pharmaceutic routines, poor cooperation ("patient failure"), or ulcer diathesis of the patient, the importance of the pathologic changes in the ulcer and surrounding area must not be overlooked. It is readily understandable why, after replacement of the muscle layers and submucosa in chronic ulcer, prevention of coaptation of the ulcer edges occurs, healing is slow, and a favorable nidus for recurrence is produced. In addition, as emphasized by Boyd,[4] inflammation, as evidenced by dilated vessels and foci of inflammatory cells, continues to occur in the ulcer bed long after the scar tissue appears quiescent and regeneration of the superficial mucosa has taken place.

Vascular changes in the local ulcer area are well described in many textbooks of pathology and treatises on the subject, but the significance of these changes, particularly in event of erosion of the vessels by the ulcer, has received little consideration. The decision for surgical intervention in the case of hemorrhage from peptic ulcer is usually based (far too often) on the degree of generalized arteriosclerosis which the patient has, the common denominator being the patient's age. It is the purpose of this study to review the local vascular changes in cases of peptic ulcer in which patients have had severe hemorrhage, in an attempt to determine whether these changes make severe hemorrhage more likely in case the vessel(s) becomes eroded by the ulcer, regardless of the presence of, or lack of, generalized sclerotic vessels.

Received for publication, Oct. 2, 1953.

*Resident in surgery at the United States Public Health Service Hospital, New Orleans.

GENERAL CONSIDERATIONS

Besides the hemodynamics and clotting power of the blood, there are obviously local factors that determine whether the blood loss in bleeding peptic ulcer will be severe. Among these may be mentioned the size or number of vessels eroded, the integrity of the neuromuscular system, and pathologic changes in the vessels which might affect contractility or smooth coaptation of the vessel intima. Anatomically, although the vessels commonly involved in fatal or severe hemorrhage from peptic ulcer are the right or left gastric arteries, or the gastroduodenal or their branches[5] (especially the superior pancreaticoduodenal), severe and even fatal bleeding may occur from the erosion of small vessels entering the ulcer bed, which may not be grossly discernible at surgery or at autopsy. Occasionally, the exact bleeding point may not be seen and may not be defined unless careful serial sections for microscopic examination are made. It is also of some importance to recall that the pylorus, although frequently the site of peptic ulcer, is rarely, if ever, the site of severe bleeding because of its relative avascularity.[6]

According to Anderson,[7] localized infections in tissues may involve an artery to produce an acute periateritis. Such a vessel may become thrombosed or weakened to the point of rupture. As a matter of fact, Lisa and Likely[8] reported cases of chronic peptic ulcer with death from exsanguinating hemorrhage in which bacterial infection of the wall of the involved vessel was demonstrated in each case. Bacterial involvement of the vessels in bleeding ulcer, however, is rarely elicited in the pathogenesis of severe hemorrhage, and was not seen in any of the cases in the present study.

THE AGE FACTOR

In most large series of cases reported, fatalities from bleeding peptic ulcer occur most frequently in the age group 45 to 60 years.[9-11] Bockus[12] reported no deaths in the 20- to 30-year age group, while Methany and Green[13] went so far as to say that bleeding ulcer in young people is a self-limited and nonfatal disease, with favorable results to be expected with conservative therapy in all cases of patients under 45 years. Such optimism is not universally held, and to make such optimism the basis for treatment is to invite disaster.

Meyer and his associates[14] reported a mortality rate of 30 per cent in patients under 45 years and 43 per cent over 45 years of age treated surgically, as compared to no mortality in the age group under 45 years and 21 per cent over 45 years treated medically. However, in evaluating any statistics regarding therapy, certain considerations must be entertained before any conclusions are made; among these we must include other factors in addition to concomitant disease processes, particularly in regard to the ability to withstand blood loss. Also, an important fact to keep in mind always in attempting to compare treatment is the amount of blood lost before surgery is finally undertaken. In hemorrhage from any source, the surgical risk rises with each hour surgery is withheld.

That age per se should not be the sine qua non in determining whether surgery should be resorted to in severely bleeding peptic ulcer is further attested by the fact that severe and fatal hemorrhage may occur in infants and children. Bird and his group[15] have reported twenty-two cases of bleeding peptic ulcer in the newborn infant. Rothwell and Strode[16] reported a case of an infant with continued bleeding from gastric ulcer in which a lifesaving gastric resection was performed.

METHODS AND FINDINGS

Twenty-five cases of bleeding peptic ulcer were reviewed, particular attention being paid to the vascular changes in the ulcer bed and immediate surrounding area and, in addition, to the morphology of the gastric and duodenal vessels remote from the ulcer area. In the fatal cases, a search for arteriosclerosis or vascular disease in other organs and tissues was made.

TABLE I. CASE SUMMARIES

CASE NO.	AGE (YR.)	ULCER LOCATION	HEMATOCRIT	TREATMENT	RESULTS	VASCULAR PATHOLOGY IN SURGICAL OR AUTOPSY SPECIMENS
1-A1621	29	Duodenum	18	Medical	Died	Marked intimal proliferation of vessels in ulcer bed; no arteriosclerosis in coronaries or aorta (Figs. 1 and 2)
2-S2887-52	63	Stomach	20	Surgical	Lived	Irregular thickening of intima of vessels in ulcer base; elsewhere evidence of arteriosclerosis in vessels remote from ulcer area (Fig. 3)
3-S1964-50	49	Stomach	24	Surgical	Lived	Obliterative endarteritis in some vessels in ulcer base; elsewhere vessels show intimal proliferation (Fig. 4)
4-S11992	29	Stomach	21	Surgical	Lived	Replacement of smooth muscle by hyaline fibrous tissue; thickening of intima (Fig. 5)
5-A2000	45	Duodenum	21	Medical	Died	Large vessel (superior pancreaticoduodenal) was eroded by ulcer; artery had "pipe-stem" appearance; intimal proliferation (Fig. 6)
6-S1271-50	47	Duodenum	20	Surgical	Lived	All vessels in ulcer bed were thickened; no large vessels in ulcer area
7-S2231-52	49	Stomach	22	Surgical	Lived	Marked intimal proliferation of all vessels in ulcer area; obliteration of elastica interna
8-S3203-52	54	Stomach	24	Surgical	Lived	Irregular intimal thickening; invasion of vessel walls by inflammatory cells
9-S40-53	62	Duodenum	20	Surgical	Lived	Vessels in ulcer bed and adjacent area show intimal proliferation; in some cases there is active fibrosis (proliferation of fibroblasts) in the media; distally from the ulcer site the vessels appear normal
10-S23751-52	26	Duodenum	16	Surgical	Lived	Small vessels in ulcer bed have thickened walls; vessels elsewhere appear normal

The cases (ten of which are summarized in Table I) fulfilled the following criteria: (1) Severe bleeding had occurred, based on a hematocrit of 25 per cent or less. (2) There was no history of hypertension or renal disease. (3) No noteworthy generalized arteriosclerosis was demonstrable on examination, at surgery, or on examination of vessels at autopsy. (4) No history of cardiac disease was elicited and none was evident at necropsy. (5) Blood vessels in the ulcer area were demonstrable in the microscopic sections.

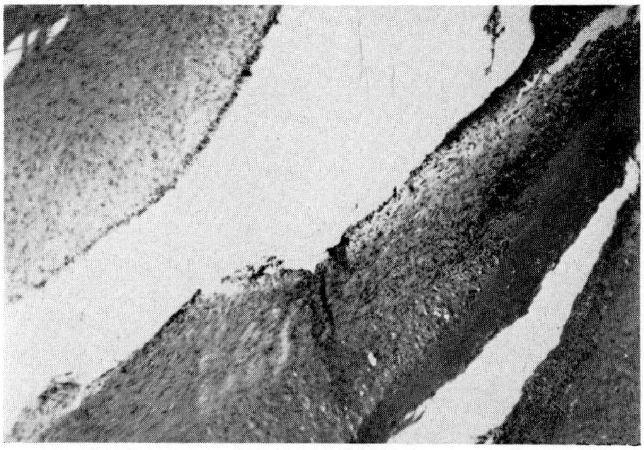

Fig. 1.—Case 1. Section of artery at site of erosion showing infiltration of inflammatory cells.

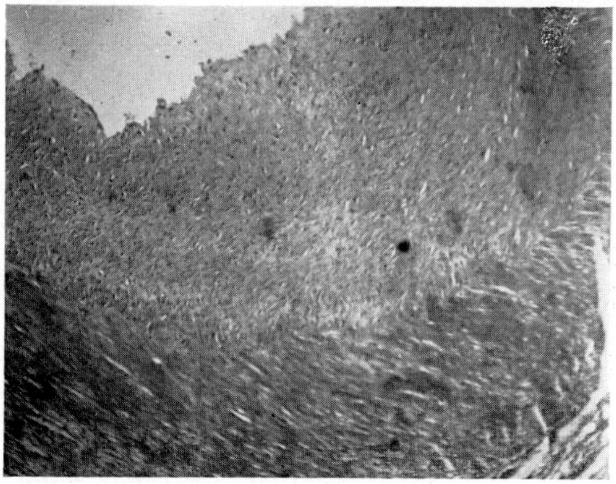

Fig. 2.—Case 1. Same vessel as in Fig. 1 remote from site of erosion. Note marked intimal proliferation.

It was found from these studies that the pathologic changes within the blood vessels were similar regardless of the age of the patient. These changes were: (1) proliferation of the intima, (2) replacement of smooth muscle of the media by fibrous tissue, and (3) varying destruction of the elastica interna. For details see Table I.

All the patients here reported had severe hemorrhage. In one-half the patients, it was the first episode of bleeding, which correlates with the findings of Shapiro and Shiff,[17] who reported that no significance in the severity of bleeding could be attached to the fact that hemorrhage had or had not occurred one or more times previously, or whether the present episode was the initial one.

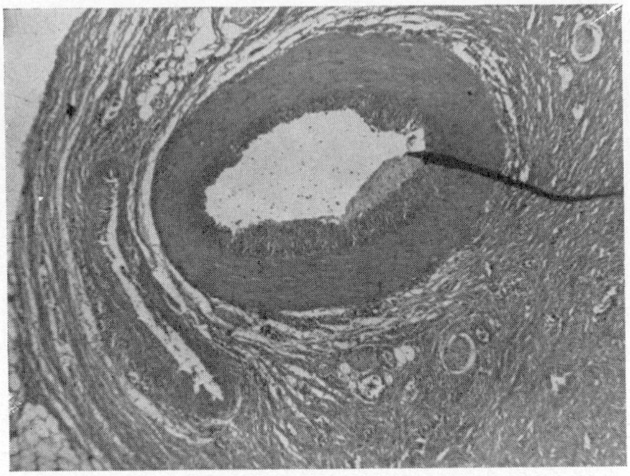

Fig. 3.—Case 2. Vessels just beneath ulcer. Both artery and vein show irregular thickening of the intima.

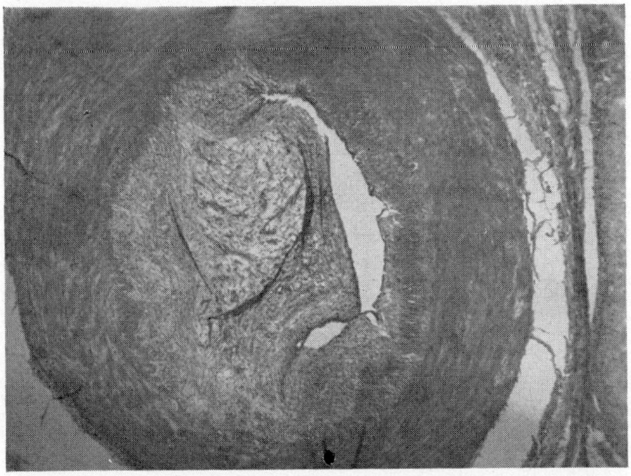

Fig. 4.—Case 3. Artery in ulcer bed showing obliterative endarteritis.

Significant also in the treatment of bleeding peptic ulcer is the possibility of recurrence of hemorrhage. Holman,[18] for example, found that of those patients who recover under conservative management, more than 50 per cent bleed again; moreover, at least one-half the patients who continue to bleed forty-eight hours after being placed on a strict medical regimen expire.

It will be noted from among the ten cases selected in this study for summary that in three of the cases, patients were under 30 years of age. The patient in Case 1 died from exsanguination after several days of intensive medical management, whereas the patients in Cases 4 and 10 were treated surgically and survived. That age, per se, may not be the important factor in ability to survive severe bleeding is also indicated by the studies of Bohrer,[19] who found a mortality rate of 20 per cent in patients under 45 years.

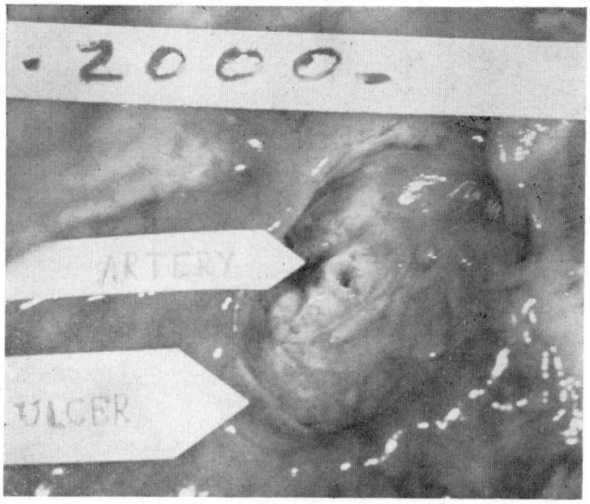

Fig. 5.—Case 5. Gross specimen showing artery from which fatal hemorrhage occurred. Microscopically, the vessel was thickened.

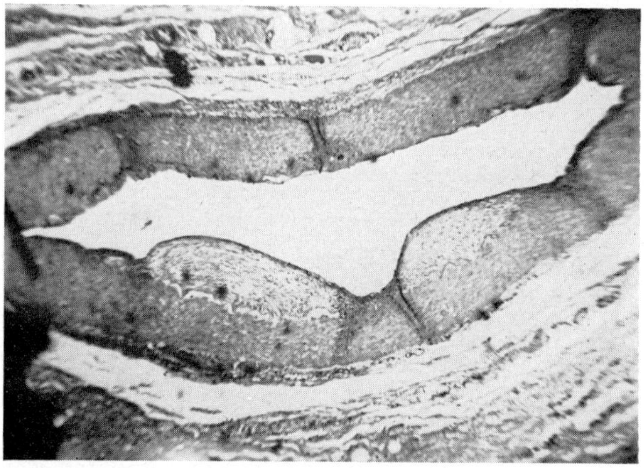

Fig. 6.—Case 7. Note beginning of intimal proliferation. Other vessels in the ulcer bed showed marked proliferation of the intima.

The surgical procedure in the cases selected in this study consisted of subtotal gastric resection of the Polya type, after immediate stoppage of the bleeding point by ligation of the major vessel, if possible, or plication of the ulcer over the vessel(s). Massive replacement of blood was attempted in each case, an average of 2,500 c.c. being given before operation was performed.

In one patient (Case 5) treated medically, 7,500 c.c. of blood was given before he expired. At autopsy, as in the other cases here selected, there was no generalized arteriosclerosis, the significant vascular changes being limited to the ulcer area.

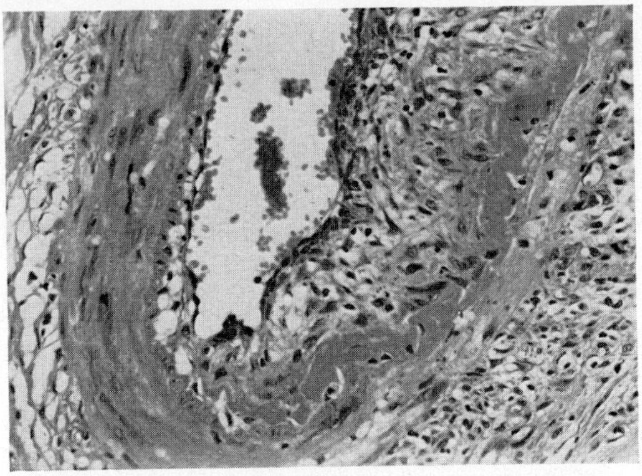

Fig. 7.—Case 4. The muscular media has been partially replaced by fibrous tissue.

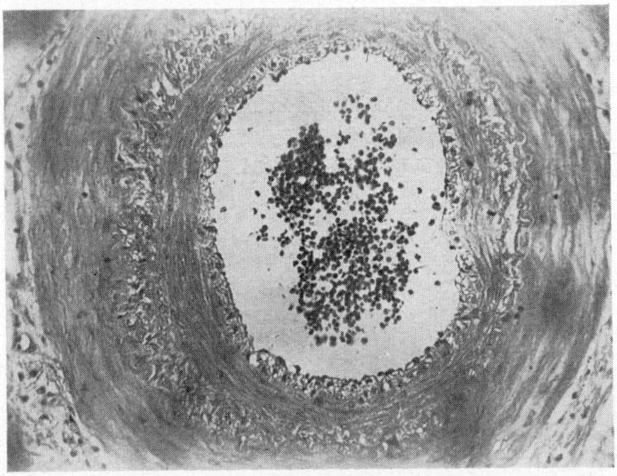

Fig. 8.—Case 8.—There is intimal proliferation, fibrosis of the media, and preservation of the elastica interna.

In a comprehensive review of severely bleeding peptic ulcer, Lewison[20] has emphasized the fact that hematemesis is indicative of severe hemorrhage, while melena alone may not be. Although some idea of the amount of blood loss may be obtained by estimating the quantity from hematemesis or melena, it must be remembered that a large volume of blood may be within the gastrointestinal tract concealed from the observer. In addition, of course, the volume of packed red blood cell determination, blood volume, red cell count, and hemoglobin all vary depending on the shift of fluid from the intracellular to extracellular space as bleeding progresses, and these laboratory determinations at the moment may not be entirely accurate in giving the exact picture of continued or severe blood loss. Repeated, frequent determinations, as well as careful clinical observation and cooperation between internist and surgeon, are essential in proper management.

The true indication of the severity of bleeding must be individualized, and it is that amount of blood necessary to restore the physiologic hemodynamics. Because of this fact, it has been suggested by Clark[21] that each case of bleeding peptic ulcer be managed as though preparing for surgery, conservative management being continued only if hemodynamics is restored by a given volume of whole blood (such as 4 or 5 units) and is maintained thereafter without further transfusions.

CONCLUSIONS

The reason for the increased mortality rate in the older individual with severely bleeding peptic ulcer, other factors being equal, has usually been attributed to arteriosclerosis of the vessel(s) eroded by the ulcer and to definitive surgical treatment being arbitrarily withheld in the patient with supposed normal, elastic blood vessels—age, a priori, being made the common denominator in conservative versus surgical management. Oöphuls[22] believed that arteriosclerosis in peptic ulcer is frequently observed and may occur as a local process in young persons. Askanazy,[23] on the other hand, observed that gross arteriosclerosis of the vessels of the celiac axis is uncommon in patients even in the fifth or sixth decade.

In the cases reviewed in this study, there was no arteriosclerosis of the vessels to the stomach or duodenum peripheral to the ulcer area. It is suggested that the vascular changes seen in peptic ulcer are secondary to inflammatory processes in the ulcer bed, and the changes seen depend on the stage seen, which, in turn, depends on the extent and duration of the inflammatory reaction, regardless of the age of the patient or vascular pathology elsewhere.

The pathologic microscopic changes included invasion of vessels by inflammatory cells, irregular proliferation of the intima (which at times was striking), replacement of smooth muscle of the media by fibrous tissue, and inconstant dehiscence of elastic fibers. It may be conjectured that the pathologic physiology may be similar to arteriosclerosis and, in the case of erosion, bleeding from the vessel is likely to be severe due to impaired contractility and poor coaptation of the intima, the former being due to replacement of smooth muscle by fibrous tissue, and the latter due to irregular intimal proliferation. Furthermore, if obliterative endarteritis occurs, it may be supposed that the resulting ischemia to the area may further delay healing of the ulcer, further scarring, and make recurrences more likely—all of which impair the success of conservative therapy.

SUMMARY

Twenty-five cases of severe hemorrhage from peptic ulcer were reviewed and ten cases were selected for summary which fulfilled the following criteria:

(1) The hematocrit was 25 per cent or lower during bleeding. (2) No severe concomitant disease was present. (3) Microscopic sections of the surgical specimen or autopsy tissues were made showing blood vessels in the ulcer area (serial sections).

No arteriosclerosis of the gastric or duodenal vessels was demonstrated. The vascular changes occurring in the vessels in the ulcer area were similar, regardless of the age of the patient, and consisted, in the main, of proliferation of the intima (irregular), varying replacement of the muscular media by fibrous tissue, inconstant changes in the elastica interna, and, in some cases, active inflammation of the vessels with invasion of the vessel walls with inflammatory cells.

Vascular changes in peptic ulcer are well known and have been frequently described; however, the significance of these changes has received little consideration, the decision for surgical treatment in the event of hemorrhage too often being based on the supposed degree of arteriosclerosis present, the common denominator being the age of the patient.

It is suggested that the pathologic changes in the vessels in peptic ulcer are secondary to the inflammatory process in the ulcer area, and that these changes render the vessels less elastic, impair their contractility, and prevent smooth coaptation of their intima; thus, in case of erosion, bleeding is likely to be severe, depending on the size or number of vessels involved. Inasmuch as these vascular changes occur regardless of the age of the patient, it is proposed that making merely the age of the patient the sine qua non in determining therapy is not valid.

REFERENCES

1. Wangensteen, O. H.: The Problem of Surgical Arrest of Massive Hemorrhage in Duodenal Ulcer, SURGERY **8**: 275, 1940.
2. Herbut, P. A.: Surgical Pathology, Philadelphia, 1948, Lea & Febiger, p. 344.
3. Eusterman, G. B.: Gastrointestinal Hemorrhage From Otherwise Symptomless Lesions, Proc. Staff. Meet., Mayo Clin. **15**: 513, 1939.
4. Boyd, W.: A Textbook of Pathology, Philadelphia, 1943, Lea & Febiger, p. 482.
5. Allen, A. W.: Acute Massive Hemorrhage From Upper Gastrointestinal Tract, SURGERY **2**: 713, 1937.
6. Berlet, K.: Ueber die Arterien des Menschlichen Magens und Ihre Beziehungen zur Aetiologie und Pathogenese des Mageneschwürs. Grankf., Ztschr. f. Path. **30**: 472, 1924.
7. Anderson, W. A. D.: Pathology, St. Louis, 1948, The C. V. Mosby Company.
8. Lisa, J. R., and Likely, D. S.: Infection as a Cause of Massive Hemorrhage in Chronic Peptic Ulcer, Arch. Surg. **40**: 15, 1940.
9. Blackford, J. M., and Allen, H. E.: Bleeding Peptic Ulcers, J. A. M. A. **120**: 811, 1942.
10. Cates, H. B.: Massive Hemorrhage From Peptic Ulcer: Prognosis and Treatment; Conclusions Drawn From a Large Series, Ann. Int. Med. **32**: 1144, 1950.
11. Allen, A. W., and Benedict, E. B.: Acute Massive Hemorrhage From Duodenal Ulcer, Ann. Surg. **98**: 736, 1953.
12. Bockus, H. L.: Gastroenterology, Philadelphia, 1944, W. B. Saunders Company.
13. Methany, D., and Green, D. M.: Exsanguinating Hemorrhage in Peptic Ulcer, West. J. Surg. **55**: 97, 1947.
14. Meyer, J., Sorter, H. K., and Nicheles, H. J.: Medical and Surgical Treatment of Hemorrhage From Peptic Ulcer: A Critical Evaluation of the Factor of Age, J. A. M. A. **120**: 813, 1942.
15. Bird, C. E., Limper, M. A., and Mayer, J. M.: Surgery in Peptic Ulcer of Stomach and Duodenum in Infants and Children, Ann. Surg. **114**: 526, 1941.
16. Rothwell, H. T., and Strode, J. E.: Personal communication.
17. Shapiro, N., and Shiff, L.: Ten Years' Experience With Bleeding Peptic Ulcer With Emphasis on 45 Fatal Cases, SURGERY **31**: 327, 1952.

18. Holman, C. W.: Treatment of Severe Bleeding From Peptic Ulcer, S. Clin. North America **30**: 421, 1950.
19. Bohrer, J. V.: Massive Gastric Hemorrhage, Ann. Surg. **144**: 510, 1941.
20. Lewison, E. R.: Collective Review: Bleeding Peptic Ulcer, Surg., Gynec. & Obst. **90**: 1, 1950.
21. Clark, J. H.: Personal communication.
22. Oöphuls, W.: The Relation of Gastric and Duodenal Ulcer to Vascular Lesions, Arch. Int. Med. **11**: 469, 1913.
23. Askanazy, M.: Ueber Bau Und Entschung des Chronischen Magengeschwürs soriue Soorpilzenbefunde, Virchows Arch. f. path. Anat. **234**: 111, 1921.

ONE-STAGE PANCREATODUODENECTOMY WITH RESECTION OF THE SUPERIOR MESENTERIC VEIN

GEORGE E. MOORE, M.D., PH.D.,* AND BARBARA URE, M.D.,**
MINNEAPOLIS, MINN.

(From the Department of Surgery, University of Minnesota)

ALLEN Whipple, in 1935, reported on three patients with carcinoma of the ampulla treated by a two-stage radical pancreatoduodenectomy, and stimulated further surgical attack on the problem of biliary tract carcinomas.

Subsequently, many reports of technically successful resections of ampullary and pancreatic neoplasms were added to the surgical literature. Reports of encouraging numbers of patients with ampullary carcinoma who, subsequent to operation, survived five years or more have been published.[2, 3] These results should be achieved as predicated by the autopsy studies of Baggenstoss, who found that in over one-third of the cases no metastases were present.

Unfortunately, a similar encouraging situation does not exist in regard to carcinoma of the pancreas. Nevertheless, increasing numbers of five-year survivals are being reported. The modified pancreatoduodenectomy procedures described herein are further attempts to achieve a satisfactory "cancer operation" in those patients in whom the disease is still localized. Descriptions of similar operations have been published.[5, 7, 9] Certainly such operations will not result in a substantial impress upon this dread disease, but in an occasional case they may mean the difference between death and survival.

A brief review (Table I) of patients with ampullary and pancreatic carcinomas between 1936 and 1951 seen at the University of Minnesota Hospitals is included to emphasize the scope of the problem at a medical center.

All cases with a definitive diagnosis of cancer of the biliary tree and pancreas are included; however, it must be remembered that a certain additional number of patients were briefly seen in the outpatient department and discharged as hopeless cases without establishment of a diagnosis. Second, undoubtedly others with this disease were considered hopeless cases by their physicians and were not referred to the University Hospitals for treatment. Therefore, the data included in graphic form cannot be interpreted as accurately reflecting the outcome of a wholly unselected group of patients with this disease.

Note that a curative procedure was attempted in only 15.4 per cent of the cases, including many extremely aggressive procedures.

Received for publication, Sept. 29, 1953.

*Presently Director, Roswell Park Memorial Institute, and Associate Professor, University of Buffalo Medical School, Buffalo, N. Y.

**Kings County Hospital, Brooklyn, N. Y.

TABLE I. CANCER OF BILIARY TREE AND PANCREAS (1936-1951)

Total cases	486	
Surgery	333	
Exploratory only		85
Palliation		173
Resection		75

CARCINOMA OF PANCREAS

There were 193 patients with carcinoma of pancreas. In 145 patients, the lesion occupied the head of the pancreas, and in 48, the body or tail.

The age incidence of these patients is depicted in Fig. 1.

It is interesting to note the predominance of men afflicted with pancreatic cancer (and carcinoma of the common duct) in contrast to the preponderance of women afflicted with carcinoma of the gall bladder (Fig. 2).

The most frequent symptoms mentioned by patients with carcinoma of the pancreas at the onset of the disease were pain 86 per cent, jaundice 29 per cent, and anorexia 15 per cent. Other prominent symptoms were diarrhea and constipation, nausea, vomiting, bloating, and belching. The duration of symptoms is indicated in Fig. 3.

Both patients with lesions of the head of the pancreas and those with lesions in the body and tail indicated that their pain was in the mid-epigastrium. Back pain, which has been considered an important diagnostic symptom, was elicited in one-third of those with lesions of the body and tail and only 6 per cent of those with tumors in the head of the pancreas. The complaints at the time of admission are summarized in Fig. 4.

Excessive weight loss has been noted by most clinicians and was confirmed in this series of patients (Fig. 5).

Despite an aggressive surgical attitude toward pancreatic cancer in the last few years, only 20 of the 193 patients were subjected to radical resection because of local extension or widespread metastases (Table II).

TABLE II. CARCINOMA OF PANCREAS (1936-1951)

Total cases	193	
No surgery	63	
Surgery	130	
Exploration		35
Palliation		75
Resection		20

Survival of these patients is extremely discouraging, as is indicated graphically in Table III.

TABLE III. SURVIVAL OF PATIENTS WITH CARCINOMA OF PANCREAS

	TOTAL	ONE MONTH	TWO MONTHS	SIX MONTHS	ONE YEAR
No surgery	63	22 (35%)	10 (16%)	5 (8%)	0
Exploration	35	12 (34%)	6 (17%)	1 (3%)	0
Palliation	75	47 (63%)	34 (45%)	7 (9%)	3*
Radical	20	14 (70%)	11 (55%)	4 (20%)	0

*Insertion of T tube, 2 cases; choledochojejunostomy, 1 case.

It must be remembered that with such a small number of cases, individual percentages are not valid and are included only to indicate the trend of survival with and without surgery.

PALLIATION

It is difficult to provide effective palliation for this tumor. Certainly, the patient and relatives are relieved to see the disappearance of jaundice and its attendant discomfort. This can be most simply provided by insertion of a T tube, but this technique has the disadvantages of loss of electrolytes and water, and the problem of continual external drainage. We prefer, if choledochojejunostomy is impossible, to insert an enterostomy tube also, which can be connected to the T tube externally, allowing the bile to be returned to the intestine. The enterostomy tube can, of course, also be used for feeding purposes.

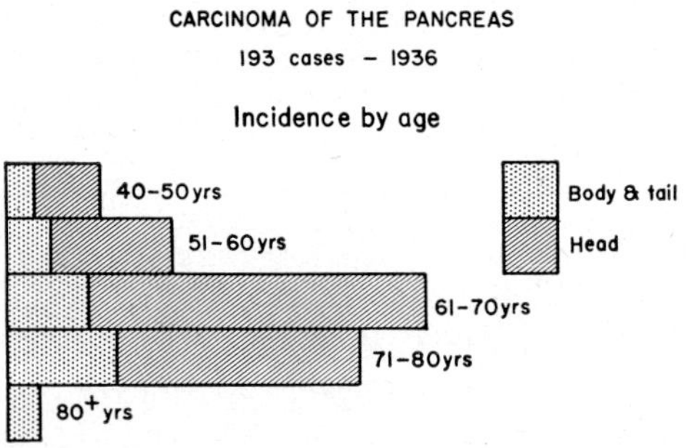

Fig. 1.

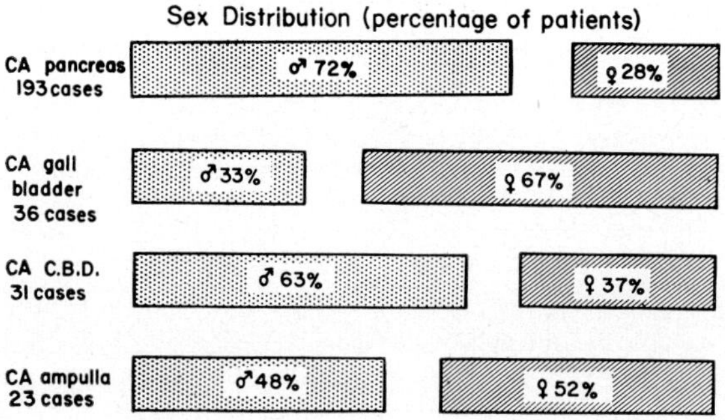

Fig. 2.

Although choledochojejunostomy is increasingly popular, our experience does not indicate that it offers an increased period of palliation. Both the loop of jejunum and the Roux Y principle have been utilized, with little difference clinically.

Finally, it should be noted that radical pancreaticoduodenectomy is not a satisfactory palliative procedure and should be used only when there is a possibility of effecting a curative excision.

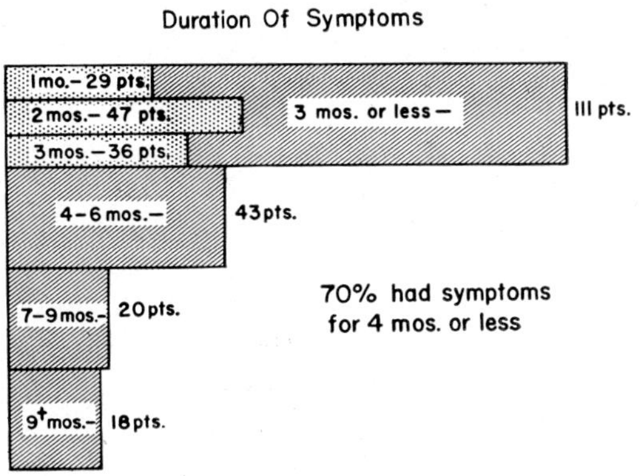

Fig. 3.

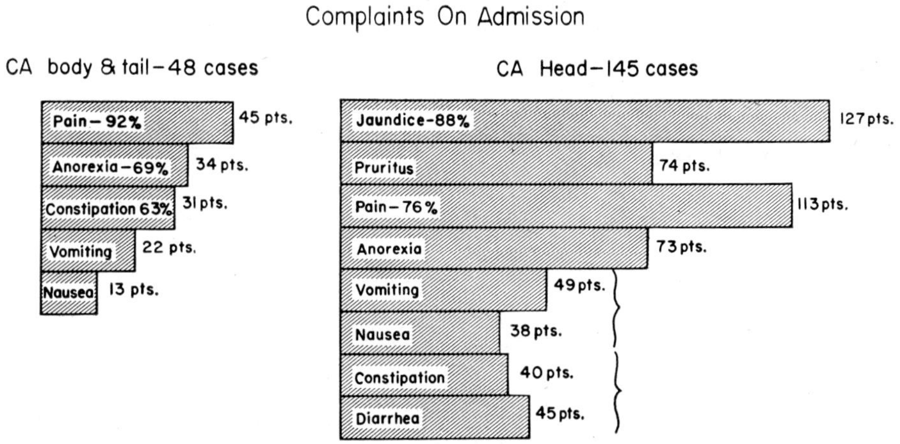

Fig. 4.

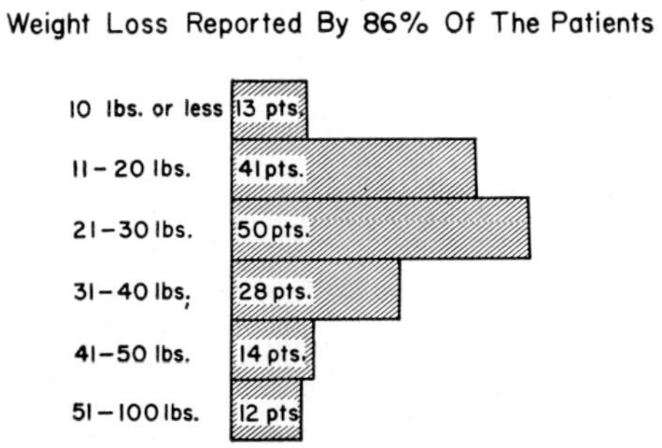

Fig. 5.

LONG-TERM SURVIVORS

Five-year survivals following resection of biliary and pancreatic neoplasms in this hospital number only two patients with carcinoma of the ampulla and one with a diagnosis of sarcoma of the body of the pancreas. All three patients are in good health.

In this regard it should be noted that a patient with pancreatic carcinoma (not included in this study) operated upon by Dr. Clarence Dennis, formerly on the University of Minnesota staff, is still alive and well. This woman was 70 years of age when first admitted to the Minneapolis General Hospital in 1943 with severe cardiac decompensation, auricular fibrillation, generalized arteriosclerosis, and hypertension. On March 28, 1945, a pancreaticoduodenostomy was performed and the patient was discharged on May 4, 1945.

The carcinoma was described as being about 3 cm. in diameter; no involved lymph nodes were noted. This patient has since survived many bouts of cardiac decompensation, and at last report was alive (eight years) without recurrence of the cancer.

EXTENSION OF THE PANCREATODUODENECTOMY PROCEDURE

In recent years, several surgical groups have reported their attempts to extend the standard one-stage Whipple procedure. Child has reported several two-stage pancreatoduodenectomies with portal vein resection,[5] and Parsons[9] and McDermott[6] have reported one-stage operations. In several of the latter cases, however, it was noted that the portal vein was partially occluded prior to resection.

Child[4, 5] carried out a series of excellent experimental and clinical studies to demonstrate the feasibility of interrupting the portal vein. Finally, he reported a successful two-stage pancreatoduodenectomy with resection of an unobstructed portal and mesenteric vein. Such a procedure makes possible an attempt to perform a curative procedure in those patients with a carcinoma of the head and/or uncinate process with extension to the portal vein. Interestingly enough, examination of our specimens with extension of the tumor to the vein did not show actual penetration of the tumor through the vein wall.

A patient with carcinoma of the pancreas and involvement of the superior mesenteric vein but without significant reduction of the lumen necessitating resection of the vein has been previously reported by us.[7] Briefly, the tumor was found to be adherent to the superior mesenteric vein and, therefore, after gently clamping both the superior mesenteric vein and artery, the pancreatic dissection was completed, a 3 cm. section of the vein resected, and reanastomosis performed. The vessels were clamped for ninety-five minutes without ill effect. Although the patient enjoyed an uneventful postoperative course, she was readmitted forty-two days later with evidence of widespread metastasis and died afterward. Autopsy examination revealed the vein anastomosis to be widely patent.

A second such operation with excision and reanastomosis of the superior mesenteric vein was performed by Dr. D. Ferguson and one of us without event. The superior mesenteric vessels were clamped for forty-three minutes (Fig. 6, *3*) without interruption of the artery.

In a third patient in whom the carcinoma was adjacent to the mesenteric vessels, reanastomosis was impossible because of the length of the involved segment. The superior mesenteric vein was dissected free of several small branches and then anastomosed end to side to the vena cava (Fig. 6, *2*). The mesenteric vessels were simultaneously clamped for forty minutes.

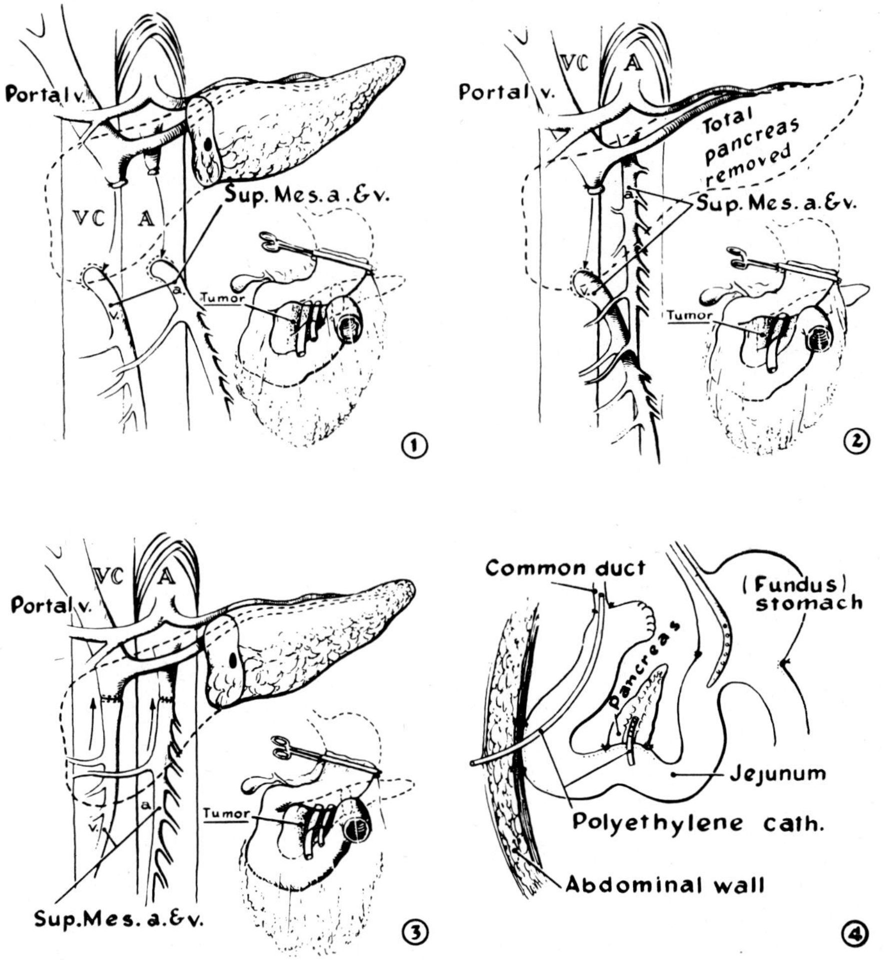

Fig. 6.—Possible modifications of radical pancreatoduodenectomy when the superior mesenteric vessels are involved by tumor.

Clinically, the tumor seemed to extend along the pancreatic duct into the body of the pancreas and, therefore, a total pancreatectomy was performed. The postoperative course was complicated by an inability to control adequately the blood sugar levels and, consequently, a normal electrolyte pattern. Several episodes of profound hypoglycemia were followed by a continuing comatose condition. The patient died thirty-six days subsequent to the operative procedure.

Post-mortem examination revealed the anastomosis of the superior mesenteric vein to the vena cava to be patent. No evidence of residual tumor was found.

Fig. 6, *4* illustrates an operative technique somewhat different from those described in the literature which is useful in special instances. The common duct should always be divided as high as possible, usually above the level of the cystic duct, since experience has shown that intramural and extramural lymphatics of the common duct are commonly involved. Division of the common duct at or immediately below the apparent junction should be avoided. Often the cystic duct forms an integral part of the common duct with a slightly reduced diameter of the common duct or a double-barreled configuration which can make the choledochojejunostomy more difficult. If the surgeon wishes to splint the anastomosis temporarily, a minute polythene tube can be used, as illustrated. Usually this technique is not necessary. Similarly, a small polythene tube with multiple perforations, as recommended by Dennis and Varco, may be used to splint the pancreatic duct jejunal anastomosis temporarily. A mucosa-to-mucosa anastomosis with a single row of interrupted sutures of 00000 silk is preferable. As has been pointed out many times, an adequate gastric resection should be peformed in order to obviate the subsequent development of marginal ulcers. This complication has been seen even in patients surviving only a short time.

Obviously, the surgical approaches outlined have a limited usefulness. The percentage of pancreatic cancer victims dying with the tumor still limited to the local area is unknown and awaits a study similar to that concerning ampulla carcinoma reported by Baggenstoss.

Further, it is evident that the rapacious character of this tumor is such that even wide dissections of the definitive tumor may fail to eradicate the tumor completely, as is amply indicated by the dearth of five-year survivals following radical surgery. This is not intended to imply that further attempts to treat this tumor surgically should be abandoned, but is merely a recognition of the severity of the problem.

DISCUSSION

The problems attendant on resection of the superior mesenteric vein are:

(1) increased operative hemorrhage from ligation of the portal vein (Child),

(2) thrombosis of the portal system resultant to temporary occlusion of the mesenteric vessels,

(3) hypoxia with subsequent injury to the intestine following prolonged clamping of the mesenteric vessels, and

(4) re-establishment of the portal circulation or performance of a portal canal shunt.

As is indicated in our abbreviated case reports, none of these problems preclude the successful accomplishment of a one-stage procedure.

In contrast to the experience of Child, no increased portal hemorrhage was encountered with temporary clamping of the portal vein during dissection even though in none of our cases was the portal vein obstructed or its lumen significantly reduced. It is interesting that McDermott, in his summary of previous clinical and experimental observations, stated that "resection of the portal vein together with the pancreas and duodenum is possible, but only after collateral channels have been developed."[6] His own excellent case report of a one-stage radical pancreaticoduodenectomy with segmental resection of the portal vein and its anastomosis to the vena cava did not indicate an unusual degree of hemorrhage; narrowing of the portal vein was not mentioned.

In regard to engorgement of the portal system during surgical treatment of the superior mesenteric vein, it is imperative that the accompanying artery be occluded simultaneously or preferably a few seconds earlier.

The threat of mesenteric thrombosis following prolonged clamping of the superior mesenteric vessel for intervals necessary to complete a block dissection of the pancreas and reanastomosis of the vessels cannot be disregarded. Fortunately, such a catastrophe was not encountered in our patients nor has it been reported by others. Undoubtedly, the fact that most patients with carcinoma of the pancreas have an obstructed biliary tract and some depression of liver function increases the margin of safety.

Experimental studies by Nelson and Kremen[8] indicated that, in the dog, either the superior mesenteric artery or vein could be safely clamped for two hours whereas occlusion for four hours was fatal in a majority of the animals. Occlusion of the superior mesenteric vein alone definitely was more lethal. They reported that preoperative administration of heparin significantly extended the period during which the vessels could be occluded.

Finally, the possible patterns of vessel resection are several. Fig. 6 depicts the procedures performed at this clinic and, in addition, a proposed scheme of resecting both the superior mesenteric vessels with their respective anastomosis to the portal vein and aorta. Similarly, it might be necessary and advisable to resect the portal vein proximal to the entrance of the splenic vein with excision of the splenic vessels and the accompanying lymphatics.

SUMMARY

1. Partial statistics concerned with diagnosis and treatment of biliary tract malignancy are presented, and several long-term survivals noted.

2. The technical feasibility of resecting the superior mesenteric vessels in order to accomplish a more adequate resection of the pancreas is demonstrated.

REFERENCES

1. Baggenstoss, A. H.: Major Duodenal Papilla: Variations of Pathologic Interest and Lesions of the Mucosa, Arch. Path. **26**: 853, 1938.

2. Brunschwig, A.: Pancreatoduodenectomy: A "Curative" Operation for Malignant Neoplasms in the Pancreatoduodenal Region, Ann. Surg. **136**: 610-617, 1952.
3. Cattell, R. B., and Warren, K. W.: Surgery of the Pancreas, chap. 8, Philadelphia, 1953, W. B. Saunders Company.
4. Child, C. G., Milnes, R. F., Holswade, G. R., and Gore, A. L.: Sudden and Complete Occlusion of the Portal Vein in the Macaca Mulatta Monkey, Ann. Surg. **132**: 475, 1950.
5. Child, C. G., Holswade, G. R., McClure, R. D., Gore, A. L., and O'Neill, E. A.: Pancreatoduodenectomy With Resection of the Portal Vein in the Mucaca Mulatta Monkey and in Man, Surg., Gynec. & Obst. **94**: 31-45, 1952.
6. McDermott, W. V., Jr.: A One-stage Pancreatoduodenectomy With Resection of the Portal Vein for Carcinoma of the Pancreas, Ann. Surg. **136**: 1012-1017, 1952.
7. Moore, G. E., Sako, Y., and Thomas, L. B.: Radical Pancreatoduodenectomy With Resection and Reanastomosis of the Superior Mesenteric Vein, SURGERY **30**: 1-4, 1951.
8. Nelson, L. E., and Kremen, A. J.: Experimental Occlusion of the Superior Mesenteric Vessels With Special Reference to the Role of Intravascular Thrombosis and Its Prevention by Heparin, SURGERY **28**: 819-826, 1950.
9. Parsons, W. B.: Discussion, Ann. Surg. **132**: 494-495, 1950.

FEMORAL HERNIOPLASTY: SUPRAPUBIC EXTRAPERITONEAL (CHEATLE-HENRY) APPROACH

William P. Mikkelsen, M.D., and Clarence J. Berne, M.D.,
Los Angeles, Calif.

(From the Department of Surgery, University of Southern California School of Medicine, and the Los Angeles County Hospital)

THE surgical correction of a femoral hernia has generally been performed through a groin incision placed either above or below the inguinal ligament. A combination of the two incisions is occasionally employed. There is no doubt but that an adequate hernioplasty can be performed through either approach, although a strangulated femoral hernia is usually better managed through an incision above the inguinal ligament. The purpose of this presentation is to emphasize the advantages of a seldom-used alternative approach and to suggest an improved technique for the actual hernioplasty.

The approach to be described is initiated by a suprapubic, abdominal incision, either vertical midline or Pfannenstiel. The incision is carried through the fascia, and from this point the dissection remains extraperitoneal and the femoral region is approached from above, behind the rectus muscle.

The advantages of the suprapubic extraperitoneal approach for the repair of femoral hernia have been stressed in several reports.[1-5] It has recently been referred to as the "Henry Operation" in the belief that Henry[3] in 1936 was the first to describe it. However, credit should be given to Cheatle for the basic concepts of this approach. In 1920,[1] he reported such a repair of a femoral hernia through a rectus muscle-splitting extraperitoneal approach on the involved side. He later[2] reported the use of a midline abdominal incision for the repair of bilateral hernias, inguinal as well as femoral.

When the suprapubic extraperitoneal approach has been used, closure of the femoral ring has been accomplished by a variety of methods. These methods have included plugging of the femoral canal with a segment of saphenous vein, elevation to Poupart's ligament of a flap of periosteum from the superior pubic ramus, or of a flap of fascia overlying the pectineus muscle, and, more commonly, simple suture of Poupart's ligament to Cooper's ligament. The hernioplasty technique presented here utilizes a doubled layer of the fused transversalis fascia and aponeurosis of the transversus muscle which is anchored to Cooper's ligament.

TECHNIQUE

The accompanying illustrations were obtained from a cadaver preparation. An actual femoral hernia is not present in this specimen, but this is not necessary for adequate illustration of the repair. The dissection demonstrates the superior exposure and the resultant ease with which the hernioplasty is

Received for publication, Oct. 5, 1953.

accomplished. The photographs are presented in serial arrangement and with their labels are self-explanatory.

DISCUSSION

During the four-year period from July, 1949, to July, 1953, 214 patients with femoral hernias were operated upon at the Los Angeles County Hospital.

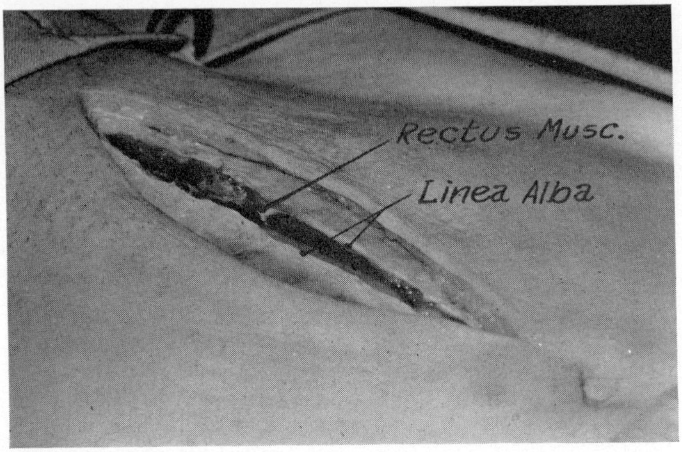

Fig. 1.—Either a vertical midline or Pfannenstiel incision may be used. Each affords equally good exposure.

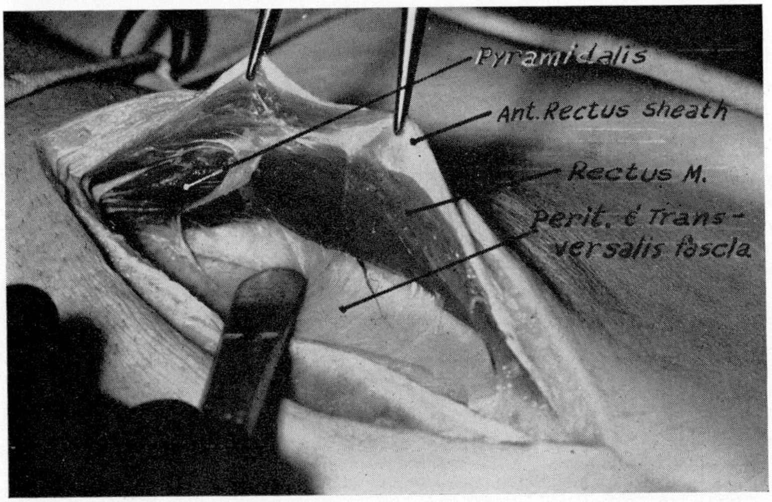

Fig. 2.—Beginning extraperitoneal dissection. This is accomplished bluntly by finger or gauze dissection.

Of this number, 113 were operated upon through the suprapubic extraperitoneal approach. No patient has returned for treatment of recurrence. This method is now preferred by the majority of the resident and attending staff of this hospital.

This approach has the obvious advantage of allowing the performance of a bilateral hernioplasty through one incision, a factor of importance since about 20 per cent of femoral hernias are overtly bilateral. We feel, however, that its

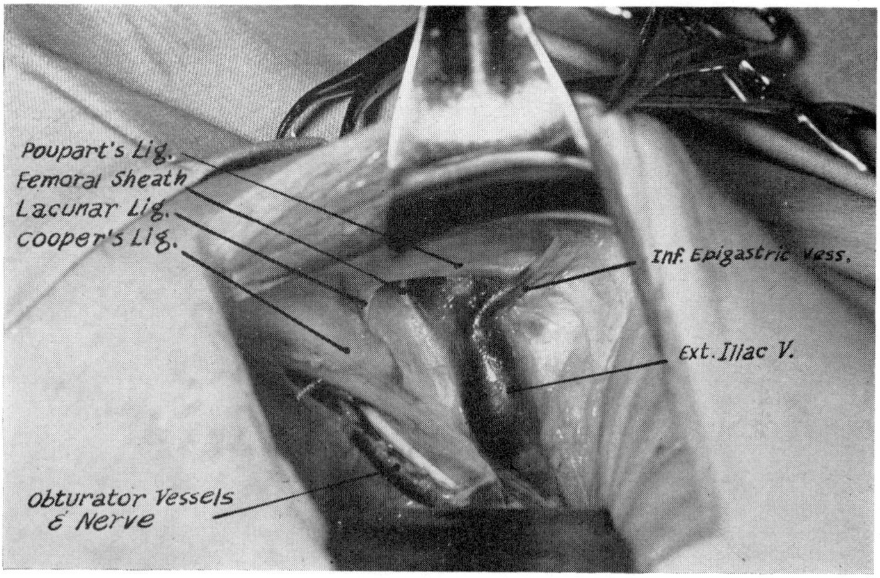

Fig. 3.—Retraction of the peritoneum superiorly and posteriorly widely exposes the femoral area. In actual practice, at this point the hernia sac is teased from the femoral ring. An accessory incision either inguinal or femoral has never been required. The close proximity of the obturator vessels and nerve is demonstrated.

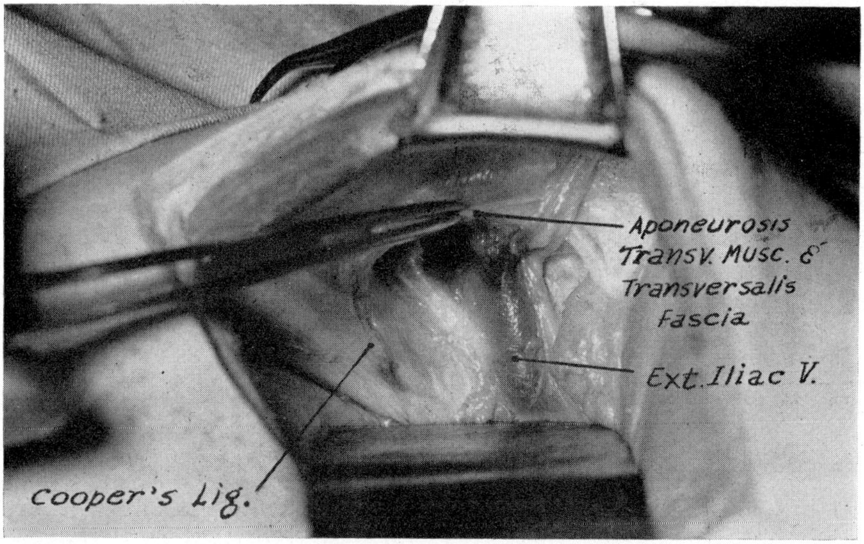

Fig. 4.—The fold of fused transversalis fascia and aponeurosis of the transversus muscle is grasped by a thumb forceps. It appears that the forceps are grasping Poupart's ligament, but actually they have grasped the fused transversalis fascia and aponeurosis of transversus muscle 1½ to 2 cm. above Poupart's ligament and are tenting them forward.

use should not be limited to bilateral hernias. In all patients with unilateral femoral hernia, the opposite side is explored. This additional exploration requires no more than two or three minutes' additional time and does not increase morbidity. In several instances a frank unsuspected hernia has been found

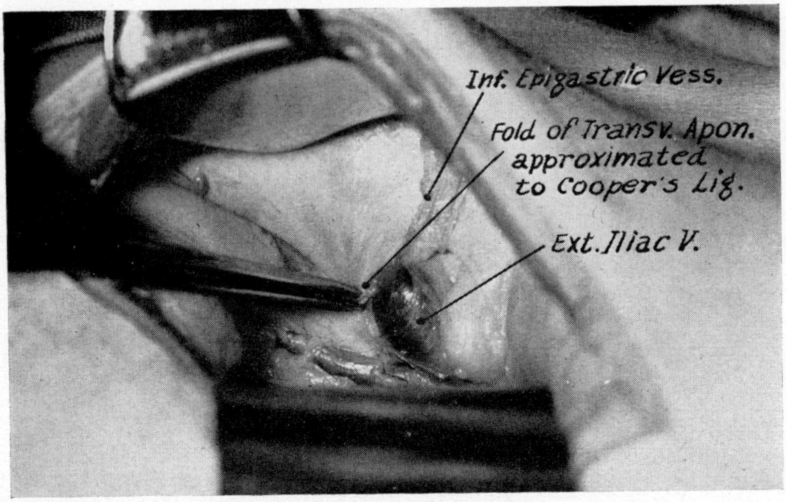

Fig. 5.—The fold of fused transversalis fascia and aponeurosis of transversus muscle is brought down to Cooper's ligament, thus obliterating the femoral ring and lying in juxtaposition to the external iliac vein.

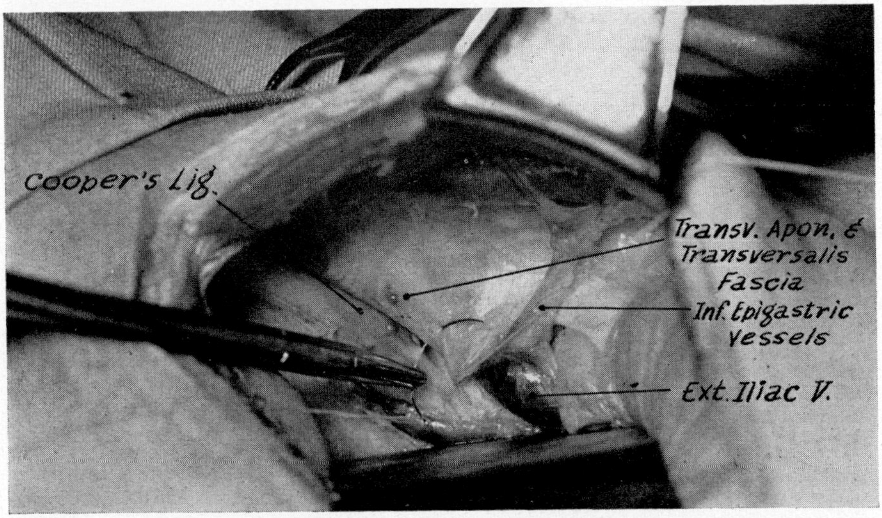

Fig. 6.—The most lateral suture has been placed, and the ease with which the hernioplasty is accomplished is shown by the placement of the second suture.

on the opposite side. More commonly, an enlarged femoral ring is encountered, which can be quickly and easily repaired if desired.

This approach is especially useful for strangulated hernias. In such instances the incarcerated bowel is released in the usual fashion by incising the lacunar ligament or Poupart's ligament if necessary. If resection or further exploration of the bowel is necessary, the peritoneal incision is extended superiorly as far as desired so as to result in a routine lower abdominal laparotomy incision.

Further advantages are apparent. An anomalous obturator vessel is readily recognized and dealt with. The possibility of injury to the external iliac vein and urinary bladder is minimized. A bilateral femoral hernioplasty can be accomplished in conjunction with any lower abdominal operation. While obesity has been cited as a contraindication,[4, 5] we believe that this factor interferes no more in this approach than it does in any abdominal operation, and we have employed this approach in several obese patients. An associated obturator hernia, one of which was encountered in this series, is readily accessible.

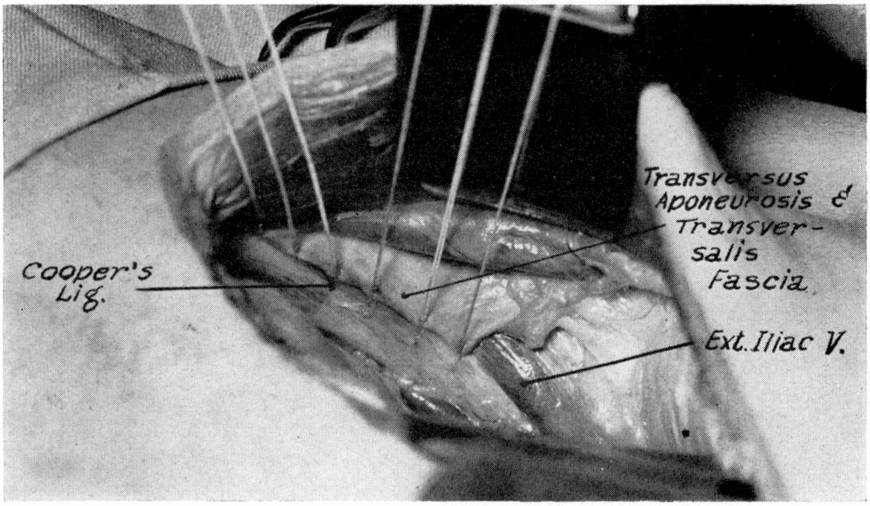

Fig. 7.—The completed hernioplasty.

While we are not here reporting or necessarily advocating the use of this approach for inguinal hernias, several such bilateral hernias, both direct and indirect, have been so repaired. In the case of the direct and large indirect inguinal hernias, a type of repair essentially the same as that which we employ for femoral hernias is carried out. In small indirect inguinal hernias, the sac is excised and the size of the internal inguinal ring is reduced by placing one or two sutures through the fused transversalis fascia and aponeurosis of the transversus muscle on the medial aspect of the ring.

From the accompanying illustrations it is seen that the femoral hernioplasty is accomplished by suturing a fold of the fused transversalis fascia and aponeurosis of the transversus muscle to Cooper's ligament. This results in a strong two-layer repair. The lateral edge of this structure lies in juxtaposition to the external iliac vein and does not result in compression of the vein such as may occur when Poupart's ligament is sutured to Cooper's ligament.

The use of a fold of this structure in place of an incised flap not only doubles the strength of the repair, but obviates a lateral triangular defect such as may occur in the routine McVay hernioplasty.

SUMMARY

Emphasis is directed to the advantages of the suprapubic extraperitoneal approach for the surgical correction of femoral hernia. A modification in the technique of the actual hernioplasty is presented. One hundred thirteen patients with femoral hernias have been successfully operated upon in this fashion at the Los Angeles County Hospital with no known recurrences.

REFERENCES

1. Cheatle, G. L.: An Operation for the Radical Cure of Inquinal and Femoral Hernia, Brit. M. J. **2**: 68, 1920.
2. Cheatle, G. L.: An Operation for Inquinal Hernia, Brit. M. J. **2**: 1025, 1921.
3. Henry, A. K.: Operation for Femoral Hernia by a Midline Extraperitoneal Approach, Lancet **230**, 531, 1936.
4. Musgrove, J. E., and McCready, F. J.: The Henry Approach to Femoral Hernia, Surgery **26**: 608, 1949.
5. Hull, H. C., and Ganey, J. B.: The Henry Approach to Femoral Hernia, Ann. Surg. **137**: 57, 1953.

THE TREATMENT OF INFECTION AFTER MEDULLARY NAILING

J. Albert Key, M.D., and Fred C. Reynolds, M.D., St. Louis, Mo.

(From the Department of Surgery, Washington University School of Medicine)

THE introduction of noncorrosive metals and the use of antibiotic drugs before and after operation render the fixation of the fragments of the fractured shaft of a long bone by means of a long heavy medullary nail a relatively safe and practical procedure. Consequently, this method of treating fractures is becoming increasingly popular. Its popularity is justified because the method lessens the periods of hospitalization and of disability, and in skillful hands yields better results than do more conservative methods.

However, treatment of major fractures by intramedullary nailing is fraught with complications, and one of the principal dangers is infection.

It is our impression that postoperative infection occurs more frequently after medullary nailing than it does after other major surgical operations. There are several reasons for this: (1) Wounds of the buttock and lower extremities are more likely to become infected than are similar ones elsewhere. (2) The skin over the operated area may be in poor condition, especially if the extremity has been in traction or in a cast for some weeks, or pressure sores may be present. (3) The tissues have been traumatized and some of them are devitalized, and the wound may contain pieces of devitalized bone. (4) The operation may be quite traumatic, and this is especially true if excessive shortening has occurred or if the operation is performed by a surgeon who is not skilled in this procedure. (5) A large foreign body is left in the wound. (6) The patient may be anemic and debilitated from hemorrhage, shock, or prolonged rest in bed, or he may be suffering from some other disease, such as malignancy, and the operation may be undertaken as a lifesaving or palliative measure. (7) The fracture may be a fresh compound fracture or one in which the wound has been closed, and may have been contaminated or even infected, or it may have been mildly infected by a previous unsatisfactory operation for open reduction with or without internal fixation. (8) Hematomas are especially likely to develop in the wound after the insertion of a medullary nail, and these may become infected. (9) A nail which is too long or one which has migrated may erode through the skin and thus become infected.

The infection may occur at the site of the fracture or near the end of the bone in the wound where the nail was introduced and may remain localized in the soft tissues or bone, or it may involve the bone throughout the track of the nail.

During the past few years we have observed a number of patients with infection following the insertion of a medullary nail, and while the majority of these were not seen by us until the bone was chronically infected, in some the nailing was carried out in our clinic and the chronic bone infection developed while the patient was under our care (Fig. 1). In each instance there were some

Received for publication, Aug. 28, 1953.

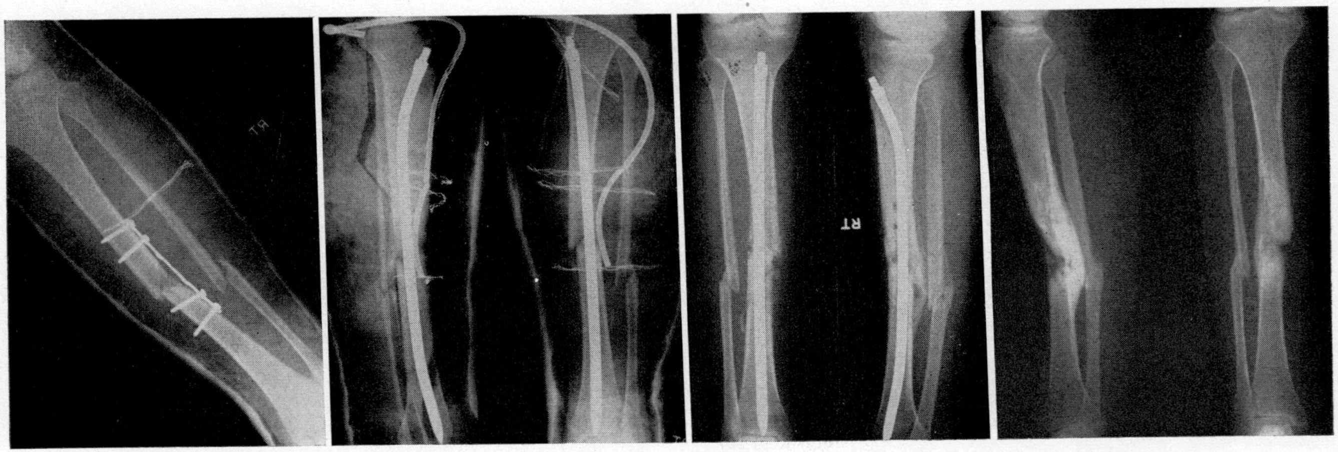

A. B. C. D.

Fig. 1.—*A*, Closed fracture of both bones of the leg treated elsewhere by reduction and inadequate plating, plus the removal of a large piece of bone. X-ray appearance on admission; wound healed and apparently clean one week after operation.

B, Following removal of the plate and insertion of a Lottes nail, infection developed. The wound was widely opened and the tube left in depth of the wound for instillation of penicillin.

C, Two months later chronic infection present, nail still in place, and fracture healing.

D, Because of persistent drainage, nail and sequestra removed. Fracture united but precarious, wound healed. The bone gradually strengthened and the patient now has full use of the leg and no drainage.

extenuating circumstances, but the result is just as bad as if there were no excuses. From this experience we have formulated some ideas concerning the treatment of infection after medullary nailing which we wish to communicate in this paper. We offer as evidence illustrations of three of the severe infections with chronic osteomyelitis.

DIAGNOSIS OF POSTOPERATIVE INFECTION

It is important that the presence of infection in an operative wound be diagnosed as soon after its onset as possible. This is because the optimum time to treat the infection is early in the process and before the bone becomes involved. Early diagnosis requires vigilance on the part of those in charge of the patient after the operation.

It is usual for the surgeon to think of fever as the first sign of infection, and certainly this is usually one of the earliest signs. However, it is not a reliable sign after medullary nailing because in most of these patients the temperature is elevated for from twenty-four to forty-eight hours after the operation. Consequently, we inspect the wound in such patients, but do not open it unless there are other signs of infection. We are suspicious of infection if the fever lasts more than forty-eight hours or if it develops after the temperature has been normal a few days. Furthermore, absence of fever is not a dependable sign that infection is not present, particularly if the patient has had antibiotic therapy.

When such a patient complains of unusual pain in the wound and especially of a throbbing pain, the surgeon should become suspicious of infection. Other symptoms are headache and general malaise. Increased pulse rate and elevation of temperature may be signs of infection, and this is more likely to be true if increase in the pulse is proportionately greater than the increase in temperature. Corroborative evidence of infection is increase in the leukocyte count, and this is more significant if there is a pronounced increase in young forms of leukocytes in the differential count (shift to the left).

The onset of infection may be ushered in by a chill with high fever, and the patient may become acutely ill within a few hours and the infection pursue a stormy course. More frequently, however, the onset is insidious, and deep infection may be present for several days and the area around the fracture be converted into an abscess cavity before there are sufficient signs and symptoms to justify opening the wound. This is especially likely to occur in patients who have been treated with antibiotics after the operation.

TREATMENT OF INFECTION

Any or all of the symptoms or signs mentioned previously demand that the dressing be removed and the wound inspected. If the tissues are red, swollen, and edematous and the skin exhibits increased heat and is unusually tender, one or two of the skin, and if necessary some of the deeper, sutures should be removed and an instrument introduced into the wound. If a hematoma is encountered and this is not large and clotted, it should be evacuated and the wound edges strapped together with adhesive and a pressure dressing applied.

If a small amount of pus is encountered in the superficial tissues (stitch abscess or small hematoma) and the surgeon is reasonably sure that the infection does not involve the deeper tissues, this should be evacuated and the area left open and covered with grease gauze and a dry dressing or a wet dressing.

If the hematoma is large and the wound contains considerable clotted blood, or if evidence of infection in the deeper tissues is encountered, it is advisable to take the patient to the operating room, administer a general anesthetic, and open the wound under aseptic conditions. There the wound is opened widely and irrigated thoroughly, and if a large hematoma is found it is evacuated and if there is no evidence of infection the wound is sutured. If a bleeding vessel is found it is ligated. If there is considerable bleeding from the bone or if there is much general oozing, a rubber tissue drain should be left in the wound and a moderate pressure dressing applied.

If there is evidence of infection, any loose fragments of bone or bone grafts which may be in the wound are removed, devitalized soft tissues are excised, and the wound is again irrigated thoroughly. This is because the loose bone fragments and grafts are not viable and, if left, will act as irritating foreign bodies which hinder healing, harbor infection, and will have to be removed later. The nail is not removed, and if it is found that it is not fixing the fragments firmly, the limb should be immobilized, preferably in a large plaster cast. Then the wound may be packed open loosely with petrolatum gauze, but we prefer to place one or two rubber tubes in the depths of the wound and pack it loosely with gauze soaked in normal salt solution (Fig. 1). Then a massive hot wet dressing as applied and a solution of penicillin is instilled into the wound every three hours, or it may be irrigated continuously with a penicillin solution. The solution used is 1,000 units of penicillin per cubic centimeter of normal salt solution. The dressing and pack are changed in twenty-four to forty-eight hours, and after seven or eight days, if the wound is clean it may be closed by secondary or delayed primary suture.

Cultures of the wound are taken when it is opened, and the organisms are tested for sensitivity to antibiotics and the appropriate drug (penicillin, streptomycin, Aureomycin, Terramycin, and so forth) is used systemically in full dosage. Until the laboratory findings are reported, the patient should be given penicillin and some broad spectrum antibiotic (streptomycin) in full dosage.

If the infection does not subside within a few days to a point where it is considered safe to suture the wound, it is probable that the bone is involved and it is possible that the infection may have entered the marrow canal and extended upward or downward along the track of the nail. In such a case the nail should not be removed until union is present, but antibiotic therapy should be continued, and the wound may be explored again for loose pieces of bone and then packed open with petrolatum gauze while the limb is immobilized, preferably in a large plaster cast.

There is still a possibility that the infection may subside, the wound heal, and the bone unite without sequestration. The wound is dressed infrequently and the petrolatum gauze pack changed at each dressing. It is thus encouraged to heal by granulation. During this period the fragments and the extremity are immobilized in a cast or splint, and the fracture has an excellent opportunity to heal. Usually under such treatment the fracture does heal unless there is diastasis or sequestra are present.

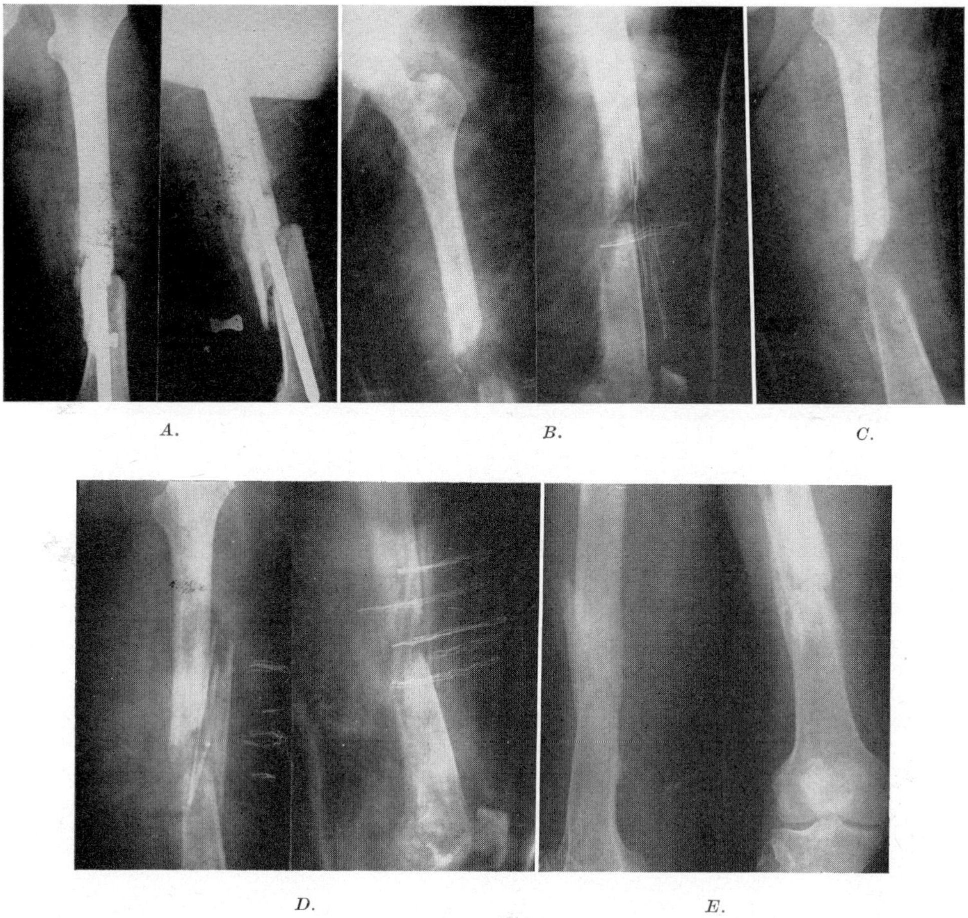

Fig. 2.—*A*, X-ray appearance on admission three and one-half months following nailing of an open fracture and wound closure as a primary single-stage operation. Débridement and drainage of the wound failed to improve its condition. The large central fragment was a sequestrum. At a second operation it was removed and the fragments pushed together with the nail still in place.

B, Following sequestrectomy the wound continued to be unfit for closure. The nail loosened and began to back out and had to be removed. The wound and medullary canal were irrigated by constant drip of penicillin with three catheters in the canal (1,000,000 units to the liter). Closure was performed two weeks later. This was complicated by a postoperative hemorrhage that required opening this wound and ligation of a vessel, followed three days later by a secondary closure. The wound healed and remained healed.

C, Appearance after a period of three months of immobilization in a cast. Wound healed.

D, Because of non-union, autogenous bone grafts used to bridge the defect.

E, Present condition of the femur: wound healed, fracture healed, but there remains considerable stiffness of the knee.

Sometimes after prolonged infection the end of one or of each fragment may become necrotic and be sequestrated as ring or cone-shaped sequestra. These and other sequestra should be removed soon after they are discovered, and the bone ends should be forced together and immobilization and free drainage continued. This is true even though the sequestrum is large and comprises an entire section of the shaft. Such sections, like ring sequestra, should be split into two

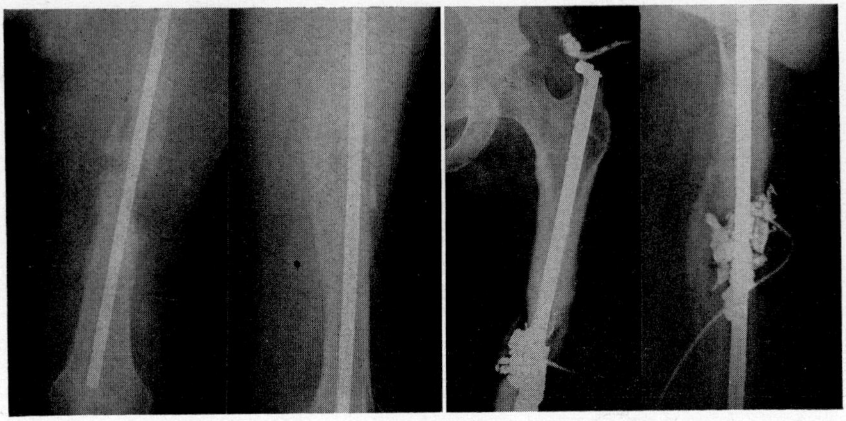

A. B.

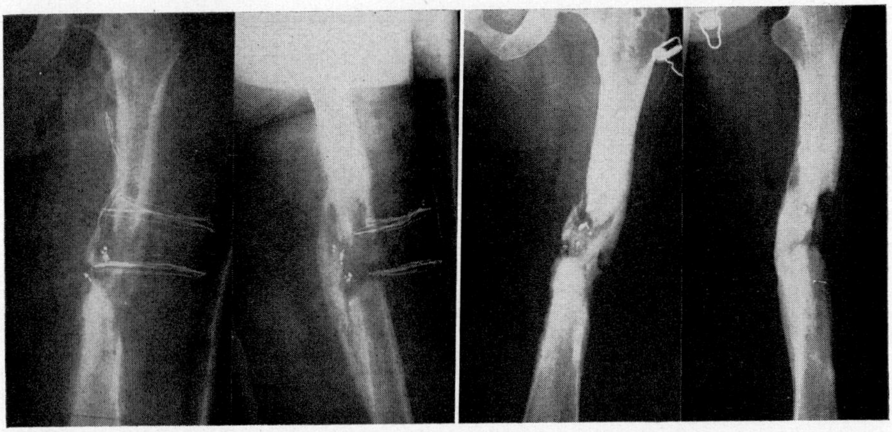

C. D.

Fig. 3.—*A*, Appearance on admission fourteen months following a closed fracture of the femoral shaft which was treated by open reduction, plating, and cast. After four months another operation was performed, the plate removed, an intramedullary nail inserted, and iliac graft implanted. Postoperative infection developed.

B, Injection of sinus tract with Lipiodol revealed extensive involvement of medullary canal. Nail was removed and canal irrigated with penicillin while wound was packed open with three catheters in the canal, immobilized in a plaster spica cast.

C, Appearance following removal of the nail; beginning of union.

D, Wound healed, union still precarious but patient walking without support. Improvement has continued.

or more sections and removed from around the nail (Fig. 2). We believe that in such instances it is good surgical judgment to accept a moderate amount of shortening rather than court a chronic infection and non-union.

Occasionally infection extends up and down the medullary canal along the entire track of the nail. In such instances it is advisable to remove the nail whether union is present or not and to remove any dead bone and infected granulation tissue which can be identified, and then the medullary canal can be irrigated and even scrubbed by running strips of gauze from the trochanter down to the fracture site, and the canal in the distal fragment can be curetted lightly and irrigated with a catheter (Fig. 3). Catheters, usually three (one in either end of the proximal fragment and one in the distal fragment), are left in the wound, and penicillin solution (1,000 units per cubic centimeter) is either instilled into the catheters every three hours or is administered by a continuous drip. The wounds are packed loosely with petrolatum gauze, and the limb is immobilized in a large plaster cast, the catheters being led out through the cast. In ten days or so it may be possible to close one or both wounds by a secondary suture (Fig. 2). If this does not seem possible, they may be permitted to heal by granulation tissue (Fig. 3).

In addition to the chronic disease of the bone and non-union of the fracture, the infected case of medullary nailing may be further complicated by infection and eventual stiffening and ankylosis of the joints above and below the fracture. This is especially likely to occur if the nail enters the joints.

In every instance where infection has occurred after a medullary nailing, the general health of the patient is a primary consideration, and he should be given supporting treatment: transfusions of whole blood, high-calorie and high-protein diet, intravenous feedings if necessary, excess vitamins, the most judicious antibiotic therapy, and careful and assiduous nursing care. At the same time, the patient should be made as comfortable as possible and pain relieved by proper attention to the wound and immobilization of the fracture, rather than by drugs.

If the fracture does not heal, autogenous bone grafts may be placed across the fracture site in order to expedite union. This is done after the infection has subsided and the wound has been closed or has healed by secondary intention. With the protection afforded by antibiotics, the bone grafting operation need not be delayed six months or more, as in the past, but can be carried out within a few weeks after the wound is healed (Fig. 2).

In exceptional cases where it seems unlikely that a useful extremity will be obtained even after further prolonged treatment, amputation is the procedure of choice. Decision to amputate the extremity is favored by advanced age of the patient, poor general condition of the patient, and failure to improve this by transfusions, high-protein diet, relief of pain, and other conservative measures, inability to eradicate the infection, failure to obtain union, excessive shortening of the extremity, damage to the nerve or blood supply of the extremity, and inability of the patient to finance prolonged hospitalization and indefinite disability. This last should not be a factor, but it cannot be ignored.

PREVENTION OF INFECTION

When one considers the difficulty which is sometimes encountered in the early diagnosis of a deep postoperative infection and the dire results which may follow if the bone becomes involved, it is evident that even without the use of antibiotics special care should be taken to avoid infection after medullary nailing. This demands not only that the procedure be performed only by qualified surgeons who are experienced in the open treatment of fractures, but that such surgeons take the care to have on hand the proper equipment before the operation is started. During the operation the tissues should be handled gently, extensive stripping of the periosteum avoided, and the nail inserted and the reduction effected with as little trauma as possible. Also, only those cases in which the fracture is suitable for this type of fixation should be treated with a medullary nail; that is, they should be simple transverse or short oblique fractures of the shaft without too much comminution and not too near the end of the bone. Likewise, some care should be exercised in selecting the patient and in preparing him for the operation. If he is in shock or impending shock the operation should be delayed until he has reacted satisfactorily. If he is debilitated or the skin is in poor condition, the operation should be postponed until these are corrected, unless fixation of the fracture is considered to be so important that the nail may be inserted as a lifesaving procedure.

In compound fractures it is a moot question whether or not the wound should be débrided and the nail inserted at the primary operation and the wound either closed or left open to be closed later by delayed primary or secondary suture. Débridement, insertion of a medullary nail, and primary suture of the wound have been carried out successfully in many instances where the tissue damage was not extensive and the compound fracture had had antibiotic therapy, and was operated upon within less than twelve hours after the injury.

However, in a compound fracture, prevention of infection and closure of the wound are the primary aims of treatment, and treatment of the fracture is secondary. With full realization of the benefit afforded by immobilization in preventing and combating infection, in promoting healing of the soft tissues and of the bone, and in adding to the comfort of the patient, we believe that in most instances internal fixation should not be applied at the primary operation, but the wound should be débrided, and after it has been closed by primary, delayed primary, or secondary suture or by secondary healing, then the medullary nail may be inserted or other internal fixation applied if indicated. In the meantime, the fracture should be immobilized by external fixation (traction or a cast, or a splint).

If postoperative infection occurs in a compound fracture after medullary nailing, the condition is treated just as described previously. We have had no experience with inserting medullary nails in the presence of frank infection in the bone; however, this has been carried out with a fair degree of success by others.[1, 2]

DISCUSSION AND SUMMARY

It is emphasized that infection is especially likely to occur after insertion of a medullary nail and that this may lead to prolonged illness and disability and even to loss of life or the limb. Consequently, the patient should be watched carefully after the operation, and at the first signs of infection the wound should be inspected and, if necessary, the wound opened widely, and loose bone, but not the nail, removed and vigorous treatment of the infection instituted. Such early treatment may abort or eradicate the infection before the bone is involved and permit the fracture to heal in the usual manner.

If the bone becomes infected, sequestra should be removed when discovered, but the nail should be left in place until union occurs because the immobilization which it affords is a valuable asset in limiting spread of the infection and promoting healing of the fracture. In such cases the treatment is similar to that now used in the treatment of chronic osteomyelitis. If the infection spreads up and down the track of the nail and this becomes loose and inefficient, it should be removed and the fracture treated as an infected compound fracture with or without union.

REFERENCES

1. Brav, E. C., and Jeffress, V. H.: J. Bone & Joint Surg. **35-A**: 141-152 (Jan.) 1953.
2. Carr, C. R., and Turnipseed, D.: J. Bone & Joint Surg. **35-A**: 153-171 (Jan.) 1953.

THE TRACTION BRACE

A New Traction Method in the Conservative Treatment of Intervertebral Disc Lesions

Luben S. Walchef, M.D., Cincinnati, Ohio

THE present concept of intervertebral disc lesions is built on the pathologic data, the operative findings, and the clinical picture which have been described in the literature during the last fifteen to twenty years. The ruptured or herniated intervertebral disc is recognized generally as a common cause of low-back disability.

Speed[1] found that 80 per cent of patients who complain of low-back pain combined with true sciatic radiation are regarded as having disc injury with probable protrusion. The syndrome occurs most commonly in young men who make their living by doing hard manual labor, such as farmers, ranchers, mechanics, and so forth. Sell[2] reported a series of 252 patients, in which 25 per cent eventually had to be operated upon.

As a practical plan, the previously mentioned authors[1, 2] recommended conservative treatment of patients who have a probable herniated disc.

The majority of patients who present the syndrome of a ruptured disc may be relieved temporarily or permanently by nonsurgical measures.

The conservative treatment consists of: (1) Complete rest on a hard bed with boards under the mattress; (2) heat diathermy (only occasionally); (3) antispasmodics, such as Tolserol (mephenesin); (4) traction for a duration of ten to twenty days, with slight flexion of the bed under the knee; (5) plaster jacket or low-back brace, in some severe cases after the traction.

The most important of all these means is the traction. It is carried out by so-called skin traction with five to ten pounds on each leg. The legs are shaved, washed with soap, and painted with tincture of benzoin. Then the skin traction is applied by means of skin plaster tapes and elastic bandages. This method of traction has the disadvantages that the plaster straps are torn frequently and the traction has to be reapplied. Furthermore, it is frequently complicated with irritation of the skin, swelling of the ankles, and, in a number of cases, allergic reaction to the plaster tapes. Dermatitis with blisters and painful sensation results, and the traction has to be removed. Instead of the specific treatment, there is treatment of dermatitis for a few days or weeks. This is time consuming and an unnecessary expense for the patient; it means loss of time from work and extended hospitalization. A large number of patients develop dermatitis and pain in the legs resulting from the skin traction. Some of the diabetic or allergic patients get very severe dermatitis. It appears on the next day approximately twenty-four to thirty-six hours after the application of the plaster tapes. It starts with itching and pain under the tapes followed by redness and swelling. The patient is very uncomfortable and asks for immediate

Received for publication, Aug. 28, 1953.

removal of the traction. When the tapes are removed, there are large areas of redness of the skin and large blister formations measuring approximately 3 to 4 cm. in diameter. Some of the blisters rupture leaving superficial ulcerations.

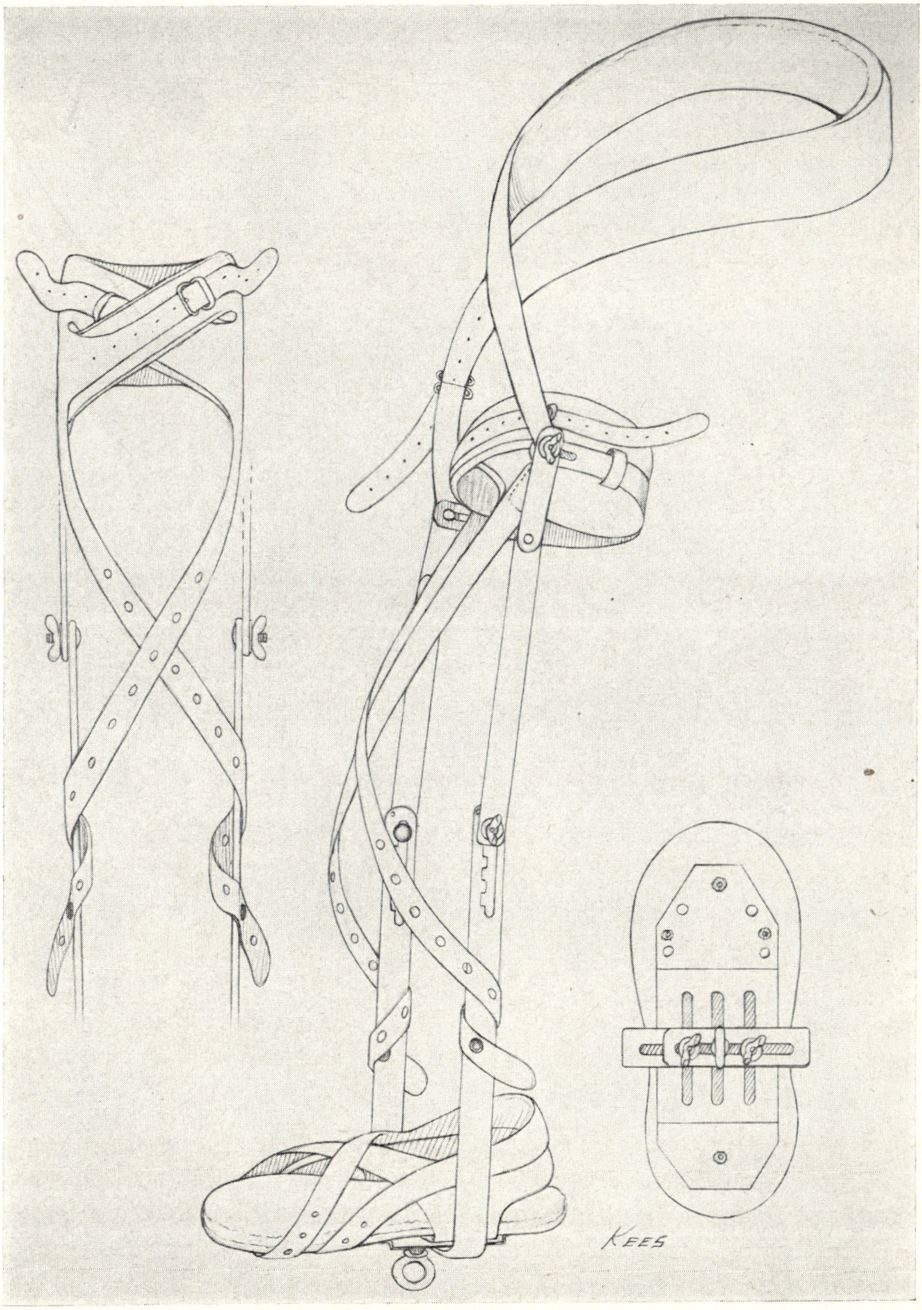

A. B. C.

Fig. 1.—Drawing of the traction brace. *A*, Front view of lateral adjustable bars and knee leather lacings. *B*, Lateral view of the traction brace as a unit. The crossed leather straps prevent slipping. *C*, Bottom view of the foot plate.

The inflammation subsides in a few days after the removal of the plaster tapes, but several days or weeks are necessary until the ulcerations heal. During this time no traction can be applied. Also, these patients develop dermatitis when the skin traction is reapplied, and therefore an adequate treatment for them is not possible.

Having in mind these defects, a brace was designed and perfected. The traction brace* is made from a light metal (aluminum), and is adjustable in length and width. This is made possible by using perforations and movable screws on the lateral bars, semicircular band, and foot plate. The foot plate is made from metal and wood, and felt-lined with foam rubber. There is a permanent knee joint which permits movement in the anterior-posterior position. The brace can be adjusted to many different contours of the lower extremities.

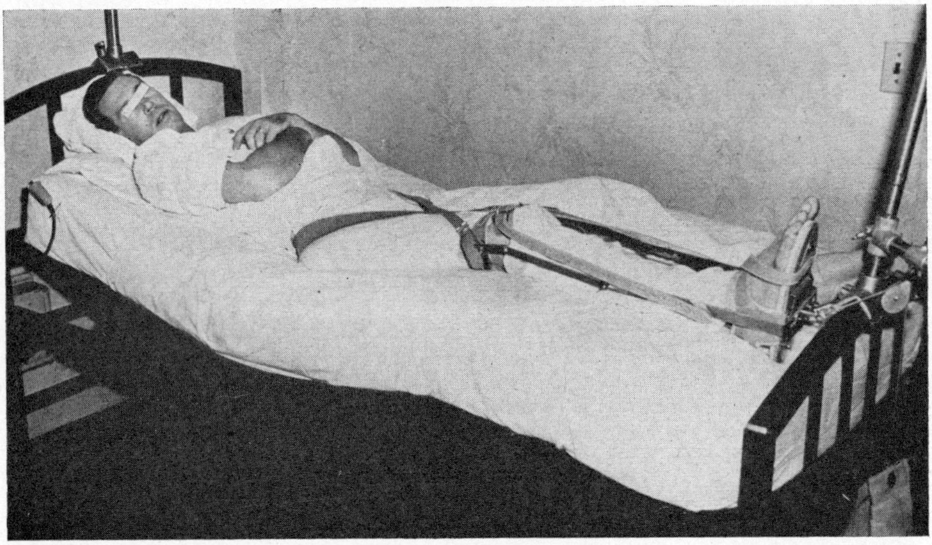

Fig. 2.—Photograph of the traction brace in use. The straps are felt-lined by foam rubber and attached to the hip, knee, and foot. It is used with five, ten, or fifteen pounds of weight. The knee is slightly flexed by breaking the bed at that level.

Leather cuffs and straps are attached to the metallic part of the brace. They are felt-lined with cemented foam rubber so that slipping and compression of the vessels and nerves are avoided. The leather cuffs over the knee are attached posteriorly on the semicircular band; they cross each other anteriorly and posteriorly around the lower portion of the thigh to prevent any slipping. They are made as tight as desired by means of buckles. Two leather straps extend down on both sides of the knee and cross over the anterior aspect of the lower leg. They are attached to the lateral bars, using small buttons, one on each side. The leather cuffs above the knee are to prevent slipping by the patella, and therefore the knee has to be slightly flexed using a pillow or breaking the bed under the knees slightly.

Two leather straps on each side of the foot cross around the heel and the dorsum of the foot and are attached to the foot plate by buttons. They hold the

*Manufactured by Max Wocher & Son Co., Cincinnati, Ohio.

foot firmly in place. The heel itself is free and elevated from the bed so that no pain or discomfort occurs. The foot plate is adjustable to the lateral bars to keep the heel free and to give the best comfort.

A leather strap fixed permanently on the upper end of one of the lateral bars goes around the hip for traction in intervertebral disc lesions and muscular spasm, or around the middle of the thigh for traction in upper femur fractures and postoperatively in hip prosthesis. It crosses the anterior aspect of the upper thigh and is attached on the opposite lateral bar by means of a buckle. These straps are also felt-lined with foam rubber cemented to the leather (Figs. 1 and 2).

The process of applying the brace is best carried out in a hospital, where supervision and care of the patient are best given. It can be used also at home by attaching any kind of weight in any way over the bed and using a pillow under the knee for slight flexion of the knee. The application is so simple that an intelligent patient will be able to do it himself after instruction by the physician. The brace as a whole may be adjusted during the application upward or downward in length and laterally in width to permit the most comfortable position for each leg. It can be used with five, ten, or fifteen pounds of weight on either the left or right leg. The time required is minimal; two or three minutes is sufficient for application as compared to fifteen or twenty minutes for the skin traction.

The orthopedic and neurosurgeons will find the traction brace especially useful in the conservative treatment of intervertebral disc lesions. It has been used with great satisfaction. The brace is one of the simplest and most variable devices. It can be used for a large number of conditions, both as an adjustable splint and as a traction brace for partial immobilization and traction on the lower extremities.

SUMMARY

1. The skin traction method is complicated by dermatitis and is time consuming.

2. A new traction brace has been described for conservative treatment of intervertebral disc lesions. The brace is made from aluminum and has a foot plate of wood, felt-lined with foam rubber. It is attached to the lower extremities by means of leather lacings and straps felt-lined with foam rubber.

3. The traction brace is adjustable, simple, and rapid to apply and gives the most comfortable and smooth traction for hospital and home use with five, ten, or fifteen pounds of weight.

4. The traction brace can be used in all conditions where traction on the lower extremities is required, such as low-back disability, pain from muscular spasm, upper femur fractures, and postoperatively in hip prosthesis.

REFERENCES

1. Speed, J. S.: Ruptured Intervertebral Disc, Pathologic, Diagnostic and Therapuetic Considerations, South. Surgeon **13:** 645-652, 1947.
2. Sell, L. S.: Misdiagnosis and Mismanagement of Early Intervertebral Disc Lesions, J. A. M. A. **150:** 987-990, 1952.

PROMINENT COSTAL CARTILAGES (TIETZE'S SYNDROME)

WILLIAM C. BECK, M.D., AND SAMUEL BERKHEISER, M.D., SAYRE, PA.

TIETZE, in 1921,[1] reported four cases of a peculiar syndrome for which he had no explanation. He described it as "swelling of costal cartilages of unknown etiology, insidious in onset, spontaneously painful, not associated with constitutional disturbances and of a prolonged fluctuating course." Since this time, there have been sporadic reports of similar cases and, in some instances, rather large series. These have been reported in the European, the British, the Canadian, and the Japanese literature. Not until June of this year, however, has a report of similar cases been seen in the American literature. In Dean Lewis' *Practice of Surgery*,[2] in the chapter on afflictions of the thoracic cage, Heuer and his associates showed two pictures which unquestionably described a similar condition. A letter from the publisher states that these photographs appeared in the original edition of Lewis' *Practice of Surgery* which was published in 1930, but that the photographs were received with the text for Chapter 5 on Oct. 6, 1927. There is no doubt that American surgeons have observed similar cases. In the last two years, we have seen four such instances which lead to this report. From our experiences with these cases, we are not certain that this is a disease of the costal cartilage at all.

Judging from published reports, there is no certainty as to the etiology, or even any exact definition of the pathology, of this condition. Only in their clinical symptomatology do these patients fall into a group.

Tietze described the syndrome as a cartilage dystrophy, probably due to wartime malnutrition. In one of his patients who was subjected to biopsy, there was no evidence of inflammatory change. Gill, Jones, and Pollak[3] reported five cases, in one of which a biopsy was performed. In none of these was malnutrition a factor. In Geddes'[4] series of thirty cases, all of which occurred in Canadian soldiers, there was no evidence of any malnutrition. Some authors have noted an associated respiratory tract infection. In many other cases, however, this was not present.

The clinical signs of the syndrome are consistently uniform. In most of the reported cases, as well as in ours, a healthy, usually young adult of either sex reports to the physician because of a painful swelling situated over one of the costal cartilages. The most frequently affected cartilage is the second, more often on the left than on the right. Less frequently, the third left costal cartilage or, rarely, one of the other costal cartilages is involved. The lesion is usually limited to one costal cartilage but in rare cases has been reported simultaneously present in two or three. There is a minimal amount of pain, usually described as a dull aching pain deep in the chest beneath the prominent cartilage. The pain appears to precede the appearance of the cartilaginous swelling or protrusion. It is rarely severe enough even to require the mildest of anodynes. The

Received for publication, Aug. 31, 1953.

pain is fluctuant in its course and may disappear, only to reappear after a time. The patient and, indeed, the surgeon often fear that this might represent a tumor of some sort. There are no constitutional symptoms.

In almost all series reported, occasional biopsies have been taken. In Geddes' rather large series of thirty cases, one patient was subjected to biopsy. Rather surprisingly, in none of the reported cases have we found that the entire cartilage was removed. Of the biopsies which are reported, one can only say that they all apparently have had the appearance of normal costal cartilage, and in none was there any evidence of tumor formation. In some of the reports there is mention of hyperplasia of the cartilage and occasionally mention of calcification or bone formation. In our opinion these reports are consistent with the finding of normal cartilage.

We must admit that until the article by Motulsky and Rohn[5] appeared we had seen only the report in Lewis' *Practice of Surgery,* most of the previous articles in the literature having been buried under the terminology of Tietze's syndrome. Therefore, in the four cases reported herein, the rib cartilage was removed. This has resulted in our acceptance of a different concept of the syndrome than is general.

The second costal cartilage was involved in all four of our cases. The clinical history was identical with reports in the literature: a painful swelling appearing at variable times in the region of the second costal cartilage.

Physical examination revealed a marked and definite prominence at this point, which was mildly tender to palpation and to percussion. There were no constitutional symptoms. The x-ray examination was entirely negative in all of the patients. At operation, the cartilage was found to be approximately normal in size and thickness. It was, however, buckled forward in an acute angle. Immediately subadjacent to the cartilage, heavy ligamentous fibrous tissue bands were visible. These were neither incised nor resected. Histologic study of the removed cartilages proved them to be entirely normal.

It appears to us, therefore, that the disease is not specifically one of the costal cartilage, but that some other process causes the buckling. It is interesting to note that in the one patient in Tietze's series who was subjected to surgical intervention, the surgeon described the cartilage as being "buckled forward" (vorgebückelt).

It is noteworthy that this condition affects the second costal cartilage oftener than any other. In the complete absence of any occupational or traumatic history in the reported cases, one must search for an anatomic reason for this peculiar localization. There is nothing in the bony blood supply or in the histologic anatomy of the second cartilage which differentiates it from any other of these cartilages. The only difference appears to be in the ligamentous fibers which surround the costal cartilage. According to Spalteholz,[6] a fibrocartilaginous layer, the interarticular chondrosternal ligament, extends from the medial end of the second cartilage to the cartilaginous or bony junction of the manubrium with the body of the sternum. This constantly divides the chondrosternal joint into two separate joint cavities. The other cartilages have somewhat similar fibrous strands, but these strands are different from the second. They lead generally to only incomplete division of the joint cavity. With such an intricate ligamentous arrangement, it is quite probable that in certain anomalous situations, a similar arrangement might take place behind the third or fourth costal cartilage. From these findings we would suggest that the disease entity described by Tietze may not be one of the cartilage at all. There may be an inflammatory reaction contracting the ligaments lying immediately behind the cartilage, producing the consequent buckling.

The therapy of this condition apparently needs little comment. The other inflammatory and noninflammatory diseases of costal cartilage need to be differentiated. If it is certain that one is dealing with such a buckling of cartilage, then reassurance of the patient is probably all that is needed. We have resected the cartilage in our patients with a cure of symptoms in all. When the cartilage is resected, we have followed the suggestion of Maier[7] to leave a cuff of perichondrium to insure healing. We have removed the cartilage and assured ourselves of a cuff of perichondrium by curetting a small portion of the cartilage away on either side.

CASE REPORTS

CASE 1.—A 22-year-old unmarried woman presented herself with a lump over the second costal cartilage which had been present for approximately four or five years. She felt that it had grown slowly during this time, especially recently, and had in recent weeks prior to admission noticed mild pain in this area. At the onset of the condition years previously, she had also noted some pain beneath the sternum. Other than the protruding mass over the second costal cartilage, the physical examination was entirely negative, with the exception of a small lump present in the left breast. Under general anesthesia, the second costal cartilage was resected and found to be buckled forward. A fibroadenoma of the left breast was also removed. The patient made an uneventful recovery. She was seen two years after the removal and had had no recurrence of symptoms.

CASE 2.—A 34-year-old woman had noticed a lump over the left second costal cartilage for approximately three years. It was occasionally painful, especially when she did excessive work, such as ironing. Physical examination revealed a mass of about 2 or 3 cm. in diameter over the second left costal cartilage. Physical examination was otherwise entirely negative. Under general anesthesia, an incision was made over this costal cartilage and it was found to be buckled forward at this point. The cartilage was removed. The patient was seen six months later and found to be entirely free of symptoms.

CASE 3.—This patient complained of a mass over the second right costal cartilage which had existed approximately two months. It was moderately painful at the time of onset, and she had noticed some pain beneath the sternum for approximately two or three weeks before the mass itself was noted. Physical examination revealed a mildly tender mass about 2 cm. in diameter over the second right costal cartilage. Physical examination was, otherwise, entirely negative. Under general anesthesia, an incision was made over the second costal cartilage. The cartilage was found to be buckled forward; it was completely resected. The postoperative course was uneventful. The patient was seen about one year later and stated that there had been no recurrence of symptoms.

CASE 4.—A boy of 11 years was seen because of a mass over the second right costal cartilage of one week's duration. There was no history of trauma. At the onset of this condition, the child had complained of a slight aching in the right chest and arm. The aching disappeared after about twenty-four hours and had not recurred. Physical examination was otherwise completely negative. At exploration, an anomalous bifid rib was found with an abnormally buckled forward costal cartilage. The cartilage was completely resected and the wound closed. The child was seen two years following surgery, and there has been no recurrence.

SUMMARY AND CONCLUSIONS

A prominence of a costal cartilage had been reported in the literature for some time as a specific syndrome under the name of Tietze's syndrome. This occurs most frequently on the second costal cartilage. We reported four cases in which the costal cartilage has been completely removed. In these we have found that the cartilage itself was not diseased, but appeared to be buckled forward. The anatomic explanation which we would like to suggest is that this is a disease of the ligament which lies subadjacent to the second costal cartilage rather than a disease of the cartilage itself, and that a contracture of this ligament causes a buckling forward of the costal cartilage.

REFERENCES

1. Tietze, A.: Ueber eine eigenartige Haüfung von Fallen mit Dystrophie der Rippenknorpel, Berl. klin. Wchnschr. **58:** 829-831, 1921.
2. Heuer, G. J., Andrus, W. DeW., Barnes, W. A., and Eckel, J. H.: Tumors and Cysts of the Thorax in Lewis, D.: Practice of Surgery, vol. 5, chapt. 5, Hagerstown, Md., 1952, W. F. Prior Company, Inc., pp. 17-18.
3. Gill, A. M., Jones, R. A., and Pollak, L.: Tietze's Disease (Non-suppurative Non-specific Swellings of Rib Cartilage), Brit. M. J. **2:** 155-156 (Aug. 8) 1942.
4. Geddes, A. K.: Tietze's Syndrome, Canad. M. A. J. **53:** 571-573 (Dec.) 1945.
5. Motulsky, A. G., and Rohn, R. J.: Tietze's Syndrome, J. A. M. A. **152:** 504-503 (June 6) 1953.
6. Spalteholz, W.: Hand Atlas of Human Anatomy, Philadelphia, 1937, J. B. Lippincott Company.
7. Maier, H. C.: Tietze's Syndrome, Surg., Gynec. & Obst. **84:** 1038-1039, 1947.

ACCURACY OF PREOPERATIVE X-RAY DIAGNOSES OF BREAST TUMORS

J. GERSHON-COHEN, M.D., HELEN INGLEBY, M.D., M. B. HERMEL, M.D., AND S. M. BERGER, M.D., PHILADELPHIA, PA.

(From the Albert Einstein Medical Center, Northern Division)

ROENTGENOLOGY must impart additive or confirmatory information if it is to attain its rightful place among procedures useful in the preoperative diagnosis of breast tumors. Following recent improvements,[1] it is now possible to make some preliminary assessment of advances afforded by roentgenography of breast tumors. This subject has been static during the past twenty-five years. Dr. George E. Pfahler attempted diagnostic x-ray studies of the breast in 1930 when he successfully demonstrated several cases of cancer to the members of the Medical Literature Club in Philadelphia.[2] He never published his findings since he felt then, as most surgeons do today, that an x-ray examination of the breast could add little to an expert clinical examination. He therefore remained satisfied to use the x-ray examination only when he believed it would help him in a differential diagnosis. Our experience has taught us, however, that the x-ray examination should be used routinely since its disclosures often come as a surprise.

METHOD AND RESULTS

The last 210 consecutive x-ray studies of breast tumors in the Albert Einstein Medical Center (Northern Division) were interpreted by three roentgenologists, twice without and finally with knowledge of the clinical findings. After these readings were analyzed for consistency among themselves, they were compared with the pathologic findings.

Of the lesions in these 210 cases, 163 were benign and 47 were malignant. During the first round of x-ray interpretations, erroneous diagnoses were made in approximately 10 per cent by all three roentgenologists. With each successive review, a slight improvement in accuracy of diagnosis occurred, chiefly because each roentgenologist gained more experience in adhering to the diagnostic criteria previously formulated.[1]

When the third session of interpretations was concluded, erroneous diagnoses had been made in only 5 per cent, chiefly because of better recognition of malignant lesions and because the clinical findings also were taken into consideration (Table I). The inconsistencies of the individual interpretations were surprising, being subject to the "human error" encountered by Garland and associates.[3]

Very encouraging was the high accuracy (approximately 97 per cent) achieved by all roentgenologists in the diagnosis of benign lesions, but the accuracy of x-ray diagnosis of malignant lesions never exceeded approximately

Received for publication, Sept. 8, 1953.

SUMMARY

A comparative review was made of the x-ray interpretations by three roentgenologists of 210 consecutive mammary lesions which were checked by the pathologist, either from biopsy or study of the whole breast sections. The x-ray diagnoses of three repeated readings were tabulated for accuracy among themselves by the same and among different radiologists and finally checked against the pathologic findings.

Of the 163 benign lesions, 97 per cent were correctly diagnosed, and of the 47 malignant lesions, 41 finally were accurately designated. Discrepancies among the x-ray diagnoses decreased with repeated interpretations, both among the repeated readings of the individual and between the readings of the several roentgenologists. Causes for errors in diagnosis of malignant lesions lurk occasionally in the complex architecture of the physiologically active breast in middle-aged women and less often among the isolated malignant, but benign-appearing, lesions of the fat postclimacteric breast. In the x-ray diagnosis of malignant lesions, careful attention must be given to technical details, diagnostic criteria, and the clinical findings. Examples of some pitfalls in diagnosis are given in this report.

REFERENCES

1. Gershon-Cohen, J., and Ingleby, H.: Carcinoma of the Breast. Roentgenographic Technic and Diagnostic Criteria, Radiology **60:** 68-76 (Jan.), 1953.
2. Pfahler, G. E.: Personal communication.
3. Garland, L. H., Miller, E. R., Zwerling, H. B., Harkness, J. T., Hinshaw, H. C., Shipman, S. J., and Yerushalmy, J.: Studies on the Value of Serial Films in Estimating the Progress of Pulmonary Disease, Radiology **58:** 161-175 (Feb.), 1952.
4. Gershon-Cohen, J., and Ingleby, H.: Roentgenography of Cancer of the Breast, Am. J. Roentgenol. **68:** 1-7 (July) 1952.
5. Gershon-Cohen, J., and Ingleby, H.: Roentgenography of Fibroadenoma of the Breast, Radiology **59:** 77-87 (July) 1952.
6. Gershon-Cohen, J., and Ingleby, H.: Secretory Disease and Plasma Cell Mastitis in the Female Breast, Surg., Gynec. & Obst. **95:** 479-504 (Oct.) 1952.
7. Gershon-Cohen, J., Ingleby, H., and Hermel, M. B.: Roentgenographic Diagnosis of Calcification in Carcinoma of the Breast, J. A. M. A. **152:** 676-677 (June 20) 1953.

TRAUMA AND CAPILLARY RESISTANCE

A Clinical and Experimental Study

Jenö Kramár, M.D., Dwaine J. Peetz, M.D., and Harry H. McCarthy, M.D., Omaha, Neb.

(From the Departments of Pediatrics and Surgery of the Creighton University School of Medicine)

In the constant endeavor to minimize the risks of surgical intervention and to render postoperative convalescence as short and undisturbed as possible, increased attention is being given to the pituitary-adrenocortical system as the principal factor in the stress phenomenon. Determination of urinary steroid excretion, of the level of the circulating eosinophils, and of the spontaneous or induced change in this level have been used as helpful adjuncts to clinical observation of the postoperative patient.

The purpose of this paper is to show that another method may be added to our armamentarium, namely, evaluation of the capillary resistance.

The resistance of the capillary wall as measured by the negative or positive pressure method and expressed in centimeters of mercury has been considered heretofore as a local phenomenon which may be influenced by many factors acting locally. This concept has changed entirely during the last three years. Clinical observations (Robson and Duthie[1, 2]) and animal experiments (Eichholtz and associates,[3] Kramár and Simay-Kramár[4]) have clearly demonstrated that capillary resistance is subject to hormonal influence. The principal hormone involved is cortisone. The correlation between capillary resistance and cortisone is so intimate that testing of the first may give information on the level of the latter. It has been shown that any decrease in the cortisone concentration in the organism (adrenalectomy, experimental depletion of the adrenal cortex in the late phases of stress response) is followed by a decrease in the capillary resistance, whereas any increase in the cortisone content of the body (administration of cortisone or ACTH, early phase of stress response) is accompanied by an increase in the capillary resistance.

It has been known since 1944 that trauma consistently causes the capillary resistance to increase after surgical interventions in the human being (Scarborough[5]), as well as following experimental crush in the rat, guinea pig, and mouse (Ungar[6]). In view of our recent knowledge of the endocrine background of the capillary resistance it seemed that a detailed study of these conditions would be highly desirable.

The present work consists of two parts. In the first, the effect of surgical intervention and of crush was studied on the capillary resistance of experimental

---

This work represents part of a project supported by the Cardiovascular Section of the Division of Research Grants of the United States Public Health Service and by the Creighton University School of Medicine.

Received for publication, Aug. 28, 1953.

animals. In the second part, the capillary resistance of human patients was observed during the postoperative course. The final aim was to correlate the results of clinical observations with the finding in the experimental animals.

METHODS

Capillary resistance was tested in both parts of this work by means of the negative pressure method. The device used consisted of a vacuum reservoir, a small transparent plastic suction cup (with an inner diameter of 7 mm.), and a mercury manometer with the necessary connecting tubing and stopcocks. Suction was supplied by an electric suction pump in the laboratory and by a two-way Potain hand aspirator in the wards. The abdominal skin was selected for the site of testing in the animals, the flexor aspect of the forearm in the human beings. The least negative pressure capable of eliciting capillary rupture and formation of petechiae was considered the value of the capillary resistance. Details of the technique, especially with regard to the precautions necessary for preventing erroneous readings or misinterpretation, have been described elsewhere (Kramár and Simay-Kramár,[4] Kramár, Peetz, and McCarthy[7]).

PROCEDURE

Part I.—Two types of experimental trauma were used, namely, surgical operations and crush of the hind limb.

1. Twenty albino rats (eleven males and nine females) of the Sprague-Dawley strain, weighing approximately 200 grams and maintained on Purina Dog Chow, were trained until they became fully accustomed to the restraint necessary for testing capillary resistance. Bilateral sham adrenalectomy was then performed under deep ether anesthesia. The lumbar approach was used and the adrenal gland was visualized but not touched. The operation was carried out in a deliberately circumstantial manner with the intention of producing an extensive and, at the same time, relatively standard tissue injury. For this purpose, muscle layers were cut through instead of being severed bluntly, length of incisions through skin and muscle, number of stitches, and duration of anesthesia and of the operation itself were standardized. A control base line of capillary resistance was determined prior to the operation, and the testing was continued at one-to-two-day intervals for about two months thereafter.

2. Five rats (two males and three females) were trained in the same manner, and then anesthetized with ether. One hind extremity was then crushed with a padded hammer. Testing of the capillary resistance was performed in the same manner as described previously.

3. Twelve rats (five males and seven females) were not subjected to the routine training procedure prior to the experiments. In addition, for testing capillary resistance they were tied to a board instead of being gently held by an assistant, as was done with the previous animals. In this way, a considerable emotional upset was created which gave rise to a typical capillary response causing the capillary resistance to drop after an initial rise and to remain at a

low level for about one week. Crush was applied during this latter period and the capillary resistance tested as described in the foregoing experiments.

Part II.—Ninety-four major surgical cases were selected at random, the criteria of selection being an anticipated hospital convalescent period of at least seven days. Forty-three men and fifty-one women, ranging in age from 17 to 78 years, were included. Eight cases were observed daily, and in eighty-six cases readings were obtained every other day. Initial readings in eighty-two cases were obtained on the day of surgery. In twelve cases, at least two daily preoperative readings were obtained. The type of anesthesia was considered relatively constant, as all patients received similar anesthesia consisting of Pentothal Sodium induction followed by ether, oxygen, and nitrous oxide mixture as required.

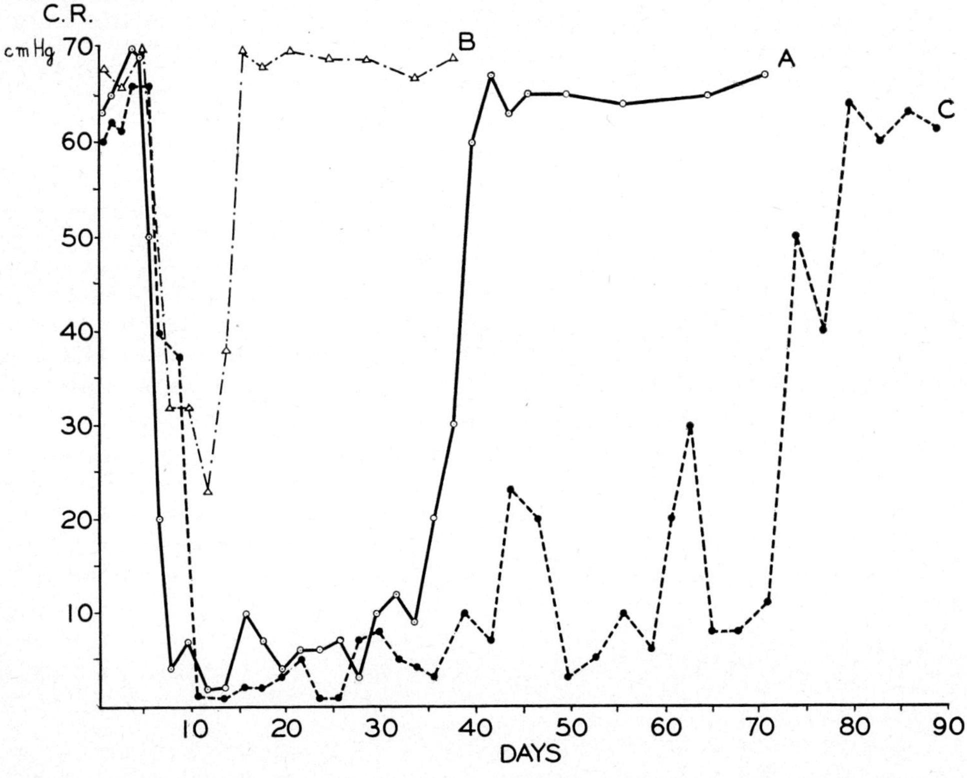

Fig. 1.—Patterns of capillary resistance change following surgical trauma (sham adrenalectomy) in the albino rat. *A*, Average pattern; *B*, accelerated or telescoped pattern; *C*, protracted pattern. The four phases of capillary response are best seen in the average pattern: initial rise, sudden drop, period of pathologically low resistance, and restoration to normal.

RESULTS

Part I (Animal Experiments).—

1. *Effect of sham adrenalectomy on previously trained rats:* As shown in Fig. 1, the changes occurring in the capillary resistance could be divided into four phases: (a) an initial rise immediately following operation, (b) a sudden

drop to pathologically low levels, (c) a period of abnormally low capillary resistance, and (d) restoration to normal. The length of the first phase was about the same in all the animals (one to two days) and the degree of rise was principally dependent on the preoperative level of the capillary resistance, as no marked increase could have occurred when the initial level was already high. Phases b, c, and d revealed more individual differences. On this basis, three patterns could be distinguished. That shown by the majority of the animals (fifteen of twenty) may be termed the *average pattern* (Curve *A* in Fig. 1).

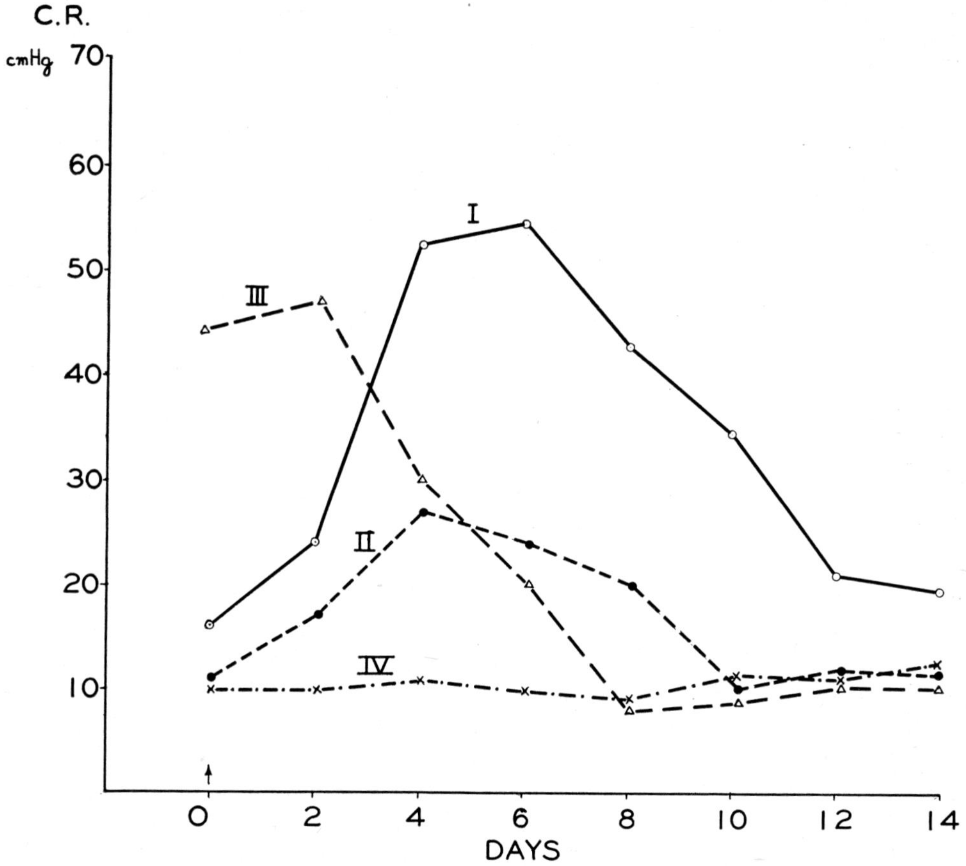

Fig. 2.—Patterns of capillary resistance change in the human being following surgery. *I*, Vigorous response (increase of capillary resistance by at least 20 cm. Hg); *II*, moderate increase (6 to 19 cm.); *III*, decrease of capillary resistance; *IV*, no change.

Here the drop of the capillary resistance was precipitous and the third phase, lasting about ten to fifteen days, was followed by rapid recuperation. The entire response had an average duration of thirty days. Three animals showed a capillary response that was shorter and less intensive. The drop in the second phase was moderate and the third phase very short. The entire duration of this *accelerated or telescoped pattern* was about ten days (Curve *B* in Fig. 1). Two rats disclosed another extreme in their capillary response: here the third phase was of extremely long duration and the recuperation was interrupted by frequent relapses. The entire response lasted seventy to seventy-five days (*protracted pattern,* Curve *C* in Fig. 1).

2. *Effect of crush on previously trained rats:* The experiments in this category brought a uniform result. All five rats showed a change in the capillary resistance which was essentially similar to that seen after sham adrenalectomy. There was, however, some difference in the details. The first phase of the response was strikingly long (three to five days), during which time the capillary resistance was constantly at its highest level. The third phase, on the other hand, was much shorter, and recuperation took place very rapidly, hence, the entire response lasted, despite the longer first phase, only fifteen to twenty days.

3. *Effect of crush on untrained animals:* The low capillary resistance of these rats brought about by means of emotional stress prior to crush, rendered the first phase of the capillary response following crush very spectacular. The capillary resistance rose within the first twenty-four hours, the rise amounting to 20 to 60 cm. The duration of this high capillary resistance level, however, was very short and was followed by a typical drop in the second phase. In the course of the third and fourth phases, four rats disclosed an average pattern, whereas six rats had a protracted pattern. In one rat, the capillary resistance decreased only slightly after the marked initial rise, and thus the resulting pattern was rather ill defined. Similar ''rudimentary'' patterns were sometimes encountered following forced muscular exercise or cold stress (Kramár[8]).

Part II (Clinical Observation).—Although every case responded in an individual manner, all could be placed in one of four groups depending on the type and degree of change or changes found in the capillary resistance (Fig. 2). Group I included those cases in which an increase of at least 20 cm. Hg was noted in the capillary resistance during the observed period of the postoperative course. Group II was characterized by an increase of from 6 to 19 cm. Hg in capillary resistance. Group III included those cases in which the last recorded capillary resistance was lower than the initial reading and in which no pronounced increase of resistance was observed during the postoperative period. Group IV encompassed those cases in which there was no change in capillary resistance.

According to this classification, the distribution of our ninety-four cases was as follows:

Group	*Number of cases*	*Per cent*
I	33	(35)
II	31	(33)
III	15	(16)
IV	15	(16)

Having found that all the patients could be placed into four basic groups, an attempt was made to determine whether age, sex, and extent of the surgical procedure were causally related to the four groups.

The age of the patients was first correlated with the response, and it was found that no significant correlation could be made. However, when the sex of the individual was correlated with type and degree of response, some interesting facts became evident (Table I). The majority of the male patients (51.3 per cent) were in Group I, the vigorous response category, whereas the largest percentage (45.3 per cent) of women fell into the less vigorously responding Group II. In contrast, Groups III and IV failed to reveal any sex difference.

TABLE I. CORRELATION OF TYPE OF CAPILLARY RESPONSE WITH SEX

GROUP	NUMBER OF PATIENTS	♂	♀
I	33	22	11
II	31	8	23
III	15	7	8
IV	15	6	9

Equally significant was the correlation of the degree of surgical intervention and type of capillary response (Table II). Arbitrarily, three degrees of surgical intervention were distinguished, depending on the amount of tissue disturbed at operation. Forty-nine cases of herniotomy, hysterectomy, and cholecystostomy were considered to have been subjected to the least traumatic type of intervention ("minor" in Table II). Twenty-eight patients were subjected to gastric or intestinal resection, pulmonary lobectomy, suprapubic prostatectomy, gastroenterostomy, and amputation, that is, interventions assumed to be connected with a moderately severe degree of tissue damage ("moderate" in Table II). Seventeen patients were subjected to the most severe and extensive surgical procedures, such as combined abdominoperineal resection, radical mastectomy, arthroplasty, spinal fusion, and any other type of procedure followed by unusual complications ("marked" in Table II).

TABLE II. CORRELATION OF TYPE OF CAPILLARY RESPONSE WITH DEGREE OF SURGICAL INTERVENTION

DEGREE OF TISSUE TRAUMA	NUMBER OF PATIENTS	TYPE OF CAPILLARY RESPONSE			
		GROUP I	GROUP II	GROUP III	GROUP IV
Minor	49	10 20.4%	22 44.9%	10 20.4%	7 14.3%
Moderate	28	14 50.0%	4 14.4%	5 17.8%	5 17.8%
Marked	17	9 52.9%	5 29.4%	—	3 17.7%

It is seen that whereas the dominant type of response among our patients subjected to minor degree of tissue trauma was that of Group II, the majority of patients inflicted with a moderate or marked degree of tissue damage showed the Group I type of response. It is interesting to note that 14 to 18 per cent of patients exhibit no definite increase in the capillary resistance regardless of the type of surgery performed.

DISCUSSION

The change in the capillary resistance found in the experimental part of this work following two kinds of tissue injury, surgical operation and crush, was similar to that encountered in previous works after cold stress, forced muscular exercise (Kramár[8]), and after severe emotional upset (Kramár, Peetz, and McCarthy[7]). This uniformity of response suggests that we are dealing with a nonspecific phenomenon that may have a common, nonspecific underlying mechanism. It is believed that this capillary response with its four well-defined phases is part of the general stress syndrome as described by Selye.[9] In view of the previous work discussed in the introduction of this paper concerning the hormonal regulation of the capillary resistance, it seems that the initial phase of this response, the rise in the capillary resistance, is the result of ACTH discharge and consecutive adrenocortical activation, whereas the second and third phases, termed "capillary crisis," are due to a hypofunction of the adrenal cortex, presumably caused by its nonresponsiveness (depletion?). The fourth phase, then, may represent one of the many manifestations of the restoration process taking place in the organism.

The clinical part of this work demonstrates that the change in the capillary resistance following surgery is much more complicated than as described by Scarborough.[5] On the basis of two readings, one three hours preoperatively, the other twenty-four hours postoperatively, this author stated that all the twenty-three cases observed evidenced a definite increase in the capillary resistance. He further maintained that this increase appeared to be independent of the age and sex of the patient as well as of the nature of the operation performed.

While observing a greater number of patients during a longer period of time, it was found, first, that this capillary response is subject to great individual variations. In the final analysis, four patterns could be established that would encompass all these variations. Second, a definite sex difference was found in that men are prone to develop more vigorous response to the same degree of tissue damage. Third, a definite relationship was found between type of response and kind of surgical intervention. In general, as the amount of tissue involved increases, the more marked becomes the increase in the capillary resistance.

Before any attempt is made to evaluate the meaning and significance of these findings, it seems necessary to correlate them with the results of the experimental study. The comparison shows a common feature and a discrepancy.

There is a tendency, in both human being and experimental animal, to develop certain patterns in the capillary response. There is no doubt that capillary response may be influenced by many factors. In experimental animals subjected to other types of stress (cold, forced muscular work), these factors have been fairly well established (Kramár[8]). We know that it is not so much the type of stress as its intensity that is decisive and, furthermore, that previous diet, repetition of stress (training), and individual differences are also modifying factors. The effect of some of these factors was seen in the present work. The role of individual differences was well demonstrated in the experimental part in which rats were subjected to sham adrenalectomy. Despite carefully standardized experimental conditions, these animals displayed three patterns of response. The individual differences were also seen in the clinical material. The patients, although subjected to the same kind of operations, exhibited four patterns of response. On the other hand, the influence of the intensity of stress, that is, of the type of operation involving various degrees of tissue damage, upon the capillary response was also demonstrable: the greater the stress, the higher the number of patients with Group I (very pronounced) response.

The discrepancy between clinical and experimental observations lies in the fact that whereas the majority of experimental animals disclosed a typical change in the capillary resistance with four well-defined phases, this "full-blown" capillary response was only exceptionally encountered in the human being. As a rule, the postoperative patient showed only fragments of the change displayed by the experimental animal, although these fragments are well recognizable. The Group I and II type of response represents the first phase of the capillary response in the rat; Group III corresponds to the second and third phases. No match was encountered in the present animal experiments for the nonresponsive Group IV of the patients. Nevertheless, as this refractory type was repeatedly found in other stress experiments it may also be expected following trauma provided that a greater number of animals is used than in the present work.

It is believed that this difference between clinical and experimental observations has a phylogenetic basis. The albino rat, the animal used in these experiments, has a sheltered life and is hardly exposed to any serious stress. Consequently, its pituitary adrenocortical axis is very sensitive and its response to stress prompt and alarming, in sharp contrast to the well-trained system and, therefore, more sluggish response in the human being.

In reviewing the recent surgical literature, one gathers the impression that a prompt pituitary-adrenocortical response has been regarded as obligatory for a satisfactory and uneventful postoperative recovery. In our series of ninety-four cases we fail to recognize this direct relationship. Apparently, some 14 to 18 per cent of individuals do not exhibit increased pituitary-adrenocortical activity as measured by capillary resistance but, nevertheless, make a very uneventful recovery. On the other hand, excessively high capillary resistance values may be found in patients whose postoperative course is far from satisfactory. Two cases serve as examples.

A 45-year-old woman was subjected to gastric resection. No elevation in the capillary resistance occurred through the convalescence. On the tenth postoperative day a standard Thorn test was performed with entirely negative results. The postoperative course of this patient was completely uneventful.

A 78-year-old man, following a combined abdominoperineal resection, exhibited a marked increase ($>$ 70 cm. Hg) in capillary resistance. For six weeks the capillary resistance remained high, and the postoperative course was very complicated. The wound disrupted on the fifth postoperative day; repeated episodes of partial bowel obstruction requiring Levin suction further clouded the issue, and a pre-existing asthma continued to flare. On the thirty-fourth postoperative day a marked fall in the capillary resistance (from 70 to 28 cm. Hg) occurred; two days later a generalized edema appeared and the patient expired rapidly.

We are far from implying that no correlation exists between postoperative recovery and pituitary-adrenocortical function. We wish to emphasize solely that such a correlation is more complex than is generally appreciated. There are several reasons for the difficulty encountered in the evaluation of this correlation.

The first concerns the pituitary-adrenocortical function per se, irrespective of the method of testing. We really do not know what is the most favorable type of postoperative pituitary-adrenocortical response. Our still limited knowledge of the basic mechanism of wound healing and the capacity of the organism to meet stress may fully account for this shortcoming.

In addition, there are other reasons originating in the particular method used in this work for testing pituitary-adrenocortical function. We do not know yet whether cortisone is the sole hormone regulating capillary resistance or, as on the basis of some current work it may be suspected (Kramár[10]), whether the level of the capillary resistance reflects the balance of several hormonal functions. We also begin to realize that both low and high capillary resistance may have more than one interpretation. Assuming that cortisone alone is responsible for the actual level of the capillary resistance, a low resistance may, for instance, indicate that adrenocortical function is at its leisure because there is no need for increased activity, but also that the adrenal cortex is incapable of increased activity. By the same token, a high level in the capillary resistance may herald a vigorous adrenocortical function resulting from stimuli favorable for the organism (for example, physical activity after long sedentary occupation, effect of sunshine after a long, gloomy winter, recreation), but also a desperate struggle against a stress of abnormal intensity and duration. A sudden drop of the resistance in this latter condition may mean that the stress ceased to exist but also that the organism, owing to adrenocortical exhaustion, is unable to cope with it.

SUMMARY

The effect of trauma on the capillary resistance was studied in animal experiments and on surgical patients in the postoperative convalescence.

Groups of albino rats were subjected to surgical operation, others to crush. A uniform response was found consisting of four phases: initial rise of the capillary resistance, sudden drop, a period of abnormally low level, and restoration to normal. In view of the similarity of this response to that encountered after various other types of stress, the described change in the capillary resistance is considered a part of the nonspecific stress syndrome. An attempt has been made to evaluate these changes with reference to our recent knowledge of the endocrine regulation of the capillary resistance.

Patients during the postoperative convalescence showed the full-blown rat-pattern of the capillary resistance change only exceptionally. Most of them exhibit only fragments, that is, one or the other phases of the response typical of the rat. A phylogenetic explanation is given for this difference.

The capillary response in the human being following surgery is related to the amount of tissue involved in the procedure, sex of the patient, and individual characteristics.

The question of correlation of the capillary response to the clinical picture of the recovery phase is still open to discussion and requires further investigations.

Acknowledgment.—We are indebted to Dr. C. M. Wilhelmj of the Creighton University School of Medicine for his constant interest and valuable assistance.

REFERENCES

1. Robson, H. N., and Duthie, J. J. R.: Capillary Resistance and Adrenocortical Activity, Brit. M. J. **2:** 971, 1950.
2. Robson, H. N., and Duthie, J. J. R.: Further Observations on Capillary Resistance and Adrenocortical Activity, Brit. M. J. **1:** 994, 1952.
3. Eichholtz, F., Staab, A., and Taugner, R.: Weitere pharmakologische Wirkungen von Nebennieren-Rindenhormon, Arch. internat. pharmcodyn. **86:** 407, 1951.
4. Kramár, J., and Simay-Kramár, M.: The Effect of Adrenalectomy, Surgical Trauma and Ether Anesthesia Upon the Capillary Resistance of the Albino Rat, Endocrinology **52:** 453, 1953.
5. Scarborough, H.: The Effect of Surgical Operation Upon Capillary Resistance, Edinburgh M. J. **51:** 335, 1944.
6. Ungar, G.: The Effect of Trauma on Bleeding Time and Capillary Resistance, J. Physiol. **103:** 18, 1944.
7. Kramár, J., Peetz, D. J., and McCarthy, H. H.: Capillary Response to Emotion, Psychosom. Med. In press.
8. Kramár, J.: Stress and Capillary Resistance, Am. J. Physiol. **175:** 69, 1953.
9. Selye, H.: A Syndrome Produced by Diverse Nocuous Agents, Nature, London **138:** 32, 1936.
10. Kramár, J.: Hormonal Regulation of the Capillary Resistance, XIX Internat. Physiological Congress, Montreal, Canada, September, 1953.

BLOOD CULTURE STUDIES IN NORMAL DOGS AND IN DOGS IN HEMORRHAGIC SHOCK

RUSSELL M. NELSON, M.D.,* AND HOWARD E. NOYES, M.S.,
WASHINGTON, D. C.

(From the Division of Surgery, Army Medical Service Graduate School, Walter Reed Army Medical Center)

INTEREST in the interrelationships between shock and infection has been reactivated with the recent reports of a rapid shocklike state produced by bacteremia in animals[1, 2] and in human beings,[3-5] the observation that the mortality rate from a standard hemorrhagic shock procedure is reduced in dogs by oral pretreatment with aureomycin or neomycin,[6] and the finding that, in shock, there is an increased blood level of a specific bacterial toxin initially placed in the intact intestine of a dog.[7] Such data suggest that bacteria may play a role in profound shock, even within the breadth of time ordinarily considered too brief for bacterial complications.

In the present study, blood cultures were taken from dogs during the course of experiments on hemorrhagic shock. This communication reports the results obtained from initial and terminal blood cultures in dogs in shock and in control dogs not in shock.

METHODS

Animal Preparation.—This experiment utilized seventy-three mongrel dogs, not selected for sex, and weighing approximately ten kilograms. Twenty-four dogs served as controls, and forty-nine were subjected to a state of hemorrhagic hypotension. Prior to experimentation, the dogs were held for thirty days for standardization of environment, deworming, and immunization against canine distemper. Experiments were then performed in an air-conditioned operating room. Each dog was lightly anesthetized with ether. The skin of the groin was shaved and prepared with surgical detergent and alcohol, and the femoral vessels were surgically exposed, employing strict aseptic precautions. Heparin (6 mg. per kilogram) was injected intravenously, and all initial blood cultures were taken from the exposed femoral artery. In the control dog, the femoral artery was ligated, and in the dog to be bled, a 13 gauge cannula was inserted into the right femoral artery and connected to a sterile reservoir system, as described elsewhere.[7] The animals were then allowed to recover from anesthesia, and no further ether was employed. The control dogs were returned to the cage for later sampling, and the "shock" dog was bled until the pressure in the system was 30 to 40 mm. Hg. The mean volume of blood withdrawn to produce this state of hypotension was 52 ml. per kilogram, which figure is consistent with

Received for publication, Sept. 29, 1953.

*Cancer trainee, National Institutes of Health. Present address: Department of Surgery, University of Minnesota Hospitals, Minneapolis, Minn.

that reported by other investigators in this type of preparation.[8] Duration of the period of hypotension ranged from one hour to six hours, with the period in twenty-four of the forty-nine dogs extending beyond five hours. Final blood culture was taken in the shock dogs from the femoral artery, just prior to death in most instances. Final samples were withdrawn through the surgically prepared skin from the cubital or jugular vein of the control dogs at a corresponding time.

Bacteriologic Methods.—Two cultures were obtained from each dog, an initial and a final specimen. Therefore, ninety-seven cultures were from dogs not in shock (including forty-nine initial specimens from the shock group) and forty-nine cultures were from dogs in hemorrhagic shock. Ten milliliters of blood was injected into a sterile rubber-stoppered vaccine bottle containing 50 ml. of trypticase soy broth with 0.1 per cent sodium citrate and 0.1 per cent agar. Samples for staining and isolation were removed after one, two, seven, and fourteen days of incubation at 35° C. These samples were inoculated into thioglycollate medium for the cultivation of microaerophilic and anaerobic organisms, and streaked on blood agar and trypticase soy agar plates for the cultivation of aerobic organisms. Specimens of bacterial growth in thioglycollate broth were streaked on blood agar plates which were incubated in anaerobe jars for forty-eight hours. Identification was based on standard criteria.*

RESULTS

The incidence of positive blood cultures for the initial and terminal samples for the two groups is summarized in Table I.

TABLE I. INCIDENCE OF POSITIVE BLOOD CULTURES

GROUP	INITIAL	FINAL
Control dogs (24)	4 (16.7%)	8 (33.3%)
Shock dogs (49)	9 (18.4%)	11 (22.3%)

Inasmuch as the initial samples from the shock group were drawn from dogs still in a control state, these cultures can be grouped with the cultures from the dogs in the control group in order to determine the incidence of sterile versus positive cultures in control and shock states. This analysis is presented in Table II.

TABLE II. INCIDENCE OF STERILE AND POSITIVE BLOOD CULTURES

GROUP	STERILE	POSITIVE
Dogs not in shock (97 cultures)	76 (78.3%)	21 (21.6%)
Dogs in shock (49 cultures)	38 (77.6%)	11 (22.3%)

**Escherichia coli* and *Paracolobactrum aerogenoides* were identified by Gram stain and characteristic biochemical reactions.

Corynebacterium species were identified by the characteristic appearance of the colonies on tellurite serum agar.

Actinomyces species were identified by microscopic appearance and morphology in thioglycollate broth and on blood agar plates.

Micrococci and streptococci were identified by colony morphology and Gram stain. No attempt was made to type according to Lancefield classification.

Clostridium perfringens was identified by Gram stain and double zone of hemolysis on blood agar.

Table II demonstrates an essentially identical incidence of sterile and positive blood cultures between samples drawn from dogs in shock and those in a control state.

Only in four (16.7 per cent) of the twenty-four control dogs and in five (10 per cent) of the forty-nine shock dogs was the final culture positive when the initial culture was negative, indicating no greater predilection for subsequent positive blood cultures in the state of shock.

Analysis of bacteria isolated from the positive blood cultures is presented in Table III.

TABLE III. BACTERIA ISOLATED FROM BLOOD CULTURES

	CONTROL CULTURES		SHOCK CULTURES	
	NUMBER	PER CENT OF 21 POSITIVE CULTURES*	NUMBER	PER CENT OF 11 POSITIVE CULTURES†
Clostridium perfringens	7	33	5	45
Corynebacterium species	5	24	2	18
Micrococcus pyogenes var. *albus*	1	5	2	18
Hemolytic streptococcus	1	5	0	0
Nonhemolytic streptococcus	3	14	1	9
Escherichia coli	2	10	2	18
Paracolobactrum aerogenoides	3	14	1	9
Bacillus subtilis	1	5	0	0
Actinomyces species	1	5	0	0

*Total exceeds 100 per cent because two species of organisms were isolated from three cultures.

†Total exceeds 100 per cent because two species of organisms were isolated from two cultures.

In a small number of cultures of mesenteric lymph nodes, intestinal organisms were found which were not present in the peripheral blood of the same animal.

DISCUSSION

The bacteria cultured, as shown in Table III, were predominantly *Clostridium perfringens* and Corynebacterium species (diphtheroids). The flora isolated from the two groups were similar.

The finding of a similar incidence of positive blood cultures in shock and control states, of course, does not necessarily indicate that bacteria may not play a role in potentiating the pathophysiology of shock. The gross technique of blood culture yields only an index as to the presence of living bacterial cells, and not to the toxins or products of bacteria, which are the agents responsible for the deleterious consequences of infection. In this regard, we previously found that the concentration of a specific bacterial toxin, initially placed in the intact intestine, was higher in the peripheral blood of dogs in shock than in control dogs.[7] At least it would appear from these data that the incidence of bacteremia in shock is no greater than in normal dogs, so that further investigation into the role of bacteria in shock will require more specialized techniques capable of measuring toxins.

The application of these data to the problem of shock in human beings is precluded because the bacteriology of the dog is vastly different from that of the human being. While bacteria can be cultured from the liver of dogs in

35 per cent of biopsies, for example, less than 2 per cent of human liver biopsies are positive.[9]

SUMMARY

Of ninety-seven bacterial cultures taken from the peripheral circulation of control dogs 21.6 per cent were positive. Similarly, 22.3 per cent of forty-nine cultures taken from dogs in terminal hemorrhagic shock were positive. The predominant organisms cultured from both groups were *Clostridium perfringens* and Corynebacterium species (diphtheroids). Interpretation of these data is limited by the difference in the bacteriology of the dog from that of other mammalian species, and by the inadequacy of blood culture to provide a means by which the harmful effects of bacteria may be measured.

Acknowledgment.—We are indebted to Lieutenant Colonel E. J. Pulaski, Lieutenant Derwin Ashcraft, and Mrs. Jane S. Poole for their valuable aid in this study.

REFERENCES

1. Nelson, R. M.: Metabolic Effects of Paracolon Bacteremia, Ann. Surg. **134**: 885, 1951.
2. Furr, W. E., Bourdeau, R. V., Roach, H. D., and Laugman, H.: In Vivo Effects of Clostridium Welchii Lecithinase, Surg., Gynec. & Obst. **95**: 465, 1952.
3. Pittman, M.: A Study of Bacteria Implicated in Transfusion Reactions and of Bacteria Isolated From Blood Products. In press.
4. Borden, C. W., and Hall, W. H.: Fatal Transfusion Reactions From Massive Bacterial Contamination of Blood, New England J. Med. **245**: 760, 1951.
5. Wise, R. I., Shaffer, J. M., and Sping, W. W.: The Syndrome of Vascular Collapse Due to Gram-negative Bacteria: Its Management With l-Norepinephrine and Antibiotics, J. Lab. & Clin. Med **40**: 961, 1952.
6. Fine, J.: Etiology and Mechanisms of Shock. V. Irreversible Shock, Symposium on Shock. Nat. Res. Council and Army Med. Serv. Grad. School, Washington, D. C., May 7, 1951.
7. Nelson, R. M., and Noyes, H. E.: Permeability of the Intestine to Bacterial Toxins in Hemorrhagic Shock, Proc. Surg. Forum, Clin. Congress Am. Coll. Surgeons, 1952, Philadelphia, 1953, W. B. Saunders Company, p. 474.
8. Fine, J.: Personal communication, 1953.
9. Sborov, V. M., Morse, W. C., Giges, B., and Jahnke, E. J.: Bacteriology of the Human Liver, J. Clin. Investigation **31**: 986, 1952.

GALL BLADDER TRACTION

Anthony V. Migliaccio, M.D., Providence, R. I.

A MARKEDLY thickened, edematous gall bladder, or one which is filled solid with stones, is rather difficult to apply traction to with the usual clamps. The clamp will invariably cut through, resulting in a spillage of considerable bile or pus, or the clamp will slip off.

As traction is extremely important in attaining adequate exposure of the cystic common duct area, some other means had to be found.

Application of figure-of-eight sutures at different levels in the gall bladder seemed quite satisfactory. This has been carried out in a fairly large series of cases during the past two years and has proved to be even superior to clamps.

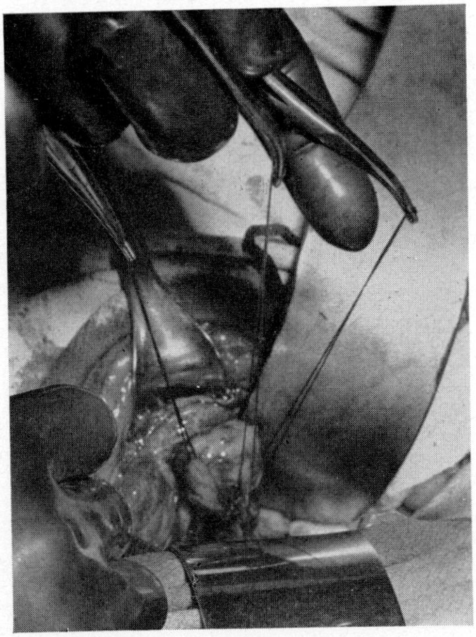

Fig. 1.

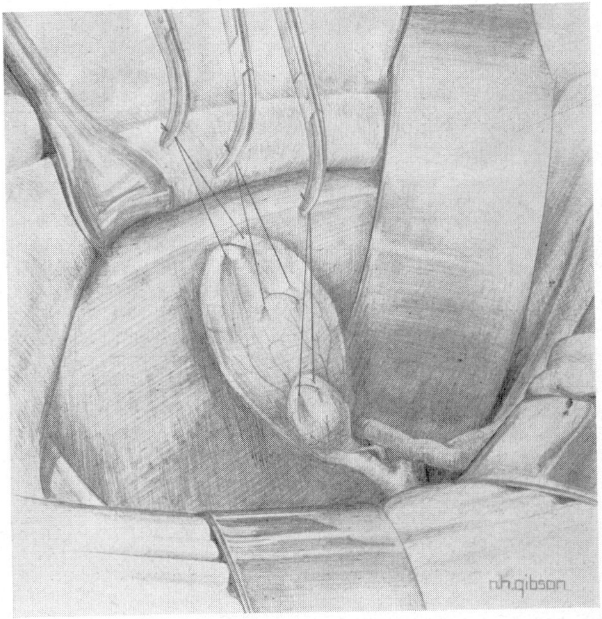

Fig. 2.

The amount of spillage due to the needle holes is minimal and rarely of any serious danger. The photograph and picture demonstrate the technique.

The No. 0 chromic suture is preferred over silk or cotton, as it is less likely to cut through the wall of the gall bladder. The lower suture offers an excellent means of pulling a dilated Hartmann's pouch away from the common duct, thus lessening the danger of injury to the common duct.

Received for publication, Sept. 22, 1953.

Case Reports

SPLENIC HEMANGIOMA WITH SUBSEQUENT FATAL HEMANGIOSARCOMA

Ralph D. Whitley, M.D., and Theodore Winship, M.D., Washington, D. C.

HEMANGIOMAS are probably the most common primary benign tumors of the spleen, but their incidence cannot be determined accurately because of the variable terminology used in reporting cases. Vascular splenic lesions have been grouped together as hamartomas, endotheliomas, or angiomatous cysts; however, none of these classifications is entirely satisfactory, for investigators have collected case reports according to their individual interpretation, and cases are so rare that few have reported more than a single instance.[1-6]

Splenic hemangiomas are extremely uncommon, and most of them are found at autopsy. Schottenfeld and Wolfson[7] found four angiomas of the spleen in 2,800 autopsies, and Thiele[8] discovered three splenic angiomas in 19,000 autopsies. In 1942, Pines and Rabinovitch[9] were able to collect only forty-two cases, and 52 per cent of these were discovered incidentally at autopsy. Most of the previously reported vascular lesions of the spleen were benign histologically, and the majority were single and small.[10-12] Doubt has been expressed that vascular lesions in the spleen and elsewhere should be referred to as tumors since it cannot be proved that they are not congenital vascular abnormalities which became clinically significant because of infectious, hormonal, or mechanical factors. Splenic angiomas are of no clinical importance unless they are malignant or of sufficient size to enlarge the organ. The size of the spleen, the multiplicity of the lesions, and the histologic appearance of the tissue warrant the use of the term tumor in the case to be described.

CASE REPORT

A 23-year-old Negro woman was admitted to Garfield Memorial Hospital on Nov. 15, 1949, having been referred from the Obstetrical Clinic for investigation of a mass in the upper left quadrant of the abdomen and a nodule in the right supraclavicular fossa. She was five and one-half months pregnant.

Roentgenograms revealed clear lung fields, enlarged mediastinal lymph nodes, and an enlarged spleen which extended nearly to the iliac crest. Bone marrow and numerous clinical laboratory examinations were reported to be within normal limits. Needle biopsy of the spleen yielded only fibrous tissue, blood, and a small amount of normal lymphoid tissue.

Removal of the right supraclavicular mass was attempted, but it was found to be a thin-walled, fluid-containing cystic structure which was evacuated and only partially removed. This proved to be a cystic hygroma which, as seen on microscopic examination, was lined by a thin, hyalinized, fibrous membrane. Outside of this was an incomplete layer of fibrofatty tissue supporting small aggregates of lymphocytes and lymphatic channels lined by flattened endothelial cells.

Received for publication, July 27, 1953.

Because of the roentgenographic findings in the mediastinum and the enlarged spleen, a presumptive diagnosis of lymphoma was made, and a histologic diagnosis could not be established except by thoracotomy. A test dose of irradiation was administered, and the patient received a calculated tumor dose of 1,100 r over the mediastinum between Dec. 27, 1949, and Jan. 10, 1950. Roentgenograms taken on Jan. 31, 1950, showed no essential change in the size of the mediastinal masses.

On March 2, 1950, the patient gave birth to a normal, living male infant after eight hours of labor. No difficulty was encountered in the delivery, and she was discharged on the fourth post-partum day.

Three months later, May 2, 1950, the patient was readmitted and the spleen was removed through a left rectus incision. Exploration of the abdominal cavity at the time of operation revealed no adhesions about the spleen, no accessory splenic tissue, and no other gross abnormalities. The patient made an uneventful recovery and was discharged from the hospital on the eighth postoperative day.

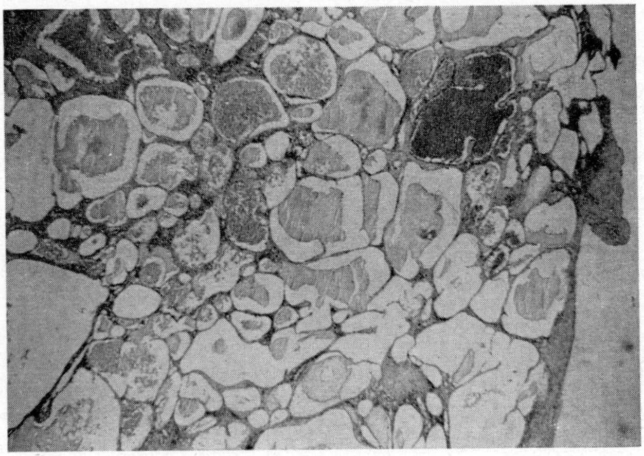

Fig. 1.—Photomicrograph of a typical area of hemangioma of the spleen. (Hematoxylin and eosin. ×75; reduced ½.)

The spleen weighed 3,065 grams and measured 36 by 23 by 12 cm. The surface was nodular because of numerous soft subcapsular dark red masses measuring from 0.5 cm. to 3 cm. in diameter. Cut section of the spleen showed a honeycombed structure composed of blood-filled cysts separated by thin, dark red, fibrous strands. The cysts varied in size from 0.1 cm. to 5 cm. and contained either blood or amber fluid. No recognizable splenic tissue was present in any part of the organ.

Microscopic sections of blocks removed from numerous parts of the spleen showed a similar structure. The tissue was composed almost entirely of blood-filled spaces separated by wide bands of hyalinized, fibrous tissue and supporting strands of lymphoid cells devoid of germinal centers. The blood-filled spaces varied greatly in size, and the larger ones were multiloculated. All the spaces were lined by normal, flattened endothelial cells.

The patient was readmitted Feb. 12, 1952, complaining of hemoptysis and substernal pain of four months' duration. Physical examination was essentially negative except for dullness and moist râles over the entire left lung. Bronchoscopy showed that the blood was coming from the left lower lobe, and bronchial washings were negative for acid-fast organisms and tumor cells. Roentgenograms showed the left hilar mass to be essentially unchanged and the right paratracheal lymph nodes to have increased in size slightly. Bronchograms demonstrated a slight narrowing of the left main bronchus due to pressure from the mediastinal mass. No areas of ulceration were demonstrated to account for the pulmonary hemorrhage.

Laboratory procedures were helpful only in revealing anemia, which was combated by repeated transfusions.

On Feb. 28, 1952, a left pneumonectomy was performed,* and two groups of mediastinal nodes were removed. The lung weighed 520 grams. Its surface was smooth except for numerous soft, dark red, bullous nodules averaging 1 cm. in diameter. On cut section the bronchi were blood-filled and the normal spongy lung tissue was almost completely replaced by irregularly shaped, blood-filled cysts, some of which communicated with the small bronchi. The mediastinal lymph nodes, which averaged 3 cm. in greatest dimension, collapsed when sectioned, and were composed of large, thin-walled cysts containing blood or yellow fluid.

Most of the blood-filled cysts in the lungs were microscopically similar to those in the previously removed spleen, and were lined with normal endothelium.

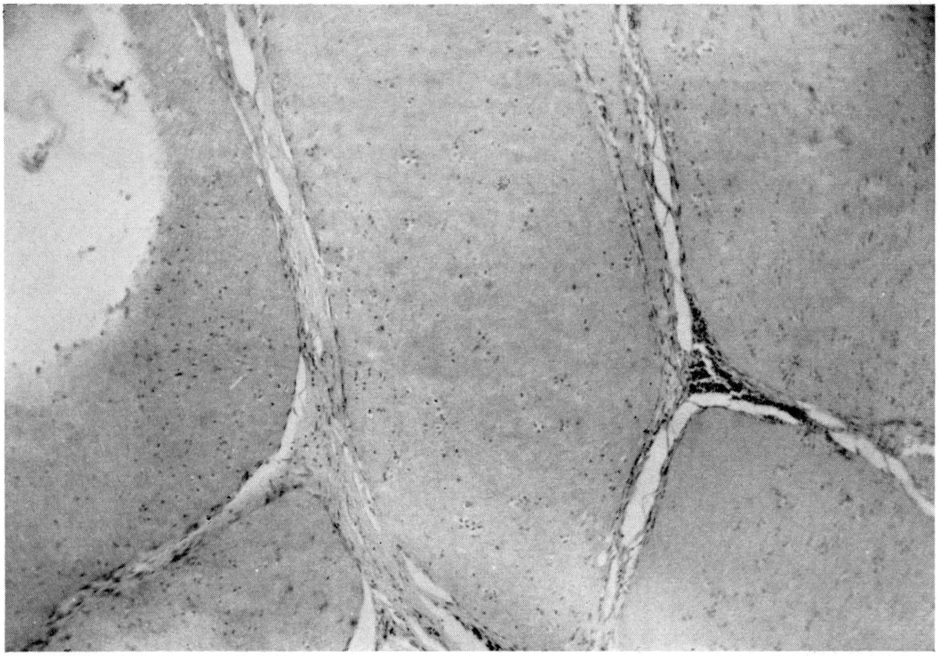

Fig. 2.—Photomicrograph of a mediastinal lymph node showing an area of hemangioma. (Hematoxylin and eosin. ×175; reduced ¼.)

Much of the lung parenchyma separating the vascular cysts was replaced by hyalinized fibrous tissue. In addition to the cavernous hemangiomas, numerous cystic structures, composed of a distinctly different type of tissue, were scattered throughout the lung. These cysts were small, irregular, and lined by large, cuboidal hyperchromatic cells. There was a suggestive papillary structure in some areas, and numerous rounded groups of enlarged endothelial cells projected into the lumina of the small, endothelial-lined spaces. Mitoses were present but extremely rare. The adjacent fibrous stroma showed widespread invasion by malignant cells, forming poorly differentiated blood vessels devoid of blood.

The resected mediastinal lymph nodes were composed almost entirely of cysts similar to those in the lung. Some of the cysts were surrounded by thick bands of fibrous tissue and were lined by normal, flattened epithelium, while in other adjacent cysts the lining cells were obviously malignant.

Postoperative roentgenograms showed numerous ill-defined masses in the right lung and slight enlargement of the mediastinal nodes on the right. Following the operation, the

*By Dr. R. G. Klepser.

patient continued to have hemoptysis, and expired on the third postoperative day. At autopsy the right lung weighed 910 grams. Its appearance was similar to that of the excised left lung. Bullouslike, dark red, soft, subpleural nodules and the blood-filled cysts occupied approximately one-half the lung parenchyma. There were many enlarged, ovoid mediastinal and periaortic lymph nodes composed mainly of bloody cysts. The liver weighed 1,550 grams and its surface was scattered with subcapsular multilocular cysts containing blood. Similar structures, present throughout the entire liver, averaged 1 cm. in diameter. In both ovaries there were small, soft, dark red, compressible areas measuring up to 1 cm. Cut section showed these to be blood-filled cysts. There was no involvement of the brain, bones, or any of the remaining viscera by the angiomatous process.

Microscopic sections of the right lung, liver, ovaries, and mediastinal and periaortic lymph nodes showed both benign and malignant vascular tumors similar to those described in the excised left lung and mediastinal nodes.

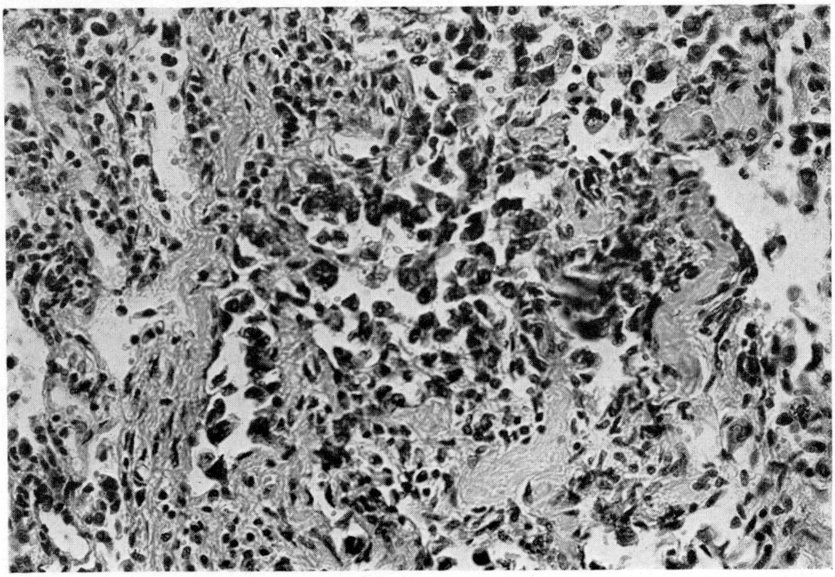

Fig. 3.—Photomicrograph of the same lymph node as in Fig. 2 showing angiosarcoma. (Hematoxylin and eosin. ×175; reduced ⅓.)

DISCUSSION

It is difficult to evaluate all aspects of the disease in this case and to classify it properly. Most of the vascular lesions of the spleen are benign cavernous hemangiomas, but occasionally, as in the case being reported, they are more complex lesions and are associated with benign or malignant vascular lesions elsewhere. Our case demonstrates some features similar to those reported in earlier cases. In one other reported case, metastases were found in lymph nodes,[13] and metastatic tumor was present in the ovaries in one instance.[14] One patient was pregnant at the time of the discovery of the splenic tumor.[15] The size of the splenic tumors in the comparable cases reported has varied from a few centimeters to a tumor occupying the entire organ and weighing as much as 5,800 grams.[16]

This condition is not always fatal, for several patients with angiosarcoma of the spleen were reported to be living after splenectomy, but very few have been followed for an adequate period.

Numerous explanations of the disease process in this case are possible, but none is entirely satisfactory. The primary site of the angiosarcoma is not known.

The case is reported as a hemangioma of the spleen despite the fact that only sixteen sections, taken at random in a very large organ, were examined histologically. It is recognized that malignant portions might have been present in areas not examined microscopically. A thorough gross examination did not reveal tissue different from that selected for microscopic examination. It could be postulated that the primary site of the tumor was in the spleen and was not included in the numerous sections taken for microscopic examination. This viewpoint is attractive, for the widespread angiosarcoma could be considered as metastatic tumor. However, this does not explain the presence of benign hemangiomas in some organs involved by angiosarcoma and the fact that the liver was grossly uninvolved at the time of splenectomy. Furthermore, there is roentgenographic evidence that mediastinal lymph nodes were involved two years before death, and the thick, hyalinized walls of the blood-filled spaces in all of the involved organs indicate that the benign hemangiomas had been present for a long time.

There is insufficient evidence to consider the liver as the primary site of the angiosarcoma because of the small, multiple foci of tumor in this organ and also because it would be difficult to explain the presence of metastatic tumor in the abdominal lymph nodes. Primary angiosarcoma of multiple lymph nodes may be a possibility, but does not appear probable in this case, and no report of such a case was found in the literature.

The lungs are dismissed as the primary site of the tumor for they were the organs least affected by the malignant process, and were clinically the last organs to become involved.

Probably the most logical diagnosis is multiple visceral cavernous hemangiomas with simultaneous malignant transformation of certain portions of the lesions in numerous organs.

There is no satisfactory explanation for all of the features of the disease in this case, for none can be proved, and most of the previously reported cases have a similarly questionable primary site. The confusing aspects of this bizarre disease cannot be clarified until a larger number of similar cases are reported or until more is known about the etiology of cavernous hemangiomas and angiosarcomas.

SUMMARY

A case of fatal angiosarcoma is reported in which the malignant disease became apparent two years after the removal of a large splenic hemangioma.

The literature relative to hemangiomas of the spleen is reviewed and discussed briefly.

REFERENCES

1. Langhans, T.: Palsirende cavernose Geschwulst der Milz mit metastatischen Knoten in der leber, Arch. f. path. Anat. **75**: 273, 1879.
2. Jores, V. L.: Ein Fall von sarkomatösem Angiom der Milz und Leber, Centralbl. f. allg. Path. u. path. Anat. **19**: 662, 1908.
3. Garlock, J. H.: Primary Angiosarcoma of the Spleen, J. Mt. Sinai Hosp. **6**: 319, 1940.
4. Wright, A. W.: Primary Malignant Hemangioma of the Spleen With Multiple Liver Metastases, Am. J. Path. **4**: 507, 1928.
5. De Navasques, S.: Angioblastoma of the Spleen With Metastases in the Liver, J. Path. & Bact. **42**: 651, 1936.
6. Dowd, C. N.: Cavernous Angioma of the Spleen, Ann. Surg. **62**: 177, 1915.
7. Schottenfeld, L. E., and Wolfson, W. L.: Cavernous Hemangioma of the Spleen, Arch. Surg. **35**: 867, 1937.
8. Thiele: Ueber Angiome und sarkomatose Angiome der Milz, Virchows Arch. f. path. Anat. **178**: 296, 1904.
9. Pines, B., and Rabinovitch, J.: Hemangioma of the Spleen, Arch. Path. **33**: 487, 1942.
10. Gibson, D. M., and Wyatt, W. M.: Angiomata of the Liver, Spleen and Mesentery, J. Kansas M. Soc. **51**: 417, 1950.
11. Hodge, G. B., and Wilson, D. A.: Benign Cavernous Hemangiomas of the Spleen, SURGERY **21**: 343, 1947.
12. Smith, C. E., and Rusk, G. Y.: Endothelioma of the Spleen, Arch. Surg. **7**: 371, 1923.
13. Bauer, D. de F., and Stanford, W. R.: Splenic Hemangiosarcoma, Arch. Path. **41**: 668, 1946.
14. Shennan, T.: Histologically Non-malignant Angioma With Numerous Metastases, J. Path. & Bact. **19**: 139, 1914-15.
15. Reich, W. W., and Van Tassell, L. R.: Cystic Hemangioma of Spleen, Am. J. Surg. **75**: 840, 1948.
16. Zeno, A., and Cid, J. M.: Hémangio-endothéliome de la rate, Ann. d'anat. path. **7**: 583, 1930.

ABDOMINAL PREGNANCY WITH FETAL AND MATERNAL SURVIVAL

Report of a Case

M. H. Harris, M.D., Newport, Ark.

THE survival of the mother and a normal child following abdominal pregnancy is sufficiently rare to justify the report of another case.

Broomes[1] reviewed 343 cases of abdominal pregnancies, including his own case, and reported that there were only 85 cases in which both mother and child survived, and of these, only 33 children showed no demonstrable evidence of neurological or mental disturbances.

Jarrett[2] stated that 565 cases of abdominal pregnancies were recorded between 1809 and 1946. He added two cases, with the survival of both mothers and one child.

Review of recent literature[3-15] showed 24 additional cases with survival of 22 mothers and 13 infants, with 12 of the latter normal in all respects.

The management of the placenta varied. It was completely removed, or it was marsupialized and cavity-packed, and the abdomen was then drained, or no attempt was made to remove the placenta with closure without drainage. The most satisfactory results were obtained in the cases where it was possible to remove the placenta completely. In several cases it was necessary to perform a supravaginal hysterectomy in removing the placenta.[3, 5, 7, 11]

CASE REPORT

N. W., aged 36 years, a Negro housewife, was first seen June 15, 1950, complaining of irregular menstruation for two months and moderate swelling of the lower extremities. She gave a history of one previous pregnancy, about ten years previously, which terminated spontaneously in the third month of pregnancy. On examination the uterus was found to be enlarged to the size of about a three months' pregnancy, with a small mass palpable above and to the right of the uterus. A diagnosis was made of ovarian cyst on the right, or fibroid uterus. Examination again on July 27, 1950, revealed the uterus to be larger, and positive breast changes. Although she continued to have irregular bleeding, a diagnosis was made of pregnancy, and the expected date of delivery was set for about Feb. 2, 1951. The prenatal course was uneventful except for continued menstruation at irregular intervals. She maintained a normal blood pressure, normal weight gain, and negative urine throughout. On Nov. 26, 1950, she was admitted to the hospital with the diagnosis of premature labor. Labor pains were excellent for over twenty-four hours without any dilation of the cervix. After about twenty-seven hours of continuous labor, it was decided to terminate the pregnancy by cesarean section. A low midline incision was made, under general anesthesia, and on opening the peritoneum a large amount of thin, flaky, yellowish fluid escaped. An incision was made in what was thought to be the uterus, but was later found to be the placenta. Bleeding was controlled with pressure until the female fetus was delivered with the aid of forceps. The baby, who weighed 5 pounds, cried immediately. The placenta was attached by a pedicle to the dome of the uterus and the right broad ligament. The placenta was removed entirely, with bleeding from the attachment sites controlled with transfixing sutures. The abdomen was closed without drainage. The

Received for publication, Aug. 3, 1953.

postoperative course was uneventful, and the mother and the baby were discharged from the hospital on the seventh postoperative day. The baby was normal in every respect. Follow-up in April, 1953, revealed the mother to be pregnant again, and the child developing normally.

REFERENCES

1. Broomes, E. L. C.: Full Term Abdominal Pregnancy With Delivery of Living Child, Report of Case and Review of Literature, J. Indiana M. A. **44**: 127-129 (Feb.), 1951; J. A. M. A. **145**: 399-401 (Feb. 10), 1951.
2. Jarrett, J. C.: A Report of Two Cases of Late Abdominal Pregnancy, Ohio State M. J. **48**: 219-221 (March), 1952.
3. MacGregor, A. S.: Abdominal Pregnancy, Am. J. Surg. **82**: 365-371 (Sept.), 1951.
4. Burleson, R. J., and Bragg, J. C.: Full Term Abdominal Pregnancy, Report of Case, J. A. M. A. **147**: 1349-1350 (Dec. 1), 1951.
5. Webster, B. J., and McCain, T. J.: Delivery of Living Child From an Abdominal Pregnancy, Northwest Med. **51**: 404 (May), 1952.
6. Siegal, H. A.: Advanced Abdominal Pregnancy With Fetal and Maternal Survival, J. Internat. Coll. Surgeons **18**: 77-85 (July), 1952.
7. Troconis, R.: Abdominal Pregnancy Proceeding to Term With Birth of Living Fetus, Rev. obst. y. ginec., Caracas **10**: 100, 1950; Brennan, J. W.: Internat. Abstr. Surg., Surg., Gynec. & Obst. **92**: 479 (May), 1951.
8. Brainard, H. H.: Full Term Abdominal Pregnancy With Intestinal Obstruction, Arizona Med. **8**: 39-41 (Feb.), 1951.
9. Bourgeois, G. A., and Morris, W. S.: Abdominal Pregnancy Secondary to Rupture of Accessory Uterus With Survival of Mother and Infant, Report of a Case, New England J. Med. **247**: 84-87 (July), 1952.
10. Pearson, E. A.: Abdominal Pregnancy, West. J. Surg. **58**: 712-713 (Dec.), 1950.
11. Posner, A. C., and Beer, M. A.: Full Term Pregnancy With Living Mother and Child, New York J. Med. **51**: 1185-1186 (May 1), 1951.
12. Bowen, G. L.: Abdominal Pregnancy With Living Baby Delivered Near Term, Am. J. Obst. & Gynec. **61**: 455-457 (Feb.), 1951.
13. Abdominal Pregnancy Terminating in a Living Child and Complete Removal of Placenta, Am. J. Obst. & Gynec. **63**: 908-910 (April), 1952.
14. Douglas, G. F., Douglas, G. C., and Douglas, G. F., Jr.: Ectopic Pregnancy, J. Internat. Coll. Surgeons **15**: 28-37 (Jan.), 1951.
15. Steptoe, P.: Case of Abdominal Pregnancy, J. Obst. & Gynaec. Brit. Emp. **57**: 949-952 (Dec.), 1950.

HERNIA THROUGH FORAMEN OF WINSLOW

Report of a Case With Preoperative Roentgen Diagnosis and Successful Surgical Management

Alan L. Dorian, M.D.,* and George N. Stein, M.D.,**
Philadelphia, Pa.

(From the Department of Surgery and the Department of Radiology of the Graduate Hospital and the Graduate School of Medicine, University of Pennsylvania)

Hernia through the foramen of Winslow is not a common occurrence. According to Lavarde and Chevret,[1] there have been less than seventy cases reported in the world literature, and of these, there were but six in which the preoperative diagnosis was suggested. Recently, Hollenberg[2] and Cimmino[3] recorded cases in which such a diagnosis was made. It is the purpose of this paper to present an unusual case of this rare internal hernia in which the diagnosis of herniation of the large intestine through the foramen of Winslow was made by roentgen studies and confirmed at operation.

ANATOMY AND PATHOLOGY

The foramen of Winslow or epiploic foramen is a potential canal connecting the general peritoneal cavity with the omental bursa. It is bounded anteriorly by the border of the lesser omentum with the common bile duct, hepatic artery, and portal vein. Posteriorly is the peritoneum overlying the inferior vena cava. Superiorly is the peritoneum covering the duodenum.[4] From a knowledge of these anatomic relationships, it can be seen that the surgical management must be accomplished with the utmost regard for the vital structures concerned.

Moynihan and Dobson[5] have postulated that one or more of the following conditions must be present for herniation to occur: (1) a common mesentery for the entire intestinal tract, (2) absence of secondary fusion of the ascending colon to the parietal abdominal wall, (3) an abnormally large foramen of Winslow, and (4) an abnormally long mesentery allowing undue mobility of the small bowel. Several authors including Cimmino have suggested that a large right lobe of the liver may also predispose to hernia in that a funnel-like approach to the foramen is thus formed.

SYMPTOMATOLOGY

Silverstone[6] has stated that cases of herniation may be either acute or long standing in nature. The acute cases are characteristically heralded by the signs and symptoms of intestinal obstruction, varying with the level at which obstruction has occurred. Usually this obstruction is precipitous in

Received for publication, Aug. 27, 1953.

*Formerly senior resident in surgery, Surgical Service of H. R. Hawthorne, M.D., Graduate Hospital.

**Associate in radiology, Graduate School of Medicine, and associate radiologist, Graduate Hospital.

onset, although occasionally symptoms may be present for some days before the patient consults a physician. Infrequently, however, herniation may be present for a long time before actual obstruction intervenes. Indeed, Dewis[7] presented a case in which the history and roentgen findings suggested that herniation had been present for some seventeen years prior to complete obstruction and sudden death.

CASE REPORT

Mrs. A. W., a 54-year-old white woman, was admitted to the Graduate Hospital Medical Service on Nov. 18, 1952, complaining of epigastric fullness, pain in the right upper quadrant, and intermittent vomiting. Her past history was of interest in that for the previous five years she had been under treatment for giant follicle lymphoblastoma, for which she had received both roentgen and nitrogen mustard therapy.

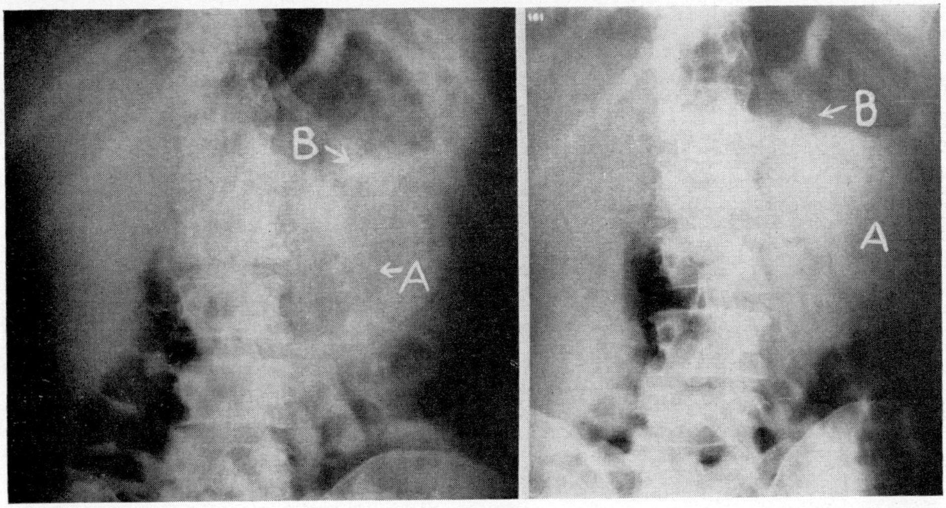

Fig. 1.—Anteroposterior recumbent (*left*) and erect (*right*) films of abdomen on admission. Large collection of gas (*B*) to left of midline just below diaphragm exhibits fluid-air level in erect position. This lies medial to stomach (*A*) and represents the cecum and ascending colon herniated into the lesser omental sac.

The patient dated the onset of the present difficulties to three weeks prior to admission, when for the first time she noticed a sense of upper abdominal fullness following each meal. This sensation would persist for several hours, with slight relief being obtained by the ingestion of large quantities of water. Gradually, the patient had restricted her diet entirely to fluids. One week prior to admission she began to have occasional vomiting. She denied hematemesis. Associated with the vomiting was an increasingly severe ''griping'' pain beneath the left anterior costal margin. On Nov. 16, 1952, the pain was more constant, requiring injection of morphine by her physician. On this date she had a small, formed bowel movement, but no further passage of flatus or feces was noted until admission.

Physical examination revealed a moderately dehydrated patient lying quietly in bed, not appearing in any acute distress. Temperature was 100° F. rectally, pulse 90 per minute, blood pressure 144 mm. Hg systolic and 80 mm. Hg diastolic. The primary findings were confined to the abdomen, which was slightly protruberant but quite soft to examination. The liver was palpable to a point slightly below the level of the umbilicus. A globular, solid mass was present in the epigastrium and left upper quadrant which was interpreted as spleen. No tenderness was elicited; by auscultation, peristalsis was not obstructive. The rectum was empty of feces.

Laboratory data on admission were reported as: hemoglobin 12.1 Gm., white blood cells 5,000 cells per millimeter with a normal differential, blood sugar 103 mg. per 100 ml., blood urea nitrogen 8 mg. per 100 ml. Electrolytes were all within normal limits; the urine presented no albumen or sugar. Liver function tests were normal.

On the day following admission, survey films of the abdomen made in the anteroposterior recumbent and erect positions (Fig. 1) failed to demonstrate any evidence of intestinal obstruction. An unusual, large radiolucent shadow which exhibited an air-fluid level in the erect position was noted medial to the stomach. This evidently represented the cecum and ascending colon in the lesser peritoneal sac, but its significance was not appreciated at this time. Because of the inability to make a definitive diagnosis from the survey films, and since there was no roentgen or clinical evidence of obstruction, it was recommended that the patient be given a barium mouth meal.

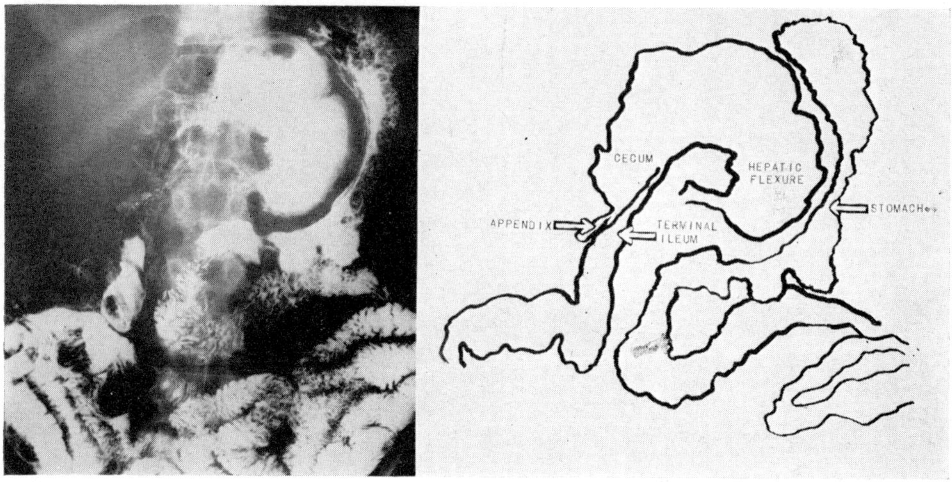

A. *B.*

Fig. 2.—Anteroposterior film (*A*) following barium meal with schematic drawing (*B*) showing stomach and entire small intestine filled with barium. Large collection of barium medial to stomach is in the herniated cecum and ascending colon.

The next day (Nov. 20, 1953) the patient was given six ounces of a barium-water mixture by mouth. In fifteen minutes the barium had passed through the jejunum and most of the ileum; the head of the column was directed cephalad and medially, where the barium seemed to enter a pouch located medial and posterior to the stomach. Shortly after this, when the appendix filled with barium, it became apparent that this pouch represented the cecum, ascending colon, and the hepatic flexure, which were herniated into the lesser sac (Figs. 2 and 3). In order to determine accurately how much of the colon was involved in the hernia, a small barium enema was then given. Almost complete obstruction to the flow of barium was encountered in the proximal transverse colon (Fig. 4).

On the evening of this examination, the patient complained of cramping, upper abdominal pain, but had no vomiting, temperature, or pulse elevation and was passing flatus by rectum. Physical examination was unchanged and peristalsis was not obstructive. However, on the morning of Nov. 22, 1953, the pain began to increase in frequency and severity. Present in the epigastrium was a tympanitic, fluctuant, tender mass. The abdomen was generally distended, and peristalsis was high pitched and obstructive in nature. Temperature was 99° F. orally, pulse 120 per minute. Clinically, the patient appeared acutely ill. A survey film of the abdomen at this time revealed a large amount of barium in the herniated proximal colon in the same position as demonstrated on previous films.

No barium was seen in the distal half of the colon. There was no evidence of small intestinal obstruction.

A surgical consultation was requested. The roentgen diagnosis of hernia of the large bowel into the lesser sac was concurred, and immediate exploration was decided upon. On opening the abdomen through a long upper midline incision, there was release of about 500 c.c. of clear, odorless, straw-colored fluid from the peritoneal cavity. The right lobe of the liver was greatly enlarged, extending into the right lower quadrant and presenting

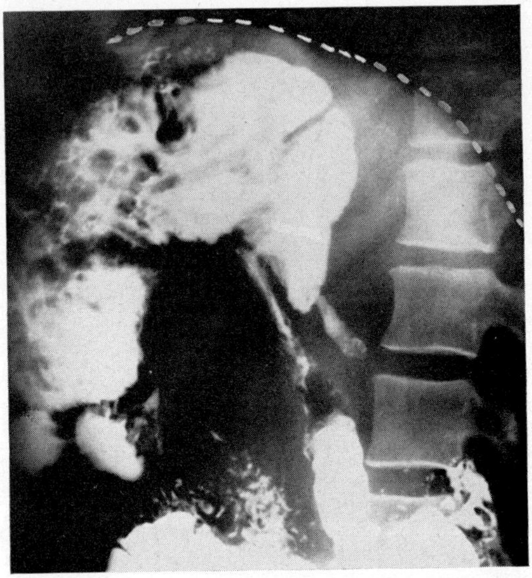

Fig. 3.—Lateral view showing position of hernia. White dotted line represents dome of diaphragm.

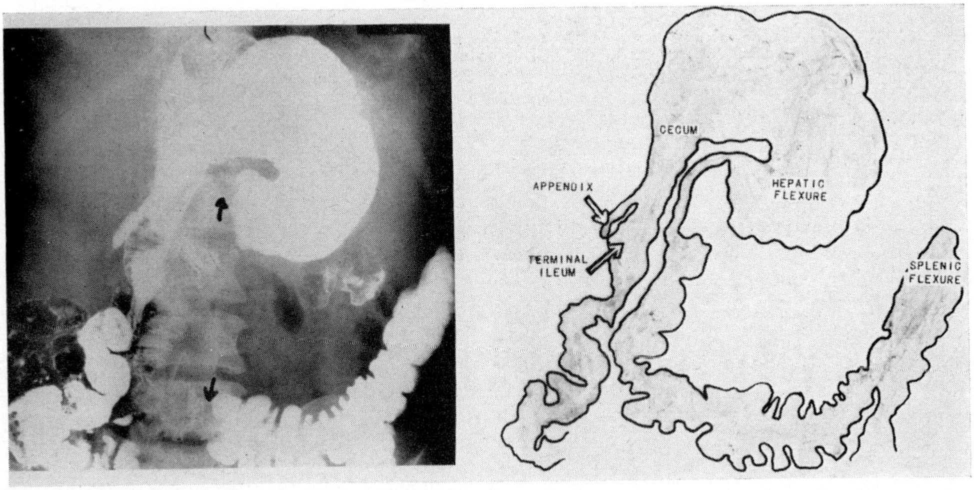

A. B.

Fig. 4.—Anteroposterior recumbent film (*A*) and schematic drawing (*B*) following combined barium meal and cautious barium enema, demonstrating amount of colon in the hernia and partial obstruction in proximal transverse colon indicated by black arrows.

a very hard mulberry-like appearance suggestive of far-advanced cirrhosis. A wedge biopsy was taken of this lobe. The spleen was enlarged to about three times normal size; it was soft and mushy to palpation. Immediately below the incision was a large, distended, markedly inflamed, tense loop of large bowel. With further exploration, it was evident

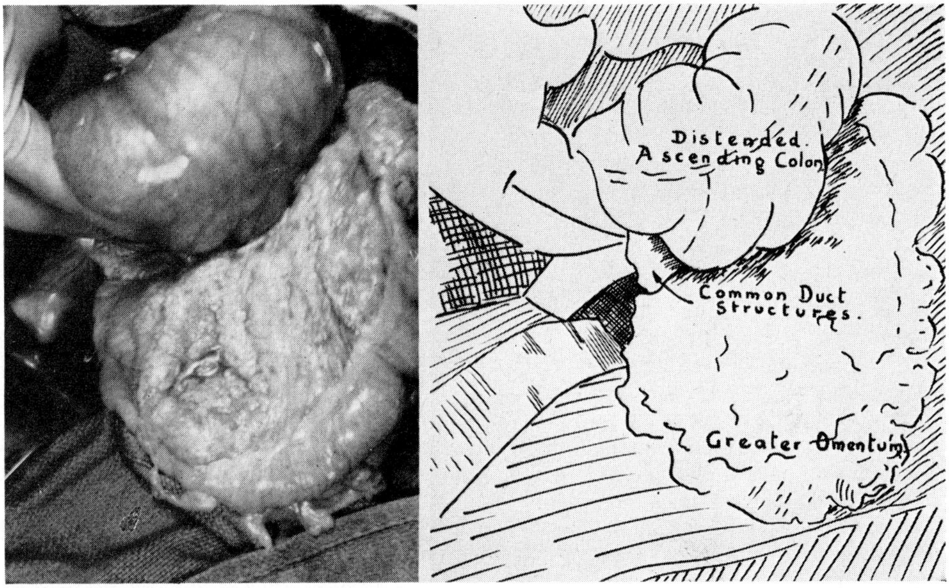

Fig. 5.—Photograph and accompanying diagram demonstrating the appearance of the herniated bowel as it presented through the tear in the gastrohepatic omentum.

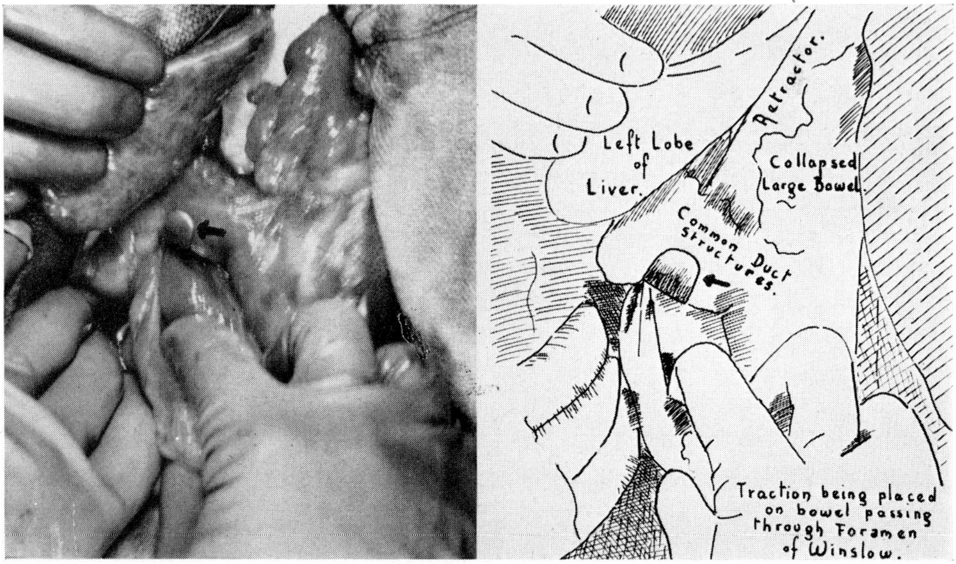

Fig. 6.—Appearance of bowel following aseptic enterotomy as traction is being exerted to reduce through the foramen of Winslow. A retractor is seen elevating the common duct structures. Arrow indicates retractor in the foramen of Winslow.

that this represented the entire ascending colon to a point just distal to the hepatic flexure, which was presenting through a large rent in the gastrohepatic omentum (Fig. 5). The mode of entry was apparent with the finding of a slightly distended loop of terminal ileum and collapsed transverse colon tightly compressed at the foramen of Winslow. Efforts to reduce the hernia by gentle manipulation were unsuccessful; an aseptic enterotomy was performed and severeal hundred cubic centimeters of thick semisolid barium was aspirated, with collapse of the involved bowel. Following this, the enterotomy was closed. At the completion of this procedure, it was possible to reduce the bowel through the gastrohepatic omentum with gentle traction and thence through the foramen of Winslow without difficulty (Fig. 6). Within a short time, the bowel appeared viable.

Two fingers could be slipped easily through the foramen of Winslow. The rent in the gastrohepatic omentum was closed with interrupted sutures of cotton, following which two interrupted sutures of the same material were used to suture the periductal fat loosely along the common duct structures to the peritoneum overlying the inferior vena cava in an effort to obliterate the portal through which herniation had occurred. The ascending colon was then returned to its normal position in the right lower quadrant, and several fat tabs sutured to the lateral peritoneal wall to hold it in place. The abdomen was closed.

The immediate postoperative period was uneventful. However, forty-eight hours after operation the abdomen became quite distended, and it was apparent that there was definite fluid in the flanks. The liver biopsy taken at the time of surgery was reported to represent "far-advanced portal cirrhosis." Twenty-four hours later, spontaneous drainage of clear ascitic fluid began to occur from the lower angle of the incision, which continued intermittently for several days. Nine days postoperatively, all liver function tests were normal with the exception of a Bromsulphalein retention of 27.3 per cent However, clinically the patient did very well and there was no further evidence of intestinal obstruction. She was placed on a liver protection program of dietary supplement and parenteral proteins, and subsequently transferred to the Gastrointestinal Service for further treatment. A roentgen examination of the intestinal tract on Jan. 15, 1953, revealed no evidence of abnormality.

However, the cirrhosis failed to respond to the most intensive therapy, and three months following surgery (Feb. 9, 1953) she rapidly went into congestive heart failure and expired.

DISCUSSION

All of the roentgen signs of herniation through the foramen of Winslow concern themselves with the demonstration of air in the lesser sac. Case and Upson[8] stated that the demonstration of small intestine anterior to the hepatic flexure or first part of the transverse colon is necessary to establish the diagnosis. This sign is obviously not applicable when these portions of the colon are herniated in association with the small bowel, nor as in this case in which the small bowel did not enter the hernia. Hollenberg[2] emphasized the importance of gas in the lesser omental sac in association with obstruction in the transverse colon as demonstrated by barium enema. He made what he believed the first preoperative roentgen diagnosis of lesser sac hernia. Cimmino[9] has pointed out the roentgen findings in perforation into the lesser sac. In a later report[3] he described a case in which gas in the lesser sac due to hernia differed from the gas noted in perforation. We believe that once the presence of gas in the lesser sac can be determined with certainty, then the diagnosis rests between a perforation into the lesser sac or a hernia. We agree with Cimmino that if the fluid levels do not conform to the anatomic recesses of the sac or if the actual wall of the bowel can be demonstrated, then the specific diagnosis of herniation into the lesser sac can be made without subjecting the patient to barium studies.

SUMMARY

1 A case of herniation of the ascending colon and portion of the transverse colon through the foramen of Winslow which was diagnosed preoperatively and successfully treated surgically is presented.

2. The roentgen findings are discussed.

REFERENCES

1. Lavarde, J., and Chevret. R.: Contributions a l'étude radiologique des occlusions hernie étrangleé de l'hiatus de Winslow, Presse méd. **57**: 562, 1949.
2. Hollenberg. M. S.: Radiographic Diagnosis of Hernia Into Lesser Peritoneal Sac Through Foramen of Wins!ow; Report of Case, SURGERY **18**: 498, 1945.
3. Cimmino, C. V.: Lesser Sac Hernia via the Foramen of Winslow, Radiology **60**: 57-59 (Jan.) 1953.
4. Gray, H.: Anatomy of the Human Body, ed. 25, Philadelphia, 1948, Lea & Febiger, pp. 1201.
5. Moynihan, B. G. A., and Dobson, J. F.: On Retroperitoneal Hernia, ed. 2, London, 1906, Baillière, Tindall & Cox.
6. Silverstone, M.: Hernia Through the Foramen of Winslow, Lancet **2**: 786, 1939.
7. Dewis, J. W., and Miller, R. H.: Hernia Through the Foramen of Winslow, Surg., Gynec. & Obst. **45**: 95, 1927.
8. Case, J. T., and Upson, W. O.: Roentgenologic Aspects of Various Types of Hernia, J. A. M. A. **87**: 891-898 (Sept.) 1926.
9 Cimmino, C V., and Sholes, D. M.: Gas in the Lesser Sac in Perforated Peptic Ulcer, Am. J. Roentgenol. **68**: 19-21 (July) 1952.

BENIGN STRICTURE OF HEPATICODUODENOSTOMY: ITS TREATMENT

Report of Two Cases

John D. Koucky, M.D., and W. Forrester Maley, M.D., Chicago, Ill.

(From the Department of Surgery, Lutheran Deaconess Hospital)

THE procedure described in this report has been successfully employed in the treatment of two cases of benign stricture of hepaticoduodenostomy. The following two cases are reported.—

Case 1.—A 49-year-old white woman in 1931 had a cholecystectomy for cholecystitis and cholelithiasis elsewhere. During this operation an accidental excision of the extrahepatic biliary tract was made. At the second operation, no part of the hepatic and common bile ducts was found. This defect was repaired by anastomosing the adjacent duodenum to an opening in the liver at the hilus, through which much "white bile" was obtained. A 10 cm. piece of 24 Fr. rubber catheter, with a cuff, was used as a splint. Five months later this splint was removed by transpyloric forceps manipulation through a gastrotomy.

The patient remained well for six years (1937) when she developed evidence of gradually increasing obstruction of the biliary tract. Surgery was postponed too long chiefly because of the realization of the difficulties of exposing the site of obstruction. When finally relief became imperative, the liver was so large that exposure of the anastomosis at the hilus was technically near impossible.

Operation: A right upper rectus incision was used. The second portion of the duodenum was mobilized for 8 cm. The mobilized duodenum was opened longitudinally so as to expose the previous hepaticoduodenostomy. The stoma would just admit a 1 mm. probe. This opening was dilated to 30 Fr., using urethral sounds. Exploration of the intrahepatic ducts by probe, scoops, and catheter irrigation revealed twenty-five soft calculi up to 1 cm. in diameter. These calculi were removed. A 15 cm. piece of 24 Fr. rubber catheter, with a cuff, was inserted about 6 cm. up into the liver through the dilated stoma. The opening in the duodenum was closed transversely. The abdomen was closed in layers with one Penrose drain. The postoperative course was uneventful, and recovery from the obstructive jaundice was rapid.

During the past sixteen years the patient has been examined at least once a year and has been in good health. The liver has remained above the right costal margin. The patient has gained 25 pounds in weight and has been free of jaundice. In 1939 she experienced several episodes of chilliness, nausea, and epigastric pain during a two-week period. This patient was last seen on March 17, 1953.

Case 2.—In 1946, Mrs. L. H. had a cholecystectomy performed elsewhere. During this operation an accidental excision of the hepatic duct, from just at the junction of the right and left hepatic ducts, and the common bile duct was made. Approximately one month later, this was repaired by a hepaticoduodenostomy. Following an uneventful convalescence the patient continued well until 1948, when evidence of benign recurrent obstruction of the biliary tract developed. The patient was prepared for surgery.

Operation: Through a right upper rectus incision, an enlarged liver was revealed. The duodenum was found attached high up into the hilus of the liver and was rather easily

Received for publication, Sept. 1, 1953.

mobilized in spite of the adhesions and the huge liver. The duodenum was opened longitudinally opposite the anastomosis. The hepaticoduodenostomy stoma, narrowed to 1 mm., was readily located with a fine probe. It was dilated to 26 Fr., using common duct dilators. When this opening was dilated, a considerable amount of turbid bile, containing many soft calculi up to 3 mm. in diameter, poured out. A section of 24 Fr. rubber catheter, with a cuff, was introduced high into the intrahepatic ducts. Approximately six inches of the catheter extended down into the duodenum. The opening in the duodenum was closed transversely. A Penrose drain was inserted down to the operative area.

The postoperative course was uneventful, with an immediate abatement of symptoms. The patient has continued in good health to the present time.

DISCUSSION

The technique described in this report offers a rational, simplified surgical approach to a definite, although limited, group of cases of biliary obstruction in adults.

Walters and Phillips,[1] reporting on 165 patients with strictures of the extrahepatic bile ducts, listed forty-two cases of hepaticoduodenostomy with 52 per cent recurrence of biliary obstruction.

Walters and Kelly,[2] reporting on an additional 100 cases from 1948 through 1951, listed forty-six cases of anastomosis of hepatic duct to duodenum, of which thirty-two cases were traced with a recurrence of stricture in 34.4 per cent.

Lahey and Pyrtek,[3] in discussing the operative management of 280 strictures of the bile ducts, reported that of forty-five patients with biliary-intestinal anastomosis (jejunum and duodenum) from 1940 to 1948, eleven developed recurrence of biliary obstruction.

Cole, Reynolds, and Ireneus[4] have stated, "The tendency to recurrence of stenosis in patients without any duct at the hilus has become the greatest single obstacle to a successful outcome, and attempts to prevent this stenosis have represented the major part of all recent surgical effort in this field."

In the past, reconstructive or plastic types of operation upon the stricture have been the common practice.[5-7]

The seriousness of these recurrent benign strictures of the common hepatic duct is realized since Longmire and Sanford[8, 9] have recommended intrahepatic cholangiojejunostomy with partial hepatectomy for their treatment.

Borrowing a principle from the urologist, namely, that an acquired benign stricture of a mucosa-lined tube can be dilated and will remain patent, it was applied to these cases of benign stricture of a hepaticoduodenostomy with excellent results in both cases.

The potential complications which may be anticipated are that a duodenal fistula may develop or the stoma may not be found due to marked narrowing or complete obliteration. These complications have not occurred in the reported cases. The risk of development of a duodenal fistula is no greater in this operation than in the usual reconstructive or plastic type of procedure. Certain advantages are apparent, but will be mentioned for completeness. In this operation, certain important anatomic structures, namely, the portal vein, hepatic artery, and inferior vena cava, are avoided by opening into the duodenum and making a transduodenal dilation of the stricture.

Technically, this operation is less difficult. It may be performed by the less skilled surgeon. The facility with which the pathology in these cases was corrected is evident from the two reported cases. In comparison with the arduous reconstructive or plastic type of operation, this procedure involves less risk for the severely ill patient.

Another suggested advantage is that this operation may be utilized in those patients who are beginning to show evidence of recurrence of a stricture, whereas one would hesitate to perform the greater-risk reconstructive or plastic-type operation at this time By having this lower-risk operation available, the patient can be treated earlier and is in better condition for surgery.

This procedure should be of value in benign stricture of choledochoduodenostomy and choledochojejunostomy.

The results obtained in these two cases have been very satisfactory. One patient has been asymptomatic and in good health for five years. The other patient has remained in good health for sixteen years with the exception of one two-week period of recurrent episodes of epigastric pain, nausea, and chilliness.

SUMMARY

1. A low-risk operation for the treatment of benign stricture of a hepaticoduodenostomy is presented.

2. This operation has been used in the two reported cases with satisfactory results.

3. The possible complications and advantages are discussed.

REFERENCES

1. Walters, W., and Phillips, S. K.: Physiologic Aspects of Repaired Stricture of the Extrahepatic Bile Ducts: Report on 165 Cases, Proc. Staff Meet., Mayo Clin. **24:** 13 (Jan. 5) 1949.
2. Walters, W., and Kelly, A. H.: Surgical Treatment of Strictures of the Common and Hepatic Bile Ducts, Arch. Surg. **66:** 418, 1953.
3. Lahey, F. H., and Pyrtek, L. J.: Experience With the Operative Management of 280 Strictures of the Bile Ducts With a Description of a New Method and Complete Follow-up Study of the End Results in 229 of the Cases, Surgical Practice of the Lahey Clinic, Philadelphia, 1951, W. B. Saunders Company, p. 525.
4. Cole, W. H., Reynolds, J. T., and Ireneus, C., Jr.: Strictures of the Common Bile Duct, Advances Surgery **1:** 115, 1949.
5. Ravdin, I. S.: Reconstruction of Common Bile Duct, Pennsylvania M. J. **53:** 807-810 (Aug.) 1950.
6. Walters, W.: Physiologic Studies in Cases of Stricture of the Common Bile Duct, Ann. Surg. **130:** 451, 1949.
7. Walters, W., and Phillips, S. K.: Physiologic Aspects of Repaired Strictures of the Extrahepatic Bile Ducts: Report of 165 Cases, Proc. Staff Meet., Mayo Clin. **24:** 15 (Jan. 5) 1949.
8. Longmire, W. P., Jr., and Sanford, M. C.: Intrahepatic Cholangiojejunostomy, SURGERY **24:** 264, 1948.
9. Longmire, W. P., Jr., and Sanford, M. C.: Intrahepatic Cholangiojejunostomy for Biliary Obstruction: Further Studies, Ann. Surg. **130:** 455, 1949.

SPONTANEOUS RUPTURE OF THE NORMAL URINARY BLADDER

Report of One Case

Hyman Hershman, M.D.,* and Herman L. Allen, M.D.,** Boston, Mass.

(From the Surgical and Urological Services, Beth Israel Hospital)

SPONTANEOUS rupture of the urinary bladder is defined as rupture of the bladder without antecedent trauma. The purpose of this paper is to add an interesting case report to the literature of this relatively rare entity. The first comprehensive report on spontaneous rupture of the urinary bladder was that of Stone[1] in 1931, who collected forty cases in the literature up to that time and added two cases of his own. Since then, nineteen more cases have been recorded and reviewed by Crastnopol[2] in 1950.

Spontaneous rupture of the bladder is usually associated with (1) inflammation of the bladder wall, (2) malignant disease of the bladder, or (3) overdistention of the urinary bladder secondary to obstruction or due to alcohol depression of the sensorium. Spontaneous rupture of a normal bladder is rare. Barnes and Steele[3] reported the occurrence of spontaneous rupture in a normal bladder.

Prompt diagnosis of rupture of the bladder and institution of proper therapy is imperative in order to keep the mortality rate from this condition at a minimum. Diagnosis is usually difficult because of the rarity of this entity and because the patient usually presents the signs and symptoms of an acute intra-abdominal process. Therapy in the following case was delayed because of the difficulty in establishing a diagnosis and correlating the urologic radiographic findings with the clinical condition of the patient. The working diagnosis in this case was a perforated peptic ulcer. A diagnostic paracentesis demonstrated spermatozoa which directed our attention to the urologic tract.

CASE REPORT

A Negro male chef, aged 61 years, entered our Emergency Ward at 1:30 P.M. on March 11, 1953, with the chief complaint of severe generalized abdominal pain. The history was obtained from the patient and his wife. It was stated that the patient had had intermittent episodes of epigastric nonradiating pain for many years. The pain occurred usually between meals and occasionally woke the patient up at night. The pain was relieved by the ingestion of food and medication given by his local physician. The patient had been told that he had a "nervous stomach." The patient stated that he had been able to maintain his daily work and got along fairly well except for the three months prior to admission, when he had onset of increasing weakness, and he had noted a loss of fifteen pounds during this period. One week prior to admission the patient had onset of severe epigastric pain and generalized malaise. He stayed home from work and at bed rest. The symptoms of malaise persisted with intermittent epigastric pain until 5:30 A.M. on the morning of admission, when he was awakened from his sleep with severe epigastric pain associated with retching without the production of much vomitus. The patient stated

Received for publication, Sept. 8, 1953.

*Resident in Urology, Beth Israel Hospital.

**Intern, Surgical Service, Beth Israel Hospital.

that the retching was quite severe. During the episode of retching the patient noted the exaggeration of the epigastric pain, which was more severe than anything he had noted before. The epigastric pain subsided, and then the patient began to complain of generalized abdominal pain predominantly in both lower quadrants. He had a normal bowel movement twenty-four hours before his admission and had passed flatus on the morning of admission.

There were no genitourinary symptoms. Past history revealed that the patient had an appendectomy and right herniorraphy in 1932, and he had had gonorrhea and syphilis in 1918. He was treated with arsphenamine for the latter. There was no history of tuberculosis, diabetes mellitus, or neurological disorders.

Physical examination revealed a thin, anxious Negro male who was in acute distress and appeared slightly disoriented. Pulse was 100 and regular, respirations were 22, blood pressure 186/90, and the temperature was 100° F. rectally. Both pupils were fixed. Examination of the abdomen revealed a slightly distended abdomen with an absence of bowel sounds. The abdomen was generally rigid and approached a boardlike abdomen, with marked tenderness in the right lower quadrant. Rectal examination was negative. Neurological examintion was entirely negtive except for the fixed pupils.

Admission laboratory studies revealed a hemoglobin of 16.6 Gm., a white blood cell count of 15,600, nonprotein nitrogen was 81, bilirubin was 0.6, CO_2 was 46 volumes per cent, chloride was 102 meq. per liter, potassium was 5.5 meq. per liter, sodium was 147 meq. per liter, and serum amylase was 95. A catheterized urine specimen was yellow in color, had 3+ turbidity, a reaction of 4.5, a specific gravity of 1.021, albumin, sugar, acetone, and bile were absent and there were 0 to 2 white blood cells per high-power field and 100 red blood cells per high-power field. A chest film demonstrated plate atelectasis on the right. Recumbent and upright films of the abdomen revealed some gas-filled, slightly dilated small intestinal loops and gas in the colon. The roentgenographic impression was that this represented an acute abdomen, possibly secondary to peritonitis with probable atony of the small intestine. A possible diagnosis of perforated peptic ulcer was made, and the patient was watched carefully. Eight hours after admission the patient's temperature, pulse, respirations, and x-ray film of the abdomen were the same as on admission. The patient still had a semirigid abdomen, but he was in only moderate distress. The white blood cell count had not changed and the urinalysis was essentially the same except that it had 20 to 30 red blood cells per high-power field.

A diagnostic paracentesis was performed in the right gutter using a No. 18 needle and 50 c.c. syringe. The paracentesis was performed in the right lower quadrant 4 cm. medial from the superior iliac spine. The bladder was first evacuated by catheterization. The paracentesis produced 3 L. of a thin, smoky fluid. Immediately after withdrawal of this fluid the patient became much more comfortable, the abdomen became softer instantaneously, and there was marked subjective relief of pain. The fluid had a uriniferous odor and had a pH of 7.5. It contained 100 red blood cells per high-power field and 5 to 10 spermatozoa per high-power field. After the finding of the spermatozoa in the paracentesis fluid, the patient was again immediately catheterized to determine the character of the bladder urine. The bladder urine was yellow in color and had a pH of 4.5. The working diagnosis was now changed to intra-abdominal perforation of a large bladder diverticulum with a ball-valve type of opening. The patient was placed on constant drainage. He was now completely asymptomatic, and the abdominal findings had disappeared. The vital signs remained stable, as did the white blood cell count throughout the first hospital day.

The morning of the second hospital day the patient was still asymptomatic and an intravenous pyelogram revealed a normal upper urinary tract and bladder. There was no evidence of perforation of the bladder or of diverticulum of the bladder. A cystogram was performed by filling the bladder with sodium iodide through a urethral catheter. During the time the cystogram was being taken the patient complained of no pain in the abdomen and there was no change in the abdominal findings. Not all the sodium iodide that was placed into the bladder returned through the catheter. The cystogram revealed a smoothly outlined normal bladder with a saccular pouch formation behind it that was interpreted as being a large diverticulum or possibly an intraperitoneal rupture of the bladder. The patient continued to be asymptomatic and the abdominal findings were negative, and although the possibility of an intra-abdominal rupture of the urinary bladder was considered, the abdominal findings following the paracentesis did not correlate with this diagnosis. It was decided to observe the patient further in order to establish a more positive diagnosis.

The following day the patient had a cystoscopic examination and another cystogram, and a definite diagnosis of intraperitoneal rupture of the bladder was made. On the posterior wall of the bladder there was a small hole, the edges of which were normal and did not seem inflamed. The cystogram definitely revealed an intraperitoneal rupture of the bladder. During the cystoscopy the patient had no discomfort and there was no change in the abdominal findings. All the fluid that was introduced into the bladder, however, did not return. The patient was immediately prepared for surgery and an exploratory laparotomy revealed a normal urinary bladder without signs of inflammation or tumor. There was no bladder neck obstruction. There was a small opening in the posterior aspect of the dome of the bladder immediately above the trigone that connected with the intraperitoneal cavity. The area around the pin-point opening was slightly injected. Tissue taken from this area for biopsy was reported as normal bladder tissue with some hemorrhage in it. Although the intraperitoneal cavity contained some free fluid, the abdomen was remarkably free of any signs of inflammation. The area of rupture was sutured and the patient was placed on cystotomy and urethral drainage. The patient was treated with penicillin and streptomycin postoperatively. His course after surgery was entirely benign. The nonprotein nitrogen returned rapidly to normal, and the patient's urine became free of red blood cells. Evaluation of the patient's syphilitic state revealed a negative serum Hinton serologic test, but the cerebrospinal fluid serology was positive with a paretic colloidal gold curve. On the nineteenth postoperative day the patient had a repeat cystogram and cystometry study, which were both normal.

DISCUSSION

This represents a case of spontaneous rupture of a normal urinary bladder. Although spontaneous rupture of the urinary bladder associated with tumors, infections, or obstruction is rare, the occurrence of rupture in a normal bladder is rarer still, and without explanation.

It is postulated that this patient's bladder had been perforated intraperitoneally for sixteen hours before the paracentesis was performed and he was placed on constant drainage. This duration of the perforation was long enough for the patient to dialyze his own urine to a neutral pH and to produce a state of acute uremia. Although the bladder had been perforated for this protracted period, the patient's vital signs were normal and the abdomen was free of any signs of peritonitis at the time of operation. Immediately upon evacuation of the abdominal fluid on the night of admission, the patient's abdominal pain and rigidity disappeared.

The high mortality rate reported in the literature is due to (1) the preponderance of cases in the preantibiotic era and (2) the fact that the correct diagnosis was not made in many cases. It was fortuitous in this case that the patient's urine was sterile despite the lack of antibiotic therapy preoperatively. Cultures of the urine and the paracentesis fluid were negative.

Diagnosis and therapy in this case were delayed, paradoxically, not because the correct entity was not considered but because the patient's good clinical condition did not correlate with the diagnosis of intraperitoneal rupture of the urinary bladder. Although the first cystogram indicated the possibility of an intraperitoneal rupture of the bladder, the patient had no abdominal pain or signs of peritoneal irritation while the cystogram was being taken. The diagnosis was finally established when the perforation was visualized cystoscopically.

Intensive investigation of the patient's home life and social background rules out the possibility of trauma as the etiology of the bladder rupture. Direct visualization and biopsy of the bladder rules out obstruction, tumor, or inflammation as the cause of the rupture. Despite the finding of a positive cerebrospinal fluid Hinton test, the only syphilitic neurological manifestations were fixed pupils. Cystoscopy and cystometry ruled out the possibility of a neurogenic bladder secondary to syphilis.

Most cases of spontaneous rupture of the urinary bladder are misdiagnosed as rupture of an intra-abdominal viscus. This was the primary diagnosis on this patient because of his past "ulcerlike" history. Evaluation of the patient's gastrointestinal tract did not demonstrate the cause of the gastrointestinal complaints.

It is interesting to speculate as to whether the patient's retching without the production of vomitus created increased abdominal pressure of such a magnitude as to cause a rupture of a full normal urinary bladder. A review of the literature did not reveal a case report of any rupture of the bladder secondary to increased abdominal pressure produced by the physiologic process of vomiting.

SUMMARY

1. A case report of spontaneous rupture of a normal urinary bladder is presented.

2. The possibility of the effect of increased abdominal pressure due to vomiting on a full urinary bladder as an etiological factor is postulated.

REFERENCES

1. Stone, R.: Spontaneous Rupture of the Urinary Bladder, Arch. Surg. **23**: 129-144, 1931.
2. Crastnopol, P., Artz, R., and Rosett, L.: Recurrent Spontaneous Rupture of the Urinary Bladder, Arch. Surg. **60**: 1093-1101, 1950.
3. Barnes, R. W., and Steele, A. A.: Spontaneous Intraperitoneal Rupture of the Urinary Bladder, J. A. M. A. **105**: 1758, 1935.

CONGENITAL EVENTRATION OF THE DIAPHRAGM IN INFANCY

Ernest E. Arnheim, M.D., New York, N. Y.

(From the Surgical and Pediatric Services, the Mount Sinai Hospital)

EVENTRATION of the diaphragm is defined as an abnormally high position of one leaf of the intact diaphragm. From a study of the etiology of this condition, Beck[1] concluded that all the evidence points to the fact that eventration of the diaphragm is a congenital lesion. The true incidence of congenital eventration of the diaphragm can be determined only by the routine use of roentgenologic studies of the newborn child. In this manner, Beck and Motsay[2] found that about 4 per cent of 2,500 newborn children had some diaphragmatic weakness, but in only three was the condition productive of severe respiratory difficulty.

The feasibility of surgical correction of congenital eventration of the diaphragm in infancy was first demonstrated by Bisgard[3] in 1947, who reported an operative cure in an infant 6 weeks old. Subsequently, State[4] Butsch and Leahy,[5] and Shellito and Bartlett[6] each reported an operative cure in an infant with this condition. In a group of fifteen infants requiring surgery for congenital anomalies of the diaphragm, Koop and Johnson[7] reported three cures in infants with eventration.

The following case is that of the youngest patient yet reported with congenital eventration of the diaphragm treated successfully by surgical repair.

CASE REPORT

History.—L. G., a white female infant aged 8 days, was admitted to the Mount Sinai Hospital on July 3, 1952. The patient had been born at full term, by forceps delivery. Pregnancy was uncomplicated except for some fever at three months. The family history was irrelevant. Dyspnea and cyanosis had been noted since the fifth day of life. The respiratory difficulty increased, requiring inhalations of oxygen.

Physical Examination.—The infant was well developed and well nourished, weighing 7 pounds, 4 ounces. The temperature was 99.6° F., the pulse rate 120, and the respiratory rate 58. Some dyspnea and cyanosis were noted. There were no abnormalities of the head, extremities, abdomen, or genitals. Examination of the chest revealed dullness to percussion and diminished breath sounds at the left base. The heart sounds were maximal in the right chest.

The hemoglobin content was 20 Gm.; the leukocyte count was 5,000, with polymorphonuclear leukocytes 51 per cent, lymphocytes 45 per cent, monocytes 2 per cent, and eosinophils 2 per cent. Urinalysis was normal.

Roentgenograms of the chest and abdomen revealed the left diaphragm to be elevated to the level of the third rib posteriorly; loops of colon filled with radiopaque material were noted in the left chest below the level of the diaphragm (barium had been administered prior to admission); the heart was markedly displaced to the right side (Fig. 1). Fluoroscopic examination revealed slight respiratory motion of the left diaphragm.

Operation was performed on the day of admission. Under ether anesthesia, a left oblique subcostal incision was made. The stomach and loops of small and large intestine

Received for publication, Sept. 8, 1953.

were visible in the abdomen. The left lobe of the liver, the spleen, and the splenic flexure of the colon were located in the thorax. The left leaf of the diaphragm was high in the chest, and was represented by a thin translucent membrane, through which the pericardium and the left lower lobe of the lung were visible. The anterior edge of the diaphragm at its attachment to the chest wall showed a thin cuff of muscle. There were no muscular components in the remainder of the diaphragm, which continued as a thin membrane to its attachments to the lateral costal margin and the crura. The esophageal hiatus was visualized, and presented no abnormalities.

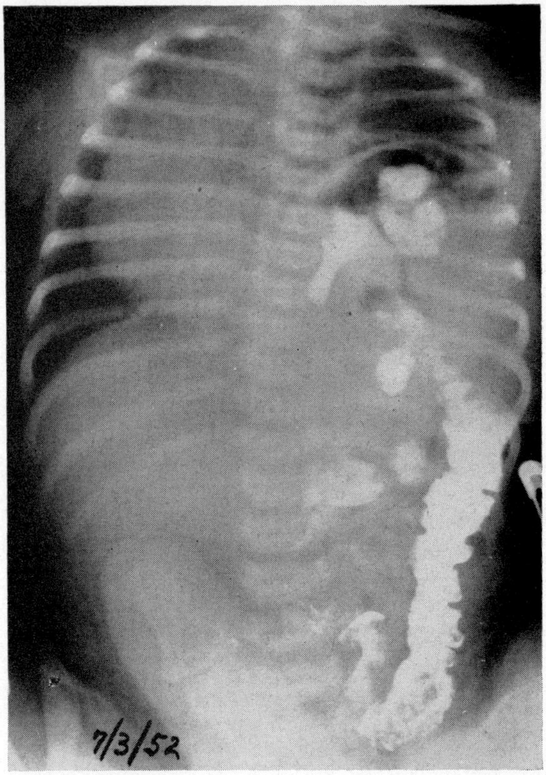

Fig. 1.—Roentgenogram of the chest and abdomen showing elevation of the left diaphragm, barium-filled splenic flexure of the colon beneath it, and displacement of the heart to the right side.

The left lobe of the liver, the spleen, and the splenic flexure of the colon were mobilized and brought down to the level of the abdominal wound. Babcock forceps were applied to the atrophic diaphragm, which was withdrawn from the chest into the abdomen The diaphragm was reconstructed by using plication mattress sutures of silk applied so as to bring various layers of the diaphragm in approximation with each other, and at the same time lowering the position of the diaphragm. The margin of the diaphragm was then sutured to the thoracic wall and renal fascia. The abdominal wall was closed with sutures of fine steel wire.

Pathologic Report.—A specimen of diaphragm was composed mainly of fibrous tissue covered on both surfaces by mesothelial cells.

Course.—An intravenous infusion of 5 per cent dextrose in saline solution and 100 c.c. of citrated blood was given during the operation. The infant was placed in an oxygen

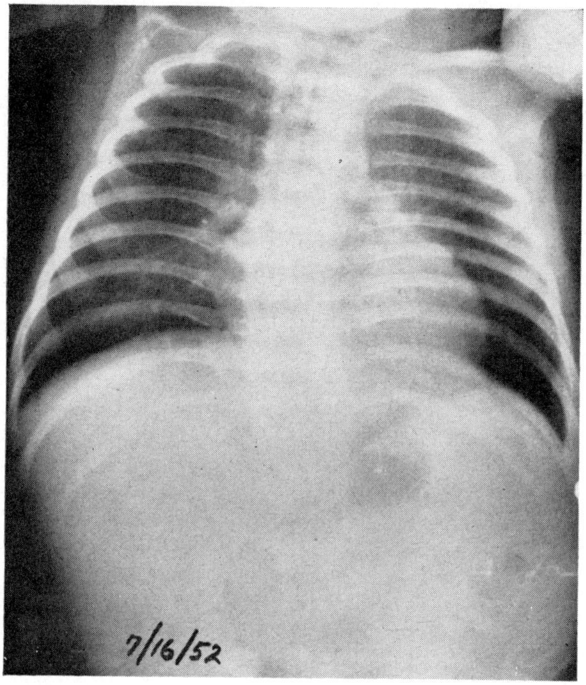

Fig. 2.—Roentgenogram of the chest taken thirteen days after the operation showing complete aeration of the lungs, and normal position of the diaphragm and heart.

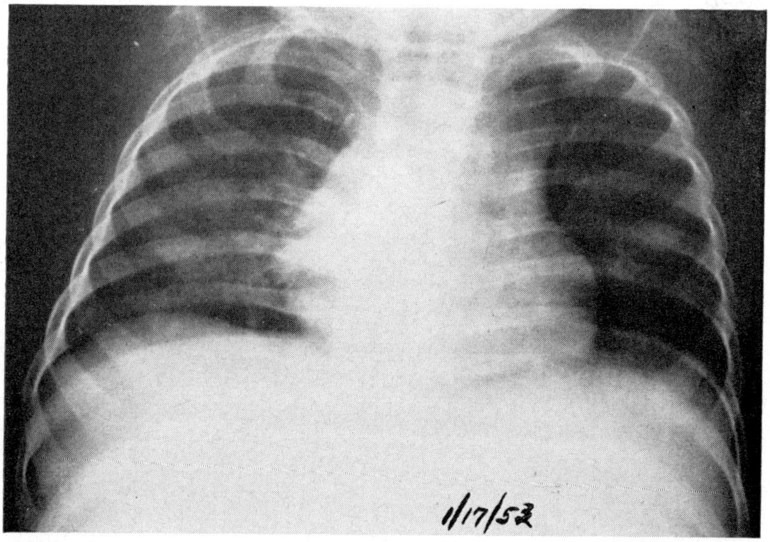

Fig. 3.—Roentgenogram of the chest taken six months after the operation, showing normal appearance of the diaphragm, heart, and lungs.

cubicle, the indwelling Levin tube was attached to a suction apparatus, parenteral fluids were continued, and penicillin was started.

The temperature remained normal throughout the postoperative course. Upon returning from the operating room the pulse was of good quality and the respiratory rate 50. There was no respiratory distress or cyanosis. Examination of the chest revealed slight dullness on percussion and diminished breath sounds in the lower part of the left side. The heart was in its normal position. During the first postoperative day, feedings were well tolerated, and there were normal bowel movements. Gastric siphonage and administration of intravenous fluids and oxygen were discontinued. Examination of the chest revealed no abnormalities on the second day. A roentgenogram of the chest, on the fifth day, showed good aeration of the lungs, a small effusion in the left costophrenic sinus, and normal position of the diaphragm and heart. Fluoroscopic examination revealed slightly diminished excursion of the left leaf of the diaphragm. The wound healed by primary union. Penicillin was discontinued on the seventh day; a total of 2.4 million units had been administered. A roentgenogram of the chest, on the thirteenth day, showed no abnormalities (Fig. 2). The infant was discharged in excellent condition on the fourteenth postoperative day, weighing 7 pounds, 9 ounces.

At follow-up examination six months after operation, the weight was 15 pounds and the height twenty-six inches. There were no complaints, and no abnormalities were noted on physical examination. A roentgenogram of the chest revealed normal position of both sides of the diaphragm; the heart and lungs appeared normal (Fig. 3). Fluoroscopic examination of the chest showed slightly diminished excursion of the left side of the diaphragm. Subsequent examination, one year after operation, revealed continued growth and development, the weight being 23 pounds, 4 ounces and the height thirty-two inches. A roentgenogram of the chest was normal.

DISCUSSION

The surgical management of congenital eventration of the diaphragm in infancy has rarely been the subject of published reports (seven cases in the literature[3-7]). Experience with one case prompted a review of the literature, and an analysis of these cases will be presented.

The age of the patients at operation varied from 8 days to 13 months as follows: 8 to 9 days in two, 6 weeks to 5 months in five, and 13 months in one.

There were six boys and two girls.

The symptoms of congenital eventration of the diaphragm in infancy were mainly respiratory, with varying degrees of dyspnea and cyanosis. These were either constantly present or made their appearance only when the respiratory reserve was needed, as during crying, respiratory infections, or fever from other causes. When symptoms continued beyond the newborn period, difficult nursing and poor weight gain were noted.

On examination of the chest there were dullness or tympany on percussion and diminished or absent breath sounds at the base of the chest posteriorly on the affected side, depending on the organs immediately under the diaphragm. Bowel sounds were heard in the chest in one infant in whom loops of intestine were in the thorax on the side of the eventration. Increased inspiratory divergence of the costal margin from the midline due to the unopposed action of the intercostal muscles (Hoover's sign) was noted in one infant. The signs of displacement of the heart to the opposite side were present.

The signs and symptoms of congenital eventration and hernia of the diaphragm may be exactly alike, although usually not so severe in eventration as in diaphragmatic hernia. The roentgenologic and fluoroscopic examinations furnish the only means of differentiation, but most often the differential diagnosis is established at operation. The roentgenologic finding of a high position of the diaphragm presenting as an unbroken curved convex line from the lateral wall of the chest to the mediastinum, with the abdominal contents beneath, is usually diagnostic of eventration. In congenital diaphragmatic hernia, the diaphragm is difficult to outline, and the portion that is visible is not elevated. The irregularity in density in the thorax on the affected side, the pattern of which suggests gas-filled loops of intestine, and the displacement of the heart and mediastinum to the contralateral side are noted in both congenital eventration and hernia of the diaphragm.

Paralysis of the diaphragm in the newborn child, producing respiratory difficulty due to phrenic nerve injury, may simulate congenital eventration of that organ (Schifrin[8]). This condition may or may not be associated with brachial plexus paralysis. Well-defined paradoxic movement of the elevated diaphragm on fluoroscopic examination of the chest is indicative of a paralysis of the phrenic nerve. The movement of the diaphragm is usually diminished in congenital eventration.

As in congenital hernia of the diaphragm, congenital eventration of that structure is more common on the left side than on the right. In the eight infants treated by operation, five were on the left side and three on the right. The strength of the affected side of the diaphragm is considerably reduced, and the diaphragm is elevated by the intra-abdominal pressure. The result on the left side is elevation in varying combinations of the stomach, the splenic flexure of the colon, the small intestine, the spleen, and the left lobe of the liver, and on the right side, elevation of the right lobe of the liver. The intra-abdominal viscera in the thorax displace the heart and mediastinal structures to the opposite side.

It is difficult to explain the difference in the structure of the diaphragm in the eight infants with congenital eventration treated by operation. In the right-sided cases, the diaphragm, although high in position, seemed to be normally developed with muscular tissue, whereas in the left-sided cases the diaphragm appeared as a thin translucent membrane.

The treatment of congenital eventration of the diaphragm is determined by the severity of the symptoms. Prompt surgical treatment should be carried out if dyspnea and cyanosis are severe. This has become the accepted practice in congenital hernia of the diaphragm, with a resultant marked reduction in mortality, particularly in the newborn period. Before transportation to the operating room, inhalation of oxygen should be supplied through an incubator or cubicle, the stomach emptied through a Levin tube, and the necessary fluids administered through a cut-down intravenous infusion in an ankle vein. The latter is utilized for transfusion of blood during operation.

Positive pressure anesthesia is helpful and is given through a small closed system using a tightly fitting face mask.

In the eight infants treated surgically, the operative technique consisted essentially in pulling the diaphragm down to the level of the margin of the diaphragmatic attachments, with or without excision of a portion of the diaphragm, and plication of the diaphragm with superimposed rows of interrupted mattress sutures of silk. In one infant, a method of tenting the diaphragm caudadward was used. Following these procedures, the newly constructed diaphragm was fixed to the thoracic wall, crus of the diaphragm, and renal fascia. The operative approach was thoracic in four infants, abdominal in three, and thoracoabdominal in one.

There was no operative mortality, and cure of the condition was effected in the recorded instances of congenital eventration of the diaphragm in infants treated surgically.

SUMMARY

The pathologic and clinical features, diagnosis, and treatment of congenital eventration of the diaphragm in infancy are reviewed.

An operative cure of congenital eventration of the diaphragm in an 8-day-old infant, the youngest recorded patient, is reported.

REFERENCES

1. Beck, W. C.: Etiologic Significance of Eventration of the Diaphragm, Arch. Surg. **60**: 1154, 1950.
2. Beck, W. C., and Motsay, D. S.: Eventration of the Diaphragm, Arch. Surg. **65**: 557, 1952.
3. Bisgard, J. D.: Congenital Eventration of the Diaphragm, J. Thoracic Surg. **16**: 484, 1947.
4. State, D.: The Surgical Correction of Congenital Eventration of the Diaphragm in Infancy, SURGERY **25**: 461, 1949.
5. Butsch, W. L., and Leahy, L. J.: A Technique for the Surgical Treatment of Congenital Eventration of the Diaphragm in Infancy, J. Thoracic Surg. **20**: 968, 1950.
6. Shellito, J. G., and Bartlett, W. C.: Surgical Correction of Congenital Eventration of the Diaphragm, Am. Surgeon **17**: 898, 1951.
7. Koop, C. E., and Johnson, J.: Transthoracic Repair of Ditphragmatic Hernia in Infants, Ann. Surg. **136**: 1007, 1952.
8. Schifrin, N.: Unilateral Paralysis of the Diaphragm in the Newborn Infant Due to Phrenic Nerve Injury With and Without Associated Brachial Palsy, Pediatrics **9**: 69, 1952.

BRONCHIOGENIC CYST ASSOCIATED WITH AN ANOMALOUS PULMONARY ARTERY ARISING FROM THE THORACIC AORTA

SYDNEY BRESSLER, M.D., AND DAVID WIENER, M.D., NEW YORK, N. Y.

(From Thoracic Surgical Service, Metropolitan Hospital)

ANOMALOUS pulmonary arteries were first described by Huber[1] in 1777. Until the relatively recent advent of pulmonary surgery, these aberrant vessels were only post-mortem curiosities. Up to the present time, there have been forty-two cases of an aberrant artery to the lower lobe of the lung reported in the literaure.[2, 3] The first report was made by Harris[4] in 1940; since then, Bruer, Clagett, and MacDonald,[5] Finley and Maier,[6] Tosatti and Gravel,[7] and Pryce, Sellors, and Blair[8] have all reported cases with their clinical summaries.

In 1946, Pryce and associates[8] published a comprehensive description of this congenital lung anomaly which was described as consisting of two components: part 1, the maldevelopment of a portion of the bronchial tree, and part 2, the anomalous artery from the aorta to the affected portion of the lung.

The anomaly may affect either of the lower lobes but has been found more frequently on the left, usually involving the posteromedial portion of this lobe.

Pryce's[8] hypothesis concerning this anomaly is quoted as follows: "A persistent artery from the dorsal aorta, instead of the ventral aorta, to the pulmonary anlage, attaches itself to one of the bulbous growing tips of the budding bronchi and then enters into competition with the developing pulmonary artery. As the embryo grows and straightens, and as the lung shifts to a more cephalad position, the captive bulb is gradually torn away and isolated (sequestered) producing rests from which cysts may develop. The anomalous artery usually has many of the physical characteristics of a pulmonary artery and these render it a relatively fragile vessel to carry blood at a systemic pressure."

CASE REPORT

R. C., a Negro boy, aged 6 years, was admitted to the Metropolitan Hospital on Nov. 28, 1952, for the repair of an umbilical hernia.

The mother furnished the past history that the child had been admitted to another hospital at 6 months of age for "difficulty in breathing" of four months' duration. A report from this hospital showed that the infant had an unexplained atelectasis of the left upper lobe which cleared after six weeks of hospitalization. A definite etiological diagnosis was not made, but there was complete re-expansion of the lung prior to discharge.

The physical examination at Metropolitan Hospital was negative except for a large, easily reducible umbilical hernia and several small, hard, discrete submaxillary, axillary, and inguinal lymph nodes. The hemogram revealed a hemoglobin of 11.8 Gm., 4,670,000 red blood cells, and 7,900 leukocytes with a normal differential count. Urinalysis and sedimentation rate were normal. On a routine roentgenogram of the chest (Fig. 1), a round

Received for publication, Sept. 17, 1953.

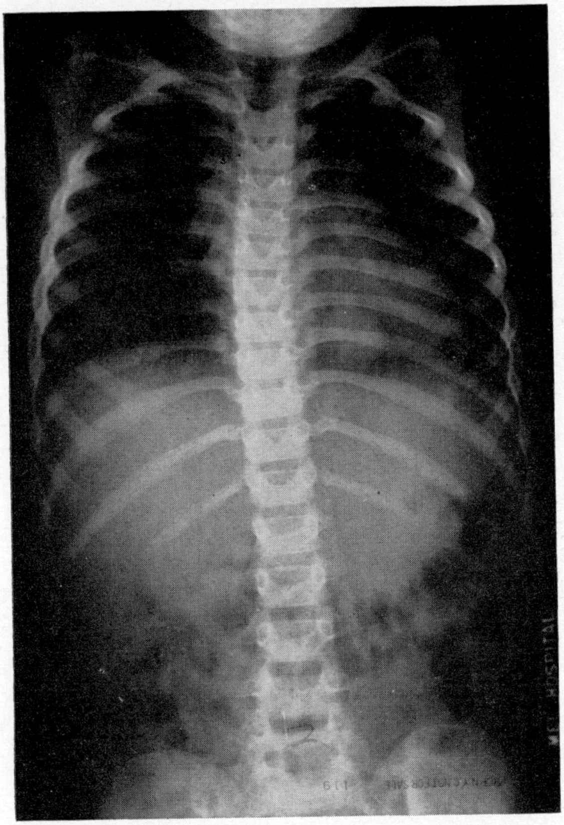

Fig. 1.—A rounded mass is visualized at the level of the left ninth rib in the paravertebral region.

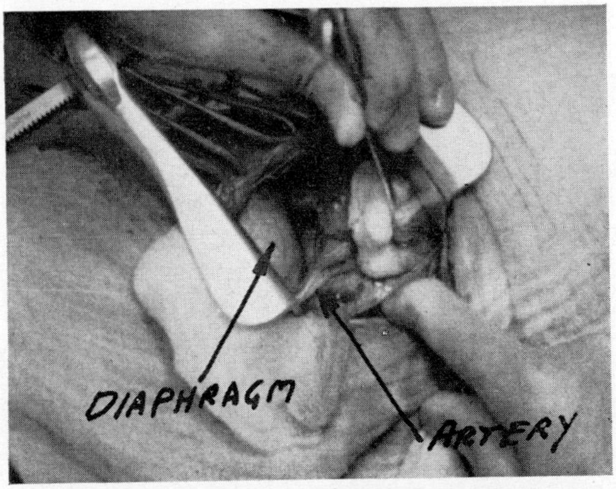

Fig. 2.—Operative exposure demonstrating the anomalous artery entering the lung.

Fig. 3.

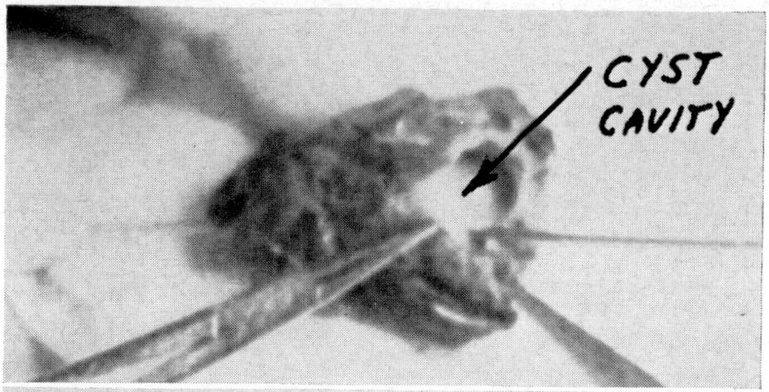

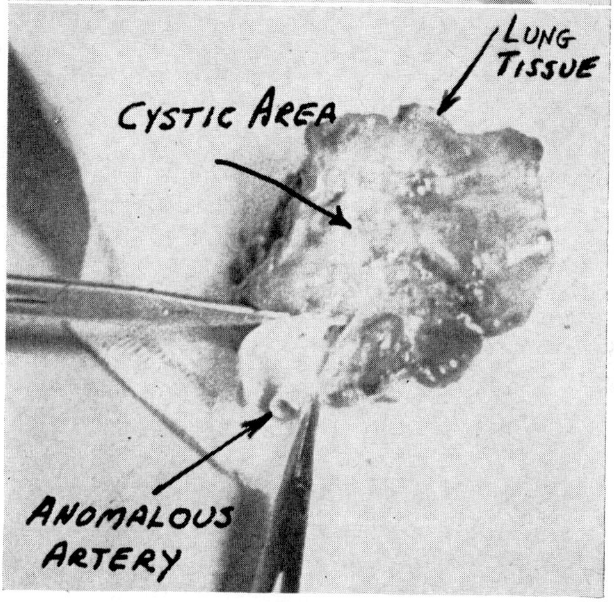

Fig. 4.

Fig. 3.—The operative specimen opened, demonstrating the cystic cavity.
Fig. 4.—Another view of the operative specimen, demonstrating the anomalous artery.

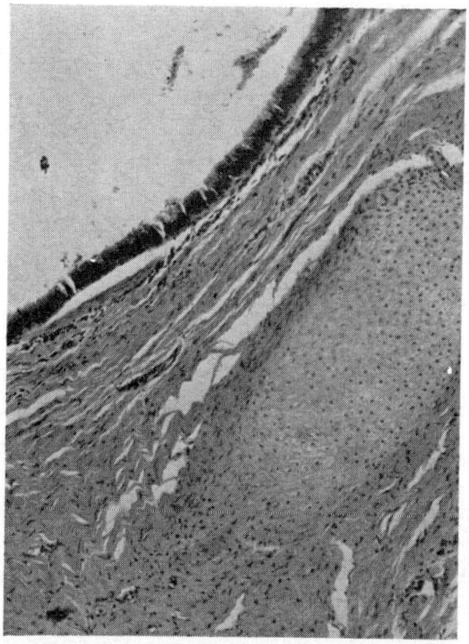

Fig. 5.—A photomicrograph showing a section of the cyst wall lined by ciliated columnar epithelium, fibrous tissue, and cartilage.

"quarter-sized" dense shadow was seen in the left lower lung field at the level of the ninth posterior rib. Lateral and oblique films showed that the shadow was posterior.

Because of this incidental finding of a lesion in the left chest, surgery for the hernia was postponed. The diagnosis of a posterior mediastinal tumor, probably neurogenic in origin, was considered. Operation for excision of this tumor was advised because of the known malignant potentiality of neurogenic tumors.[9]

Operation was performed on Dec. 29, 1952, under endotracheal anesthesia. Because of the preoperative diagnosis of posterior mediastinal tumor, an extrapleural approach was used. An oblique incision was made over the ninth rib, and a short posterior segment of this rib was removed subperiosteally. Since no tumor mass was found in the posterior mediastinum, the incision was lengthened, a longer segment of the ninth rib was removed, and the pleural cavity was entered through this rib bed. The posterior aspect of the left lower lobe was found adherent to the chest wall by thin bands of adhesions. These were separated, and an artery, approximately 6 mm. in diameter, was found arising from the anterior side of the aorta just above the diaphragm (Fig. 2). This artery coursed to the lung and entered the lower lobe on the lateral aspect of the posterior basal segment. The mass which had produced the abnormal x-ray shadow was found in this portion of the lung. It was rounded, walnut-sized, and rubbery in consistency. The anomalous artery was temporarily occluded, and as it produced no untoward symptoms, it was ligated and divided. A wedge resection of the portion of lung containing the tumor was then performed. On sectioning of the specimen, it was found to consist of a cyst containing thick, creamy, odorless material. Culture of this material later proved sterile.

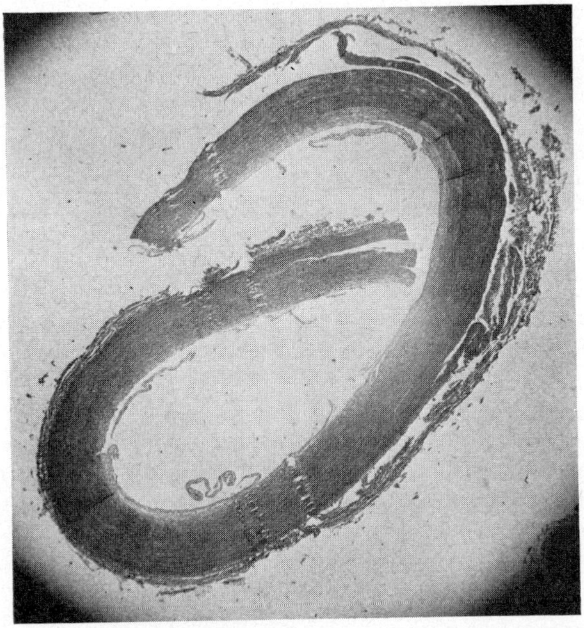

Fig. 6.—The anomalous artery in cross section.

The postoperative course was uneventful except for gastric distention, which was relieved by suction. There was complete re-expansion of the lung. The underwater catheter drain was removed in twenty-four hours. The incision healed solidly. The patient was discharged after fifteen days with instructions to return one month later for repair of the umbilical hernia.

The pathologic report was as follows: On gross examination the specimen was a section of lung tissue which measured 6.5 by 5 by 3 cm., containing in its center a cystic area 2 cm. in diameter (Fig. 3). This was lined by a smooth grayish white membrane containing odorless inspissated material. Surrounding the cyst there were several large blood vessels which were tributaries of an artery 6 mm. in diameter which entered the parenchyma at one end of the specimen (Fig. 4).

Microscopic examination showed the cyst to be lined by columnar ciliated epithelium of respiratory type (Fig. 5). The cystic cavity was surrounded by fairly dense fibrous tissue. Cartilage was also present. The vessel showed all the coats of a large-sized artery (Fig. 6).

SUMMARY

A case of bronchiogenic cyst associated with an anomalous artery has been presented. The hypothesis for the origin of this anomaly is quoted from Pryce.[8] This case differs from Pryce's description in that the anomalous artery actually had the characteristics of a systemic rather than those of a pulmonary vessel. It also differs from all of the case reports reviewed[2-8, 10] in that this patient had no respiratory symptoms, except in infancy, whereas the cases from the literature all refer to the symptomatology of chronic cough, sputum, frank pus, and hemoptysis.

REFERENCES

1. Huber, J. J., quoted by McCotter, R. E.: On the Occurrence of Pulmonary Arteries Arising From the Thoracic Aorta, Anat. Rec. **4:** 291-297, 1910.
2. Colee, F. H., Alley, F. H., and Jones, R. S.: Aberrant Systemic Arteries to the Lower Lung, Surg., Gynec. & Obst. **93:** 589-596, 1951.
3. King, J. C., and Harris, L. C., Jr.: Congenital Lung Cyst, J. A. M. A. **108:** 274, 1937.
4. Harris, H. A., and Ivor, L.: Anomalies of the Lung With Special Reference to the Dangers of the Abnormal Vessels in Lobectomy, J. Thoracic Surg. **9:** 666-671, 1940.
5. Bruer, A., Clagett, O. T., and MacDonald, J. R.: Anomalous Arteries to the Lung Associated With Congenital Pulmonary Abnormalities, J. Thoracic Surg. **19:** 957-972, 1950.
6. Finley, C. W., and Maier, H. C.: Anomalies of the Pulmonary Artery and Their Surgical Significance, SURGERY **29:** 604, 1951.
7. Tosatti, E., and Gravel, J. A.: Two Cases of Bronchiogenic Cyst Associated With Anomalous Pulmonary Arteries Arising From the Thoracic Aorta, Thorax **6:** 82-88, 1951.
8. Pryce, D. M., Sellors, T. H., and Blair, L. G.: Intralobar Sequestration of the Lung Associated With Abnormal Pulmonary Artery, Brit. J. Surg. **35:** 18-29, 1947.
9. Kent, E. M., Blades, B., Valle, A. R., and Graham, E. A.: Intrathoracic Neurogenic Tumors, J. Thoracic Surg. **13:** 116-161, 1944.
10. Case Records, New England J. Med. **243:** 383-387, 1950.

Editorial

A Note on Spinal Anesthesia and Its Relationship to a Larger Problem

THESE observations deal with a nonmedical limitation of spinal anesthesia and are concerned more with a principle underlying the practice of medicine as a whole than with spinal anesthesia. In one sense, my comments merely report a skirmish in a brush-filled hollow, but their implications relate to a larger and noisier battle now in progress.

At the moment I am not going to speak of the arguments between those who find spinal anesthesia useful and valuable and those who say it is akin to malpractice.

In this instance I can point to two items—and one seems to spring from the other—which are pertinent to the immediate subject: The first is an article written three years ago by the late Dr. Foster Kennedy and his associates.[1] In that article, which had wide coverage in the lay press, Dr. Kennedy, then near the end of a long and distinguished career in neurology, described twelve tragic cases of injury resulting from spinal anesthesia. Rebuttal to this was made:[2] ". . . to say that bad things can follow spinal anesthesia is to state the truth. What we all want to know is how often accidents occur (with spinal in comparison with other technics) . . . we are left in the dark as to how many spinal anesthesias were in the pool from which these 12 serious complications drained." It was pointed out that an equal number of serious neurological complications as a consequence of open-drop ether could be assembled.

Notwithstanding what seemed to me to be a fundamental defect in the Kennedy article (the failure to provide data on incidence of the accidents reported), it unquestionably had great influence. Some institutions promptly considered barring spinal anesthesia altogether. A recent extensive survey[3] of all the anesthesias in ten university hospitals scattered over the entire country, and made during a five-year period, demonstrated the surprising fact that spinal anesthesia accounts in these hospitals for less than 9 per cent of all anesthesias and is still declining in use. (Incidentally, in the same study, the death rate from spinal anesthesia appears to be low. It is impossible to consider this in direct comparison with other techniques, for the spinal technique is not generally used for difficult thoracic surgery, for example, which accounts for some of the bad news with other procedures.)

So much for the first point and the decline in use of spinal anesthesia. The second point is that insurance companies are, in some regions, refusing to protect physicians against damage suits when spinal anesthesia is employed. This brings us to the crux of these remarks: Are the techniques employed in the practice of medicine to be determined by competent physicians themselves, or are outside pressure groups going to do it? If spinal anesthesia is not useful in proportion to its dangers, it should be eliminated by those skilled in its use. (Many, including myself, believe it to be valuable and important for certain purposes.)

Not long ago, a judgment of $160,000 was awarded and collected in the case of a patient who had been injured by spinal anesthesia, although considerable recovery of function had occurred in that case. Clearly, no individual physician can face such a threat with equanimity. This financial hazard can be accepted only if the institutions involved assume liability in the case of suit, while the medical profession itself decides whether it will retain or reject the technique of spinal anesthesia. The alternative is to allow insurance companies to determine the nature of medical practice in this instance, and thus allow further encroachment on the freedom of the physician.

—*Henry K. Beecher*

REFERENCES

1. Kennedy, F., Effron, A. S., and Perry, G.: The Grave Spinal Cord Paralyses Caused by Spinal Anesthesia, Surg., Gynec. & Obst. **91**: 385, 1950.
2. Beecher, H. K.: Spinal Anesthesia (Correspondence), Surg., Gynec. & Obst. **92**: 256, 1951.
3. Beecher, H. K., and Todd, D. P.: A Study of the Deaths Associated With Anesthesia and Surgery. In press.

Recent Advances in Surgery

Conducted by Alfred Blalock, M.D.

CARCINOMA OF THE ESOPHAGUS: A NEW CONCEPT IN THERAPY

Sixty Collected Cases, Using the Polyethylene Tube; Report of Ten (Selected)

Edgar F. Berman, M.D., Baltimore, Md.

(From the Department of Surgery, Sinai Hospital)

IN BROAD perspective, the results of esophageal surgery for malignancy do not lead to undue optimism. In the past two decades, the progress which has been made in the attempted cure of this disease can be attributed primarily to the newer adjuvant measures generally applicable to surgery; that is, modern anesthesia, antibiotics, and multiple transfusions, and the now well-grounded basic principles of thoracic surgery.

Some of the reports of large series which have been in the literature recently have been extremely discouraging. Parker[1] and his associates have had 170 cases of cancer of the esophagus, of which 114 were inoperable. Of the fifty-six which were operable, only thirty were resectable. The operative mortality averaged 60 per cent, and only three patients were alive at ten months, with one living for three years. There have been no recent five-year cures reported at The Johns Hopkin's Hospital, according to Ravitch.[2] Sweet[3] reported 254 cases of carcinoma of the esophagus and cardia in a twelve-year period ending Jan. 1, 1951. The operative mortality in his hands was 24.3 per cent for midthoracic lesions. Of the total (107) of midthoracic patients operated on, only one survived five years. The number of five-year cures in the literature is relatively negligible.

A situation such as this calls for a thorough reappraisal of both disease and method. First, in the evaluation, two factors must be made clear; one is that carcinomas around the cardia and lower portion of the esophagus are in essence slow-growing adenocarcinomas, in contradistinction to malignancies above this point, which are extremely swiftly growing epidermoid carcinomas. Humphreys[4] deems this distinction necessary in any statistical analysis of longevity. Another factor which must be considered is that reports of large series usually come from medical centers with a high degree of specialization and experience with esophageal surgery. In reckoning mortality, it must be understood that every general surgeon does resect one or two cases of esophageal carcinoma each year, and from personal inquiry at smaller general hospitals, I find that the true mortality is well above the ghastly aforementioned figures.

Received for publication, Oct. 9, 1953.

We have reached our zenith in the techniques commonly used, but our results have not paralleled our technical facility.

Every portion of the esophagus has now been rendered available to surgical attack. The most popular method of maintaining continuity has been the esophagogastrostomy. Esophagojejunostomy and the antithoracic procedures have been almost generally abandoned for obvious reasons. The extent of the procedure of choice has grown to the point where the stomach may now be anastomosed to the esophagus in the neck. However, the rationality of this extensive procedure must be questioned, for the increase in extent of resection has been only in a vertical fashion. In a disease which seems to spread as rapidly laterally (both nodal and direct extension) as it does longitudinally, it is sheer delusion to suppose that our results will better with the increased length of esophagus resected. With a disease which frequently extends beyond its natural boundaries before symptoms occur, in a location which prohibits block or complete nodal dissection, it is extremely dubious that our present methods will better our present results.

It is highly improbable from the foregoing that the progress in this disease has been real. Concerning the postoperative course of the conventional procedure, the morbidity has been excessive. The number of leaks with empyema and fistulas are entirely too high for practicality. Esophagitis, ulcers, and strictures at the anastomotic site are not unusual before the final demise, because in this procedure the cardiac sphincter is obviated, with the anastomosis being constantly bathed in gastric juice. Obstructive recurrent malignancies at or near the anastomotic site are definite potential hazards. The vagotomized stomach in the chest predisposes to pulmonary complications.

In this disease, if most patients are to live only one year or two, one of the prime requisites of an operation should be a smooth posthospital course. However, even if the patient overcomes the hazard of morbid complication, he is usually still uncomfortable with the stomach in the chest. The quantity of food to be taken at each meal is restricted. There is usually postprandial dyspnea and palpitation. There is acid regurgitation with substernal burning and a frequent feeling of fullness in the chest.

With these facts before us, it can readily be seen that the present-day operative procedures have failed to prove themselves in any way in a trial period of over a decade and a half. The mortality is still tremendous, the longevity short, the morbidity excessive, and the comfort of the patient minimal. The procedure has taken on the aspect of a tour de force. However, any surgical tour de force for malignancy is valid only when a modicum of good is done or when the method by constant usage may lead to variations and embellishments to a procedure which will be in the realm of practicality as to figures and comfort. This has not been the case.

The procedure which we deem more rational for this disease, namely, the substitution of a plastic tube for the resected portion of the esophagus, is offered only in the light that the same extent of resection can be carried out with a greatly decreased operative mortality and morbidity, the same longevity, and advantages to the patient of comfort and normal eating. We feel, after a short collected experience comprising some sixty cases, that the "plastic esophagus" is the temporal answer to the question of procedure in malignancies of this organ. The following data substantiate our feelings.

Material and Experimental Work.—The polyethylene plastic is extremely tissue-compatible with negative water absorption, is nonporous, and easily sterilized. The tubes are unchanged when buried in human tissue. There is no foreign body reaction. They conduct heat poorly, and durability under ordinary body conditions has been very satisfactory. The tube may be left in permanently. Substituting this tube (Fig. 1) by the simple technique which I previously described for resected portions of esophagus has shown that a new fibrous sheath forms, in both animals and human beings, around the tube, which eventually (sixty to ninety days) becomes epithelized, giving a new esophagus without musculature.[5-7] This lack of musculature does not impede the flow of ingested material, as will be shown in Case 1 (previously reported), where the tube was removed by esophagoscopy after one year. Extracting the tube is not advised in cases of malignancy.

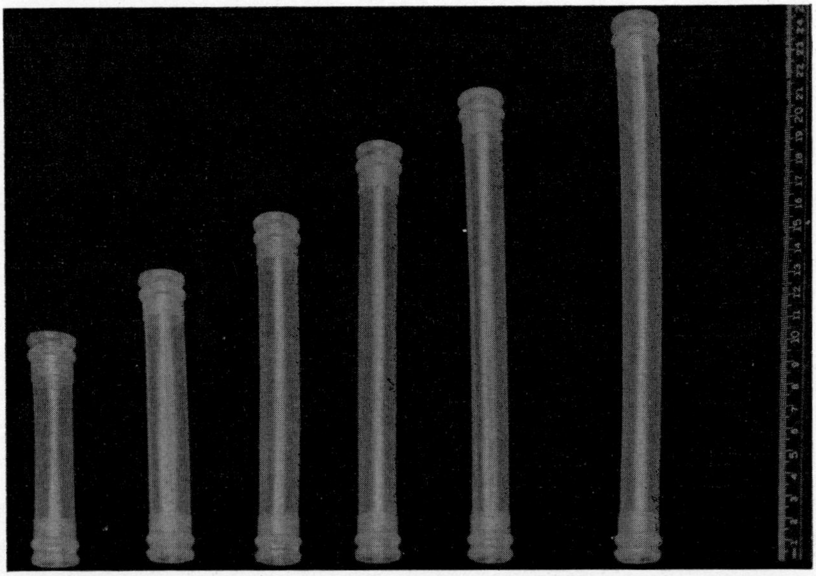

Fig. 1.—The set of six polyethylene tubes used, measuring from four to nine inches in length. After resection of the lesion, the tube is approximated for length, making sure that the full cuff is covered with esophagus. Every size should be available at each procedure.

Technique (Fig. 2).—The simplicity of this procedure allows any surgeon familiar with the thorax to perform the operation without undue risk. This is an extremely important consideration. The right chest alone is utilized for the approach, with no disturbance of the diaphragm or other intra-abdominal structures. It is unnecessary to extend the incision into the abdomen, for if there is intra-abdominal extension, the procedure is simply palliative. The aorta does not impede. There are no time-consuming, minute anastomoses necessary. There is no question of suture-line tensions. As much of the esophagus as is necessary (from the cervical region to the stomach) (Cases 1, 2, 3, and 4) may be resected, just substituting a longer tube. No case is inoperable, for when extension of the tumor has occurred, the primary growth may be removed, leaving some malignancy on the surrounding vital structures, but replacing the defect with a tube. The operating time for these elderly malnourished patients is approximately one and one-half to two hours. This procedure is not carried out with palliative intent, and should be as curative as any other procedure for the disease. A newer,* safer, and simple technique with which we are working will be presented soon as an alternate to the original one.

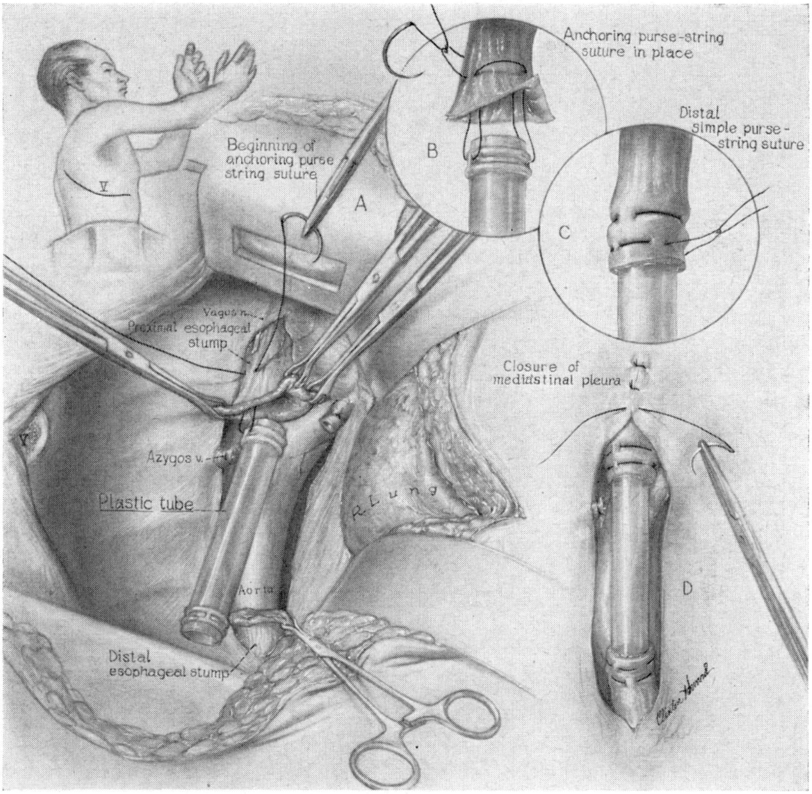

Fig. 2.

Mortality.—In the collected sixty cases, there has been less than 10 per cent operative mortality. All cases which I handled are deemed operable. There were five deaths. There is no shocking devascularization and mobilization of the stomach. There is no great blood replacement necessary with concomitant disturbances in hemodynamics. The deaths that we have had within the first four weeks postoperatively have been from coronary thrombosis, massive pleural effusion, atelectasis, cerebral hemorrhage, and one empyema.

*By August, 1953, only the newer tubes will be on the market. These will be distributed by the Murray-Baumgartner Surgical Instrument Co., 5 West Chase Street, Baltimore, Md.

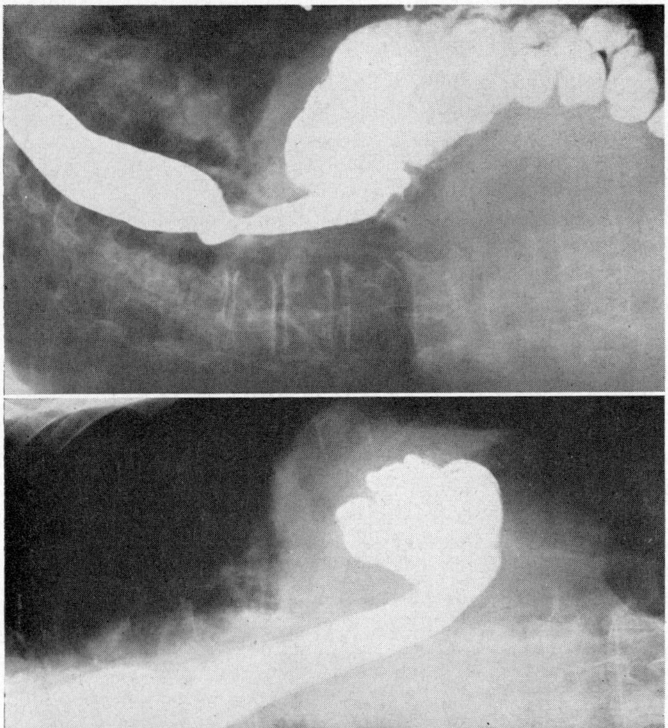

A. B. C.

Fig. 3 (Case 1).—*A*, Preoperative barium swallow showing a defect in the lower end of the esophagus measuring 3 cm. in length. *B*, Six months postoperatively the continuity of the barium flowing through the tube and stomach is shown. *C*, Twelve months postoperatively barium swallow shows the ability of the new esophagus formed around the plastic tube after the tube had been removed by esophagoscopy.

Morbidity.—It is inconceivable that any untoward pulmonary complications would be expected when the mediastinum is closed tightly over this plastic prosthesis, which is of the same diameter as the normal esophagus. In the sixty cases reported, there have been three leaks which have closed within one week, and one empyema which was fatal. There were two cases of loculated fluid collections cured by antibiotics and aspiration. There have been no mediastinal abscesses. One tube slipped into the stomach postoperatively and was retrieved.

Longevity and Comfort.—We do not expect these patients to live any longer than the average patient treated by other methods. Having handled these cases for the past two and one-half years, our longest survival has been twenty months, with maximum comfort. These have been no symptoms of acid regurgitation, stricture, or esophageal ulceration. Three patients have died of metastases. At post-mortem, two showed the tube entirely encased by epithelized fibrous tissue; one was encased in tumor tissue with no obstruction. Every patient has eaten normal meals perfectly well and comfortably until his demise.

CASE REPORTS

CASE 1.—I have previously reported this case in detail. A. G., aged 75 years, was admitted with carcinoma of the lower end of the esophagus, and had a resection of the lower 6 cm. of the esophagus and the uppermost portion of the stomach. A plastic tube, 12 cm. in length, was inserted. At operation, lymph node metastasis was present. The patient ate comfortably and lived for thirteen months. One month before his demise, the tube was extracted with an esophagoscope, and he had no difficulty in eating after this. A post-mortem was not obtained. The cause of death was generalized metastases (Fig. 3).

CASE 2.—E. C., aged 46 years, was admitted to the hospital with a complaint of dysphagia and regurgitation, with substernal burning for six months. On admission, the patient had lost thirty pounds in weight. He complained of pain in the right elbow, which later turned out to be a metastatic lesion from the esophagus. X-ray film and biopsy confirmed the diagnosis of squamous cell carcinoma of the esophagus. At operation, a lesion, approximately 6 cm. in length, was found with lymph node metastasis. The lower end of the esophagus and the cardia of the stomach were resected, pulling the stomach up through the hiatus, and a six-inch plastic tube was inserted. Postoperatively, the patient had a somewhat stormy course for a few days with a left lower lobe pneumonia, but was discharged one month postoperatively, eating practically a normal diet. He went back to work two months postoperatively. The patient had no complaints, but gradually lost weight and died of generalized metastases, corroborated by post-mortem thirteen months postoperatively. Post-mortem revealed the plastic tube lying loose but snug within an entirely new epithelial sheath (Fig. 4).

Comment.—An interesting point in this case was symptomatic evidence of metastasis of the right elbow at the time of the original symptoms.

CASE 3.—J. P., aged 65 years, was admitted to the hospital with a history of dysphagia of one year's duration and forty-pound weight loss. X-ray film revealed a lesion in the mid-portion of the esophagus, confirmed by biopsy. At operation, a 7 cm. mass tightly adherent to the aorta and right main-stem bronchus was resected with accompanying lymph nodes. A seven-inch plastic tube was inserted. This patient's convalescence was extremely smooth, and he was discharged in two and one-half weeks. He is still living and well, and eating perfectly normally (Fig. 5).

A. B.

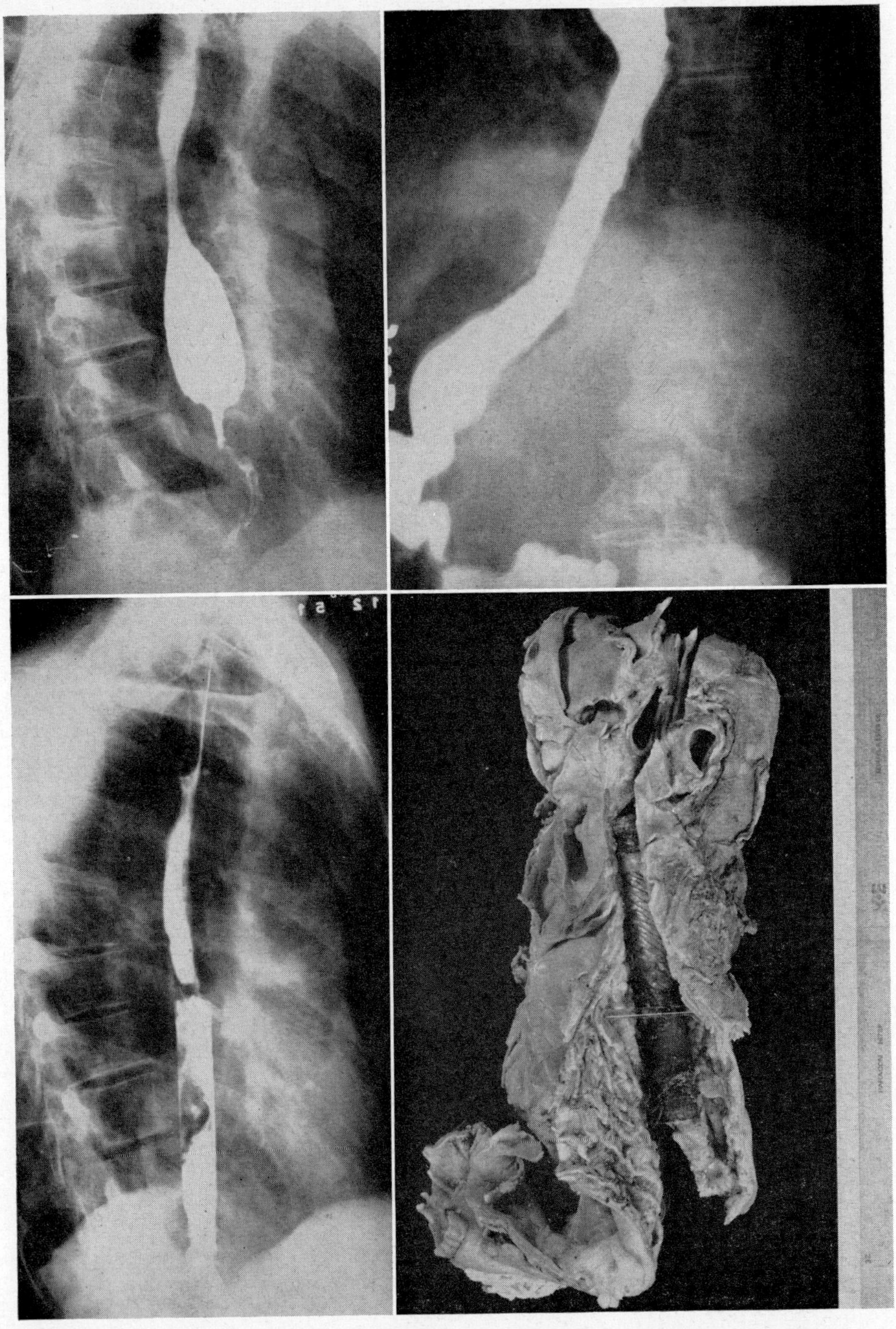

C. D.

Fig. 4 (Case 2).—*A,* The lesion is shown at the lower end of the esophagus. *B,* Fourteen days postoperatively, barium is seen going through the proximal esophagus, the tube, and into the stomach. *C,* Barium swallow, seven months postoperatively. *D,* At post-mortem ten months postoperatively, the tube is seen completely surrounded by fibrous tissue; however, there was no obstruction.

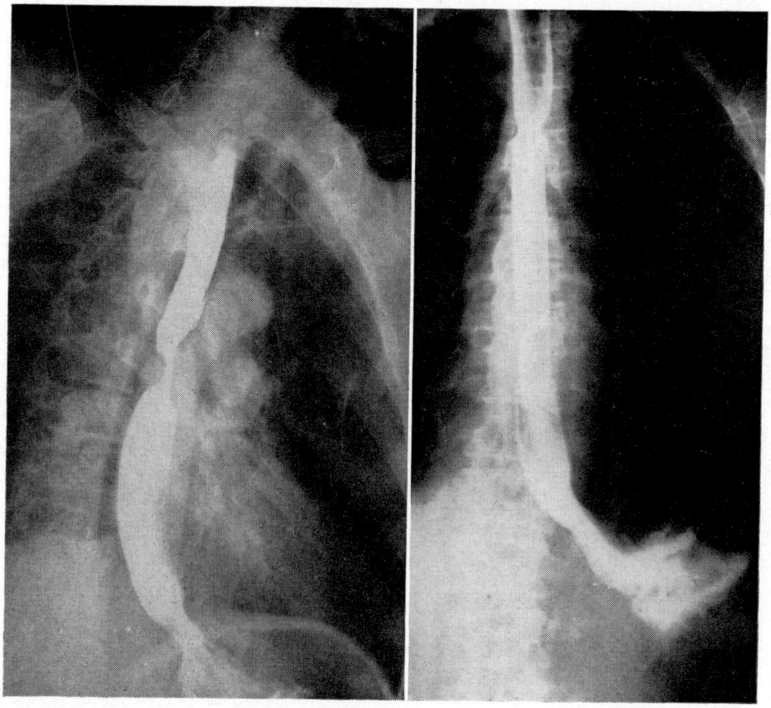

A. B.

Fig. 5 (Case 3).—*A,* The malignant obstruction in the mid-esophagus. *B,* The polyethylene tube is shown in place three weeks after resection.

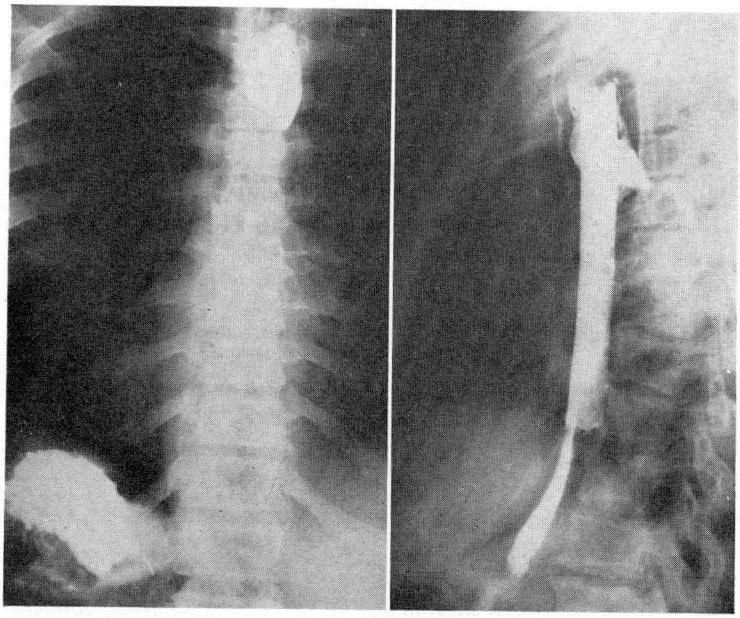

A. B.

Fig. 6 (Case 4).—*A,* A high malignant obstruction is seen in the esophagus. *B,* The barium-filled tube is shown with some of the opaque material around the tube but within the new sheath.

Case 4.—R. S., aged 49 years, was admitted with dysphagia and "food sticking in his throat" with no relief without vomiting. Esophagoscopy showed a squamous cell carcinoma in the upper middle third of the esophagus. At operation, the malignancy involved the left main-stem bronchus, some of which was left attached. A seven-inch plastic tube was inserted. The patient was discharged from the hospital in fifteen days with an excellent follow-up five months postoperatively (Fig. 6).

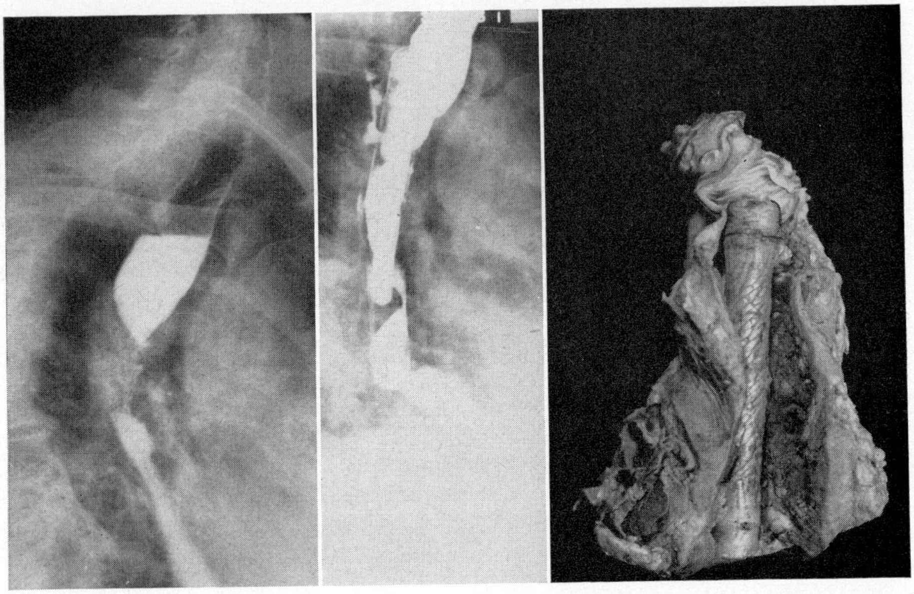

A. B. C.

Fig. 7 (Case 5).—*A*, Roentgenogram revealing an obstructive lesion in the upper one-third of the thoracic esophagus in a patient with an extreme dorsal kyphosis. *B*, Postoperative barium swallow shows the tube conforming to the curvature of the spine with barium passing through. *C*, Seven months postoperatively post-mortem shows the tube completely surrounded by fibrous tissue.

Case 5.—C. W., a 66-year-old physician, was admitted with a history of dysphagia for four months following a total laryngectomy for carcinoma. Barium swallow and biopsy revealed a squamous cell carcinoma of the middle third of the esophagus. The patient had an extreme dorsal kyphosis. At operation, a carcinoma, measuring 5 cm. and adherent to both the carina and aorta, was found with regional metastases. This was resected, leaving a portion of malignancy on the aorta, and a seven-inch plastic tube was inserted. The patient received irradiation to the area of resection postoperatively. He had a relatively smooth postoperative course and went back to his practice. Approximately seven months postoperatively, the patient had a severe hemorrhage from the lung, and post-mortem revealed that the carcinoma of the esophagus had ruptured into the main-stem bronchus.

Comment.—This case was interesting in that it was possible for the patient to speak as clearly as before by the esophageal voice method. It is doubtful that he would have had speech with a high stomach anastomosis. Second, the perforation was probably abetted by the postoperative x-ray therapy to the site of lesion (Fig. 7).

Case 6.—J. S., a 70-year-old man, had a carcinoma of the upper end of the middle third of the esophagus, which was resected, and a 14 cm. tube was inserted. The patient was dis-

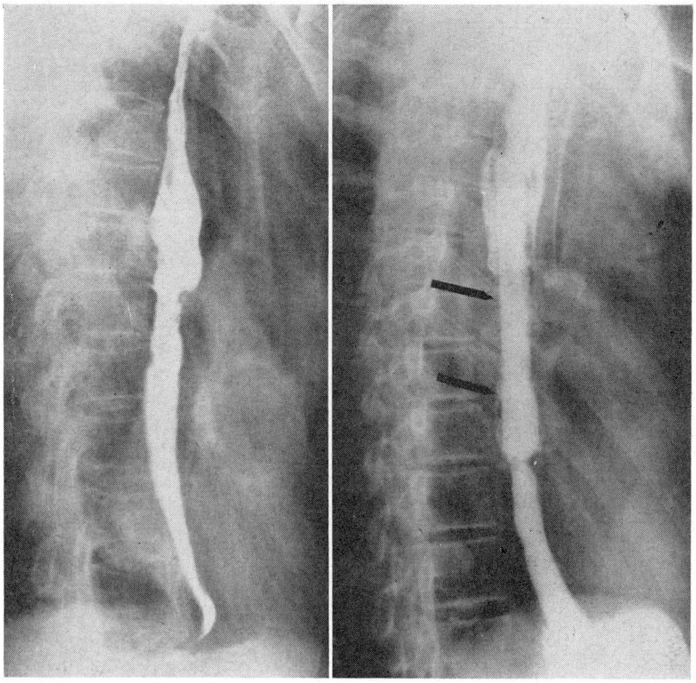

A. B.

Fig. 8 (Case 6).—*A,* Carcinoma of the midthoracic esophagus is easily seen. *B,* Five weeks postoperatively, the plastic tube is seen carrying the barium down to the stomach.

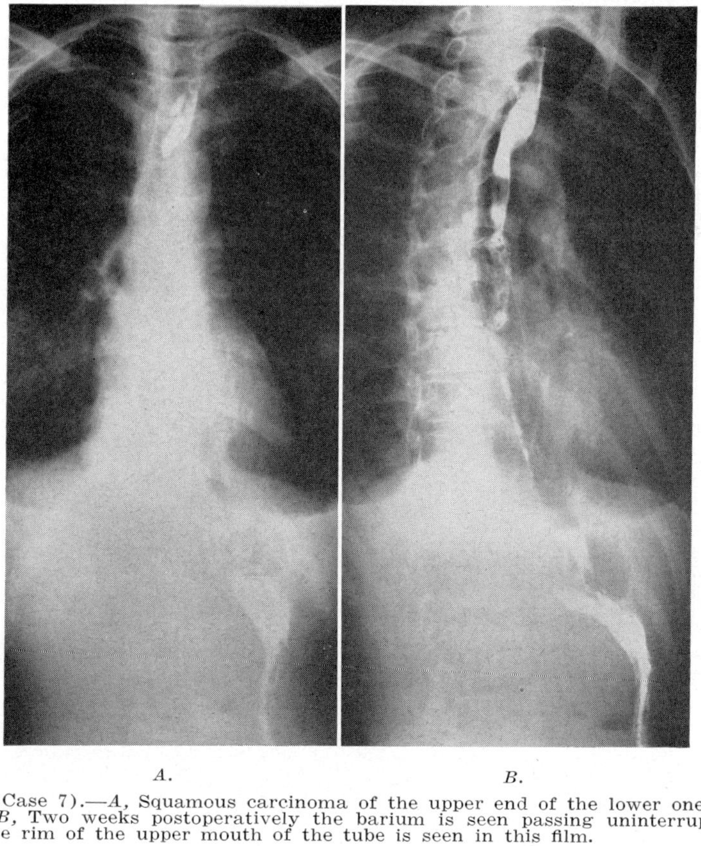

A. B.

Fig. 9 (Case 7).—*A,* Squamous carcinoma of the upper end of the lower one-third of the esophagus. *B,* Two weeks postoperatively the barium is seen passing uninterrupted into the stomach. The rim of the upper mouth of the tube is seen in this film.

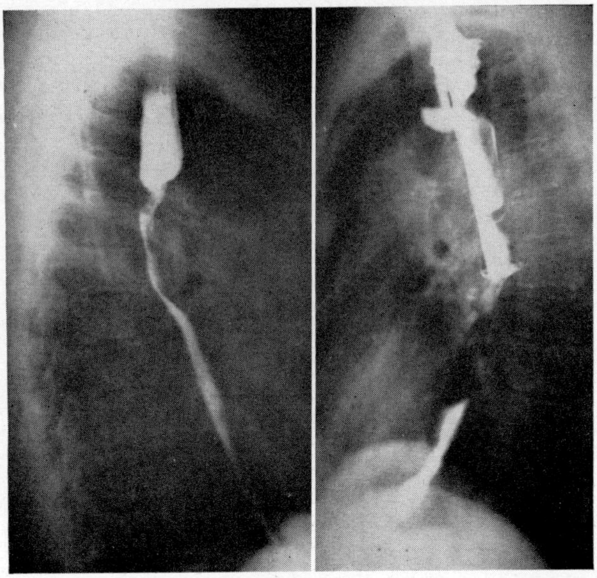

A. B.

Fig. 10 (Case 8).—*A,* A large infiltrative squamous lesion in the middle one-third of the esophagus. *B,* Barium shown going readily through the tube and into the stomach. Much malignancy was left on the surrounding structures in this case. Barium may be seen outside the tube but within the new sheath enveloping the tube.

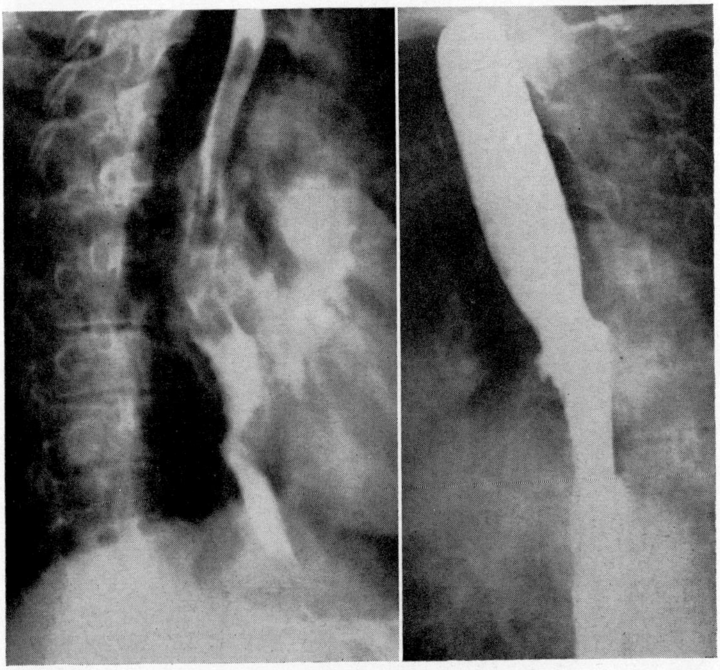

A. B.

Fig. 11 (Case 9).—*A,* The lesion seen extended from above the azygos vein down to the cardia. *B,* The barium is shown going through the nine-inch tube postoperatively. The lower anastomosis is to the stomach.

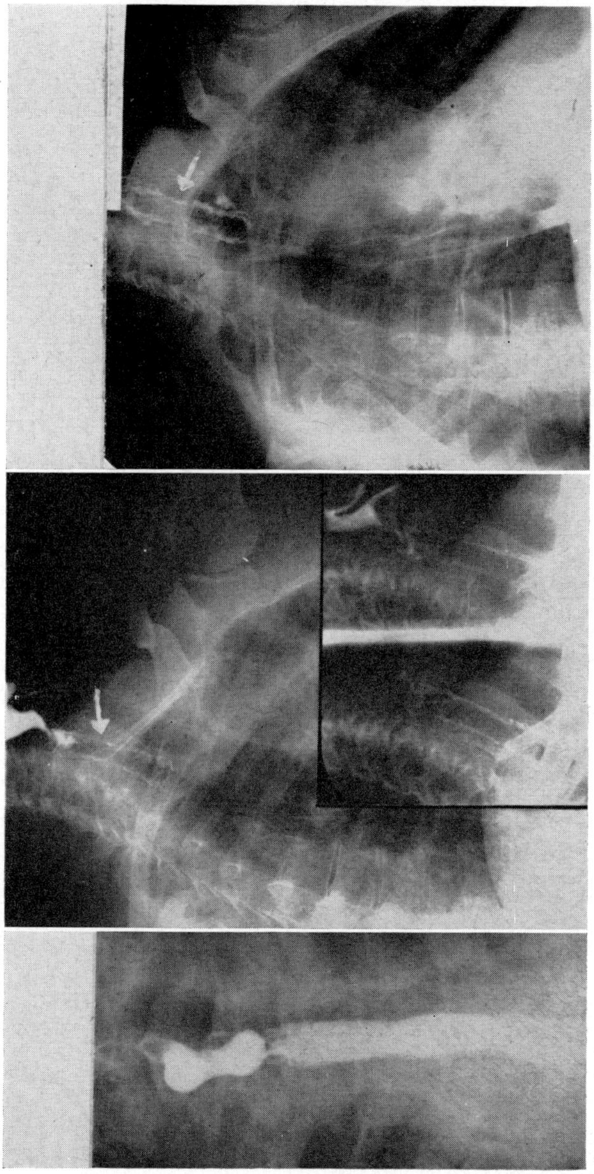

A. B. C.

Fig 12 (Case 10).—*A*, Initial lesion is nonradiographic. This film denotes spasm at the site of biopsy in the cervical region. *B*, Six weeks postoperatively, the barium is shown going through the plastic tube into the thoracic esophagus (with insert). *C*, Lipiodol swallow shows the tube and the anastomotic areas.

charged eating practically a full diet, and is still living twelve months postoperatively (Fig. 8).

Case 7.—C. C., a 52-year-old white woman, was admitted with dysphagia and symptoms of substernal obstruction for a period of eight months. Biopsy revealed squamous cell carcinoma of the upper end of the lower third of the esophagus. An exploratory laparotomy showed widespread abdominal metastasis. A thoracotomy revealed a large extensively invasive carcinoma, which was removed, and a seven-inch plastic tube was inserted. The patient is still living and eating well five months postoperatively.

Case 8.—G. H., aged 52 years, was admitted to The Johns Hopkins Hospital with a complaint of substernal discomfort while eating coarse foods. This progressed to dysphagia and regurgitation and a ten-pound weight loss. At this time, it was felt by the surgeon that the patient was inoperable, and a first stage antithoracic jejunal loop was brought up with a gastrostomy. The loop became nonviable. The jejunal loop was taken down and the chest wall drained. Two weeks later, the patient was again taken to the operating room, and a large infiltrative lesion with definite evidence of metastases in every direction was removed at about the fourth dorsal vertebra, leaving malignancy behind. He ate well on the seventh postoperative day and was discharged eighteen days postoperatively. There was no follow-up.

Comment.—This case shows that even in the most extensive lesion, and as a last resort, with the patient in an extremely bad condition, palliation is extremely simple with the tube method (Fig. 10).

Case 9.—The history of A. D., aged 68 years, began seven months prior to admission with dysphagia and weight loss. Esophagogram revealed an extensive lesion of the middle and lower third, proved by biopsy to be carcinoma. This patient was quickly becoming worse at the time of operation, with nutrition being maintained solely by the intravenous route. At operation, a tremendous lesion was found extending from the azygos vein to the cardia, and it was resected. The hiatus was enlarged by finger dissertion, and a portion of the stomach was drawn through for the lower anastomosis. The patient did extremely well and was discharged on a regular diet. A four-week check revealed the tube to be functioning well, but the patient was still losing weight (Fig. 11).

Case 10.—A. G., aged 52 years, complained that some months prior to admission he had swallowed a chicken bone which seemed to stick in his throat. Since that time he had had a sticking sensation in the neck, with some dysphagia. X-ray film was inconclusive, but esophagoscopy revealed a tiny 5 mm. lesion in the cervical esophagus which was biopsied and showed a squamous carcinoma. X-ray film (Fig. 12, *A*) shows the spasm at site of biopsy. At operation through a left cervical incision at The Johns Hopkins Hospital, the site of lesion was barely palpable, but a wide resection of the esophagus was performed, and a special (lesser diameter) three-inch plastic tube was anastomosed to either end of the esophagus. The patient has eaten perfectly well since then, with his only symptom being excessive salivation six months postoperatively.

SUMMARY

With the results as stated by different authors in large series, it seems that in concentrating our attack on the disease, the regard for the patient has become secondary. In the lapsed period of trial of almost two decades with all modern aids, a re-evaluation of the present methods of maintaining continuity after resection of portions of the esophagus for malignancy finds them sadly lacking. As reflected in the mortality, the conventional procedure is of too great a magnitude for the average patient in this group. The high morbidity attests to the imperfections in the usual technique. The short survival makes us reflect on the fact that the intrinsic nature and the anatomic relationship of this disease make it not suitable for true cancer surgery. And, last, if the patient clings so tenaciously to life so as to overcome these obstacles, he deserves a better fate, in his score or so of remaining months, than the miserable one (if it is a mid or high lesion) that most of these patients are destined for.

The polyethylene prosthesis in our short collected experience seems to offer hope, but not for the principal factor, that of increased survival time with possibility of cure. Every surgeon familiar with thoracic technique can use this method with relative safety. However, a word of caution should be interjected. Although the success of this new and rather unconventional procedure requires no undue skill, the few fundamentals of the procedure, previously alluded to, should be adhered to, and some animal or cadaver rehearsal should be carried out before the first procedure. However, if used correctly, it will allow many more patients a few years' survival by dint of the low operative mortality. There will be a decreased and less hectic postoperative course, with fewer complications. Most important, to these unfortunates who are doomed, their remaining years will be comfortable, and they will have the ability to eat whatever and as much as they want with no concomitant distress.

REFERENCES

1. Parker, E. F., Hanna, C. B., and Postlethwait, R. W.: Carcinoma of the Esophagus, Ann. Surg. **135:** 697, 1952.
2. Ravitch, M. M., Bahuson, H. T., and Johns, T. N. P.: Carcinoma of the Esophagus—A Consideration of Curative and Palliative Procedures, J. Thoracic Surg. **24:** 256, 1952.
3. Sweet, R. H.: The Results of Radical Surgical Extirpation in the Treatment of Carcinoma of the Esophagus and Cardia With Five Year Survival Statistics, Surg., Gynec. & Obst. **94:** 46, 1952.
4. Humphreys, G. H., II, and Moore, R. L.: Carcinoma Involving the Esophagus, S. Clin. North America **33:** 389-400 (April) 1953.
5. Berman, E. F.: The Experimental Replacement of Portions of the Esophagus by a Plastic Tube, Ann. Surg. **135:** 388, 1952.
6. Berman, E. F.: The Plastic Esophagus, J. Internat. Coll. Surgeons **18:** 695, 1952.
7. Berman, E. F.: A Plastic Prosthesis for Resected Esophagus, Arch. Surg. **65:** 916, 1952.

Book Reviews

Nash's Surgical Physiology. Revised and edited by Brian Blades, M.D., professor of surgery, George Washington University School of Medicine. Pp. 686. Springfield, 1953, Charles C Thomas, Publisher. $12.50.

The second edition of *Nash's Surgical Physiology* represents a considerable revision and edition by Brian Blades and his associates of the George Washington University School of Medicine of the earlier work. This new edition contains considerably more material presented in a more readable format along with an increased number of illustrations. Basically, the book deals with practical physiologic considerations as applied to clinical surgery. The material is grouped according to the major body systems, dealing successively with the cardiovascular system, burns and tissue repair, the respiratory system, the gastrointestinal system, the body fluids, the kidneys, the endocrine system, and the nervous system.

The effective stimulus of cardiac surgery to an increased interest in physiology by surgeons is reflected in this work by a chapter concerning recent advances in cardiovascular surgery. A similar expansion is seen in the treatment of physiology of the adrenal gland in the light of the recent tremendous expansion in this field. The authors make considerable reference to current articles on the subject matter.

As is inevitable when attempting to sort and organize the tremendous volume of physiologic data with reference to the equally enormous subject matter of general surgery, there is a tendency to present some controversial material in a dogmatic fashion as well as to retain a few outmoded concepts. Nevertheless, the authors have succeeded in covering a vast scope of material in a concise fashion without becoming entangled in a web of details.

While the book cannot be claimed to be a ''royal road'' to an easy and complete grasp of the subject matter (as, indeed, in this field no book can!), it does arrange the vast array of physiologic data along the path of interest of the clinical surgeon such that he may see it easily in respect to his field of interest.

This work should be of particular interest to the student, intern, and surgical resident, as well as to the practicing surgeon who wishes to refamiliarize himself with physiology in a broad sense as applied to the field of surgery.

Praktikum der Chirurgie. Ein Leitfaden für Studenten und Ärzte. By Prof. Dr. Med. Hans Hellner. Pp. 720. Munich-Berlin, 1952, Urban & Schwarzenberg.

This is the textbook of surgery written by the late O. Nordmann, revised for the seventh edition by Hellner. As in previous editions, the chief emphasis is laid on indications for surgical treatment, technique of emergency operations, pre- and postoperative care, and recognition of postoperative complications.

The book is written mainly from the personal experience of the authors, and no references are given. Since all the subspecialties of surgery are covered, treatment of many topics is necessarily brief. The surgery of heart disease is represented only by a short discussion of penetrating wounds and of pericarditis. Vagotomy is not mentioned in the section on treatment of peptic ulcer. The discussion of hernia repair takes no account of the newer knowledge of anatomy.

This volume is of interest as a reflection of current German practice, but it is of little value compared to the best books available in English.

SURGERY

VOL. 35 JUNE, 1954 No. 6

Original Communications

SIMPLIFICATION OF THE BILLROTH I GASTRIC RESECTION

KOMEI NAKAYAMA, M.D.,* CHIBA, JAPAN

FOREWORD

ALTHOUGH various operative methods have been employed to treat duodenal ulcer radically, the ulcer is not usually removed by techniques commonly employed. This is due to the surgical problems of dissection in the location of the ulcer with a consequent increased mortality. Hence, gastrectomy without removal of the ulcer, or gastroenterostomy, has been the common operative management of duodenal ulcer in the past.

The development of a proper operative method preventing the recurrence of preoperative complaints and peptic ulcer has been the hope of surgeons for many years.

We have devised a new technique of excision of the duodenal ulcer with a low operative mortality and recurrence rate.

OPERATIVE METHOD

The procedure is performed using spinal anesthesia through an upper midline abdominal incision. First, the greater curvature of the stomach is cleared by ligating the gastrocolic ligament in three or four places. The axis of the right gastroepiploic artery and Mayo's vein are ligated. Almost all duodenal ulcers are located in the duodenal cap, and frequently cause adhesion formation to surrounding organs. Freeing of the adherent and thinned portion of the duodenum is reserved as the final stage of resection. The uninvolved serosa is located distal to the ulcer and mobilization from surrounding tissues is proceded with, in the direction of the gastric pylorus. The portion invaded by the degenerating ulcer process and normal tissue can be clearly differentiated.

The lesser curvature of the stomach is mobilized to the cardiac end of the stomach, and the line of resection is determined. Subtotal gastrectomy (more than two-thirds of the stomach) is preferred in our clinic. My gastric clamp is then placed at the line of resection to amputate the stomach (Fig. 1). The upper portion of the gastric remnant is closed by continuous Lembert sutures. The distal posterior wall of the gastric pouch is fixed to the head of the pancreas

Received for publication, Sept. 30, 1953.
*Professor of surgery, School of Medicine, Chiba University.

by three interrupted silk sutures (Fig. 2,*A* and *B*). Tension on the anastomosis is thereby completely eliminated. The forceps which was placed on the duodenal remnant is removed at this juncture. The ulcer is cicatrix can be further removed when necessary so that normal mucosa is available for anastomosis to the gastric remnant. When the cicatrix extends toward the posterior wall of the duodenum, special attention is required to avoid incising the pancreas.

Many cases present problems which demand a special approach. 1. When the ulcer has penetrated adjacent structures, the base of the ulcer must be excised. Almost all of the ulcer can be removed with the resected stomach, leaving the base adherent to the adjacent organ. The remaining base must be curetted and covered by normal gastric serosa at the completion of the anastomosis. 2. When stenosis is found in the descending portion of the duodenum, a longitudinal incision is made in the duodenum to enlarge the cut end, making it more suitable for anastomosis with the gastric pouch (Fig. 2, *C*).

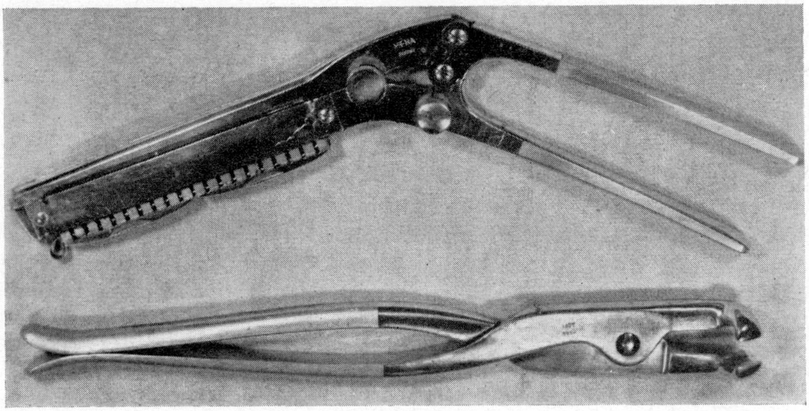

Fig. 1.—My clip placer, an instrument adapted from the V. Petz suturing apparatus. These are removal cartridges into which the clips are placed. The écraseur type of instrument shown is used to drive the clips home. The clip placer has a dorsal groove into which a knife blade is inserted to divide the tissues which are to be separated.

Over 90 per cent of duodenal ulcers can be excised by these means. Reestablishment of gastrointestinal continuity is made by a gastroduodenal anastomosis. The posterior wall of the anastomosis is a single continuous suture (Fig. 2, *D*). The anterior wall anastomosis is performed in two layers, using an Albert mucosal suture covered by a row of Lembert sutures. The upper and lower ends of the anastomosis have sutures which pass through the gastric serosa and pancreas to the duodenal serosa, thereby reinforcing the weakest portion of the anastomosis. The head of the pancreas plays a role as splint between the stomach and duodenum (Fig. 2, *D*). The anastomosis is drawn to the left by this operative technique, but the head of the pancreas is pulled with the duodenum, and tension of the anastomosis is avoided. The anastomosis usually lies to the left of the vertebral column. The operation is completed by covering the anastomosis with greater omentum and closing the abdominal wall.

A rubber tube (Levin tube) is left in the stomach for two or three days after the operation to prevent distention. The patient is discharged from the hospital on the twelfth or thirteenth postoperative day. The operative time for this procedure which requires a minimum of manipulation is usually thirty minutes.

OPERATIVE RESULTS

Since August, 1946, 687 patients have been operated upon by this technique.

There have been three hospital deaths following the operation, a mortality rate of 0.4 per cent.

A.

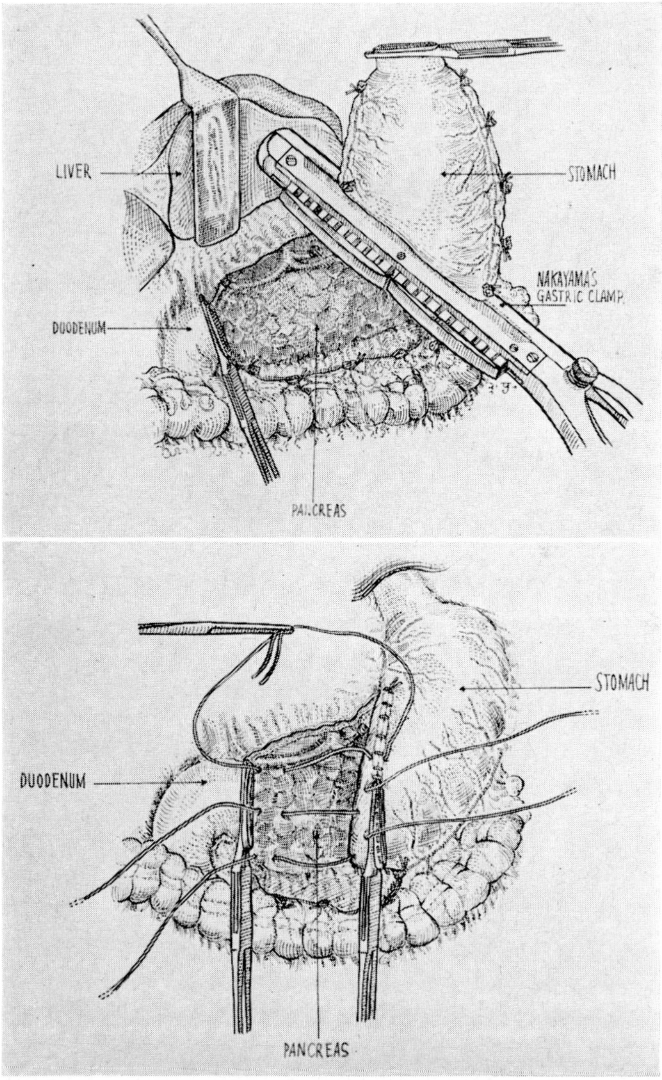

B.

Fig. 2, *A* and *B*.—My technique of gastric resection by the Billroth I method. *A*, The segment of stomach to be removed. The duodenal ulcer is excised in 90 per cent of instances. *B*, Partial closure of the lesser curvature; placement of anchoring sutures between the posterior gastric wall and the pancreatic capsule behind the duodenum.

C.

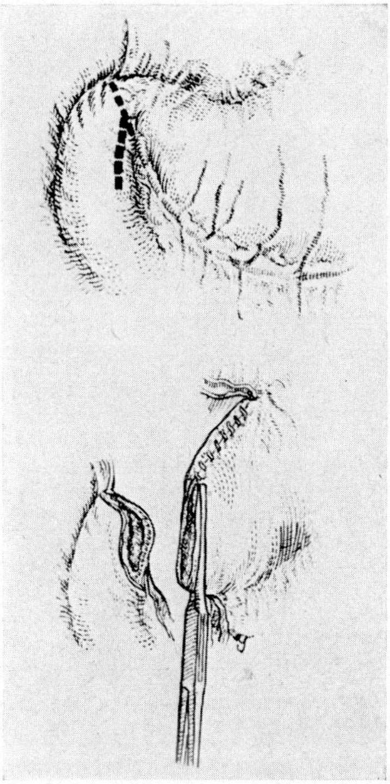

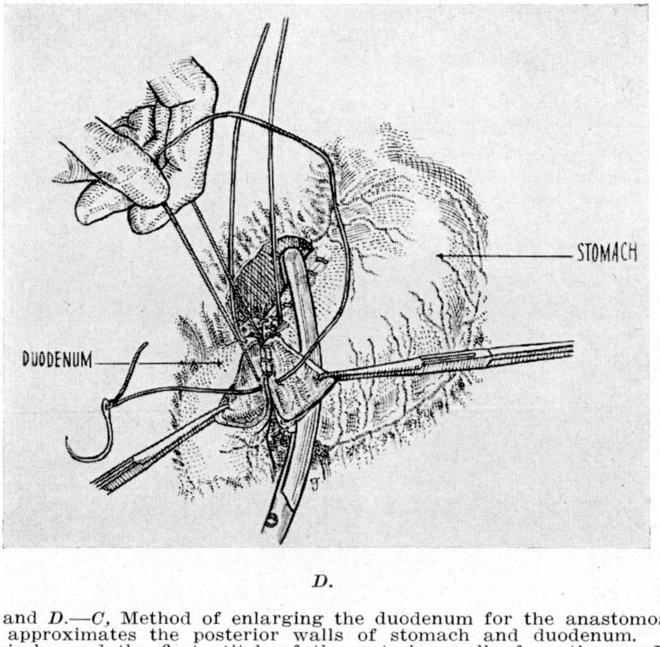

D.

Fig. 2, *C* and *D*.—*C*, Method of enlarging the duodenum for the anastomosis. *D*, A continuous suture approximates the posterior walls of stomach and duodenum. This suture is continued anteriorly, and the first stitch of the anterior wall of continuous Lembert suture has been placed previously. Posteriorly, this continuous Albert suture is employed only, for the purpose of anchoring sutures.

The proportion of duodenal ulcer to gastric ulcer in Japan is quite different from that in the United States. Of the patients mentioned, 258 had a duodenal ulcer, or only 37.6 per cent of the series of gastroduodenal ulcers. The rate of resectability of all gastroduodenal ulcers was 99.0 per cent, a higher figure than is usually seen in the larger Japanese hospitals.

A.

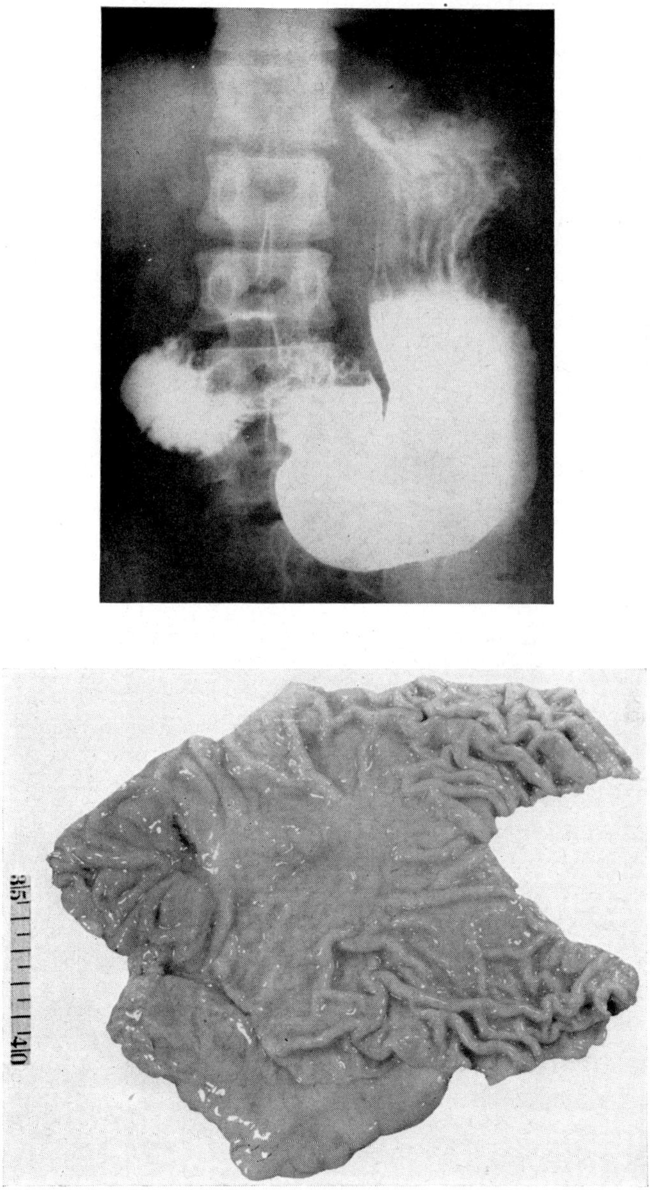

B.

Fig. 3, *A* and *B*.—Clinical data in a resection case. *A*, Roentgenogram before operation. *B*, The excised stomach.

The pancreatic function of these patients was carefully studied, and no abnormalities were found (Fig. 2, *D*). Hepatic function has shown no changes.

In an illustrative case of duodenal ulcer managed by the previously outlined technique, preoperative roentgenograms were as illustrated in Fig. 3, *A*. The removed specimen is illustrated in Fig. 3, *B*. Fig. 3, *C* shows the postoperative course of the patient. Fig. 3, *D* illustrates the postoperative roentgenogram of the patient.

C.

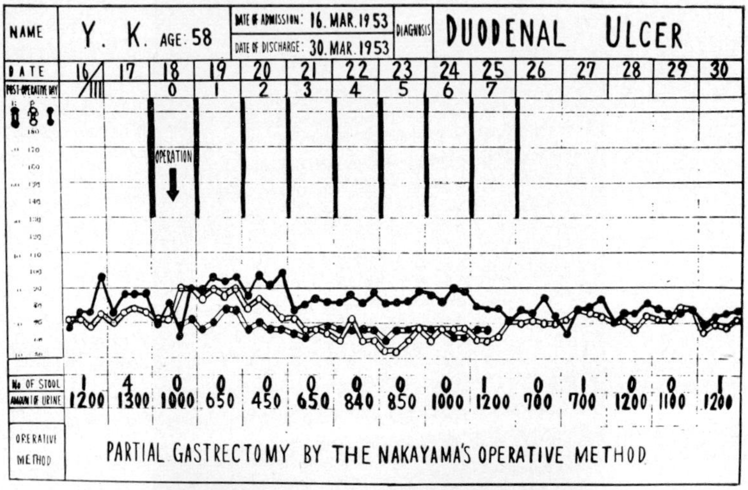

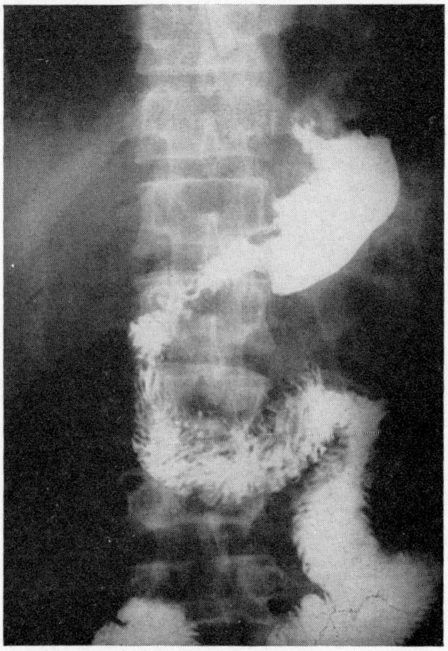

D.

Fig. 3, *C* and *D*.—*C*, The postoperative fever chart. *D*, Postoperative roentgenogram.

CLINICAL INVESTIGATION AT THE TIME OF FOLLOW-UP

Excluding the patients who died of accidental or unrelated causes, all patients were gainfully employed in their normal occupation by six months postoperatively. Routine clinical examination is normal in most cases. No anemia was found; most patients were gaining weight at this time. No recurrent peptic ulcers or bleeding has been encountered.

Complaints after the operation have been carefully studied, and nothing of a severity to require a change or discontinuance of occupation was found. No ulcer pain was seen following the operation. Abdominal pain due to ascariasis was encountered, but disappeared on treatment of the ascariasis. Vomiting has occurred since surgery in 8.4 per cent of cases. Constant vomiting was seen in 2.8 per cent. Sixteen per cent of all patients operated on by this method have diarrhea. In most patients this was not severe (two bowel movements a day). This difficulty ameliorates with passage of time.

No objective evidence of recurrence exists in these patients, and the general condition of the patients is satisfactory.

SUMMARY

The radical surgical treatment of duodenal ulcer by this operative method, that is, Billroth I gastrectomy with the alterations in technique suggested by me, gives good results; in fact, the postoperative condition of patients subjected to this operation compared very favorably with other surgical procedures. The operative technique is quite simple. Normal alimentary continuity is re-established.

CONCLUSIONS

1. In the radical surgical treatment of the duodenal ulcer, the ulcer as the source of the complaints should be removed, together with more than two-thirds of the stomach.
2. It has been thought that subtotal gastrectomy can be performed safely by the employment of a Billroth II gastrectomy. However, this operative method prevents the removal of the duodenal ulcer with the stomach.
3. I have modified the technique of the Billroth I gastrectomy, introducing a new thought in re-establishment of the alimentary tract. We fix the posterior wall of the stomach to the head of the pancreas, moving the gastroduodenal anastomosis to the left; thus we have succeeded in removing a sufficiently large amount of stomach as well as the duodenal ulcer, something which is difficult or impossible in many Billroth II resections.
4. We have treated 687 cases of gastroduodenal ulcers by this method; 285 were duodenal ulcers, all of which were cured. We have not experienced a single case of suture insufficiency, the most dangerous factor when a direct gastroduodenal anastomosis is performed after the subtotal gastrectomy.
5. Follow-up studies fail to disclose any recurrences.

A STAINLESS STEEL CANNULA FOR THE CREATION OF GASTROINTESTINAL FISTULAS

S. FRANK REDO, M.D., AND WILLIAM A. BARNES, M.D., NEW YORK, N. Y.

(From the Department of Surgery, Cornell University Medical College, and the New York Hospital)

GASTRIC fistulas have been used by many investigators for the study of gastric secretion. These have been formed (1) directly as a gastrostomy,[1, 2] (2) by interposing a segment of ileum between the stomach and skin,[3] or (3) by using a cannula. Pavlov[4] described a spool-shaped cannula, the lumen of which was blocked by a cork stopper when samples were not being taken. Dragstedt and Ellis[5] used a gold-plated cannula that was brought out to the skin.

This paper describes a spool-shaped cannula that has been found to be useful in creating gastric fistulas in dogs. Its chief advantages are that it is leakproof, well tolerated by the animals, and causes no skin reaction about its point of exit.

Description.—The cannula, made of stainless steel, consists of a central hollow cylinder internally threaded, with a flange at each end. The flanges are perforated near the periphery so that they may be sutured to the stomach and skin. This helps to stabilize the cannula. However, it has been found unnecessary to suture the flange to the skin. A stainless steel screw inserts into the central hollow cylinder to prevent leakage (Fig. 1). When gastric specimens are desired, the screw is removed and samples are readily obtained.

Specifications of Cannula.—Length is 2.5 cm., diameter of flanges 3 cm., diameter of central hollow cylinder (lumen) 0.6 cm. There are eight perforations near the periphery of the flange, each with a diameter of 1 mm. and spaced 1 cm. apart. A modification of this cannula is shown in Fig. 2. This type of cannula has a single flanged end which fits into the stomach. The central hollow cylinder is threaded on the inside and on the outside. The inner threads are for the stainless steel screw. The skin flange screws over the outside of the central hollow cylinder. A second smaller nut is then screwed down over this to prevent the flange from being accidentally unscrewed. This is superior to the original model (although slightly more expensive) since it allows for variation in thickness of the abdominal wall. In addition, the opening in the skin need be only large enough to accommodate the central cylinder.

The cannula is easily inserted, as follows: An incision is made through the wall of the stomach. The cannula is inserted and the stomach closed about it by a purse-string suture or interrupted inverting sutures of nonabsorbable material. Several sutures are then placed through all layers of the stomach and through the perforations in the gastric flange. This anchors the flange within the stomach. A piece of omentum is wrapped around the central cylinder. A

Aided by a grant from the Wyeth Foundation and Mrs. Percy Strauss.
Received for publication, Oct. 6, 1953.

stab wound is made through the abdominal wall, and the free flange of the cannula is brought through this to the surface of the skin. It is not necessary to anchor this flange to the skin.

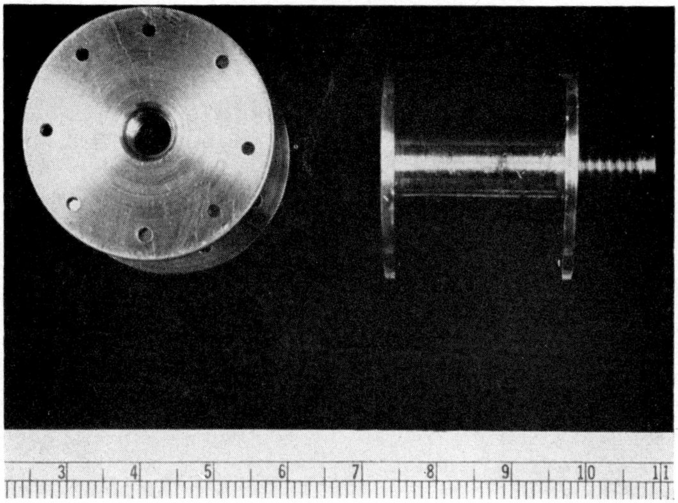

Fig. 1.—Cannula for creation of gastrointestinal fistula. Specifications are listed in the text.

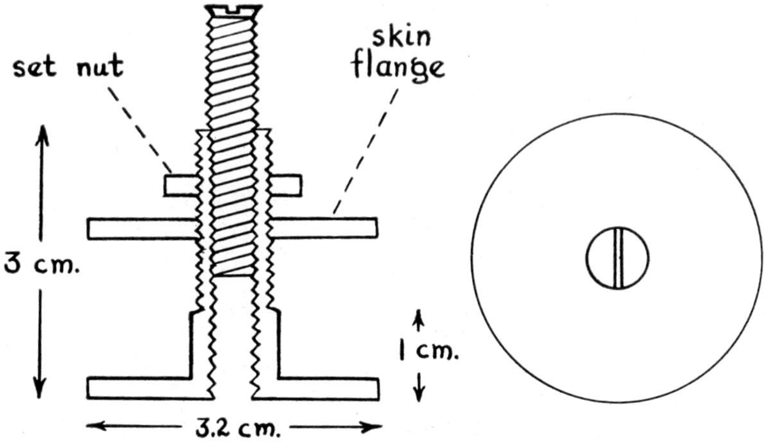

Fig. 2.—Modified cannula (cross-section and end-on views).

The cannula described has been used to create gastric fistulas in twenty dogs. There was no leakage and no maceration or infection of the skin. All animals tolerated the cannula well, several for more than six months (Fig. 3). They exhibited no interest in it and did not attempt to bite or remove it. Gastric specimens were obtained by removing the central screw and collecting the secretions in a small beaker held beneath the skin flange.

Modifications of this cannula can be used for many types of gastrointestinal fistulas. At present, work is in progress to evaluate its use in colostomy. In this connection, absence of leakage following irrigation and prevention of stricture may be among its advantages.

A.

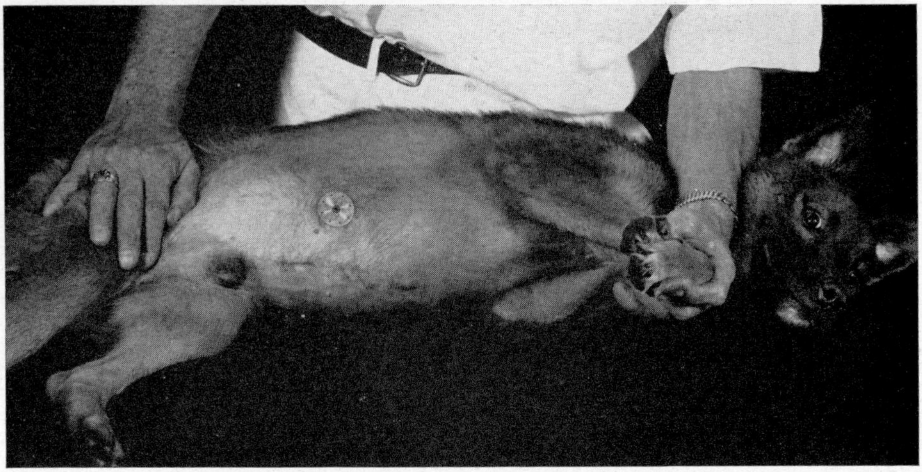

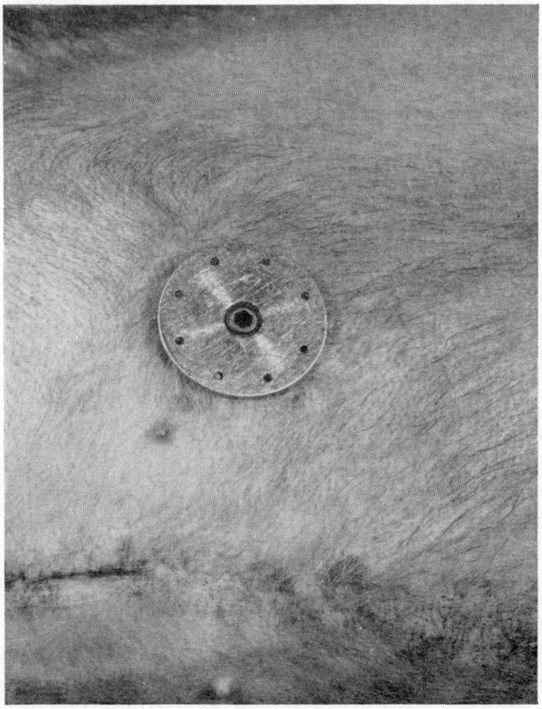

B.

Fig. 3, *A* and *B*.—Cannula two months after insertion in the stomach of a dog. Note the absence of changes in the skin about the cannula.

SUMMARY

1. A modified spool-shaped cannula for the creation of various types of gastrointestinal fistulas is described.

2. The cannula has been used in twenty dogs and has been tolerated well. There has been no leakage or maceration or infection of the skin about the site of exit.

REFERENCES

1. Markowitz, J.: Experimental Surgery, Baltimore, 1949, Williams & Wilkins Company, p. 113.
2. Gould, A. H.: Technic of Operations Upon the Intestines and Stomach, Philadelphia, 1906, W. B. Saunders Company.
3. Goldberg, S. L., and Mann, F. C.: Preparing Pouches of the Fundus of the Stomach, Ann. Surg. **94**: 1953, 1931.
4. Pavlov, I. P.: The Work of the Digestive Glands, ed. 2, London, 1910, Chas. Griffin & Co.
5. Dragstedt, L. R., and Ellis, J.: Fatal Effect of Total Loss of Gastric Juice, Proc. Soc. Exper. Biol. & Med. **26**: 305, 1929.

RETURN OF SODIUM LOADS IN NORMAL SUBJECTS FOLLOWING RESTRICTED SODIUM INTAKE

J. U. Schlegel, M.D., Rochester, N. Y.

(From the University of Rochester, School of Medicine and Dentistry, and the Department of Surgery, Buswell Urological Research Laboratory)

The prevention of sodium retention is a subject of great interest since a successful correction of this is important for the treatment of a great number of pathologic conditions. We have been studying this phenomenon, especially as it occurs following severe trauma, such as burns, and certain major operations. It was found that the increase in adrenal activity occurring in seriously burned patients does not necessarily diminish the ability to excrete sodium. In fact, it was observed that when sufficient amounts of hypertonic sodium chloride were given relatively soon following the trauma, the return of subsequent loads of sodium was higher than that found in normal persons.[1] It was also found that the urinary pH can only exhibit normal fluctuations when base excretion (sodium and potassium) is above approximately 100 microequivalents per minute, provided that titratable acidity is within a normal range of 10 to 25 microequivalents per minute.[2] The amount of hypertonic sodium chloride initially given the burned patients was, therefore, considered sufficient only when urinary pH fluctuations were maintained or restored.

Because this method of treatment is based upon the assumption that sodium retention did not exist prior to the trauma,[3] we must be very careful to rule out an unsuspected pre-existing condition of this sort. Black, Platt, and Stanbury[4] have shown that normal persons who have been on a low-sodium diet for five days would retain sodium when subjected to a load of intravenously administered 5 per cent sodium chloride. This observation seems to suggest that patients preoperatively occasionally might exhibit sodium retention, since their intake often may be low, or an actual loss might have been encountered by vomiting, diarrhea, or other routes. Since surgery in itself will lead to sodium retention, a pre-existing condition of this sort may even be exaggerated by the operation. This study is an attempt to evaluate the time necessary for establishing a sodium retention.

EXPERIMENTAL PROCEDURES AND METHODS

Twenty-one male medical students were used. Eleven of these received a low-sodium diet containing approximately ½ Gm. of sodium chloride and 3 Gm. of potassium chloride daily. The daily sodium intake in milliequivalents for each student represented in alphabetic order is given in Table I. The first

This investigation was supported with funds from the Dr. Henry C. Buswell Memorial and the Office of Naval Research.

The excellent technical assistance of Mr. William R. Johnson, Miss Patricia Bryant, and Miss Sally Fox is gratefully acknowledged.

Received for publication, Oct. 11, 1953.

five (A, B, C, D, and E) received, in addition, 3 Gm. of sodium chloride (a total of 60 meq.) on the first day of the experiment.

The return of an oral sodium load was in all cases calculated as the percentage return over a twenty-four hour period (8:00 A.M. to 8:00 A.M.) of the total amount of sodium given during the daytime of that period. A water load was given to several of the students. This is indicated in Table I by +. All the water loads given to these as well as other of the students amounted to 800 c.c. per square meter of surface area. The return was then calculated on a four-hour basis, and most of the patients had their weights followed prior to and after the water load. Since a sodium load of a magnitude given to the first five students did not exceed the amount of sodium they had lost during that period (Fig. 1), two students, F and G, were put on a low-sodium diet for eight days and were then given 15 Gm. of sodium chloride over one day. One of these (F) was given a second sodium load of the same magnitude the next day. The same procedure, except for the sodium load, was followed for two other students (H and I), who received a water load on the ninth day of their low sodium intake. J is a control study where a normal individual was subjected to a low sodium intake for eleven days. K was also subjected to a low-sodium diet, and received on the ninth day an acid load in the form of 15 Gm. of ammonium chloride. This was done to try to simulate the effect of a sudden acid load on an individual who had been on a low-sodium diet, and was thought to be somewhat comparable to the situation which may arise when a patient who has been on a low sodium intake is subjected to a sudden stress. This individual received a water load on the eleventh day.

The low-sodium diet is considerably less acid than most normal diets. It was found in all the students on this diet that the amount of titratable acid they excreted was greatly diminished.

To try to simulate the conditions of a patient preoperatively, where some degree of acidosis might be present, six students were given a low-sodium diet and, in addition, a varying amount of ammonium chloride daily. Three of these were subjected to a water load and three to an oral salt load. Since, however, the loss of sodium was very extensive in these individuals, and since for practical reasons not much more than an additional amount of 15 Gm. of sodium chloride could be given daily, they were given identical consecutive loads on the two following days, as can be seen in Table I (O, P, and Q). Also in Table I can be seen the exact amount of ammonium chloride (in grams) that was given daily. It will be noted here that some received an increasing amount of ammonium chloride, while two received an amount which did not change after the fourth day.

To evaluate the effect of starvation, four students were finally subjected to complete starvation from three to four days. Two of these received a water load and two an oral sodium load at the end of the starvation.

Serum sodium, potassium, chloride, and Co_2 were determined in all students prior to the experiment and on the last day. The group which received am-

TABLE I. EXPERIMENTAL PROCEDURE*

DAY OF EXPERIMENT		LOW SODIUM DIET ONLY											LOW SODIUM DIET AND AMMONIUM CHLORIDE						STARVATION			
		A	B	C	D	E	F	G	H	I	J	K	L	M	N	O	P	Q	R	S	T	U
		K. H.	S. D.	J. G.	J. M.	R. B.	S. D.	J. MC.	P. M.	K. H.	J. C.	R. H.	R. P.	J. M.	R. E.	W. L.	W. C.	R. M.	P. M.	R. M.	W. C.	J. B.
	Na	60	60	60	60	60	9	9	9	9	9	9	9	9	9	9	9	9	0	0	0	0
1	NH_4Cl												15	15	15	15	15	15				
	H_2O																					
	Na	60	9	9	9	9	9	9	9	9	9	9	9	9	9	9	9	9	0	0	0	0
2	NH_4Cl												15	15	15	15	15	15				
	H_2O		+																			
	Na		60	9	9	9	9	9	9	9	9	9	9	9	9	9	9	9	0	0	265	0
3	NH_4Cl												15	15	15	15	15	15				
	H_2O			+															+			
	Na			60	9	9	9	9	9	9	9	9	9	9	9	9	9	9		0		265
4	NH_4Cl												10	10	10	10	10	10				
	H_2O				+															+		
	Na				60	9	9	9	9	9	9	9	9	9	9	9	9	9				
5	NH_4Cl												10	10	10	10	10	10				
	H_2O					+																
	Na					60	9	9	9	9	9	9	9	9	9	265	265	265				
6	NH_4Cl												10	15	15	15	15	10				
	H_2O												+	+	+							
	Na						9	9	9	9	9	9		9	9	265	265	265				
7	NH_4Cl													20	20	20	20	10				
	H_2O																					
	Na						9	9	9	9	9	9		9	9	265	265	265				
8	NH_4Cl													20	20	20	20	10				
	H_2O													+	+							
	Na						265	265	9	9	9	9										
9	NH_4Cl											15										
	H_2O								+	+												
	Na						265	9	9	9	9	9										
10	NH_4Cl																					
	H_2O																					
	Na										9	9										
11	NH_4Cl																					
	H_2O											+										

*For each student is given the daily intake of sodium expressed in milliequivalents. In the group (L to Q) which received ammonium chloride, the daily intake is expressed in grams. The students who received a water load can be found in the table where + indicates the day in the experiment on which the water load was given.

monium chloride and the group which was subjected to starvation had blood chemistry determined daily. In addition, blood chemistry was determined prior to and following sodium loads as well as water loads.

The day prior to the experiment, every day during the experiment, and one day following, the urine was collected hourly from 8:00 in the morning until

Fig. 1.

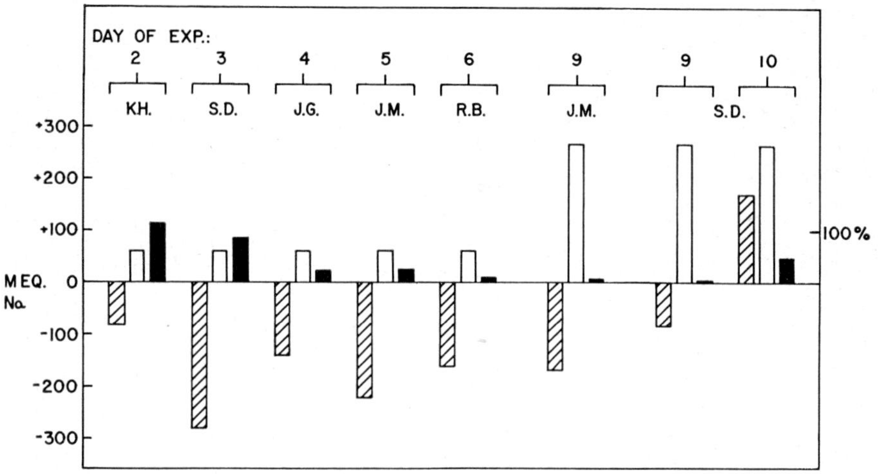

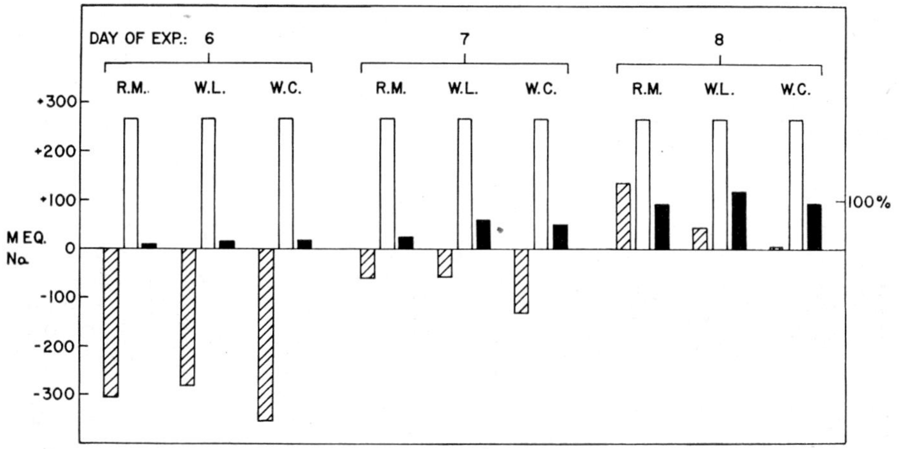

Fig. 2.

Fig. 1.—Crosshatched column: Cumulative urine sodium excretion in excess of intake from beginning of experiment until time of sodium load (milliequivalents). White column: Sodium load (milliequivalents). Black column: Return of sodium following sodium load (per cent in twenty-four hours).

The students included in this figure were on a low-sodium diet for a varying number of days. It will be noticed that the percentage return of a sodium load is lower the longer the low sodium intake has lasted. This drop in percentage return (black column) is apparently independent of the total amount of sodium lost (crosshatched column) and of the size of the sodium load (white column).

Fig. 2.—Crosshatched column: Cumulative urine sodium excretion in excess of intake from beginning of experiment until time of sodium load (milliequivalents). White column: Sodium load (milliequivalents). Black column: Return of sodium following sodium load (per cent in twenty-four hours).

The three students presented in this figure received, in addition to a low-sodium diet, varying amounts of ammonium chloride (see text for details). It will be noticed that the return of a sodium load (white column) did not reach 100 per cent before the third consecutive day of sodium loading.

4:00 in the afternoon. On these hourly collected urine samples, the pH, the specific gravity, and the volume were determined. The hourly samples were then pooled and analyzed for sodium, potassium, ammonia, titratable acidity, and chloride. The urine voided from 4:00 in the afternoon until 8:00 the next morning was also pooled and subjected to the same analyses.

The students were weighed prior to the experiment and every day during the experiment at 8:00 A.M. and 4:00 P.M.

All the experiments were carried out during winter and spring, and a routine of physical activity was established to minimize extrarenal sodium loss by sweating. The methods used for the determination of the different electrolytes in serum as well as urine have been dealt with in earlier publications, to which the reader is referred.[2]

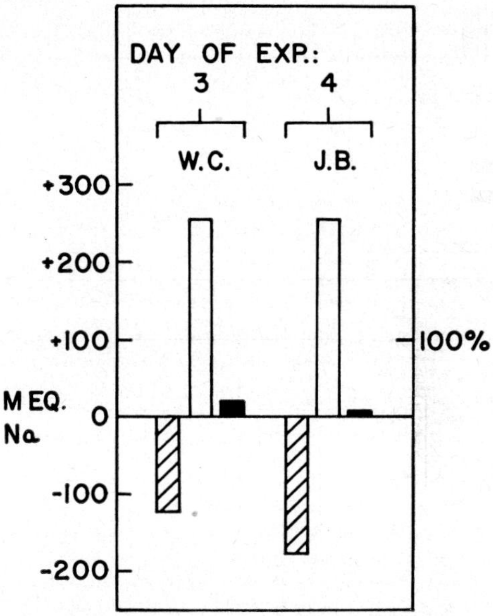

Fig. 3.—Crosshatched column: Cumulative urine sodium excretion in excess of intake from beginning of experiment until time of sodium load (milliequivalents). White column: Sodium load (milliequivalents). Black column: Return of sodium following sodium load (per cent in twenty-four hours).

The two students presented in this figure were on the third and fourth day of starvation, respectively, when they received an oral sodium load (white column). The percentage return (black column) in both cases is down, but again the one who has been deprived of sodium the longest has the lowest return following a sodium load.

RESULTS

Some of the results of sodium loading are seen in Figs. 1, 2, and 3. For each individual is shown the total urinary loss of sodium in excess of the intake in milliequivalents from the beginning of the experiment until the time the sodium load was started (crosshatched column). The negativity of the sodium balance prior to the sodium load, however, is not known exactly, since the amount of sodium lost by other routes than through the urine was not determined. Consequently, the crosshatched column can only be the smallest negative balance possible. Since, however, the daily excretion on the low-sodium diet was very close to the intake, we can assume that the amount lost by other routes was negligible.

The white column indicates the size of the sodium load in milliequivalents and the black column shows a twenty-four hour return of this load in percentage.

In Fig. 1 are represented the students on known and low-sodium diet (A to G in Table I) who were given an oral sodium load. It can readily be seen that the percentage return (black column) drops gradually in accordance with the length of time the subjects received a low sodium intake. The percentage return seems completely independent of the total sodium loss in the urine (cross-hatched column) and of the magnitude of the load (white column).

Subject S. D. (F in Table I), who received a sodium load on the ninth day of the experiment, was subjected to a second load on the tenth day. Since on the ninth day he retained practically all 265 meq. of sodium given, he probably was in positive balance on the tenth day. On this day, the percentage return was considerably higher, but he still retained more than one-half the amount given and thus increased his retention. His weight increased 600 grams on the ninth and another 600 grams on the tenth day. Serum sodium, potassium, chloride, and CO_2 did not change significantly during the entire experiment in any of these individuals.

The effect of an oral sodium load on three consecutive days given individuals who have received a low-soduim diet as well as ammonium chloride is depicted in Fig. 2. It will be seen in Table I that the subjects found under the letters O (W. L.), P (W. C.), and Q (R. M.) received, during the time they were subjected to the sodium load, ammonium chloride in different dosages. Subjects W. L. and W. C. received increasing amounts of ammonium chloride, while subject R. M. was unchanged on a 10 Gm. daily intake after the fifth day. The total amount of sodium lost in the urine in excess of the intake is considerably higher than that which is found in the individuals who were on a low-sodium diet only. The amount of potassium lost was equally high and also much greater than that found in the persons who received a low-sodium diet only. The percentage return in the student who received the lowest dosage of ammonium chloride is somewhat of the same magnitude as the one found in the subject receiving a low-sodium diet only for the same number of days. However, the weight increase was considerably higher, amounting to 1,100 Gm. The two students receiving an increasing amount of ammonium chloride both showed a slightly higher return of the sodium load; the weight increase for Subject W. L., however, also amounted to 1,100 Gm., while Subject W. C. showed a weight gain of only 400 Gm. It will be noted in Fig. 2 that the sodium load given on the sixth day was in all three cases too small to replace the total amount of sodium lost in the urine in excess of the intake. Increased return was found on the seventh day, and on the eighth day it was approximately 100 per cent in all three individuals. R. M. showed a weight increase, on the seventh day, of 800 Gm. Subject W. L. exhibited a weight gain of 300 Gm. and Subject W. C. of

600 Gm. In both of these latter cases, the return of sodium was such that it practically equaled the total amount of sodium the subjects had lost in the urine during the entire experiment in excess of the intake, while R. M. had a positive balance of approximately 135 meq. The following day, a third sodium load of the same magnitude was given the same three individuals, the result of which is seen in the third section of Fig. 2. Only Subject R. M. showed a slight weight increase of 100 grams, while Subject W. L. lost 900 grams and Subject W. C. 1,300 grams.

Serum sodium and potassium in those individuals who received a low-sodium diet as well as a daily intake of ammonium chloride were practically unchanged during the whole experiment. The CO_2 dropped steadily and was, on the last day, 18 and 19 meq. per liter in Subjects W. L. and W. C., respectively, and 24 meq. per liter in Subject R. M.

The effect of an oral sodium load given two individuals who had starved for two and three days, respectively, is finally shown in Fig. 3. Subject W. C. (T in Table I) received on the third day of starvation a sodium load, which, as can be seen, was considerably higher than the total amount of sodium lost in the urine in excess of the intake. The percentage return of the sodium load was only approximately 20 per cent. In J. B. (U in Table I), who received a similar amount of sodium, the return was even less than one-half of that seen in Subject W. C. Both of these subjects lost 1,100 grams.

The students who were on starvation showed practically no change in serum sodium or potassium during the period of the experiment. In none of the individuals who were given a water load (Table I) was any difficulty found in inducing water diuresis. However, it should be emphasized that water loads were only given prior to sodium loads or after signs of sodium retention had ceased.

Finally, one subject, K (Table I), was, after eight days of a low sodium intake, given 15 Gm. of ammonium chloride during one day. The serum sodium prior to this ammonium chloride load was identical with the serum sodium found on the day the experiment started (137 meq. per liter). However, the next day it had dropped to 132 meq. per liter and the following day it dropped to 123 meq. per liter. The minute amount of sodium excreted in the urine on the day of the ammonium chloride load was practically unchanged. while the following day it increased 9 meq. The potassium excretion, however, increased 37 meq. The excretion per minute the day following the ammonium chloride load was for sodium, 26 microequivalents per minute, which was an increase of 23 microequivalents per minute, and for potassium 94 microequivalents per minute, which was an increase of 41 microequivalents per minute.

DISCUSSION AND CONCLUSION

The results obtained in this study seem to confirm the observation by Black, Platt, and Stanbury[4] pointing to an obligatory sodium retention in persons who have been on a low-sodium diet for a certain length of time. The results obtained here, however, also seem to indicate clearly that the percentage return decreases gradually as time goes on. It is, however, very important to notice that the return is down to approximately 20 per cent after only two days of low sodium intake.

It is of interest also to notice that as little as two to three days of starvation is sufficient to decrease the percentage return of a sodium load to something in the order of 10 to 20 per cent. This again may mean that a patient can very easily run the risk of developing a sodium retention prior to an operation.

It is difficult to explain why the percentage return of a sodium load is higher as the ammonium chloride load is increased. Since, however, the ammonia excretion in the urine, which in these cases is already high, does not rise immediately, and since the chloride excretion gradually increases, one may suggest that sodium and potassium are excreted possibly in order to neutralize the excess acid until the ammonia production is adequate to prevent further loss of base. Although only one student was given an ammonium chloride load on the ninth day of his low sodium intake, this experiment seemed to indicate that when no adaptation has taken place, such a sudden acid load can lead to a rather dramatic drop in serum sodium. The mechanism which brings this about is probably to be found in derangement in the cells, since neither the weight change (decrease) nor the sodium excretion can explain such a drop in serum sodium. The increased excretion of potassium, which was in excess of the increase in sodium excretion, also seems to indicate an exchange of potassium for sodium in the cells. Although such an exchange may also take place when a person on a normal diet is given ammonium chloride, it seems as if adequate amounts of sodium are available to prevent any drop in serum sodium. However, this might not be the case in a person who has been on a low-sodium diet for some period of time.

It is surprising to notice that the weight increase found following a sodium load when the percentage return is low is in no way equal to the amount of sodium retained. For instance, S. D. (Fig. 1, F in Table I) on the ninth day of the low-sodium diet was given 265 meq. of sodium, of which he retained practically everything, yet the weight increase was only 600 grams. Since there was no considerable increase in potassium excretion, it must be concluded that the greater amount of sodium must have been deposited in cells or extracellular solids in such a way that it has been deprived of its osmotic activity.

In conclusion, it can be said that if a person is subjected to a restricted sodium intake, his ability to excrete sodium diminishes rapidly, leaving him after a couple of days in a condition where he may be unable to excrete larger amounts of sodium. Unless one is forced to restrict sodium, as in cases of hypertension or heart conditions, it would seem very undesirable to restrict the sodium intake of a patient preoperatively for any length of time, since this may only aggravate a possible postoperative salt retention. On the contrary, it seems indicated to make certain that a patient preoperatively is getting adequate amounts of sodium (as well as potassium) since this may also prevent any extensive drop in serum sodium induced by the stress itself.

SUMMARY

Sodium deficiency was established in twenty-one male medical students.

The first group of students received a low-sodium diet for a varying number of days.

The second group of students received in addition to a low sodium diet a daily intake of 10 to 20 Gm. of ammonium chloride.

The third group of students was starved for three to four days.

The percentage return of an oral sodium load in all three groups showed a gradual drop depending on the length of time they had been subjected to a low sodium intake. The return was independent of the magnitude of the sodium load as well as of the total amount of sodium lost in the urine prior to the load.

It is emphasized that only two days of starvation is sufficient to lower the return of a sodium load to 25 per cent of the normal. The possible significance of these findings for the surgeon in the preparation of a patient for surgery is discussed.

REFERENCES

1. Schlegel, J. U., Anderson, F. W., Madsen, P. O., and Betheil, J. J.: The Altered Response to Sodium Loading in Several Severely Burned Individuals After Initial Treatment With Hypertonic Sodium Containing Fluids. To be published.
2. Schlegel, J. U., Parry, W. L., Betheil, J. J., and Bloch, A. L.: A Study of the Relationship Between pH of the Urine and Sodium and Potassium Excretion, Proc. Soc. Exper. Biol. & Med. **84**: 223, 1953.
3. Schlegel, J. U.: A New Approach to the Treatment of Electrolyte Disturbances in Shock and Severe Stress, Surgery **35**: 449, 1954.
4. Black, D. A. K., Platt, R., and Stanbury, S. W.: Regulation of Sodium Excretion in Normal and Salt-Depleted Subjects, Clin. Sc. **9**: 205, 1950.

THE USE OF ARFONAD IN A MODIFICATION OF THE TECHNIQUE OF CONTROLLED HYPOTENSION

DAVID M. LITTLE, JR., M.D., L. JENNINGS HAMPTON, M.D., AND DORIS C. GROSSKREUTZ, M.D., NEW HAVEN, CONN.

(From the Section on Anesthesiology, Yale University School of Medicine, and the Department of Anesthesiology, Grace-New Haven Community Hospital)

THE problem of excessive bleeding during surgical interventions is scarcely a new one, and for many years a number of anesthetists and surgeons have found a solution in the use of chloroform anesthesia, high spinal analgesia, or the meticulous posturing of the patient so that the operative site might remain superior. In 1946 Gardner[1] introduced the technique of arteriotomy, whereby blood is withdrawn from the patient preoperatively via the arterial route, and then replaced, in part or in toto, by the same manner at the end of surgery. Such preoperative reduction of the total circulating blood volume by the removal of from 500 to 3,000 c.c. of blood serves to lower the arterial pressure to a systolic level of 50 to 90 mm. Hg, and at the same time produces peripheral vasoconstriction[2]; when combined with the proper positioning of the patient, the net result is a reduction of bleeding at the site of surgery. Arteriotomy thus exactly approximates a state of hemorrhagic shock. A more physiologic approach to the problem was contained in Gillies' classic studies in 1948 on total sympathetic blockade.[3] In this method, the blood pressure is reduced to a level of 70 mm. Hg or below by the use of spinal anesthesia to achieve paralysis of the entire efferent sympathetic outflow, with lesser degrees of sensory and motor blockade. Gillies has admitted that even this technique is without doubt "physiologic trespass,"[4] but has assumed that the arteriolar dilatation so produced guarantees normal oxygenation of the tissue cells, and that the decreased cardiac output inherent in the technique is compensated for by the decreased peripheral resistance and, therefore, the decreased work of the heart. Proper posturing of the patient is again an essential feature for the control of bleeding as it is, indeed, in all methods of "controlled hypotension." The introduction of easily injectable ganglionic-blocking agents in the form of the methonium compounds in 1948[5, 6] led to the widespread usage of hexamethonium and, to a lesser extent, pentamethonium, to lower the blood pressure to systolic levels of 50 to 60 mm. Hg and thus control excessive vascular bleeding in the operative field.[7, 8]

There can be little doubt, from the alarming warnings which have been sounded on the subject,[9-12] that certain fatal and nonfatal complications resulting from the use of the technique have been far more common than was previously supposed. Hampton and Little, polling the anesthetists of Great

We wish to express our gratitude to the Medical Department of Hoffmann-La Roche Inc., Nutley, New Jersey, for the generous supplies of the Arfonad employed in these studies.

Received for publication, Aug. 5, 1953.

Britain and Ireland, obtained reports of over 21,000 cases of controlled hypotension in anesthesia. The results of this questionnaire form the basis of a separate report,[15] but suffice it to say for the present that there was a total of 653 complications and forty-six associated mortalities among the 21,000 cases reported. Furthermore, it has become very clear that the morbidities and mortalities associated with the use of these techniques have been directly related to the extent of the reduction of the blood pressure from the preoperative normal.

Nevertheless, there also can be no doubt that there are valuable contributions to patient welfare to be derived from controlled hypotension, and that when wisely employed, in the carefully selected case. for an urgent and rational indication, the technique may prove markedly beneficial for the individual patient. Certain definite advantages may accrue from the use of controlled hypotension in anesthesia. Blood loss is tremendously reduced and the patient's own blood thereby conserved, mitigating the need for transfusions with the attendant risks of reaction. Control of vascular ooze provides the surgeon with a clear, almost dry, operating field: this is of utmost concern in an operation such as the Lempert fenestration procedure, in which one drop of blood during the critical maneuver of shaping the fenestra may obscure the entire operative field and prevent a successful result. Finally, the control of hemorrhage, in such operations as the excision of highly vascular intracranial lesions and in certain radical dissections elsewhere in the body, may be essential to surgical success, and operation may be totally unfeasible in the absence of such control.

A MODIFIED CONCEPT OF CONTROLLED HYPOTENSION

Certain important facets of the problem of induced hypotension have been elucidated from the growing body of clinical experience presently extant. First, it has become evident that the level of systolic arterial pressure which must be obtained in order to provide a relatively bloodless operative field varies tremendously with the individual patient, and the exact level to which the blood pressure must be lowered, therefore, cannot be foretold with any degree of accuracy prior to actual operation. It has frequently been advocated that the blood pressure be lowered to, say, 70 mm. Hg in order to prevent vascular ooze in the operative site. Yet in point of fact, in a given patient the blood loss may be controlled only when the arterial pressure has been reduced to 65 mm. Hg; or, conversely, it may be controlled with an arterial pressure as high as 100 mm. Hg. The level that it is necessary to attain can be determined only under conditions of actual operation after suitable posturing of the patient and by direct observation of the bleeding, or lack of it, in the operative field itself. Second, as has just been suggested, this level of optimal pressure is often much higher than the dangerously low systolic pressures of 50 to 60 mm. Hg sought by the earlier workers in this field. Indeed, a significant reduction of the blood loss from the surgical wound is frequently noted at pressures of 90 to 100 mm. Hg, which may represent a lowering of the arterial pressure of only 10 to 20 mm. Hg from the preoperative reading. This is of some considerable importance, inasmuch as the major complications of deliberately induced hypotension—suppression of kidney function, thromboses of various essential arterial supplies, and reactionary hemorrhage—would not be expected to occur in the absence of profound reductions of arterial pressures. Third, it is essential that the anesthetist be capable of exerting sufficient control over this deliberately produced hypotension to permit its maintenance with some degree of constancy, and yet at the same time to permit the rapid termination of hypotension at the end of surgery or the rapid abandonment of the technique in the face of inadvertent hemorrhage and similar surgical contingencies.

ARFONAD

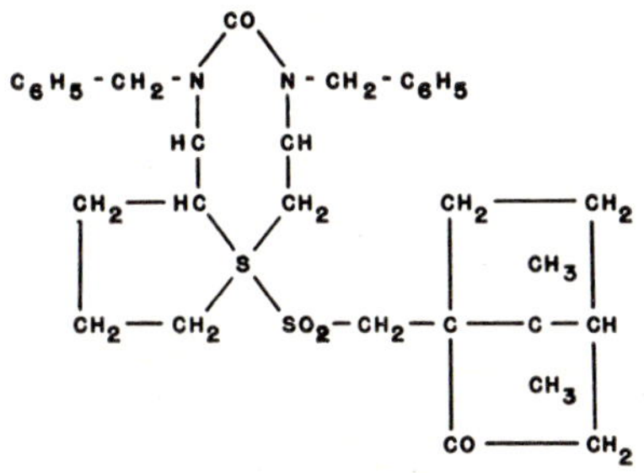

d-3,4 (1',3'-DIBENZYL-2'-KETO-IMIDAZOLIDO)-1,2-TRIMETHYLENE THIOPHANIUM d-CAMPHOR SULFONATE

Fig. 1.—Arfonad (RO 2-2222).

It is apparent, therefore, that by modifying the current practices in regard to controlled hypotension, it should be possible to obtain the advantages of reduced bleeding during operation without courting the dangers which previously have marred the clinical employment of the technique. There has been lacking a method of sufficient controllability to allow the blood pressure to be lowered gradually during the early moments of the operative procedure, so that the optimal level of the blood pressure at which bleeding in the wound was controlled could be ascertained by direct vision and then maintained by regulating the administration of the hypotensive agent at the necessary rate. This would assure utilization of the maximal level of blood pressure at which excessive bleeding could be controlled.

The introduction of Arfonad, a thiophanium compound with potent ganglionic-blocking activity, has provided the anesthetist with a thoroughly controllable and rapidly reversible method for the induction of hypotension during anesthesia. Chemically, this drug is d-3, 4 (1′3′-dibenzyl-2′-keto-imidazolido)-1, 2-trimethylene thiophanium d-camphor sulphonate (Fig. 1); it is generally referred to by the code number, RO 2-2222, or the trade name,

Arfonad. Randall, Peterson, and Lehmann[13] have reported on the ganglionic blockade and subsequent reduction of arterial pressure produced by this drug in anesthetized dogs and cats, and Sarnoff, Goodale, and Sarnoff[14] have described its use in human beings to produce peripheral vasodilatation and a graded reduction of arterial pressure in the treatment of acute pulmonary edema. It has been shown that Arfonad in single intravenous doses of 0.1 or 0.2 mg. per kilogram of body weight will produce a prompt but evanescent depressor response of the arterial pressure,[14] and it is thus possible to employ the drug by a continuous intravenous infusion technique.

TECHNIQUE

In the present study, Arfonad has been employed in surgical patients to induce a modified form of controlled hypotension for the production of a relatively bloodless surgical field. General anesthesia has been established and endotracheal intubation has been accomplished to assure a patent airway and adequate oxygenation. The endotracheal catheter, in most instances, has then been attached to a nonrebreathing valve to guarantee the removal of all excessive carbon dioxide, the accumulation of which is in itself a potent factor in the causation of excessive bleeding. Following the completion of the anesthetic induction and intubation, the patient has been positioned on the table with meticulous care to place the operative site superiorly, in order to promote venous drainage by gravity from the wound and thus check the amount of bleeding during the surgical procedure. Such posturing of the patient serves the further purpose of pooling the blood in the dilated vessels of the dependent parts of the body, and therefore provides the advantages of bloodless phlebotomy without at the same time incurring the dangerous concomitant of peripheral vasoconstriction. At this juncture the Arfonad infusion in a 0.1 per cent concentration has been started and run at a sufficiently rapid rate to evoke a substantial fall in arterial pressure. The infusion rate necessary to elicit this depressor response, and the extent of the blood pressure fall, effectively establish immediate criteria as to the general susceptibility or resistance of the patient to the drug in the individual case. Furthermore, as the arterial pressure is being lowered, repeated blood pressure readings may be correlated with the degree of vascular ooze visible in the wound in order to ascertain the all-important level of pressure which will provide control of excessive bleeding during operation. The infusion rate may then be regulated to maintain this blood pressure throughout that part of the operation during which it is desirable to control the amount of bleeding.

CLINICAL OBSERVATIONS

The assessment of these facts early in the anesthetic course is well illustrated in Fig. 2: the record of the blood pressure is depicted at the top of the chart, and that of the infusion rate below. It will be seen that three minutes after the Arfonad infusion was begun at a rate of 8 mg. per minute, the systolic pressure had been lowered from 118 mm. Hg to 74 mm. Hg, indicating a substantial susceptibility to the drug. It became clear that excessive vascular oozing was stemmed during this initial depression of the blood pressure, and the infusion rate was therefore decreased to permit the blood pressure to rise slowly. When the pressure had reattained a systolic level just above 85 mm. Hg, bleeding was once again noted in the operative site; hence, the optimal pressure was established as 85 mm. Hg. The infusion rate was subsequently regulated to maintain this level of blood pressure in order to provide a continuous dry operative field. Nine minutes later, by way of illustrating the prompt resumption of normotension, the Arfonad infusion was discontinued: it is to be noted that preoperative blood pressure had been restored within a ten- to twelve-minute interval.

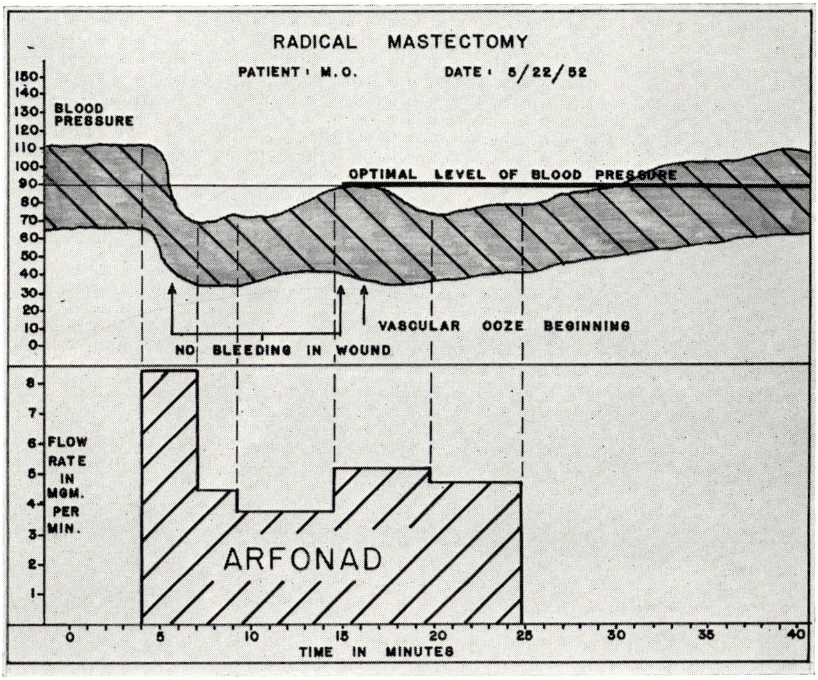

Fig. 2.—Estimation of the optimal blood pressure level at which vascular ooze can be prevented during operation. The blood pressure is lowered slowly by the administration of a dilute intravenous infusion of Arfonad until there is no further bleeding in the operative site, and is then permitted to rise slowly (by decreasing the rate of Arfonad administration) to demonstrate the level of blood pressure at which bleeding recommences.

Such controllability is depicted vividly in Fig. 3. During the initial induction of hypotension, it became evident that bleeding was well controlled at a systolic pressure of 80 mm. Hg. An attempt, therefore, was made to maintain this arterial pressure by regulating the rate of the infusion and thus in effect titrating the patient against the drug: as the infusion rate of the Arfonad solution was increased, the blood pressure fell promptly to lower levels; conversely, as the amount of Arfonad administered was decreased, there was a corresponding and prompt return of the blood pressure toward higher levels. In this manner, it was possible to achieve minute-to-minute control of both the degree and the duration of the hypotension.

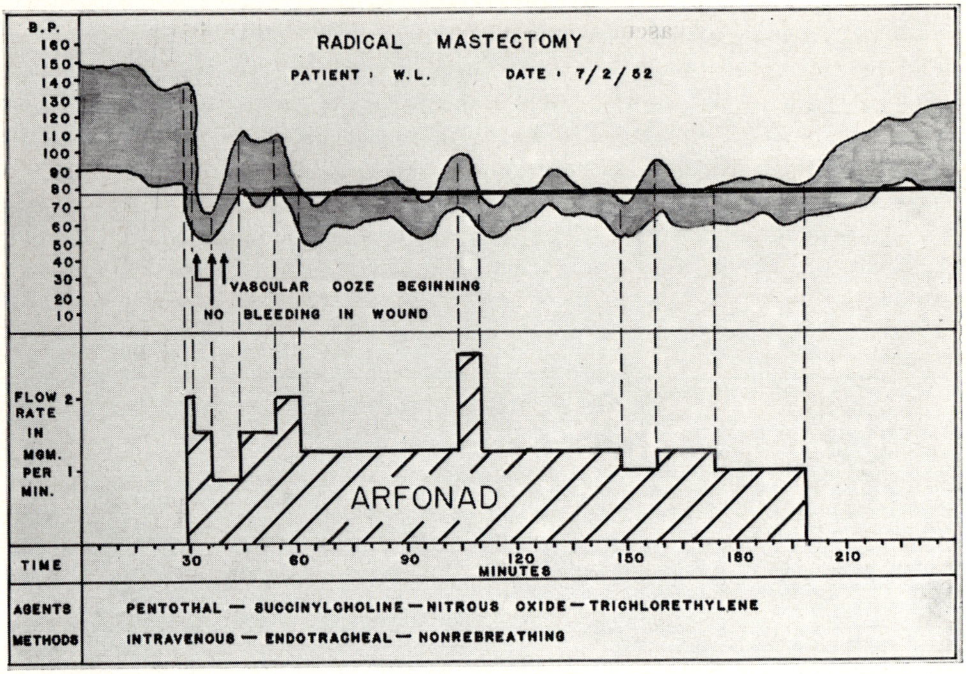

Fig. 3.—The minute-to-minute control of the level of the blood pressure is accomplished by increasing or decreasing the rate of administration of a dilute intravenous infusion of Arfonad.

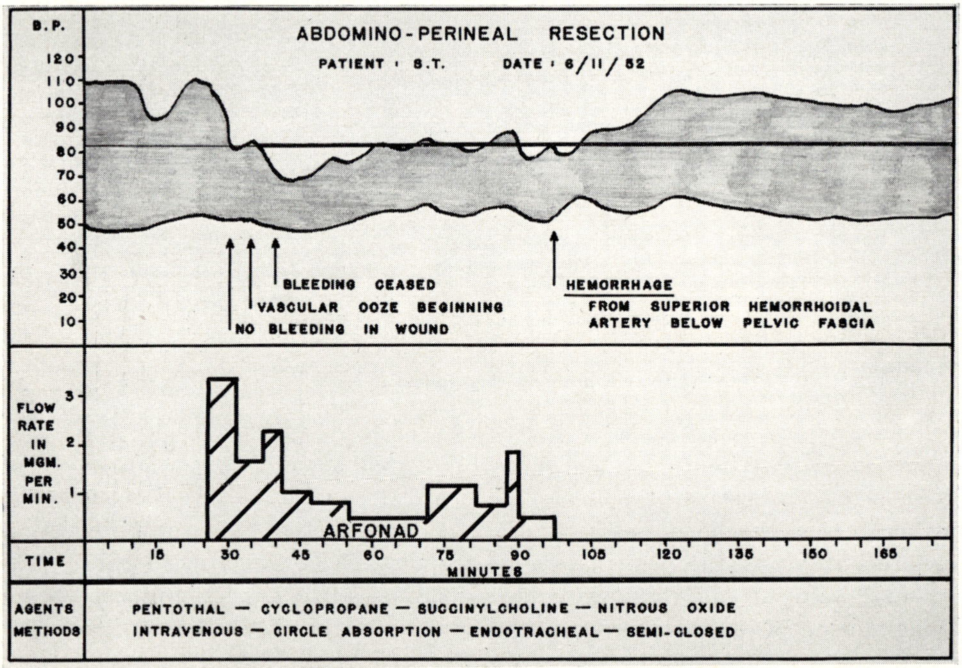

Fig. 4.—The administration of a dilute intravenous infusion of Arfonad may be terminated at the end of surgery or at any other time during operation in the event of hemorrhage or similar surgical exigency, permitting the rapid restoration of normotension.

The termination of this case reveals the advantage of such controllability at the end of surgery, when the need for the hypotensive state has passed and it is desirable to regain normotensive levels. When the infusion was discontinued, there was a prompt rise toward the preoperative blood pressure level. A similar but more dramatic aspect of the advantage of this controllability in facilitating the abandonment of the hypotensive state when necessary is illustrated in Fig. 4. Hypotension was induced, and 95 mm. Hg found to be the optimal level of the blood pressure below which excessive

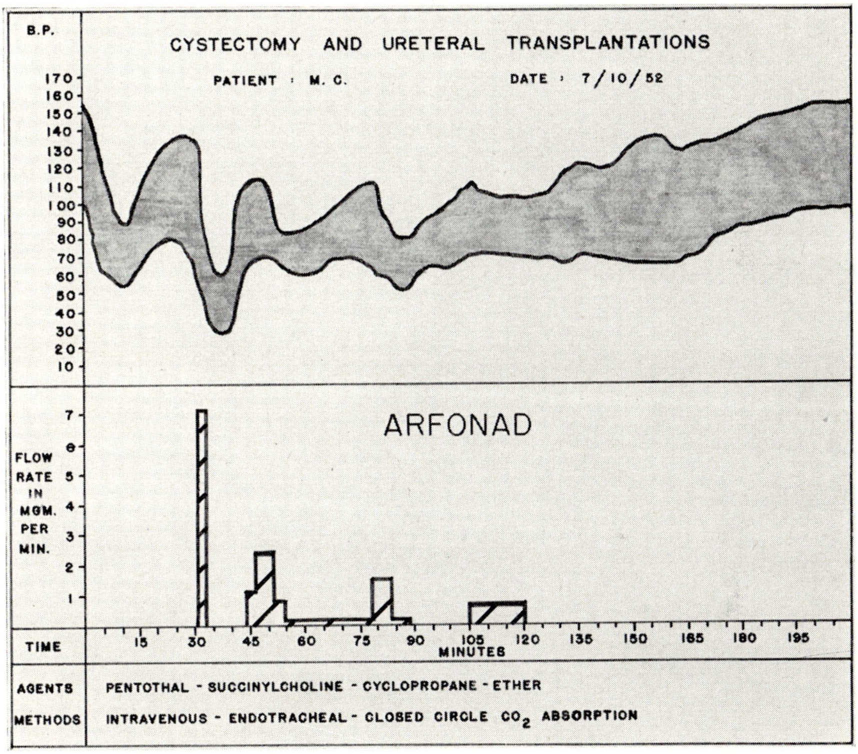

Fig. 5.—Certain patients are extremely susceptible to the intravenous administration of even dilute infusions of Arfonad, to the extent that wide and presumably dangerous swings in blood pressure occur and control becomes difficult.

vascular ooze was well controlled. This level was therefore achieved, and maintained fairly well throughout the first hour of operation. At this point, brisk hemorrhage was encountered from the superior hemorrhoidal artery. The technique of controlled hypotension assumes additional dangers in the presence of hemorrhage, since blood loss is occurring in the presence of generalized arteriolar dilatation and, hence, in the absence of the body's compensatory cardiovascular reflexes. The Arfonad infusion was therefore discontinued, the blood pressure began to rise within five minutes, and the preoperative systolic level of 110 mm. Hg was achieved within twenty minutes.

DISADVANTAGES OF ARFONAD

There are certain disadvantages to the use of Arfonad, some of which are unique to the drug itself, and some of which it shares in common with other methods of autonomic ganglion blockade employed for controlled hypotension. The inherent capacity for catastrophe that is the hallmark of all forms of induced hypotension during surgery has already been mentioned in some detail, and without question applies to the technique herein described as it does to all others. The higher blood pressure ranges utilized in this modified technique, however, and the more absolute controllability possible with Arfonad, reduce these dangers to a very considerable extent.

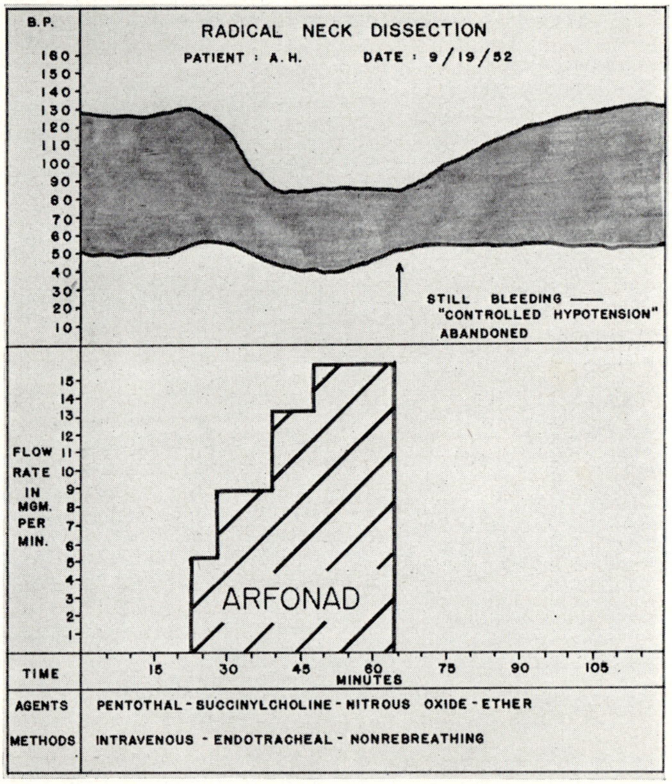

Fig. 6.—Marked resistance to the hypotensive effects of the administration of dilute intravenous infusions of Arfonad has been noted in some patients, and large amounts of the drug may fail to lower the blood pressure sufficiently below normal to effect a diminution of bleeding in the operative site.

Extreme susceptibility to the drug occurred in certain individual patients, just as it does to the methonium compounds, and such extreme susceptibility may exaggerate the technical difficulties to a marked degree. In one instance (Fig. 5), the patient's extreme susceptibility rendered control difficult, and produced wide and presumably dangerous swings in blood pressure.

On the other hand, marked degrees of resistance were encountered also, to the extent that it was occasionally impossible to induce a satisfactory degree of hypotension and concomitant control over the degree of bleeding in the operative site. Such instances of resistance have been noted frequently to the methonium compounds, particularly in the young and robust, and it remains to determine the exact incidence of such resistance to the employment of Arfonad. During the course of one operation (Fig. 6), a very rapid infusion rate and a total dosage of 500 mg. of Arfonad failed to lower the blood pressure to any marked degree or to achieve any visible reduction of the amount of bleeding in the operative site, and the technique was subsequently abandoned in this instance.

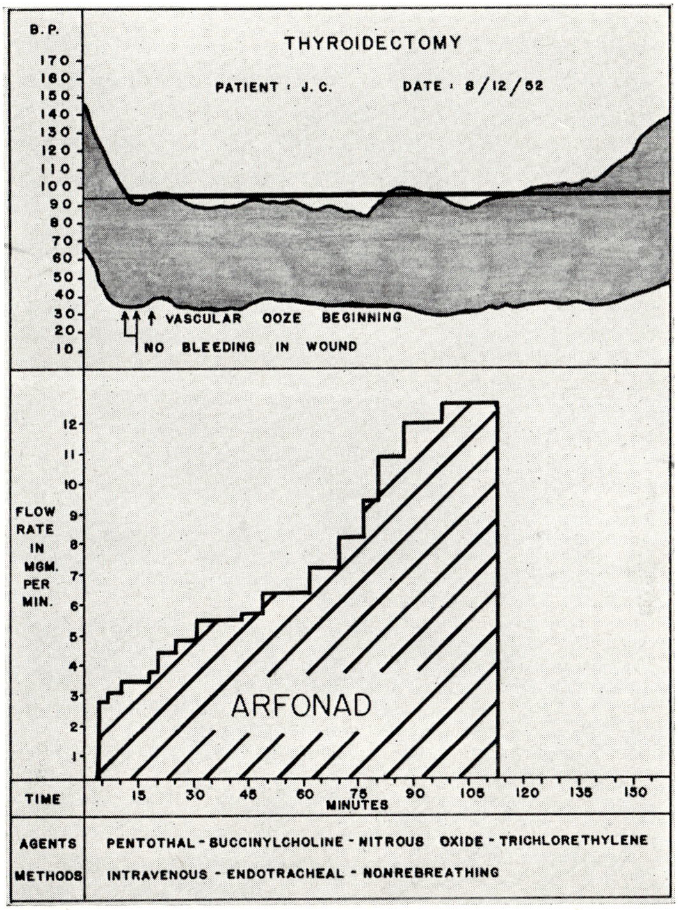

Fig. 7.—Tachyphylaxis has occurred during the intravenous administration of dilute infusions of Arfonad employed to achieve controlled hypotension. In such instances, the optimal level of blood pressure, or below, has been maintained throughout operation, but increasing dosages of the drug have been required to accomplish this.

A final disadvantage to the use of Arfonad was the development of tachyphylaxis on four occasions (Fig. 7). The initial induction of the hypotensive state, and the elucidation of the optimal blood pressure level necessary to control bleeding, were accomplished satisfactorily, but the maintenance of that level required increasingly more rapid infusion rates and hence higher total dosage of Arfonad. Such tachyphylaxis has not yet progressed to the point at which the blood pressure could not be maintained at the desired level, but this is at least a theoretical possibility.

CONCLUSIONS

Controlled hypotension to provide a bloodless operative field must be assumed to be a gravely dangerous technique, and it has become very clear that the morbidities and mortalities associated with its use are directly related to the extent of the reduction of the blood pressure from the preoperative normal. However, the use of these techniques of induced hypotension in certain specific surgical procedures has permitted successful operative intervention that would not have been possible under other circumstances.

A modified form of controlled hypotension has been evolved whereby a relatively bloodless operative field is produced at higher, and therefore presumably safer, levels of blood pressure than those that have been advocated in the past. The use of Arfonad, which possesses potent but evanescent ganglionic-blocking activity, provides a method of ascertaining the level of the systolic blood pressure at which bleeding is controlled during surgery, and further provides a means of maintaining that level with marked controllability. At the completion of surgery, or in the presence of hemorrhage or similar surgical exigency, this controllability will permit rapid reversal of arteriolar dilatation and the hypotensive state.

REFERENCES

1. Gardner, W. J.: The Control of Bleeding During Operation by Induced Hypotension, J. A. M. A. **132**: 572-573 (Nov. 9) 1946.
2. Hale, D. E.: Controlled Hypotension by Arterial Bleeding During Operation and Anesthesia, Anesthesiology **9**: 498-505 (Sept.) 1948.
3. Griffiths, H. W. C., and Gillies, J.: Thoraco-lumbar Splanchnicectomy and Sympathectomy, Anesthesia **3**: 134-146 (Oct.) 1948.
4. Gillies, J.: Physiologic Trespass in Anesthesia, Proc. Roy. Soc. Med. **45**: 1-6 (Jan.) 1952.
5. Barlow, R. B., and Ing, H. R.: Curare-like Action of Polymethylene bis-Quarternary Ammonium Salts, Nature **161**: 718 (May 8) 1948.
6. Paton, W. D. M., and Zaimis, E. J.: Curare-like Action of Polymethylene bis-Quarternary Ammonium Salts, Nature **161**: 718 (May 8) 1948.
7. Davison, M. H. A.: Pentamethonium Iodide in Anesthesia, Lancet **1**: 252-255 (Feb. 11) 1950.
8. Enderby, G. E. H.: Controlled Circulation With Hypotensive Drugs and Posture to Reduce Bleeding in Surgery, Lancet **1**: 1145-1147 (June 24) 1950.
9. Editorial, Anesthesia **7**: 65 (April) 1952.
10. Complications of Controlled Hypotension, Lancet **2**: 25 (July 5) 1952.
11. Davison, M. H. A.: Hypotension, Anesthesia **7**: 116-118 (April) 1952.
12. Editorial: Methonium-Controlled Hypotension in Surgery, J. A. M. A. **151**: 129 (Jan. 10) 1953.
13. Randall, L. P., Peterson, W. G., and Lehmann, G.: The Ganglionic Blocking Action of Thiophanium Derivatives, J. Pharmacol. & Exper. Therap. **97**: 48-57 (Sept.) 1949.
14. Sarnoff, S. J., Goodale, W. T., and Sarnoff, L. C.: Graded Reduction of Arterial Pressure in Man by Means of a Thiophanium Derivative, Circulation **6**: 63-73 (July) 1952.
15. Hampton, L. J., and Little, D. M., Jr.: The Results of a Questionnaire Concerning the Use of Controlled Hypotension in Anesthesia, Lancet **1**: 1299-1300 (June 27) 1953.

TRANSPLANTATION OF THE SAPHENOUS VEIN FOR POSTPHLEBITIC STASIS

RICHARD WARREN, M.D.,* AND THEODORE R. THAYER, M.D.,**
BOSTON, MASS.

(From the Veterans Administration Hospital, Boston)

IN RECENT years, vigorous surgical attacks have been made on various parts of the venous system of the lower extremity in order to improve the lot of individuals suffering from postphlebitic stasis. Superficial femoral vein interruption,[1] popliteal vein interruption,[2] interruption or ligation of communicating veins,[3] or of elements of the saphenous system, alone or in combination, have been recommended with varying degrees of reported success. Femoral vein interruption, although still advocated by some, was the subject of a lukewarm supplementary report by its original supporters,[4] and the initial reports on popliteal vein interruption have not been enthusiastic. Favorable results of such surgery have been reported by Linton,[5] who, using a combination of attacks in increasingly radical operations, has found a large percentage of ulcers to have healed. A significant part of his recommended therapy, however, is the provision of adequate elastic support following surgery.

The concept of removal or interruption of damaged veins arises from the commonly observed excellent results afforded by obliteration of the saphenous veins of patients with varicosities of that system but with intact deep veins. It is entirely possible, however, that deep veins with incompetent valves may not permit such unimpeded backflows as occur in valveless superficial skin veins. Furthermore, it has been suggested that, despite a marked degree of insufficiency during diastole of the "venous heart of the lower extremity" (muscular relaxation of the calf), the integrity of continuity of a principal deep vein may still be important to the lower extremity, since no other main channel may exist for outflow during the systolic calf contraction.

Venous pressures in the skin veins of the calf do not decrease more markedly in postphlebitic syndrome after superficial femoral vein interruption than before it,[6, 7] and in certain instances the postinterruption pressures have been found to have altered in an unfavorable direction.

In light of the unpredictable results following such surgical procedures as have been listed, it seems logical to search for a means of attack which would provide new or improved channels of venous return rather than to concentrate entirely on destruction of possibly useless, but probably harmless, ones already existing. In March, 1949, therefore, a transplantation of the saphenous vein was performed to the muscular compartment of the thigh of

Received for publication, Oct. 13, 1953.

*Chief, Surgical Service, Veterans Administration Hospital, West Roxbury, Mass., and Lecturer on Surgery, Harvard Medical School, Boston.

**Resident in Surgery, Veterans Administration Hospital, Boston.

a 48-year-old man apparently suffering from postphlebitic syndrome as a result of phlebitis following a back injury six months before. The saphenous vein was completely freed throughout the thigh, all branches being divided, leaving it, however, attached to the femoral vein above and to its connections to the calf below. It was then buried over as great an extent as possible beneath the deep aponeurosis of the medial aspect of the thigh. Following the procedure the walking venous pressure showed improved function by a 14 cm. further fall during walking over the preoperative value, and phlebography showed the vein to have remained patent. Despite the fact that in this case a later phlebogram disconcertingly revealed a relatively normal original femoral vein, it is believed that the patient's steady clinical improvement since that time was at least partially due to his ability to use more effectively the saphenous transplant in the thigh. It is assumed that the area of greatest postphlebitic damage in this patient was in the calf veins. Since that time thirteen additional similar operations have been performed.

TECHNIQUE

An incision is made on the medial face of the thigh from groin to knee over the course of the previously identified internal saphenous vein. The vein is carefully freed from all its attachments other than those to the femoral vein above and to the calf veins below. All branches are ligated flush with the main vein.

In the cases reported, one of two general forms of operation was then undertaken. In the first form, the saphenous vein, so freed, was transplanted to the muscular compartment of the thigh without surgical manipulation (Fig. 1, *A*). In the second form, the same transplantation was accomplished but, in addition, the vein was divided at the knee and an anastomosis performed between the proximal segment of the saphenous and the distal segment of the divided popliteal vein (Fig. 1, *B*).

Incision of the aponeurosis between the adductor muscles of the thigh and the extensors of the knee exposes the femoral vessels and permits the saphenous vein to be transplanted to lie alongside them. The aponeurosis is closed over it taking care to avoid kinks in the transplant. In the last three of the seven transplants which were performed without an anastomosis, the sartorius muscle was divided and resutured over the transplanted vein, thereby allowing the latter to be buried over a longer distance in the thigh than in the earlier cases. In the case of the transplants with anastomosis, the freed long saphenous vein was divided at the level of the knee and the distal cut end of the proximal segment drawn through under the sartorius muscle into the popliteal space, where, having dissected out and divided the popliteal vein, an anastomosis between the distal cut end of the proximal segment of the saphenous vein and the proximal cut end of the distal segment of the popliteal vein was carried out. In five of the seven cases in which this was done, the remaining saphenous vein in the calf was excised either by stripping or by direct excision. In the other two cases, the proximal cut end of the distal segment was simply ligated. The distal cut end of the proximal segment of the popliteal vein was ligated in all cases. The transplanted saphenous vein was in most of the cases brought around, or medial to, the tendon of the adductor magnus rather than through the muscular canal, where there seemed to be little room for it unless created by a traumatic dissection. The popliteal vein in all cases

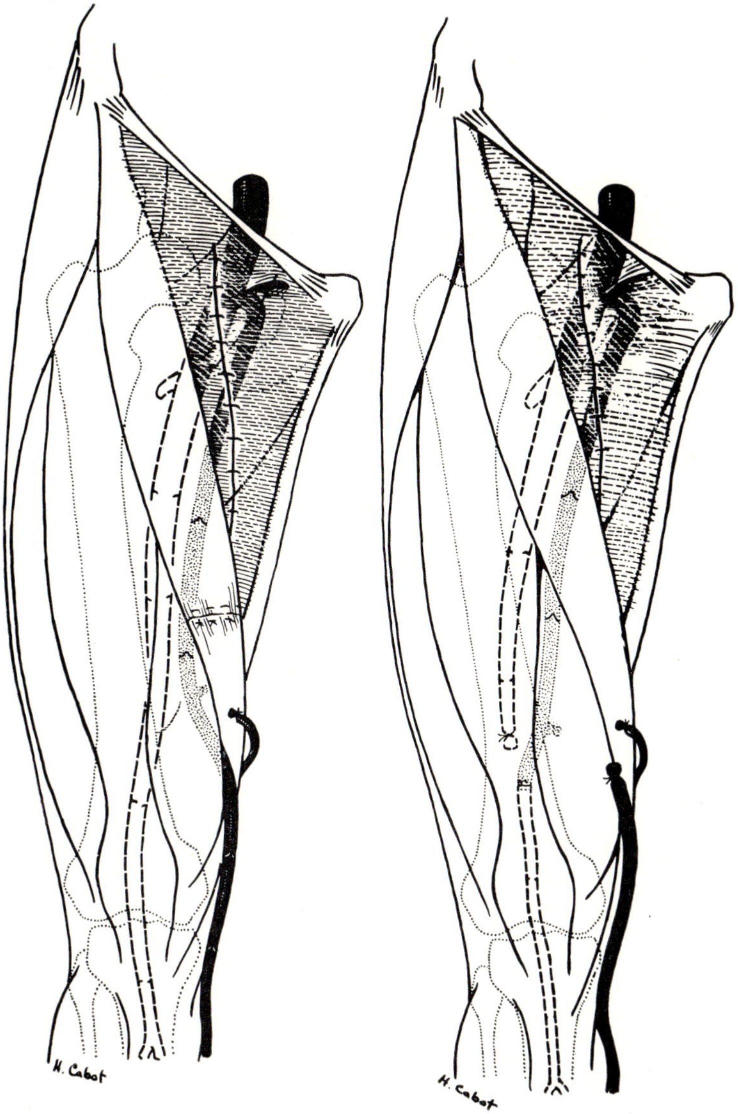

A. *B.*

Fig. 1.—Diagram of disposition of saphenous vein following transplant. *A*, Without saphenopopliteal anastomosis. *B*, With saphenopopliteal anastomosis.

showed evidence of recanalization, a feature which made the anastomosis difficult and may be a reason for failure in some. In all instances but one, the saphenous vein was anastomosed to the whole circumference of the popliteal vein, which in its recanalized state presented two or more lumens. In one

Table I. Case Summaries of Saphenous Vein Transplants: Operative Details

Patient	Sartorius muscle divided	Saphenopopliteal anastomosis	Femoral vein divided	Popliteal vein divided	Saphenous vein excised in calf	Regional heparinization	Length of follow-up (mo.)	Clinical result	Walking venous pressure result	Venographic result
J. M. D.	0	0	0	0	0	0	48	Improved	Improved	Open
T. V.	0	0	+	0	0	0	48	Unimproved*	Worse	Open
E. F. W.	0	0	+	0	0	0	42	Improved	Not carried out	Open
E. F. G.	0	0	0	0	0	0	6	Improved†	Improved	Open
J. J. B.	+	0	+	0	0	0	6	Improved‡	Improved	Open
E. E. M.	+	0	+	0	0	0	6	Improved§	Improved	Open
J. E. McA.	+	0	0	0	0	0	30	Unimproved‖	Improved	Open
C. A. M.	0	+	0	+	0	+	27	Improved	Same	Open
A. McG.	0	+	0	+	+	+	24	Improved	Improved	Questionable
D. M.	0	+	+	+	+	+	23	Unimproved¶	Improved	Not visualized
A. R.	0	+	0	+	0	+	22	Improved	Improved	Not visualized
A. A.	0	+	0	+	+	+	17	Improved	Same	Questionable
H. R. C.	0	+	+	+	+	+	15	Unimproved¶	Improved	Not visualized
F. J. I.	0	+	+	+	+	+	12	Improved	Worse	Not visualized

*Recently (April 23, 1953) had further surgery—saphenopopliteal anastomosis and excision of calf varices.
†Died of "cerebral hemorrhage" ten months postoperatively.
‡Further (three-year) follow-up report (patient not seen) is that he is working full time in restaurant.
§Died twenty-two months postoperatively—coronary heart disease with myocardial infarction.
‖Recently (Feb. 24, 1953) had further surgery—saphenopopliteal anastomosis and excision of calf varices.
¶Femoral vein divided at previous operation.

case, a thick partition separated a large lumen from a very small one, and here the saphenous vein was sutured to the large lumen alone, the smaller lumen being obliterated by sutures.

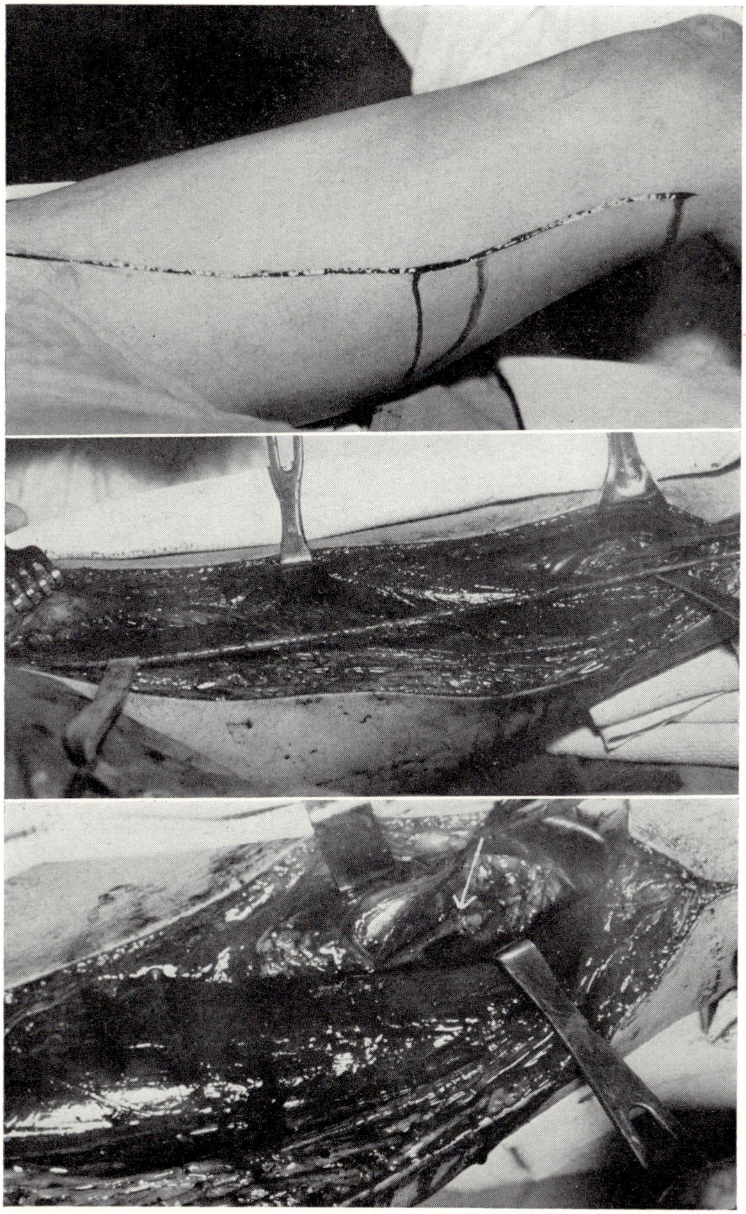

A.

B.

C.

Fig. 2.—Photographs of operative procedure with saphenopopliteal anastomosis. *A*, Incision. *B*, Prepared saphenous vein. *C*, Anastomosis of saphenous and popliteal veins.

Regional heparinization was used in all the seven patients in whom an anastomosis was performed. One hundred milligrams of heparin in a twenty-four hour period (approximately one-third the amount necessary to maintain systemic "heparinization") was dripped into a polyethelene catheter tied into the short saphenous vein near the popliteal vein. This twenty-four hour ration was in most cases given in 1,500 c.c. of fluid.

RESULTS

A summary of the results is provided in Table I.

Evaluation of Clinical Results.—Ten of the fourteen patients demonstrated improvement at the time of follow-up examination in that those who had had ulcers showed them to be still healed or, having recurred, had done so with less severity and often a longer period of freedom than had been the case preoperatively. In those who had not suffered from ulcers, the criteria for improvement were diminution in dermatitis or edema. No patient was cured.

The good clinical results were distributed evenly between the two types of operation. The results in the group with anastomosis are open to some criticism as an evaluation of the transplanting procedure itself, since procedures other than transplantation were carried out at the same time. Popliteal vein division was, of course, performed in all seven, and in the majority the saphenous vein in the calf was simultaneously excised because of the existence of large varices. Furthermore, one might state that in the cases in which the transplanted vein was not proved to be patent an effect similar to obliteration of that vein was produced, a matter which would appeal to the supporters of obliteration operations.

TABLE II. WALKING VENOUS PRESSURE BEFORE AND AFTER SAPHENOUS TRANSPLANTATION

PATIENT	PREOPERATIVE VALUE* (CM.)	POSTOPERATIVE VALUE (CM.)	CHANGE (CM.)	RESULT
J. M. D.	+2	-20	-22	Improved
T. V.	-3	+5	+8	Worse
E. F. W.	-7	Not carried out		
E. F. G.	-10	-25	-15	Improved
J. J. B.	-14	-28	-14	Improved
E. E. M.	-1	-14	-13	Improved
J. E. McA.	-16	-19	-3	Same
C. A. M.	-1	0	+1	Same
A. McG.	+3	0	-3	Same
D. M.	-5	-23	-18	Improved
A. R.	-3	-19	-16	Improved
A. A.	-8	-8	0	Same
H. R. C.	-3	-8	-5	Improved
F. J. I.	-7	0	+7	Worse

*The figures represent the change in pressure in the saphenous vein of the calf during walking from that existent when the individual was standing quietly erect.

Evaluation of Walking Venous Pressures.—Table II lists the values for walking venous pressures observed pre- and postoperatively. Pressures were recorded in the internal saphenous venous system as described by one of us (R. W.) and co-workers in 1949.[6] In seven of the cases, the changes in walking venous pressure toward improvement or unimprovement conformed with the clinical results observed. In seven cases in all, the changes were in the direction of improvement. It is to be noted that in Table II no case was classified

A.

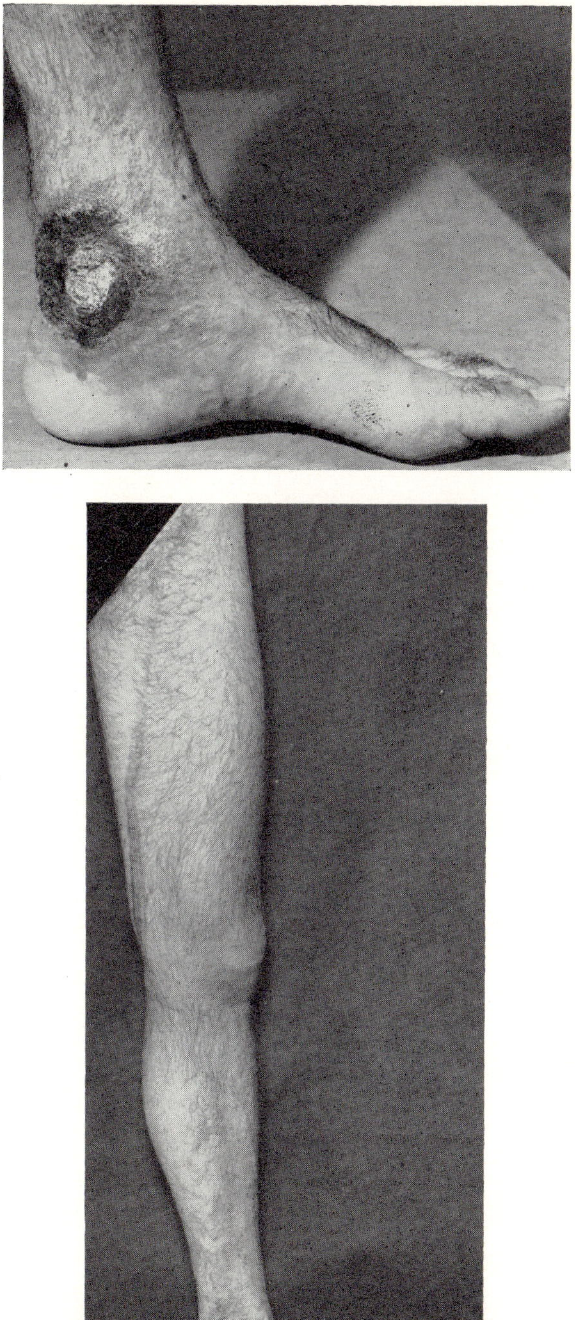

B.

Fig. 3. (Case C. A. M.).—*A*, Ulceration of medial aspect of left ankle before operation. *B*, Healed incision and area of healed ulcer twenty-seven months after saphenous transplant with saphenopopliteal anastomosis.

as improved or unimproved unless the change over the preoperative value was more than 5 cm. It is our opinion that the walking venous pressure test, being an objective means of evaluation, is more indicative of the function of the venous return of the extremity than is the clinical result, which can be affected by the activity of the patient and the care with which he uses elastic support.

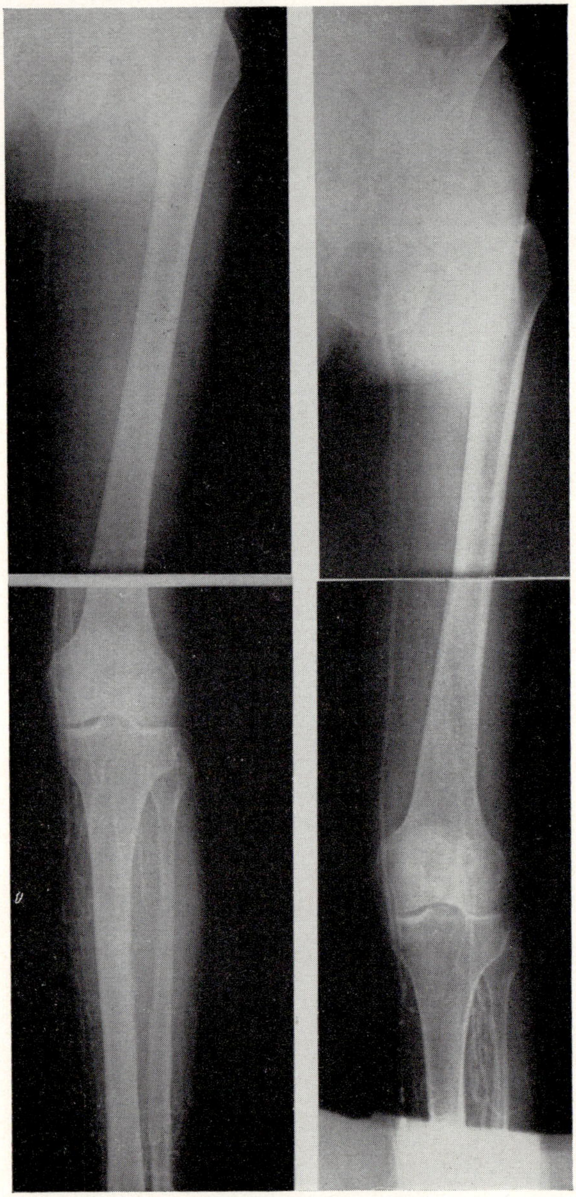

A. B.

Fig. 4 (Case E. F. W.).—Transplantation of saphenous vein without anastomosis. *A*, Preoperative phlebogram. *B*, Postoperative phlebogram illustrating transplanted saphenous vein.

Evaluation of Phlebograms.—Pre- and postoperative phlebograms were made in all cases. In the seven patients who had saphenous transplants without anastomosis, the transplants were readily recognized as being patent postoperatively in all (Fig. 4). In the seven patients who had transplants with anastomosis, the phlebograms were equivocal. In patients with venous stasis, many skin veins exist in the popliteal area, any one of which may be mistaken for the transplanted vein. In some of the patients with anastomosis, an apparently patent saphenous transplant was seen, but the area of the anastomosis was narrow or invisible. In only one of the seven can it be said that a definitely patent anastomosis was seen.

Complications.—In two patients, there were major complications. In one, the medial skin flap became necrotic over a strip 10 cm. long and 3 cm. wide. Eventual healing without disability occurred. In another patient, the symptoms and signs of venous stasis became acutely worse shortly after discharge from the hospital twenty-one days after operation. Dilated skin veins and massive edema appeared. It is probable that a recurrence of deep phlebitis with extension into collaterals has supervened. This patient is one of our poor late results on all counts.

COMMENT

The principle of the operation described is not a new one. Katzenstein[8] in 1911 stated that he had for two years been performing an operation which transplants the largest veins into the deep lying musculature, and stated that an Italian surgeon had been performing a similar one. Apparently Katzenstein contrived a channel in the sartorius muscle by folding its edges together. He stated that the symptomatic results were very good even when the calf veins did not entirely disappear. It is apparent from the article that he did not differentiate between disease of the saphenous system alone and that which resulted from disease of the deep system. Numbers of cases are not given, and later reports have not been discovered.

It is appropriate to discuss the possible directions in which future progress in this field might be made. Since the disease in many patients lies more in the calf than in the thigh, thought should be directed toward applying the principle of this type of operation at points more distal than has been done in the cases described. Since an important concept behind the operation as performed is that in postphlebitic syndrome the majority of saphenous trunks in the thigh maintain their valves, further attempts should be made to ascertain whether this is so. Heretofore, fear of thrombosis has deterred manipulation or injection of the transplant to an extent which would provide this information. If such is not the case, free transplantation of healthy valved veins from elsewhere in the body must be considered. The problem of maintaining rapid blood flow through the anastomosis is a real one. More rapid infusion with dilute heparin solution than has been reported should, we believe, be used.

SUMMARY

1. A report is made of fourteen patients with postphlebitic syndrome who were treated by transplantation of the internal saphenous vein of the thigh

from the subcutaneous to the subaponeurotic area. In one-half of the patients, concomitant anastomosis of the lower end of the saphenous vein to the popliteal vein was carried out, and in some of these, also, the saphenous vein was excised from the calf.

2. Ten of the fourteen patients were clinically improved.

3. Objective evaluation of the patients has been difficult. All the transplants without saphenopopliteal anastomosis were shown to be patent at phlebographic follow-up study. This was true of only one of seven patients having transplantation with anastomosis. A fair correlation between these facts and clinical and ambulatory venous pressure improvement was evident.

4. Suggestions as to causes for failure and comments on possible lines of future progress are made.

REFERENCES

1. Buxton, R. W., Ferris, J. M., Moyer, C. A., and Coller, F. A.: Surgical Treatment of Long-standing Deep Phlebitis of the Leg, SURGERY **15**: 749-756, 1944.
2. Bauer, G.: Division of Popliteal Vein in the Treatment of So-called Varicose Ulceration, Brit. M. J. **2**: 318-321 (Aug. 5) 1950.
3. Linton, R. R., and Keeley, J. K.: Postphlebitic Varicose Ulcer; Surgical Treatment With Special Reference to Communicating Veins of Lower Leg, Am. Heart. J. **17**: 27-39 (Jan.) 1939.
4. Buxton, R. W., and Coller, F. A.: Surgical Treatment of Long-standing Deep Phlebitis of the Leg. II. A Supplementary Report, SURGERY **18**: 663-669, 1945.
5. Linton, R. R.: Modern Concepts in the Treatment of Postphlebitic Syndrome With Ulceration of the Lower Extremities, Angiology **3**: 431-440 (Dec.) 1952.
6. Warren, R., White, E. A., and Belcher, C. D.: Venous Pressures in the Saphenous System in Normal, Varicose, and Postphlebitic Extremities, SURGERY **26**: 435-445 (Sept.) 1949.
7. DeCamp, P. T., Schramel, R. J., Ray, C. J., Feibleman, N. D., Ward, J. A., and Ochsner, A.: Ambulatory Venous Pressure Determinations in Postphlebitic and Related Syndromes, SURGERY **29**: 44-70, 1951.
8. Katzenstein: Berucht über die verhandlungen der deutsche gesellschaft für chirurgie XL kongress, Zentralbl. f. Chir. **38**: 116-117, 1911.

A TECHNIQUE FOR FACILITATING THE STRIPPING OF LARGE-BORE VARICOSE VEINS USING CONVENTIONAL STRIPPERS

NORMAN ROSENBERG, M.D., NEW BRUNSWICK, N. J.

(From the Vascular Services, St. Peter's General Hospital and Middlesex General Hospital)

THE technique of high ligation of the greater saphenous vein and its tributaries with stripping of the vein from groin to ankle is widely accepted at present as the preferred treatment for most patients with varicose veins of the lower extremities. When carried out in the usual case without difficulty, this technique permits the avulsion of the entire length of vein between upper and lower incisions. Quite often, because of undue tortuosity or catching of the stripping instrument in a valve or at a bifurcation, the employment of auxiliary incisions and successive segmental stripping maneuvers becomes necessary.

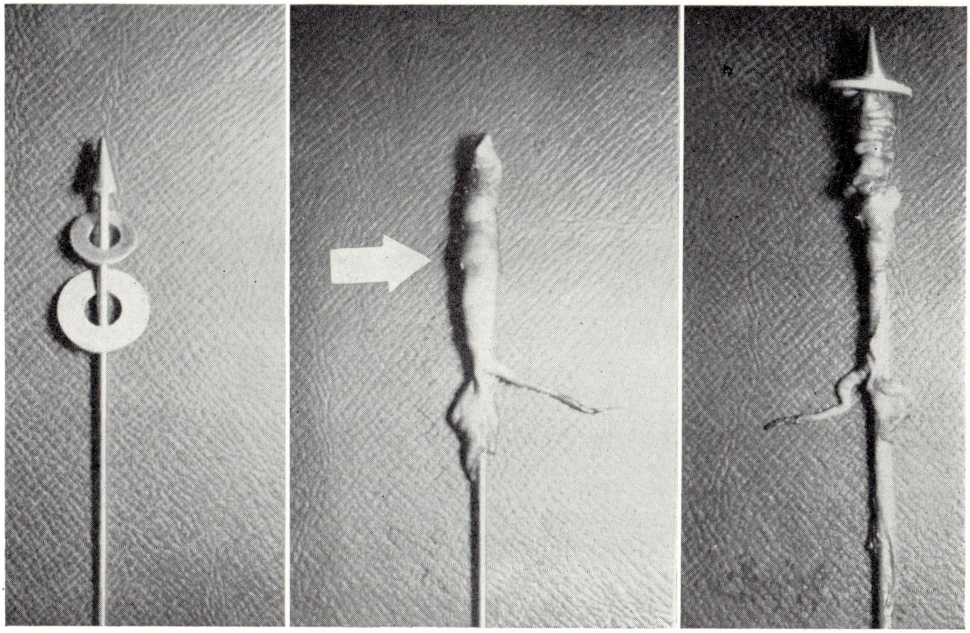

A. *B.* *C.*

Fig. 1.—

A, Babcock type of intraluminal vein stripper with metal "washers" in place near larger end of the instrument.

B, Inversion of large-bore vein by Babcock stripper (without metal washer), as instrument is pulled into lumen. Further traction (in vivo) would lead to tearing of vein. *Arrow* points to head of instrument inside vein.

C, Pleating of large-bore vein on stripping instrument with inversion of vein prevented by metal washer.

An important difficulty arises in the case of "large-bore" veins when the stripping instrument, instead of pleating the vein on itself as traction is begun, inverts the vein as the head of the instrument slips through the large,

Received for publication, Oct. 26, 1953.

distensible lumen (see Fig. 1, *B*). This may occur even though the vein is securely ligated to the instrument. Further traction, in such an eventuality, results in tearing of the vein wall, usually at the point of entrance of a tributary vein or where the wall of the vein is thin, and the stripper is drawn through with only one or two inches of vein attached. As seen in Fig. 1, *C*, this is not likely to occur if pleating of the vein along the stripper takes place, since the weakest point now becomes the tributary branch rather than the varicosed saphenous vein.

There are some stripping instruments made with detachable metal tips so that large-bore veins may be properly stripped by affixing a tip of suitable diameter. However, a conventional vein stripper of the Babcock or Linton type may also be modified by the use of ordinary metal "washers" of various sizes, which may be placed on the stripper before its introduction into the vein (see Fig. 1, *A*). Pleating of the vein is thereby assured and the likelihood of inversion obviated. These washers should preferably be of stainless or chromium-plated steel.

In a number of clinical cases with large varices this technique has proved satisfactory.

SUMMARY

A technique is described for facilitating the stripping of large-bore varicose veins, using conventional strippers.

A SUITABLE TECHNIQUE FOR TOTAL ARTERIALIZATION OF THE DOG LIVER

BERNARD FISHER, M.D.,* CLEM RUSS, PH.D., AND HARRY UPDEGRAFF, M.D.,**
PITTSBURGH, PA.

(From the Department of Surgery and the Addison H. Gibson Laboratory, Univerity of Pittsburgh)

IN ORDER to study the effects of both increased blood flow and oxygen tension on hepatic regeneration in the dog, it became necessary to evolve a technique for total arterialization that accomplished these functions satisfactorily and was relatively easy and safe to perform.

Several investigators have reported on their efforts to anastomose the hepatic artery to the portal vein, or one of its major tributaries.[1-3] For the most part, they have been unsuccessful. The most recent report of this maneuver, by Schilling,[4] indicates good results in four animals. Here, portal blood is not diverted away from the liver, so that some dilution takes place with that from the hepatic artery. To date, no quantitative data have been presented to indicate by what magnitude hepatic blood flow is actually increased by this method.

Shortly before the publication of a technique for arterialization by Cohn,[5] we began to use the method to be described here to eliminate all venous blood flow through the liver and to supply it with an increased flow of arterial blood.

TECHNIQUE

The day preceding arterialization, under Nembutal anesthesia, the left jugular vein is removed. As much length as possible is obtained (average 6 cm.). It is then stored in the icebox, in a sterile stoppered flask containing Ringer's solution and penicillin, until used.

Mongrel dogs of both sexes, ten to fifteen kilograms in weight, are anesthetized with either drop ether or intravenous Nembutal (depending on the capabilities of the anesthetist). A small sandbag, or its equivalent, is placed under the back of the animal just below the costal margin to thrust the vena cava and portal vein forward. For the best exposure, a large incision beginning at the midline below the xiphoid is extended in a gentle curve laterally to just beyond the right nipple line, and then caudad. To simplify the procedure, an adequate incision is essential. Wide retraction of the incision with a self-retaining retractor is helpful. The small and large intestines are wrapped in the duodenal mesentery and packed off to the left, thus exposing the portal vein and inferior vena cava.

Aided by Public Health Grant No. A-369.
Received for publication, Nov. 5, 1953.
*John and Mary Markle Foundation Scholar.
**Resident in surgery, Veterans Hospital, Aspinwall, Pa.

The portal vein is completely mobilized from the point of its bifurcation at the liver hilus to its origin at the junction of the superior mesenteric and splenic veins. Almost invariably, only two branches need be ligated, the coronary vein which usually enters the portal close to the hilus just below the bifurcation, and a very small fine tributary entering at about the middle of the course of the portal vein. If this is not tied, annoying bleeding is likely to occur. With proper exposure and retraction, the entire portal vein may be mobilized from its bed in a few minutes.

Temporarily, the portal vein is gently retracted to the left. This is done so as not to obstruct the flow through it or the hepatic artery. The hepatorenal ligament is severed, and the right liver lobes are retracted laterally, usually by an assistant's fingers over a sponge. The liver must not be traumatized during this procedure. The vena cava, now in full view, is clamped between the right renal vein and the liver by a Satinsky or any other partial occlusion clamp. After an opening is made in the occluded portion of the vena cava and sutures are placed at either end, the mobilized portal vein is once more exposed and severed between bulldog clamps, leaving adequate cuffs of vein beyond both the proximal and distal clamps. The distal lumen of the portal is then approximated to the orifice in the vena cava and, using 00000 silk on No. 9 atraumatic needles, an anastomosis is effected with over-and-over continuous stitches. With the release of the caval and bulldog clamps, there is immediate restoration of the normal pink color of the intestines, which become congested during portal occlusion. The portal vein is usually not occluded for more than ten to twelve minutes. In our hands, the success of this entire operation, just as in total hepatectomy, depends on the facility with which the portacaval shunt can be carried out. Bleeding from the anastomotic line is readily controlled in a few minutes by gentle packing of sponge gauze against it.

Next, the previously removed vein graft is anastomosed to the proximal end of the portal vein. This is accomplished by dividing into four parts the lumen of the portal and anastomosing the vein to it, interrupting the continuous sutures in four places so that little or no purse stringing occurs. As the external jugular vein of the dog has two and sometimes three sets of valves, it is important that the vein be placed so that valvular action will permit the flow of blood toward the liver. Finally, the aorta just below the renal arteries is easily mobilized by spreading the parietal peritoneum and preaortic connective tissue. It is dissected free for a length of approximately 3 cm. Usually, one pair of lumbar arteries must be ligated and severed. In close proximity to the aorta at this level are large lymphatic vessels which cannot be easily separated from the aorta without being torn. They are clamped and ligated wherever possible, although no great effort is made to do this, as invariably the flow of lymph will cease by the end of the operation. The aorta is then clamped by two rubber-shod hemostats which have had their serrated surfaces filed smooth. A slit is made between the occluding clamps about one-half inch long, and small elliptical snips are removed from each side to make the opening ovoid. The distal end of the graft is now anastomosed to the aorta, using similar suture material and the same technique as for the portacaval shunt.

Upon completion of the graft-aorta anastomosis, first the bulldog clamp is removed from the proximal portal vein, then the distal aorta clamp and, last, the proximal clamp are released. At once, the vein graft is seen to become distended with blood and, on occasion, to pulsate. A thrill is always obtained by gently compressing the graft between the thumb and index finger. Leaks in suture lines are repaired, and the operation is terminated. The completed procedure is diagrammatically demonstrated in Fig. 1.

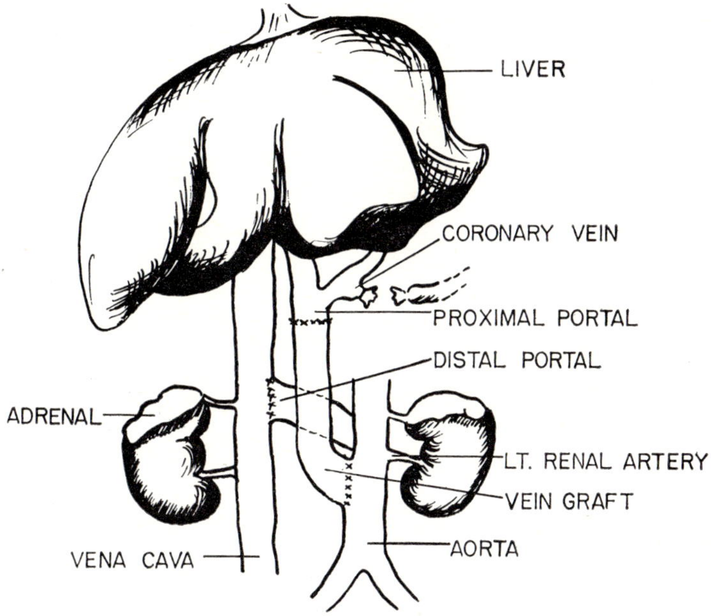

ARTERIALIZATION OF THE DOG LIVER

Fig. 1.—Diagrammatic presentation of technique for arterialization of dog liver.

The liver immediately becomes orange-red in color, and the edges are slightly rounded with the interlobar fissures becoming more prominent. In no instance in our experience has the liver pulsated.

The entire operative procedure takes from one to one and one-half hours, during which time the animal receives approximately 150 to 200 ml. of saline solution and whole blood replacement for any blood loss. This is usually small, and under 100 ml.

DISCUSSION

By the method presented, the total blood supply to the liver is arterial. Furthermore, an increase in total hepatic blood flow occurs.

The method described by Cohn has, in our hands, resulted in several technical difficulties. Here, the vein graft is passed through the diaphragm and anastomosed to the thoracic aorta. Frequently we encountered kinking of the graft with blocking of free flow of blood through it, in spite of satisfactory anastomoses. Furthermore, as the graft went through the diaphragm it would occasionally be pinched off by respirations. Third, in our experience at least, partial occlusion clamps applied to the dog's aorta are unsatisfactory, as they do not permit an adequate cuff for a clean anastomosis. Thus, it is necessary to clamp the aorta completely while anastomosing the graft to it. Total occlusion of the thoracic aorta frequently results in hind leg paralysis

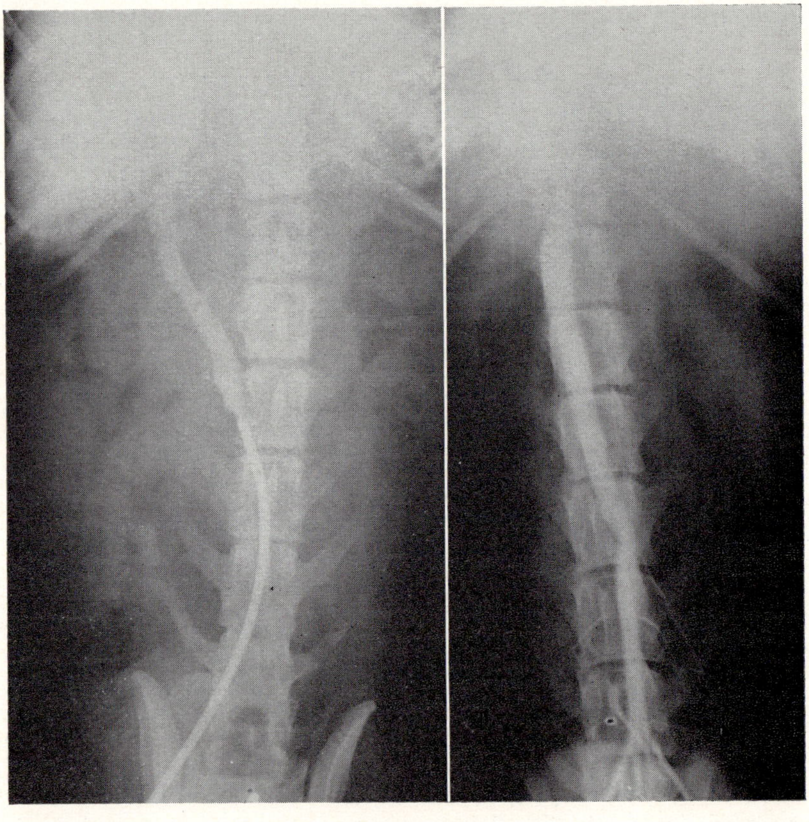

A. *B.*

Fig. 2.—Angiograms demonstrating patent channel after (*A*) four weeks, (*B*) six weeks, (*C*) six weeks, and (*D*) eight weeks. (Note constriction at junction of graft and portal.)

of the dog, as has been amply demonstrated by Blalock[6] and Gross[7] in their early studies on the surgical treatment of coarctation. This has been our experience when the aorta at this level is totally clamped for as short a time as fifteen minutes. Clamping the aorta between the renal arteries and trifurcation in twenty-three dogs for from ten to twenty-eight minutes, with an average time of eighteen minutes, has resulted in paralysis or weakness of the hind legs in no instance. The average time of occlusion in the most recent fifteen animals is twelve minutes, but in earlier operations, occlusion was effected for longer periods of time.

In twenty-seven attempts to carry out this technique, success was obtained in twenty-three animals. In the last fifteen operations, there was only one death, which was due to kinking of the portal vein following portacaval shunt, resulting in portal block and death within eight hours. The cause of death in the other three was hemorrhage in two in the immediate postoperative period and undetermined in one, when the animal was found dead in its cage seventy-two hours after operation.

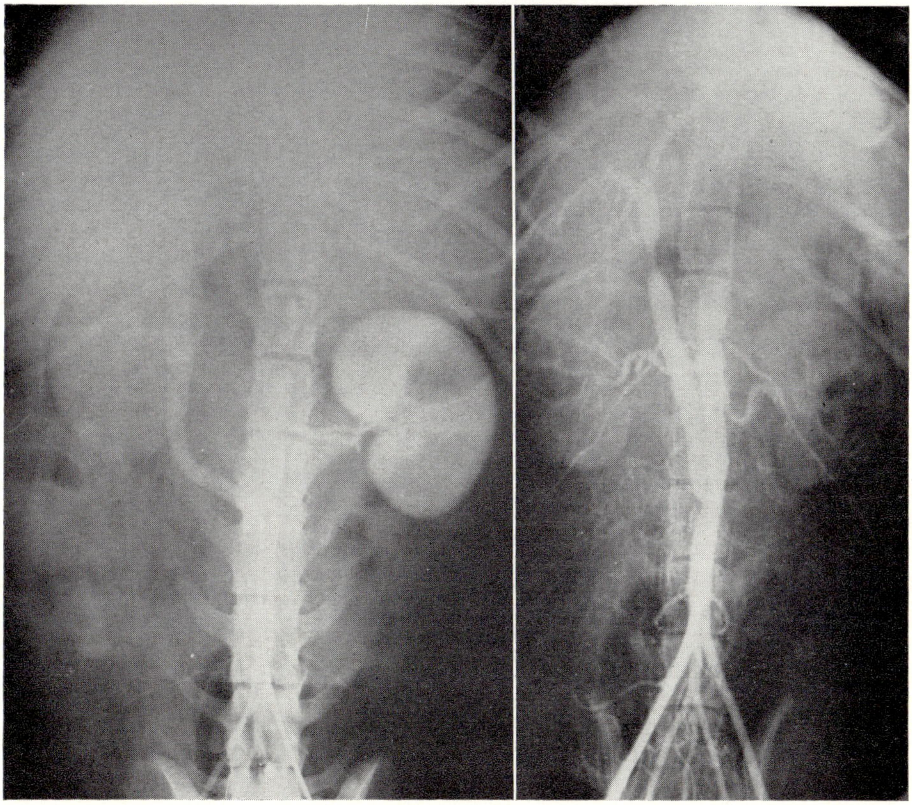

Fig. 2, *C* and *D*. (*For legend see opposite page.*)

In no animals observed did there occur postoperatively dilatation of the vein graft, but some ballooning of the proximal portal vein was common, occurring almost immediately after operation.

Angiograms were made. Fig. 2 shows representative examples demonstrating the new channel. One of the earlier operations, Fig. 2, *D* shows a marked stricture at the graft portal junction after eight weeks, but still permitting blood to travel through it.

Fig. 3 shows a specimen from an animal autopsied two months post-arterialization.

Blood flow studies, oxygen utilization of the liver under these conditions, effects on regeneration, and other studies will be presented subsequently.

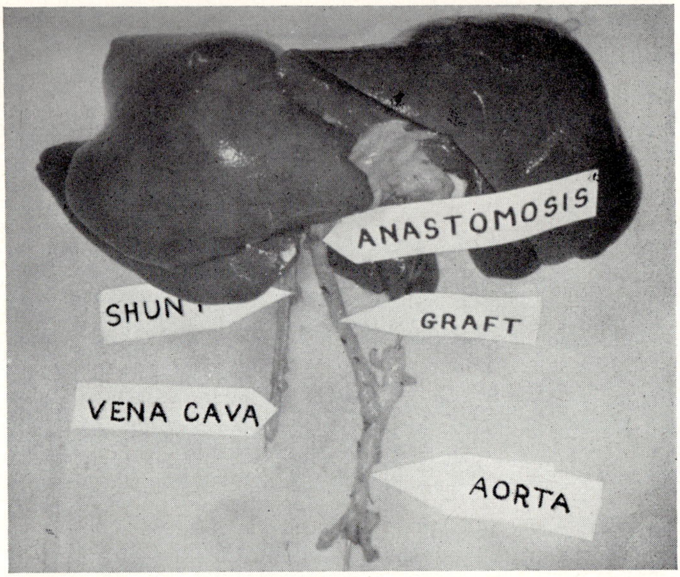

Fig. 3.—Autopsy specimen two months postarterialization.

CONCLUSION

A method for complete arterialization of the dog liver, with low mortality (under 10 per cent in the last fifteen animals) and no morbidity, is presented. This technique is serving as a useful tool for studying the effects of increased blood flow and oxygen environment on the liver.

REFERENCES

1. Narath, A.: Ueber Entstehung der anamischen Lebernekrose nach Unterbindung der Arteria hepatica und ihre Verhutung durch arterio-portale Anastomose, Deutsche Ztschr. f. Chir. **135**: 305-379, 1916.
2. Naegeli, T., and Meythaler, F.: Experimentelle Untersuchungen über arterio-venöse Gefässanastomosen der Lebergefässe, Deutsche Ztschr. f. Chir. **240**: 88-91, 1933.
3. Markowitz, J., Rappaport, A., and Scott, A. C.: Prevention of Liver Necrosis Following Ligation of Hepatic Artery, Proc. Soc. Exper. Biol. & Med. **70**: 305, 1949.
4. Schilling, J. A., McKee, F. W., and Wilt, W.: Experimental Hepatic-Portal Arteriovenous Anastomoses, Surg., Gynec. & Obst. **90**: 473-480, 1950.
5. Cohn, R., and Herrod, C.: Some Effects Upon the Liver of Complete Arterialization of Its Blood Supply, SURGERY **32**: 214-218, 1952.
6. Blalock, A., and Park, E. A.: Surgical Treatment of Experimental Coarctation of the Aorta, Ann. Surg. **119**: 445, 1944.
7. Hufnagel, C. A., and Gross, R. E.: Coarctation of the Aorta. Experimental Studies Regarding Its Correction, New England J. Med. **53**: 287, 1945.

RENAL COMPLICATIONS FROM AORTOGRAPHY*

Gerald M. Miller, M.D., Edwin J. Wylie, M.D., and Frank Hinman, Jr., M.D.,
San Francisco, Calif.

(From the Departments of Urology and Surgery, University of California School of Medicine)

DAMAGE to the kidney from translumbar aortography has been observed in seven patients in the last two years. During this time, approximately 250 aortograms have been taken on the combined University of California services, of which over 90 per cent were made by the surgeons of the vascular disease group. The seven known instances of renal complications thus represent an incidence of almost 3 per cent.

Since Dos Santos'[1] original warnings about the possibility of renal damage, no serious complications have been reported from aortography, particularly as far as the kidneys are concerned. Minor complications were described in 1952 by Larsson and Palmlöv,[2] who stated that renal injury might result if all or most of the solution were injected into one renal artery. They discussed a patient in whom this was done with subsequent temporary fall in renal function. Another patient received an excess of dye in the renal arteries without apparent damage. Melick and Vitt[3] reported injecting the media directly into the left renal artery, which caused temporary pain and microscopic hematuria, but renal function was subsequently normal.

This report is an analysis of cases of serious renal injury and of data from animal experiments, in an attempt to find the factors causing damage following aortography and the methods for avoiding injury.

From a theoretical standpoint and from an analysis of the clinical data, the cases fall into two main groups: I, direct trauma, and II, indirect damage. These have been further divided:

- I. Direct trauma (unilateral or bilateral)
  - A. Misdirected needle
  - B. Excessive pressure/volume
  - C. Chemical irritation from radiopaque media
- II. Indirect damage (bilateral, ? reflex)
  - A. Drug toxicity and/or idiosyncrasy (Diodrast, iodine)
  - B. Neurogenic factors?

Clinical Series.—

I. On analysis, three of our seven patients fit into Group I. The damage in all of these was unilateral. Another patient appears to have been affected by agents common to both groups but will be described with the second.

Case 1.—J. B., a 45-year-old man, gave a five-year history of severe leg cramps, which were due to marked narrowing of the abdominal aorta just above the bifurcation.

Received for publication, Oct. 26, 1953.
*Supported in part by the Christine Breon Fund for Medical Research.

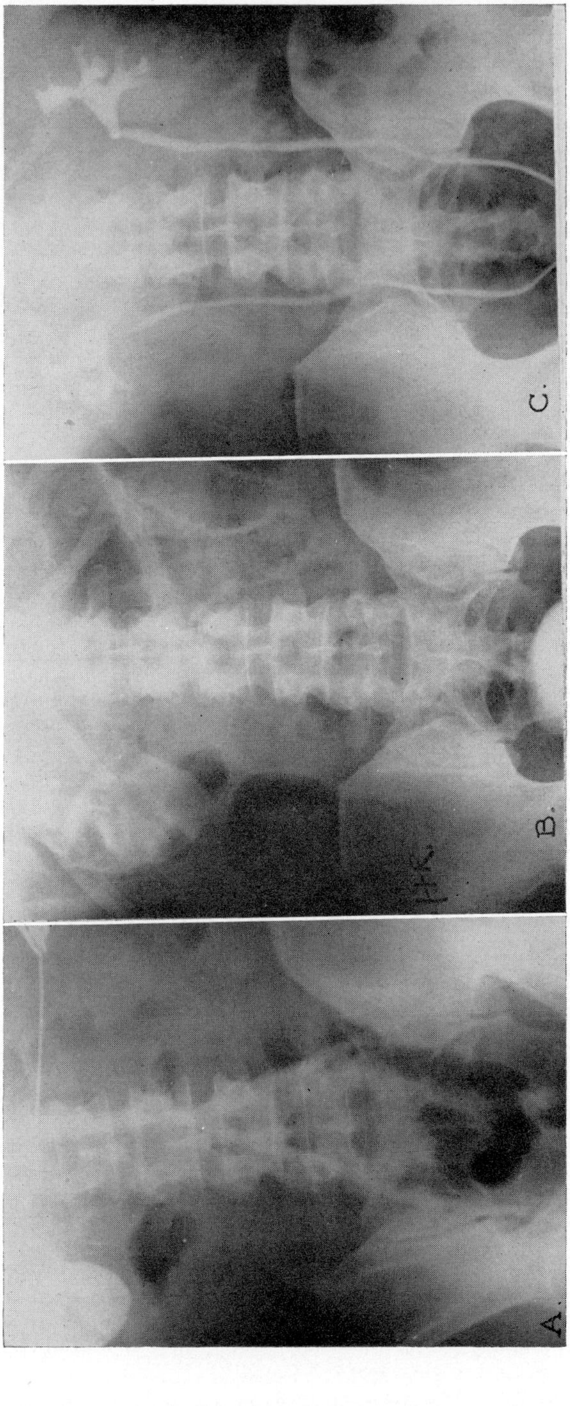

Fig. 1.—*A*, Aortogram. Direct injection into ostium of right renal artery (with gas-pressure machine). *B*, Delayed nephrogram (six hours). Residual dye proves interstitial extravasation; renal swelling. *C*, Retrograde pyelogram (3 months). Atrophy, right renal parenchyma with compensatory left hypertrophy.

On Feb. 26, 1952, translumbar aortography was carried out by the vascular surgeon under intravenous Pentothal anesthesia using 50 c.c. of 70 per cent Diodrast injected with a gas-driven machine which gives a pressure of 70 pounds per square inch. X-ray films showed that most of the dye was injected directly into the right renal artery (Fig. 1, *A*). A few hours later, the patient began to have rather severe right flank and costovertebral angle pain and tenderness. An x-ray film (Fig. 1, *B*) showed that an intense nephrogram was still present on the right. The patient developed nausea and vomiting, with fever to 103° F. The urine was grossly bloody.

The next day, retrograde study with No. 6 ureteral catheters in each renal pelvis demonstrated the following differential function:

Intravenous phenolsulfonphthalein	Right (injured)	Left (normal)
Appearance time	12 min.	2½ min.
15 min.	10 c.c. trace	15 c.c. 17.5%
Specific gravity	1.012	1.028

The patient continued to have nausea and vomiting and mild right flank pain and fever for three more days and then all of the symptoms subsided. He was discharged from the hospital on the eighth day postaortography. Total P.S.P. excretion at this time was 35 per cent in thirty minutes.

Four months later, retrograde urologic study was repeated:

Intravenous phenolsulfonphthalein	Right	Left
Appearance time	12 min.	2½ min.
15 min.	10 c.c. trace	15 c.c. 25.0%
Urine chloride	1.8 Gm./L. (31 meq./L.)	5.9 Gm./L. (100 meq./L.)
Gross appearance	Watery	Bright yellow
pH	6.5 - 7	5.5 - 6
Special gravity	1.012	1.018

Pyelograms (Fig. 1, *C*) at this time showed some atrophy of the right kidney with fairly normal calyceal pattern, and with compensatory hypertrophy on the left. No renal difficulties appeared after a successful thromboendarterectomy of the distal abdominal aorta.

CASE 2.—B. M., a 53-year-old male patient, had a two-year history of severe leg cramps. Aortography was carried out on Dec. 31, 1952, under general anesthesia, with local procaine infiltration, using 50 c.c. of 70 per cent Diodrast injected with the gas-pressure machine. Aortograms showed obstruction of the lower abdominal aorta starting just below the renal arteries and becoming complete at the level of the third lumbar vertebra (Fig. 2, *A*). The inferior portion of the right kidney showed dense opacification still present five minutes after injection (Fig. 2, *B*). It appeared that a high proportion of the charge was injected directly into an aberrant artery going from the aorta to the lower pole of the kidney.

The patient had no apparent untoward effects from this injection and two days later underwent an extensive thromboendarterectomy. No follow-up studies on the right kidney are available, but the patient has had no further symptoms.

CASE 3.—L. C., a 47-year-old man, had teeth extracted on July 24, 1952, and that evening developed acute pain in the left lower leg and foot with numbness and cyanosis, for which two lumbar sympathetic blocks were made. Blood pressure at that time was 170/88. Five days later, translumbar aortography was carried out with a two-needle technique; 70 c.c. of 70 per cent Diodrast was injected. Aortography revealed that one of the needles was directed toward the lumen of the right renal artery and the other needle was outside

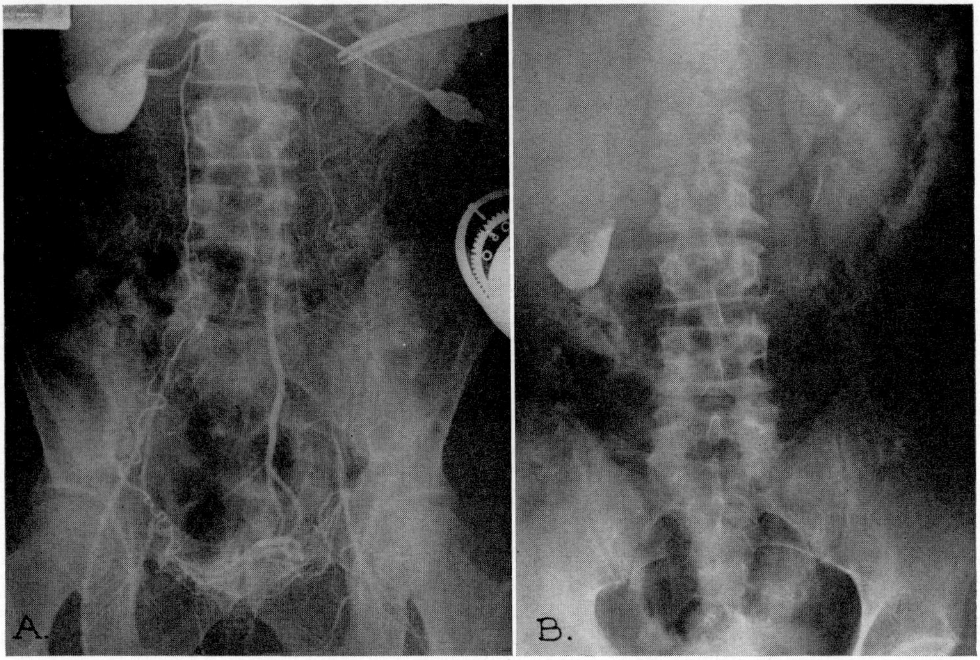

Fig. 2.—*A,* Aortogram. Direct injection into anomalous artery to lower pole of right kidney with interstitial and subcapsular extravasation.

B, Nephrogram. Persistent extravasation.

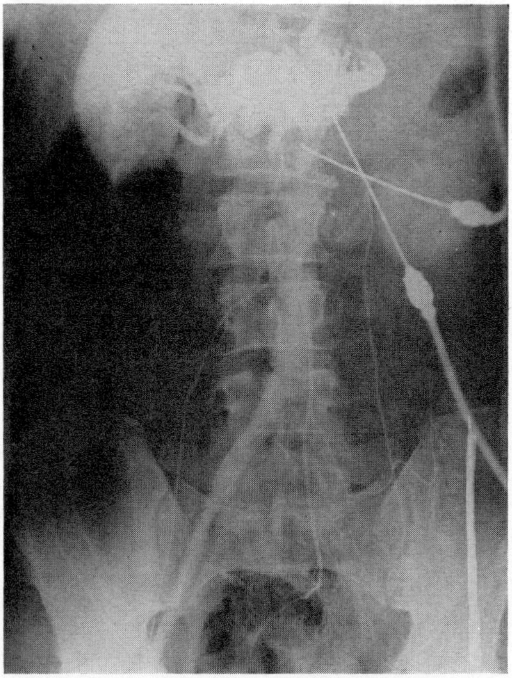

Fig. 3.—Aortogram. Periaortic extravasation and direct injection into right renal artery, resulting in temporary nonfunctioning kidney with hypertension.

the lumen of the aorta (Fig. 3). The patient thus had excessive injection into the right kidney, with extravasation around the renal artery. The arterial supply on the right appeared normal.

A few days following this procedure, the patient's blood pressure increased to 220/110. Three weeks later, bilateral iliac endarterectomy and lumbar sympathectomy were performed. In ten days, the patient began to manifest signs and symptoms of severe hypertensive retinopathy. The blood pressure had risen to 230/120. Seven weeks after aortography, intravenous urograms showed no function of the right kidney with normal function of the left. Retrograde study showed a trace of P.S.P. excretion in fifteen minutes from the right kidney, 25 per cent excretion on the left, with pyelograms demonstrating normal renal outlines.

The patient was followed without further therapy, and within the next six weeks his symptoms disappeared, the blood pressure returned to 140/90 mm. Hg, and intravenous urograms were normal, with good function on the right.

In these three cases, renal damage resulted from direct trauma at the time of aortography. Not only was the needle misdirected in each instance, but the complicating factors of excessive injection pressure, large volumes of dye, and possible irritation by the media were also present. Pressure and volume are interrelated factors, with the medium causing damage by being forced out of the capillaries or by direct irritation because of high concentration. As a result, one patient developed an atrophic kidney, and a second had a temporarily nonfunctioning kidney with severe hypertension which spontaneously reverted to normal within three months. High aortic block is particularly likely to dam back dye and promote renal damage.

II. The remaining four patients fall into the indirect classification. In each of them, the injury was bilateral.

Case 4.—H. V., a 45-year-old man, had intermittent claudication due to almost complete obstruction of the aorta just below the renal arteries. An aortogram, under spinal anesthesia, was made on Jan. 3, 1952 (Fig. 4), after a previous attempt two and one-half months before had shown merely the mesenteric vessels. A total of 100 c.c. of 70 per cent Diodrast in two divided portions of 50 c.c. each was injected. The patient developed severe headache and a transient urticarial reaction after the first injection. He was given 50 mg. of Benadryl and 100 mg. of Demerol intravenously with relief of the urticaria, but not of the headache. The second injection was accompanied by severe back and abdominal pain, followed by nausea and vomiting. Blood pressure, which was initially 130/80 mm. Hg, rose to 240/90. It remained elevated for thirty minutes, then dropped to 80/50, where it remained for a few hours. It began to rise slowly after a blood transfusion was started. The patient was completely anuric for two days and then became oliguric with twenty-four-hour output varying between 125 c.c. and 470 c.c. A diagnosis of lower nephron nephrosis was made. By the tenth day, the nonprotein nitrogen had risen to 161 mg. per 100 c.c. The patient was treated by careful balance of fluid and electrolytes and of body weight.[4] On the eleventh day, diuresis began and the patient went on from there to complete recovery. On the twenty-second day, the P.S.P. excretion, which had been less than 1 per cent during the period of lower nephron nephrosis, was 24 per cent in one hour. Eight months later, P.S.P. excretion was 65 per cent in one hour, and a successful thromboendarterectomy was performed. The patient had an uneventful postoperative course with no renal difficulties. Of interest is the fact that impotency present before surgery was completely relieved.

Case 5.—T. C., a 64-year-old man, gave a three-year history of pain, numbness, and tingling in both legs. Aortography was carried out on July 2, 1952 (Fig. 5), under intravenous Pentothal and Demerol anesthesia, after sensitivity test to Diodrast showed no reaction. A total of 60 c.c. of 70 per cent Diodrast was injected through two needles.

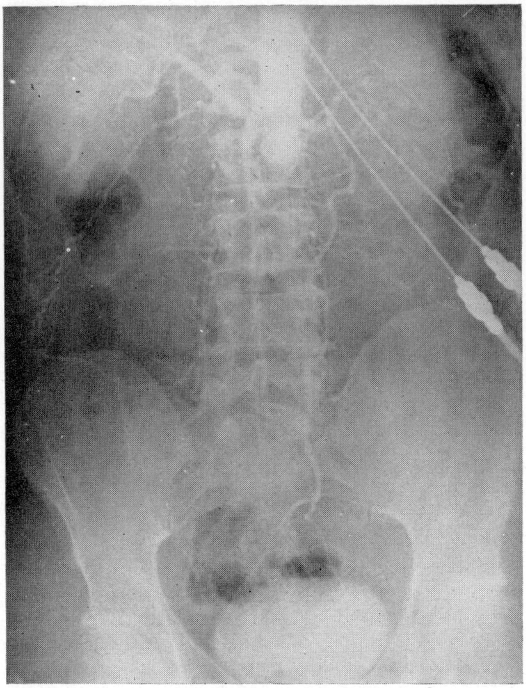

Fig. 4.—Aortogram. Large injection (50 c.c. twice) above high aortic block, resulting in lower nephron nephrosis.

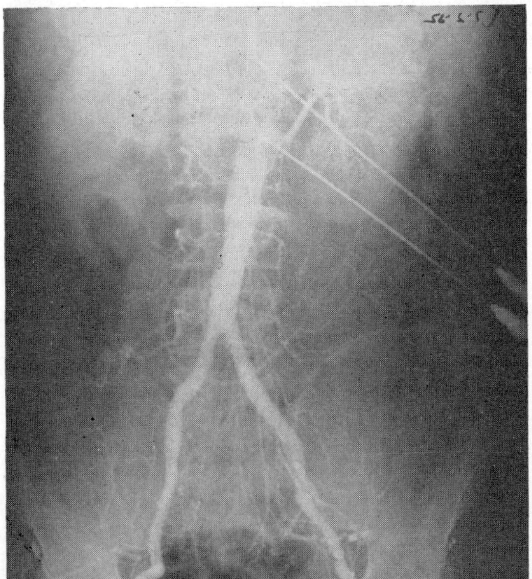

Fig. 5.—Aortogram. Patient developed I_2 sensitivity with rash and rhinorrhea, and lower nephron nephrosis.

On his way home the next day, the patient began to have severe nausea and vomiting, so that four days later he was hospitalized near his home. Examination showed a severe iodide reaction with rhinorrhea, hoarseness, and a typical eruption over the skin of the face, neck, and chest. Urinary output was scant, and N.P.N. was 101 mg. per 100 c.c. He then became anuric and the N.P.N. rose further. Hiccups and vomiting were intractable. He was treated by balance of fluids and electrolytes, and by the tenth day postaortography he began to put out urine in large amounts, with a gradual return of renal function toward normal. One month later, N.P.N. was 33 mg. per 100 c.c. and P.S.P. excretion 45 per cent in 10 minutes.

CASE 6.—N. H, a 60-year-old female patient, had a two-year history of left leg cramps due to narrowing of the aorta starting below the level of the renal vessels and marked obstruction of the right common iliac artery.

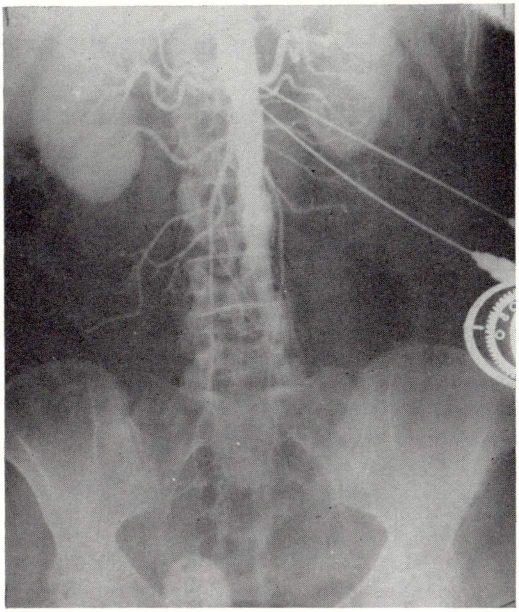

Fig. 6.—Aortogram. Large injection into aorta above stenosis, resulting in lower nephron nephrosis.

Aortography was carried out in Dec. 30, 1952, under Pentothal anesthesia with 70 c.c. of 70 per cent Diodrast, using the two-needle technique (Fig. 6). The patient was discharged from the hospital the following day, but three days later was admitted to another hospital near her home because of severe vomiting and back pain which had started twenty-four hours after the aortogram. She was found to be markedly oliguric, putting out 30 c.c. of urine in twenty-four hours. She was treated conservatively and remained oliguric until the eleventh day, when diuresis began. The N.P.N., which had risen to 111 mg. per 100 c.c., fell by the twentieth day to 28.

CASE 7.—L. M., a 58-year-old man, had an abdominal aneurysm and arteriosclerotic constriction of the iliac arteries. On Feb. 13, 1953, translumbar aortography was carried out under Pentothal anesthesia with 50 c.c. of 70 per cent Diodrast injected through a single needle with the pressure machine. (Fig. 7.) There was an intense nephrogram at eight seconds. No immediate untoward effects were noted and there was no evidence of iodine sensitivity. The patient was discharged the following morning, but that afternoon had continuous hiccups. The following morning, he noted that the urine looked like water and that his eyes were a little puffy. Three days later, he consulted a local doctor because his urine output seemed low; asparagus that he had eaten three days before had given no odor to the urine. At that time, he was found to have gained eight pounds, and serum creatinine level was 13 mg. per 100 c.c. Fluids were restricted and salt was withheld. By the tenth day, the urine output increased in amount and the patient made an uneventful recovery.

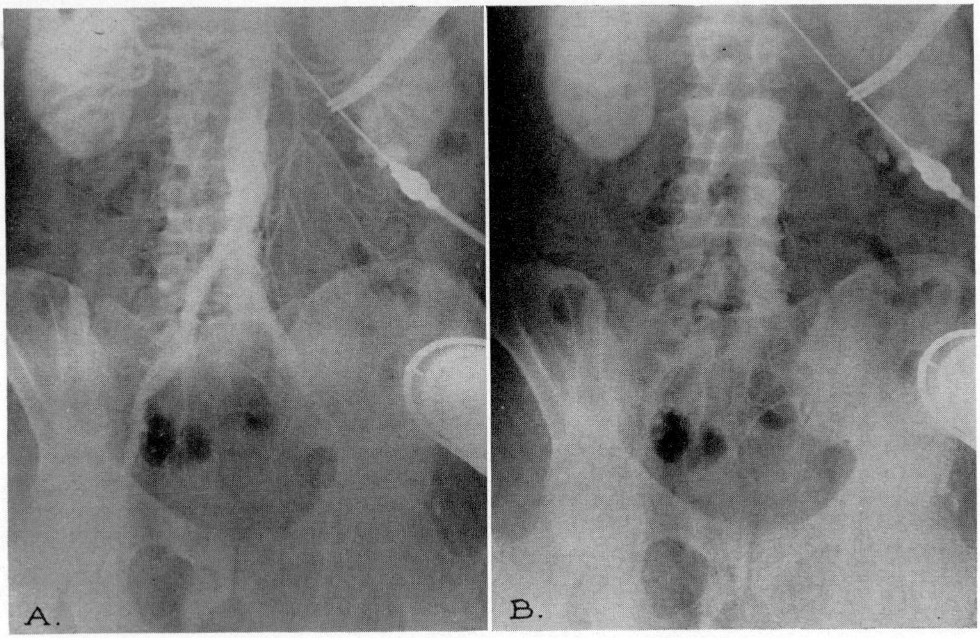

Fig. 7.—*A*, Aortogram. Injection with gas-pressure machine. *B*, Nephrogram. Followed by lower nephron nephrosis.

Four patients developed reversible renal failure after aortography (Fig. 8). In three cases, the two-needle technique was used and over 60 c.c. of dye injected. In the other, the gas-pressure machine was used; the patient appeared to have immediate parenchymal damage bilaterally. All recovered completely, after periods of oliguria of ten or eleven days. Two of the four had evidence of Diodrast idiosyncrasy.

That contrast media can cause change in renal function is illustrated in another patient who was subjected to translumbar aortography with the needle placed below the right and above the left renal arteries. Fig. 9, *A* shows the left nephrogram two seconds after injection with no filling of the right kidney, indicating that the dye went only to the left kidney. Twenty-five minutes later (Fig. 9, *B*), the right side showed a normal urogram, whereas the left side showed calyceal spasm and poor filling with persistent nephrogram indicative of at least temporary arrest of the normal tubular transport mechanism.

Experimental Findings.—To test the significance of excessive pressure in terms of renal damage, we performed two types of experiments on dogs.

Type 1. Direct injection of contrast media + India ink into renal artery: After exposure of the dog's left renal artery, 20 c.c. of 70 per cent Diodrast and

5 c.c. of dilute buffered India ink were injected with great force, using a hand-driven lever apparatus[5] directly into the artery. The kidney was immediately removed and perfused. Radiographs showed subcapsular and interstitial extravasation (Fig. 10, *A*), similar to that seen in Cases 1 and 2. The density of the India ink particles in the parenchyma after the kidney was fixed in formalin and cleared by the Spalteholz technique (R. Skarda) is shown in Fig. 10, *B*.

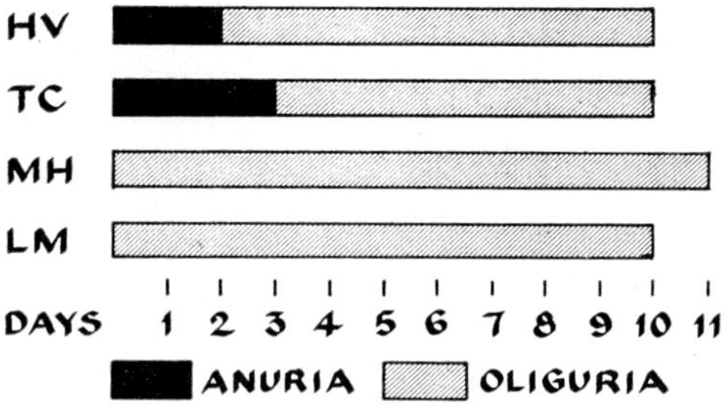

Fig. 8.—Duration of anuria and oliguria in four cases of bilateral injury.

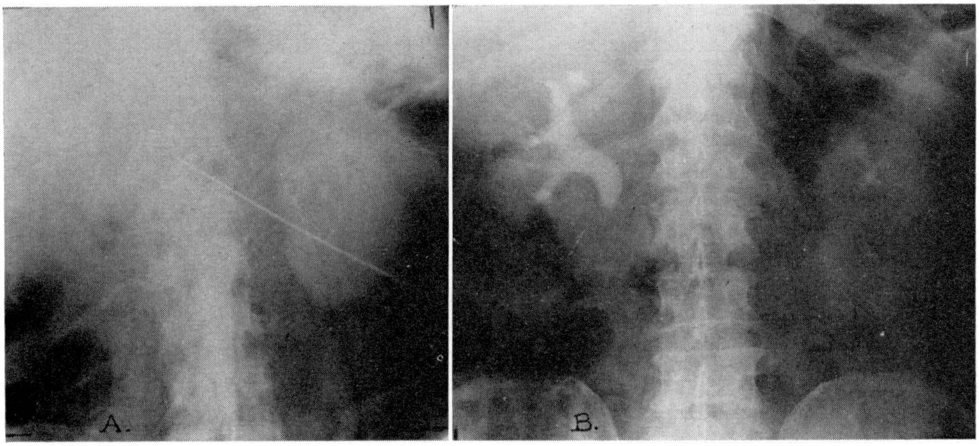

Fig. 9.—*A*, Left nephrogram. Needle inserted below right renal artery.
B, Urogram, twenty-five minutes later. Left nephrogram still present, with calyceal spasm. Normal right urogram.

Type 2. Forceful injection of Diodrast and India ink into the aorta occluded just below the renal arteries:

(A) To study immediate effects, the dog's aorta was exposed transperitoneally and occluded manually above and below the origin of the left renal artery during forceful injection of 20 c.c. of 70 per cent Diodrast and 5 c.c. of dilute buffered India ink. The kidney was removed and perfused and a radiograph was taken. Extravasation into the cortex was evident (Fig. 10, *C*), although less extreme than in the first experiment. After fixation and

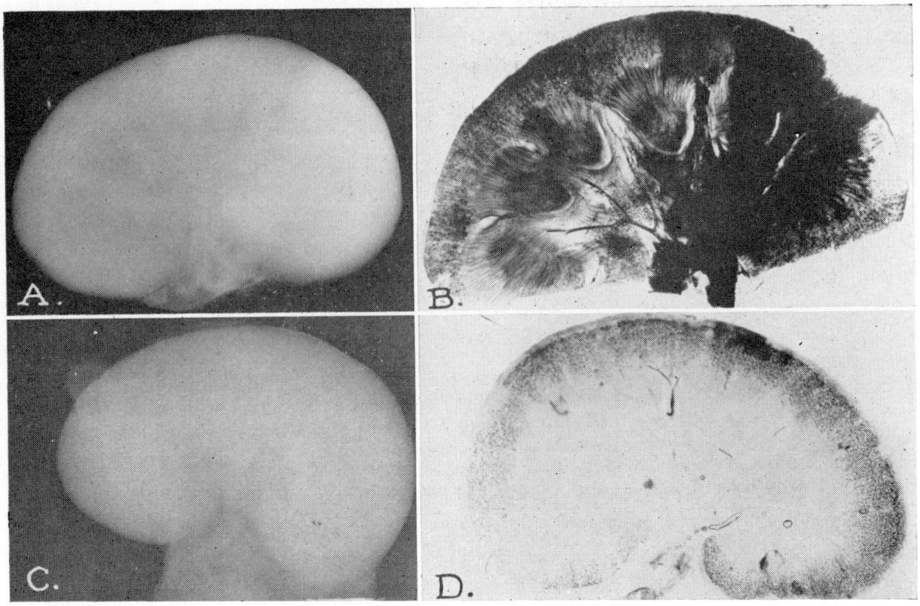

Fig. 10.—*A,* Radiograph of dog kidney showing interstitial and subcapsular extravasation after direct arterial injection of Diodrast and India ink.

B, Cleared sagittal section of same kidney.

C, Radiograph of dog kidney showing interstital extravasation after forceful injection of aorta.

D, Cleared sagittal section of same kidney. Note intercapillary filling of Bowman's space.

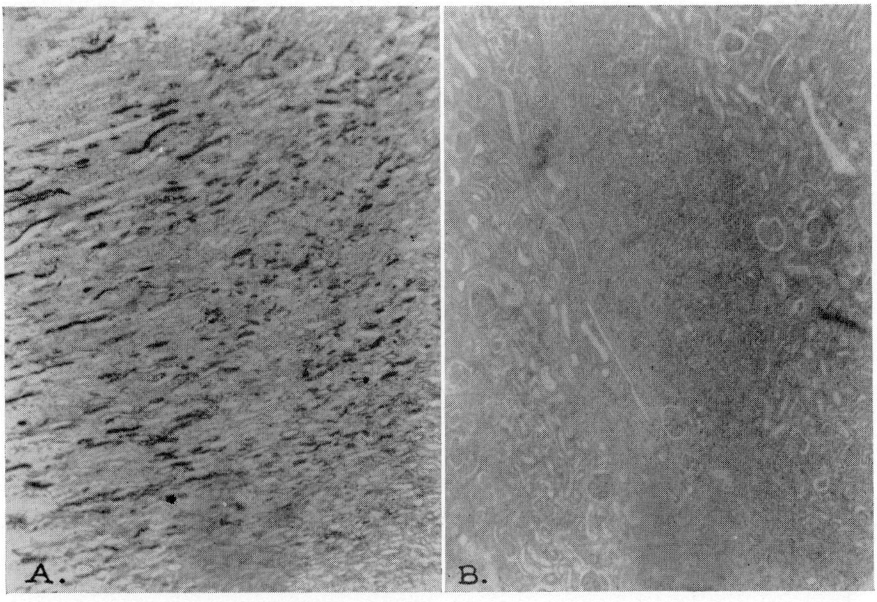

Fig. 11.—*A,* Photomicrograph (×100; reduced ⅕) of dog kidney shown in Fig. 10, *C* and *D.* Particles can be seen in the tubules and interstitially.

B, Photomicrograph (×100; reduced ⅕) of dog kidney removed three weeks after forceful injection. Note patchy interstitial fibrosis.

clearing, the kidney still showed extravasation of India ink in Bowman's space (intercapillary) and in the tubules and intertubular spaces (Figs. 10, *D* and 11, *A*).

(B) To study the delayed effects, a similar injection was made and the kidney left in situ. At the end of three weeks, microscopic examination showed patchy areas of interstitial fibrosis (Fig. 11, *B*).

Although these experiments could be amplified, they illustrate a way whereby forceful injection of a substance may cause extravasation into the renal parenchyma, which results in renal damage.

DISCUSSION

These clinical and experimental results indicate that renal damage may be caused by high pressures combined with a volume of media sufficient to generate such pressure, or by irritation of the contrast media itself if the pressure-volume relationship produces a sufficiently high concentration. The damage appears to come either from mechanical damage to the renal blood vessels with extravasation or from excessively high concentrations of the dye as it passes through the kidney.

To insure against such damage following aortography, certain limitations in technique appear desirable. If the whole aortic tree must be filled (as before vascular surgery), then at least 50 c.c. of dye is needed. To prevent excessive pressure (or the danger of trauma by too large a needle), it has been found advisable to use two smaller 17 or 18 gauge needles and inject by hand with two syringes. To avoid direct injection of the renal vessels (or other aortic branches, for that matter), the needle tips should be angulated sharply upward so that they enter the aorta just below the diaphragm and 2 to 3 cm. above the renal vessels. Long needles are required.

For urologic purposes, such large volumes of media are not needed, although the 12 c.c. volume advocated by Parke Smith[6] has not been enough in many cases to show the renal vascular pattern. We have found 25 c.c. to be adequate. But this quantity of dye injected directly into the renal artery, even by hand pressure, could be damaging, so we advocate, especially for the occasional operator, the making of a scout film after injection of 5 c.c. of dye to determine the position of the tip of the needle. It may then be moved should it lie within the lumen of the renal artery or mesenteric vessels, or should there be extravasation. This precaution might have obviated the complications in at least three of the reported cases.

These smaller volumes used to visualize just a segment of the aorta and the renal vascular tree can be conveniently injected under local anesthesia. The use of local anesthesia avoids some of the dangers inherent in general anesthesia, particularly when given away from the operating rooms, and avoids the need of an anesthetist and additional personnel. The patient is heavily premedicated with barbiturates and intravenous Demerol, and a single 17 gauge needle is inserted by local infiltration of 1 per cent procaine. Once the aorta is entered, an additional 20 c.c. of procaine is injected directly into the aorta to avoid vasospasm in the distal vessels. With 70 per cent Diodrast there has occasionally been a sudden movement by the patient from the "shock" of the injection, but this was controlled with adhesive taping. Since using 70 per cent Urokon, we have not seen this sudden movement.

SUMMARY

1. Renal damage following translumbar aortography has been observed in seven patients.

2. The direct forceful injection of a sizable amount of dye into a single renal artery produced unilateral damage in three of these patients. The high pressure produced visible extravasation of an irritating medium.

3. Bilateral renal injury followed by reversible renal failure occurred in four other patients. Two of the four had evidence of Diodrast sensitivity; three of the four had at least 60 c.c. of media injected, and the fourth had 50 c.c. injected under high pressure.

4. Animal experiments showed that high injection pressures caused interstitial extravasation of the medium, leading to late renal fibrosis.

5. A safer plan for aortography is proposed, using lower pressures and smaller volumes.

We acknowledge the asistance of Dr. John W. Schulte, who prepared the detailed data on patient No. 1, and we thank him for his interest and his valuable suggestions.

REFERENCES

1. Dos Santos, R.: Med. contemp. **47**: 93, 1929; quoted by Melick and Vitt.[3]
2. Larsson, H., and Palmlöv, A.: Abdominal Aortography, With Special Reference to Its Complications, Acta radiol. **38**: 111-124, 1952.
3. Melick, W. F., and Vitt, A. E.: The Present Status of Aortography, J. Urol. **60**: 321-334, 1948.
4. Lyon, R. P.: Lower Nephron Nephrosis, Am. Pract. & Digest Treat. **2**: 1023-1027, 1951.
5. Hinman, F., Jr.: A Simple Injector for Aortography and Intravenous Angiography, J. Urol. **70**: 119-120 (July) 1953.
6. Smith, P. G., Rush, T. W., and Evans, A. T.: An Evaluation of Translumbar Aortography, J. Urol. **65**: 911-921, 1951.

PROSTATIC CANCER

IX. Value of Transurethral Biopsy in Search of Early Prostatic Carcinoma

Perry B. Hudson, M.D., Alex L. Finkle, M.D., Aristides Trifilio, M.D., and Casimir T. Wolan, M.D., New York, N. Y.

(From the Department of Urology, Francis Delafield Hospital, Institute of Cancer Research, Columbia University, College of Physicians and Surgeons)

Current trends in cancer therapy are such that the early detection of adenocarcinoma of the prostate gland is receiving renewed interest and attention.[1, 2] The inadequacy of rectal palpation diagnosis has been demonstrated, particularly in regard to the detection of malignancies at a stage in their development preceding spread from the original focus to other parts of the body.[3] Tissue diagnosis assumes greater importance in the absence of definitive points in the medical history or of diagnostic signs which are suggestive of prostatic cancer.

Three methods for obtaining tissue from the prostate gland are utilized to detect curable cancer. Cytologic study of the expressed prostatic secretion smear is the newest of these techniques.[4] A second method involves the use of a needle[5] or punch instrument[6] which is introduced through a small perineal stab incision to obtain a core of posterior prostatic tissue. Open perineal dissection for direct wedge biopsy of the posterior lamella is the third method.[7, 8]

There has been no experience with the prostatic smear technique in this institution. Objections to the method center about the inadvisability of massaging adenocarcinomas, which are known to spread in perineural lymphatic spaces, as well as the statement by Peters and her associates[4] that there is a definite percentage of false positive impressions of cancer which are gained from a series of examinations of this sort. In addition, Colby[9] has found that only 40 per cent of his series of 100 cases of operable prostatic cancer yielded a positive diagnosis from the prostatic smear examination. There is the further theoretical objection that early prostatic cancer often may not have an anatomic connection with the ducts emptying into the prostatic urethra, thereby making it impossible to express cancer cells from a small focus in the posterior prostate. While the punch biopsy technique is useful in documenting cases of more advanced carcinoma, it does not compare favorably with the open surgical biopsy technique in cases of early prostatic cancer.[10] Open perineal prostatic biopsy appears, then, to be the most reliable method for detecting early prostatic cancer, which is thought to develop in 85 per cent of such malignancies in the posterior portion of the gland.[11-14]

This study was supported by the New York City Cancer Committee and in part by an institutional grant of the American Cancer Society to Columbia University.

Received for publication, Oct. 14, 1953.

It is mainly in an attempt to detect the 15 per cent of early carcinomas which originate in the periurethral portion of the prostate gland that transurethral prostatic biopsy has been employed.

CLINICAL STUDIES

During an evaluation of over 300 men by various methods and techniques designed to detect early prostatic cancer,[15] a transurethral prostatic biopsy has been included in the study for fifty-nine consecutive patients. In each instance, open surgical perineal prostatic biopsy was performed concurrently with transurethral biopsy.

The technique for transurethral prostatic biopsy is as follows: After anesthesia is instituted, a No. 28 Fr. Stern-McCarthy electrotome sheath is introduced through the urethra. Three areas of the prostate are routinely sampled, namely, the floor of the prostatic urethra and a mid-section of each lateral prostatic lobe. Specimens measure approximately 2 cm. in length and from 0.5 to 1.0 cm. in depth. Whenever a median lobe enlargement is encountered, a central core of median tissue is excised. Bleeding is controlled by electrocoagulation. The entire amount of tissue is removed within five minutes, obviously involving less time and tissue than in a therapeutic resection.

The specimens are fixed in Bouin's solution, made into paraffin blocks, sectioned at 5 microns, stained with hematoxylin and eosin, and studied microscopically.

The surgical pathologic material upon which evaluation of transurethral prostatic biopsy is based consists of fifty-nine consecutive transurethral prostatic biopsies, fifty-nine concurrently obtained open perineal biopsies of the posterior prostate, and forty-five final surgical specimens obtained from definitive surgical procedures upon the prostates of these patients.

RESULTS

Among the fifty-nine patients evaluated, there were forty-three in whom a benign tissue diagnosis was finally established. Of these, all forty-three were correctly diagnosed by both the open perineal biopsy and by the transurethral biopsy techniques. In the case of carcinoma, there were sixteen positive cases revealed by final pathologic diagnosis upon surgical specimens. Of the sixteen, eight cases, or 50 per cent, were unsuspected carcinoma and

TABLE I. ANALYSIS OF FIFTY-NINE TRANSURETHRAL RESECTION AND PERINEAL PROSTATIC BIOPSIES

Number of cases biopsied by both routes	59
Number of benign lesions	43
1. Correctly diagnosed by transurethral resection biopsy	43
2. Correctly diagnosed by perineal biopsy	43
Number of prostatic cancers	16
1. Correctly diagnosed by transurethral resection biopsy	8
2. Correctly diagnosed by perineal biopsy	8*

*The eight cases of prostatic cancer detected by transurethral resection biopsy were in known metastatic instances. The prostate was biopsied only for tissue confirmation of the clinical diagnosis.

eight were cases in which metastases were known to exist prior to the biopsy. All sixteen of the cancers were revealed by open perineal biopsy method. Of the eight cases of advanced cancer, the transurethral biopsy was positive. Of the eight early unsuspected carcinomas, none yielded a positive transurethral biopsy finding (Table I).

DISCUSSION

The results of this investigation suggest that little likelihood exists of diagnosing early prostatic cancer with a resectoscope. A more extensive resection than the one utilized might yield a higher diagnostic rate for malignancy. However, there are objections to extensive transurethral resections for this purpose. The fact that irrigating fluid almost always enters the blood stream during extended prostatic resection is well established.[16] It is probable that prostatic cancer cells are introduced into the blood stream in precisely the same way. In addition, extensive resection would "make the prostatic remnant unsuitable for total perineal extirpation unless it were done within 24 hours."[17]

It is probable that tumors detected during examination of transurethral prostatic curettings are those which originate in the posterior prostate, and then grow toward the urethra to a point at which they have invaded periurethral glandular hyperplasia. Such tumors are beside the subject under consideration, namely, the detection of early prostatic cancer. Suffice it to state that the resectoscope is useful for the documentation of advanced prostatic cancer when a tissue diagnosis has not previously been obtained, but with the clear knowledge of the risk of tumor spread in mind.

It should be emphasized that the modern electrotome does not alter the morphology of the specimens in such a way that distortion is a prime factor in hindering accurate microscopic appraisal.

Other studies from this institution have indicated that clinical accuracy for the detection of early prostatic cancer by the open perineal prostatic biopsy method is 89 per cent.[2, 3, 8, 10, 15] The results cited in this communication indicate that transurethral biopsy will rarely, if ever, yield a positive diagnosis of prostatic cancer while the disease is in its earlier phases of growth. Because it is technically dangerous, if not impossible, to include posterior prostatic tissue in a transurethral resection biopsy, the likelihood of missing posterior prostatic cancer—the commonest form—is extremely high.

The superiority of open perineal prostatic biopsy over transurethral biopsy seems definite. The discrepancy between the diagnostic values of the two techniques is so great that the transurethral method may reasonably be abandoned as a device for establishing the tissue diagnosis of unsuspected early prostatic carcinoma.

SUMMARY

1. A series of fifty-nine consecutive patients subjected to concurrent transurethral and open perineal surgical biopsy of the prostate is presented.

2. Sixteen adenocarcinomas were found, eight of which were known metastatic cases, and eight of which were totally unsuspected malignancies.

3. Transurethral biopsy yielded a diagnosis of cancer only in the eight known metastatic cases.

4. Transurethral biopsy yielded an erroneous diagnosis of benign prostatic tissue in all eight of the early, unsuspected cancers.

5. All of the sixteen cancers were detected by open perineal biopsy.

6. Transurethral biopsy may reasonably be abandoned as a means of detecting early prostatic cancer.

REFERENCES

1. Edwards, C. N., Steinthorsson, E., and Nicholson, D.: An Autopsy Study of Latent Prostatic Cancer, Cancer **6**: 531-554 (May) 1953.
2. Hudson, P. B., Finkle, A. L., Trifilio, A., Jost, H. M., Sproul, E. E., and Stout, A. P.: Prostatic Cancer. VIII. Detection of Unsuspected Adenocarcinoma in the Aging Male Population, J. A. M. A., 1954. In press.
3. Totten, R. S., Heinemann, M. W., Hudson, P. B., Sproul, E. E., and Stout, A. P.: Microscopic Differential Diagnosis of Latent Carcinoma of Prostate, Arch. Path. **55**: 131-141 (Feb.) 1953.
4. Peters, H., and Frank, I. N.: The Cytologic Interpretation of the Prostatic Smear, Surg., Gynec. & Obst. **94**: 69-76 (Jan.) 1952.
5. Pierson, E. L., and Nickerson, D. A.: Biopsy of the Prostate With the Silverman Needle, New England J. Med. **228**: 675-678 (May 27) 1943.
6. Veenema, R. J.: A Simplified Prostatic Perineal Biopsy Punch, J. Urol. **69**: 320-322 (Feb.) 1953.
7. Henline, R. B.: Early Diagnosis and Treatment of Prostatic Carcinoma, New York Med. **3**: 17 (Nov. 5) 1947.
8. Hudson, P. B., and Finkle, A. L.: Prostatic Cancer. II. Regional (Pudendal Plexus) Block Anesthesia for Open Perineal Surgical Biopsy of the Prostate Gland, Surgery **33**: 308-311 (Feb.) 1953.
9. Colby, F. H.: Carcinoma of the Prostate: Results of Total Prostatectomy, J. Urol. **69**: 797-806 (June) 1953.
10. Hudson, P. B., Finkle, A. L., Jost, H. M., Trifilio, A., and Stout, A. P.: Prostatic Cancer. X. Comparison of Open and "Punch" Biopsy Techniques, Arch. Surg., 1954. In press.
11. Moore, R. A.: The Morphology of Small Prostatic Carcinoma, J. Urol. **33**: 224-234 (March) 1935.
12. Moore, R. A.: Benign Hypertrophy and Carcinoma of the Prostate. Occurrence and Experimental Production in Animals, Surgery **16**: 152-167 (July) 1944.
13. Gaynor, E. P.: Zur Frage des Prostatakrebses, Virchows Arch. f. path. Anat. **301**: 602-652 (March) 1938.
14. Mulligan, R. M.: Syllabus of Human Neoplasms, Philadelphia, 1951, Lea and Febiger, p. 170.
15. Hudson, P. B., Finkle, A. L., Hopkins, J. A., Sproul, E. E., and Stout, A. P.: Early Prostatic Cancer Diagnosed by Arbitrary Open Perineal Biopsy Among 300 Unselected Patients, Cancer, 1954. In press.
16. Creevy, C. D.: Observations on Hemolysis During Transurethral Resection: The Effects of Urea, J. Urol. **68**: 324-328 (July) 1952.
17. Creevy, C. D.: Personal communication.

MIXED TUMORS IN UNUSUAL SITES

BÉLA HALPERT, M.D., AND HAROLD J. BRELSFORD, M.D., HOUSTON, TEXAS

(From the Department of Pathology and the Department of Surgery, Baylor University College of Medicine, and the Veterans Administration Hospital)

MIXED tumors of anlage origin, the so-called mixed tumors of the salivary glands, have a structure mimicking an organ. They usually occur in or near the parotid or submandibular glands, and occasionally in or near the sublingual glands, or elsewhere along the lines of embryonal facial fissures. In rare instances, they have been observed in parts distant from the head. The frequency with which these mixed tumors occur in unusual sites is as yet undetermined. Information is accumulating, however, revealing that they occur more often than was formerly believed. In this paper, six such tumors are presented, one in each of the following locations: the scalp, the lower eyelid, the hard palate, the lower lip, the back, and the testis. That on the back is believed to be the second such growth recorded in this location. The growth in the testis is included even though other observers may interpret it as a teratoma.

CASE REPORTS

CASE 1.—A. M. C., a 58-year-old white man, was admitted to the Veterans Administration Hospital, Houston, Texas, July 6, 1953, for treatment of painful varicose veins. On examination a freely movable, slightly tender mass, 2 cm. in diameter, was noted in the right temporal region just above the auricle. The patient said that the mass had been present for many years, that it seemed to vary in size, and was sometimes tender, but never painful. Following removal, the wound healed and there was no recurrence.

The specimen (S-1331-53) consisted of a thin-walled multiloculated sac, 1.5 by 1.5 by 0.6 cm., the locules containing a tan transparent coagulum. Microscopically, various-sized spaces contained a pale pink coagulum and were lined with low columnar cells, with the nuclei heaped into several rows. The septa were delicate, with occasional projections. Some of these had a stroma of embryonal connective tissue partly hyalinized. In it were acinar tubular structures lined by cuboidal cells and endothelial-lined slitlike spaces (Fig. 1).

CASE 2.—A. R. T., a 53-year-old white man, was admitted to the Veterans Administration Hospital, Houston, Texas, Nov. 15, 1949, with a mass on the left lower eyelid of about five years' duration. It had developed slowly, and during the previous year there had been mild conjunctivitis. At the time of admission, the mass was 1 cm. medial to the lateral canthus and was 0.3 cm. in diameter. Following removal, the wound healed promptly, and there has been no recurrence to date.

The specimen (S-764-49) consisted of a wedge of tissue, 0.5 by 0.3 cm., partly covered with skin, that had a raised area 0.2 cm. wide. Microscopically, in the corium, beneath a delicate layer of stratified squamous epithelium, there

Received for publication, Nov. 30, 1953.

was a fairly well-circumscribed field of strands of epithelial cells that enclosed various-sized lumina, empty or filled with pink amorphous substance. The cell strands had a lacelike pattern, with palisading at the periphery. There were lobules of adipose tissue cells within the loose connective tissue stroma (Fig. 2).

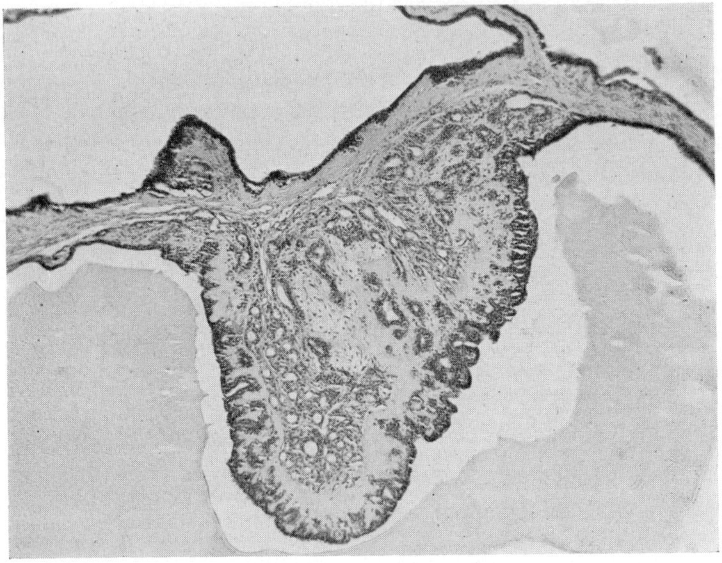

Fig. 1.—Mixed tumor from the right temporal region of a man aged 58 years (Case 1). In the stroma are stellate embryonal connective tissue cells. (×85.)

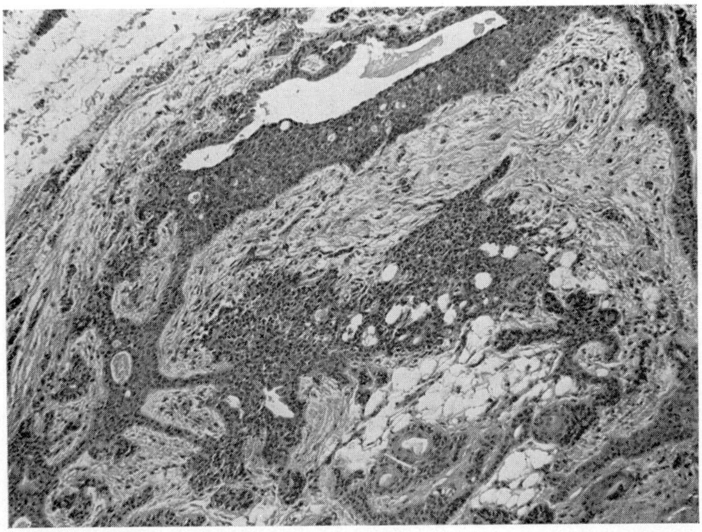

Fig. 2.—Mixed tumor from the left lower eyelid of a man aged 53 years (Case 2). In the stroma are scattered adult adipose tissue cells. (×80.)

Case 3.—C. L. J., a 58-year-old white man, was admitted to the Veterans Administration Hospital, March 13, 1952, with a painless tumor of the hard palate for eight years. At the time of admission there was a firm bulging mass, 4 by 3 cm., in the hard palate on the left that extended posteriorly for 1 cm. into the soft palate (Fig. 3). The mass was excised and found to be limited to the soft tissues of the palate. Following operation, a naso-oral fistula developed that healed spontaneously. There has been no recurrence to date.

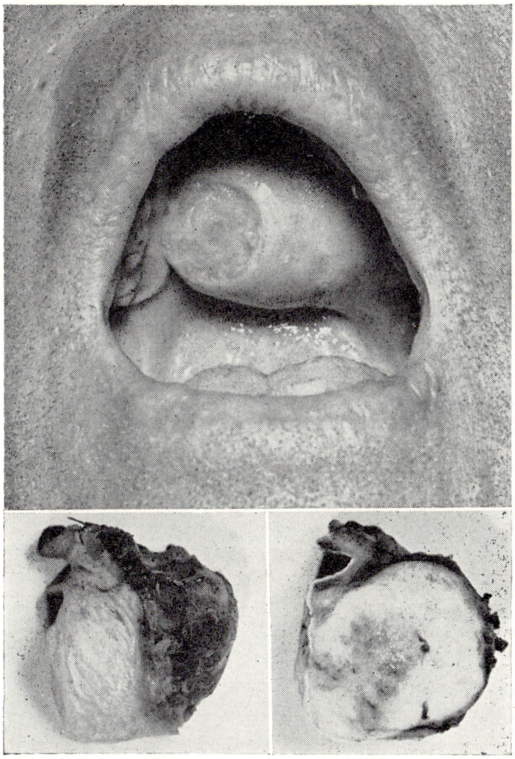

Fig. 3.—Mixed tumor in the palate of a man aged 58 years (Case 3). The growth is seen in situ, and the external and cut surfaces of the removed specimen are also shown.

The specimen (S-491-52) consisted of a globular mass of firm tissue, 3.5 by 3 by 3 cm. One surface was partly covered by mucous membrane eroded in an area measuring 1.5 cm. The cut surfaces were yellow-gray, mottled with red (Fig. 3). Microscopically, strands and nests of epithelial cells, some in a concentric pattern with central keratinization and frayed borders, were within a loose or more dense and hyalinizing connective tissue stroma. In the latter, lobules of adult adipose tissue cells were conspicuous (Fig. 4).

Case 4.—G. C. S., a 62-year-old white man, was admitted to the Veterans Administration Hospital, May 28, 1952, for arthritis. On examination, a nodule, 1 cm. in diameter, was noted on the inner surface of the left lower lip, which was said to have been present for six years. At the time of excision it appeared encapsulated. When the patient was last seen, May, 1953, there had been no recurrence.

The specimen (S-987-52) consisted of a globular portion of tissue, 1 by 0.8 by 0.4 cm., partly covered by mucous membrane, measuring 2 by 0.3 cm.

The cut surfaces revealed a solid nodule within a delicate capsule. Microscopically, there was a well-circumscribed area of compactly arranged, varying sized epithelial cells in a streamlike pattern. The cells had vesicular nuclei

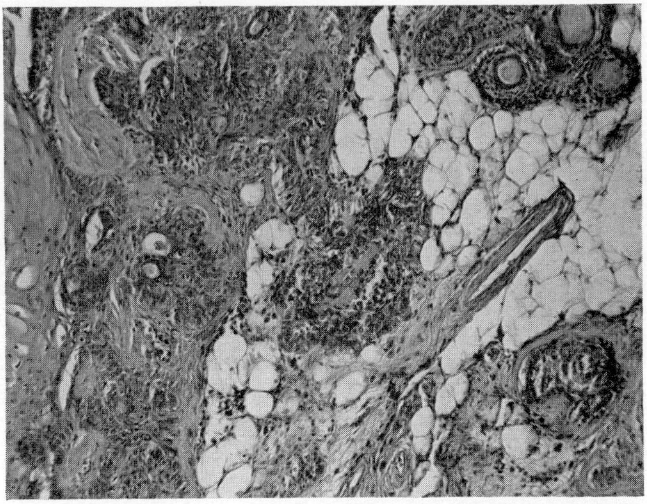

Fig. 4.—Microscopic structure of the growth shown in Fig. 3. The adult adipose tissue cells in the stroma are believed to be an intrinsic part of the neoplasm. (×75.)

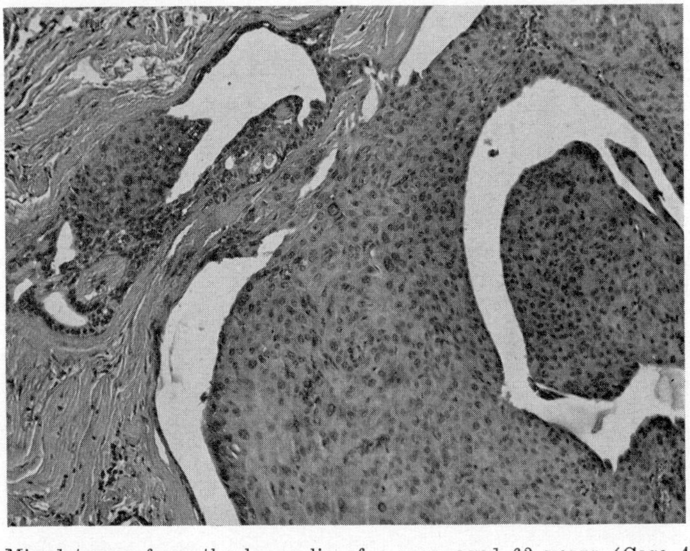

Fig. 5.—Mixed tumor from the lower lip of a man aged 62 years (Case 4). The compactly arranged epithelial cells have a streamlike pattern. Elsewhere cuboidal cells line acinar or elongated spaces. (×80.)

in abundant pink or lavender cytoplasm. Elsewhere cuboidal cells lined minute lumina or elongated spaces. The connective tissue stroma was scanty in places and elsewhere abundant, dense, and hyalinizing (Fig. 5).

CASE 5.—J. C. B., a 62-year-old white man, was admitted to the Veterans Administration Hospital, March 27, 1951, with osteoarthritic pain. On examination, a tumor mass,

10 by 5 cm., was discovered in the left lumbar region. The mass was under the skin, freely movable, and slightly tender. The patient stated that a similar mass was removed from his back during World War I. He believed that the growth recurred in the same region about three years later. It had enlarged slowly during the previous thirty years. The growth was excised, the wound healed, and when the patient was seen one year later there had been no recurrence.

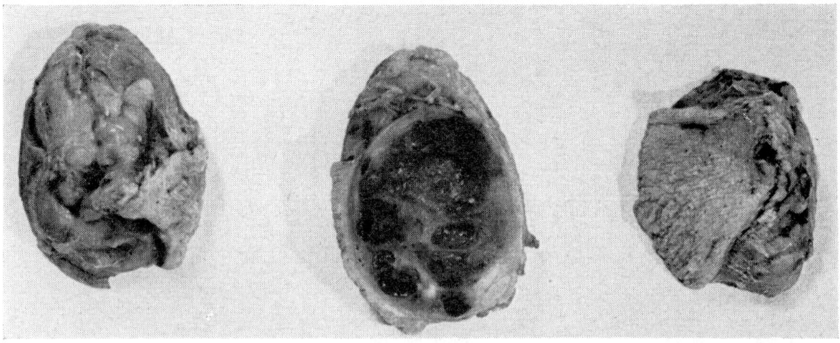

Fig. 6.—Mixed tumor from the left lumbar region of a man aged 62 years (Case 5). Cystic spaces filled with dark liquid are seen on the cut surface of the removed specimen.

The specimen (S-650-51) consisted of a firm mass, 4 by 2.8 cm., attached to an ellipse of white skin, 7 by 3 cm. On section, shiny brown and yellow tissue contained cystic spaces filled with dark liquid (Fig. 6). Microscopically, the neoplastic area was deep in the corium beneath the level of hair follicles and sweat glands. It was delimited by a fairly dense hyalinized fibrous connective tissue capsule. Inside the capsule there were acinar tubular structures lined by low cuboidal cells. There were also large spaces lined by flat cells and filled by pink coagulum. Some of these contained many large mononuclear cells with foamy cytoplasm. These epithelial cell groups were in a scanty loose or dense connective tissue stroma, with occasional broad bands of hyalinized connective tissue. Elsewhere, in loose fibrillar tissue, epithelial cell nests in an acinar pattern faded into connective tissue. Interspersed were fields of young connective tissue with a loose streamlike arrangement of the cells and fibrils (Fig. 7).

Case 6.—A. J., a 42-year-old white man, was admitted to the Psychiatric Service of the Veterans Administration Hospital, March 14, 1952. On physical examination a small nodule was noted in the right testicle. The patient had discovered the nodule about six weeks prior to admission. At operation, a nodule about 1 cm. in diameter was removed from inside the tunica albuginea of the right testicle. Several months following excision there had been no recurrence of the growth.

The specimen (S-548-52) consisted of a portion of gray-white tissue, 1.2 by 1.0 by 0.8 cm. Microscopically, nests and strands of epithelial cells with deep blue nuclei and hardly any cytoplasm were unevenly distributed in a pale fibrillar and vacuolated ground substance (Fig. 8). At one margin there were a few seminiferous tubules which were lined by Sertoli cells and contained no sperms.

COMMENT

The neoplasms herein recorded are essentially similar in their microscopic structure. While they resemble closely those arising in and about the salivary glands, they are of less complex pattern, and the epithelial elements usually

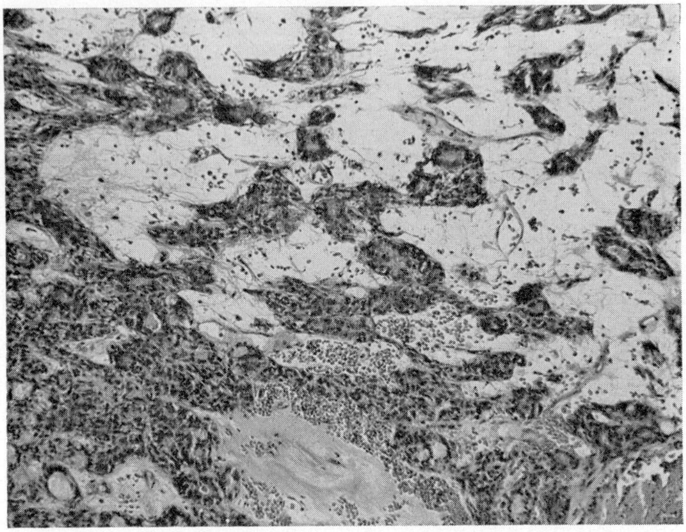

Fig. 7.—Microscopic structure of the growth shown in Fig. 6. In a loose fibrillar substance epithelial cell nests in an acinar pattern fade into connective tissue. (×80.)

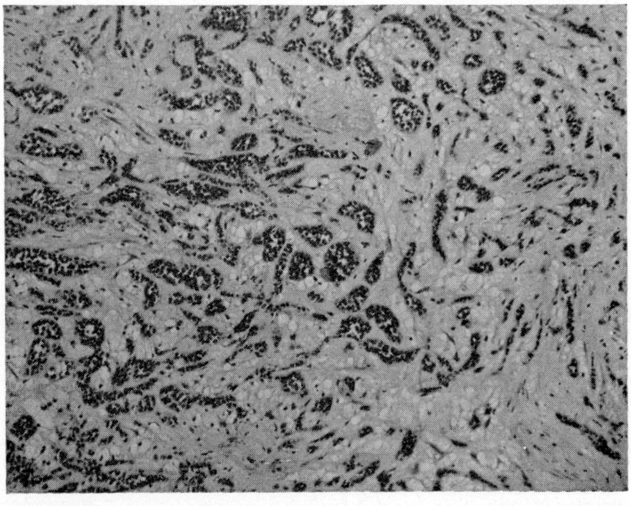

Fig. 8.—Mixed tumor from the right testicle of a man aged 42 years (Case 6). Nests and strands of epithelial cells are unevenly distributed in a pale fibrillar and vacuolated ground substance. (×75.)

predominate. These mixed tumors are fairly common about the oral cavity and the face, at some distance from the large salivary glands. They are more often observed in the palate[1-6] and in the upper lip[7] than elsewhere about the oral cavity. They have been reported about the nose,[8] on the lower lip,[9] on the eyelids,[8, 10] on the cheek,[8, 11] on the eyebrows,[8, 10] and, less frequently, in the tongue,[12] the tonsillar fossa,[13] larynx,[14] the pterygomaxillary space,[15] and the nasal septum.[16] They have been observed also on the scalp,[17, 18] on the ear,[19, 20] on the postauricular region, and on the neck.[17] Among those located distant from the head, fourteen were recorded as occurring on the upper extremities,[8, 10, 20, 21] eight on the lower extremities,[8] two each in the mammary gland and over the sternum,[10] and one each on the back, inguinal region, vulva,[10] vagina,[22] and buttock.[8]

An understanding of the morphologic features and clinical behavior of these neoplasms is of utmost importance in the approach to a rational therapy.[23] The close similarity in their microscopic structure and behavior suggests a common derivation. It has been inferred that they are derived of ectoderm, the anlage having separated at a stage when the cells as yet had not acquired their dominant characteristics as ectodermal or mesodermal cells.[24] The proportion of ectodermal and mesodermal elements may vary considerably, with at times the mesodermal elements predominating. The testicle itself is a mesodermal structure, hence both the epithelial and nonepithelial elements of the growth are likewise derived of mesoderm. Placing this growth into the group of mixed tumors of anlage origin is therefore not inconsistent with the previously proposed theory of their origin.[24]

SUMMARY

Mixed tumors of anlage origin, the so-called mixed tumors of salivary gland type, occasionally occur on the face and head where salivary glands are not usually present. They have also been observed at sites distant from the head. Observations are recorded on six such tumors, one each of the following locations: the scalp, the lower eyelid, the hard palate, the lower lip, the back, and the testis. That on the back is believed to be the second such growth recorded in this location, while that in the testis may also be interpreted as a teratoma.

REFERENCES

1. Sonnenschein, R.: Mixed Tumors in the Soft Palate. Report of Two Cases and Survey of the Recent Literature, Arch. Otolaryng. **11:** 137-150, 1930.
2. Abshier, A. B.: Mixed Tumors of the Palate, Arch. Dermat. & Syph. **32:** 622-625, 1935.
3. Barroux, P., and Blaquiere, G.: Étude anatomo-cliniques des tumeurs mixtes du voile du palais, Rev. de laryng. **63:** 145-174, 1942.
4. Gidall, S. H.: Mixed Tumors of the Soft Palate, Arch. Otolaryng. **38:** 166-168, 1943.
5. Cutler, M.: Mixed Tumors of the Palate, Am. J. Roentgenol. **61:** 82-90, 1949.
6. Wild, C., and Blenck, J. P.: Volumineuse tumeur mixte du voile du palais. opération guérison, Strasbourg méd. **2:** 790-792, 1951.
7. Bernier, J. L.: Mixed Tumors of the Lip, J. Oral Surg. **4:** 193-202, 1946.
8. Lennox, B., Pearse, E., and Richards, H. G. H.: Mucin-secreting Tumors of the Skin: With Special Reference to the So-called Mixed-salivary Tumor of the Skin and Its Relation to Hidradenoma, J. Path. & Bact. **64:** 865-880, 1952.
9. Eggers, H. E.: Mixed Tumors of the Lip, Arch. Path. **26:** 348-353, 1938.
10. Halpert, B., and Hackney, V. C.: Anlage Tumors of the Salivary Gland Type in Unusual Sites, SURGERY **27:** 609-615, 1950.
11. Grether, A., and Tetu, J.: Tumeur mixte sous-muqueuse de la joue, Revue de stomatologie **52:** 349-352, 1951.
12. Coker, W. G.: Mixed Tumors of the Tongue, Bowman Gray School of Med. **4:** 49-55, 1946.

13. Bates, C. E. H.: Mixed Salivary Tumor in the Right Tonsil Fossa With Narcolepsy and Cataplexy, Ann. Otol., Rhin. & Laryng. **54**: 812-817, 1945.
14. Liu, J. T., Wu, Y. K., and Liu, Y.: Mixed Tumors Occurring in Regions Unassociated With Salivary Glands; A Report of Seven Cases, Chinese M. J. **68**: 211-216, 1950.
15. Ehrlich, H.: Mixed Tumors of the Pterygomaxillary Space, Oral Surg., Oral Med. & Oral Path. **3**: 1366-1371, 1950.
16. Gabriel, G. E.: A Case of Mixed Salivary Tumor of the Nasal Septum, J. Laryng. & Otol. **66**: 329-330, 1952.
17. Geschickter, C. F., and Koehler, H. P.: Ectodermal Tumors of the Skin, Am. J. Cancer **23**: 804-836, 1935.
18. Gates, O., Warren, S., and Warvi, W. N.: Tumors of Sweat Glands, Am. J. Path. **19**: 591-626, 1943.
19. Mark, I., and Rothberg, M.: Mixed Tumor of Skin of External Auditory Canal, Arch. Otolaryng. **53**: 556-559, 1951.
20. Morehead, R. P.: Mixed Tumors of the Skin; Report of Cases, With a Consideration of the Histogenesis of Mixed Tumors of Organs Derived From the Ectoderm, Arch. Path. **40**: 107-113, 1945.
21. Simard, L. C.: Tumor of the Palm Having the Structure of a Mixed Tumor of the Salivary Glands, Am. J. Cancer **33**: 182-195, 1938.
22. Brown, C. E.: Mixed Epithelial Tumor of the Vagina, Am. J. Clin. Path. **23**: 237-240, 1953.
23. Brown, J. B., McDowell, F., and Fryer, M. P.: Direct Operative Removal of Benign Mixed Tumors of Anlage Origin in the Parotid, Surg., Gynec. & Obst. **90**: 257-268, 1950.
24. Halpert, B., and Tool, C. D.: Anlage Tumors of the Salivary Glands, Cancer Research **7**: 346-350, 1946.

A MODIFICATION OF THE HUNTERIAN LABORATORY ANESTHESIA APPARATUS FOR EXPERIMENTAL SURGERY

Harvey N. Lippman, M.D., Paul A. Johnson, Jr., B.A., and Kent A. Flygare, Los Angeles, Calif.

(From the Department of Surgery, School of Medicine, University of California Medical Center)

HANLON, Johns, and Thomas,[1] in 1950, described an apparatus which is used in the Surgical Hunterian Laboratory of the Johns Hopkins Medical School for providing anesthesia in experimental thoracic surgery. This apparatus consists of a motor-driven valve which periodically interrupts a stream of compressed air or oxygen passing over an ether reservoir into an endotracheal tube. The source of air or oxygen, the ether reservoir (a one-liter Woulfe bottle), and the interrupter valve are interconnected by means of suitable lengths of rubber tubing. The concentration of ether vapor in the anesthetic mixture may be varied by partially diverting the stream of air which passes over the ether fluid. This is accomplished by the application of one or two hand clamps at particular points on the rubber tubing which connects the ether reservoir to the other units of the system (Fig. 1).

For the past two years we have used a modified form of this apparatus in the Experimental Surgical Laboratory of the University of California Medical Center at Los Angeles. It has provided satisfactory anesthesia for use in both thoracic and prolonged abdominal procedures. The modifications which we have imposed upon the original model have proved to be of sufficient value to warrant their description. These modifications consist of: (1) an air reservoir which is interposed in the line between the air or oxygen supply and the ether reservoir (Fig. 2), (2) a multiple foot pedal device, which replaces the hand clamps, for varying the ether concentration (Figs. 2 to 5), and (3) a blowoff valve which eliminates the expired gases from a point just proximal to the endotracheal catheter (Figs. 2 and 6).

Air Reservoir.—As the interrupter valve rotates, it periodically opens and closes the circuit leading into the endotracheal tube (Fig. 1, *3*). Inasmuch as the flow of compressed air or oxygen is constant, the pressure in the system proximal to the interrupter alternately increases and decreases with the closing and opening of the valve. Hanlon and associates[1] noted that this increase in pressure is dissipated by the expansion of the rubber tubing and compression of the vapor in the ether reservoir (Fig. 1, *5*). Elimination of this cushioning effect by completely diverting the Woulfe bottle (clamps applied at *10* and *11*, Fig. 1) may cause respiratory distress or separation of the connections proximal to the clamps. While, admittedly, a minimal amount of ether vapor will flow through the interrupter valve if only one of the two

Received for publication, Oct. 19, 1953.

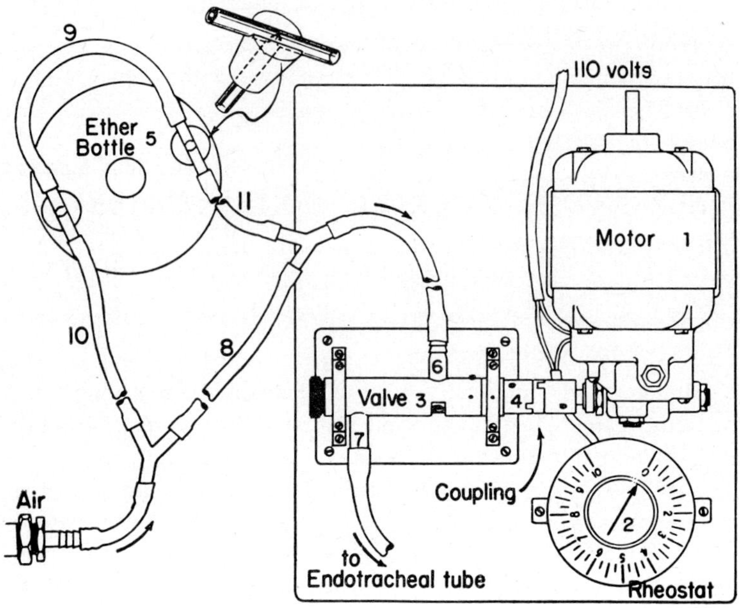

Fig. 1.—Diagram of original apparatus described by Hanlon, Johns, and Thomas.[1] (From Hanlon, Johns, and Thomas.[1])

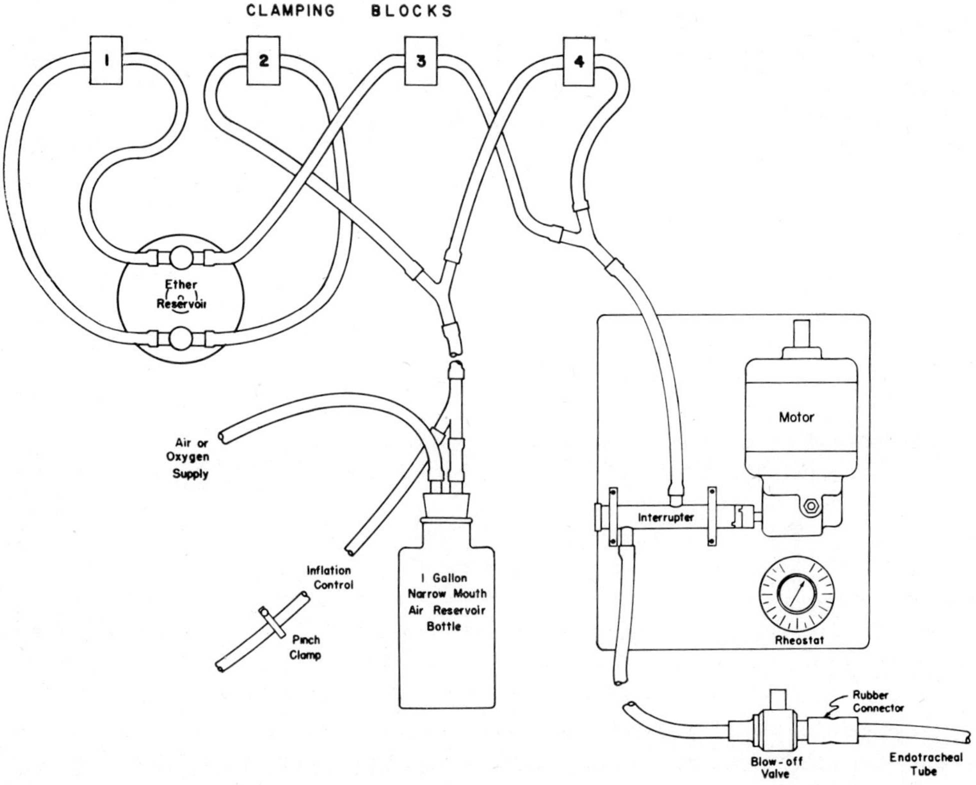

Fig. 2.—Diagram of modified apparatus showing relationships of air reservoir bottle, clamping blocks of foot pedal control mechanism, and blowoff valve. Note lung inflation control in airline.

tubes leading from the Woulfe bottle is occluded, we have found that by interposing an air reservoir (a one-gallon narrow-mouthed bottle) into the system, as indicated in Fig. 2, a separate expansion chamber is provided, so that if the ether reservoir should be completely diverted by compression of both tubes at the same time (at clamping blocks *2* and *3*, Fig. 2), the increase in pressure is absorbed by the compression of air in the reservoir bottle. By this simple device, delivery of ether-free air or oxygen may be accomplished and the apparatus may be used to additional advantage as an air or pure oxygen insufflator or resuscitator.

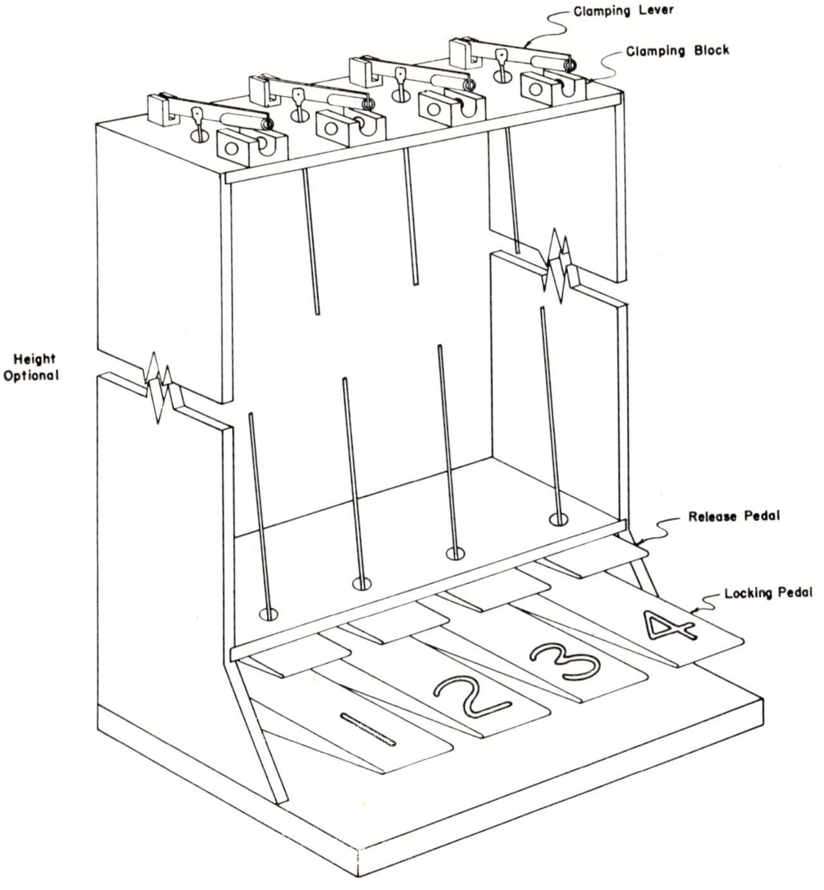

Fig. 3.—Isometric diagram of foot pedal control device (see also Figs. 4 and 5). By pressing down upon any of the four locking pedals, tension is applied to the connecting rod, which in turn lowers the clamping lever. When the foot pedal attains the required pressure (adjustable in the connecting rod), the locking latch is engaged. This maintains the depressed position of the clamping lever until the release pedal is pressed. The release pedal disengages the locking latch, which allows the locking pedal to be pulled up to its original position by the return spring.

In Fig. 2, a safety valve has been inserted in the air line to control the degree of lung inflation. If the tubing and pinch clamp are sterilized and brought into the operative field, this valve may be adjusted by the operator or his assistant as required during the procedure.

Foot Pedal Control.—The addition of a mechanical foot pedal device for the purpose of varying the ether concentration has been the direct outgrowth of a need to conserve the number of unscrubbed assistants engaged in any particular procedure. This innovation allows the surgeon or his assistant, without contaminating himself, to change the concentration of the ether mixture by a simple movement of his foot. The foot pedal control mechanism has been installed at the head of the table directly beneath the anesthesia apparatus. It is constructed in such a way as to permit compression of one or a combination of tubes which connect the ether reservoir to the other units of the system in exactly the same manner as would ordinarily be accomplished by the hand clamps. A diagram of the apparatus with details of the working parts is represented in Figs. 3, 4, and 5.

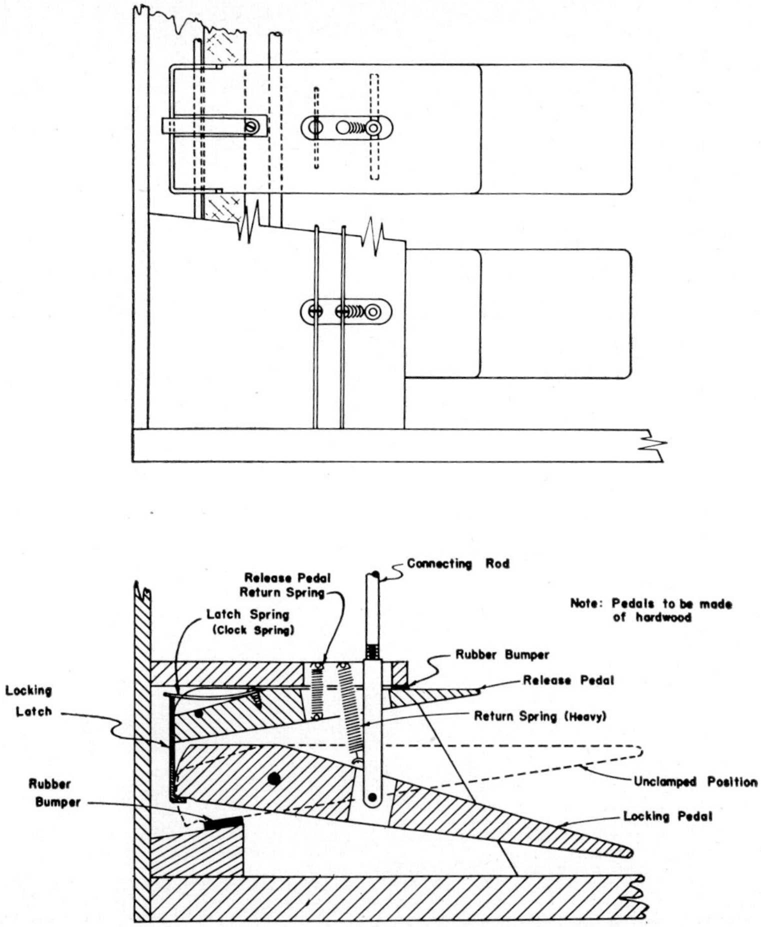

Fig. 4.—Projection drawing in two views showing locking and release pedal details of foot pedal control device (see legend, Fig. 3).

The concentration of ether vapor in the anesthetic mixture may be varied by engaging the four locking pedals of the controlling device singly or in combination, as follows:

Pedals 2 and 3	Ether-free air or oxygen
Pedals 2 or 3	Minimal ether vapor
All pedals released	Moderate ether vapor (usual maintenance level)
Pedals 1 or 4	Heavy ether vapor
Pedals 1 and 4	Maximal anesthetic effect

Blowoff Valve.—The interrupter valve allows for exhaustion of expired gases with each revolution of its cylinder from an opening immediately opposite the intake port (Fig. 1, *6*). The greater the length of tubing which conducts the ether mixture from the apparatus to the animal, the greater the volume of dead space in the system. To avoid this problem, we have inserted

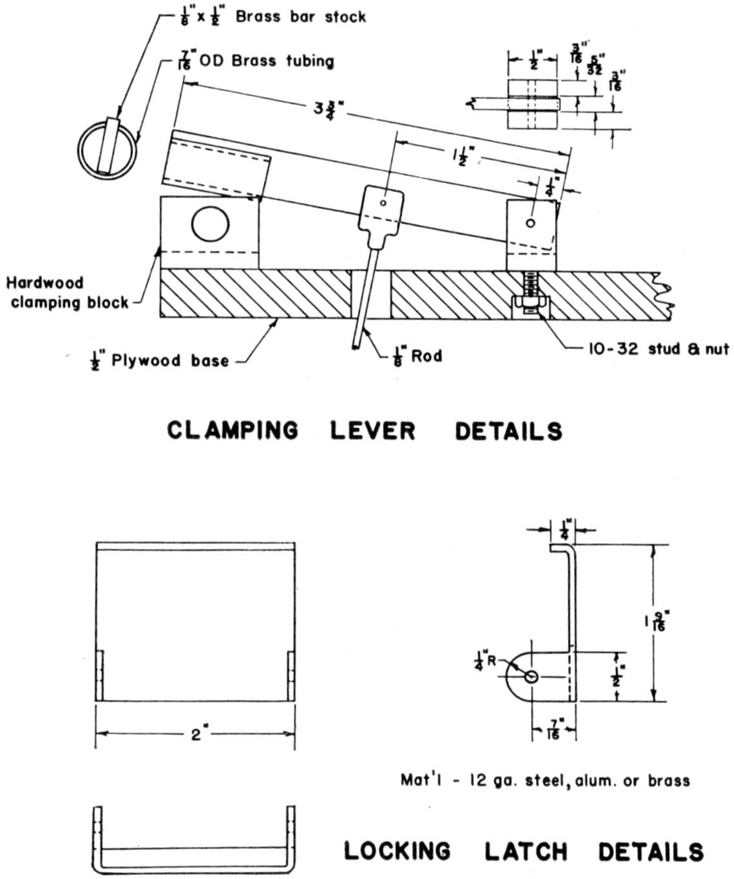

Fig. 5.—Drawing showing clamping lever and locking latch details of foot pedal control device (see legend, Fig. 3).

a simple blowoff valve of our own design just proximal to the endotracheal catheter. This valve is similar in principle to those used by clinical anesthetists. While it is the most recent of the innovations which we have applied to the apparatus, the blowoff valve has already proved to be of considerable value in controlling the amount of carbon dioxide which the animal is required to rebreathe. A detailed drawing of this valve is seen in Fig. 6.

DISCUSSION

It has been our practice to induce anesthesia, after suitable medication with morphine and atropine, with an intravenous injection of 2½ per cent thiopental sodium or parenteral pentobarbital sodium. We have found this to be much simpler than the use of open drop ether. After the endotracheal catheter is passed and the cuff inflated, connection is established with the interrupter valve, the required settings for rate and depth of respiration are made,

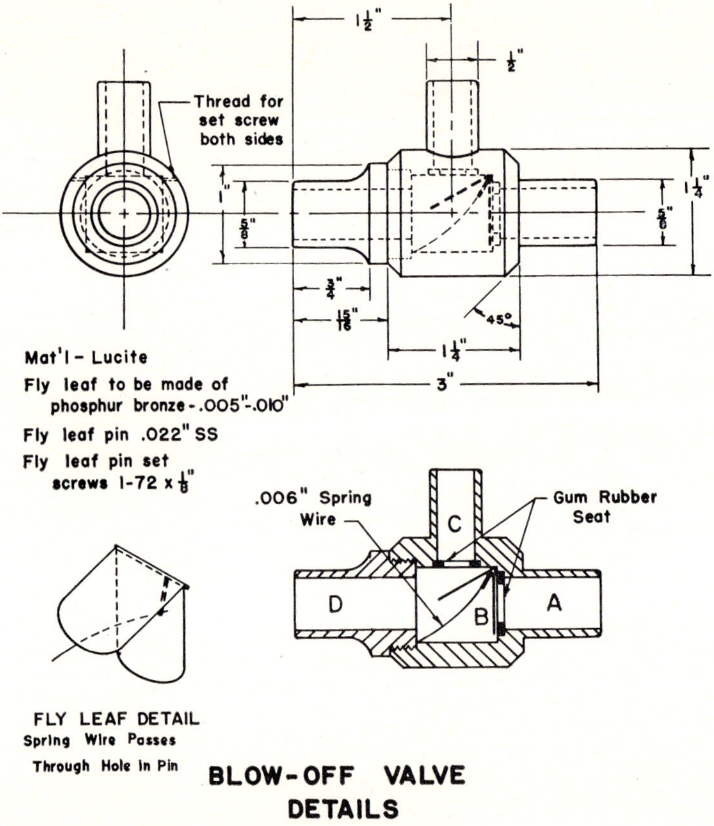

Fig. 6.—Drawing showing details of blowoff valve. When positive pressure is applied through opening at *A*, the spring-loaded butterfly valve (*B*) is forced open, and simultaneously the exhaust port at *C* is closed. This allows the anesthetic mixture to pass through *D* into the endotracheal tube. When the positive pressure is interrupted, the spring-loaded valve (*B*) resumes its resting position, closing intake port at *A* and opening the exhaust port at *C*. This permits the expired gases to escape.

and the foot pedals are set to provide a suitable mixture of ether vapor and compressed air or oxygen. If the shorter-acting barbiturate is used for induction, rapid saturation with ether is encouraged. If pentobarbital sodium is used, saturation with ether is accomplished more slowly. Shifting of the foot pedals provides any necessary change in concentration of ether vapor, depending on the depth of anesthesia required.

SUMMARY

Three modifications which have been applied to the Hunterian Laboratory anesthesia apparatus for experimental surgery have been described.

These modifications are: (1) an air reservoir which is inserted in the line between the air or oxygen supply and the ether reservoir, (2) a multiple foot pedal device for controlling the ether concentration, and (3) a blowoff valve for eliminating the expired gases.

A brief description of our anesthetic practice in experimental surgery has been presented.

Acknowledgment.—The original suggestion for the anesthesia blowoff valve described in this article was made by William H. Muller, Jr., M.D., associate professor of surgery, University of California Medical Center at Los Angeles, in whose laboratory this device was developed.

REFERENCE

1. Hanlon, C. R., Johns, T. N. P., and Thomas, V.: An Apparatus for Anesthesia in Experimental Thoracic Surgery, J. Thoracic Surg. 19: 887-890, 1950.

DIAGNOSTIC PARACENTESIS IN THE ACUTE ABDOMEN

CLARENCE T. THOMPSON, M.D., NEW ORLEANS, LA., AND DONALD R. BROWN, M.D., CHARLOTTETOWN, PRINCE EDWARD ISLAND, CANADA

(From the Tulane University of Louisiana School of Medicine and Charity Hospital of Louisiana at New Orleans)

DIAGNOSTIC paracentesis is not a new procedure. It has been used on occasion in the differentiation of the various types of peritonitis and ascites. Although there were sporadic reports of diagnostic taps in the early part of the century, the first comprehensive report was by Neuhof and Cohen in 1926.[1]

The value of diagnostic paracentesis has long been recognized in the differentiation of primary peritonitis from the peritonitis of perforated bowel, particularly in infants and children.[2] Later, its value in the diagnosis of strangulated bowel was emphasized.[3] Keith, Zollinger, and McCleery[5] stressed the importance of amylase determinations on peritoneal fluid in the diagnosis of late acute pancreatitis.

The present report stems from extensive experience over the past three years from the Tulane Surgical Service at Charity Hospital of New Orleans, La. This service includes a large group of acute abdominal cases, both traumatic and otherwise.

We have found diagnostic paracentesis to be of immense value in several groups of patients encountered. Its greatest use is in preoperative evaluation of blunt abdominal injuries, the differentiation of the various types of peritonitis, and in the diagnosis of many of the various abdominal catastrophies. The prime value, in addition to being of diagnostic import, is that it frequently averts an unnecessary laparotomy.

Blunt Abdominal Injuries.—It is generally recognized that penetrating wounds of the abdomen are an indication for laparotomy. However, the diagnostic difficulties of many of the closed injuries are well known. These injuries primarily include ruptures of the liver and spleen. The hollow viscera are not so commonly ruptured by blunt injuries, although an occasional case may be seen.

There are many patients in whom the diagnosis of severe intra-abdominal injury is obvious. These cases present no problem inasmuch as laparotomy is clearly indicated as soon as shock is combated adequately.

The patients presenting with minimal abdominal signs and symptoms frequently make the decision for or against laparotomy quite difficult. In early rupture of the spleen and liver, there is often a well-known latent period before the onset of shock. We have found that our method of paracentesis is frequently the deciding factor in these equivocal cases.

Patients are commonly seen in our emergency room with multiple severe injuries. Those with head injuries and crushing injuries of the chest are

Received for publication, Dec. 21, 1953.

particularly difficult to evaluate for possible abdominal injuries. Those with head injuries are frequently unconscious or stuporous and therefore unable to cooperate for an adequate examination. We have seen patients with known head injuries who remained in shock with no physical reasons apparent. Peritoneal aspiration revealed blood which did not clot. We use this finding as a clear-cut indication for laparotomy. Ruptures of the liver and spleen are frequently seen in blunt injuries of the chest, particularly with fractures of the lower rib cage. In all of these patients, a moderate degree of upper abdominal pain and splinting is encountered. Inasmuch as these patients with severe chest injuries are poor risks from an anesthetic viewpoint, caution must be exercised in the decision for a laparotomy. Paracentesis in these cases has been invaluable in making that decision in that frequently it reveals nonclotting blood in the peritoneal cavity indicating intra-abdominal injury of a major nature.

When clotted blood is obtained from the needle, we assume that the needle has probably damaged a vessel in the abdominal wall. Blood in the general peritoneal cavity has been sufficiently defibrinated so that it will not clot.

Many patients were submitted to laparotomy with minimal or no evidence of abdominal injury other than a positive diagnostic tap. In only one patient was an unnecessary laparotomy performed. This patient was stuporous due to a head injury. Repeated needle aspiration revealed partially clotting blood from the right lower quadrant. Subsequent laparotomy revealed three needle holes in a very low right lobe of the liver extending to the iliac crest.

We know of no patient in this group over a three-year period in whom the tap was negative, who subsequently revealed major abdominal pathology.

Acute Abdominal Conditions Accompanied by Shock (Exclusive of Injuries).—A number of patients are seen here in peripheral collapse with a rigid, distended, silent abdomen, generally of recent onset. Frequently, no underlying pathology is apparent. Abdominal paracentesis has been of value in this group because it frequently distinguishes a clearly operable condition from one which is not. This pertains particularly to the differentiation of acute hemorrhagic pancreatitis from strangulated bowel.

It has been emphasized by Keith, Zollinger, and McCleery[5] that amylase levels on peritoneal fluid generally remain high after the serum amylase has fallen to normal levels in acute pancreatitis. We have had three cases in which the diagnosis of acute hemorrhagic pancreatitis was established by paracentesis with the finding of typical sanguinous, dark fluid. In these cases, all had markedly elevated amylase levels in the peritoneal fluid but had perfectly normal serum amylase levels. In these three cases, laparotomy was fortunately averted.

The hemorrhagic peritoneal fluid is likewise encountered when nonviable gut is present in the abdominal cavity. The fluids in these two abdominal emergencies are quite similar, and the amylase determination is therefore quite significant in differentiation.

The classical fluid obtained in perforated ulcer is cloudy or purulent with flecks of amorphous fibrinous material. However, the clinical picture is usually diagnostic without resort to paracentesis.

Peritonitis of Unknown Etiology.—The literature reviewed has stressed the importance of diagnostic paracentesis primarily in this group of patients. In our hands its value has been in the differentiation of so-called primary bacterial peritonitis from generalized peritonitis due to ruptured viscera in infants and children. The consensus of opinion is that smears of peritoneal exudates revealing gonococcus, pneumococcus, Staphylococcus, and Streptococcus are an indication for conservative management.

When purulent or cloudy fluid is obtained by paracentesis, a smear is indicated for the differential diagnosis. If leukocytes are present with Staphylococcus, Streptococcus, pneumococcus, or gonococcus, the diagnosis of so-called primary peritonitis is established and laparotomy is not indicated. If leukocytes alone are obtained, with or without gram-negative rods, laparotomy is performed. If numerous organisms of all types are obtained without leukocytes, it may be assumed that the needle has been in the lumen of the bowel. If the bowel is inadvertently punctured, this, per se, is not an indication for laparotomy.

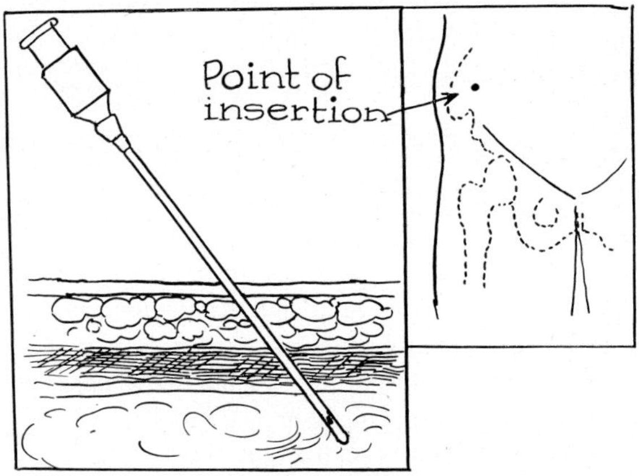

Fig. 1.—Technique.

Miscellaneous.—Clear, serous fluid has been encountered in mild pancreatitis and nonstrangulated obstructions. This type is found in ascites due to cirrhosis, heart failure, carcinomatosis, and tuberculous peritonitis, all of which are of little surgical importance. Centrifuged fluid and cell-block examinations are necessary to distinguish some of these fluids, and are out of the scope of this paper.

TECHNIQUE

The technique we use is simple. The Potter needle is probably more suitable because it is blunt and the opening is on the side, thereby not plugging as easily. However, the procedure has been carried out successfully with an ordinary 22 gauge spinal needle.

The skin is prepared in both lumbar quadrants of the abdomen and, with or without local anesthesia, the needle is inserted into the peritoneal cavity. The site of puncture is usually about 3 cm. superior and medial to the anterior superior iliac spine. The needle is directed medially into the peritoneal cavity.

The obturator of the needle is removed and, if fluid is not obtained immediately, a syringe is applied and gentle suction employed. The direction and depth of the needle may be changed without danger in an attempt to encounter fluid. The patient should be tilted so that the side of the tap is most dependent to facilitate fluid drainage. In case of a negative result, a similar procedure is used on the opposite side at the same level.

COMPLICATIONS

Needle perforations of the intestine are rare and, when they do occur, are of no consequence. In approximately 300 of these abdominal punctures, no complications have ensued. One mistaken diagnosis has been described in which an unnecessary laparotomy was performed.

CONCLUSIONS

1. Abdominal paracentesis is an important adjunct in the diagnosis of the acute abdomen.
2. In blunt injuries of the abdomen which are difficult to evaluate, paracentesis may present a concrete indication for laparotomy. This is particularly important in patients with concomitant head injuries and crushing chest injuries.
3. Patients severely ill with an acute abdominal emergency may be spared an unnecessary and even contraindicated laparotomy if the diagnosis of acute pancreatitis or primary peritonitis can be established. Evaluation of the peritoneal fluid frequently makes the diagnosis.
4. In 300 cases of diagnostic abdominal paracenteses, no complications have resulted.

REFERENCES

1. Neuhof, H., and Cohen, I.: Abdominal Puncture in the Diagnosis of Acute Intraperitoneal Diseases, Ann. Surg. **83**: 454-462, 1926.
2. Denzer, B. S.: Abdominal Puncture in the Diagnosis of Peritonitis in Childhood, J. Pediat. **8**: 741-747, 1936.
3. Hill, F. C.: Peritoneal Aspiration in Diagnosis of Strangulated Bowel, Surg., Gynec. & Obst. **74**: 121-123, 1942.
4. Campbell, H. E.: Abdominal Puncture, Rocky Mountain M. J. **43**: 305-307 (April) 1946.
5. Keith, L. M., Jr., Zollinger, R. M., and McCleery, R. S.: Peritoneal Fluid Amylase Determinations as an Aid in Diagnosis of Acute Pancreatitis, Arch. Surg. **61**: 930-936, 1950.

Case Reports

CANCER OF THE STOMACH: TWENTY-YEAR CURES

Report of Two Cases

George T. Pack, M.D., New York, N. Y.

(From the Gastric Service of the Memorial Cancer Center)

THE ANECDOTE

UNTIL 1930, the therapeutic activities of the Memorial Hospital were more greatly occupied with radium and x-ray treatment of cancers. Laparotomies, except for gynecologic procedures, were seldom employed. A gastric service functioned largely as an outpatient clinic, with one or two patients seen weekly, and they were receiving only medical treatment for vague dyspepsia. In the previous decade, only three gastrectomies had been performed in the institution, and then with fatal terminations. The radical surgical treatment of cancer was frowned upon as a policy. In January, 1931, I was given the post as chief of this department, which was more nominal than actual; my status at that time and during the succeeding six months was Resident Surgeon and Fellow in Cancer Surgery. As an insurance against inexperience in technique and judgment, the one contingency on the appointment was the requirement that a senior surgeon of the hospital be in attendance as a preceptor at each abdominal operation during the first year of my incumbency.

Case 1.—The first case was of a patient with a gastric cancer, which showed no outward evidence of dissemination. At the operation, the senior consultant, who was serving as first assistant and arbiter, advised a gastroenterostomy, despite my plea for gastrectomy. His arguments were several: (a) although no hepatic metastases were seen, the cancer was unquestionably incurable; (b) gastrectomy most likely would be fatal; (c) in the presence of pyloric obstruction, gastroenterostomy would do just as well in enabling the patient to live comfortably for a few months. Accordingly, a retrocolic posterior gastroenterostomy was performed.

Twelve weeks later the senior consultant left for Europe on a vacation; with the temporary loss of surgical restriction, the patient was immediately readmitted to the hospital. A second operation was performed, consisting of a distal sleeve resection of the stomach, after the method of Billroth II. The report of the pathologist was: "Tubular adenocarcinoma. Tumor throughout thickness of wall and is growing in serosa. Not a resection case with idea of cure." Convalescence was uneventful. The patient, now 80 years of age, is living and well except for arthritis; this represents a definitive cure period of survival for twenty-two years.

Received for publication, Sept. 30, 1953.

The case illustrates several points, both factual and moral: (a) The first gastrectomy for cancer performed on the newly organized gastric service of the Memorial Hospital resulted in a twenty-two-year cure. (b) A "second look" performed twelve weeks after a gastroenterostomy revealed the cancer to be still operable and permitted a second stage gastrectomy. (c) In retrospect and with regard to this one case, one might well ask which benefits the cancer patient more: the conservative attitude and greater experience of an older surgeon, or the lesser experience and more aggressive point of view of a younger surgeon? (d) The advice of Polonius to his son or the oft-quoted homily of the Golden Rule finds suitable application in this dilemma. (e) The definition of operability was established so definitively in the mind of the operator, together with the inevitable fatality without resection, that he was willing to risk censure and professional retardation if the gastrectomy had resulted in death. The subject was an indigent clinic patient. (f) The judgments of the senior surgeon with regard to operability and the pathologist with regard to curability were both incorrect, as proved by the survival of the patient for twenty-two years.

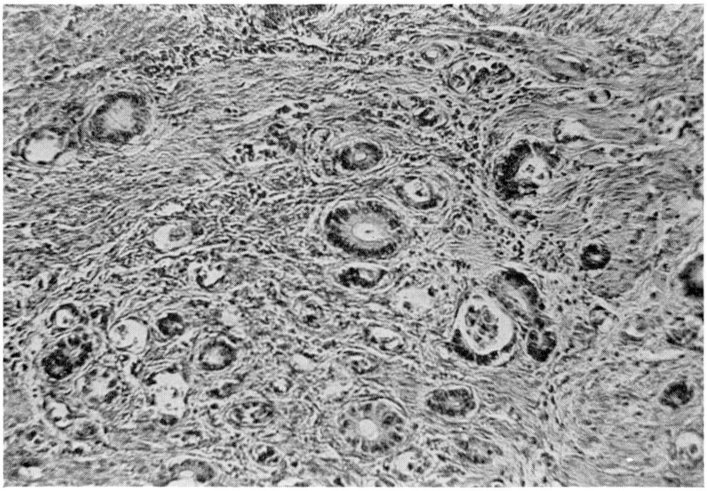

Fig. 1 (Case 1).—Tubular adenocarcinoma of stomach; twenty-two-year cure.

FORMAL CASE REPORT

J. Z., a 58-year-old man, sometime blacksmith helper and later janitor, applied to the Gastric Service of the Memorial Hospital on May 11, 1931. His past history was relatively normal except for bilateral herniorrhaphy in 1916 at the Hospital for the Ruptured and Crippled. His normal weight was 169 pounds.

Present History.—He had been in excellent health until January, 1930, at which time he developed regurgitation of bitter, hot fluid, eructation of gas, upper abdominal distress, and pain, occurring two to three hours after meals. Six hours after supper he was usually awakened with severe epigastric pain radiating from left to right, accompanied by loud gurgling. Vomiting occurred about once every two weeks. The symptoms had increased steadily since the date of onset. In December, 1930, gastrointestinal x-ray studies made elsewhere were reported as normal. On the date of application he weighed 121 pounds with a loss of 48 pounds in sixteen months since the onset of symptoms.

Physical Examination.—The patient gave evidence of weight loss, anemia, and cachexia. No tumor mass could be felt in the abdomen. The chest was normal to physical examination. There were no palpable masses in the pelvic cul-de-sac.

Gastrointestinal x-ray series made on May 12, 1931, revealed obstruction of the pylorus with an irregular filling defect and a marked gastric retention in six hours after the barium ingestion. The diagnosis was carcinoma of the prepyloric gastric segment.

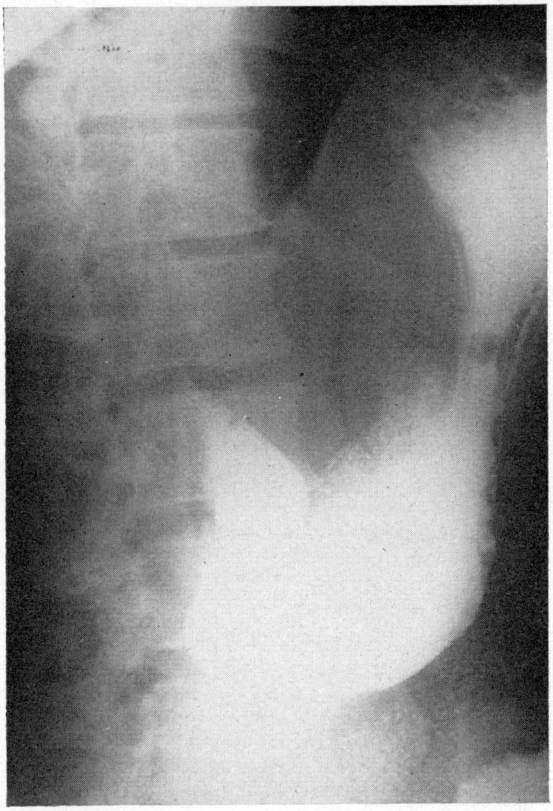

Fig. 2 (Case 2).—Roentgenogram of stomach showing early polypoid carcinoma.

Operative Procedure.—On May 29, 1931, a laparotomy was performed. The tumor was found to be confined to the distal third of the stomach. The serosa was involved, but there were no demonstrable metastases to the liver or other abdominal viscera. A retrocolic posterior gastrojejunostomy was performed. Convalescence was uneventful. After the patient was discharged from the hospital, he received some high-voltage x-ray therapy to the left epigastrium anteriorly and posteriorly, cross-firing at the distal segment of the stomach, employing 199 kv., ½ mm. of copper filter, 70 cm. target skin distance, portals 12 by 10 cm., 420 roentgens at a dose, treatment being given once every four days alternating between the anterior and posterior fields, for a total dose of 1,260 roentgens to the anterior port, and 840 roentgens to the posterior field.

The patient did not gain weight in the interval, but did have some relief of the symptoms of gastric retention due to pyloric obstruction.

He was readmitted to the hospital, and on Aug. 5, 1931, the segment of stomach distal to the previous and superiorly placed posterior gastrojejunostomy was removed, together with a liberal segment of the duodenum. This constituted a second stage Billroth II procedure. Convalescence from the second operation was uneventful.

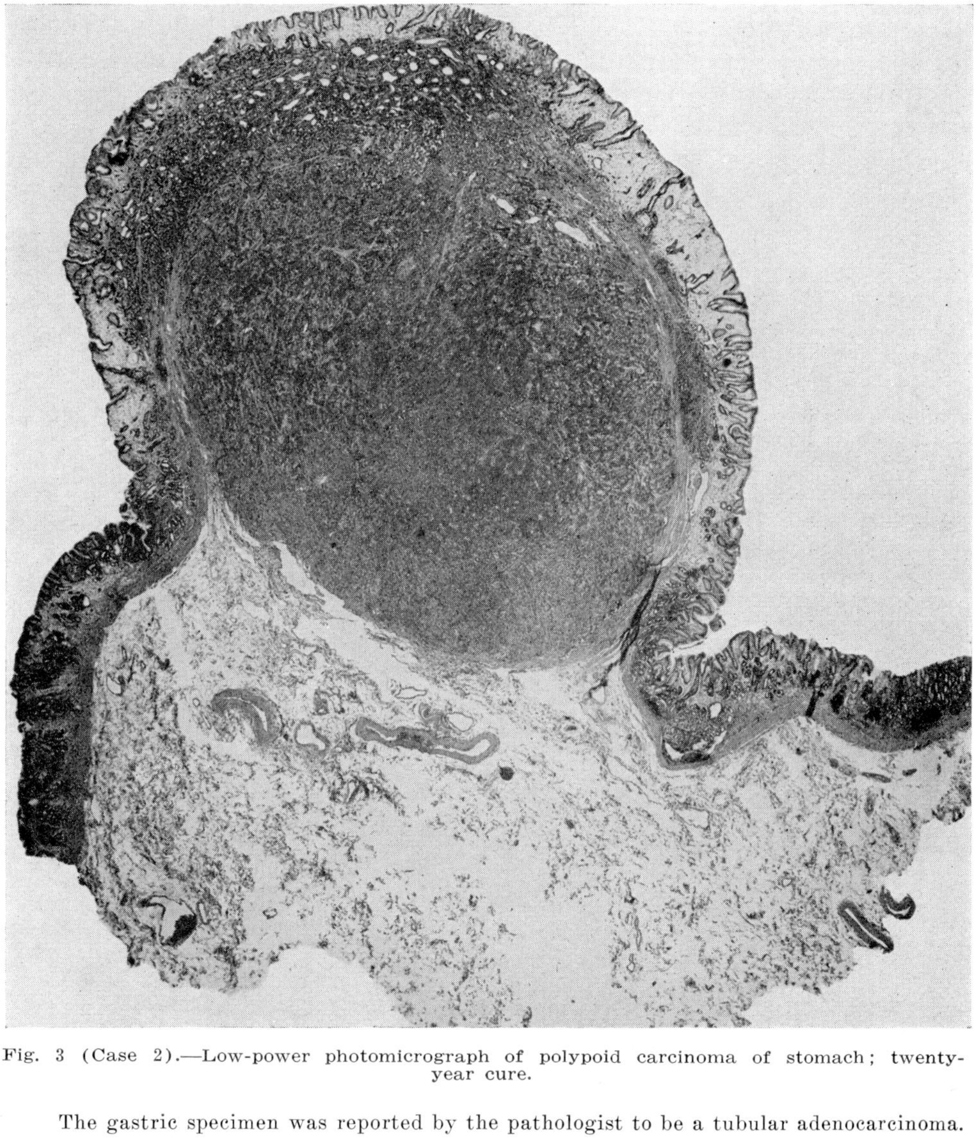

Fig. 3 (Case 2).—Low-power photomicrograph of polypoid carcinoma of stomach; twenty-year cure.

The gastric specimen was reported by the pathologist to be a tubular adenocarcinoma. In the intervening years this patient has been in good condition, except as he approached the age of 80 years he had increasing arthritis in the knees which caused him some disability. His weight increased from 121 to 144 pounds. He has had no gastric complaints, and remains in good general health for an octogenarian.

CASE 2.—Twenty to twenty-one years ago, Dr. Harry Hauser, then a Fellow of the Memorial Hospital, conducted a series of x-ray examinations of the gastrointestinal tract in male patients over 40 years of age, who had no gastric complaints. The purpose was to ascertain, if possible, any tumors, ulcers, or other physical abnormalities which might be present in the absence of suspicious symptoms. This experiment antedated by many years the more detailed surveys recently published from numerous sources in which one patient of 800 so examined was found to have an asymptomatic gastric cancer. Dr. Hauser examined less than 100 patients and in this group discovered a single polypoid gastric tumor in one patient. Immediate surgical intervention was carried out and the tumor, an early gastric cancer, was resected. The patient is living and free of evidence of recurrence after twenty years.

FORMAL CASE REPORT

K. C. T., a 41-year-old man, was superintendent of an estate. His employer, who had endowed a bed at Memorial Hospital, sent him to the hospital for a physical examination. Since his appendectomy at age 16 years, he had taken bran, Caroid, and bile salts intermittently to regulate his bowel movements. He had a good appetite and had lost no weight. There was no nausea or vomiting. Fluoroscopy and gastrointestinal x-ray series on June 28, 1933, revealed a small circular filling defect, measuring 1.5 cm. in diameter, situated on the anterior wall of the pars media. There was no gastric residue of the barium ingesta. Gastric analysis using histamine revealed complete anacidity and no occult blood in all specimens. Laparotomy was performed on July 11, 1933, and the polypoid tumor was resected. Dr. James Ewing gave the following report: adenocarcinoma, Grade II. The patient is living and free of evidence of gastric cancer on Sept. 1, 1953, more than twenty years later.

PERFORATION OF THE STOMACH IN THE NEWBORN INFANT

A Case Report

R. O. Northway, M.D., Saginaw, Mich., R. H. DeLano, M.D., Grand Forks, N. D., and A. A. Claytor, M.D., Saginaw, Mich.

ALTHOUGH perforation of the stomach in the newborn infant has been a recognized entity for one-quarter of a century, only twenty-two cases have been reported. The first survival was recorded by Leger, Ricard, Leonard, and Piette in 1950.[1] Although the case herein discussed represents the twenty-third reported case and the second survival, we assume the condition is more prevalent than reported.

In the majority of the reported cases of gastric perforation in the newborn infant, the lesion is usually secondary to ulcer, mechanical injury from gavage, congestion due to asphyxia and septicemia, and, finally, congenital defects in the musculature of the gastric wall.[2] The latter was reported by Herbut[3] in 1936. Ruptures are found to occur in all portions of the stomach wall, having no one prominent location. Race does not appear to be an important factor.

Greene and Gase[4] reported the twenty-first and twenty-second cases in 1953, the first being secondary to gastric ulcer, the other to pyloric atresia. The only other report of gastric perforation secondary to pyloric atresia was made by Burnett and Halpert[5] in 1947.

CASE REPORT

C. T., a newborn Negro boy weighing 5 pounds, 8 ounces, was born at Saginaw General Hospital, Nov. 23, 1952. The infant was the product of a normal pregnancy of eight months' gestation. The mother was 23 years old, gravida iiii, para iii with negative serology. Labor lasted seven hours and resulted in a spontaneous delivery. The infant cried spontaneously and immediately.

Initial physical examination revealed a normal infant with the exception of a high-pitched cry; temperature was 98° F. rectally. He was noted to nurse poorly at first feeding. Normal meconium stools were passed on the first and second day. At 5 A.M. on the third day, dark red blood was noted in the stools, abdominal distention was first noted, and respirations became labored and shallow. Three hours later another bloody stool was passed and surgical consultation was obtained. Physical findings revealed the patient to be a dyspneic Negro male infant with increased, shallow respirations, appearing acutely ill. The lungs were normal to percussion and auscultation. The abdomen was distended and silent, but soft. On percussion, no liver dullness was detected. There were no palpable masses. Laboratory findings at this time were: white blood cells 2,700, red blood cells 7.33 million, hemoglobin 22.5 Gm., 155 per cent. Blood group was O Rh positive. Blood Kahn test was negative. Microscopic urine examination showed a rare hyalin cast and one to two white blood cells per low-powered field. At 8:45 A.M. a scout film of the abdomen in supine and upright positions revealed a large amount of air in the area of the stomach and beneath the diaphragm, suggestive of a perforated viscus.

Received for publication, Sept. 28, 1953.

Intubation was carried out, without relief of the distention and without return flow of injected saline solution. While preparing for surgery, x-ray contrast studies of the upper intestinal tract were carried out, using a small amount of Lipiodol injected into the Levin tube. The Lipiodol was seen to spread diffusely throughout the abdomen through a rent on the greater curvature of the stomach.

Eight hours following onset of distention and five hours after passage of bloody stools, the infant was operated upon.

Under drop ether anesthesia, with protective warm water bottles about the body for maintenance of temperature, the infant was draped and prepared in the usual manner. Celiotomy was carried out through a right transrectus incision centered midway between the xiphoid process and umbilicus. On opening the peritoneal cavity, a large amount of bile-colored fluid was noted. A rent, about 2 cm. in length, was found along the greater curvature of the stomach and midway between the cardia and pylorus. There was no inflammatory reaction about the rent suggestive of gastric ulcer. The rent, we felt, was due to a congenital defect in the musculature of the stomach wall. The perforation was closed with a running 00 chromic catgut suture to include all layers, followed by a second seromuscular inverting layer of silk. Following closure of the stomach, the Levin tube was injected with 10 c.c. of sterile water, and no leakage occurred, confirming the presence of but one gastric defect. It was also found that the water inserted into the stomach could be expressed into the duodenum and jejunum, ruling out a congenital atresia of the duodenum. The entire gastrointestinal tract was then examined to rule out the presence of other anomalies. The wound was closed in layers, using interrupted sutures of fine silk throughout. The infant received 50 c.c. of whole blood during the procedure and was returned to the ward in good condition.

Postoperatively, the Levin suction was continued for two days, following which small amounts of 5 per cent glucose in water were given by mouth. Boiled skim milk was started on the third postoperative day with gradual increase in the formula to twenty calories per ounce. Fluid and electrolyte balance were maintained throughout, using 5 per cent glucose in water, Ringer's solution, and whole blood. Vitamin supplements of vitamin K, ascorbic acid, and Poly-vi-sol were given. Temperature remained 97° to 99° F. rectally throughout the hospital course, and the wound healed per primam. The white blood count gradually increased from 2,700 preoperatively to a peak of 27,200 on Dec. 4, 1952. Upon discharge, the white blood count was 14,700, hemoglobin 14.8 Gm., or 102 per cent. The infant was discharged on the twenty-seventh postoperative day weighing 5 pounds, 9½ ounces.

Although perforation of the stomach is uncommon, it does occur, and we consider the mortality and morbidity to be directly dependent upon early diagnosis and prompt surgical intervention. In the usual case, the infant appears entirely normal on examination at birth only later to develop feeding difficulties, melena, abdominal distention, and marked lethargy. Although the abdomen may be soft, it is distended, and the absent bowel sounds bespeak peritoneal irritation and soilage. The onset has been reported to occur from twelve hours to eleven days after birth. Diagnosis is made by the history, examination, and, most important, x-ray studies, especially upright films of the abdomen revealing free air beneath the diaphragm. We feel the use of Lipiodol advisable in contrast studies in the avoidance of complications of aspiration during and after surgery, and believe Lipiodol to offer less peritoneal reaction than barium sulfate. Injection and distention of the stomach with water after closure of the perforation avoids overlooking a second perforation and/or atresia of the duodenum, both of which have been reported.

Thorough examination of the remainder of the gastrointestinal tract is advised to rule out the presence of other anomalies.

SUMMARY

A case report of spontaneous perforation of the stomach in the newborn child, believed to represent the twenty-third occurrence of gastric perforation in the newborn infant, the second case with survival, is presented. Suggestions as to diagnosis and treatment are outlined. The mortality and morbidity depend on the rapidity of surgical intervention.

REFERENCES

1. Leger, J. L., Ricard, P. M., Leonard, C., and Piette, J.: Union méd. du Canada **79:** 1277-1280, 1950.
2. Tow, A., and Ross, H.: J. A. M. A. **111:** 1178, 1938.
3. Herbut, P. A.: Arch. Path. **36:** 91, 1936.
4. Greene, W. W., and Gase, D. F.: Am. J. Dis. Child. **85:** 47-51, 1953.
5. Burnett, H. A., and Halpert, B.: Arch. Path. **44:** 318, 1947.
6. Pendergrass, E., and Booth, R.: Am. J. Roentgenol. **56:** 590, 1946.

RETROPERITONEAL RUPTURE OF THE DUODENUM DUE TO NONPENETRATING ABDOMINAL TRAUMA

Presentation of a Case and Review of the Literature

Captain John J. Stransky, Medical Corps, United States Air Force*

RETROPERITONEAL rupture of the duodenum as a result of nonpenetrating abdominal trauma is an injury which occurs rarely. This injury carries a mortality of from 20 to 50 per cent although recent articles[1, 2] emphasize the fact that accurate diagnosis and early treatment will reduce the mortality almost to 0. A recent opportunity to treat such an injury successfully, coupled with the marked discrepancy between the actual and the attainable mortality in this condition, prompts this review of the subject.

CASE REPORT

K. R. A. (No. 10,898), a 29-year-old white airman, was admitted to Shaw Air Force Base Hospital, South Carolina, on April 15, 1953, following an automobile accident. He was under the influence of alcohol at the time of admission, and the history was very incomplete. Details made available during postoperative convalescence revealed that the patient was thrown against the steering wheel of his automobile at the time of the accident and that he was unconscious for a short period of time. Examination on admission was negative except for multiple contusions and abrasions about the face and knees.

I first saw the patient some ten hours after admission. At this time he complained of abdominal pain and difficulty in breathing. The abdominal pain was steady, moderately severe, and present in both lower quadrants, but most marked on the right side. The difficult breathing was attributable to right anterior chest pain, which was accentuated with chest motion. Examination was negative except for the chest, abdomen, and vital signs. The temperature was 100.4°, the pulse 124, and respirations 20. There was tenderness over the third and fourth right ribs anteriorly. Abdominal examination revealed moderate spasm of both recti in the lower quadrants, most marked on the right. There was associated tenderness without rebound in the right lower quadrant. Auscultation revealed hypoactive bowel sounds.

The white blood cell count was 23,700. Urinalysis was negative. Skull films were negative. The chest roentgenogram revealed a fracture of the right fourth rib anteriorly, and the presence of air beneath the right diaphram (Fig. 1). Scout films of the abdomen showed air retroperitoneally in the right perirenal area, sharply outlining the right kidney and having a characteristic alveolar pattern (Fig. 2). During the period of radiologic examination, the patient had two episodes of hematemesis and shortly thereafter went into shock. He was immediately given intravenous fluids and whole blood, and prepared for surgery.

Exploratory laparotomy was performed under nitrous oxide, oxygen, and ether anesthesia, with succinylcholine chloride being employed for adequate muscular relaxation. The abdomen was entered through a right paraumbilical, paramedial incision. In freeing the right rectus muscle from its fascia, a 3 by 3 cm. area of muscle contusion and softening was noted in the superior pole of the wound. A moderate amount of serosanguineous fluid was present in the abdominal cavity. Systematic examination of the abdominal viscera was negative except for these findings (Fig. 3): (1) a 10 by 10 cm. hematoma in the ascending mesocolon,

Received for publication, Nov. 3, 1953.

*Present address: Watertown, S. D.

(2) a 1 by 2 cm. area of fat necrosis on the posterior parietal peritoneum in the angle formed by the medial border of the cecum and the inferior segment of the root of the small bowel mesentery, (3) multiple serosal tears in the ascending colon, and (4) emphysema and crepitation in the retroperitoneal tissues overlying the right kidney. The entire right retroperitoneal space was exposed by incising the peritoneum on the lateral border of the ascending colon and displacing the ascending colon and its mesocolon medially (Fig. 4). The retroperitoneal tissues immediately inferior to the duodenum were bile stained. Examination of the duodenum revealed a transverse tear in the third portion of the duodenum at the point where it crosses the vertebral column (Fig. 4).

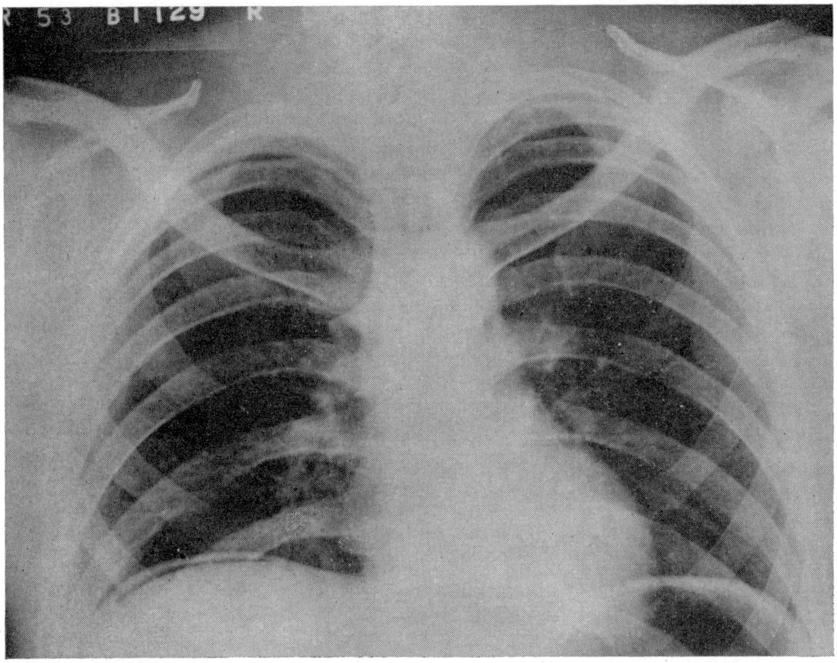

Fig. 1.—Chest roentgenogram showing air beneath the right diaphragm and fracture of the right fourth rib anteriorly.

The tear was 3 cm. in length and extended about one-half the circumference of the duodenum on its anterior-inferior surface. The tear was closed in two layers using a continuous inverting stitch of 000 catgut (Connell stitch) for the first layer and reinforcing this with a second layer of interrupted silk Lembert stitches. A Penrose drain was placed in the retroperitoneal space and brought out through a right flank stab wound. The hematoma was then evacuated from the ascending mesocolon, and the serosal tears were repaired. The colon was replaced in its anatomic position, and a layer closure of the abdominal incision was then effected. The patient received 1,000 c.c. of whole blood during the operation.

Postoperatively, the patient was treated with continuous nasogastric suction, intravenous fluids, and parenteral streptomycin and Terramycin. Oral fluids were started on the fifth postoperative day. Removal of the retroperitoneal drain was begun on the seventh postoperative day and completed on the thirteenth. On the ninth postoperative day, a partial disruption of the abdominal wound occurred. This involved the skin, subcutaneous tissues, and the anterior fascial layer; the posterior fascia and peritoneum were intact. The wound disruption was repaired under local anesthesia (bilateral intercostal nerve block with Novocain), effective closure being secured with interrupted through-and-through wire sutures.

Gastrointestinal study three and one-half weeks after operation showed a normal duodenum without evidence of constriction at the operative site (Fig. 5). The patient was discharged from the hospital at this time and returned to full military duty following two weeks of convalescent leave.

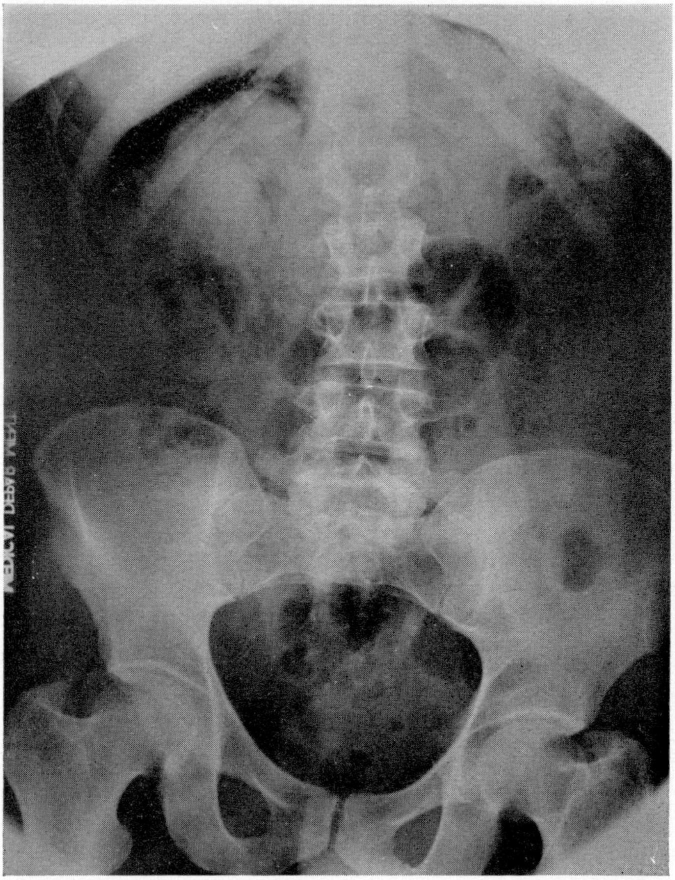

Fig. 2.—Scout film of the abdomen showing air retroperitoneally in the right perirenal area. The right kidney is sharply outlined and the air is distributed in a characteristic alveolar pattern.

INCIDENCE

Subcutaneous rupture of the intestine without penetrating injury occurs not infrequently, but duodenal involvement is rather uncommon. Siler[1] cited a review of 1,183 cases of subcutaneous rupture of the intestine in which 113 or approximately 10 per cent involved the duodenum. Maingot[3] stated that only 30 per cent of the duodenal ruptures involve the retroperitoneal portion of the duodenum. Johnson[4] reviewed the world literature from 1916 to 1944 and was able to find only fifty-two bona fide cases of retroperitoneal rupture of the duodenum. Of these patients, twenty-six survived. Also of interest is the fact that in seven of the fifty-two cases, the lesion was not discovered at the time of surgery. Cohn[2] has tabulated the cases reported from 1944 to 1952, but some of the twenty-five cases which he listed do not involve the retroperitoneal portion of the duodenum (Siler, Case IV).

ETIOLOGY

Subcutaneous traumatic rupture of the duodenum is usually the result of blunt trauma to the abdominal wall but may also occur following blast, crushing, or run-over accidents. One of the more common mechanisms of injury is seen in automobile accidents. With rapid deceleration, the driver is forcefully thrown forward against the steering wheel, thus causing impingement of the duodenum against the vertebral column.

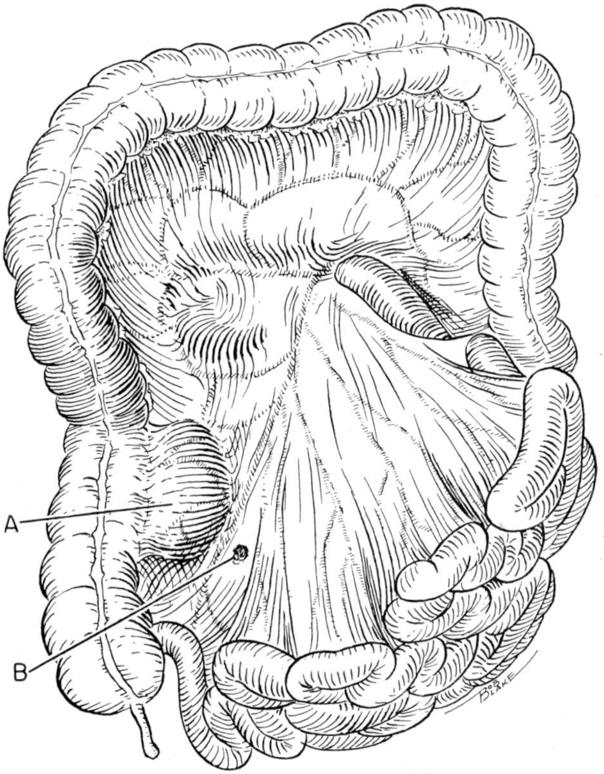

Fig. 3.—Findings at exploratory laparotomy. The following intraperitoneal lesions were indicative of retroperitoneal pathology: *A*, large hematoma in the ascending mesocolon, *B*, 1 by 2 cm. area of fat necrosis on the posterior parietal peritoneum in the angle formed by the medial border of the cecum and the inferior segment of the root of the small bowel mesentery.

MORTALITY

The case mortality rate has shown a progressive decrease over the years. Schumacher[5] in 1910 and Miller[6] in 1916 presented forty-six cases of retroperitoneal duodenal rupture with a mortality of 89 per cent. In the most recent series of cases reported,[2] the mortality rate was 20 per cent. Moreover, in this series there were no fatalities in the sixteen patients operated on between 1947 and 1952.

DIAGNOSIS

Signs and Symptoms.—When retroperitoneal rupture of the duodenum occurs as an isolated injury, the diagnosis can often be suspected from the history alone. Following abdominal injury there is a period of several hours during which the patient is asymptomatic. This asymptomatic phase is due to the fact that following the injury some time must elapse before sufficient duodenal contents spill into the retroperitoneal tissues to cause symptoms.

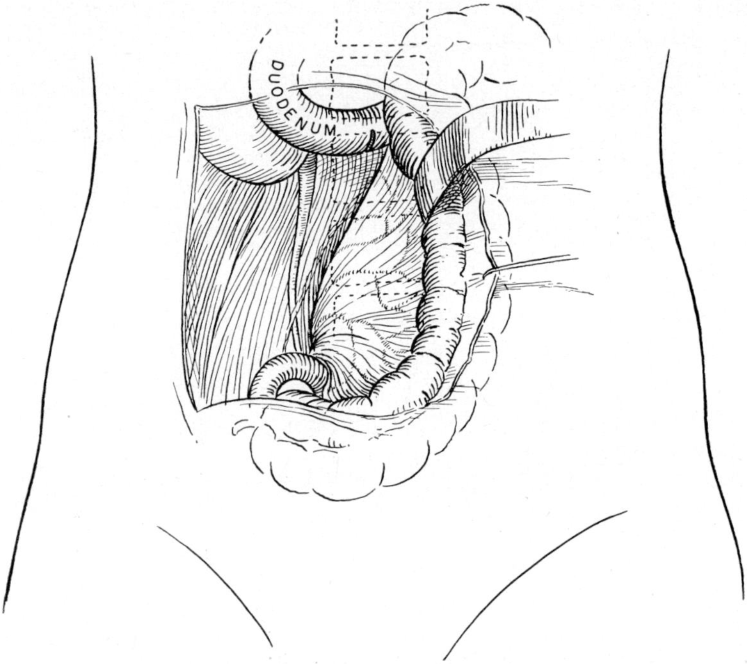

Fig. 4.—Method of exposure of the right retroperitoneal space. The peritoneum on the lateral border of the ascending colon is incised from the cecum to the hepatic flexure. The colon and its mesocolon are freed from the underlying retroperitoneal structures and displaced medially. This results in excellent exposure of the right kidney and ureter as well as the entire retroperitoneal portion of the duodenum. The duodenal tear is apparent at the point where the duodenum crosses the vertebral column.

Abdominal pain begins when sufficient duodenal leakage has occurred. This pain is steady, severe, and becomes progressively more intense. It may be localized in the right upper quadrant, in the right lumbar back area, or in the right lower quadrant.

Nausea and vomiting may or may not occur after the onset of the pain. At times, the vomitus may contain blood, although this is not a constant finding.

Irritation of the retroperitoneal tissues may include the testicular nerves, and when this occurs, testicular pain results. Testicular pain as a symptom of retroperitoneal duodenal rupture was first described by Butler and Carlson.[7] This does not appear to be a common finding, however.

Abdominal tenderness and associated muscle rigidity are usually present, and follow the course of the pain. Abdominal auscultation reveals hypoactive or completely absent bowel sounds. If the retroperitoneal escape of air from the duodenal rupture has been sufficient, emphysema and crepitation of the pelvic tissues can be detected on rectal examination.

Shock may be present and is due to the original trauma, to the leakage of duodenal contents into the retroperitoneal tissues, or to blood loss secondary to the duodenal rupture.

Laboratory Findings.—Leukocytosis is present and may vary from 10,000 to 40,000. The hemoglobin and red blood cell count are helpful in determining the amount of blood loss.

The serum amylase may be elevated as a result of traumatic pancreatitis; a moderate elevation of the serum amylase may also occur as a result of the spillage of duodenal contents retroperitoneally.

Roentgenographic Findings.—Radiologic examination of the abdomen and gastrointestinal tract is of great help in establishing a diagnosis of duodenal rupture.

Scout films of the abdomen may reveal the presence of a pneumoperitoneum. While this ordinarily suggests the rupture of an intraperitoneal hollow viscus, it may also be seen with retroperitoneal duodenal rupture. A more constant finding, as first pointed out by Sperling and Rigler,[8] is the collection of air about the right kidney and adjacent retroperitoneal tissues.

There is no unanimity of thought regarding the use of barium or Lipiodol to demonstrate duodenal rupture. Siler[1] recommended the use of barium whenever the diagnosis is in doubt.

TREATMENT

Preoperative.—In the usual case of retroperitoneal duodenal rupture, the diagnosis will not be made immediately upon admission. Radiologic studies and repeated clinical observation are required, and these take time. During this period of diagnostic work-up and observation, the patient should be at bed rest and should receive nothing by mouth. Whole blood should be available and given as indicated. Water and electrolyte balance should be maintained by parenteral administration. Continuous nasogastric suction should be instituted. Once the diagnosis has been established, operative treatment is accomplished.

Operative.—Abdominal exploration must be thorough since multiple injuries may be present. It must be remembered that there may be no intraperitoneal evidence of the retroperitoneal rupture. The following signs have been reported as suggestive of retroperitoneal duodenal rupture: (1) hematoma or bile extravasation in the ascending or transverse mesocolon, or in the retroperitoneal tissues, (2) fat necrosis of the posterior parietal peritoneum or in the ascending or transverse mesocolon, (3) crepitation or emphysema of the retroperitoneal tissue, especially in the region of the right kidney.

When any of these findings suggest duodenal exploration, the remainder of the intraperitoneal exploration should be completed first, and any lesions thus found should be treated. The duodenum should then be exposed and carefully examined. In lesions involving the second portion of the duodenum, this may easily be accomplished by dividing the posterior parietal peritoneum along the lateral border of the duodenum and then displacing the duodenum

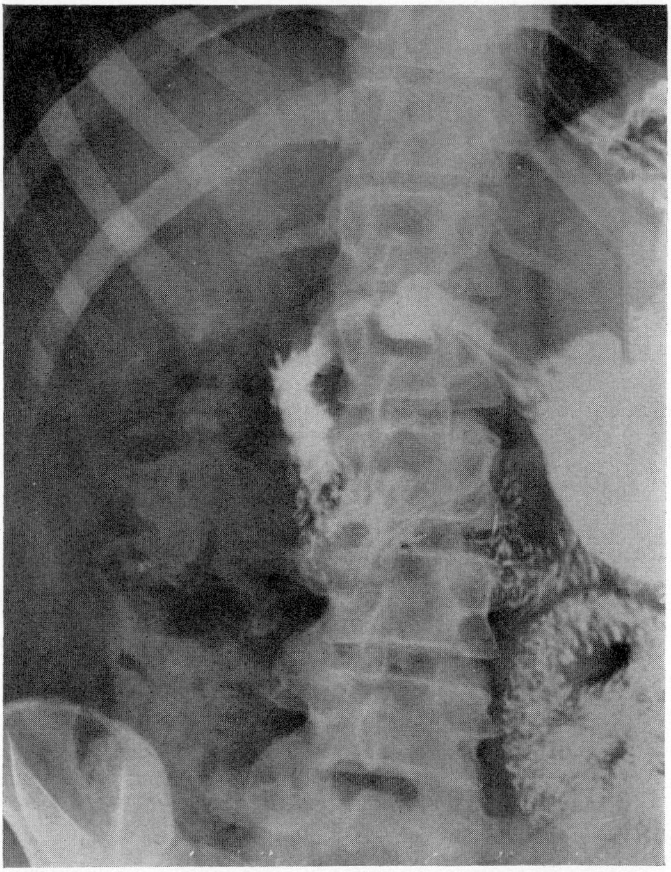

A.

Fig. 5.—Gastrointestinal x-ray study three and one-half weeks postoperatively. The site of duodenal repair is apparent, but there is no evidence of constriction or obstruction at the operative site.

to the left. In those cases involving the third and fourth portions of the duodenum, and in those cases in which the exact nature and extent of the retroperitoneal injury is not immediately apparent, greater exposure seems desirable. Complete exposure of the right retroperitoneal space, including the entire retroperitoneal portion of the duodenum, is easily obtained by incision of the peritoneum on the lateral border of the ascending colon and displacement of the colon and its mesocolon medially (Fig. 4).

The local treatment of the duodenum will depend on the nature and extent of the perforation. Whenever feasible, simple suture of the perforation should be accomplished. Such closure is best obtained with a Connell type inner layer closure with catgut, reinforced with an outer layer of nonabsorbable Lembert or Halsted sutures. When such closure would result in stricture

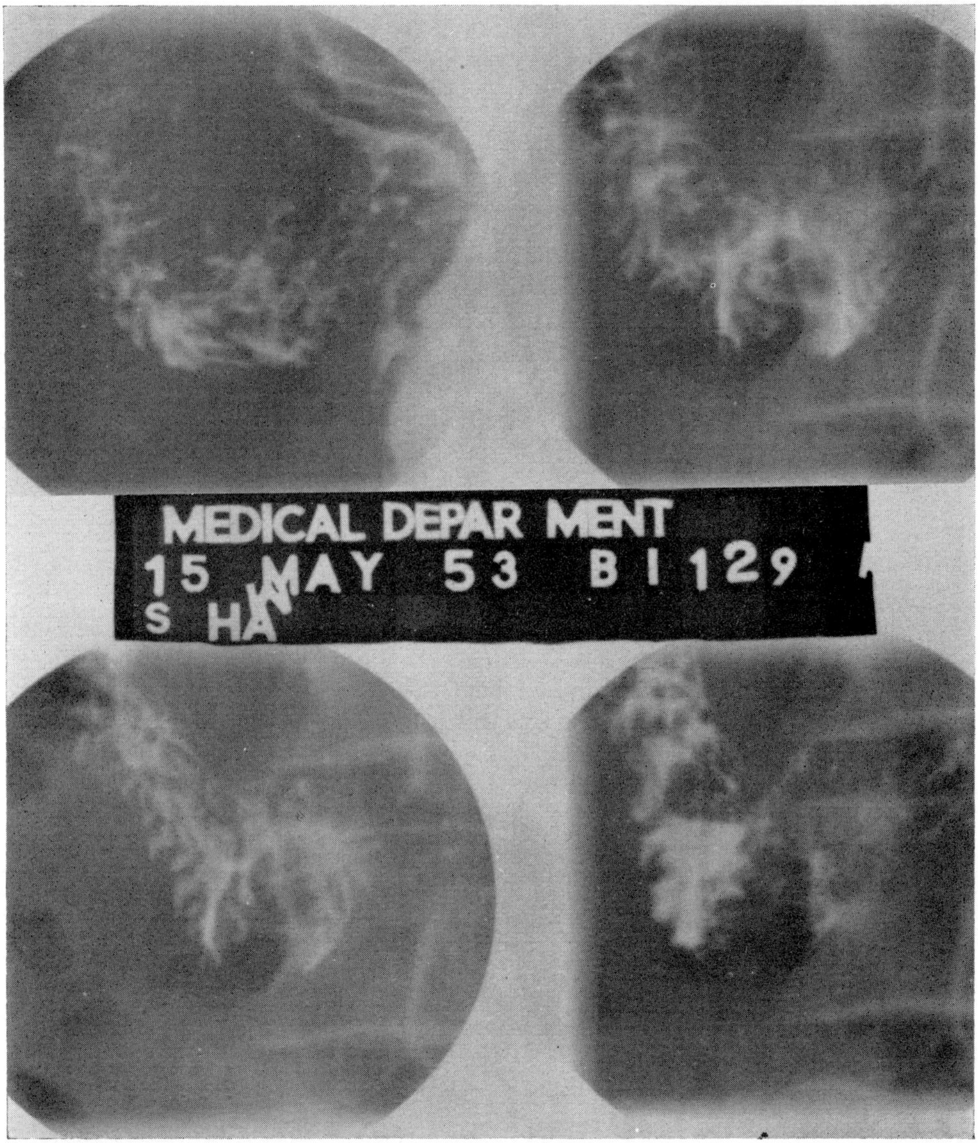

B.

Fig. 5*B*. (*For legend see opposite page.*)

at the site of repair, the choice of treatment lies between the following: (1) complete division of the duodenum with end-to-end anastomosis, (2) complete division of the duodenum, closure of both ends, and gastrojejunostomy, (3) division of the duodenum, closure of the distal duodenal stump, and duodenojejunostomy.

Drainage of the retroperitoneal space is mandatory and is best accomplished through a stab wound in the right flank.

Postoperative.—Treatment here is similar to that following any major gastrointestinal surgery. Water and electrolyte balance are maintained by parenteral administration.

Continuous nasogastric suction is employed until the return of normal peristalsis is apparent. Parenteral streptomycin and Terramycin are used for such time as is indicated by the clinical course.

COMPLICATIONS

The most commonly encountered complications following retroperitoneal duodenal rupture are peritonitis and retroperitoneal cellulitis. Other complications include duodenal fistula, pancreatic fistula, subphrenic and subhepatic abscess.

SUMMARY

1. Retroperitoneal rupture of the duodenum due to nonpenetrating abdominal trauma is an injury which occurs rarely. The mortality rate is high unless accurate diagnosis and early surgical treatment are accomplished.

2. Diagnosis is based on an accurate history, repeated clinical observation, and radiologic findings. There are no constantly present pathognomonic signs or symptoms in this type of injury

3. At laparotomy, there may be no intraperitoneal evidence to indicate the retroperitoneal pathology. However, there are findings which when present are indicative of retroperitoneal pathology.

4. The method of treatment of the duodenal rupture is dictated by the extent of the injury. Intestinal continuity should be re-established by the simplest procedure possible. In the majority of cases, this can be accomplished by transverse closure of the duodenal tear.

5. Drainage of the retroperitoneal space is mandatory.

6. Postoperative treatment is similar to that employed following any major gastrointestinal surgery.

REFERENCES

1. Siler, V. E.: Management of Rupture of the Duodenum Due to Violence, Am. J. Surg. **78**: 715-832 (Nov.) 1949.
2. Cohn, I., Jr.: Retroperitoneal Rupture of the Duodenum in Non-Penetrating Abdominal Trauma, Am. J. Surg. **84**: 293-301 (Sept.) 1952.
3. Maingot, R.: Abdominal Operations, New York, 1948, D. Appleton-Century Company, Inc.
4. Johnson, M. L.: Traumatic Retroperitoneal Rupture of the Duodenum, Arch. Surg. **48**: 372-380 (May) 1944.
5. Schumacher, E. D.: Surgery of the Duodenum, Beitr. z. klin. Chir. **71**: 482-527, 1910.
6. Miller, R. T.: Retroperitoneal Rupture of the Duodenum by Blunt Force, Ann. Surg. **64**: 550-578 (Nov.) 1916.
7. Butler, E., and Carlson, E.: Pain in the Testicles: Symptom of Retroperitoneal Traumatic Rupture of the Duodenum, Am. J. Surg. **11**: 118-130 (Jan.) 1931.
8. Sperling, L., and Rigler, L. G.: Traumatic Retroperitoneal Rupture of Duodenum: Description of Valuable Roentgen Observation in Its Recognition, Radiology **29**: 521-524 (Nov.) 1937.

TOTAL ESOPHAGOPLASTY USING INTRATHORACIC RIGHT COLON

Earle B. Mahoney, M.D.,* and Charles D. Sherman, Jr., M.D.,**
Rochester, N. Y.

(From the Department of Surgery of the University of Rochester School of Medicine and Dentistry and the Surgical Service of the Strong Memorial and Municipal Hospitals)

THE problem of reconstruction of the esophagus following resection has remained a major difficulty since Torek[1] in 1913 reported the first successful case of resection of the thoracic esophagus. This paper reports the intrathoracic transplantation of the right and transverse colon following total thoracic esophagectomy in one patient with carcinoma of the esophagus.

The use of stomach or tubes formed from stomach has been one of the most common methods of reconstruction of the esophagus. The stomach has been transplanted subcutaneously by Jianu,[2] Fink,[3] Kirschner,[4] Beck,[5] Halpern,[6] Hirsch,[7] Kümmell,[8] and others. Modifications of this method have been reported more recently by Mes,[9] Rienhoff,[10] and Potts.[11] The first intrathoracic reconstruction using stomach following a resection of a carcinoma of the lower third of the esophagus was reported by Adams and Phemister[12] in 1938. Since then, higher and higher transplantation has been accomplished, culminating in the work of Garlock,[13] Sweet,[14] and others who have performed a gastropharyngeal anastomosis.

Antethoracic jejunal transplantation was suggested as early as 1904 by Wullstein[15] and was successfully used by Roux[16] in France and Herzen[17] in Russia during the year 1907. There have been numerous modifications of this method by many surgeons since that time either with or without a short skin tube connecting the cervical esophagus with the proximal end of the transplant. Intrathoracic jejunal transplantation has been a more recent accomplishment as reported by Rienhoff,[18] Robertson,[19] Harrison,[20] and others. The use of a subcutaneous skin tube to bridge the cervical esophagus and stomach was first proposed and utilized by Bircher in 1894.[21] This has been used intermittently to the present day. One modification was that of Esser,[22] who in 1917 described two cases in which inlay Thiersch grafts were placed on a stent in a subcutaneous tunnel. The use of intrathoracic skin tubes was accomplished by Bricker and associates[23] in 1949.

Pathologic study of carcinoma of the esophagus has demonstrated repeatedly that segmental resection is inadequate and that recurrence due to intramural spread up and down the esophagus occurs with disturbing frequency. In a recent report[24] of the experience at Memorial Center and New York Hospital, 45 per cent of a group of seventy-nine esophagectomies were inadequately resected as determined by histologic evidence of spread up and down the

Received for publication, Oct. 19, 1953.

*Associate professor of surgery.

**Instructor in surgery.

esophagus, an additional 35 per cent were inconclusive as to adequacy of resection, and in only 20 per cent was there definitely an adequate resection. Ochsner[25] collected 1,025 autopsied cases of carcinoma of the esophagus and stated that in 41 per cent the lesion had not extended outside the esophagus. Abel[26] reviewed another series of fatal cases of carcinoma of the esophagus and found that 25 per cent of these were operable. These observations seem to indicate that it is not futile to hope for some improvement in results following more extensive resections. All the published results using present methods of treatment (including radiation) show that the prognosis is so poor that there is an obvious need for improvement. Any procedure in which a very wide margin of esophagus is not taken is to be condemned. The fear of inability to reconstruct the esophagus often causes a surgeon to perform an inadequate resection. It would be of real value to have available for reconstruction some structure of adequate length with good blood supply to replace the entire esophagus. We believe that colon might serve such a purpose. It would then be possible to extend the limits of resection further by excision of parts of the trachea, or great vessels, and by radical neck dissection. Should the use of colon as a transplant stand the test of time, it should prove especially valuable for lesions of the upper esophagus, whether benign or malignant.

The chief advantage of stomach is that it is readily available. However, it is very difficult to bring it well up into the neck and there is the constant temptation to make the proximal margin of resection too close to the tumor. Furthermore, the esophagus does not tolerate gastric secretions well, and peptic esophagitis of a very serious degree may develop. The vagotomized stomach may undergo dilatation and become atonic, causing encroachment on the surrounding tissues which may embarrass pulmonary function. This is especially true in infants, where it is used for correction of atresia. These patients may regurgitate gastric juice into the pharynx and aspirate, particularly with cervical anastomosis. There have been successful cervical gastric anastomoses, but they are the exception rather than the rule.

We have had little direct experience with skin tubes, and although at first thought they would seem to be of considerable value, in reality the disadvantages are numerous. They usually require a great many stages and long hospitalizations, with numerous small failures and disappointments. Strictures and fistulas at either end are common, and at the gastric end these are particularly difficult to treat.

Because of the inadequacies of both stomach and skin tubes, the use of jejunal loops has been extended, and ingenious methods have been devised to make their use successful. The great disadvantage of using jejunum is that it is extremely difficult and often impossible to preserve a blood supply of sufficient length to nourish the transplant all the way to the neck. Despite extensive investigation to offset this disadvantage, almost everyone who has had much experience with esophagoplasty admits that the blood supply is still a major problem. Mes[9] in his review stated that more jejunal transplants perish than survive. Yudin,[27] who has probably had more experience by far than anyone else (having performed some 200 to 300 esophagojejunostomies by 1949[28]), stated, "Total intestinal plastics can be very difficult, very risky, or absolutely impossible" and "There are some cases in which the greatest skill is doomed to failure; the arcades are too short, their junctions are extremely thin, the radial trunks are in many places insufficiently developed, unequally distributed, the mesentery is too fat and easily tears." Shumacker[29] stated that the reported incidence of failure due to poor blood supply is quite high, but the real incidence is probably much higher. Other difficulties include ulcerations from intestinal secretions. If jejunum is anastomosed into the stomach distally, the incidence of jejunal ulceration is quite high; so high, in fact, that most surgeons by-pass the stomach, using a Roux Y transplant. If no food is going into the stomach, the isolated gastric pouch seems to be an invitation to peptic ulceration.[30] Yudin[27] does not feel that by-passing the stomach leads to any serious consequences, although he does not make any definite statement regarding peptic ulceration but refers rather to "metabolic disturbances," and so forth. Sweet[31] has objected to the Roux Y procedure, stating it may have all the disadvantages of a jejunostomy.

Inert tubes (rubber, plastic, and so forth) as stents to bridge the gap following esophageal resection have been used infrequently since 1922.[32, 33] Epithelization occurs around the tube, which is later passed or removed from above, leaving a patent tube. These have been essentially palliative procedures used to bridge short gaps and have not worked out as well as was hoped at first.

The use of colon is not new, dating back to the early 1900's with the work of Kelling,[34] Vulliet,[35] Roith,[36] von Hacker,[37] and others. Following improved methods of sterilizing the colon, the French surgeons have revived its use in the last three or four years. Numerous reports have been made by Orsoni,[38] Rudler,[39] Poilleux,[40] Toupet,[41] Lafargue,[42, 43] and others, but almost all of them have been palliative subcutaneous transplants. There are a few intrathoracic colon transplants to which we can make reference. Rudler[44] performed a palliative retrosternal transplant of ileum and ascending colon with distal anastomosis to jejunum. Lortat-Jacob[45] reported the use of right and transverse colon in one case of stricture with the distal anastomosis to jejunum, and Kergin[46] transplanted a short segment of transverse colon to by-pass a benign paraffinoma of the upper esophagus. There have been several discussions of the intrathoracic colon transplant and some unsuccessful cases reported in the recent literature.

The use of colon in this country has been practically negligible. Last fall, Scanlon, Morton, and co-workers[47] at Memorial Center attempted the procedure in two patients who died in the immediate postoperative period, although the bowel was viable at the time of death in both. Early in 1953 a surgeon at Children's Hospital at Los Angeles is said to have used transverse colon in the reconstruction of an infant with esophageal atresia. The results of this procedure are not available to us at the present time. Last year Wangensteen,[48] in discussing Ravitch's paper, stated that in patients under 50 years of age with an active gastric secretion, colon is probably a far better organ to use than stomach, although the technical difficulties in employing it rather than stomach are obvious. Ochsner,[49] in a review of all types of esophagoplasties, stated that of all the groups in which the operation was started and the end result stated, colon was best, with 56 per cent good results. The colon group showed the lowest mortality rate, namely, 22 per cent. Ochsner further stated that the advantage of using colon in reconstruction is the ease with which a relatively long loop, the viability of which is definite, can be secured.

The crucial factors in utilizing colon are: (1) Is the anatomy and blood supply adequate to produce a sufficiently long segment without question of viability and (2) will the colon resist gastric secretions? Both right and left colon transplants have been accomplished, and the blood supply to each has been studied. The marginal artery to the colon is fairly close to the bowel wall, as contrasted with small bowel. In about 5 per cent of cases, this artery is incomplete near the ileocecal junction, but there are usually anastomoses nearer the root of the mesentery to offset this. In a series of autopsies, Toupet[41] found that the middle colic artery will supply adequate blood to the left colon in all cases to reach the level of the pharynx. Fry[50] dissected twenty human cadavers and found adequate length of blood supply to the right colon in all. Scanlon and Morton[47] dissected sixteen cadavers and found that the left colon would always reach the pharynx. When right colon was evaluated, in four of the sixteen cases it would not reach above the clavicle, but there were unusual anatomic features present in these four cases. The right colon could not be mobilized adequately because of a large liver in three, and the fourth was a six-foot, two-inch man whose cecum lay high in the right gutter. We autopsied two infants and three adults and found that the cecum would reach to the pharynx in all after division of the ileocolic vessels. We have carried out no experimental work of our own to demonstrate resistance of colon to gastric secretion, but Dragstedt and Vaughan[51] in 1924 took a loop of dog's colon and sewed it into the stomach as a flap. After one year the colon was normal both macroscopically and microscopically. Ivy,[52] Wangensteen,[53] and Florey and Harding[54, 55] have all shown the resistance of colon to gastric secretion to be greater than that of jejunum or esophagus, and Moroney[56] has transplanted colon into stomach in twenty-two ulcer patients to act as a reservoir.

CASE REPORT

W. C. (SMH No. 355947), a 55-year-old white man, was admitted to Strong Memorial Hospital on Jan. 15, 1953, because of difficulty in swallowing. In September, 1952, he had first noted this symptom and had consulted his physician. A barium swallow was performed, and no abnormality of the esophagus was noted. Dysphagia gradually increased and he was admitted for esophagoscopy.* He had lost twenty pounds in weight but had no other symptoms. The past history and family history were noncontributory.

Physical examination was essentially negative except for evidence of weight loss. Blood pressure was 140/86. Heart and lungs were negative. Laboratory findings were: hemoglobin, 15 Gm.; hematocrit, 44 per cent; white blood count, 8,800 with normal differential; Wassermann, negative; total proteins, 6.5 Gm. per cent with normal albumin-globulin ratio; nonprotein nitrogen, 25 mg., alkaline phosphatase, 10.9; prothrombin activity, 80 per

*By Dr. C. Heatly.

cent; Na, 140 meq.; K, 4.65 meq., Cl, 108 meq., electrocardiogram normal. Barium swallow showed a filling defect in the esophagus from the level of the third to the sixth dorsal vertebrae. Esophagoscopy showed an irregular mass involving the esophageal wall at the beginning of the thoracic esophagus. Biopsy showed epidermoid carcinoma.

The preoperative preparation included large bowel preparation with Sulfathalidine and neomycin.

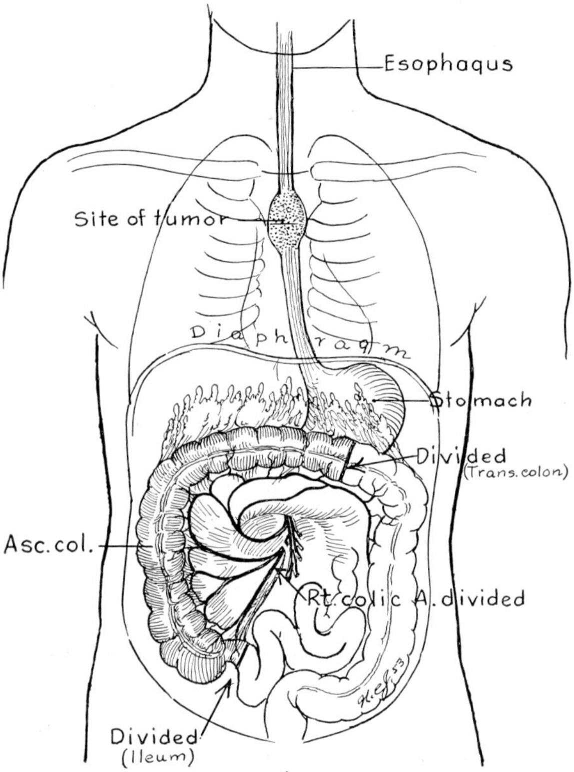

A.

Fig. 1.—*A*, Note that the marginal artery is quite close to bowel so that its length is almost equal to the length of colon it supplies. The ileocolic artery is divided near its origin. Note the point of division of ileum and transverse colon.

Operation.—Operation was performed Jan. 27, 1953. (See Fig. 1, *A*, *B*, and *C*.) Anesthesia was Pentothal Sodium and I.T. gas-oxygen-ether. The right pleural cavity was entered through the bed of the sixth rib. The carcinoma of the esophagus extended from the level of the first rib posteriorly to below the azygos vein. It was adherent to the membranous portion of the trachea. The entire esophagus was mobilized and the thoracic wound temporarily closed. The patient was turned on his back, and the abdomen was entered through a midline incision. The cecum, ascending, and transverse colons were then mobilized. After digital compression of the right ileocolic artery it was divided at its origin from the superior mesentery artery. The terminal ileum was divided and the distal end inverted. The transverse colon was divided and the continuity of the bowel restored by end-to-end ileocolostomy. The free segment of bowel maintained normal color, with the middle colic artery as its only source of blood supply. The distal end of the segment (transverse colon) was then anastomosed to the anterior wall of the stomach.

The thoracotomy wound was then reopened, the esophagus divided at the cardia, and distal end inverted with two layers of silk. The esophagus was then brought out through an incision in the neck. A tunnel was then made through the anterior mediastinum by blunt and sharp dissection, and the cecal end of the free colon segment was brought up and anastomosed to the divided esophagus in the neck. The anastomosis between the esophagus and cecum was performed with two layers of fine silk. The colon was under no tension and the color of the bowel was excellent. The wounds were closed and both pleural cavities were drained with intercostal catheters attached to water-bottle suction because of bilateral pneumothorax.

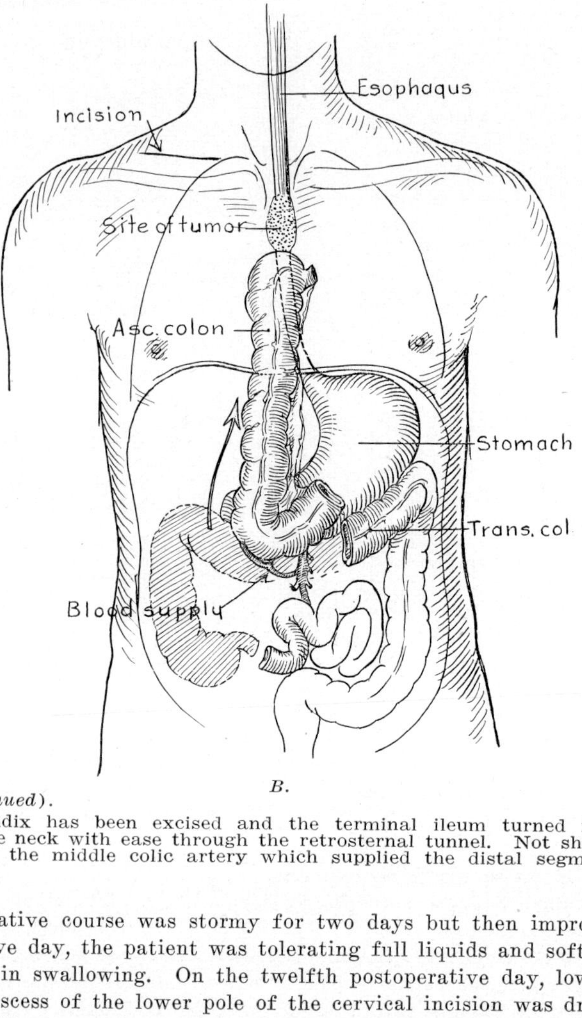

B.

Fig. 1 (*Continued*).

B, The appendix has been excised and the terminal ileum turned in. The colon is being brought to the neck with ease through the retrosternal tunnel. Not shown on the drawing is a branch of the middle colic artery which supplied the distal segment of transverse colon.

The postoperative course was stormy for two days but then improved, and by the eighth postoperative day, the patient was tolerating full liquids and soft solids by mouth with no difficulty in swallowing. On the twelfth postoperative day, low-grade fever developed and an abscess of the lower pole of the cervical incision was drained. This was due to a fistula with the esophagus. The fistula closed spontaneously within six days and the patient was again able to take full liquids. He was discharged one month after the operation.

On March 10, 1953, the patient was readmitted because of difficulty in swallowing. (See barium swallow, Fig. 2.) He had been able to take liquids and solids following discharge, but for two days had been having increasing difficulty in swallowing, and was losing weight. A feeding gastrostomy was contemplated but the colon transplant overlay the stomach; so a feeding colostomy was performed. Following this, the patient gained weight and was able to swallow liquids without difficulty, but continued having difficulty with solid food. During April he received sectional rotational x-ray therapy with the million-volt machine.

On May 14, 1953, biopsy of a subcutaneous nodule below the right scapula showed epidermoid carcinoma. The liver was enlarged at this time.

On May 20, 1953, the patient suddenly developed pain in the chest with marked dyspnea, and he expired within twenty-four hours. It was felt that the trachea had been perforated, but no autopsy could be obtained.

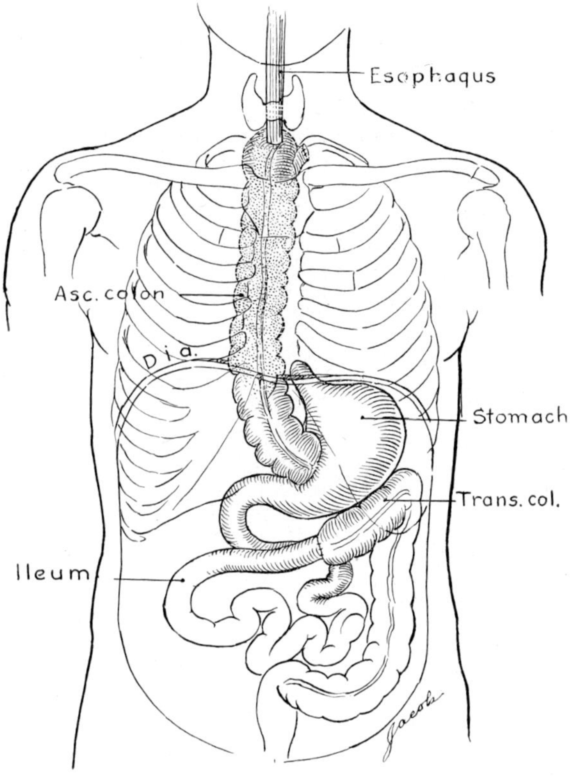

C.

Fig. 1 (*Continued*).
C, The completed operation. The entire thoracic esophagus has been excised. The cervical esophagus has been anastomosed to cecum. The proximal transverse colon has been anastomosed into the anterior wall of the stomach and an end-to-end ileotransverse colostomy has been completed. The sole blood supply to the transplanted colon comes from the middle colic artery.

DISCUSSION

This one case report supports the feasibility of using colon to replace the esophagus. In this instance the lesion had involved the trachea, and it recurred rather promptly. The patient did, however, have a postoperative period of freedom from symptoms, and during this time he was surprisingly free of digestive symptoms. In our experience, the patients usually have loss of appetite, nausea, and other distressing symptoms when the stomach is transplanted high in the chest. These symptoms may be avoided if the stomach is left in its normal position, as in this procedure.

The operative procedure involves both a thoracic and abdominal incision, but with further experience in the technical aspects, the procedure should be less formidable. The thoracic portion can be completed first, and if the patient's condition is poor, the colon replacement can be delayed as a second stage. The procedure should be especially valuable for lesions in the middle and upper thirds of the esophagus. The technical procedure is feasible, it should carry a low mortality, and the physiologic functional aspects appear superior to other procedures. The greater length of the colon which is available for transplantation should make possible more adequate resection of carcinoma of the esophagus.

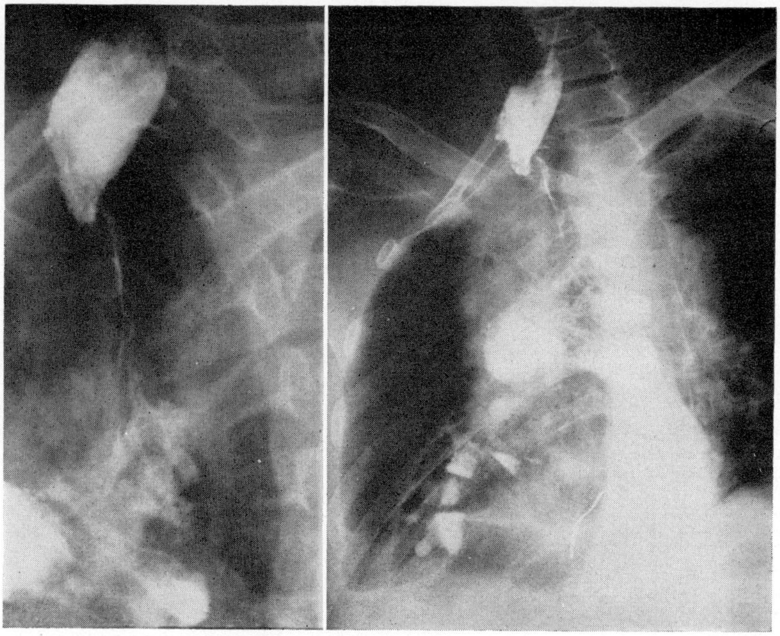

A. *B.*

Fig. 2, *A* and *B*.—Barium swallow seven weeks postoperatively. There is a partial but not complete stricture just above the clavicle at the esophagocecal anastomosis.

SUMMARY

The utilization of a retrosternal colon transplant for reconstruction of the thoracic esophagus following esophagectomy for carcinoma is reported. A brief historical review of esophagoplasty and the rationale of esophageal reconstruction with colon are presented. We feel this method has theoretical and practical advantages over other types of esophagoplasty now in use, especially for carcinoma of the upper thoracic esophagus. Further trial seems warranted.

REFERENCES

1. Torek, F.: First Successful Case of Resection of the Thoracic Esophagus, Surg., Gynec. & Obst. **16**: 614, 1913.
2. Jianu, A.: Gastrostomie und Oesophagoplastik, Deutsche Ztschr. f. Chir. **118**: 383, 1912.

3. Fink, F.: Ueber Plastischen Ersatz der Speriserohre, Zentralbl. f. Chir. **40**: 545, 1913.
4. Kirschner: Ein Neues Verfalwen der Oesophagoplastik, Arch. f. klin. Chir. **114**: 606, 1920.
5. Beck, C., and Carrell, A.: Demonstration of Specimens Illustrating a Method of Formation of a Prethoracic Esophagus, Illinois M. J. **7**: 463, 1905.
6. Halpern, J. O.: Zur Frage von der Speiserohrenplastik, Zentralbl. f. Chir. **40**: 1834, 1913.
7. Hirsch, M.: Plastischer Ersatz der Oesophagus aus dem Magen, Zentralbl. f. Chir. **38**: 1561, 1911.
8. Kümmell, H., Jr.: Ueber Intrathorakale Oesophagusplastik, Beitr. z. klin. Chir. **126**: 264-277, 1922.
9. Mes, G. M.: New Method of Esophagoplasty, J. Internat. Coll. Surgeons **11**: 270-277, 1948.
10. Rienhoff, W. F., Jr.: Antethoracal Transplantation of the Stomach in the Treatment of Congenital Atresia of the Thoracic Esophagus, Bull. Johns Hopkins Hosp. **82**: 496, 1948.
11. Potts, W. J.: Congenital Atresia of the Esophagus, J. Thoracic Surg. **20**: 681, 1950.
12. Adams, W. E., and Phemister, D. B.: Carcinoma of Lower Thoracic Esophagus; Report of Successful Resection and Esophagogastrostomy, J. Thoracic Surg. **7**: 621, 1938.
13. Garlock, J. H.: Resection of Thoracic Esophagus for Cancer Located Above Arch of Aorta. Cervical Esophagogastrostomy, SURGERY **24**: 1, 1948.
14. Sweet, R. H.: A New Method of Restoring Continuity of the Alimentary Canal in Cases of Congenital Atresia of the Esophagus With Tracheo-esophageal Fistula Not Treated by Immediate Primary Anastomosis, Ann. Surg. **127**: 757, 1948.
15. Wullstein, L.: Ueber Antethorakale Oesophago-jejunostomie und Operationen Nach gleichen Prinzip, Deutsche med. Wchnschr. **30**: 734, 1904.
16. Roux, C.: L'oesophago-jejuno-gastrostomose nouvelle opération pour rétrécissement infranchissable de l'oesophage, Semaine méd. **27**: 37, 1907.
17. Herzen, P.: Eine Modification der Rous-schen Oesophago-jejunogastrostomie, Zentralbl. f. Chir. **35**: 219, 1908.
18. Rienhoff, W. F., Jr.: Intrathoracic Esophagojejunostomy for Lesions of the Upper Third of the Esophagus, South. M. J. **39**: 928, 1946.
19. Robertson, R., and Sargeant, T. R.: Reconstruction of the Esophagus, J. Thoracic Surg. **20**: 689, 1950.
20. Harrison, A. W.: Transthoracic Small Bowel Substitution in High Stricture of the Esophagus, J. Thoracic Surg. **18**: 316, 1949.
21. Bircher, E.: Ein Beitrag zur Plastischen Bildung eines neuen Oesophagus, Zentralbl. f. Chir. **34**: 1479, 1907.
22. Esser, J. F. S.: Sogenannte Totale Oesophagusplastik aus Hautlappen nach Thiersch ohne Verwendung von Darmschlinge, Deutsche Ztschr. f. Chir. **142**: 403, 1917.
23. Bricker, E. M., Burford, T. H., and Eiseman, B.: The Use of Tubed Pedicle Graft in Cancer of the Esophagus, J. Thoracic Surg. **18**: 304, 1949.
24. Scanlon, E. F., Morton, D. R., Walker, J., and Watson, W. L.: The Case Against Segmental Resection for Esophageal Carcinoma. Presented at Central Surg. Assn., Chicago, March, 1953.
25. Ochsner, A., and DeBakey, M.: Surgical Aspects of Cancer of the Esophagus, J. Thoracic Surg. **10**: 401, 1941.
26. Abel, A. L.: The Treatment of Cancer of the Oesophagus, Brit. J. Surg. **27**: 131, 1926.
27. Yudin, S. S.: The Surgical Construction of 80 Cases of Artificial Esophagus, Surg., Gynec. & Obst. **78**: 561-583, 1944.
28. Crafoord, C.: Discussion of Reference 20.
29. Shumacker, H. B., Jr., and Battersby, T. S.: The Problem of Esophageal Replacement by Jejunum With Particular Reference to Influence Upon Circulation of Staging Division of Mesenteric Vessels, Ann. Surg. **133**: 463-471, 1951.
30. Wangensteen, O. H.: Discussion of Reference 20.
31. Sweet, R. H.: Discussion of Reference 19.
32. Neuhof, H., and Ziegler, J. M.: Experimental Reconstruction of the Esophagus by Granulation Tubes, Surg., Gynec. & Obst. **34**: 767, 1922.
33. Berman, E. F.: A Plastic Prosthesis for Resected Esophagus, Arch. Surg. **65**: 916-919, 1952.
34. Kelling, G.: Oesophagoplastik Mit Hilfe des Querkolon, Zentralbl. f. Chir. **38**: 1209, 1911.
35. Vulliet, H.: De l'oesophagoplastie et des diverses modifications, Semaine méd. **31**: 529, 1911.
36. Roith, O.: Die Einzeitige Ante-thorakale Oesophagoplastik aus dem Dickdarm, Deutsche Ztschr. f. Chir. **183**: 419, 1923-24.
37. Hacker, V. von: Ueber Oesophagoplastik im Allgemeinen und über den Ersatz der Speiserohre Durch Antethorakale Haut-Dickdarm-schlauchbildung im Besonderen, Arch. f. klin. Chir. **105**: 973, 1914.

38. Orsoni, P., and Toupet, A.: The Use of the Descending Colon and Left Part of the Transverse Colon for Prethoracic Esophagoplasty, Presse méd. **58**: 804, 1950.
39. Rudler, J. C.: Correspondence, Presse méd. **59**: 479, 1951.
40. Poilleux, F., and Frileux, C.: Two Palliative Prethoracic Esophagoplasties for Cancer of the Esoghagus, Presse méd. **58**: 1147, 1950.
41. Toupet, A.: Some Thoughts on the Blood Supply of the Colon and Its Abaissements in Surgery of the Left Colon and Rectum, Rev. de chir. **70**: 70, 1951.
42. Lafargue, P., Dufour, R., Cabanie, H., and Chavannaz, J.: Iléo-colo-oesophagoplastie, Mém. Acad. chir. **77**: 420, 1951.
43. Lafargue, P., Dufour, R., Cabanie, H., and Chavannaz, J.: Oesophagoplastie Préthoracique à l'aide du colon droit et de l'iléon terminal, Mém. Acad. chir. **77**: 362, 1951.
44. Rudler, J. C., and Monod-Broca, P.: Un cas d'oesophagoplastie palliative retrosternale avec l'ileocolon droit, Mém. Acad. chir. **77**: 747, 1951.
45. Lortat-Jacob, J. J.: Oesophagoplastie isoperistaltique transthoracomediastinale avec le colon transverse, Mém. Acad. chir. **77**: 586, 1951.
46. Kergin, F. G.: Esophageal Obstruction Due to Paraffinoma of Mediastinum, Ann. Surg. **137**: 91, 1953.
47. Scanlon, E. F., and Morton, D. R.: Personal communication.
48. Wangensteen, O. H.: Discussing M. Ravitch's paper, J. Thoracic Surg. **24**: 256, 1952.
49. Ochsner, A., and Owens, A.: Antethoracic Esophagoplasty for Impermeable Stricture of the Esophagus, Ann. Surg. **100**: 1055, 1934.
50. Fry, W.: Experimental Intrapleural Substitution of the Right Colon for the Resected Esophagus, Surg., Gynec. & Obst. **96**: 315, 1953.
51. Dragstedt, L. B., and Vaughan, A. M., quoted by Moroney.[56]
52. Ivy, A. C., Grossman, M. I., and Bachrach, W. H.: Peptic Ulcer, Philadelphia, 1950, Blakiston Company.
53. Wangensteen, O. H.: Surgical Lesions of the Esophagus, Rev. Gastroenterol. **19**: 525, 1952.
54. Florey, H. W., and Harding, H. E.: Further Observations on the Secretion of Brunner's Glands, J. Path. & Bact. **39**: 255, 1934.
55. Florey, H. W., Wright, R. D., and Jennings, M. A.: Secretions of the Intestine, Physiol. Rev. **21**: 36, 1941.
56. Moroney, J.: Colonic Replacement of the Stomach, Lancet **260**: 993, 1951.

SIMULTANEOUS ACUTE OBSTRUCTION OF THE COLON AND TERMINAL ILEUM FROM ENDOMETRIOSIS

RICHARD JOSEPH WHITE, M.D., FORT WORTH, TEXAS

ENDOMETRIOSIS is a very common disease, and the familiar picture of relative sterility, acquired dysmenorrhea, deep pelvic pain, palpable tender nodules in the vaginal fornix or cul-de-sac, frequent tender ovarian masses, and dyspareunia is known to every surgeon who is concerned with gynecology. Many of us have seen the blue or puckered spots on the lower small intestine, sigmoid, and rectum along with nodules in the cul-de-sac, hemorrhagic cysts of the ovaries, and, at times, woody adhesions of the rectum to the posterior cervix which give pause to the most ardent advocates of the routine use of complete hysterectomy, but the picture of intestinal obstruction from endometriosis is not so generally known. McGuff, Dockerty, and others[1] assembled only sixteen cases from the files of the Mayo Clinic and Colcock and Lamphier,[2] fourteen from the Lahey Clinic. A few small series have been gathered here and there, and there are a number of single case reports, but, as Dockerty pointed out, a ''literature'' of only forty cases at the time of their report emphasizes its rarity or its lack of recognition. The preponderance of these cases has been in the sigmoid or rectosigmoid, with a few in the terminal ileum. The rectum is often involved but, because of its large size, is rarely obstructed. I have found no account of acute obstruction of the terminal ileum and the sigmoid at the same time from endometriosis, and wish to report such a case.

M. B., a 44-year-old single woman, was admitted to St. Joseph's Hospital March 13, 1950. (Discharge was on May 28, 1950.)

Some eight days before admission here, this patient had been seen in a hospital in a neighboring town as an emergency with a history of cramping and vomiting and no bowel movement for several days and a gradually developing abdominal distention. Plain plate of the abdomen showed marked distention of the colon and small bowel. There had been no passage of blood or mucus by rectum, and nothing could be felt in the rectum. There was a vague sense of thickening in the vaginal vault, but because of the great distention, the uterus could not be felt. She gave a history of many attacks of abdominal cramps, severe constipation, and sometimes abdominal distention at menstrual time during the previous several years.

Endometriosis was discussed as a possibility, but I thought carcinoma of the left colon more likely. She was operated on as an emergency through a right mid-rectus incision; all the small bowel and the colon were hugely distended. A hard mass in the rectosigmoid which felt like carcinoma was palpated. A loop of transverse colon was freed and brought out over a glass rod, the wound was closed about it, a purse-string suture was placed, and through a large needle a great quantity of gas was evacuated. The next day her physician opened the colostomy with a cautery. Several days passed, and there was very little passage of gas and feces from the colostomy, and the cramps, nausea, and distention persisted, with partial relief by suction. I saw the patient again after one week, when she was transferred to St. Joseph's Hospital by ambulance. A barium enema was

Received for publication, Oct. 26, 1953.

performed on April 14, 1950, and examination of the colon by retrograde enema revealed a complete obstruction to the flow of barium at about 17 cm. from the anus. Re-examination, on April 19, 1950, by injecting barium into the distal colostomy loop showed that the mucosa was normal to the area of the previously described obstructing mass. Here, loops were rather redundant, but actual malignancy could not be identified. Bowel filled distal to this and the rectum was normal. From the general appearance, it was felt that this was inflammatory; however, perforated carcinoma could not be ruled out.

A day or two later there was profuse drainage of thin fecal contents through the colostomy with marked recession of symptoms, but this was short lived. Gradually increasing signs of complete small bowel obstruction developed, and re-exploration was carried out on April 19, five days after admission, through a long left rectus incision because of infection in the original incision. Enormous loops of dilated small bowel were encountered. A purse-string suture was placed, and through a stab wound a trocar was inserted; by suction and pleating of the bowel, a large quantity of gas and bowel content was evacuated. The bowel was traced down practically to the ileocecal junction. Dense fibrous scar was encountered in the pelvis which did not feel like malignant tissue, and since it seemed certain that an attempt at dissecting loose the last three or four inches of the terminal ileum involved in this mass would result in a perforation of the bowel and a massive spill, a lateral anastomosis to the now collapsed cecum was performed with two layers of Dulox sutures. The mass in the rectosigmoid was re-examined, and it felt like a carcinoma. No gross evidence of metastatic spread was seen. The patient's condition was poor at the end of this procedure, but she rallied and soon began to have profuse bowel movements through the colostomy. After she was convalescent, a proctoscopic examination was made and a rather tight stricture in the lower sigmoid was encountered which could not be passed. The mucosa seemed intact, and no gross evidence of carcinoma could be seen. She was allowed to recuperate from the almost fatal double obstruction until May 5, 1950, and after proper preparation with sulfasuxidine and bowel cleansing, she was operated on for the obstructing tumor of the rectosigmoid. After separation of inflammatory adhesions, massive woody-feeling plaques were found in the pelvis, so that it seemed impossible to make a safe dissection to clear the pelvic floor for consideration of an abdominoperineal resection. The tumor of the rectosigmoid felt very hard and was constricting, but extending from it and continuous with it for about one and one-half inches outside the bowel down over the right sacrum was a woody, hard, stringlike mass. Since it seemed impossible to consider a wide resection if the lesion were malignant, it was decided to try to remove the obstructing lesion and perform an end-to-end anastomosis, preserving the superior hemorrhoidal vessels, if possible. The mass was resected very close to the bowel wall. There was fair bleeding from both bowel ends. End-to-end anastomosis was performed, and she had an uneventful recovery.

*Pathologic Report.**—Gross sectioning of a segment of large bowel some 11 cm. in length revealed the mucosa to be intact. Deep within the mid-part of the wall was felt a firm, elastic tumor mass, and gross sectioning of this revealed an unencapsulated grayish white tumor with radially arranged strands. Deep within the mass was a yellowish white mottled area within the fatty mesentery, within which short yellowish white masses were found. Sections showed dense fibrous tissue as forming the major portion of the blocks. This was practically hyaline in areas, with the strands cut in all directions and cut at various angles. Bits of intestinal muscularis were recognized. Deep within were found gland tubules lined with low to tall cells resembling those from endometrium. Elsewhere and within the yellow portion mentioned previously was seen marked fibroplastic tissue infiltration, with numbers of lymphocytes and a smaller number of leukocytes. There was much congestion here.

Diagnosis was endometrioma of bowel.

---

*By Dr. Sim Hulsey.

Three weeks later the transverse colostomy was closed. When the patient had recovered from this, she was given a sterilizing dose of x-ray. She made a rapid recovery, and except for two minor episodes of abdominal cramping has been well since.

SUMMARY

1. The rarity of bowel obstruction from endometriosis is discussed.

2. A case, believed to be unique, of simultaneous acute obstruction of the terminal ileum and rectosigmoid from endometriosis is presented.

REFERENCES

1. McGuff, P., Dockerty, M. B., et al.: Endometriosis as a Cause of Intestinal Obstruction, Surg., Gynec. & Obst. **86**: 273-288 (March) 1948.
2. Colcock, B. P., and Lamphier, T. A.: Endometriosis of the Large and Small Intestine, SURGERY **28**: 997-1004 (Dec.) 1950.
3. Owen, J. G., and Stone, C. S.: Endometriosis of the Bowel, Bull. Mason Clin. **3**: 20-28 (Dec.) 1949.

NECROTIZING PANARTERITIS FOLLOWING REPAIR OF COARCTATION OF AORTA

Report of Two Cases

Paul H. Lober, M.D.,* and C. Walton Lillehei, M.D.,**
Minneapolis, Minn.

(From the Departments of Pathology and Surgery, University of Minnesota)

THE occurrence of periarteritis nodosa is generally considered a phenomenon related to hypersensitivity.[1] Lesions resembling those of periarteritis nodosa in man have been produced in experimental animals by many methods, including those involving chiefly increased arterial blood pressure.[2] That hypertension may play an important role in human periarteritis nodosa has been suggested.[3] Two clinical cases are reported here in which lesions of necrotizing panarteritis indistinguishable from periarteritis nodosa developed following the surgical repair of a coarctation of the aorta. One of these cases has come to autopsy. The distribution of the lesions in vessels subjected to suddenly increased pressure has suggested the possibility that vascular strain is important in their production.

CASE REPORTS

Case 1.—A white boy, 12 years of age, was first seen at the University Hospitals on June 4, 1953, with complaints of prominent pulsations in the neck and aching in the legs following exercise. There were histories of asthma, hypertension, and rheumatic fever in his family. The patient had had no serious illness or evidence of hypersensitivity.

Physical examination showed prominent pulsations in the lower anterior neck to the right of the midline. There was a blowing systolic murmur over the precordium. The blood pressure in the arms was elevated to 160/98. Femoral pulses were barely palpable. Fluoroscopy showed left ventricular enlargement and bilateral rib notching. The leukocyte count showed 6,000 cells, of which 70 per cent were neutrophils, 23 per cent lymphocytes, 3 per cent monocytes, 2 per cent eosinophils, and 2 per cent basophils. The hemoglobin was 14.0 Gm. per 100 c.c. Urinalysis was negative; body temperature was normal.

On June 26, 1953, under Pentothal Sodium anesthesia, a coarctation of the aorta was excised and an end-to-end anastomosis made. The operation was uneventful and required three hours. No intercostal aneurysms were seen. The patient was given customary amounts of penicillin preoperatively, and penicillin and streptomycin postoperatively. He required only occasional doses of codeine and morphine for chest pain. He did well for the first three days.

On the fourth postoperative day the patient began to complain of diffuse epigastric pain, which was never well localized. Temperature ranged up to 101° F. On the sixth day, penicillin and streptomycin were discontinued and Terramycin was started. On the eighth day, the abdomen became distended. Hyperactive bowel sounds could be heard throughout this period upon auscultation. X-ray films of the chest and abdomen showed no significant

This work was supported by the following two grants: National Heart Institute, Contract H-830, and the Minnesota Heart Association.

Received for publication, Dec. 14, 1953.

*Department of Pathology, University of Minnesota.

**Department of Surgery, University of Minnesota.

change. After the sixth day, the leukocyte count remained at 25,000 cells with 85 per cent neutrophils. There was no eosinophilia. Blood cultures were repeatedly negative. The blood pressure had stabilized at about 150/100, and the femoral pulses were strong. A tentative diagnosis of acute appendicitis was entertained, but laparotomy was postponed because there were no localizing signs.

On July 11, 1953, the fifteenth postoperative day, the patient suddenly became pale, dyspneic, and restless. The blood pressure fell and he lost consciousness. He was given plasma, Levophed Bitartrate and oxygen, and an emergency laparotomy was immediately performed. Massive hemoperitoneum was found, with arterial blood entering through the foramen of Winslow. It was thought, in the absence of other evident source, that aortic dissection and rupture had occurred, and the chest was reopened. The aortic anastomosis was found intact. With extension of the abdominal incision, the source of the bleeding was found to be an aneurysmal dilatation of the splenic artery which had ruptured. This was excised with removal of the spleen. On first exploration of the abdomen, it had been noted that approximately three-fourths of the small intestine was discolored and nonviable. Multiple nodular thrombosed vessels were seen in the mesentery. Approximately 300 cm. of involved intestine was now resected with end-to-end anastomosis between jejunum and ileum. The remaining bowel had a normal color although a few nodular lesions remained in the mesentery.

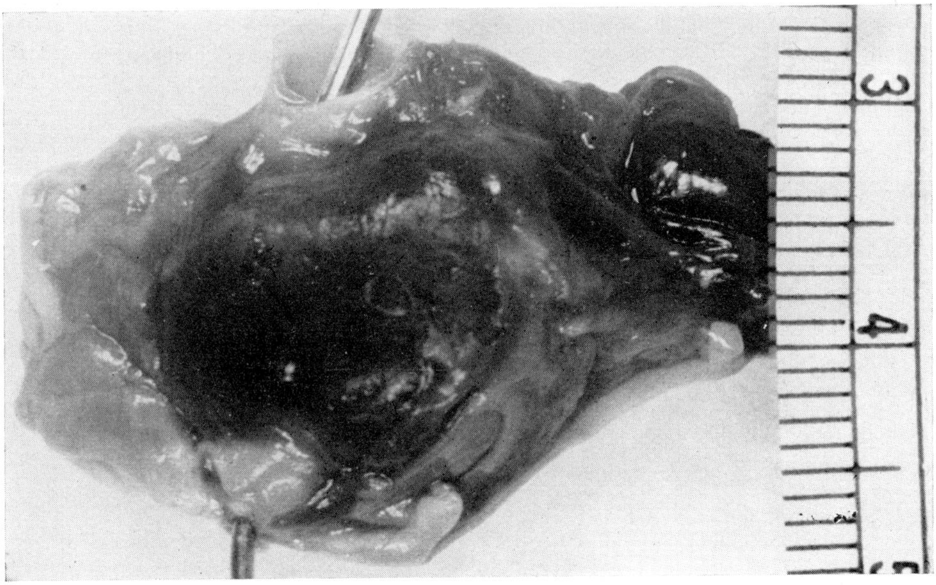

Fig. 1.—Photograph of a typical aneurysm of an intercostal artery found at autopsy in Case 1. This was located lateral to the angle of the rib. Probe is in the lumen.

Postoperatively, blood pressure again became measurable, and the patient was continued on penicillin and streptomycin with aureomycin added. Heparin was also given, but discontinued after six days because of bloody diarrhea and a fall of hemoglobin levels. Adrenocorticotrophic hormone was also begun on July 16, but on July 18 all medications were discontinued. On July 19, 1953, there was extreme respiratory distress and cyanosis which did not respond to treatment, and the patient expired with signs of pulmonary edema twenty-three days after the coarctation repair and eight days after the emergency laparotomy.

Autopsy Findings.—At autopsy there was atelectasis of the left lung and severe edema of the right, with moderate bilateral hemothorax. The heart weighed 300 grams and the aortic valve was bicuspid. The aortic anastomosis was smoothly healed with no thrombosis or narrowing. The right subclavian artery was enlarged. The intercostal arteries originating below the level of the anastomosis contained thrombosed aneurysms up to 2 cm. in size (Fig. 1). These were lateral to the angle of the rib, in contrast to those occasionally found close to the aorta in long-standing cases of coarctation, and they had an inflammatory appearance. The remaining mesentery contained nodules up to 1 cm. in size which appeared to be thrombosed vessels and small aneurysms. The intestinal anastomosis was healing and the remaining small intestine, measuring 70 cm. in length, had a normal appearance. The liver contained a yellow softened area in the left lobe, beneath which a prominent dilated vessel was occluded by adherent clot. The remainder of the gross findings were not significant.

CASE 2.—The second case is that of a 46-year-old white male who had been hospitalized in state institutions continuously since childhood because of mental retardation. In February, 1953, resection of a segment of the right upper lobe of the lung had been carried out under Pentothal Sodium anesthesia for tuberculosis at Anoka State Hospital, Anoka, Minn. The patient was noted to have blood pressure in the arms ranging up to 200/100, with absent femoral pulses. There was enlargement of the left ventricle with an apical systolic murmur.

The conclusion was reached that he was suffering from a coarctation of the aorta, and on May 6, 1953, the coarctation was resected and an end-to-end anastomosis was made under Pentothal Sodium anesthesia. Penicillin, streptomycin, and isoniazid, which he had been receiving previously, were continued postoperatively. The immediate postoperative period was uneventful.

On the eighth postoperative day the patient developed a low fever and vomited once. By the tenth day the abdomen was distended, tender, and rigid. Temperature rose to 103° F. Abdominal exploration was carried out, and free pus was found in the peritoneal cavity. Gangrenous patches were present along the ileum and distal part of the jejunum. Thirty-eight centimeters of the small intestine was resected. The vessels of the mesentery were not remarkable grossly.

Postoperatively the patient has done well except for some diarrhea, and at the time of writing he is in good physical condition, although still hospitalized at Anoka State Hospital.

MICROSCOPIC DESCRIPTION

Sections of the operative specimen of Case 1 showed the muscular arteries of the mesentery to contain areas of acute necrosis and inflammation. The muscular media showed fraying and disintegration of fibers with infiltration by leukocytes and mononuclear inflammatory cells. The internal elastic lamina frequently was preserved until the media was nearly destroyed. Collections of fibrinoid material were seen in the intima and media. The intima was frequently covered by fresh or partially organized thrombus. Polymorphonuclear leukocytes were found infiltrating the degenerating media and in the adventitia. There was some proliferation of adventitial fibrous tissue, and this contained large numbers of lymphocytes, plasma cells, and macrophages. Eosinophils were infrequently seen. In the dilated segments, the arterial wall seemed to be composed only of adventitial fibrous tissue. The necrosis of the arterial wall was often found to involve only a portion of the circumference, leaving the remaining wall intact. The smallest lesions appeared to involve the inner part of the media only (Fig. 2).

Fig. 2.

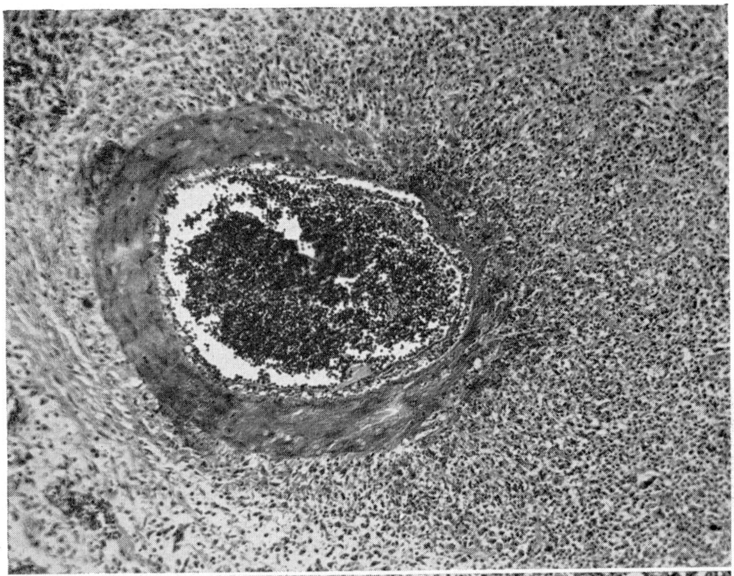

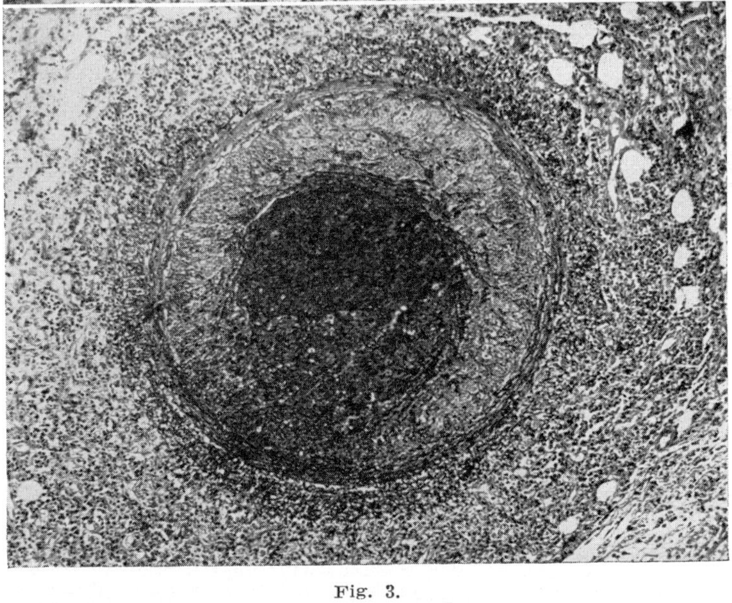

Fig. 3.

Fig. 2.—Photomicrograph of a small mesenteric artery in the surgical specimen of Case 1. Note the patch of necrosis involving only a portion of the arterial wall. (Hematoxylin and eosin stain. ×85.)

Fig. 3.—Photomicrograph of a small mesenteric artery from the surgical specimen of Case 2. The exudate and necrosis involve the entire circumference, and the lumen contains thrombotic material. (Hematoxylin and eosin stain. ×85.)

In the small arteries within the bowel wall, the changes were less intense, with less necrosis and only small collections of chronic inflammatory cells in the adventitia. Sections of the splenic artery in the region of the ruptured aneurysm showed necrosis of the wall similar to that seen in the muscular arteries of the mesentery.

Sections of the autopsy material in this case showed similar necrosis and inflammation in the mesenteric, hepatic, and intercostal arteries. Other arteries were not affected, and no arteries originating above the coarctation were involved. Sections of the liver showed a progressive infarction. There was central lobular ischemic necrosis throughout the liver, with some bile duct proliferation. Sections of the lung showed inflammatory exudate and edema fluid in the alveoli. Sections of the kidney and other organs showed nothing of note.

Examination of the histologic sections of the surgical specimen of Case 2 showed similar changes in the mesenteric arteries. Necrosis of the media with infiltration of the wall by inflammatory cells was found. The involvement of only portions of the arterial walls was again seen. The entire inflammatory process appeared to be less extensive than in the first case. Relatively more polymorphonuclear leukocytes appeared in the adventitial exudate, with few eosinophils. Small amounts of fibrinoid material were found in the necrotic vessels. Aneurysmal dilatation of the arteries was not marked, and there appeared to be less fibrous proliferation (Fig. 3).

The histologic differences seen in the two cases might represent a difference in time interval from the coarctation repair to the resection of the bowel. This interval was fifteen days in the first case and ten days in the second. No evidence of pre-existing arterial disease was found in either case.

COMMENT

It has been noted that the lesions of periarteritis nodosa seldom affect vessels having a low intravascular pressure, such as the pulmonary arteries,[4] and the veins generally. Persons having elevated pressure in the pulmonary arteries may develop lesions,[5] and they may be produced in arterialized veins.[6] Many of the experimental means used to produce lesions resembling those of human periarteritis nodosa in animals involve the marked elevation of the blood pressure.[2, 4, 7] Vessels protected from increased intravascular pressure do not develop necrotic changes.[7]

There is much evidence that lesions of necrotizing arteritis may be produced by methods involving hypersensitivity.[8] Zeek, Smith, and Weeter attempted to distinguish the lesions of hypersensitivity from those of periarteritis nodosa proper, which they stated is primarily related to intravascular pressure and strain.[4] Hopps and Wissler[9] have suggested that arterial spasm in hypersensitivity reactions may cause localization of the lesions at similar points of strain.

Although both of the patients reported here received antibiotics and other medications, there was no overt evidence of hypersensitivity at any time in the clinical course. The onset of the abdominal pain in the immediate postoperative period in both cases seemed to relate the changes directly to events of the surgery. The most striking event affecting the vascular system was the sudden introduction of pulsatile elevated systemic blood pressure to that portion of the circulation which had never previously been subjected to that stress. It seemed significant that the vascular lesions in the autopsy case, and, as far as can be determined, in the second case also, were limited to those vessels which originated distal to the coarctation repair.

The lesions of periarteritis nodosa in a normal circulatory system may also be limited to vessels of certain organs or regions.[10] The distribution of the lesions in the present cases corresponded to those classified by Zeek[4] as periarteritis nodosa rather than to those considered to be hypersensitivity angiitis. The histologic appearance and distribution of the lesions was not that of the arterial and arteriolar necrosis seen typically in malignant hypertension.

Sealy[11] has mentioned a case clinically similar to those reported here. At autopsy, lesions of a "peculiar thrombosing vascular disease confined to the body area below the coarctation" were found.

The sudden increase in intravascular strain appears to have been the precipitating influence in producing the arteritis in these cases. It is evident that the changes in arterial blood pressure after coarctation repair must be accompanied by an abnormal response of the patient to produce a necrotizing arteritis. Hypersensitivity may be one factor in this altered response.

SUMMARY

Two cases of necrotizing panarteritis indistinguishable from periarteritis nodosa occurring immediately after surgical repair of coarctation of the aorta are presented. The lesions produced infarction of the intestine in both cases, with death of one patient. The lesions at autopsy were limited to the arteries supplied by the aorta below the coarctation. The possible significance of the sudden increase in blood pressure in precipitating the lesions of periarteritis nodosa is discussed.

We wish to acknowledge the assistance of Dr. F. John Lewis of the Department of Surgery, and of Dr. E. G. Evans of the Department of Pathology, who performed the autopsy reported.

REFERENCES

1. Rich, A. R.: The Role of Hypersensitivity in Periarteritis Nodosa, Bull. Johns Hopkins Hosp. **71**: 123-135, 1942.
2. Byrom, F. B., and Dodson, L. F.: The Causation of Acute Arterial Necrosis in Hypertensive Disease, J. Path. & Bact. **60**: 357-368, 1948.
3. Zeek, P. M.: Periarteritis Nodosa and Other Forms of Necrotizing Arteritis, New England J. Med. **248**: 764-773 (April 30) 1953.
4. Zeek, P. M., Smith, C. C., and Weeter, J. C.: Studies on Periarteritis Nodosa. III. The Differentation Between the Vascular Lesions of Periarteritis Nodosa and of Hypersensitivity, Am. J. Path. **24**: 889-918, 1948.
5. Symmers, W. St. C.: Necrotizing Pulmonary Arteriopathy Associated With Pulmonary Hypertension, J. Clin. Path. **5**: 36-41, 1952.

6. Rather, L. J., and Cohn, R.: Some Effects Upon the Liver of Complete Arterialization of Its Blood Supply. III. Acute Vascular Necrosis, SURGERY **34**: 207-210 (Aug.) 1953.
7. Wilson, C., and Pickering, G. W.: Acute Arterial Lesions in Rats With Experimental Renal Hypertension, Clin. Sc. **3**: 343-351, 1938.
8. Rich, A. R., and Gregory, J. E.: The Experimental Demonstration That Periarteritis Nodosa Is a Manifestation of Hypersensitivity, Bull. Johns Hopkins Hosp. **72**: 65-88, 1943.
9. Hopps, H. C., and Wissler, R. W.: The Experimental Production of Generalized Arteritis and Periarteritis (Periarteritis Nodosa), J. Lab. & Clin. Med. **31**: 939-957, 1946.
10. Harris, W. A., Lynch, G. W., and O'Hare, J. P.: Periarteritis Nodosa, Arch. Int. Med. **63**: 1163-1182, 1939.
11. Sealy, W. C.: The Indications for Surgical Treatment of Coarctation of the Aorta, Surg., Gynec. & Obst. **97**: 301-306 (Sept.) 1953.

VENOUS THROMBOSIS OF THE UPPER EXTREMITY COMPLICATED BY PULMONARY EMBOLUS

Case Report

First Lieutenant Arthur H. Aufses, Jr., Medical Corps, United States Army,* New York, N. Y.

(From the Surgical Service, 320th General Hospital, A.P.O. 180)

VENOUS thrombosis of the upper extremity is a relatively uncommon condition, constituting but a small percentage of all cases of venous thrombosis. Barker and his associates,[1] in a review of 1,260 cases of thrombosis, found that in only 1.7 per cent of the patients did thrombosis originate in the upper extremity. DeCamp and his associates,[3] in reporting a group of ninety cases of "spontaneous thrombophlebitis," cited only one case in which the upper extremity was involved. Because of the unusual onset of symptoms and because of the many problems involved in management, the following case of thrombosis of the left axillary vein complicated by pulmonary embolism is reported in detail.

CASE REPORT

A 35-year-old Negro man (Reg. No. 410-11) was admitted to the 320th General Hospital, A.P.O. 180, on Jan. 11, 1953, with the chief complaint of pain and swelling of the left arm. Four days prior to admission, while on board ship en route to the European theater, the patient noted the onset of tingling pain in the left arm and fingers. A history of trauma could not be elicited. At this time there was no restriction of arm motion. The day before admission, the left arm and hand suddenly became swollen and painful, and he could not flex the fingers or elbow. He had no chills or fever; there was no cough, sputum, or chest pain. The patient's past history and system review did not contribute significantly to the present illness.

Physical examination showed a muscular Negro man in moderate discomfort, with an oral temperature of 98.6° F.; the pulse rate was 80 per minute; respirations, 20 per minute; and the blood pressure, 120 mm. systolic and 80 mm. diastolic. Positive findings were limited to the neck and left upper extremity. The left side of the neck was edematous, and both the supra- and infraclavicular fossae were markedly swollen, but without palpable masses or tenderness. There was massive swelling of the left upper extremity from shoulder girdle to finger tips, with numerous dilated veins over the upper arm and shoulder girdle; the cephalic vein was distended. There was no localized tenderness, nor was there any axillary adenopathy. The left radial pulse was strong and equal to that on the right. The fingers were warm. All arm and hand movements were painful because of swelling. The physical examination was otherwise normal.

Laboratory studies on admission showed the hemoglobin to be 13.2 Gm.; the red blood cell count was 3,950,000; the white blood cell count was 7,100, with neutrophils 66 per cent, lymphocytes 26 per cent, monocytes 2 per cent, and eosinophils 6 per cent. Urinalysis was negative. Cardiolipin was negative. A roentgenogram of the chest taken on admission was within normal limits.

Received for publication, Oct. 5, 1953.

*Assistant Chief, Surgical Service. Present address: Department of Surgery, The Presbyterian Hospital, New York.

On admission it was felt that the patient had a thrombosis of the left axillary vein, and the early treatment consisted of elevation and warm packs. During the first two and one-half days of hospitalization, the patient was fairly comfortable and afebrile; the swelling of the hand and forearm decreased remarkably, but the enlargement of the upper arm persisted.

At 10 P.M. on the third hospital day, the patient suddenly complained of severe, unremitting pain, pleuritic in nature, in the left lower chest and the left upper quadrant of the abdomen, associated with the onset of a nonproductive cough. There was no sputum or hemoptysis. He became extremely dyspneic and apprehensive, and thought that he was dying. Temperature was 99° F. orally; the pulse rate, 88 per minute; and the blood pressure, 180 mm. systolic and 70 mm. diastolic. He appeared to be in severe discomfort. The chest showed splinting of the left side with shallow respirations. There were persistent râles in the left lower chest laterally. There was no friction rub. The white blood cell count was 9,400, with 66 per cent neutrophils. Ten hours after the onset of pain, a roentgenogram of the chest was normal. The clinical impression was that of pulmonary embolus of the lower lobe of the left lung.

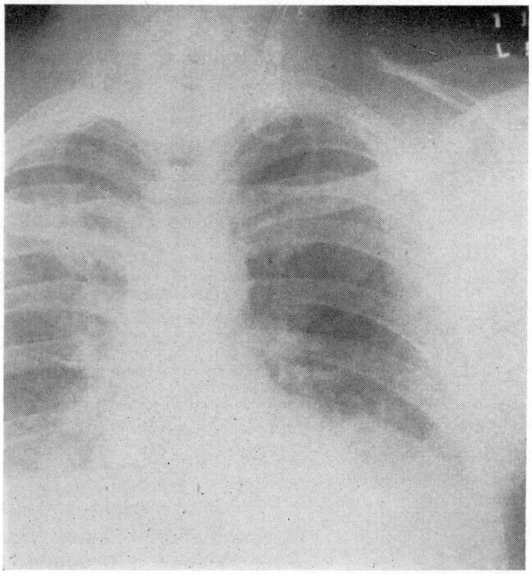

Fig. 1.—Roentgenogram revealing a definite infiltration in the lower lobe of the left lung.

At this time, ten hours after the onset of pain, anticoagulation therapy was begun, using both heparin and Dicumarol. The heparin was discontinued after seventy-two hours, when an effective Dicumarol level was attained. During the succeeding three days, the patient remained acutely ill, with severe chest and abdominal pain, dyspnea, and tachycardia. He was placed in an oxygen tent, and notable relief was obtained.

Sixty hours after the onset of pain, bronchial breathing was noted in the left axillary line anteriorly. At this time, a roentgenographic examination revealed a definite infiltration in the lower lobe of the left lung (Fig. 1). Temperature rose to 101° F. orally, and then returned to normal within seven days.

Eight days after admission (six days after embolization) the administration of oxygen was discontinued. Steady improvement followed, although the patient occasionally complained of pain in the lower left side of the chest, without objective evidence of further embolic phenomena. The swelling of the arm gradually decreased; however, the shoulder girdle and the clavicular fossae remained edematous, and evidence of collateral circulation was manifest throughout the hospital stay. Dicumarol therapy was continued for five and one-half weeks; a prothrombin level of from 11 to 35 per cent of normal was maintained.

On the twenty-fourth hospital day, infrared photographs were obtained which demonstrated persistence of the collateral circulation over the shoulder girdle (Fig. 2). The thickened axillary vein could be readily palpated at this time.

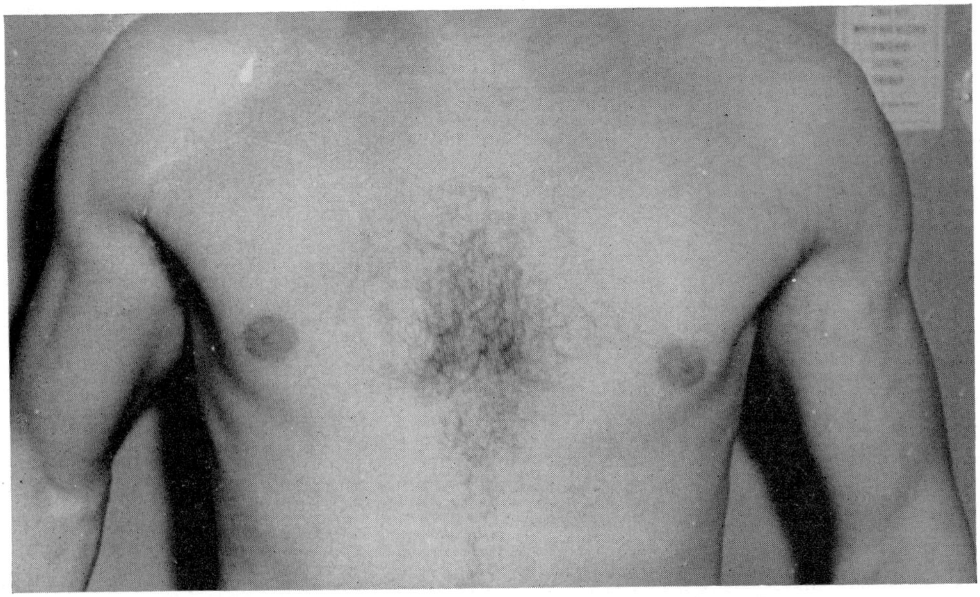

Fig. 2.—Photograph demonstrating persistence of the collateral circulation over the shoulder girdle.

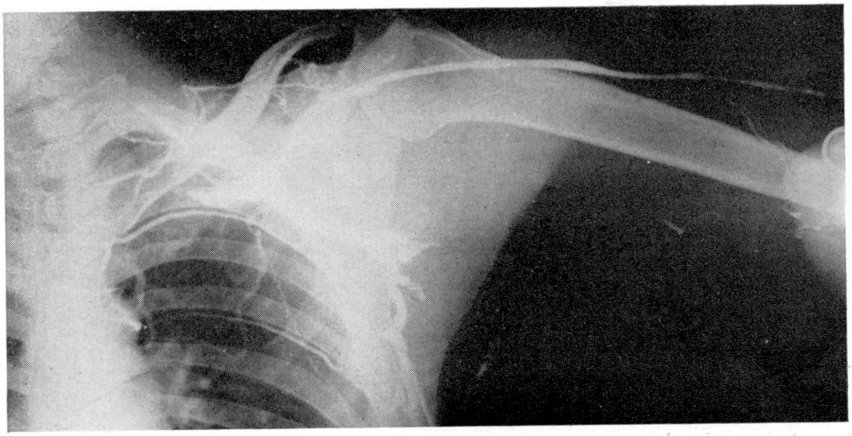

Fig. 3.—Phlebogram taken with the arm in the horizontal position showing no dye passing through the axillary vein proximal to the axilla.

On the forty-sixth hospital day, phlebograms were taken with the arm at the side. Injection of 20 c.c. of Neo-Iopax demonstrated a block of the axillary vein deep in the axilla, with collateral circulation passing over the shoulder girdle and down the long thoracic vein, entering the intercostal vessels. Phlebograms were repeated eight days later with the arm in the horizontal position, and again showed no dye passing through the axillary vein proximal to the axilla (Fig. 3). Following phlebography, the patient experienced pain and discomfort in the arm, associated with thrombosis of the antecubital veins at the site where the dye was injected. This responded rapidly to warm applications.

Eight weeks after admission, the patient was asymptomatic, and the only abnormal physical findings were the palpable axillary vein, the dilated collateral vessels, and the thrombosed antecubital veins which had been noted previously. It was felt that this man was not qualified for duty in an overseas theater, and he was therefore returned to the United States for further treatment and disposition.

DISCUSSION

Most cases of upper extremity thrombosis generally follow either mild repetitive trauma, congestive heart failure, or obstructing neoplasm.[8, 9] In the case presented here, we were unable to establish an etiology; there was no history of trauma, and there was no evidence of either cardiac failure or neoplasm. It may well be that this represents a case of so-called "spontaneous thrombophlebitis."

The diagnosis of axillary vein thrombosis was made on admission. Anticoagulants were not administered immediately because it was felt that pulmonary embolus rarely, if ever, occurs in this type of thrombosis. In 1949, Hughes[4] reviewed 320 reported cases of upper extremity thrombosis and concluded that no case of this syndrome had ever ended fatally. He stated that "it is doubtful whether nonfatal pulmonary embolism has ever occurred." Kleinsasser[5] likewise was of the opinion that there was practically no tendency to embolization in effort thrombosis.

In a study of fifty-eight cases of axillary and subclavian vein thrombosis reported by Veal and Cotsonas,[8] there were seventeen cases of pulmonary embolism. All emboli occurred, however, in stasis thrombosis secondary to congestive heart failure. Barnett and Levitt,[2] in 1951, described what they believed to be the first reported case of pulmonary embolism following effort thrombosis of the axillary vein. Tomlin[7] later re-emphasized the serious nature of thrombophlebitis of the upper extremity by presenting in detail five cases complicated by pulmonary embolism. Wright[9] has stated that the incidence of pulmonary embolus is lower in upper extremity thrombosis than in other types of thrombosis, but that it does occasionally occur. It would seem, therefore, that anticoagulants should be included in the initial therapy of upper extremity thrombosis in an attempt to prevent embolization.

The prognosis following upper extremity thrombosis is relatively poor. Residual fatigue is common, even after the subsidence of edema[6]; and repeated attacks of thrombosis are prone to occur.[9]

SUMMARY AND CONCLUSIONS

1. A case of venous thrombosis of the left upper extremity complicated by pulmonary embolus is presented in detail.

2. Pulmonary embolus complicating upper extremity thrombosis occurs more frequently than is supposed, and this fact must be borne in mind.

3. Anticoagulant therapy is recommended in the early treatment of all cases of upper extremity thrombosis.

REFERENCES

1. Barker, N. W., Nygaard, K. K., Waters, W., and Priestly, J. T.: A Statistical Study of Postoperative Venous Thrombosis and Pulmonary Embolism. Location of Thrombosis: Relation of Thrombosis and Embolism, Proc. Staff Meet., Mayo Clin. **16:** 33, 1941.
2. Barnett, T., and Levitt, L. M.: Effort Thrombosis of the Axillary Vein With Pulmonary Embolism, J. A. M. A. **146:** 1412, 1951.
3. DeCamp, P. T., Landry, R. M., Ochsner, A., and DeBakey, M. E.: Spontaneous Thrombophlebitis, SURGERY **31:** 43, 1952.
4. Hughes, E. S. R.: Venous Obstruction in the Upper Extremity, Internat. Abstr. Surg. **88:** 89, 1949.
5. Kleinsasser, L. J.: Effort Thrombosis of the Axillary and Subclavian Veins: Analysis of 16 Personal Cases and 56 Cases Collected From the Literature, Arch. Surg. **59:** 258, 1949.
6. Matas, R., quoted by Wright.[9]
7. Tomlin, C. E.: Pulmonary Infarction Complicating Thrombophlebitis of the Upper Extremity, Am. J. Med. **12:** 411, 1952.
8. Veal, J. R., and Cotsonas, N. J., Jr.: Diseases of the Superior Vena Caval System With Special Consideration of Pathology and Diagnosis, SURGERY **31:** 1, 1952.
9. Wright, I. S.: Vascular Diseases in Clinical Practice, Chicago, 1948, The Year Book Publishers, Inc., pp. 423-426.

Editorial

Biologic Behavior of Carcinoma of the Lung

WHATEVER the predisposing and inciting causes may be, carcinoma of the lung is on the increase. It is more common in the male than in the female and occurs more often in the white person than in the Negro. The order of frequency is white male, Negro male, white female, and Negro female. Irrespective of sex or race, the age incidence appears to be the same, most commonly the sixth decade of life.

All carcinomas of the lung originate in the mucosa of the bronchial tree near a bifurcation. The cells lining the alveoli are not likely to produce a carcinoma of the lung in man. About one-half of the carcinomas are located in a main bronchus, often close to the bifurcation of the trachea, or near the opening of a bronchial branch that leads to a lobe of the lung. The remainder originate more peripherally in a bronchial branch to a lobe or in a bronchial twig to a segment of a lobe. From the bronchial mucosa where it originates, the carcinoma grows outward away from the bronchial wall. Usually, at first it does not ulcerate or protrude into the lumen nor does it encircle the wall of the bronchus. The growth expands away from the bronchial wall and infiltrates the near-by tissue, lymph, and blood spaces. Before the carcinoma protrudes into the lumen and obstructs it, a considerable portion of the lung tissue adjacent to the bronchus is already involved.

Like other carcinomas, those of the lung infiltrate locally and metastasize to regional lymph nodes and to other organs. The over-all cellular pattern of each carcinoma of the lung as it exists throughout the growth is usually reproduced in all the distant sites to which the cells are transported and where they become implanted. A small primary growth may produce a distant metastasis many times its own size. Distant metastases from carcinoma of the lung have a predilection for the liver, the suprarenal glands, and the brain, in that order. Metastasis to the brain occurs in one of three patients with carcinoma of the lung. The cell type bears no relation to the frequency of intracranial metastasis.

The biologic features just enumerated appear to be common to all carcinomas of the lung. This might be expected, since all carcinomas of the lung, whatever their cellular structure, originate from the same ancestor cell, the reserve cell. The reserve cells, that appear to be the parent cells of all carcinomas of the lung, are at the bottom of the epithelial cell layer lining the bronchial tree. They are the only epithelial cells here still capable of multiplication. The reserve cells replenish the columnar and goblet cells when they are spent or injured. In the process of cell division, and presumably under the influence of some carcinogenic agent, one or more reserve cells acquire malignant properties and become cancer cells. Under such circumstances the reserve cell may differentiate into cancerous columnar cells or cancerous squamous cells, or it may multiply into undifferentiated cancer cells. Accordingly, carcinomas of the lung may be grouped into columnar cell carcinomas, squamous cell carcinomas, and undifferentiated, that is, reserve cell carcinomas. About 50 per cent of the carcinomas of the lung are squamous cell carcinomas, less than 30 per cent are reserve cell carcinomas, and less than 20 per cent are columnar cell carcinomas. The rest are mixed columnar cell and squamous cell carcinomas, with occasionally all three cell types represented in the same growth. While multicentric origin of carcinoma of the lung has been observed, two carcinomas of the lung, each having a different microscopic structure, rarely occur in the same individual.

Within each histologic group, there is a range of variations in cellular pattern, degree of differentiation, rapidity of growth, and the amount and kind of stroma induced. Regardless of the cell type, carcinoma of the lung may grow slowly or rapidly. The speed of growth is apparently governed by factors other than the cellular pattern.

It is as yet undetermined under what influence or influences the dividing reserve cell gives rise to cancer cells. If the reserve cell that divides into cancer cells has progressed toward differentiation into columnar cells, the carcinoma is of the columnar cell type. If the reserve cell divides into cancer cells when its potential to become a squamous cell is dominant, the carcinoma is of the squamous cell type. If the reserve cell divides into cancer cells while it is uncommitted, it reproduces itself, and the resulting carcinoma is of the reserve cell type (that is, undifferentiated). Thus, the cellular pattern appears to depend on the direction and the degree of differentiation of the reserve cell at the time it gives rise to cancer cells.

Under physiologic conditions, the reserve cell multiplies for the purpose of replacing the top cells lining the bronchial mucosa. The same factors or agents that accelerate or interfere with the normal multiplication of reserve cells may be responsible for the carcinogenesis. The behavior of the carcinoma thus induced seems to depend not on the particular pattern formed by the cells but on inherent characteristics of the cancer cell. This concept of the cellular origin of carcinoma of the lung may aid in comprehending its biologic behavior.

—*Béla Halpert*

Recent Advances in Surgery

Conducted by Alfred Blalock, M.D.

A STUDY OF PATIENTS FOLLOWING TOTAL AND NEAR-TOTAL GASTRECTOMY

William D. Kelly, M.D., Lloyd D. MacLean, M.D., John F. Perry, M.D., and Owen H. Wangensteen, M.D., Minneapolis, Minn.

(From the Department of Surgery, University of Minnesota Medical School)

Until recent years, total gastrectomy has been considered an operation justifiable only in cases in which a lesser procedure is not possible. With the great improvements which have attended advances in pre- and postoperative care and in anesthesia, a number of reports[1-3] show that in skilled hands total gastrectomy may be accomplished with no greater hazard than for partial gastrectomy. At best, partial gastrectomy can be considered only a compromise between the principles of cancer surgery and the consequences of total extirpation of the stomach. In view of the more favorable mortality attending total gastrectomy now, several surgeons[1-3] feel that total gastrectomy should be considered in the routine treatment of gastric cancer of all types. Although the survival rates have not been encouraging following total gastrectomy for cancer, much of this is undoubtedly due to the type of case for which this procedure his been reserved.

Another deterrent to the use of total gastrectomy has been the impression that these patients are more likely to have nutritional difficulties of a severe degree than do patients who undergo lesser resections of the stomach.

This study was undertaken to give further information regarding the condition of human beings following total or near-total removal of the stomach.

Material and Methods.—Twenty-two individuals were studied following total gastrectomy which was performed from two months to eight years earlier. Four additional patients were studied who had undergone near-total gastrectomy (more than 90 per cent of the stomach removed) from two to six years earlier. Four patients were women, twenty-two men. The age ranged from 28 to 83 years. Seventeen of the operations were for carcinoma, four for gastric ulcers which proved to be benign, four for gastric polyps, and one for esophageal varices. Three of the patients operated on for cancer were found to have evidence of recurrence at the time of the study. The remainder showed no evidence of recurrent cancer. Following total gastrectomy, esophagoduodenostomy was performed in three instances, esophagojejunostomy plus entero-

Received for publication, Nov. 2, 1953.

enterostomy in eleven instances, and a Roux Y reconstruction in seven instances. The Hofmeister modification of the Billroth II operation was used in all four cases following near-total gastrectomy. All patients were admitted to the hospital for a period of eight to ten days, during which time the following studies were performed:

1. Routine history and physical examination with special inquiry into the patients' eating habits and gastrointestinal symptoms.

2. Determination of hemoglobin, erythrocytes, leukocytes, and differential, mean cell diameter, reticulocytes, blood urea nitrogen, and total serum protein. In some cases, blood CO_2 and chloride were determined.

3. Roentgenologic examination with barium of the esophagus and upper small bowel, as well as estimation of the transit time to the cecum in some cases.

4. Measurement of fecal fat and nitrogen excretion. Three- to four-day collection periods were used with carmine dye orally to mark the interval. A weighed diet containing 145 Gm. of carbohydrate, 80 Gm. of fat, 80 Gm. of protein with a total of 1,620 calories was offered, and the amount eaten calculated. Fecal fat was determined by the method of Fowweather[4] and fecal nitrogen by the method of Kjeldahl.[5] Fat excretion in the stool was usually reported in percentage of the ingested fat. Fecal nitrogen was reported in grams per day excreted.

5. Pancreatic function was studied by aspirating the intestinal content a short distance below the anastomosis of the esophagus to the intestine. In some instances two intestinal tubes were inserted under fluoroscopic control. One of these tubes had a balloon near the tip just proximal to the opening in the tube. This tube was positioned fluoroscopically so that it lay in the efferent jejunal loop a short distance below the enteroanastomosis. This was then inflated with about 30 to 40 c.c. of air so that the duodenal content would be dammed back and could be aspirated by the second tube placed just proximal to it. In addition, various stimuli could be injected through the distal tube into the efferent loop of jejunum, simulating the conditions present on eating but preventing contamination of the duodenal content. The volume, pH, amylase, lipase, and trypsin, and in some instances bicarbonate, were measured. The pH was determined with a glass electrode. Amylase was determined by the method of Somogyi,[6] trypsin by the method of Dorothy Anderson,[7] and lipase by a modification of the method of Cherry and Crandall.[8] Specimens were collected on ice and frozen until the determination was done.

6. Iron absorption: Serum irons were determined by the method of Barkan and Walker.[9] Iron absorption was studied by first drawing a fasting blood level, then administering 1.0 Gm. of ferrous gluconate orally, and drawing blood specimens at one-, three-, and five-hour intervals.

7. Esophagoscopy: Eleven individuals were examined by esophagoscopy at different times following total gastrectomy by an experienced esophagoscopist. The procedure was performed under general anesthesia.

Results.—The results are tabulated in detail in Tables I through VIII. The essential points may be summarized as follows:

TABLE I. WEIGHTS AFTER TOTAL AND NEAR-TOTAL GASTRECTOMY

PATIENT	AGE (YR.)	SEX	DIAGNOSIS	TYPE OF ANASTOMOSIS	NORMAL PREOPERATIVE WEIGHT	WEIGHT IMMEDIATELY POSTOPERATIVELY	PRESENT WEIGHT	INTERVAL FROM SURGERY	% OF WEIGHT LOSS FROM NORMAL
					Total Gastrectomy				
1. A*	69	M	Ca	E-D†	170	150	108	4 mo.	37
2. B	67	M	Ca	Roux Y	160	132	130	4 mo.	19
3. C	70	F	Ca	E-J‡	155	143	123	4 mo.	21
4. D	35	M	Ca	Roux Y	195	176	140	4½ mo.	28
5. E	28	F	Esophageal varices	E-J	127	118	90	5 mo.	24
6. F	75	M	Ca	E-J	200	190	152	5 mo.	24
7. G	64	M	Ca	Roux Y	140	118	103	7 mo.	27
8. H	46	F	Ca	Roux Y	120	115	93	8 mo.	22.5
9. I	60	M	Gastric polyps	E-D	215	200	140	8 mo.	35
10. J	71	M	Ca	Roux Y	165		115	9 mo.	36
11. K	67	M	Ca	E-D	200	158	154	10 mo.	23
12. L	63	M	Ca	E-J	165	140	110	14 mo.	33
13. M	74	M	Gastric ulcer	Roux Y	145	119	112	17 mo.	22.7
14. N	79	M	Gastric polyps	E-J	160	149	125	22 mo.	22
15. O	83	M	Ca	Roux Y	138	84	114	24 mo.	17.3
16. P	66	M	Ca	1st operation subtotal, Billroth II	130	116	115	26 mo.	11.5
				2nd operation total, E-J	115	104	88	14 mo.	20.8

17. Q	69	M	Gastric ulcer	E-J	160	137	133	31 mo.	16.9
18. R	68	M	Ca	E-J	170	158	138	36 mo.	25
19. S	68	M	Ca	E-J	177	115	120	41 mo.	32
20. T	28	F	Gastric polyps	First operation subtotal, Billroth II	155		145	5 yr.	6.4
				Second operation total, E-J	145		135	2 mo.	12.8
21. U	70	M	Gastric ulcer	E-J	170	149	154	6 yr., 4 mo.	15.3
22. V	68	M	Ca	E-J	145	130	116	8 yr., 9 mo.	20
					Near-total Gastrectomy				
1. W	72	M	Gastric polyps	Billroth II	152	132	118	2 yr.	22
2. X	46	M	Gastric ulcer	Billroth II	158		138	4½ yr.	13
3. Y	66	M	Ca	Billroth II	130	115	110	6 yr.	15
4. Z	65	M	Ca	Billroth II	130	128	132	6 yr.	0

Total gastrectomy: All cases average weight loss = 24 per cent; median weight loss = 23 per cent. Less than one year postoperative average weight loss = 27 per cent; median weight loss = 24 per cent. More than one year postoperative average weight loss = 22 per cent; median weight loss = 22 per cent.

Near-total gastrectomy: Average weight loss = 12.5 per cent; median weight loss = 14 per cent.

*One-half of pancreas excised.

†E-D = Esophagoduodenostomy.

‡E-J = Esophagojejunostomy with enteroanastomosis.

1. *Weight change:* The figures for twenty-two patients after total gastrectomy show an average weight loss of 24 per cent (median value = 23 per cent loss) compared to normal preoperative weight. The range was from 12.8 per cent to 37 per cent loss. One-half of this group had survived operation by less than one year at the time of observation and the remainder had survived for one year or more. The average weight loss in the former group was 27 per cent with a median value of 22 per cent. Although the number of patients is small, there is no particular difference in weight loss following total gastrectomy when the patients are compared on the basis of the type of anastomosis performed.

The four cases studied after near-total gastrectomy showed an average weight loss of 12.5 per cent with a median value of 14 per cent.

2. *Eating habits and gastrointestinal symptoms:* Fifteen of eighteen patients eat more frequent meals than normal. None of the patients felt they were able to eat as much at one time as they normally had prior to the onset of illness. The average intake at one meal was about two-thirds of the preoperative normal quantity. There was considerable variation in this regard, the quantity intake ranging from 20 to 25 per cent up to 90 to 95 per cent of the normal quantity.

TABLE II. GASTROINTESTINAL SYMPTOMATOLOGY

PATIENT	POSTOPERATIVE INTERVAL	NUMBER OF MEALS* PER DAY	QUANTITY† OF INTAKE (%)	DYSPHAGIA‡	NAUSEA OR VOMITING‡	DISTRESS OR PAIN‡	WEAKNESS‡
1. A	4 mo.	3 M, 3 S	50	+	0	0	1+
2. B	4 mo.	3 M, 2 S	50	0	0	1+	2+
3. C	4 mo.	6	33	0	0	2+	0
4. D	4½ mo.	5	50	0	0	+	0
5. E	5 mo.			0	2+	1+	2+
6. F	5 mo.	4-5	50	+	0	0	1+
7. G	7 mo.			0	1+	1+	1+
8. H	8 mo.	6	50	+	1+	0	2+
9. I	8 mo.			0	1+	1+	2+
10. J	9 mo.			0	1+	2+	3+
11. K	10 mo.	4	85	0	0	0	0
12. L	14 mo.		20-30	+	0	1+	2+
13. M	17 mo.			0	0	1+	1+
14. N	22 mo.	3-4	90-95	0	0	0	0
15. O	24 mo.	3 M, 2 S	85	0	0	0	1+
16. P	26 mo.	Numerous	25	+	1+	1+	3+
17. Q	31 mo.	3	66-75	Occasional	0	0	0
18. R	36 mo.	Very frequent	Small amounts	+	1+	1+	3+
19. S	41 mo.	8	66	Slight	0	0	1+
20. U	6 yr., 4 mo.	3 M, 3 S	90	0	0	0	1+
21. V	8 yr., 9 mo.	3	90-95	0	0	0	0
1. W	2 yr.	6	50	0	0	1+	1+
2. X	4½ yr.	3 M, 2 S	75	0	0	0	0
3. Y	6 yr.	3 M, 1 S	75	0	0	0	0
4. Z	6 yr.		80	0	0	0	0

*M = meal, S = snack.
†Normal meal when well = 100 per cent.
‡0-4 + scale.

Dysphagia was a complaint in eight patients. In one patient it was present only occasionally, and in a second patient the difficulty was very slight.

Three patients complained of mild difficulty in swallowing and three experienced moderate to severe difficulty. All of the patients except one who complained of dysphagia had roentgenologic evidence of narrowing at the anastomosis roughly proportional to the severity of the complaint. The one patient who was negative radiographically had very mild dysphagia of an intermittent type.

Of the three cases of moderate to severe dysphagia, two were apparently due to benign stricture and one to recurrent carcinoma.

Mild distress in the epigastrium and nausea and/or vomiting were present in about one-third of the entire group after meals. Weakness was present in nearly two-thirds of the group, being severe in three of twenty-two patients.

3. *Fecal fat and nitrogen excretion:* Fourteen patients with a total gastrectomy were studied and the value reported in terms of percentage of the ingested fat which was excreted in the stool. The figures range from 5.8 to 20.5 per cent with a mean value of 11.5 per cent on a diet containing 85 Gm. of fat per day. Normal values for fat excretion in the feces are given by various authors[10-12] as from 5 to 10 per cent of the dietary intake. Taking 10 per cent as the upper limit of normal, only eight of the fourteen patients showed an increased excretion of fat. Using 5 per cent as the upper limit of normal, all fourteen showed an increased excretion of fat. Two additional cases showed values of 4.9 Gm. and 2.7 Gm. of fecal fat per day. Both of these may be considered normal.

TABLE III. FAT AND NITROGEN EXCRETION AFTER TOTAL AND NEAR-TOTAL GASTRECTOMY

PATIENT	AGE (YR.)	SEX	POSTOPERATIVE INTERVAL	TYPE OF ANASTOMOSIS	FAT*	NITROGEN (GM. PER DAY)
				Total		
1. A	69	M	4 mo.	E-D	11.6%	0.7
2. B	67	M	4 mo.	Roux Y	7.0%	1.2
3. C	70	F	4 mo.	E-J	5.8%	0.7
4. D	35	M	4½ mo.	Roux Y	15.5%	0.2
5. E	28	F	5 mo.	E-J	4.9 Gm. per day	1.1
6. G	64	M	7 mo.	Roux Y	9.0%	0.5
7. H	46	F	8 mo.	Roux Y	10.8%	0.4
8. I	60	M	8 mo.	E-D	12.0%	1.75
9. J	71	M	9 mo.	Roux Y	8.7%	1.17
10. L	63	M	14 mo.	E-J	2.7 Gm. per day	0.7
11. M	74	M	17 mo.	Roux Y	20.5%	0.3
12. O	83	M	24 mo.	Roux Y	12.2%	0.2
13. Q	69	M	31 mo.	E-J	13.3%	2.1
14. R	68	M	36 mo.	E-J	33% dry wt.	1.2
15. T	28	F	5 yr.	E-J	6.0%	0.5
16. U	70	M	6 yr., 4 mo.	E-J	20.4%	1.0
17. V	68	M	8 yr., 9 mo.	E-J	8.6%	1.6
				Near-total		
1. W	72	M	2 yr.	Billroth II	3.6%	1.49
2. X	46	M	4½ yr.	Billroth II	1.5%	1.34

*Percentage of ingested fat excreted in feces, unless otherwise indicated, with dietary intake of 80 Gm. of fat per day.

Two patients with near-total gastrectomy both show values of less than 5 per cent excretion of dietary fat. Therefore, of sixteen patients with total or near-total gastrectomy, only eight showed mildly increased fecal excretion

TABLE IV. PANCREATIC FUNCTION STUDIES

PATIENT	POSTOPERATIVE INTERVAL	TYPE OF SPECIMEN	VOLUME (C.C.)	pH	MEQ. PER L. OF HCO_3	AMYLASE (SOMOGYI UNITS)	LIPASE (C.C. OF 0.05N NaOH)	TRYPSIN (TUBES LIQUEFIED)
		After Total and Near-total Gastrectomy						
1. B	4 mo.	Fasting	0.2	7.0	0	103,600	0.0	0
		Fasting	4.5	7.45	0	151,500	0.1	5-9
		Secretin	25	7.36	0	75,150	0	6-9
		Secretin	11	8.3	0	46,300	0	6-9
		Secretin	17.0	7.7	0	77,250	0.3	6-9
2. C	4 mo.	Fasting	16	7.5	8.9	39,200	0.4	5-9
		Milk	31	6.9	0	40,500	0.2	5-9
		Eggnog	45	7.0	13.7	13,500	3.5	6-9
		0.1N HCl	105	7.1	8.9	9,900	0.3	6-9
3. G	7 mo.	Fasting	8.0	7.55	0		0.2	6-9
		Fasting	15.0	7.36	0		0.6	5-9
		Secretin	4.0	7.11	0		Insufficient quantity	5-9
		Secretin	8.0	8.05	2.0		0.1	6-9
		Secretin	15.0	7.64	3.0		0.1	6-9
4. I	8 mo.	Fasting	17.5	7.56	14.4	29,800	0.3	4-9
		Fasting	47.0	7.01	12.3	28,000	0.4	5-9
		Secretin	50.0	7.64	38.8	27,000	0.5	5-9
		Secretin	97.0	7.69	29.7	35,500	0.4	6-9
		Secretin	35.0	7.28	21.5	35,800	0.2	4-9
5. J	9 mo.	Fasting	12.0	7.8	3	30,100	0.2	8-9
		Fasting	22.0	7.6	0	45,800	0.7	5-9
		Secretin	2.0	8.0	0	33,200	0	0
		Secretin	27.0	7.7	30	51,800	0.1	8-9
		Secretin	12.5	8.0	22	55,400	0	5-9
6. L*	14 mo.	Fasting				53,600	0	5-9
		Skim milk				Insufficient quantity	0.2	6-9
		0.1N HCl				73,400	0	4-9
		Secretin				38,600	0	4-9
7. N	22 mo.	Fasting	5.0	Insufficient quantity		Insufficient quantity	0.1	7-9
		Skim milk	8.0	7.65		14,050	0.1	5-9
		0.1N HCl	20.0	7.6		15,900	19.8	5-9
8. Q	31 mo.	Fasting	8.0			3,850		0
		Skim milk	17.0	8.2		7,900		5-9
		Eggnog	26.0	8.05		2,400	10.47	8-9
		0.1N HCl	35.0			3,550	22.65	8-9
9. S	41 mo.	Fasting	15	7.6		7,400	0	5-9
		Eggnog	125	7.1		7,000	20.98	4-9
		0.1N HCl	54	7.0		28,100	17.28	5-9
		Secretin	71	7.45		36,900	7.91	5-9
10. T	5 yr., 2 mo.	Fasting	49	7.6		13,700	3.78	3-9
		Skim milk	36	7.05		7,400	0.78	5-9
		Eggnog	52	7.2		8,100	1.75	5-9
		Dilute HCl	88	7.5		7,900	22.0	5-9
		Secretin	47	7.7		9,600	21.6	5-9
11. U	6 yr., 4 mo.	Eggnog	37	6.7	0	11,200	20.98	3-9
		Dilute HCl	71	7.3	0	4,700	13.37	6-9
12. V	8 yr., 9 mo.	Fasting	11	7.5		8,400	0.1	5-9
		Dilute HCl	28	6.35		12,700	12.38	5-9
		Secretin	29	7.2		6,950	12.97	4-9
13. W	2 yr.	Fasting	37	7.75	5.0	48,800	0.44	7-9
		Skim milk	36	7.45	0.3	34,800	0.19	4-9
		Eggnog	68	7.4	0.3	21,800	1.68	2-9
		Dilute HCl	93	7.35	5.0	14,200	0.82	5-9
14. X	4½ yr.	Fasting	20	7.25	0	16,200	0.66	5-9
		Skim milk	16	7.6	5.0	31,600	0	6-9
		Eggnog	35	7.45	5.0	9,600	0.72	6-9
		Dilute HCl	54	8.0	23.0	14,800	0	5-9

TABLE IV—CONT'D

PATIENT	POSTOPERATIVE INTERVAL	TYPE OF SPECIMEN	VOLUME (C.C.)	pH	MEQ. PER L. OF HCO_3	AMYLASE (SOMOGYI UNITS)	LIPASE (C.C. OF 0.05N NaOH)	TRYPSIN (TUBES LIQUEFIED)
15. Y	6 yr.	Fasting	28	7.05		75,800	4.0	4-9
		Eggnog	105	6.98		72,800	19.2	2-9
		Dilute HCl	186	7.55		69,000	0	5-9
		Secretin	105	7.75		52,600	0	5-9
16. Z	6 yr.	Fasting	34	7.2	0	1,800	0	6-9
		Skim milk	27	7.8	4.5	1,800	18.9	4-9
		Eggnog	75	7.2	4.5		19.8	4-9
			Normals					
1. B. M.		Fasting 30′	10	6.8		24,400	0.2	4-9
		After 20′	38	7.1	22	16,200	0.2	4-9
		Secretin 40′	18	7.7	4	11,500	0.2	5-9
		60′	37	7.0	4			6-9
2. F. S.		Fasting 30′	121	2	0	------	---	Negative
		After 20′	44	9	64	20,000	0.2	2-9
		Secretin 40′	117	8	57	12,700	0.05	6-9
		60′	61	7	34	12,900	0.3	6-9
3. M. E.		Fasting 30′	16	6.9	---	11,150	0.2	3-9
		After 20′	20	7.3	45			
		Secretin 40′	7.5	8.0	36	17,450	0.5	3-9
		60′	0.4	8.3	0			
4. K. S.		Fasting 30′	15.5	7.5	0	8,400	---	3-9
		After 20′	13	7.7				
		Secretin 40′	33	7.6	28	15,200	0.38	4-9
		60′	27	8.1				
5. C. L.		Fasting 30′	95	6	10	0	---	0
		After 20′	20	8	12.5			
		Secretin 40′	50	8	21	16,550	---	6-9
		60′	40	8	30			

*One-half pancreas excised.

of fat if 10 per cent is used as the upper limit of normal. Again, there is no significant difference in fat excretion in comparing the three types of anastomosis used.

Protein excretion as measured by the nitrogen content of the feces was not significantly elevated in any of the nineteen patients. Two grams of nitrogen in the feces per day was used as the upper limit of normal.

4. *Pancreatic function* (Table IV): Pancreatic function was studied in sixteen patients. Twelve patients were studied in regard to their response to various stimuli such as skim milk, eggnog, and dilute HCl, as well as secretin in some instances. Four patients had secretin tests only. Five normal individuals were also studied using the secretin test. None of the patients show changes which could indicate a change in pancreatic function.

5. *Hematology* (Table V): Values are given for twenty-two patients after total gastrectomy and for four patients after near-total gastrectomy. Six of the twenty-two (Cases 6, 17, 20, 22, 25, and 26) have previously treated blood abnormalities. One of these (Case 6) was diagnosed as pernicious anemia shortly before a carcinoma of the stomach was discovered. Three patients (Cases 22, 25, and 26) developed severe anemia eight years, five years, and six years postoperatively, respectively. All three cases proved to be megaloblastic anemia on hematologic study. One patient (Case 20) developed megaloblastic anemia fifteen months after subtotal gastrectomy performed for bleeding gas-

TABLE V. BLOOD PICTURE AFTER TOTAL AND NEAR-TOTAL GASTRECTOMY

PATIENT	AGE (YR.)	SEX	INTERVAL SINCE SURGERY	PREOPERATIVE HEMOGLOBIN (GM.)	PRESENT HEMOGLOBIN (GM.)	R.B.C. (MILLIONS)	HCT (%)	RETICULOCYTES (%)	MEAN CELL DIAMETER (μ)	MCV (μ^3)	MCH ($\gamma\gamma$)	MEAN CORPUSCULAR HEMOGLOBIN CONCENTRATION (%)	BUN (MG. %)	CO_2 (MEQ./L.)	Cl (MEQ./L.)	TSP (GM. %)
1. A	69	M	4 mo.	15.0	14.4	5.22	44	1.0	7.4	84	27.6	32.7				
2. B	67	M	4 mo.	13.6	12.1	3.62	38.5	0.3		106	34	31	11	24	106	5.9
3. C	70	F	4 mo.	10.4	13.5	3.75	43	1.0	8.0	114.7	36	31.4	10	27	113	6.5
4. D	35	M	4½ mo.	11.7	15.0	5.36	47	1.4	7.2				22			6.6
5. E	28	F	5 mo.	9.4	14.0	4.87	44						13	25	107	6.0
6. F	75	M	5 mo.	9.9	13.4	4.18	41	0.6	7.8	99	30.6	33.3	24			7.0
7. G	64	M	7 mo.	9.8	11.8	4.26	39	1.0	7.3	91.5	27.7	30.3	32	28	105	6.6
8. H	46	F	8 mo.	14.8	13.2	4.36										
9. I	60	M	8 mo.	15.7	14.5	4.33				102	34	33	12	30	104	6.2
10. J	71	M	9 mo.	8.0	14.6	3.70	42.5	0.8		114.8	39.4	34.3	17	28	101	7.3
11. K	67	M	10 mo.	12.1	14.3	5.38	46	0.8	7.8	86	27	31	19			6.4
12. L	63	M	14 mo.	15.3	15.7	4.37	43.5	0.5	7.4	99	33	36	15	24	98	6.2
13. M	74	M	17 mo.	14.7	13.3								14			5.9
14. N	66	M	22 mo.	9.2	11.4		34						19	27	104	4.2
15. O	83	M	24 mo.	11.5	13.3	3.25	42	0.9	8.0							
16. P	79	M	26 mo.	8.9	12.5	3.51	37	0.3	7.1	105	35	33.8	33			7.1
17. Q	69	M	31 mo.	14.0	12.3	3.35	35	0.8	8.8	106	36.7	34.6	19	26	105	5.9
18. R	68	M	36 mo.	13.1	12.6	3.35	39	1.2					13	25	107	6.0
19. S	68	M	41 mo.		7.2	1.92	22.3	2.3	9.4	116	37.5	32.7	11			6.0
20. T	28	F	6 yr., 2 mo.		13.9	3.94	43.4	0.7	7.4	110.2	35.2	32	10			6.8
21. U	70	M	6 yr., 4 mo.	14.7	14.7	3.55	42.4	1.2					17	26	108	5.9
22. V*	68	M	8 yr., 9 mo.	10.7	14.3	3.2	45.0	1.2	8.4	140.6	44.7	31.8	22	28	105	7.3
Near-total Gastrectomy																
23. W	72	M	2 yr.	12.3	14.5	4.86	44	0.5	6.8	90.3	29	31.6	25			6.2
24. X	46	M	4½ yr.	16.3	18.5	5.06	50	0.8	6.8	98.8	36.6	37	21			7.1
25. Y	66	M	6 yr.	11.5	13.1	3.78		1.1	7.6				12			6.4
26. Z	65	M	6 yr.	15.0	10.1	2.43							18	26	109	5.8

*Treated blood abnormality.

tric polyps. She subsequently had a total gastrectomy because of residual polyps with continued bleeding. The sixth patient (Case 17) showed only macrocytosis. He had been taking liver injections regularly, although no definite history of anemia could be obtained.

Three additional cases showed macrocytosis as the only abnormality.

Three other patients were anemic at the time of this study. One of these (Case 19) was a typical megaloblastic anemia occurring three years and five months after a total gastrectomy for carcinoma. The other two were hypochromic anemias.

All cases of megaloblastic anemia responded satisfactorily to the usual methods of treatment.

Therefore, excluding the one case in which it was known that a blood abnormality was present prior to gastrectomy, eleven of twenty-six patients showed some type of blood abnormality when examined at varying intervals following total or near-total gastrectomy. Five of these abnormalities were megaloblastic anemias occurring at intervals of one and one-fourth, three and one-fourth, five, five, and six years following operation, respectively. Two of the abnormalities were mild hypochromic anemia, and the remaining four abnormalities consisted of macrocytosis. Of eleven patients alive two years or longer after gastrectomy, five developed a megaloblastic anemia.

Blood urea nitrogen, CO_2, chlorides, and total serum protein showed no consistent deviation from normal.

6. *Iron tolerance test:* None of the patients studied showed fasting serum iron levels significantly altered from normal. Six of eleven patients showed strikingly little change in the serum iron level after the oral administration of 1 Gm. of ferrous gluconate.

TABLE VI. IRON ABSORPTION AFTER TOTAL AND NEAR-TOTAL GASTRECTOMY

PATIENT	POSTOPERATIVE INTERVAL	SERUM IRON* (γ/100 C.C.)			
		FASTING	1 HR.	3 HR.	5 HR.
1. A	4 mo.	75	67	77	72
2. C	4 mo.	54	98	103	67
3. E	5 mo.	62	118	100	
4. F	7 mo.	145	125	180	135
5. G	8 mo.	65	65	65	68
6. K	22 mo.	107			
7. O	41 mo.	192	195	170	166
8. P	5 yr., 2 mo.	110	140	115	65
9. F. H.†	2 yr.	52	56	66	83
1. S	2 yr.	122	149	100	392
2. T	4½ yr.	138	150	125	107
3. V	6 yr.	176		202	213

*1.0 Gm. ferrous gluconate given orally after fasting specimen taken.
†Not included in other tables.

7. *Roentgenologic studies:* Seven of seventeen patients showed some narrowing at the site of anastomosis of the esophagus to the intestines. Six of these were symptomatic, but only two were severe enough to interfere with

alimentation seriously. One of these was successfully dilated with restoration of normal swallowing. The other patient was uncooperative and refused further dilatation after one failure due to technical difficulties.

TABLE VII. X-RAY STUDIES IN CASES OF TOTAL AND NEAR-TOTAL GASTRECTOMY

PATIENT	AGE (YR.)	SEX	POSTOPERATIVE INTERVAL	NARROWING ANASTOMOSIS (0-4 + SCALE)	SMALL BOWEL PATTERN	PASSAGE TIME TO CECUM
				Total		
1. A	69	M	4 mo.	+ + +	N	4 hr.
2. C	70	F	4 mo.	0	Enlargement and coarsening of folds in jejunum	7 hr.
3. E	28	F	5 mo.	+	N	
4. F	75	M	5 mo.	+ +	Decreased motility retention of Ba in upper jejunum 2 hr. after ingestion	
5. H	46	F	8 mo.	+	N	1⅔ hr.
6. I	60	M	8 mo.	0	Small bowel empties rapidly	
7. J	71	M	9 mo.	0	N	4 hr.
8. K	67	M	10 mo.	0	N	2 hr.
9. L	63	M	14 mo.	+	N	4 hr.
10. N	79	M	22 mo.	0	N	4 hr.
11. O	83	M	24 mo.	0	N	½ hr.
12. P	66	M	14 mo.	+ + +	Spastic areas	
13. Q	69	M	31 mo.	0	N	7 hr.
14. R	68	M	36 mo.	+	N	
15. T	28	F	5 yr.	0	N	
16. U	70	M	6 yr., 9 mo.	0	N	3 hr.
17. V	68	M	8 yr., 9 mo.	0	Moderate dilatation of proximal jejunum with moderate delay in emptying	
				Near-total		
1. W	72	M	2 yr.	0	N	Gastric pouch emptied 2 hr.
2. X	46	M	4½ yr.	0	N	Gastric pouch emptied 1 hr., transit to colon 3 hr.
3. Z	65	M	6 yr.	0	N	Pouch empties with extreme rapidity; 5-6 hr. for Ba to reach colon

Three cases showed some dilatation and stasis in the upper jejunum. The total transit time through the small intestine was in the normal range in nine of the twelve cases in which it was determined.

8. *Esophagitis:* Eleven patients were examined by esophagoscopy. Two of these showed a mild esophagitis in the distal esophagus as evidenced by increased reddening and tendency to bleed on contact. One patient had an esophagoduodenal anastomosis and the other a Roux Y type of reconstruction. A third patient showed a moderate esophagitis as evidenced by more pronounced redness of the mucosa. This patient had an esophagojejunal anastomosis with enteroanastomosis. The interval since operation was ten months,

seven months, and two months, respectively. A third patient wtih an esophagojejunostomy and enteroanastomosis showed a questionable esophagitis when examined forty-one months following operation.

TABLE VIII. ESOPHAGITIS AFTER TOTAL AND NEAR-TOTAL GASTRECTOMY

PATIENT	POSTOPERATIVE INTERVAL	TYPE OF ANASTOMOSIS	ESOPHAGITIS
1. G	7 mo.	Roux Y	Mild
2. H	8 mo.	Roux Y	None
3. K	10 mo.	Esophagoduodenostomy	Mild
4. M	17 mo.	Roux Y	None
5. O	24 mo.	Roux Y	None
6. S	41 mo.	Esophagojejunostomy	Questionable
7. T	2 mo.	Esophagojejunostomy	None
8. U	6 yr., 4 mo.	Esophagojejunostomy	None
9. V	8 yr., 9 mo.	Esophagojejunostomy	None
10. TQ*	6 mo.	Esophagojejunostomy	None
11. AB*	3 mo.	Esophagojejunostomy	Moderate

*Not included in other tables.

DISCUSSION

Disturbances in nutrition and hemopoiesis are the main categories of undesirable side effects which may occur following gastrectomy.

Disturbances in Nutrition.—Weight loss and weakness are the usual manifestations of nutritional insufficiency. In the cases under consideration in this report, weight loss was moderate to marked with apparently little improvement with the passage of time. Many reports[3, 13-16] indicate that there is a gain in weight following partial or total gastrectomy. These figures are of less importance in assessing the nutritional status of the patient than are figures which compare the postoperative weight to the normal preoperative weight. Wells and Welbourn[17] reported that patients treated by total gastrectomy showed an average of fourteen pounds' weight loss before operation and another sixteen pounds' after operation. Brain and Stammers[18] stated that after total gastrectomy patients look like the inmates of a concentration camp. Everson,[19] in a collective review, noted that only three of forty patients treated by total gastrectomy regained normal preoperative weight. The remainder were below normal weight by an average of twenty-six pounds. In the experimental animal, total gastrectomy is frequently followed by moderate to severe weight loss.[20] Ivy and associates,[23] however, reported that if dogs are fed about twice the normal amount after total gastrectomy they will remain in good nutrition.

In many patients, the so-called normal preoperative weight represents moderate to severe obesity, so that it might be argued that the reduction in weight after total gastrectomy still leaves the patient in the normal range for his age and height. Using the Metropolitan Life Insurance Company tables for average weight correlated to height, body build, and sex, we find that three of nine patients with total gastrectomy fall in the normal range given. The remaining six fall below average optimum weight by an average of 12 per cent (median = 12 per cent). However, two-thirds of the patitents in this report complained of weakness, suggesting the likelihood of true impairment of nutrition.

In general, the major factors involved in weight loss must be (1) inadequate intake, (2) inadequate assimilation of the ingested food, or (3) a combination of the two factors.

1. *Inadequate intake:* The obvious factors involved here are (a) anorexia or (b) pain, a sense of fullness or discomfort or disagreeable sensations commonly termed the "dumping syndrome" which may occur after the ingestion of a relatively small amount of food. The dumping syndrome has been well described after partial gastrectomy. Most investigators[16, 17, 39, 40, 42, 43] agree that the sudden filling of some portion of the upper gastrointestinal tract with food is responsible for the early symptoms. Gholiger[63] reported that 100 per cent of patients with total gastrectomy have the dumping syndrome. The impression gained from careful questioning of the patients in this study is that dietary intake is generally reduced moderately to markedly when compared to the normal preoperative quantity. Furthermore, nearly one-half of the patients regularly experienced distress or pain following meals which, although generally mild, undoubtedly results in a reduction of food intake.

2. *Inadequate assimilation:* Much importance has been attached to the impaired assimilation of dietary fat as an etiological factor in poor nutrition after total gastrectomy. Everson[19] reported impaired fat assimilation in twenty-one of thirty-three collected patients, and impaired protein assimilation in six of fourteen patients. Of fifteen dogs studied, all showed increased fecal fat excretion, and fifteen of sixteen reported dog studies showed increased protein loss in the stool. Brázda[15] reported the excretion of 12 to 37 per cent of the ingested fat (107 Gm. per day) in ten patients with total gastrectomy with a mean value of 28.5 per cent. Our own figures of 5.8 to 20 per cent fat excretion with a mean of 11.5 per cent in fourteen patients represents only a mild abnormality in assimilation of fat (diet of 80 Gm. per day). Protein assimilation was normal. There was no correlation with the interval since operation. The commonly suggested etiological factors in the impaired assimilation of dietary fat following gastrectomy are (a) deficient pancreatic secretion secondary to inadequate stimuli, vagotomy, and absence of sufficient hydrochloric acid to activate the secretin mechanism, (b) inadequate mixing of the food with the biliary and pancreatic secretions, and (c) increased rate of transit of food through the small intestine.

The role of bile and pancreatic juice in the digestion and absorption of fat is well known. Annis and Hallenbeck[24] noted in dogs after partial gastrectomy that the volume, total bicarbonate, total nitrogen, and trypsin activity of the pancreatic juice were greatly reduced. Howard and co-workers[25] found, in studying a patient with a pancreatic fistula following a bullet wound, that a test meal introduced by intestinal tube into the jejunum produced only slight stimulation of pancreatic secretion, whereas introduction of the same meal into the duodenum caused a much greater flow of juice. A maximal response was obtained when the meal was eaten. This suggests the importance of the passage of food through the duodenum in eliciting pancreatic secretion. Vagotomy in itself is said by some authors,[26, 27] to decrease pancreatic secretion, but a more recent work favors the opinion that no significant alteration occurs.[28, 29] Shingleton[30] reported that after vagotomy the fasting volume of duodenal content is increased but the pancreatic enzyme content is decreased. The impression obtained from the study of pancreatic secretion after total gastrectomy in the present paper is that the pancreas is capable of normal secretion.

Inadequate stimulation and poor mixing secondary to by-passing the duodenum, delayed secretory response, and increased rate of passage of the ingested food are probably of greater importance in the etiology of impaired fat and protein assimilation than any primary decrease in pancreatic secretion.

Wollaeger[31] reported the mean fecal fat excretion to be 8.7 Gm. per day in the normal individual, 12.3 Gm. per day after the Billroth I type of gastrectomy, and 19.9 Gm. per day after the Billroth II gastrectomy when the patient is on a high fat diet (200 Gm. per day). The difference was found to be statistically significant, and he concluded that Billroth I gastrectomy is followed by less gastrointestinal disturbance than Billroth II. Bohmansson[32] came to the same conclusion, which he attributed to better mixing with bile and pancreatic juice when food traversed the duodenum plus more normal emptying after Billroth I. Everson[33] found that dogs excreted more of the dietary nitrogen after total gastrectomy with esophagojejunal anastomosis than with esophagoduodenal anastomosis. Calabi and associates[34] studied a patient with an esophagodermojejunoplasty, who also had a gastrostomy because of esophageal stenosis. They found that fat assimilation was normal when the diet was given by gastrostomy but abnormally decreased when fed orally, by-passing the stomach and duodenum. They attributed the difference to the storage function of the stomach and the gradual emptying in small prepared amounts of food from the stomach. Dragstedt[35] showed in the dog that removal of 80 to 90 per cent of the pancreas did not alter the normal assimilation of fat and protein. However, ligation of the pancreatic ducts or pancreatectomy causes excessive excretion of fat and protein in the stool, approximately 60 per cent of the fat and 40 per cent of the protein ingested being lost in this way. Similarly, diversion of all bile from the upper intestinal tract in dogs causes them to excrete quite constantly 60 per cent of their dietary fat.[36, 37] Large doses of ox bile extracts or bile salts were necessary for complete fat absorption. Since vagal control and hormonal regulation from the duodenum are known physiologic mechanisms in biliary tract emptying, a situation exists parallel to the pancreas, which can help explain alterations in the assimilation of dietary fat after gastrectomy. Here again inadequate stimuli, delayed response, and poor mixing appear to be likely factors.

As mentioned earlier, changes in the rate of passage of food through the gut may cause poor mixing with the digestive juices and decreased absorption of the ingested diet. Freeman[21] showed in monkeys following total gastrectomy that barium passed rapidly through the upper small intestine but underwent compensatory slowing in the lower ileum. Bruusgaard[41] found in human beings after partial gastrectomy for peptic ulcer that evacuation of the small intestine is accelerated in the proximal 30 to 50 cm. while passage through the whole small intestine is little changed from normal. Wells and Welbourn,[17] who studied 300 cases after gastrectomy, asserted that the rapid entrance of a large bulk of food into the jejunum stimulates active peristalsis, which transports the food down the small bowel very rapidly. In many cases, the increased activity affects the jejunum only and there is a compensatory slowing in the ileum. After total gastrectomy this effect is exaggerated. Farris, Ransom, and Coller[14] noted that all gastric operations may be followed by transient increased motility. Ingested powdered charcoal may appear on the stool in twelve hours. They cited two long-term survivors after total gastrectomy in whom barium studies show, if anything, slightly decreased motility. Two of twenty of our patients showed this delayed emptying with puddling in the jejunum, two patients showed rapid emptying of the entire small bowel, and the remainder were in the normal range. Weigen and co-workers[44] found no consistent change in gastric emptying or intestinal transit by means of roentgenologic studies after total pancreatectomy in dogs. Alvarez[45] noted hyperirritability of the small bowel as a constant finding after vagotomy in rabbits. To summarize, there is evidence suggesting that after gastrectomy there is alteration in gastrointestinal motility, particularly in the upper small bowel, with quickened transit. The importance of this in the etiology of assimilation disturbances is apparent and has been discussed previously.

Disturbances in Hemopoiesis.—Following the epic work of Minot and Castle in elucidating much of the problem of pernicious anemia, a great deal of attention was given to experimental work in an effort to produce this disease in animals. Petri and Jensenius[46, 47] and Jacobsen and Plum[48] reviewed much of this work and concluded that gastrectomy alone or combined with extirpation of various segments of the intestinal tract has not been successful in producing the typical picture of pernicious anemia. Gastrectomy in dogs, swine, cats, monkeys, and rats is followed frequently by a more or less pronounced anemia, usually hypochromic in variety. Other features seen are inhibition of growth, emaciation, changes in the skin and hair, and sometimes disturbances in bone calcification. Several authors[48] have shown that extracts from the liver of gastrectomized animals have no therapeutic effect in human pernicious anemia. This suggests, of course, that storage of antipernicious anemia principle is greatly reduced, but the fact that a typical anemia does not occur in the animal would seem to indicate that some absorption is still taking place.

Numerous reports have been made on the appearance of megaloblastic anemia occurring after total gastrectomy and also partial gastrectomy and gastroenterostomy.[2, 19, 49-53] In the main, this anemia closely resembles pernicious anemia. Beebe and Meneeley,[54] in reporting such a case, surveyed the literature and found fifty-five reported cases of pernicious anemia following total or partial gastrectomy. These occurred from two to five years after operation.

MacDonald,[55] in 1947, reviewed the literature on forty-six patients surviving total gastrectomy by three years or more. In twelve of these cases the blood findings resembled pernicious anemia and in five others the findings were doubtful. Of the remainder, many had been receiving liver therapy, although no definite history of anemia could be determined. Macrocytosis has been noted as the only abnormality after total gastrectomy; Brain and Stammers[18] reported this condition in eleven of forty patients following total or near-total gastrectomy. Schwartz and Legere[56] studied fifty-four patients with pernicious anemia, and found that following complete cessation of liver therapy it took from two to thirty-eight months for hematologic relapse to occur. Landboe-Christensen[57] recently found evidence suggesting that the human duodenum may contain a small amount of intrinsic factor. If this is proved, it would help to explain the long interval apparently necessary before megaloblastic anemia occurs after total gastrectomy in the human being. Since comparatively few patients who have required total gastrectomy have survived for the requisite length of time, it is not too surprising that megaloblastic anemia is encountered relatively infrequently. However, the likelihood of megaloblastic anemia developing after total gastrectomy need have no influence on the decision to employ this procedure, as the anemia is readily managed by the same methods used in the treatment of pernicious anemia.

Hypochromic microcytic anemia is more commonly encountered after gastrectomy. Many reports have been made, with most figures ranging from 10 to 20 per cent. Women have a higher incidence, and when considered separately are seen to have from two to three times as many anemias. Bruusgaard[41] found that after partial gastrectomy 44 per cent of the women and 28 per cent of the men were anemic. The difference in these figures is accounted for by the higher incidence in the menstruating female, the women under 40 showing an incidence of 59 per cent, whereas those over 40 had an incidence of 28 per cent, the same as for men.

Lyngar[58] found that the serum iron was low in patients with hypochromic anemia after gastrectomy. Iron absorption studies showed poor absorption in some cases. All patients responded eventually to iron therapy, although some finally required intravenous administration.

The absence of HCl, which frees combined iron and reduces it to the ferrous state necessary for absorption, the by-passing of the duodenum in many cases, which is the most active site in iron absorption, and increased motility through the upper intestines are all factors which can explain inadequate iron absorption.

Starkenstein[59] found that maximal utilization of iron complexes was obtained when they were administered per os with the addition of fats. Vannotti and Delachaux[60] suggested that this may indicate that the duodenal absorption of iron is effected with the help of bile. Disturbances in regard to the secretion of the latter have been mentioned earlier.

In our series of cases, megaloblastic anemia has been more frequent than hypochromic.

To recapitulate briefly, after total or near-total gastrectomy, megaloblastic anemia may be expected to occur frequently when patients survive for a long enough period of time. This anemia is apparently the same as the spontaneously occurring pernicious anemia, and responds to the same management. Hypochromic microcytic anemia is also seen and is apparently secondary to inadequate iron absorption. Treatment with iron orally or parenterally is uniformly successful.

Iron absorption as seen by the iron tolerance test is suggestively impaired in six of eleven of the patients studied in the group reported herein.

Recent studies by Ferguson and associates[61] and Cross and Wangensteen[62] have shown the great sensitivity of the esophageal mucosa to gastric juice and, to a lesser extent, to bile and pancreatic juice. That regurgitation of bile and pancreatic juice occurs after total gastrectomy is known. Regurgitation would probably be most likely after esophagoduodenostomy and less so after esophagojejunostomy with esophagoenterostomy or the Roux Y procedure. While esophagitis has been little noted in the literature, we found mild to moderate esophagitis in three of eleven cases, plus one questionable case. None of these patients had symptoms, however. The importance of this observation remains to be determined.

SUMMARY AND CONCLUSION

Twenty-two patients with total gastrectomy and four patients with near-total gastrectomy were studied at varying intervals of two months to eight years, nine months after operation. Information was obtained in regard to weight loss, eating habits, gastrointestinal symptoms, roentgenologic study of the upper gastrointestinal tract, pancreatic function, fecal fat and nitrogen, iron absorption, hematology, and esophagitis. This information is tabulated in detail and discussed in brief form. The present study indicates that total gastrectomy is regularly followed by loss of weight and, not uncommonly, weakness of a mild degree. While loss of dietary fat in the feces is somewhat increased, on the average the amount involved is not sufficient to account for the degree of weight loss. The more likely explanation is reduced food intake secondary to loss of the storage function of the stomach and the occurrence of distress after eating more than a small amount of food at one time.

Anemia may be expected to occur frequently, particularly if the patient survives for a long enough period of time after operation. This anemia presents no particular problem in management and should not influence the decision to use the procedure. Dietary regulation using a high-caloric, high-protein, high-fat diet with small frequent meals would appear to offer the most logical approach to management. Supplemental medication, such as pancreatin, Tween 80, atropine, and so forth, has been recommended by various authors and may be worthy of trial in difficult cases.

REFERENCES

1. Lahey, F.: Total Gastrectomy for All Patients With Operable Cancer of the Stomach, Editorial, Surg., Gynec. & Obst. **90**: 246, 1950.
2. Lahey, F., and Marshall, S. F.: Should Total Gastrectomy Be Employed in Early Cancer of the Stomach? Ann. Surg. **132**: 540, 1950.
3. Scott, H. W., and Longmire, W.: Total Gastrectomy, SURGERY **26**: 488, 1949.
4. Fowweather, F. S., cited by Peters, J. P., and Van Slyke, D. D.: Methods, vol. 2, Baltimore, 1932, Williams & Wilkins Company.
5. Kjeldahl, J., cited by Peters, J. P., and Van Slyke, D. D.: Methods, vol. 2, Baltimore, 1932, Williams & Wilkins Company.
6. Somogyi, M.: Micromethods for the Estimation of Diastase, J. Biol. Chem. **125**: 399, 1938.
7. Anderson, D. H., and Early, M. U.: Method of Assaying Trypsin Suitable for Routine Use in Diagnosis of Congenital Pancreatic Deficiency, Am. J. Dis. Child. **63**: 891-896, 1942.

8. Cherry, I. S., and Crandall, L. A., Jr.: Specificity of Pancreatic Lipase: Its Appearance in Blood After Pancreatic Injury, Am. J. Physiol. **100:** 266-273, 1932.
9. Barkan, G., and Walker, B.: Determination of Serum Iron and Pseudohemoglobin Iron With o-Phenanthroline, J. Biol. Chem. **135:** 37-42, 1940.
10. Wollaeger, E. E., Comfort, M. W., and Osterberg, A. E.: Total Solids, Fat and Nitrogen in the Feces. A Study of Normal Persons Taking a Test Diet Containing a Moderate Amount of Fat, Gastroenterology **9:** 272, 1947.
11. Wollaeger, E. E., Comfort, M. W., Weir, J. F., and Osterberg, A. E.: The Total Solids, Fat and Nitrogen in the Feces: A Study of Normal Persons and of Patients With Duodenal Ulcer on a Test Diet Containing Large Amounts of Fat, Gastroenterology **6:** 83, 1946.
12. Wollaeger, E. E., Comfort, M. W., and Weir, J. F.: The Total Solids, Fat and Nitrogen in the Feces: A Study of Persons Who Had Undergone Partial Gastrectomy With Anastomosis of the Entire Cut End of the Stomach and the Jejunum (Polya Anastomosis), Gastroenterology **6:** 93, 1946.
13. Church, R. E., and Hinton, J. W.: Follow-Up Results in Subtotal Gastric Resection for Ulcer, Am. J. Digest. Dis. **9:** 317, 1942.
14. Farris, J. M., Ransom, H. K., and Coller, F. A.: Total Gastrectomy; Effects Upon Nutrition and Hematopoiesis, Surgery **13:** 823, 1943.
15. Brázda, B.: Sur les troubles de métabolisme des graisses, Presse méd. **58:** 642, 1950.
16. Palumbo, L. T., Paul, R. E., and Westley, G. T.: Partial Gastrectomy With and Without Vagus Resection in the Treatment of Duodenal Ulcer, Arch. Surg. **64:** 756, 1952.
17. Wells, C., and Welbourn, R.: Postgastrectomy Syndromes, Brit. M. J. **1:** 546 (March 17), 1951.
18. Brain, R. H. F., and Stammers, F. A. R.: Sequellae of Radical Gastric Resections, Lancet **1:** 1137, 1951.
19. Everson, T. C.: Nutrition Following Total Gastrectomy With Particular Reference to Fat and Protein Assimilation, Surg., Gynec. & Obst. **95:** 209, 1952.
20. Bussbarger, R. A., and Jung, F. T.: Dietary and Hematologic Studies After Gastrectomy in the Rat, Am. J. Physiol. **117:** 59, 1936.
21. Freeman, S., Hough, V., Wigodosky, H., and Ivy, A. C.: The Effect of Gastrectomy Upon Growing Monkeys, Gastroenterology **1:** 199, 1943.
22. Kelly, W. D., and Wangensteen, O. H.: Unpublished data.
23. Ivy, A. C., Morgan, J. E., and Farrell, J. I.: The Effects of Total Gastrectomy: Experimental Achylia Gastrica in Dogs With the Occurrence of a Spontaneous Anemia and Anemia of Pregnancy, Surg., Gynec. & Obst. **53:** 611, 1931.
24. Annis, D., and Hallenbeck, G. A.: The Effects of Partial Gastrectomy on Canine External Pancreatic Secretion, Surgery **31:** 517, 1952.
25. Howard, J. M., James, E. L., and Evans, S. S.: Physiological Studies on the External Pancreatic Secretion in Man, Proc. Surg. Forum, Clin. Congress Am. Coll. Surgeons, Philadelphia, 1951, W. B. Saunders Company, p. 577-582.
26. Crider, J. O., and Thomas, J. E.: Secretion of Pancreatic Juice After Cutting Extrinsic Nerves, Am. J. Physiol. **141:** 730, 1944.
27. Pincus, I. J., Thomas, J. E., and Lachman, P. O.: The Effect of Vagotomy on the Secretion of Pancreatic Juice After the Injection of Various Food Stuffs (Preliminary Report), Fed. Proc. VII-I: 94, 1948.
28. Routley, E., Mann, F. C., Bollman, J. L., and Grindlay, J. H.: Effects of Vagotomy on Pancreatic Secretion, Proc. Staff Meet., Mayo Clin. **25:** 218, 1950.
29. Routley, E., Mann, F. C., Bollman, J. L., and Grindlay, J. H.: Effects of Vagotomy on Pancreatic Secretion in Dogs With Chronic Pancreatic Fistula, Surg., Gynec. & Obst. **95:** 529, 1952.
30. Shingleton, W. W., Fawcett, B., and Vetter, J. S.: Pancreatic Secretion and Response to Secretin After Vagotomy and Sympathectomy, Postgraduate Gastroenterology, Philadelphia, 1950, W. B. Saunders Company, p. 155.
31. Wollaeger, E.: Disturbances of Gastrointestinal Function Following Partial Gastrectomy, Postgrad. Med. **8:** 251, 1950.
32. Bohmansson, G.: Studien über die chirurgische Behandlung von Gastroduodenalgeschwüren mit besonderer Berücksichtigung der Operations-anatomie und der postoperativen Digestions physiologie nebst einem Beitrag zur Frage der chirurgischen Behandlung akuter Ulkusblutungen, Acta chir. Scandinav. (supp. 7) **60:** 78-79, 126, 1926.
33. Everson, T. C.: The Effect of Esophagoduodenostomy on Fecal Fat and Nitrogen Loss Following Total Gastrectomy, Proc. Surg. Forum, Clin. Congress Am. Coll. Surgeons, Philadelphia, 1951, W. B. Saunders Company, p. 68.
34. Calabi, V., Paolini, A. M., and Pliteri, S.: On the Importance of Gastric Transit in the Utilization of Alimentary Lipids, J. internat. chir. **9:** 79, 1951.
35. Vermeulen, C., Owens, F. M., and Dragstedt, L. R.: Effect of Pancreatectomy on Fat Absorption From Intestines, Am. J. Physiol. **138:** 792-796 (April) 1943.

36. Searle, G. W., and Annegers, J. H.: Correction of Steatorrhea in Bile Fistula Dogs by Duodenal and Oral Administration of Bile, Gastroenterology **19:** 558, 1951.
37. Linke, C.: The Effect of Diversion of Bile to Various Parts of the Intestine, Proc. Surg. Forum, Clin. Congress Am. Coll. Surgeons, Philadelphia, 1951, W. B. Saunders Company, p. 179.
38. Emery, E. S., Jr.: The Cause of Faulty Digestion in Dogs Without Stomachs, Am. J. Digest. Dis. **2:** 599, 1935.
39. Watson, A. B.: Partial Gastrectomy for Simple Ulcer, Brit. J. Surg. **34:** 353, 1947.
40. Smith, F. H., and Jordan, S. M.: Gastric Ulcer: A Study of 600 Cases, Gastroenterology **11:** 575, 1948.
41. Bruusgaard, C.: The Operative Treatment of Gastric and Duodenal Ulcer, Acta chir. scandinav. (supp. 117) **94:** 1, 1946.
42. Bohmansson, G.: Prophylaxis and Therapy in Late Postgastrectomy Complications, Acta med. scandinav. (supp. 246), p. 37, 1950.
43. Machella, T. E.: Experience With the ''Dumping'' Syndrome, Postgraduate Gastroenterology, Philadelphia, 1950, W. B. Saunders Company.
44. Weigen, J. F., Pendergrass, E. P., Ravdin, I., and Machella, T. E.: A Roentgen Study of the Effect of Total Pancreatectomy on the Stomach and Small Intestine in the Dog, Radiology **59:** 92, 1952.
45. Alvarez, W. C.: An Introduction to Gastroenterology, New York, 1948, Paul B. Hoeber, Inc.
46. Petri, S., Norgaard, F., and Jensenius, H.: Experimental Studies on the Production of Pernicious Anemia by Operation on the Digestive Tract. Part II, Acta med. scandinav. **107:** 506, 1941.
47. Petri, S., and Jensenius, H.: Experimental Studies on the Production of Pernicious Anemia by Operation on the Digestive Tract. Part III, Acta med. scandinav. **107:** 532, 1941.
48. Jacobsen, E., and Plum, C. M.: The Effect of Gastrectomy on the Blood Picture and on the Ripening Index of Reticulocytes in Rats, Acta med. scandinav. (supp. 213), p. 209, 1948.
49. Conway, N. S., and Conway, H.: Vitamin B-12 and Folic Acid in Megaloblastic Anemia After Total Gastrectomy, Brit. M. J. **1:** 158 (Jan. 27) 1951.
50. Inglefinger, F. J.: The Late Effects of Total and Subtotal Gastrectomy, New England J. Med. **231:** 321, 1944.
51. Ransom, H. K.: Total Gastrectomy, Arch. Surg. **55:** 13, 1947.
52. Meyer, K. A., Schwartz, S. O., and Weissman, L. H.: Pernicious Anemia Following Total Gastrectomy, Arch. Surg. **42:** 18, 1941.
53. Goldhamer, S. M.: The Pernicious Anemia Syndrome in Gastrectomized Patients, Surg., Gynec. & Obst. **57:** 257, 1933.
54. Beebe, R. T., and Meneeley, J. K.: Pernicious Anemia Following Gastrectomy, New York State J. Med. **49:** 2437, 1949.
55. MacDonald, R. M., Inglefinger, F. J., and Belding, H. W.: Late Effects of Total Gastrectomy in Man, New England J. Med. **237:** 887, 1947.
56. Schwartz, S. O., and Legere, H.: Relapses in Pernicious Anemia, J. A. M. A. **124:** 637, 1944.
57. Landboe-Christensen, E., Berk, L., and Castle, W. B.: Observations on the Etiologic Relationship of Achylia Gastrica to Pernicious Anemia. XIV. Intrinsic Factor Activity of Desiccated and Defatted Human Fundus, Duodenum and Jejunum, Am. J. M. Sc. **224:** 1, 1952.
58. Lyngar, E.: Blood Changes After Partial Gastrectomy for Ulcer, Acta med. scandinav. (supp. 247), 1-132, 1950.
59. Starkenstein, E.: Eisen. Handb. d. Exper. Pharmakologie III/2, Berlin, 1934, Springer-Verlag, pp. 682-1284.
60. Vannotti, A., and Delachaux, A.: Iron Metabolism and Its Clinical Significance, London, 1949, Frederick Muller, Ltd.
61. Ferguson, D. J., Sanchez-Palomera, E., Sako, Y., Clatworthy, H. W., Jr., Toon, R. W., and Wangensteen, O. H.: Studies on Experimental Esophagitis, SURGERY **28:** 1022-1039, 1950.
62. Cross, F. S., and Wangensteen, O. H.: Role of Bile and Pancreatic Juice in Production of Esophageal Erosions and Anemia, Proc. Soc. Exper. Biol. & Med. **77:** 862-866, 1951.
63. Gholiger, J. C., and Riley, T. R.: Incidence and Mechanism of Early Dumping Syndrome After Gastrectomy, Lancet **1:** 630-636, 1952.

INDEX TO VOLUME 35

AUTHORS INDEX*

In this index, following the author's name, the title of the subject is given as it appeared in the JOURNAL. Editorials are also included in the list and are indicated by (*E.*).

A

ABEATICI, S. (*See* Dogliotti and Abeatici), 503
ACKERMAN, LAUREN V. (*See* Lieberman and Ackerman), 350
ALLEN, HERMAN L. (*See* Hershman and Allen), 805
ALLEN, M. SHANNON. Mechanism of omental migration, 249
AMSPACHER, WILLIAM H. (*See* Davis, Kuhn, Shaffer, and Amspacher), 434
ARIEL, IRVING M., JEROME, ANTHONY P., AND PACK, GEORGE T. Treatment of tumors of the parotid salivary gland, 124
ARNHEIM, ERNEST E. Congenital eventration of the diaphragm in infancy, 809
ATERMAN, K. Hyaluronidase and experimental exophthalmos, 443
AUFSES, ARTHUR H., JR. Venous thrombosis of the upper extremity complicated by pulmonary embolus, 957

B

BACON, HARRY E., LOWELL, EDWARD J., JR., AND TRIMPI, HOWARD D. Villous papillomas of the colon and rectum, 77
—. (*See* McElwain, Bacon, and Trimpi), 513
BADER, MORTIMER E. (*See* Bader, Bader, Kim, and Cournand), 366
BADER, RICHARD A., BADER, MORTIMER E., KIM, SOON WON, AND COURNAND, ANDRE. Comparative studies, in normotensive man, of the effectiveness, retention, and elimination of various plasma expanders, 366
BARNES, WILLIAM A. (*See* Redo and Barnes), 844
BARR, L. H. (*See* Donato, Mayo, and Barr), 719
BEACONSFIELD, PETER. (*See* Messent and Beaconsfield), 382
BECK, WILLIAM C., AND BERKHEISER, SAMUEL. Prominent costal cartilages (Tietze's syndrome), 762
BEECHER, HENRY K. A note on spinal anesthesia and its relationship to a larger problem, 820 (*E.*)
BERGER, S. M. (*See* Gershon-Cohen, Ingleby, Hermel, and Berger), 766
BERKHEISER, SAMUEL. (*See* Beck and Berkheiser), 762
BERMAN, EDGAR F. Carcinoma of the esophagus: a new concept in therapy, 822
BERNE, CLARENCE J. (*See* Mikkelsen and Berne), 743
BERRY, FRANK B. The Research and Development Board, 290 (*E.*)
BIGGANE, CHARLES F., JR. (*See* Lilly, Smith, Biggane, and Jana), 1
BILL, ALEXANDER H., JR., AND POPE, WILLIAM M. Congenital duodenal diaphram, 482
BOWERS, RALPH F. Choledochojejunostomy en Roux Y, 159
BREA, MARIO M. J. Primary carcinoma of the lung, 167
BRELSFORD, HAROLD J. (*See* Halpert and Brelsford), 901
BRESSLER, SYDNEY, AND WIENER, DAVID. Bronchiogenic cyst associated with an anomalous pulmonary artery arising from the thoracic aorta, 815
BRIZZOLARA, LOUIS G., AND GERACI, CHARLES L. Esophageal leiomyoma, 465
BROWN, DONALD R. (*See* Thompson and Brown), 916
BRUNSCHWIG, ALEXANDER, AND LÜSCHER, MARIE. Hyperchloremic acidosis following anterior partial and complete pelvic exenteration, 197
BURCH, B. H., TRAPHAGEN, D. W., FOLKMAN, M. J., ROSENBAUM, D. A., AND MUELLER, E. C. Temporary aortic occlusion in abdominal surgery, 684

C

CANCELMO, JOHN B. (*See* Ulin and Cancelmo), 640
CARVER, GORDON M., JR., AND PATTERSON, W. Transorbitocranial foreign body, 475

*January, pp. 1-166; February, pp. 167-334; March, pp. 335-502; April, pp. 503-672; May, pp. 673-836; June, pp. 837-1002.

CATE, W. R., JR., AND CULLEY, T. S. The mixing of material injected into pulsatile and nonpulsatile streams: application to regional heparinization, 411

CLAGETT, O. THERON. (*See* Wierman, McDonald, and Clagett), 335

CLAYTOR, A. A. (*See* Northway, DeLano, and Claytor), 925

COHEN, MORLEY, AND MOORE, GEORGE E. Malignant lesions of the thyroid, 62

COURNAND, ANDRE. (*See* Bader, Bader, Kim, and Cournand), 366

CRILE, GEORGE, JR. Dangers of conservative surgery in abdominal emergencies, 122 (*E.*)

CULLEY, T. S. (*See* Cate and Culley), 411

D

DAVIS, JOHN H., KUHN, LUDWIG R., SHAFFER, JOSEPH R., AND AMSPACHER, WILLIAM H. Preoperative preparation of the bowel with neomycin, 434

DEBAKEY, MICHAEL E. (*See* Halpert, Fields, and DeBakey), 346

DELANO, R. H. (*See* Northway, DeLano, and Claytor), 925

DERBES, VINCENT J., AND HARAN, THOMAS. Rib fractures from muscular effort with particular reference to cough, 294

DOGLIOTTI, A. M., AND ABEATICI, S. Transparietal splenoportal roentgenography and research on portal hypertension, 503

DONATO, HENRY, MAYO, HENRY W., JR., AND BARR, L. H. The effect of peroral barium in partial obstruction of the small bowel, 719

DORIAN, ALAN L., AND STEIN, GEORGE N. Hernia through foramen of Winslow, 795

E

ELKIN, D. C. (*See* Shea, Robertson, and Elkin), 698

ENGELBERG, JOSEPH. (*See* Gimbel and Engelberg), 645

ENTERLINE, HORATIO T. (*See* Zintel, Enterline, and Rhoads), 612

F

FARMER, DOUGLAS A., AND SMITHWICK, REGINALD H. The effect of partial exclusion of bile and pancreatic juice on the acidity of the gastric contents in the postgastrectomy patient, 557

FEY, WILLIAM P. (*See* Tucker and Fey), 213

FIELDS, WILLIAM S. (*See* Halpert, Fields, and DeBakey), 346

FINKLE, ALEX L. (*See* Hudson, Finkle, Trifilio, and Wolan), 897

FISHER, BERNARD, RUSS, CLEM, AND UPDEGRAFF, HARRY. A suitable technique for total arterialization of the dog liver, 879

FITTS, WILLIAM T., JR., KEUHNELIAN, JOHN G., RAVDIN, I. S., AND SCHOR, STANLEY. Swelling of the arm after radical mastectomy, 460

FITZPATRICK, HUGH. (*See* Humphreys, Powers, Fitzpatrick, and Lanman), 9

FLYGARE, KENT A. (*See* Lippman, Johnson, and Flygare), 909

FOLKMAN, M. J. (*See* Burch, Traphagen, Folkman, Rosenbaum, and Mueller), 684

FRIEDGOOD, CHARLES E. (*See* Ripstein, Friedgood, and Solomon), 98

G

GENTSCH, THOMAS O., WATERS, LEVIN L., AND GLENN, WILLIAM W. L. The influence of acute hypervolemia on the freeze-dry homologous aortic graft, 30

GERACI, CHARLES L. (*See* Brizzolara and Geraci), 465

GERSHON-COHEN, J., INGLEBY, HELEN, HERMEL, M. B., AND BERGER, S. M. Accuracy of preoperative x-ray diagnoses of breast tumors, 766

GILFILLAN, RUTHERFORD S., STEINFELD, JESSE L., AND LEEDS, FRANK H. The syndrome of peripheral arterial insufficiency with partial occlusion of the iliac artery, 598

GIMBEL, NICHOLAS S., AND ENGELBERG, JOSEPH. Blood oxygenators: theory and studies in design, 645

GLENN, WILLIAM W. L. (*See* Gentsch, Waters, and Glenn), 30

GOLDSMITH, RALPH. (*See* Sterling and Goldsmith), 624

GOLLAN, FRANK, HAMILTON, EDWARD C., AND MENEELY, GEORGE R. Consecutive survival of open-chest, hypothermic dogs after prolonged by-pass of heart and lungs by means of a pump-oxygenator, 88

GRAFF, SAMUEL. (*See* May, Hines, Weintraub, Scudder, and Graff), 191

GROSSKREUTZ, DORIS C. (*See* Little, Hampton, and Grosskreutz), 857

H

HALPERT, BÉLA. Biologic behavior of carcinoma of the lung, 962 (*E.*)

—, AND BRELSFORD, HAROLD J. Mixed tumors in unusual sites, 901

—, FIELDS, WILLIAM S., AND DEBAKEY, MICHAEL E. Intracranial metastasis from carcinoma of the lung, 346
HAMILTON, EDWARD C. (*See* Gollan, Hamilton, and Meneely), 88
HAMPTON, L. JENNINGS. (*See* Little, Hampton, and Grosskreutz), 857
HARAN, THOMAS. (*See* Derbes and Haran), 294
HARDIN, CREIGHTON A. (*See* Werder and Hardin), 405
HARDY, JAMES D. (*See* Neely, Wilson, Milnor, Hardy, and Wilson), 22
HARKINS, HENRY N. (*See* Knopp and Harkins), 493
HARRIS, M. H. Abdominal pregnancy with fetal and maternal survival, 793
HARVEY, W. PROCTOR. (*See* Hufnagel, Harvey, Rabil, and McDermott), 673
HAY, LYLE J. (*See* Lehmann and Hay), 401
—. (*See* Thomas and Hay), 635
HAYES, MARK A. Shock and the adrenocortex, 174
HERMEL, M. B. (*See* Gershon-Cohen, Ingleby, Hermel, and Berger), 766
HERSHMAN, HYMAN, AND ALLEN, HERMAN L. Spontaneous rupture of the normal urinary bladder, 805
HILL, MALCOLM R., JR., AND KIPEN, CHARLES S. Laryngocele: an unusual tumor of the neck, 273
HINES, MARGUERITE. (*See* May, Hines, Weintraub, Scudder, and Graff), 191
HINMAN, FRANK, JR. (*See* Miller, Wylie, and Hinman), 885
HINTON, J. WILLIAM. The mechanism of action of ergotamine in hyperthyroidism, 491 (*E.*)
HOLCOMB, GEORGE W., JR., AND MATSON, DONALD D. Thoracic neurenteric cyst, 115
HUDSON, PERRY B., FINKLE, ALEX L., TRIFILIO, ARISTIDES, AND WOLAN, CASIMIR T. Prostatic cancer. IX. Value of transurethral biopsy in search of early prostatic carcinoma, 897
HUFNAGEL, CHARLES A., HARVEY, W. PROCTOR, RABIL, PIERRE J., AND MCDERMOTT, THOMAS F. Surgical correction of aortic insufficiency, 673
HUGHES, CARL W. (*See* Seeley, Hughes, and Jahnke), 421
HUMPHREYS, GEORGE H., II, POWERS, SAMUEL, FITZPATRICK, HUGH, AND LANMAN, BEN MARR. Pulmonary valvulotomy, 9
HURLEY, ANSON G. (*See* Moore and Hurley), 283

I

INGLEBY, HELEN. (*See* Gershon-Cohen, Ingleby, Hermel, and Berger), 766
ISAACSON, NORMAN H., AND MCCARTY, DENNIS. Recurring myxomatous cutaneous cyst, 621

J

JAHNKE, EDWARD J., JR. (*See* Seeley, Hughes, and Jahnke), 421
JANA, JOSEPH T., JR. (*See* Lilly, Smith, Biggane, and Jana), 1
JENSEN, RODERICK E. Evaluation of a method for the study of burn healing, 390
JEROME, ANTHONY P. (*See* Ariel, Jerome, and Pack), 124
JOHNSON, PAUL A., JR. (*See* Lippman, Johnson, and Flygare), 909

K

KELLY, WILLIAM D., MACLEAN, LLOYD D., PERRY, JOHN F., AND WANGENSTEEN, OWEN H. A study of patients following total and near-total gastrectomy, 964
—. (*See* MacLean, Perry, Kelly, Mosser, Mannick, and Wangensteen), 705
KEUHNELIAN, JOHN G. (*See* Fitts, Keuhnelian, Ravdin, and Schor), 460
KEY, J. ALBERT, AND REYNOLDS, FRED C. The treatment of infection after medullary nailing, 749
KIM, SOON WON. (*See* Bader, Bader, Kim, and Cournand), 366
KIPEN, CHARLES S. (*See* Hill and Kipen), 273
KIRILUK, LAWRENCE B., AND MERENDINO, K. ALVIN. The comparative sensitivity of the mucosa of the various segments of the alimentary tract in the dog to acid-peptic action, 547
—, AND —. An elucidation of the intestinal sensitivity factor and the distance factors in the incidence of stomal ulcer in the Billroth II type gastrectomy, 538
—, AND —. An experimental study of the buffering capacity of the contents of the upper small bowel, 532
—. (*See* Merendino and Kiriluk), 590
KNOPP, LAWRENCE M., AND HARKINS, HENRY N. Traumatic rupture of the normal spleen, 493
KOONTZ, AMOS R. Surgical anesthesia, 643 (*E.*)
KOUCKY, JOHN D., AND MALEY, W. FORRESTER. Benign stricture of hepaticoduodenostomy: its treatment, 802
KRAMÁR, JENÖ, PEETZ, DWAINE J., AND MCCARTHY, HARRY H. Trauma and capillary resistance, 772

KUHN, LUDWIG R. (*See* Davis, Kuhn, Shaffer, and Amspacher), 434

L

LANMAN, BEN MARR. (*See* Humphreys, Powers, Fitzpatrick, and Lanman), 9

LAUFMAN, HAROLD. (*See* Roach and Laufman), 45

LEEDS, FRANK H. (*See* Gilfillan, Steinfeld, and Leeds), 598

LEHMANN, ARNOLD L., AND HAY, LYLE J. A controlled pressure plastic dressing for skin grafting, burns, and thrombophlebitis, 401

LIEBERMAN, ZELIG, AND ACKERMAN, LAUREN V. Principles in management of soft tissue sarcomas, 350

LILLEHEI, C. WALTON. (*See* Lober and Lillehei), 950

LILLY, GEORGE D., SMITH, DONALD W., BIGGANE, CHARLES F., JR., AND JANA, JOSEPH T., JR. An evaluation of "high" lumbar sympathectomy in arteriosclerotic circulatory insufficiency of the lower extremities, 1

LIPPMAN, HARVEY N., JOHNSON, PAUL A., JR., AND FLYGARE, KENT A. A modification of the Hunterian Laboratory anesthesia apparatus for experimental surgery, 909

—. (*See* Shore, Lippman, and Weber), 633

LISA, JAMES R. (*See* Pack and Lisa), 277

LITTLE, DAVID M., JR., HAMPTON, L. JENNINGS, AND GROSSKREUTZ, DORIS C. The use of Arfonad in a modification of the technique of controlled hypotension, 857

LOBER, PAUL H., AND LILLEHEI, C. WALTON. Necrotizing panarteritis following repair of coarctation of aorta, 950

LOWELL, EDWARD J., JR. (*See* Bacon, Lowell, and Trimpi), 77

LUGER, NORTON M. (*See* Surks and Luger), 104

LUKE, JOSEPHUS C. The management of recurrent varicose veins, 40

LÜSCHER, MARIE. (*See* Brunschwig and Lüscher), 197

LYONS, CHAMP. Cardiac arrhythmia as a predictable surgical risk, 292 (*E.*)

M

MACKAY, CALVIN R. The significance of local vascular changes in bleeding peptic ulcer, 724

MACLEAN, LLOYD D., PERRY, JOHN F., KELLY, WILLIAM D., MOSSER, DONN G., MANNICK, ANGELINE, AND WANGENSTEEN, OWEN H. Nutrition following subtotal gastrectomy of four types (Billroth I and II, segmental, and tubular resections), 705

—. (*See* Kelly, MacLean, Perry, and Wangensteen), 964

MAHONEY, EARLE B., AND SHERMAN, CHARLES D., JR. Total esophagoplasty using intrathoracic right colon, 937

MALEY, W. FORRESTER. (*See* Koucky and Maley), 802

MANNICK, ANGELINE. (*See* MacLean, Perry, Kelly, Mosser, Mannick, and Wangensteen), 705

MATSON, DONALD D. (*See* Holcomb and Matson), 115

MATTICK, WALTER L., AND STREUTER, MILTON A. Carcinoma of the maxillary antrum, 236

MAY, LEOPOLD, HINES, MARGUERITE, WEINTRAUB, LEONARD, SCUDDER, JOHN, AND GRAFF, SAMUEL. Some physical-chemical properties of polyvinylpyrrolidone, 191

MAYO, HENRY W., JR. (*See* Donato, Mayo, and Barr), 719

MCCARTHY, HARRY H. (*See* Kramár, Peetz, and McCarthy), 772

MCCARTY, DENNIS. (*See* Isaacson and McCarty), 621

MCCLURE, JOHN N., JR. Rupture of the pregnant uterus due to nonpenetrating abdominal trauma, 487

MCDERMOTT, THOMAS F. (*See* Hufnagel, Harvey, Rabil, and McDermott), 673

MCDONALD, JOHN R. (*See* Wierman, McDonald, and Clagett), 335

MCELWAIN, JACK W., BACON, HARRY E., AND TRIMPI, HOWARD D. Lymph node metastases: experience with aortic ligation of inferior mesentery artery in cancer of the rectum, 513

MCGOWAN, JOHN M. (*See* Sarkisian and McGowan), 565

MENEELY, GEORGE R. (*See* Gollan, Hamilton, and Meneely), 88

MERENDINO, K. ALVIN, AND KIRILUK, LAWRENCE B. Human measurements involved in tracheobronchial resection and reconstruction procedures, 590

—. (*See* Kiriluk and Merendino), 532, 538, 547

MESSENT, DAVID, AND BEACONSFIELD, PETER. Circulatory changes in the lower limb following lumbar sympathectomy, 382

MIGLIACCIO, ANTHONY V. Gall bladder traction, 786

MIKKELSEN, WILLIAM P., AND BERNE, CLARENCE J. Femoral hernioplasty: suprapubic extraperitoneal (Cheatle-Henry) approach, 743

MILLER, GERALD M., WYLIE, EDWIN J., AND HINMAN, FRANK, JR. Renal complications from aortography, 885

MILNOR, J. PERVIS. (*See* Neely, Wilson, Milnor, Hardy, and Wilson), 22

MOORE, DANIEL C. Complications following the use of Efocaine, 109

MOORE, GEORGE E., AND URE, BARBARA. One-stage pancreatoduodenectomy with resection of the superior mesenteric vein, 734

—. (*See* Cohen and Moore), 62

MOORE, HORACE G., JR. The midline incision for surgery of the gall bladder and common bile duct, 440

MOORE, THOMAS C., AND HURLEY, ANSON G. Congenital duplication of the gall bladder, 283

MOSSER, DONN G. (*See* MacLean, Perry, Kelly, Mosser, Mannick, and Wangensteen), 705

MOYER, CARL A. (*See* Robinson and Moyer), 690

MUELLER, E. C. (*See* Burch, Traphagen, Folkman, Rosenbaum, and Mueller), 684

MULLINS, DAVID M. (*See* Riddell and Mullins), 270

N

NAKAYAMA, KOMEI. Approach to midthoracic esophageal carcinoma for its radical surgical treatment, 574

—. Simplification of the Billroth I gastric resection, 837

NARDI, GEORGE L. Urinary loss of amino acids after surgery, 378

NEELY, WILLIAM A., WILSON, FRANK C., JR., MILNOR, J. PERVIS, HARDY, JAMES D., AND WILSON, HARWELL. Cardiac output: a clinical comparison of the direct Fick, dye, and ballistocardiographic methods, 22

NELSON, RUSSELL M., AND NOYES, HOWARD E. Blood culture studies in normal dogs and in dogs in hemorrhagic shock, 782

NORTHWAY, R. O., DELANO, R. H., AND CLAYTOR, A. A. Perforation of the stomach in the newborn infant, 925

NOYES, HOWARD E. (*See* Nelson and Noyes), 782

P

PACK, GEORGE T. Cancer of the stomach: twenty-year cures, 920

—, AND LISA, JAMES R. Mesenchymoma, 277

—. (*See* Ariel, Jerome, and Pack), 124

PATTERSON, W. (*See* Carver and Patterson), 475

PEETZ, DWAINE J. (*See* Kramár, Peetz, and McCarthy), 772

PELTIER, LEONARD F. Eponymic fractures: Abraham Colles and Colles' fracture, 322

PERRY, JOHN F. (*See* Kelly, MacLean, Perry, and Wangensteen), 964

—. (*See* MacLean, Perry, Kelly, Mosser, Mannick, and Wangensteen), 705

POPE, WILLIAM M. (*See* Bill and Pope), 482

POWERS, SAMUEL. (*See* Humphreys, Powers, Fitzpatrick, and Lanman), 9

R

RABIL, PIERRE J. (*See* Hufnagel, Harvey, Rabil, and McDermott), 673

RAINEY, ROBERT. The association of lymphogranuloma inguinale and cancer, 221

RASCH, GEORGE C., AND STRANGE, DEMPSEY C. Mucocele of inverted appendiceal stump following appendectomy, 629

RAVDIN, I. S. (*See* Fitts, Keuhnelian, Ravdin, and Schor), 460

REDO, S. FRANK, AND BARNES, WILLIAM A. A stainless steel cannula for the creation of gastrointestinal fistulas, 844

REYNOLDS, FRED C. (*See* Key and Reynolds), 749

RHOADS, JONATHAN E. (*See* Zintel, Enterline, and Rhoads), 613

RIDDELL, DOUGLAS H., AND MULLINS, DAVID M. Appendicitis in the newborn infant, 270

RIPSTEIN, CHARLES B., FRIEDGOOD, CHARLES E., AND SOLOMON, NATHAN. A technique for the production of hypothermia, 98

ROACH, H. DAVID AND LAUFMAN, HAROLD. The use of intravenous trypsin in experimental pulmonary embolism, 45

ROBERTSON, ROY L. (*See* Shea, Robertson, and Elkin), 698

ROBINSON, JOHN R., AND MOYER, CARL A. Comparison of late sequelae of common and superficial femoral vein ligations, 690

ROSENBAUM, D. A. (*See* Burch, Traphagen, Folkman, Rosenbaum, and Mueller), 684

ROSENBERG, NORMAN. A technique for facilitating the stripping of large-bore varicose veins using conventional strippers, 877

RUSS, CLEM. (*See* Fisher, Russ, and Updegraff), 879

RUTENBURG, ALEXANDER M. (*See* Schweinburg, Sylvester, and Rutenburg), 204

S

SARKISIAN, S. ALBERT, AND MCGOWAN, JOHN M. The relation of bacteria in the bile to biliary dynamics, cholangitis, and postcholecystectomy syndrome, 565

SCHLEGEL, JØRGEN U. A new approach to the treatment of electrolyte disturbances in shock and severe stress, 449
—. Return of sodium loads in normal subjects following restricted sodium intake, 848
SCHOR, STANLEY. (*See* Fitts, Keuhnelian, Ravdin, and Schor), 460
SCHWEINBURG, FRITZ B., SYLVESTER, ELSIE M., AND RUTENBURG, ALEXANDER M. The relation of the in vitro sensitivity test to the clinical response to Aureomycin therapy, 204
SCUDDER, JOHN. (*See* May, Hines, Weintraub, Scudder, and Graff), 191
SEELEY, SAM F., HUGHES, CARL W., AND JAHNKE, EDWARD J., JR. Major vessel damage in lumbar disc operation, 421
SHAFFER, JOSEPH R. (*See* Davis, Kuhn, Shaffer, and Amspacher), 434
SHEA, PATRICK C., JR., ROBERTSON, ROY L., AND ELKIN, D. C. An effective clinical method for determining coagulation time of blood, 698
SHERMAN, CHARLES D., JR. (*See* Mahoney and Sherman), 937
SHORE, SAMUEL, LIPPMAN, HARVEY N., AND WEBER, ROBERT A. Ascariasis of the comon bile duct, 633
SMITH, DONALD W. (*See* Lilly, Smith, Biggane, and Jana), 1
SMITHWICK, REGINALD H. (*See* Farmer and Smithwick), 557
SOLOMON, NATHAN. (*See* Ripstein, Friedgood, and Solomon), 98
STEIN, GEORGE N. (*See* Dorian and Stein), 795
STEINFELD, JESSE L. (*See* Gilfillan, Steinfeld, and Leeds), 598
STERLING, JULIAN A., AND GOLDSMITH, RALPH. Total transplant of thyroid gland using vascular anastomoses, 624
STRANGE, DEMPSEY C. (*See* Rasch and Strange), 629
STRANSKY, JOHN J. Retroperitoneal rupture of the duodenum due to nonpenetrating abdominal trauma, 928
STREUTER, MILTON A. (*See* Mattick and Streuter), 236
SURKS, SYLVAN N., AND LUGER, NORTON M. Clinical use of levo-arterenol during cyclopropane anesthesia, 104
SYLVESTER, ELSIE M. (*See* Schweinburg, Sylvester, and Rutenburg), 204

T

THAYER, THEODORE R. (*See* Warren and Thayer), 867
THIEME, E. T. The empiric use of gastric resection in the treatment of upper gastrointestinal hemorrhage, 56
THOMAS, JOHN V., AND HAY, LYLE J. Adenocarcinoma of the esophagus, 635
THOMPSON, CLARENCE T., AND BROWN, DONALD R. Diagnostic paracentesis in the acute abdomen, 916
TRAPHAGEN, D. W. (*See* Burch, Traphagen, Folkman, Rosenbaum, and Mueller), 684
TRIFILIO, ARISTIDES. (*See* Hudson, Finkle, Trifilio, and Wolan), 897
TRIMPI, HOWARD D. (*See* Bacon, Lowell, and Trimpi), 77
—. (*See* McElwain, Bacon, and Trimpi), 513
TUCKER, JAMES W., AND FEY, WILLIAM P. The management of perforating injuries of the colon and rectum in civilian practice, 213
TURELL, ROBERT. Long-acting drugs for avoidance of posthemorrhoidectomy pain: a negative report, 243

U

ULIN, ALEX W., AND CANCELMO, JOHN B. Stress syndrome and perforated peptic ulcer, 640
UPDEGRAFF, HARRY. (*See* Fisher, Russ, and Updegraff), 879
URE, BARBARA. (*See* Moore and Ure), 734

W

WALCHEF, LUBEN S. The traction brace, 758
WANGENSTEEN, OWEN H. (*See* Kelly, MacLean, Perry, and Wangensteen), 964
—. (*See* MacLean, Perry, Kelly, Mosser, Mannick, and Wangensteen), 705
WARREN, RICHARD, AND THAYER, THEODORE R. Transplantation of the saphenous vein for postphlebitic stasis, 867
WATERS, LEVIN L. (*See* Gentsch, Waters, and Glenn), 30
WAWRO, N. WILLIAM. The case for de novo origin of late recurrence of cancer of the female breast, 470
WEBER, ROBERT A. (*See* Shore, Lippman, and Weber), 633
WEINTRAUB, LEONARD. (*See* May, Hines, Weintraub, Scudder, and Graff), 191
WELCH, KEASLEY. A method for exposure of midline lesions of the brain: craniotomy on the "down side," 430
WERDER, ALVAR A., AND HARDIN, CREIGHTON A. The effect of splenectomy on the survival rate of homologous skin grafts in C.F.W. mice, 405
WHITE, RICHARD JOSEPH. Simultaneous acute obstruction of the colon and terminal ileum from endometriosis, 947
WHITLEY, RALPH D., AND WINSHIP, THEODORE. Splenic hemangioma with subsequent fatal hemangiosarcoma, 787

WIENER, DAVID. (*See* Bressler and Wiener), 815
WIERMAN, WILLIAM H., MCDONALD, JOHN R., AND CLAGETT, O. THERON. Occult carcinoma of the major bronchi, 335
WILSON, FRANK C., JR. (*See* Neely, Wilson, Milnor, Hardy, and Wilson), 22
WILSON, HARWELL. (*See* Neely, Wilson, Milnor, Hardy, and Wilson), 22
WINSHIP, THEODORE. (*See* Whitley and Winship), 787
WOLAN, CASIMIR T. (*See* Hudson, Finkle, Trifilio, and Wolan), 897
WYLIE, EDWIN J. (*See* Miller, Wylie, and Hinman), 885

Z

ZINTEL, HAROLD A., ENTERLINE, HORATIO T., AND RHOADS, JONATHAN E. Benign cystadenoma of pancreas, 612

SUBJECT INDEX*

Book reviews are indicated by (*B. Rev.*); editorials by (*E.*).

A

Abdomen, acute, diagnostic paracentesis in (Thompson and Brown), 916
mechanism of omental migration (Allen), 249
Abdominal diseases, acute, roentgen examinations in, 165 (*B. Rev.*)
emergencies, dangers of conservative surgery in (Crile), 122 (*E.*)
pain; traumatic rupture of normal spleen (Knopp and Harkins), 495
pregnancy with fetal and maternal survival (Harris), 793
procedures; modification of Hunterian Laboratory anesthesia apparatus for experimental surgery (Lippman et al.), 909
surgery, temporary aortic occlusion in (Burch et al.), 684
trauma, nonpenetrating, retroperitoneal rupture of duodenum due to (Stranksy), 928
rupture of pregnant uterus due to (McClure), 487
Acid-peptic action, comparative sensitivity of mucosa of various segments of alimentary tract in dog to (Kiriluk and Merendino), 547
Acidity of gastric contents in postgastrectomy patient, effect of partial exclusion of bile and pancreatic juice on (Farmer and Smithwick), 557
Acidosis, hyperchloremic, following anterior partial and complete pelvic exenteration (Brunschwig and Lüscher), 197
Adenocarcinoma of esophagus (Thomas and Hay), 635
treatment of tumors of parotid salivary gland (Ariel et al.), 135
Adhesions; mechanism of omental migration (Allen), 249
Adrenocortex, shock and (Hayes), 174
Alimentary tract in dog, comparative sensitivity of mucosa of various segments of, to acid-peptic action (Kiriluk and Merendino), 547
American Goiter Association (announcement), 502
Amino acids, urinary loss of, after surgery (Nardi), 378
Ammonium chloride; return of sodium loads in normal subjects following restricted sodium intake (Schlegel), 849
Anastomoses, vascular, total transplant of thyroid gland using (Sterling and Goldsmith), 624
Anastomosis, esophagogastric; approach to midthoracic esophageal carcinoma for its radical surgical treatment (Nakayama), 574
Anatomy, Morris' human, 330 (*B. Rev.*)
Anemia; traumatic rupture of normal spleen (Knopp and Harkins), 496
Anesthesia apparatus, Hunterian Laboratory, for experimental surgery, modification of (Lippman et al.), 909
conduction, 332 (*B. Rev.*)
cyclopropane, clinical use of levo-arterenol during (Surks and Luger), 104
spinal, and its relationship to larger problem, note on (Beecher), 820 (*E.*)
surgical (Koontz), 643 (*E.*)
use of Arfonad in modification of technique of controlled hypotension (Little et al.), 857
Anesthetic; long-acting drugs for avoidance of posthemorrhoidectomy pain: negative report (Turell), 243
Angiosarcoma; splenic hemangioma with subsequent fatal hemangiosarcoma (Whitley and Winship), 787
Announcements, 166, 334, 502, 672
Anorectal disease; association of lymphogranuloma inguinale and cancer (Rainey), 224
operations; long-acting drugs for avoidance of posthemorrhoidectomy pain: negative report (Turell), 243
Antibiotic; preoperative preparation of bowel with neomycin (Davis et al.), 434
Antrum, maxillary, carcinoma of (Mattick and Streuter), 236
Aorta, coarctation of, necrotizing panarteritis following repair of (Lober and Lillehei), 950
thoracic, bronchiogenic cyst associated with anomalous pulmonary artery arising from (Bressler and Wiener), 815
Aortic graft, freeze-dry homologous, influence of acute hypervolemia on (Gentsch et al.), 30
insufficiency, surgical correction of (Hufnagel et al.), 673
ligation of inferior mesentery artery in cancer of rectum, experience with: lymph node metastases (McElwain et al.), 513
occlusion, temporary, in abdominal surgery (Burch et al.), 684
Aortography, renal complications from (Miller et al.), 885

*January, pp. 1-166; February, pp. 167-334; March, pp. 335-502; April, pp. 503-672; May, pp. 673-836; June, pp. 837-1002.

Appendiceal stump, inverted, mucocele of, following appendectomy (Rasch and Strange), 629
Appendicitis in newborn infant (Riddell and Mullins), 270
Arfonad, use of, in modification of technique of controlled hypotension (Little et al.), 857
Arm, swelling of, after radical mastectomy (Fitts et al.), 460
Arrhythmia, cardiac, as predictable surgical risk (Lyons), 292 (*E.*)
Arterial insufficiency, peripheral, with partial occlusion of iliac artery, syndrome of (Gilfillan et al.), 598
Arterialization, total, of dog liver, suitable technique for (Fisher et al.), 879
Arteriosclerosis; significance of local vascular changes in bleeding peptic ulcer (MacKay), 726
Arteriosclerotic circulatory insufficiency of lower extremities, evaluation of "high" lumbar sympathectomy in (Lilly et al.), 1
Artery, anomalous pulmonary, arising from thoracic aorta, bronchiogenic cyst associated with (Bressler and Wiener), 815
  gastric; approach to midthoracic esophageal carcinoma for its radical surgical treatment (Nakayama), 574
  iliac; major vessel damage in lumbar disc operation (Seeley et al.), 421
  inferior mesentery, experience with aortic ligation of, in cancer of rectum: lymph node metastases (McElwain et al.), 513
  renal complications from aortography (Miller et al.), 885
Ascariasis of common bile duct (Shore et al.), 633
Aureomycin therapy, relation of in vitro sensitivity test to clinical response to (Schweinburg et al.), 204
Autonomic nervous system, anatomy of, 163 (*B. Rev.*)

B

Back; mixed tumors in unusual sites (Halpert and Brelsford), 901
Bacteria in bile, relation of, to biliary dynamics, cholangitis, and postcholecystectomy syndrome (Sarkisian and McGowan), 565
Ballistocardiographic methods, clinical comparison of direct Fick, dye, and: cardiac output (Neely et al.), 22
Barium, peroral, effect of, in partial obstruction of small bowel (Donato et al.), 719
Benign cystadenoma of pancreas (Zintel et al.), 612
  epithelial tumors; treatment of tumors of parotid salivary gland (Ariel et al.), 124
  stricture of hepaticoduodenostomy: its treatment (Koucky and Maley), 802
Bile duct, common, ascariasis of (Shore et al.), 633
    midline incision for surgery of gall bladder and (Moore), 440
  and pancreatic juice, effect of partial exclusion of, on acidity of gastric contents in postgastrectomy patient (Farmer and Smithwick), 557
  relation of bacteria in, to biliary dynamics, cholangitis, and postcholecystectomy syndrome (Sarkisian and McGowan), 565
Biliary tract; one-stage pancreatoduodenectomy with resection of superior mesenteric vein (Moore and Ure), 734
Billroth I gastric resection, simplification of (Nakayama), 837
  and II, segmental, and tubular resections; nutrition following subtotal gastrectomy of four types (MacLean et al.), 705
Billroth II resection; cancer of stomach: twenty-year cures (Pack), 920
  type gastrectomy, elucidation of intestinal sensitivity factor and distance factors in incidence of stomal ulcer in (Kiriluk and Merendino), 538
Biologic behavior of carcinoma of lung (Halpert), 962 (*E.*)
Biopsy, transurethral; prostatic cancer (Hudson et al.), 897
Bladder, normal urinary, spontaneous rupture of (Hershman and Allen), 805
Bleeding peptic ulcer, significance of local vascular changes in (MacKay), 724
Blood culture studies in normal dogs and in dogs in hemorrhagic shock (Nelson and Noyes), 782
  effective clinical method for determining coagulation time of (Shea et al.), 698
  flow; suitable technique for total arterialization of dog liver (Fisher et al.), 879
  loss; use of Arfonad in modification of technique of controlled hypotension (Little et al.), 857
  oxygenators: theory and studies in design (Gimbel and Engelberg), 645
Bone, tumors of, roentgenographic atlas, 164 (*B. Rev.*)
Book reviews, 163, 329, 501, 670, 836
Bowel, preoperative preparation of, with neomycin (Davis et al.), 434
  small, effect of peroral barium in partial obstruction of (Donato et al.), 719
  upper small, experimental study of buffering capacity of contents of (Kiriluk and Merendino), 532
Brace, traction (Walchef), 758
Brain, midline lesions of, method for exposure of: craniotomy on "down side" (Welch), 430
Breast, female, case for de novo origin of late recurrence of cancer of (Wawro), 470

Breast—Cont'd
tumors, accuracy of preoperative x-ray diagnoses of (Gershon-Cohen et al.), 766
Brock technique; pulmonary valvulotomy (Humphreys et al.), 9
Bronchi, major, occult carcinoma of (Wierman et al.), 335
Bronchiogenic cyst associated with anomalous pulmonary artery arising from thoracic aorta (Bressler and Wiener), 815
Buffalo Surgical Society (announcement), 166
Buffering capacity of contents of upper small bowel, experimental study of (Kiriluk and Merendino), 532
Burn healing, evaluation of method for study of (Jensen), 390
Burns, skin grafting, and thrombophlebitis, controlled pressure plastic dressing for (Lehmann and Hay), 401
By-pass, prolonged, of heart and lungs by means of pump-oxygenator, consecutive survival of open-chest, hypothermic dogs after (Gollan et al.), 88

C

Calf; circulatory changes in lower limb following lumbar sympathectomy (Messent and Beaconsfield), 382
Cancer, association of lymphogranuloma inguinale and (Rainey), 221
Congress, Sixth International (announcement), 166
of female breast, case for de novo origin of late recurrence of (Wawro), 470
malignant lesions of thyroid (Cohen and Moore), 62
prostatic (Hudson et al.), 897
of rectum, experience with aortic ligation of inferior mesentery artery in: lymph node metastases (McElwain et al.), 513
of stomach: twenty-year cures (Pack), 920
Cannula, stainless steel, for creation of gastrointestinal fistulas (Redo and Barnes), 844
Capillary resistance, trauma and (Kramár et al.), 772
Carbon dioxide elimination; blood oxygenators: theory and studies in design (Gimbel and Engelberg), 647
Carcinoma of esophagus: new concept in therapy (Berman), 822
total esophagoplasty using intrathoracic right colon (Mahoney and Sherman), 937
of lung, biologic behavior of (Halpert), 962 (*E.*)
intracranial metastasis from (Halpert et al.), 346
of maxillary antrum (Mattick and Streuter), 236
Carcinoma—Cont'd
midthoracic esophageal, approach to, for its radical surgical treatment (Nakayama), 574
occult, of major bronchi (Wierman et al.), 335
one-stage pancreatoduodenectomy with resection of superior mesenteric vein (Moore and Ure), 734
primary, of lung (Brea), 167
prostatic cancer (Hudson et al.), 897
treatment of tumors of parotid salivary gland (Ariel et al.), 125
Cardiac arrhythmia as predictable surgical risk (Lyons), 292 (*E.*)
output: clinical comparison of direct Fick, dye, and ballistocardiographic methods (Neely et al.), 22
surgery; technique for production of hypothermia (Ripstein et al.), 98
Cartilages, prominent costal (Tietze's syndrome) (Beck and Berkheiser), 762
C.F.W. mice, effect of splenectomy on survival rate of homologous skin grafts in (Werder and Hardin), 405
Cheatle-Henry, suprapubic extraperitoneal, approach: femoral hernioplasty (Mikkelsen and Berne), 743
Chest, Third International Congress on Diseases of (announcement), 672
Childhood, surgery of infancy and, its principles and techniques, 502 (*B. Rev.*)
Chlorpromazine; technique for production of hypothermia (Ripstein et al.), 98
Cholangitis, biliary dynamics, and postcholecystectomy syndrome, relation of bacteria in bile to (Sarkisian and McGowan), 565
Choledochojejunostomy en Roux Y (Bowers), 159
Circulation; blood oxygenators: theory and studies in design (Gimbel and Engelberg), 645
shock and adrenocortex (Hayes), 174
Circulatory changes in lower limb following lumbar sympathectomy (Messent and Beaconsfield), 382
insufficiency, arteriosclerotic, of lower extremities, evaluation of "high" lumbar sympathectomy in (Lilly et al.), 1
Clinical orthopaedics, 330 (*B. Rev.*)
response to Aureomycin therapy, relation of in vitro sensitivity test to (Schweinburg et al.), 204
Clotting, intravascular; effective clinical method for determining coagulation time of blood (Shea et al.), 698
Coagulation time of blood, effective clinical method for determining (Shea et al.), 698
Coarctation of aorta, necrotizing panarteritis following repair of (Lober and Lillehei), 950
Colles, Abraham, and Colles' fracture: eponymic fractures (Peltier), 322

Colon, intrathoracic right, total esophagoplasty using (Mahoney and Sherman), 937
and rectum, management of perforating injuries of, in civilian practice (Tucker and Fey), 213
villous papillomas of (Bacon et al.), 77
and terminal ileum, simultaneous acute obstruction of, from endometriosis (White), 947
Colostomy; association of lymphogranuloma inguinale and cancer (Rainey), 221
hyperchloremic acidosis following anterior partial and complete pelvic exenteration (Brunschwig and Lüscher), 197
Common and superficial femoral vein ligations, comparison of late sequelae of (Robinson and Moyer), 690
Conduction anesthesia, 332 (*B. Rev.*)
Congenital duodenal diaphragm (Bill and Pope), 482
duplication of gall bladder (Moore and Hurley), 283
eventration of diaphragm in infancy (Arnheim), 809
Congress of Pan-Pacific Surgical Association, Sixth (announcement), 672
Conservative surgery, dangers of, in abdominal emergencies (Crile), 122 (*E.*)
Costal cartilages, prominent (Tietze's syndrome) (Beck and Berkheiser), 762
Cough, rib fractures from muscular effort with particular reference to (Derbes and Haran), 294
Cranial wound; transorbitocranial foreign body (Carver and Patterson), 475
Craniotomy on "down side": method for exposure of midline lesions of brain (Welch), 430
Crepitation; rib fractures from muscular effort with particular reference to cough (Derbes and Haran), 312
Crush; trauma and capillary resistance (Kramár et al.), 772
Cutaneous cyst, recurring myxomatous (Isaacson and McCarty), 621
Cyclopropane anesthesia, clinical use of levoarterenol during (Surks and Luger), 104
Cylindroma; treatment of tumors of parotid salivary gland (Ariel et al.), 135
Cyst, bronchiogenic, associated with anomalous pulmonary artery arising from thoracic aorta (Bressler and Wiener), 815
recurring myxomatous cutaneous (Isaacson and McCarty), 621
thoracic neurenteric (Holcomb and Matson), 115
Cystadenoma, benign, of pancreas (Zintel et al.), 612
Cystic duct; congenital duplication of gall bladder (Moore and Hurley), 283
Cysts; laryngocele: unusual tumor of neck (Hill and Kipen), 273

D

Desmoid tumors; principles in management of soft tissue sarcomas (Lieberman and Ackerman), 350
Dextran; comparative studies, in normotensive man, of effectiveness, retention, and elimination of various plasma expanders (Bader et al.), 366
Diagnostic paracentesis in acute abdomen (Thompson and Brown), 916
Diaphragm, congenital duodenal (Bill and Pope), 482
eventration of, in infancy (Arnheim), 809
Diodrast; renal complications from aortography (Miller et al.), 885
Disc lesions, intervertebral; traction brace (Walchef), 758
operation, lumbar, major vessel damage in (Seeley et al.), 421
Dog, comparative sensitivity of mucosa of various segments of alimentary tract in, to acid-peptic action (Kiriluk and Merendino), 547
liver, suitable technique for total arterialization of (Fisher et al.), 879
Dogs, blood culture studies in normal, and in dogs in hemorrhagic shock (Nelson and Noyes), 782
effect of peroral barium in partial obstruction of small bowel (Donato et al.), 719
elucidation of intestinal sensitivity factor and distance factors in incidence of stomal ulcer in Billroth II type gastrectomy (Kiriluk and Merendino), 539
experimental study of buffering capacity of contents of upper small bowel (Kiriluk and Merendino), 532
influence of acute hypervolemia on freeze-dry homologous aortic graft (Gentsch et al.), 31
mixing of material injected into pulsatile and nonpulsatile streams: application to regional heparinization (Cate and Culley), 413
open-chest, hypothermic, consecutive survival of, after prolonged by-pass of heart and lungs by means of pump-oxygenator (Gollan et al.), 88
stainless steel cannula for creation of gastrointestinal fistulas (Redo and Barnes), 844
technique for production of hypothermia (Ripstein et al.), 98
temporary aortic occlusion in abdominal surgery (Burch et al.), 684
use of intravenous trypsin in experimental pulmonary embolism (Roach and Laufman), 45
Dressing, controlled pressure plastic, for skin grafting, burns, and thrombophlebitis (Lehmann and Hay), 401
Drugs, long-acting, for avoidance of posthemorrhoidectomy pain: negative report (Turell), 243

Duct, common bile, ascariasis of (Shore et al.), 633
midline incision for surgery of gall bladder and (Moore), 440
cystic; congenital duplication of gall bladder (More and Hurley), 283
Duodenal diaphragm, congenital (Bill and Pope), 482
ulcer; simplification of Billroth I gastric resection (Nakayama), 837
Duodenum, retroperitoneal rupture of, due to nonpenetrating abdominal trauma (Stransky), 928
Duplication of gall bladder, congenital (Moore and Hurley), 283
Dye, direct Fick, and ballistocardiographic methods, clinical comparison of: cardiac output (Neely et al.), 22

E

Edema; evaluation of method for study of burn healing (Jensen), 391
Editorials, 122, 290, 292, 491, 643, 820, 962
Efocaine, complications following use of (Moore), 109
Electrolyte disturbances in shock and severe stress, new approach to treatment of (Schlegel), 449
Embolism, experimental pulmonary, use of intravenous trypsin in (Roach and Laufman), 45
Embolus, pulmonary, venous thrombosis of upper extremity complicated by (Aufses), 957
Endometriosis, simultaneous acute obstruction of colon and terminal ileum from (White), 947
Epithelial malignancy; carcinoma of maxillary antrum (Mattick and Streuter), 236
tumor, benign; villous papillomas of colon and rectum (Bacon et al.), 77
tumors; treatment of tumors of parotid salivary gland (Ariel et al.), 124
Eponymic fractures: Abraham Colles and Colles' fracture (Peltier), 322
Ergotamine, mechanism of action of, in hyperthyroidism (Hinton), 491 (*E.*)
Esophageal carcinoma, midthoracic, approach to, for its radical surgical treatment (Nakayama), 574
leiomyoma (Brizzolara and Geraci), 465
Esophagoplasty, total, using intrathoracic right colon (Mahoney and Sherman), 937
Esophagoscopy; study of patients following total and near-total gastrectomy (Kelly et al.), 965
Esophagus, adenocarcinoma of (Thomas and Hay), 635
carcinoma of: new concept in therapy (Berman), 822
Eventration, congenital, of diaphragm in infancy (Arnheim), 809
Exenteration, pelvic, anterior partial and complete, hyperchloremic acidosis following (Brunschwig and Lüscher), 197
Exophthalmos, experimental, hyaluronidase and (Aterman), 443
Expanders, various plasma, comparative studies, in normotensive man, of effectiveness, retention, and elimination of (Bader et al.), 366
Experimental surgery, modification of Hunterian Laboratory anesthesia apparatus for (Lippman et al.), 909
Extremities, lower, arteriosclerotic circulatory insufficiency of, evaluation of "high" lumbar sympathectomy in (Lilly et al.), 1
Extremity, upper, venous thrombosis of, complicated by pulmonary embolus (Aufses), 957
Eyelid, lower; mixed tumors in unusual sites (Halpert and Brelsford), 901

F

Facial nerve; treatment of tumors of parotid salivary gland (Ariel et al.), 139
Fecal fat; study of patients following total and near-total gastrectomy (Kelly et al.), 965
Femoral hernioplasty: suprapubic extraperitoneal (Cheatle-Henry) approach (Mikkelsen and Berne), 743
vein ligations, comparison of late sequelae of common and superficial (Robinson and Moyer), 690
Fetus and newborn, pathology of, 329 (*B. Rev.*)
Fibrosarcoma; principles in management of soft tissue sarcomas (Lieberman and Ackerman), 350
Fick, dye, and ballistocardiographic methods, clinical comparison of direct: cardiac output (Neely et al.), 22
Fistulas, gastrointestinal, stainless steel cannula for creation of (Redo and Barnes), 844
Foam oxygenator; blood oxygenators: theory and studies in design (Gimbel and Engelberg), 646
Foot; circulatory changes in lower limb following lumbar sympathectomy (Messent and Beaconsfield), 382
Foramen of Winslow, hernia through (Dorian and Stein), 795
Fracture; treatment of infection after medullary nailing (Key and Reynolds), 749
Fractures, eponymic: Abraham Colles and Colles' fracture (Peltier), 322
rib, from muscular effort with particular reference to cough (Derbes and Haran), 294
Freeze-dry homologous aortic graft, influence of acute hypervolemia on (Gentsch et al.), 30

G

Gall bladder, congenital duplication of (Moore and Hurley), 283
midline incision for surgery of, and common bile duct (Moore), 440
traction (Migliaccio), 786
Gastrectomy, Billroth II type, elucidation of intestinal sensitivity factor and distance factors in incidence of stomal ulcer in (Kiriluk and Merendino), 538
experimental study of buffering capacity of contents of upper small bowel (Kiriluk and Merendino), 532
subtotal, nutrition following, of four types (Billroth I and II, segmental, and tubular resections) (MacLean et al.), 705
total and near-total, study of patients following (Kelly et al.), 964
Gastric contents, effect of partial exclusion of bile and pancreatic juice on acidity of, in postgastrectomy patient (Farmer and Smithwick), 557
resection, Billroth I, simplification of (Nakayama), 837
in treatment of upper gastrointestinal hemorrhage, empiric use of (Thieme), 56
vessels; approach to midthoracic esophageal carcinoma for its radical surgical treatment (Nakayama), 574
Gastrointestinal fistulas, stainless steel cannula for creation of (Redo and Barnes), 844
Gesunde und kranke wirbelsäule in röntgenbild und klinik, 164 (*B. Rev.*)
Gingivitis in military personnel with special reference to ulceromembranous gingivitis, 501 (*B. Rev.*)
Gland, parotid salivary, treatment of tumors of (Ariel et al.), 124
thyroid, total transplant of, using vascular anastomoses (Sterling and Goldsmith), 624
Glandular metaplasia; adenocarcinoma of esophagus (Thomas and Hay), 635
Graft, freeze-dry homologous aortic, influence of acute hypervolemia on (Gentsch et al.), 30
Grafting, skin, burns, and thrombophlebitis, controlled pressure plastic dressing for (Lehmann and Hay), 401
Grafts, homologous skin, in C.F.W. mice, effect of splenectomy on survival rate of (Werder and Hardin), 405
Grenzen des normalen und anfänge des pathologische im röntgenbilde des skelettes, 671 (*B. Rev.*)
Guinea pigs; hyaluronidase and experimental exophthalmos (Aterman), 443

H

Hand injuries, surgery of repair as applied to, 501 (*B. Rev.*)
Heart; blood oxygenators: theory and studies in design (Gimbel and Engelberg), 645
and lungs, prolonged by-pass of, by means of pump-oxygenator, consecutive survival of open-chest, hypothermic dogs after (Gollan et al.), 88
Hemangioma, splenic, with subsequent fatal hemangiosarcoma (Whitley and Winship), 787
Hemoglobin saturation; blood oxygenators: theory and studies in design (Gimbel and Engelberg), 646
Hemorrhage, upper gastrointestinal, empiric use of gastric resection in treatment of (Thieme), 56
Hemorrhagic shock, blood culture studies in normal dogs and in dogs in (Nelson and Noyes), 782
Heparinization, application to regional: mixing of material injected into pulsatile and nonpulsatile streams (Cate and Culley), 411
Hepaticoduodenostomy, benign stricture of: its treatment (Koucky and Maley), 802
Hernia through foramen of Winslow (Dorian and Stein), 795
Hernioplasty, femoral: suprapubic extraperitoneal (Cheatle-Henry) approach (Mikkelsen and Berne), 743
Homologous aortic graft, freeze-dry, influence of acute hypervolemia on (Gentsch et al.), 30
skin grafts in C.F.W. mice, effect of splenectomy on survival rate of (Werder and Hardin), 405
Human anatomy, Morris', 330 (*B. Rev.*)
measurements involved in trachebronchial resection and reconstruction procedures (Merendino and Kiriluk), 590
Hunterian Laboratory anesthesia apparatus for experimental surgery, modification of (Lippman et al.), 909
Hyaluronidase and experimental exophthalmos (Aterman), 443
Hyperchloremic acidosis following anterior partial and complete pelvic exenteration (Brunschwig and Lüscher), 197
Hypertension, portal, transparietal splenoportal roentgenography and research on (Dogliotti and Abeatici), 503
Hyperthyroidism; malignant lesions of thyroid (Cohen and Moore), 65
mechanism of action of ergotamine in (Hinton), 491 (*E.*)
Hypervolemia, acute, influence of, on freeze-dry homologous aortic graft (Gentsch et al.), 30
Hypotension, controlled, use of Arfonad in modification of technique of (Little et al.), 857
Hypothermia, technique for production of (Ripstein et al.), 98

Hypothermic dogs, open-chest, consecutive survival of, after prolonged by-pass of heart and lungs by means of pump-oxygenator (Gollan et al.), 88

I

Ileum, terminal, simultaneous acute obstruction of colon and, from endometriosis (White), 947
Iliac artery; major vessel damage in lumbar disc operation (Seeley et al.), 421
  syndrome of peripheral arterial insufficiency with partial occlusion of (Gilfillan et al.), 598
In vitro sensitivity test, relation of, to clinical response to Aureomycin therapy (Schweinburg et al.), 204
Incision, midline, for surgery of gall bladder and common bile duct (Moore), 440
Infancy and childhood, surgery of, its principles and techniques, 502 (*B. Rev.*)
  congenital eventration of diaphragm in (Arnheim), 809
Infant, newborn, appendicitis in (Riddell and Mullins), 270
  perforation of stomach in (Northway et al.), 925
Infection after medullary nailing, treatment of (Key and Reynolds), 749
Inflammation; mechanism of omental migration (Allen), 249
Injuries, perforating, of colon and rectum, management of, in civilian practice (Tucker and Fey), 213
International Cancer Congress, Sixth (announcement), 166
  Congress on Diseases of Chest, Third (announcement), 672
Intervertebral disc lesions; traction brace (Walchef), 758
Intestinal sensitivity factor and distance factors in incidence of stomal ulcer in Billroth II type gastrectomy, elucidation of (Kiriluk and Merendino), 538
Intracardiac surgery; blood oxygenators: theory and studies in design (Gimbel and Engelberg), 645
Intracranial metastasis from carcinoma of lung (Halpert et al.), 346
Intrathoracic right colon, total esophagoplasty using (Mahoney and Sherman), 937
Intravascular clotting; effective clinical method for determining coagulation time of blood (Shea et al.), 698
Intravenous trypsin, use of, in experimental pulmonary embolism (Roach and Laufman), 45
Iron absorption; study of patients following total and near-total gastrectomy (Kelly et al.), 965
Irradiation; treatment of tumors of parotid salivary gland (Ariel et al.), 154
Isotope therapy; malignant lesions of thyroid (Cohen and Moore), 68

J

Joint, temporomandibular, 165 (*B. Rev.*)

K

Kidney; renal complications from aortography (Miller et al.), 885
Klapp'sche kriechverfahren, 501 (*B. Rev.*)

L

Laryngocele: unusual tumor of neck (Hill and Kipen), 273
Leiomyoma, esophageal (Brizzolara and Geraci), 465
Lesions, malignant, of thyroid (Cohen and Moore), 62
  midline, of brain, method for exposure of: craniotomy on "down side" (Welch), 430
Levo-arterenol, clinical use of, during cyclopropane anesthesia (Surks and Luger), 104
Ligation, aortic, of inferior mesentery artery in cancer of rectum, experience with: lymph node metastases (McElwain et al.), 513
Ligations, common and superficial femoral vein, comparison of late sequelae of (Robinson and Moyer), 690
Limb, lower, circulatory changes in, following lumbar sympathectomy (Messent and Beaconsfield), 382
Lip, lower; mixed tumors in unusual sites (Halpert and Brelsford), 901
Liposarcoma; principles in management of soft tissue sarcomas (Lieberman and Ackerman), 350
Liver, dog, suitable technique for total arterialization of (Fisher et al.), 879
Lobectomy; primary carcinoma of lung (Brea), 169
Lumbar disc operation, major vessel damage in (Seeley et al.), 421
  sympathectomy, circulatory changes in lower limb following (Messent and Beaconsfield), 382
    "high," in arteriosclerotic circulatory insufficiency of lower extremities, evaluation of (Lilly et al.), 1
Lung, biologic behavior of carcinoma of (Halpert), 962 (*E.*)
  carcinoma of, intracranial metastasis from (Halpert et al.), 346
  primary carcinoma of (Brea), 167
Lungs, prolonged by-pass of heart and, by means of pump-oxygenator, consecutive survival of open-chest, hypothermic dogs after (Gollan et al.), 88
Lymph node metastases: experience with aortic ligation of inferior mesentery artery in cancer of rectum (McElwain et al.), 513
  nodes; treatment of tumors of parotid salivary gland (Ariel et al.), 140

Lymphogranuloma inguinale and cancer, association of (Rainey), 221

M

Malignancy; carcinoma of esophagus: new concept in therapy (Berman), 822
  occult carcinoma of major bronchi (Wierman et al.), 335
Malignant lesions of thyroid (Cohen and Moore), 62
Mastectomy, radical, swelling of arm after (Fitts et al.), 460
Maxillary antrum, carcinoma of (Mattick and Streuter), 236
Measurements, human, involved in tracheobronchial resection and reconstruction procedures (Merendino and Kiriluk), 590
Medullary nailing, treatment of infection after (Key and Reynolds), 749
Mesenchymoma (Pack and Lisa), 277
Mesenteric vein, superior, one-stage pancreatoduodenectomy with resection of (Moore and Ure), 734
Mesentery artery, inferior, experience with aortic ligation of, in cancer of rectum: lymph node metastases (McElwain et al.), 513
Metabolism; nutrition following subtotal gastrectomy of four types (Billroth I and II, segmental, and tubular resections) (MacLean et al.), 705
Metaplasia, glandular; adenocarcinoma of esophagus (Thomas and Hay), 635
Metastases, lymph node: experience with aortic ligation of inferior mesentery artery in cancer of rectum (McElwain et al.), 513
  malignant lesions of thyroid (Cohen and Moore), 63
  treatment of tumors of parotid salivary gland (Ariel et al.), 130
Metastasis, intracranial, from carcinoma of lung (Halpert et al.), 346
Mice, C.F.W., effect of splenectomy on survival rate of homologous skin grafts in (Werder and Hardin), 405
Midline incision for surgery of gall bladder and common bile duct (Moore), 440
  lesions of brain, method for exposure of: craniotomy on "down side" (Welch), 430
Midthoracic esophageal carcinoma, approach to, for its radical surgical treatment (Nakayama), 574
  esophagus; esophageal leiomyoma (Brizzolara and Geraci), 465
Morris' human anatomy, 330 (*B. Rev.*)
Mucocele of inverted appendiceal stump following appendectomy (Rasch and Strange), 629
Mucoepidermoid carcinoma; treatment of tumors of parotid salivary gland (Ariel et al.), 136
Mucosa, esophageal; adenocarcinoma of esophagus (Thomas and Hay), 635
  of various segments of alimentary tract in dog, comparative sensitivity of, to acid-peptic action (Kiriluk and Merendino), 547
Muscular effort, rib fractures from, with particular reference to cough (Derbes and Haran), 294
Myelitis, transverse; complications following use of Efocaine (Moore), 110
Myocardium; surgical correction of aortic insufficiency (Hufnagel et al.), 673
Myxomatous cutaneous cyst, recurring (Isaacson and McCarty), 621

N

Nailing, medullary, treatment of infection after (Key and Reynolds), 749
Nash's surgical physiology, 836 (*B. Rev.*)
Neck, unusual tumor of: laryngocele (Hill and Kipen), 273
Necrotizing panarteritis following repair of coarctation of aorta (Lober and Lillehei), 950
Neomycin, preoperative preparation of bowel with (Davis et al.), 434
Neoplasia; association of lymphogranuloma inguinale and cancer (Rainey), 221
Nerve, facial; treatment of tumors of parotid salivary gland (Ariel et al.), 139
Neurenteric cyst, thoracic (Holcomb and Matson), 115
Neuritis; complications following use of Efocaine (Moore), 110
Neurological surgery, principles of, 329 (*B. Rev.*)
Neurology and psychiatry, physiological foundations of, 670 (*B. Rev.*)
Newborn infant, appendicitis in (Riddell and Mullins), 270
  perforation of stomach in (Northway et al.), 925
  pathology of fetus and, 329 (*B. Rev.*)
Nitrogen excretion; study of patients following total and near-total gastrectomy (Kelly et al.), 965
Node, lymph, metastases: experience with aortic ligation of inferior mesentery artery in cancer of rectum (McElwain et al.), 513
Nodes, lymph; treatment of tumors of parotid salivary gland (Ariel et al.), 140
Nonpulsatile streams, mixing of material injected into pulsatile and: application to regional heparinization (Cate and Culley), 411
Normotensive man, comparative studies in, of effectiveness, retention, and elimination of various plasma expanders (Bader et al.), 366
Nurses, surgery for, 670 (*B. Rev.*)

Nutrition following subtotal gastrectomy of four types (Billroth I and II, segmental, and tubular resections) (MacLean et al.), 705

O

Obstruction, partial, of small bowel, effect of peroral barium in (Donato et al.), 719
 simultaneous acute, of colon and terminal ileum from endometriosis (White), 947
Occlusion, partial, of iliac artery, syndrome of peripheral arterial insufficiency (Gilfillan et al.), 598
 temporary aortic, in abdominal surgery (Burch et al.), 684
Omental migration, mechanism of (Allen), 249
Open-chest, hypothermic dogs, consecutive survival of, after prolonged by-pass of heart and lungs by means of pump-oxygenator (Gollan et al.), 88
Orbitocranial wound; transorbitocranial foreign body (Carver and Patterson), 475
Orthopädische konstruktionen, 501 (*B. Rev.*)
Orthopaedics, clinical, 330 (*B. Rev.*)
Oxygen tension; suitable technique for total arterialization of dog liver (Fisher et al.), 879
Oxygenators, blood: theory and studies in design (Gimbel and Engelberg), 645
Oxypolygelatin; comparative studies, in normotensive man, of effectiveness, retention, and elimination of various plasma expanders (Bader et al.), 366

P

Pain, posthemorrhoidectomy, long-acting drugs for avoidance of: negative report (Turell), 243
Palate, hard; mixed tumors in unusual sites (Halpert and Brelsford), 901
Panarteritis, necrotizing, following repair of coarctation of aorta (Lober and Lillehei,) 950
Pancreas, benign cystadenoma of (Zintel et al.), 612
Pancreatic function; nutrition following subtotal gastrectomy of four types (Billroth I and II, segmental, and tubular resections) (MacLean et al.), 705
 study of patients following total and near-total gastrectomy (Kelly et al.), 965
 juice, effect of partial exclusion of bile and, on acidity of gastric contents in postgastrectomy patient (Farmer and Smithwick), 557
Pancreatitis; choledochojejunostomy en Roux Y (Bowers), 159
Pancreatoduodenectomy, one-stage, with resection of superior mesenteric vein (Moore and Ure), 734
Pan-Pacific Surgical Association, Sixth Congress of (announcement), 672
Papillary mass; benign cystadenoma of pancreas (Zintel et al.), 616
Papillomas, villous, of colon and rectum (Bacon et al.), 77
Paracentesis, diagnostic, in acute abdomen (Thompson and Brown), 916
Parotid salivary gland, treatment of tumors of (Ariel et al.), 124
Parturition; rib fractures from muscular effort with particular reference to cough (Derbes and Haran), 297
Pathologie vasculaire, medicale et chirurgicale, 333 (*B. Rev.*)
Pathologische physiologie der frischen geschlossenen hirnverletzungen, insbesondere hirnerschütterung: klinische, anatomische und experimentelle befünde, 163 (*B. Rev.*)
Pathology of fetus and newborn, 329 (*B. Rev.*)
Pelvic exenteration, anterior partial and complete, hyperchloremic acidosis following (Brunschwig and Lüscher), 197
Peptic, acid-, action, comparative sensitivity of mucosa of various segments of alimentary tract in dog to (Kiriluk and Merendino), 547
 ulcer, bleeding, significance of local vascular changes in (MacKay), 724
  perforated, stress syndrome and (Ulin and Cancelmo), 640
Perforating injuries of colon and rectum, management of, in civilian practice (Tucker and Fey), 213
Perforation of stomach in newborn infant (Northway et al.), 925
Peripheral arterial insufficiency with partial occlusion of iliac artery, syndrome of (Gilfillan et al.), 598
Peristalsis; mechanism of omental migration (Allen), 256
Peritoneum; mechanism of omental migration (Allen), 249
Peritonitis; diagnostic paracentesis in acute abdomen (Thompson and Brown), 916
pH determination; experimental study of buffering capacity of contents of upper small bowel (Kiriluk and Merendino), 533
Physiology, Nash's surgical, 836 (*B. Rev.*)
Plasma expanders, various, comparative studies, in normotensive man, of effectiveness, retention, and elimination of (Bader et al.), 366
 extender; some physical-chemical properties of polyvinylpyrrolidone (May et al.), 191
Plastic surgery award (announcement), 334
Pneumonectomy; primary carcinoma of lung (Brea), 168

Polyethylene tube; carcinoma of esophagus: new concept in therapy (Berman), 822
Polyvinylpyrrolidone; comparative studies, in normotensive man, of effectiveness, retention, and elimination of various plasma expanders (Bader et al.), 366
some physical-chemical properties of (May et al.), 191
Portal hypertension, transparietal splenoportal roentgenography and research on (Dogliotti and Abeatici), 503
Posthemorrhoidectomy pain, long-acting drugs for avoidance of: negative report (Turell), 243
Postoperative pain; complications following use of Efocaine (Moore), 109
Postphlebitic stasis, transplantation of saphenous vein for (Warren and Thayer), 867
Praktikum der chirurgie. Leitfaden für studenten und ärtze, 836 (*B. Rev.*)
Pregnancy, abdominal with fetal and maternal survival (Harris), 793
Pregnant uterus, rupture of, due to nonpenetrating abdominal trauma (McClure), 487
Prematurity; appendicitis in newborn infant (Riddell and Mullins), 270
Preoperative preparation of bowel with neomycin (Davis et al.), 434
Prostatectomy: method and its management, 333 (*B. Rev.*)
Prostatic cancer (Hudson et al.), 897
Prosthesis, polyethylene; carcinoma of esophagus: new concept in therapy (Berman), 822
surgical correction of aortic insufficiency (Hufnagel et al.), 674
Psychiatry, physiological foundations of neurology and, 670 (*B. Rev.*)
Pulmonary artery, anomalous, arising from thoracic aorta, bronchiogenic cyst associated with (Bressler and Wiener), 815
embolism, experimental, use of intravenous trypsin in (Roach and Laufman), 45
embolus, venous thrombosis of upper extremity complicated by (Aufses), 957
valvulotomy (Humphreys et al.), 9
Pulsatile and nonpulsatile streams, mixing of material injected into: application to regional heparinization (Cate and Culley), 411
Pump-oxygenator, prolonged by-pass of heart and lungs by means of, consecutive survival of open-chest, hypothermic dogs after (Gollan et al.), 88

R

Rabbits; evaluation of method for study of burn healing (Jensen), 390
Radiation; carcinoma of maxillary antrum (Mattick and Streuter), 238
Radical mastectomy, swelling of arm after (Fitts et al.), 460
surgical excision; mesenchymoma (Pack and Lisa), 278
treatment, approach to midthoracic esophageal carcinoma for its (Nakayama), 574
Rats; trauma and capillary resistance (Kramár et al.), 773
Reconstruction procedures, tracheobronchial resection and, human measurements involved in (Merendino and Kiriluk), 590
surgery and traumatology, 164 (*B. Rev.*)
Rectum; association of lymphogranuloma inguinale and cancer (Rainey), 221
cancer of, experience with aortic ligation of inferior mesentery artery in: lymph node metastases (McElwain et al.), 513
management of perforating injuries of colon and, in civilian practice (Tucker and Fey), 213
villous papillomas of colon and (Bacon et al.), 77
Recurrence, late, of cancer of female breast, case for de novo origin of (Wawro), 470
Renal complications from aortography (Miller et al.), 885
Repair of coarctation of aorta, necrotizing panarteritis following (Lober and Lillehei), 950
surgery of, as applied to hand injuries, 501 (*B. Rev.*)
Research and Development Board (Berry), 290 (*E.*)
Resection, Billroth I gastric, simplification of (Nakayama), 837
cancer of stomach: twenty-year cures (Pack), 920
gastric, in treatment of upper gastrointestinal hemorrhage, empiric use of (Thieme), 56
and reconstruction procedures, tracheobronchial, human measurements involved in (Merendino and Kiriluk), 590
of superior mesenteric vein, one-stage pancreatoduodenectomy with (Moore and Ure), 734
total esophagoplasty using intrathoracic right colon (Mahoney and Sherman), 937
Resections, Billroth I and II, segmental, and tubular; nutrition following subtotal gastrectomy of four types (MacLean et al.), 705
Respiratory infections; thoracic neurenteric cyst (Holcomb and Matson), 115
Retention, sodium; return of sodium loads in normal subjects following restricted sodium intake (Schlegel), 848

Retroperitoneal rupture of duodenum due to nonpenetrating abdominal trauma (Stransky), 928
Rhabdomyosarcoma; principles in management of soft tissue sarcomas (Lieberman and Ackerman), 350
Rib fractures from muscular effort with particular reference to cough (Derbes and Haran), 294
Roentgen diagnosis, preoperative; hernia through foramen of Winslow (Dorian and Stein), 795
  examinations in acute abdominal diseases, 165 (*B. Rev.*)
Roentgenography, transparietal splenoportal, and research on portal hypertension (Dogliotti and Abeatici), 503
Röntgenuroscopie, 165 (*B. Rev.*)
Roux Y, choledochojejunostomy en (Bowers), 159
Rupture of pregnant uterus due to nonpenetrating abdominal trauma (McClure), 487
  retroperitoneal, of duodenum due to nonpenetrating abdominal trauma (Stransky), 928
  spontaneous, of normal urinary bladder (Hershman and Allen), 805
  traumatic, of normal spleen (Knopp and Harkins), 493

S

Salivary gland, parotid, treatment of tumors of (Ariel et al.), 124
Saphenous vein; management of recurrent varicose veins (Luke), 41
  transplantation of, for postphlebitic stasis (Warren and Thayer), 867
Sarcomas, soft tissue, principles in management of (Lieberman and Ackerman), 350
Scalp; mixed tumors in unusual sites (Halpert and Brelsford), 901
Segmental, Billroth I and II, and tubular resections; nutrition following subtotal gastrectomy of four types (MacLean et al.), 705
Septal defect; pulmonary valvulotomy (Humphreys et al.), 13
Shock and adrenocortex (Hayes), 174
  clinical use of levo-arterenol during cyclopropane anesthesia (Surks and Luger), 104
  hemorrhagic, blood culture studies in normal dogs and in dogs in (Nelson and Noyes), 782
  and severe stress, new approach to treatment of electrolyte disturbances in (Schlegel), 449
Shoulder lesions, 164 (*B. Rev.*)
Sialography; treatment of tumors of parotid salivary gland (Ariel et al.), 129
Skin grafting, burns, and thrombophlebitis, controlled pressure plastic dressing for (Lehmann and Hay), 401
  grafts, homologous, in C.F.W. mice, effect of splenectomy on survival rate of (Werder and Hardin), 405
Sneezing; rib fractures from muscular effort with particular reference to cough (Derbes and Haran), 296
Society for Vascular Surgery issue, 1-55
Sodium loads, return of, in normal subjects following restricted sodium intake (Schlegel), 848
  retention; new approach to treatment of electrolyte disturbances in shock and severe stress (Schlegel), 449
Somatic tissues; mesenchymoma (Pack and Lisa), 277
Spinal anesthesia and its relationship to larger problem, note on (Beecher), 820 (*E.*)
Spinning disk oxygenator; blood oxygenators: theory and studies in design (Gimbel and Engelberg), 645
Spleen, normal, traumatic rupture of (Knopp and Harkins), 493
Splenectomy, effect of, on survival rate of homologous skin grafts in C.F.W. mice (Werder and Hardin), 405
Splenic hemangioma with subsequent fatal hemangiosarcoma (Whitley and Winship), 787
Splenoportal roentgenography, transparietal, and research on portal hypertension (Dogliotti and Abeatici), 503
Squamous carcinoma; treatment of tumors of parotid salivary gland (Ariel et al.), 136
  cell; occult carcinoma of major bronchi (Wierman et al.), 335
Starvation; return of sodium loads in normal subjects following restricted sodium intake (Schlegel), 849
Stasis, postphlebitic, transplantation of saphenous vein for (Warren and Thayer), 867
Stedman packing oxygenator; blood oxygenators: theory and studies in design (Gimbel and Engelberg), 645
Stenosis; pulmonary valvulotomy (Humphreys et al.), 9
Stomach, cancer of: twenty-year cures (Pack), 920
  perforation of, in newborn infant (Northway et al.), 925
  study of patients following total and near-total gastrectomy (Kelly et al.), 964
Stomal ulcer in Billroth II type gastrectomy, elucidation of intestinal sensitivity factor and distance factors in incidence of (Kiriluk and Merendino), 538
Streams, pulsatile and nonpulsatile, mixing of material injected into: application to regional heparinization (Cate and Culley), 411
Stress, severe, new approach to treatment of electrolyte disturbances in shock and (Schlegel), 449
  syndrome and perforated peptic ulcer (Ulin and Cancelmo), 640
Stricture, benign, of hepaticoduodenostomy: its treatment (Koucky and Maley), 802

Stripping of large-bore varicose veins using conventional strippers, technique for facilitating (Rosenberg), 877
Superficial femoral vein ligations, comparison of late sequelae of common and (Robinson and Moyer), 690
Surgical anesthesia (Koontz), 643 (*E.*)
physiology, Nash's, 836 (*B. Rev.*)
Swelling of arm after radical mastectomy (Fitts et al.), 460
Sympathectomy, "high" lumbar, in arteriosclerotic circulatory insufficiency of lower extremities, evaluation of (Lilly et al.), 1
lumbar, circulatory changes in lower limb following (Messent and Beaconsfield), 382
Synovial sarcoma; principles in management of soft tissue sarcomas (Lieberman and Ackerman), 350

T

T-tube drainage; relation of bacteria in bile to biliary dynamics, cholangitis, and postcholecystectomy syndrome (Sarkisian and McGowan), 565
Temperatures, subcutaneous; evaluation of method for study of burn healing (Jensen), 390
Temporomandibular joint, 165 (*B. Rev.*)
Test, in vitro sensitivity, relation of, to clinical response to Aureomycin therapy (Schweinburg et al.), 204
Testis; mixed tumors in unusual sites (Halpert and Brelsford), 901
Tetany; total transplant of thyroid gland using vascular anastomoses (Sterling and Goldsmith), 624
Therapy, Aureomycin, relation of in vitro sensitivity test to clinical response to (Schweinburg et al.), 204
Thoracic aorta, bronchiogenic cyst associated with anomalous pulmonary artery arising from (Bressler and Wiener), 815
neurenteric cyst (Holcomb and Matson), 115
surgery; modification of Hunterian Laboratory anesthesia apparatus for experimental surgery (Lippman et al.), 909
Thoracotomy; primary carcinoma of lung (Brea), 167
Thrombophlebitis, controlled pressure plastic dressing for skin grafting, burns, and (Lehmann and Hay), 401
Thrombosis, venous, of upper extremity complicated by pulmonary embolus (Aufses), 957
Thyroid gland, total transplant of, using vascular anastomoses (Sterling and Goldsmith), 624
malignant lesions of (Cohen and Moore), 62
Tietze's syndrome; prominent costal cartilages (Beck and Berkheiser), 762
Tissue, soft, sarcomas, principles in management of (Lieberman and Ackerman), 350
Tissues, somatic; mesenchymoma (Pack and Lisa), 277
Tracheobronchial resection and reconstruction procedures, human measurements involved in (Merendino and Kiriluk), 590
Traction brace (Walchef), 758
gall bladder (Migliaccio), 786
Translumbar aortography; renal complications from aortography (Miller et al.), 885
Transorbitocranial foreign body (Carver and Patterson), 475
Transparietal splenoportal roentgenography and research on portal hypertension (Dogliotti and Abeatici), 503
Transplant, total, of thyroid gland using vascular anastomoses (Sterling and Goldsmith), 624
Transplantation of saphenous vein for postphlebitic stasis (Warren and Thayer), 867
Transurethral biopsy; prostatic cancer (Hudson et al.), 897
Trauma and capillary resistance (Kramár et al.), 772
nonpenetrating abdominal, retroperitoneal rupture of duodenum due to (Stransky), 928
rupture of pregnant uterus due to (McClure), 487
return of sodium loads in normal subjects following restricted sodium intake (Schlegel), 848
Traumatic rupture of normal spleen (Knopp and Harkins), 493
Traumatology, reconstruction surgery and, 164 (*B. Rev.*)
Trypsin, intravenous, use of, in experimental pulmonary embolism (Roach and Laufman), 45
Tube, polyethylene; carcinoma of esophagus: new concept in therapy (Berman), 822
(d)-Tubocurarine chloride; long-acting drugs for avoidance of posthemorrhoidectomy pain: negative report (Turell), 243
Tubular resections, Billroth I and II, segmental, and; nutrition following subtotal gastrectomy of four types (MacLean et al.), 705
Tumor, benign epithelial; villous papillomas of colon and rectum (Bacon et al.), 77
mesenchymoma (Pack and Lisa), 277
of neck, unusual: laryngocele (Hill and Kipen), 273
Tumors of bone, roentgenographic atlas, 164 (*B. Rev.*)
breast, accuracy of preoperative x-ray diagnosis of (Gershon-Cohen et al.), 766

Tumors—Cont'd
desmoid; principles in management of soft tissue sarcomas (Lieberman and Ackerman), 350
mixed, in unusual sites (Halpert and Brelsford), 901
of parotid salivary gland, treatment of (Ariel et al.), 124

U

Ulcer, bleeding peptic, significance of local vascular changes in (MacKay), 724
duodenal; simplification of Billroth I gastric resection (Nakayama), 837
empiric use of gastric resection in treatment of upper gastrointestinal hemorrhage (Thieme), 57
perforated peptic, stress syndrome and (Ulin and Cancelmo), 640
stomal, in Billroth II type gastrectomy, elucidation of intestinal sensitivity factor and distance factors in incidence of (Kiriluk and Merendino), 538
Ulceromembranous gingivitis, gingivitis in military personnel with special reference to, 501 (*B. Rev.*)
Urinary bladder, normal, spontaneous rupture of (Hershman and Allen), 805
loss of amino acids after surgery (Nardi), 378
Urine; hyperchloremic acidosis following anterior partial and complete pelvic exenteration (Brunschwig and Lüscher), 197
Uterus, pregnant, rupture of, due to nonpenetrating abdominal trauma (McClure), 487

V

Valvular defect; surgical correction of aortic insufficiency (Hufnagel et al.), 673
Valvulotomy, pulmonary (Humphreys et al.), 9
Varicose veins, large-bore, technique for facilitating stripping of, using conventional strippers (Rosenberg), 877
recurrent, management of (Luke), 40
Vascular anastomoses, total transplant of thyroid gland using (Sterling and Goldsmith), 624
changes, local, in bleeding peptic ulcer, significance of (MacKay), 724
Vein ligations, common and superficial femoral, comparison of late sequelae of (Robinson and Moyer), 690
saphenous, transplantation of, for postphlebitic stasis (Warren and Thayer), 867
superior mesenteric, one-stage pancreatoduodenectomy with resection of (Moore and Ure), 734
Veins, large-bore varicose, technique for facilitating stripping of, using conventional strippers (Rosenberg), 877
recurrent varicose, management of (Luke), 40
Vena caval injury; major vessel damage in lumbar disc operation (Seeley et al.), 421
Venous thrombosis of upper extremity complicated by pulmonary embolus (Aufses), 957
Vessel damage, major, in lumbar disc operation (Seeley et al.), 421
Villous papillomas of colon and rectum (Bacon et al.), 77
Vomiting; rib fractures from muscular effort with particular reference to cough (Derbes and Haran), 297

W

Water metabolism; new approach to treatment of electrolyte disturbances in shock and severe stress (Schlegel), 449
Weight loss; nutrition following subtotal gastrectomy of four types (Billroth I and II, segmental, and tubular resections) (MacLean et al.), 705
study of patients following total and near-total gastrectomy (Kelly et al.), 964
Whipple type resection; benign cystadenoma of pancreas (Zintel et al.), 612
Winslow, foramen of, hernia through (Dorian and Stein), 795

X

X-ray diagnosis, preoperative, of breast tumors, accuracy of (Gershon-Cohen et al.), 766
therapy; malignant lesions of thyroid (Cohen and Moore), 67

Y

Year book of general surgery, 330 (*B. Rev.*)